NURSING DIAGNOSIS HANDBOOK

*An Evidence-Based
Guide to Planning Care*

NURSING DIAGNOSIS HANDBOOK

An Evidence-Based Guide to Planning Care

Betty J. Ackley, MSN, EdS, RN

Gail B. Ladwig, MSN, RN, CHTP

Ninth Edition

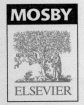

MOSBY

ELSEVIER

3251 Riverport Lane
St. Louis, Missouri 63043

Library of Congress Cataloging-in-Publication Data
Nursing diagnosis handbook : an evidence-based guide to planning care / [edited by] Betty J. Ackley,
Gail B. Ladwig. — 9th ed.
    p. ; cm.
    Includes bibliographical references and index.
    ISBN 978-0-323-07150-5 (pbk. : alk. paper) 1. Nursing diagnosis—Handbooks, manuals, etc. 2. Nursing care plans—Handbooks, manuals, etc. I. Ackley, Betty J. II. Ladwig, Gail B.
    [DNLM: 1. Nursing Diagnosis—Handbooks. 2. Evidence-Based Medicine—methods—Handbooks.
3. Patient Care Planning—Handbooks. WY 49 N9745 2010]
    RT48.6.A35 2010
    616.07'5--dc22

                                                                            2009054148

Acquisitions Editor: Sandra Clark
Senior Developmental Editor: Cindi Crismon Jones
Publishing Services Manager: Deborah L. Vogel

Project Manager: Brandi Tidwell
Designer: Karen Pauls

Printed in the United States of America

Last digit is the print number: 9 8 7 6 5 4 3 2 1

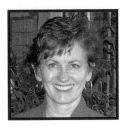

Betty Ackley has worked in nursing for 40 years in many capacities. She has been a staff nurse on a CCU unit, medical ICU unit, respiratory ICU unit, intensive care unit, and step-down unit. She has worked on a gynecological surgery floor and on an orthopedic floor, and she has spent many years working in oncology. She also has been in management, has been in nursing education in a hospital, and has spent 31 years as a professor of nursing at Jackson Community College. In 1996, she began the online learning program at Jackson Community College, offering an online course in nutrition. In 2000 Betty was named Faculty of the Year at her college.

Betty has presented conferences nationally and internationally in the areas of nursing diagnosis, nursing process, online learning, and evidence-based nursing. She has written NCLEX-RN questions for the national licensure examination four times and is an expert in the area of testing and NCLEX preparation.

Betty obtained her BSN from Michigan State University, MS in nursing from the University of Michigan, and education specialist degree from Michigan State University.

Presently Betty has her own company and serves as a nursing consultant in evidence-based nursing at Allegiance Health in Jackson, Michigan. In addition, she has written/edited *Evidence-Based Nursing Care Guidelines: Medical-Surgical Interventions, 2008*. This text is designed to help nurses utilize evidence to provide excellence in nursing care.

Her free time is spent exercising, especially spinning, Pilates, and Zumba. She is certified and teaches classes in Pilates, Zumba, and Total Control, a program to help women with urinary incontinence. In addition, she loves to travel, read, garden, spend time with her grandchildren, and learn anything new!

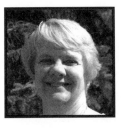

Gail Ladwig is a professor Emeritus of Jackson Community College. During her tenure, she served four years as the Department Chairperson of Nursing and as a nurse consultant for Continuing Education. She was instrumental in starting a BSN transfer program with the University of Michigan.

Gail has taught classroom and clinical at JCC in Fundamentals, Med-Surg, Mental Health, and a transfer course for BSN students. In addition, she has taught online courses in pharmacology, as well as a hybrid course (partially online) for BSN transfer students. She has also taught an online course in pathophysiology for the Medical University of South Carolina.

She worked as a staff nurse in medical-surgical nursing and intensive care for over 20 years prior to beginning her teaching career. She was a Certified Critical-Care Nurse for several years and has a Masters degree in Psychiatric Mental Health Nursing from Wayne State University. Her Masters research was published in the *International Journal of Addictions*.

She has presented nationally and internationally, including Paris, Tokyo, and Puerto Rico, on many topics, including nursing diagnosis, computerized care planning, and holistic nursing topics.

Gail is co-author of *Nursing Diagnosis: Guide to Planning Care,* which has been a very successful text for over 17 years, and she has been co-author for all editions of *Mosby's Guide to Nursing Diagnosis*, now in its third edition. She is also a co-author/editor of *Evidence-Based Nursing Care Guidelines: Medical-Surgical Interventions*. This text published in 2008 and was named AJN book of the year.

She is certified as a Healing Touch practitioner and is co-owner and founder of Holistic Choices, specializing in Alternative presentations and Healing Touch and Guided Imagery treatments. She helped to start the first "Healthy Living Day" in Jackson, Michigan.

Gail has volunteered at Saint Luke's clinic in Jackson, Michigan. This clinic serves the underserved and uninsured populations, the working poor. Gail gets a great deal of satisfaction working at this clinic.

Gail is on the Diagnosis Development Committee of NANDA-I. She was elected to this position in November 2008. She also served on the nominating committee for NANDA-I and chaired the committee.

In 2009 Gail served on the Task Force for the Development of Standards of Holistic Nursing. She also has been a reviewer for the journal *WORLDviews on EVIDENCE-BASED NURSING* for past several years.

Gail is the mother of four children and grandmother of twelve and loves to spend time with her grandchildren. She has been married to her husband Jerry for 45 years and is passionate about her family and the profession of nursing.

CONTRIBUTORS

Betty J. Ackley, MSN, EdS, RN
President and Owner
The Betty Ackley, LLC;
Consultant in Nursing Process, Evidence-Based Nursing,
 and Pilates
Jackson, Michigan
*Activity intolerance; Risk for Activity intolerance; Ineffective
 Airway clearance; Risk for Aspiration; Risk for Autonomic
 dysreflexia; Risk for imbalanced Body temperature; Ineffective
 Breathing pattern; Risk for Caregiver role strain; Acute
 Confusion; Risk for acute Confusion; Risk for Constipation;
 Risk for sudden infant Death syndrome; Impaired Dentition;
 Diarrhea; Risk for compromised human Dignity; Risk for
 Disuse syndrome; Deficient Diversional activity; Impaired
 Environmental interpretation syndrome; Readiness for enhanced
 Fluid Balance; Deficient Fluid volume; Risk for deficient
 Fluid volume; Excess Fluid volume; Risk for imbalanced
 Fluid volume; Impaired Gas exchange; Risk for complicated
 Grieving; Hyperthermia; Hypothermia; Risk for urge urinary
 Incontinence; Risk for disorganized Infant behavior; Readiness
 for enhanced organized Infant behavior; Risk for impaired
 Liver function; Dysfunctional gastrointestinal Motility; Risk
 for dysfunctional gastrointestinal Motility; Noncompliance;
 Imbalanced Nutrition: less than body requirements; Imbalanced
 Nutrition: more than body requirements; Risk for imbalanced
 Nutrition: more than body requirements; Readiness for enhanced
 Nutrition; Impaired Oral mucous membrane; Risk for Peripheral
 neurovascular dysfunction; Risk for Poisoning; Risk for
 Powerlessness; Risk for impaired Religiosity; Risk for Relocation
 stress syndrome; Disturbed Sensory perception; Chronic Sorrow;
 Risk for Spiritual distress; Risk for Suffocation; Impaired
 Swallowing; Ineffective Thermoregulation*

Nadine M. Aktan, PhD, RN, FNP-BC
Assistant Professor
Nursing Department
William Paterson University
Wayne, New Jersey
*Risk for Suffocation; Consultant in Pediatric Diagnoses and
 Interventions, Section III*

Donna L. Algase, PhD
Josephine M. Sana Collegiate Professor of Nursing
University of Michigan School of Nursing
Ann Arbor, Michigan
Wandering

Keith A. Anderson, PhD
Assistant Professor
College of Social Work
The Ohio State University
Columbus, Ohio
Readiness for enhanced family Coping

Sharon Baranoski, MSN, RN, CWCN, APN, FAAN
President
Wound Care Dynamics, Inc.
Consultant Services
Shorewood, Illinois
*Impaired Skin integrity; Risk for impaired Skin integrity; Impaired
 Tissue integrity*

Nancy Albright Beyer, RN, CEN, MS
Clinical Nurse Specialist
Emergency Center
Methodist Hospital
Minneapolis, Minnesota
*Diarrhea; Risk for impaired Liver function; Dysfunctional
 gastrointestinal Motility*

Kathaleen C. Bloom, PhD, CNM
Professor and Associate Director for Undergraduate Studies
University of North Florida
Jacksonville, Florida
*Ineffective Health maintenance; Impaired Home maintenance;
 Deficient Knowledge; Readiness for enhanced Knowledge*

Amy Brown, APRN, MSN
Assistant Professor of Nursing
Morehead State University
Morehead, Kentucky
Risk for Injury; Risk for Trauma

Lisa Burkhart, PhD, RN
Associate Professor
Marcella Niehoff School of Nursing
Loyola University Chicago
Chicago, Illinois
*Moral Distress; Impaired Religiosity; Readiness for enhanced
 Religiosity; Spiritual distress; Readiness for enhanced Spiritual
 well-being*

Emilia Campos de Carvalho, RN, PhD
Full Professor
College of Nursing
University of São Paulo at Ribeirão Preto
São Paulo, Brazil
Risk for vascular Trauma

Stacey M. Carroll, PhD, ANP-BC
Assistant Professor
Rush University College of Nursing
Chicago, Illinois
*Readiness for enhanced Communication; Impaired verbal
 Communication*

June M. Como, RN, MSA, MS, CCRN, CCNS
Faculty
Department of Nursing
College of Staten Island
The City University of New York
Staten Island, New York
Stress overload

Elizabeth A. Crago, RN, MSN
Research Associate
School of Nursing
University of Pittsburgh
Pittsburgh, Pennsylvania
Autonomic dysreflexia

Maryanne Crowther, MSN, APN, CCRN
Nurse Practitioner, Cardiology
Saint Joseph's Regional Medical Center
Paterson, New Jersey
Decreased Cardiac output; Ineffective peripheral tissue Perfusion

Ruth M. Curchoe, RN, MSN, CIC
Director, Infection Prevention
Unity Health System
Rochester, New York
Risk for Infection; Ineffective Protection

Rebecca Davis, RN, PhD
Associate Professor
Kirkhof College of Nursing
Grand Valley State University
Grand Rapids, Michigan
Chronic Confusion

Susan J. Dempsey, MN, CNS, RN-BC
Faculty
Department of Nursing
California State University, Fullerton
Fullerton, California;
Clinical Nurse Specialist
Sharp HealthCare
Chula Vista, California
Acute Pain; Chronic Pain

Mary A. DeWys, BS, RN
Infant Development and Feeding Specialist
Harmony Through Touch;
Consultant for Muskegon Intermediate School District
Muskegon and Spectrum Health
Healthier Communities Department
Grand Rapids, Michigan
Risk for Impaired Attachment; Disorganized Infant behavior

Lorraine A. Duggan, MSN, RN, APNC
Acute Care Nurse Practitioner
Cardiovascular Services
St. Joseph's Regional Medical Center
Paterson, New Jersey
Decreased Cardiac output; Ineffective peripheral tissue Perfusion

Wendy Duggleby, PhD
Nursing Research Chair, Aging and Quality of Life
Faculty of Nursing
University of Alberta
Edmonton, Alberta
Canada
Hopelessness

Shelly Eisbach, PhD, RN
Lecturer
University of Iowa
Iowa City, Iowa
Risk for compromised Resilience; Impaired individual Resilience; Readiness for enhanced Resilience

Brenda Emick-Herring, RN, MSN, CRRN
Staff Nurse
St. Luke's Hospital;
Clinical Nursing Instructor
Mount Mercy College
Cedar Rapids, Iowa
Impaired bed Mobility; Impaired physical Mobility; Impaired wheelchair Mobility; Impaired Transfer ability; Impaired Walking

Dawn Fairlie, ANP, FNP, GNP, DNS(c)
Assistant Professor
College of Staten Island
The City University of New York
Staten Island, New York
Decisional Conflict; Ineffective community Coping; Readiness for enhanced community Coping; Readiness for enhanced Decision-Making; Ineffective self Health management; Readiness for enhanced Self Health management; Ineffective family Therapeutic regimen management

Arlene T. Farren, RN, PhD, AOCN®, CTN-A
Assistant Professor of Nursing
College of Staten Island
The City University of New York
Staten Island, New York
Ineffective Coping

Teresa Ferguson, MSN, RN
Assistant Professor of Nursing
Morehead State University
Morehead, Kentucky
Ineffective infant Feeding pattern

Patricia Ferreira, RN, MSN
Professor of Nursing
Centro Universitário São Camilo SP
Universidade Federal de São Paulo (UNIFESP)
São Paulo, Brazil
Defensive Coping; Disturbed personal Identity

Debora Y. Fields, RN, BSN, MA, LICDC, CARN
Staff Nurse/Counselor
Cleveland Clinic
Cleveland, Ohio
Dysfunctional Family processes

Natalie Fischetti, PhD, RN
Assistant Professor
College of Staten Island
Staten Island, New York
Readiness for enhanced Comfort

Judith A. Floyd, PhD, RN, FAAN
Professor
College of Nursing
Wayne State University
Detroit, Michigan
*Insomnia; Sleep deprivation; Readiness for enhanced Sleep;
Disturbed Sleep pattern*

Terri A. Foster, RN, BSN, CNOR
Surgical Services Educator
Allegiance Health
Jackson, Michigan
*Risk for imbalanced Fluid volume; Risk for perioperative
positioning Injury*

Shari Froelich, MSN, MSBA, APRN, BC, ACHPN
Palliative Care Nurse Practitioner
Allegiance Health System
Jackson, Michigan
Risk for compromised human Dignity

Susanne W. Gibbons, PhD, C-ANP, C-GNP
Assistant Professor
Graduate School of Nursing
Uniformed Services University of the Health Sciences
Bethesda, Maryland
Self Neglect

Joyce Newman Giger, EdD, APRN, BC, FAAN
Professor and Lulu Wolff Hassenplug Endowed Chair
School of Nursing
University of California, Los Angeles
Los Angeles, California
Consultant in Culturally Competent Care

Marie Giordano, RN, MS
Assistant Professor
Department of Nursing
College of Staten Island
The City University of New York
Staten Island, New York
*Readiness for enhanced Decision-Making; Readiness for enhanced
Hope; Readiness for enhanced Power*

Barbara Given, RN, PhD, FAAN
University Distinguished Professor
Associate Dean for Research and Doctoral Program
College of Nursing
Michigan State University
East Lansing, Michigan
Caregiver role strain; Fatigue

Mikel Gray, PhD, CUNP, CCCN, FAANP, FAAN
Professor and Nurse Practitioner
Department of Urology
University of Virginia Health System
Charlottesville, Virginia
*Bowel incontinence; Functional urinary Incontinence; Overflow
urinary Incontinence; Reflex urinary Incontinence; Stress
urinary Incontinence; Urge urinary Incontinence; Risk for urge
urinary Incontinence; Impaired Urinary elimination; Readiness
for enhanced Urinary elimination; Urinary retention*

Pauline M. Green, PhD, RN, CNE
Professor
Division of Nursing
Howard University
Washington, DC
Contamination; Risk for Contamination

Sherry A. Greenberg, MSN, GNP-BC
Consultant
Hartford Institute for Geriatric Nursing
New York University College of Nursing
New York, New York
Risk for Falls

Jennifer Hafner, RN, BSN, TNCC
Staff Nurse, Medical/Surgical Intensive Care
Aspirus Wausau Hospital
Wausau, Wisconsin
*Risk for Electrolyte imbalance; Risk for ineffective renal Perfusion;
Risk for decreased cardiac tissue Perfusion; Risk for ineffective
cerebral tissue Perfusion; Ineffective peripheral tissue Perfusion;
Risk for Shock*

Elizabeth A. Henneman, RN, PhD, CCNS, FAAN
Associate Professor
School of Nursing
University of Massachusetts, Amherst
Amherst, Massachusetts
Impaired spontaneous Ventilation; Dysfunctional Ventilatory weaning response

Sheri Holmes, RNC, MSN, CNS-C
Service Line Administrator—Aspirus Women's Health
Aspirus Wausau Hospital
Wausau, Wisconsin
Risk for Bleeding; Risk for disturbed Maternal/Fetal dyad

Paula D. Hopper, MSN, RN
Professor of Nursing
Jackson Community College
Jackson, Michigan
Risk for unstable blood Glucose level

Teresa Howell, MSN, RN, CNE
Associate Professor of Nursing
Morehead State University
Morehead, Kentucky
Effective Breastfeeding; Ineffective Breastfeeding; Interrupted Breastfeeding

Jean D. Humphries, PhD(c), RN
Doctoral Candidate
Wayne State University
Detroit, Michigan
Insomnia; Sleep deprivation; Readiness for enhanced Sleep; Disturbed Sleep pattern

Dena L. Jarog, DNP, RN, CCNS
Clinical Nurse Specialist
Children's Hospital of Wisconsin
Wauwatosa, Wisconsin
Disabled family Coping; Risk for delayed Development; Delayed Growth and development; Risk for disproportionate Growth

Elizabeth S. Jenuwine, PhD, MLIS
Researcher
College of Nursing
Wayne State University
Detroit, Michigan
Insomnia; Sleep deprivation; Readiness for enhanced Sleep; Disturbed Sleep pattern

Rebecca A. Johnson, PhD, RN
Millsap Professor of Gerontologic Nursing and Public Policy
Sinclair School of Nursing
University of Missouri-Columbia
Columbia, Missouri
Relocation stress syndrome

Michelangelo Juvenale, BSc, MSc, PhD
Professor of Immunology, Pathology, and Microbiology
Centro Universitário São Camilo
Universidade Federal de São Paulo (UNIFESP)
Faculdade Santa Marcelina
São Paulo, Brazil
Defensive Coping; Disturbed personal Identity

Kathleen Karsten, MS, RN, BC
Assistant Professor
La Guardia Community College
The City University of New York
Long Island City, New York
Readiness for enhanced Immunization status

Joan Klehr, RNC, BS, MPH
Information Systems Analyst
Aspirus Wausau Hospital
Wausau, Wisconsin
Risk for Electrolyte imbalance; Dysfunctional gastrointestinal Motility; Risk for dysfunctional gastrointestinal Motility; Risk for ineffective renal Perfusion; Risk for decreased cardiac tissue Perfusion; Risk for ineffective cerebral tissue Perfusion; Risk for ineffective gastrointestinal tissue Perfusion; Risk for Shock

Katharine Kolcaba, PhD, RN
Associate Professor (Emeritus)
The University of Akron
Akron, Ohio;
Consultant
The Comfort Line
Chagrin Falls, Ohio
Impaired Comfort

Beverly Kopala, PhD, RN
Associate Professor
Marcella Niehoff School of Nursing
Loyola University Chicago
Chicago, Illinois
Moral Distress

Angela Kueny, PhD(c), MSN, BA
Doctoral Candidate
University of Iowa
Iowa City, Iowa
Risk for compromised Resilience; Impaired individual Resilience; Readiness for enhanced Resilience

Gail B. Ladwig, MSN, RN, CHTP
Co-Owner
Holistic Choices;
Consultant
Guided Imagery, Healing Touch, Holistic Nursing, Nursing
  Diagnosis
Hilton Head, South Carolina
*Ineffective Activity planning; Risk-prone health Behavior;
  Disturbed Body image; Readiness for enhanced Childbearing
  process; Parental role Conflict; Defensive Coping; Readiness
  for enhanced Coping; Disturbed Energy field; Adult Failure to
  thrive; Dysfunctional Family processes; Grieving; Complicated
  Grieving; Disturbed personal Identity; Impaired Parenting;
  Risk for impaired Parenting; Readiness for enhanced Parenting;
  Post-Trauma syndrome; Risk for Post-Trauma syndrome;
  Readiness for enhanced Relationship; Ineffective Role
  performance; Readiness for enhanced Self-Concept; Impaired
  Social interaction*

France Maltais, BSc, MEd
L'ordre Des Infirmières et Infirmiers du Québec
Cégep du Vieux Montréal
Montréal, Québec
Canada
Ineffective Activity planning

Ruth McCaffrey, DNP, ARNP
Associate Professor
Christine E. Lynn College of Nursing
Florida Atlantic University
Boca Raton, Florida
Anxiety; Death Anxiety; Fear

Graham J. McDougall, Jr., PhD, RN, FAAN
Professor
School of Nursing
University of Texas—Austin
Austin, Texas
Impaired Memory

Laura H. McIlvoy, PhD, RN, CCRN, CNRN
Assistant Professor
Indiana University Southeast
New Albany, Indiana
Decreased Intracranial adaptive capacity

Susan Mee, RN, PhD, CPNP
Assistant Professor
Department of Nursing
College of Staten Island
The City University of New York
Staten Island, New York
*Readiness for enhanced Immunization status; Readiness for
  enhanced Self-Care*

Noreen C. Miller, RN, MSN, ONC
Ortho/Neuro Nurse Case Manager
St. Charles Medical Center
Bend, Oregon
Risk for Peripheral neurovascular dysfunction

DeLancey Nicoll, SN
Nursing Student
Hartwick College
Oneonta, New York
*Latex Allergy response; Risk for latex Allergy response; Delayed
  Surgical recovery (Working with Leslie H. Nicoll)*

Leslie H. Nicoll, PhD, MBA, RN, BC
President and Owner
Maine Desk, LLC
Portland, Maine
*Latex Allergy response; Risk for latex Allergy response; Delayed
  Surgical recovery*

Lisa Oldham, MSN, RNC, NE, FABC, GCM
Professor
William Patterson University
Wayne, New Jersey
*Consultant in Geriatric Diagnoses and Interventions, Sections II
  and III*

Barbara J. Olinzock, RN, EdD
Associate Professor
School of Nursing
University of North Florida
Jacksonville, Florida
*Ineffective Health maintenance; Impaired Home maintenance;
  Deficient Knowledge; Readiness for enhanced Knowledge*

Peg Padnos, AB, BSN, RN
Nursing Consultant
Early On Transition Team
Muskegon County, Michigan
Risk for impaired Attachment; Disorganized Infant behavior

Kathleen L. Patusky, PhD, APRN-BC
Assistant Professor
University of Medicine and Dentistry of New Jersey
Newark, New Jersey
*Powerlessness; Self-Mutilation; Risk for Self-Mutilation; Risk for
  Suicide; Risk for other-directed Violence; Risk for self-directed
  Violence*

Laura V. Polk, PhD, RN
Professor
College of Southern Maryland
La Plata, Maryland
Contamination; Risk for Contamination

Major General (Ret) Gale S. Pollock, CRNA, MHA, FACHE, FAAN
Executive Director
Louis J. Fox Center for Vision Restoration
University of Pittsburgh
Pittsburgh, Pennsylvania
Disturbed Sensory perception

Sherry H. Pomeroy, PhD, RN
Assistant Professor
School of Nursing
University at Buffalo
The State University of New York
Buffalo, New York
Sedentary Lifestyle; Impaired physical Mobility

Lori M. Rhudy, PhD, RN
Clinical Nurse Researcher
Mayo Clinic;
Clinical Assistant Professor
School of Nursing
University of Minnesota
Rochester, Minnesota
Unilateral Neglect

Mary Jane Roth, RN, BSN, MA
Nurse Clinician
Ann Arbor VAMC
Ann Arbor, Michigan
Chronic low Self-Esteem; Situational low Self-Esteem; Risk for situational low Self-Esteem

Vanessa Sammons, MSN, APRN, BC, CNE
Assistant Professor of Nursing
Morehead State University
Morehead, Kentucky
Parental role Conflict; Interrupted Family processes; Readiness for enhanced Family processes

Marilee Schmelzer, PhD, RN
Associate Professor
School of Nursing
The University of Texas at Arlington
Arlington, Texas
Constipation; Perceived Constipation

Paula Riess Sherwood, RN, CNRN, PhD
Assistant Professor
School of Nursing
University of Pittsburgh
Pittsburgh, Pennsylvania
Autonomic dysreflexia; Caregiver role strain; Fatigue

Mary T. Shoemaker, RN, MSN, SANE
Sexual Assault Nurse Examiner
Olive Hill, Kentucky
Ineffective Denial; Risk for Loneliness; Rape-Trauma syndrome; Social isolation

Mary E. B. Stahl, RN, MSN, CEN
Faculty Specialist II
Bronson School of Nursing
Western Michigan University
Kalamazoo, Michigan
Risk for sudden infant Death syndrome; Risk for Poisoning

Elaine E. Steinke, PhD, RN, FAHA
Professor of Nursing
School of Nursing
Wichita State University
Fairmount, Wichita
Sexual dysfunction; Ineffective Sexuality pattern

Katherina A. Nikzad Terhune, MSW
Hartford Doctoral Fellow
Graduate Center for Gerontology
University of Kentucky
Lexington, Kentucky
Compromised family Coping

Janelle M. Tipton, MSN, RN, AOCN®
Oncology Clinical Nurse Specialist
University of Toledo Medical Center
Toledo, Ohio
Nausea

Diane Wardell, PhD, RN, WHNP-BC
Associate Professor
School of Nursing
The University of Texas Health Science Center Houston
Houston, Texas
Disturbed Energy field

Linda S. Williams, MSN, RN
Professor of Nursing
Jackson Community College
Jackson, Michigan
Bathing Self-Care deficit; Dressing Self-Care deficit; Feeding Self-Care deficit; Toileting Self-Care deficit

David Wilson, MS, RNC
Faculty
Langston University School of Nursing, Tulsa;
Staff
St. Francis Children's Hospital
Tulsa, Oklahoma
Neonatal Jaundice

REVIEWERS

Sharon Marie Abbate, EdD, MS, BSN, RN
Assistant Professor
University of St. Francis
Joliet, Illinois

Marianne Curia, PhD, MSN, RN
Assistant Professor
University of St. Francis
Joliet, Illinois;
Staff Nurse
University of Chicago
Chicago, Illinois

Jackie Lall Michael, PHD, ANP, WHNP-BC
Assistant Clinical Professor
School of Nursing
The University of Texas at Arlington
Arlington, Texas

Carol A. Penrosa, MS, RN
Faculty, Associate Degree Nursing
Southeast Community College
Lincoln, Nebraska

Mary Strong, RN, BSN, MSN
Professor
Health Science Department
Kirkwood Community College
Cedar Rapids, Iowa

Jo Ellen Welborn, BSN, MSN, RN
Nursing Instructor, Associate Degree
Weatherford College
Weatherford, Texas

Nancy Lynn Whitehead, MS, FNP,C, CSN
Nursing Instructor
Milwaukee Area Technical College: Mequon Campus
Mequon, Wisconsin

Tamara Lynn Wright, RN, BSN, MSN
Clinical Instructor
School of Nursing
The University of Texas at Arlington
Arlington, Texas

PREFACE

Nursing Diagnosis Handbook: An Evidence-Based Guide to Planning Care is a convenient reference to help the practicing nurse or nursing student make a nursing diagnosis and write a care plan with ease and confidence. This handbook helps nurses correlate nursing diagnoses with known information about clients on the basis of assessment findings; established medical, surgical, or psychiatric diagnoses; and the current treatment plan.

Making a nursing diagnosis and planning care are complex processes that involve diagnostic reasoning and critical thinking skills. Nursing students and practicing nurses cannot possibly memorize the extensive list of defining characteristics, related factors, and risk factors for the 201 diagnoses approved by NANDA-International. This book correlates suggested nursing diagnoses with what nurses know about clients and offers a care plan for each nursing diagnosis.

Section I, Nursing Process, Nursing Diagnosis and Evidence-Based Nursing, explains how the nurse formulates a nursing diagnosis using assessment findings, determines outcomes, writes appropriate interventions, and evaluates the plan of care. In addition there is information on evidence-based nursing care, and Quality and Safety in Nursing Education (QSEN).

In Section II, Guide to Nursing Diagnoses, the nurse can look up symptoms and problems and their suggested nursing diagnoses for more than 1450 client symptoms; medical, surgical and psychiatric diagnoses; diagnostic procedures; surgical interventions; and clinical states.

In Section III, Guide to Planning Care, the nurse can find care plans for all nursing diagnoses suggested in Section II. We have included the suggested nursing outcomes from the Nursing Outcomes Classification (NOC) and interventions from the Nursing Interventions Classification (NIC) by the Iowa Intervention Project. We believe this work is a significant addition to the nursing process to further define nursing practice with standardized language.

Scientific rationales based on research are included for most of the interventions. This is done to make the evidence base of nursing practice very apparent to the nursing student and practicing nurse.

New special features of the ninth edition of *Nursing Diagnosis Handbook: An Evidence-Based Guide to Planning Care* include the following:

- **Twenty-one** new nursing diagnoses recently approved by NANDA-I, along with deletion of six nursing diagnoses
- **Eight** revisions of nursing diagnoses made by NANDA-I in existing nursing diagnoses
- Addition of pediatric and critical care interventions to appropriate care plans
- An associated EVOLVE Course Management System that includes additional critical thinking case studies;

worksheets; PowerPoint slides; and the ability to post a class syllabus, outline, and lecture notes, share e-mail, and encourage student participation through chat rooms and discussion boards

The following features of *Nursing Diagnosis Handbook: A Guide to Planning Care* are also included:

- Suggested nursing diagnoses for more than 1450 clinical entities including signs and symptoms, medical diagnoses, surgeries, maternal-child disorders, mental health disorders, and geriatric disorders
- Labeling of nursing research as EBN (Evidence-Based Nursing) and clinical research as EB (Evidence-Based) to identify the source of evidence-based rationales
- An EVOLVE Courseware System with the Ackley Ladwig Care Plan Constructor that helps the student or nurse write a nursing care plan, including links to websites for client education
- Rationales for nursing interventions that are mostly based on nursing research
- Nursing references identified for each care plan
- A complete list of NOC outcomes on the EVOLVE website
- A complete list of NIC interventions on the EVOLVE website
- Nursing care plans that contain many holistic interventions
- Care plans written by leading national nursing experts from throughout the United States, along with international contributors, who together represent all of the major nursing specialties and have extensive experience with nursing diagnoses and the nursing process. Care plans written by experts include:
  - **Caregiver role strain** and **Fatigue** by Dr. Barbara Given and Dr. Paula Riess Sherwood
  - **Constipation** by Dr. Marilee Schmelzer
  - **Contamination** and **Risk for Contamination** by Dr. Laura V. Polk
  - **Rape-Trauma syndrome** by Mary T. Shoemaker
  - Care plans for **Spirituality** by Dr. Lisa Burkhart
  - Care plans for **Religiosity** by Dr. Lisa Burkhart
  - Care plans for **Skin integrity** by Sharon Baranoski
  - **Impaired Memory** by Dr. Graham J. McDougall, Jr.
  - Care plans for **Incontinence** by Dr. Mikel Gray
  - **Insomnia** and **Sleep deprivation** by Dr. Judith A. Floyd
  - **Decreased Intracranial adaptive capacity** by Dr. Laura H. McIlvoy
  - **Latex Allergy response** by Dr. Leslie H. Nicoll and DeLancey Nicoll
  - **Unilateral Neglect** by Dr. Lori M. Rhudy
  - **Wandering** by Dr. Donna L. Algase

- **Impaired spontaneous Ventilation** and **Dysfunctional Ventilatory weaning response** by Dr. Elizabeth A. Henneman
- **Hopelessness** by Dr. Wendy Duggleby
- **Disturbed Energy field** by Dr. Diane Wardell
- **Anxiety, Death Anxiety,** and **Fear** by Dr. Ruth McCaffrey
- **Impaired Comfort** by Dr. Katharine Kolcaba
- **Moral Distress** by Dr. Lisa Burkhart and Dr. Beverly Kopala
- **Risk for Infection** and **Ineffective Protection** by Ruth Curchoe
- **Readiness for enhanced Communication** and **Impaired verbal Communication** by Dr. Stacey Carroll
- **Sexual dysfunction** and **Ineffective Sexuality pattern** by Dr. Elaine E. Steinke
- **Defensive Coping** and **Disturbed personal Identity** revised by Dr. Michelangelo Juvenale and Dr. Patricia Ferreira

- A format that facilitates analyzing signs and symptoms by the process already known by nurses, which involves using defining characteristics of nursing diagnoses to make a diagnosis
- Use of NANDA-I terminology and approved diagnoses
- An alphabetical format for Sections II and III, which allows rapid access to information
- Nursing care plans for all nursing diagnoses listed in Section II
- Specific geriatric interventions in appropriate plans of care
- Specific client/family teaching interventions in each plan of care
- Information on culturally competent nursing care included where appropriate
- Inclusion of commonly used abbreviations (e.g., AIDS, MI, CHF) and cross-references to the complete term in Section II

We acknowledge the work of NANDA-I, which is used extensively throughout this text. In some rare cases, the authors and contributors have modified the NANDA-I work to increase ease of use. The original NANDA-I work can be found in *NANDA-I Nursing Diagnoses: Definitions & Classification 2009–2011.* Several contributors are the original submitters/authors of the nursing diagnoses established by NANDA-I. These contributors include the following:

Lisa Burkhart, PhD, RN
Impaired Religiosity; Risk for impaired Religiosity; Readiness for enhanced Religiosity; Spiritual distress; Readiness for enhanced Spiritual well-being

Brenda Emick-Herring, RN, MSN, CRRN
Impaired bed Mobility; Impaired wheelchair Mobility; Impaired Transfer ability; Impaired Walking

Laura V. Polk, PhD, RN
Contamination; Risk for Contamination

Katharine Kolcaba, PhD, RN
Impaired Comfort

Sheri Holmes, RNC, MSN, CNS-C
Risk for Bleeding; Risk for disturbed Maternal/Fetal dyad

Joan Klehr, RNC, BS, MPH
Dysfunctional Gastrointestinal Mobility; Risk for Dysfunctional Gastrointestinal Motility

Jennifer Hafner, RN, BSN, TNCC
Risk for Electrolyte imbalance; Risk for ineffective renal Perfusion; Risk for decreased cardiac tissue Perfusion; Risk for ineffective cerebral tissue Perfusion; Ineffective peripheral tissue Perfusion; Risk for Shock

Emilia Campos de Carvalho, RN, PhD (Brazil)
Risk for vascular Trauma

Shelly Eisbach, PhD, RN, Angela Kueny, PhD(c), MSN, BA
Risk for compromised Resilience; Impaired individual Resilience; Readiness for enhanced Resilience

David Wilson, MS, RNC
Neonatal Jaundice

Susanne W. Gibbons, PhD, C-ANP, C-GNP
Self Neglect

France Maltais, BSc, MEd (Québec)
Ineffective Activity planning

We would also like to thank Carole S. Homewood for her English translation from French for the care plan **Ineffective Activity planning.**

We and the consultants and contributors trust that nurses will find this ninth edition of *Nursing Diagnosis Handbook: An Evidence-Based Guide to Planning Care* a valuable tool that simplifies the process of diagnosing clients and planning for their care, thus allowing nurses more time to provide evidence-based care that speeds each client's recovery.

Betty J. Ackley
Gail B. Ladwig

ACKNOWLEDGMENTS

We would like to thank the following people at Elsevier: Sandra Clark, Acquisitions Editor, who supported us with this ninth edition of the text with intelligence and kindness; Cindi Crismon Jones, Senior Developmental Editor, who was a continual support and constant source of wise advice and who is frankly wonderful; a special thank-you to Brandi Tidwell and Jodi Willard for project management of this edition; and Brooke Bagwill, Senior Editorial Assistant, for her ongoing support and hard work.

We acknowledge with gratitude nurses and student nurses, who are always an inspiration for us to provide fresh and accurate material. We are honored that they continue to value this text and to use it in their studies and practice.

Care has been taken to confirm the accuracy of information presented in this book. However, the authors, editors, and publisher cannot accept any responsibility for consequences resulting from errors or omissions of the information in this book and make no warranty, express or implied, with respect to its contents. The reader should use practices suggested in this book in accordance with agency policies and professional standards. Every effort has been made to ensure the accuracy of the information presented in this text.

We hope you find this text useful in your nursing practice.

Betty J. Ackley
Gail B. Ladwig

ASSESS

Following the guidelines in Section I, begin to formulate your nursing diagnosis by gathering and documenting the objective and subjective information about the client.

DIAGNOSIS

Turn to Section II, Guide to Nursing Diagnoses, and locate the client's symptoms, clinical state, medical or psychiatric diagnoses, and anticipated or prescribed diagnostic studies or surgical interventions (listed in alphabetical order). Note suggestions for appropriate nursing diagnoses.

Use Section III, Guide to Planning Care, to evaluate each suggested nursing diagnosis and "related to" etiology statement. Section III is a listing of care plans according to NANDA-I, arranged alphabetically by diagnostic concept, for each nursing diagnosis referred to in Section II. Determine the appropriateness of each nursing diagnosis by comparing the Defining Characteristics and Risk Factors to the client data collected.

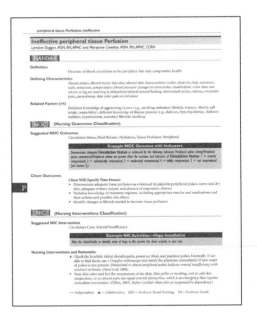

DETERMINE OUTCOMES

Use Section III, Guide to Planning Care, to find appropriate outcomes for the client. Use either the NOC outcomes with the associated rating scales, or Client Outcomes as desired.

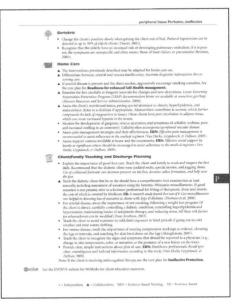

PLAN INTERVENTIONS

Use Section III, Guide to Planning Care, to find appropriate interventions for the client. Use either the NIC interventions or Nursing Interventions as found in that section.

GIVE NURSING CARE

Administer nursing care following the plan of care based on the interventions.

EVALUATE NURSING CARE

Evaluate nursing care administered using either the NOC outcomes or Client Outcomes. If the outcomes were not met, and the nursing interventions were not effective, reassess the client and determine if the appropriate nursing diagnoses were made.

DOCUMENT

Document all of the previous steps using the format provided in the clinical setting.

CONTENTS

NURSING DIAGNOSIS HANDBOOK

An Evidence-Based
Guide to Planning Care

Nursing Process, Nursing Diagnosis, and Evidence-Based Nursing

Section I offers an overview of the nursing process, including the use of evidence-based nursing care. This section provides information on how to make a nursing diagnosis and directions on how to plan nursing care.

Components of the five key steps in the nursing process:

1. **Assessing**: performing a nursing assessment
2. **Diagnosing**: making nursing diagnoses
3. **Planning**: formulating and writing outcome statements and determining appropriate nursing interventions based on appropriate evidence (research)
4. **Implementing** care
5. **Evaluating** the outcomes and the nursing care that has been implemented. Make necessary revisions in care as needed

THE NURSING PROCESS AND EVIDENCE-BASED NURSING

The nursing process is an organizing framework for professional nursing practice. It is very similar to the steps used in scientific reasoning and problem solving. Critical thinking is a key component of the nursing process.

An easy, convenient way to remember the steps of the nursing process is to use an acronym, **ADPIE:**

1. **A**ssessing: performing a nursing assessment
2. **D**iagnosing: making nursing diagnosis
3. **P**lanning: formulating and writing outcome/goal statements and determining appropriate nursing interventions based on evidence (research)
4. **I**mplementing care
5. **E**valuating the outcomes and the nursing care that has been implemented. Make necessary revisions in care as needed.

The process can be visualized as a circular, continuous process (see Figure I-1).

Basing nursing practice on evidence or research is a concept that has been added to the nursing process. This concept is called *evidence-based nursing* (EBN). EBN is a systematic process that uses current evidence in making decisions about the care of clients, including evaluation of quality and applicability of existing research, client preferences, costs, clinical expertise, and clinical settings (Fineout-Overholt & Johnson, 2005).

EBN is a problem-solving approach designed to enhance the profession of nursing and to promote quality client care (Spear, 2006). It is very much like the nursing process. EBN emphasizes asking searchable, answerable clinical questions (Fineout-Overholt & Johnston, 2005). In Section III of this text, the abbreviation **EBN** is used when interventions have

scientific rationale supported by nursing research. The abbreviation **EB** is used when interventions have scientific rationale for research that has been obtained from disciplines other than nursing.

A barrier to implementing EBN has been a lack of understanding of the process and limited knowledge of the research process (Hockenberry et al, 2006). This text utilizes both research and the nursing process. By integrating these concepts it assists the nurse in increasing the use of evidence-based interventions in the clinical setting.

There is another concept, quality control, which has been used for many years, with processes in place to ensure that the client receives appropriate care. Quality control departments have been the main change agents in health care facilities, bringing in new methods of improving care. This text includes interventions to promote quality as evidenced by the use of EBN and EB in the rationales for most interventions.

Table I-1 illustrates three problem-solving methods: nursing process, evidence-based nursing, and quality-control initiatives. The nursing process uses nursing interventions for individual clients to attain *individual* client outcomes. Evidence-based nursing and quality initiatives use nursing interventions to improve the quality of care for *large numbers* of clients to help them achieve positive outcomes.

Another initiative is emphasis on client safety. Clients come into the health care environment expecting to receive care that is safe and does not cause harm. Unfortunately research has shown that too often this may not be true. Clients may receive the wrong medications, the wrong transfusions, and sometimes have the wrong extremity removed. "Client safety is one of the most critical issues for health care today. The escalating need to decrease preventable complications serves as a signifi-

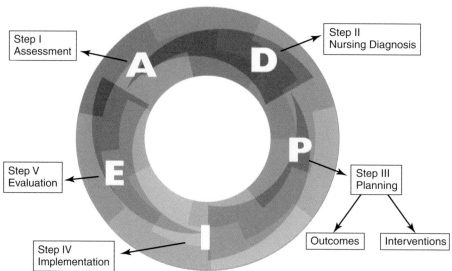

Figure I-1
Nursing process.

TABLE I-1

Comparison of the Nursing Process, Evidence-Based Nursing, and the Quality Process

Method	Components	Implementation
Nursing Process	Assessment	Collecting data about the client using physical assessment and interviewing techniques
	Diagnosis	Using client data and critical thinking skills to identify and validate an appropriate nursing diagnosis
	Planning	Writing measurable client outcomes and interventions to accomplish outcomes
	Implementation	Initiating the care plan and performing the interventions
	Evaluation	Evaluating if outcome(s) met and appropriateness of the interventions to meet client needs
Evidence-Based Nursing	Ask the clinical question	Identifying the problem and clinical question
	Searching for and critically appraising the evidence	Searching for evidence (research) applicable to the clinical question. Using critical thinking to appraise the evidence for validity, reliability, generalization, and appropriateness of the question.
	Determining outcome(s) and evidence-based interventions	Writing appropriate, measurable outcome(s) and evidence-based interventions to accomplish the outcomes
	Application of the evidence to nursing practice	Initiating care and performing the evidence-based interventions
	Evaluation of the evidence-based nursing care	Evaluating if outcome(s) met and appropriateness of the interventions to meet client needs
Quality Initiatives	Plan: Assess, identify, and plan process	Identify a quality issue of concern and plan a process improvement.
	Do: Collect data and analyze results to form conclusion	Map the current and proposed process. Collect data about the current reality and analyze results.
	Check: Establish criteria to measure progress toward solution	Propose a solution and check the results of the new process/procedure/guideline.
	Check: Initiate action and measure progress	Propose a solution and check the results of the new process/procedure/guideline.
	Act: Evaluate process and take appropriate action	Adopt, adapt, or abandon the solution.

cant catalyst to identify and use evidence-based practice (EBP) at the bedside" (Bradley & Dixon, 2009).

Client safety has to be a national priority wherever health care is given. Safety work is enforced by the Joint Commission (2009), an important accrediting agency for health care. The Joint Commission has guidelines (2009) for improving safety that include the need for increased handwashing, better client identification before receiving medications or treat-

ments, and protecting suicidal clients from harm. Many of these guidelines designed to keep clients safe from harm are incorporated into the care plans in this text.

Evidence-based nursing, safety initiatives, and quality control work together in a synergistic manner, similar to a three-legged stool, to support each other and lead to excellence in nursing care. Quality care for clients needs to be more than safe; the care should result in the best outcome possible for the client. For this to happen, the client should receive care that is based on evidence of the effectiveness of the care.

THE NURSING PROCESS

This book focuses on an essential part of the nursing process: how to make and use a nursing diagnosis. A nursing diagnosis is a clinical judgment about individual, family, or community responses to actual or potential health problems or life processes. Nursing diagnoses provide the basis for selection of nursing interventions to achieve outcomes for which the nurse is held accountable (NANDA-I, 2009).

The nursing diagnoses that are used throughout this book are taken from North American Nursing Diagnosis Association-International (NANDA-I, 2009). The complete nursing diagnosis list is on the back inside of this text, and it can also be found on the Evolve website that accompanies this text.

The diagnoses used throughout this text are listed in alphabetical order by the **diagnostic concept.** If you are looking for *impaired wheelchair mobility,* you would find it under *"mobility,"* not under *"wheelchair"* or *"impaired"* (NANDA-I, 2009).

The following is an overview and practical application of the steps of the nursing process. The steps are listed in the usual order in which they are performed.

STEP 1: ASSESSMENT (ADPIE)

Assessment: This is the data collection step. It involves performing a thorough holistic nursing assessment of the client. This is the first step needed to make an appropriate nursing diagnosis, and it is done using the assessment format adopted by the facility or educational institution in which the practice is situated. Several organizational approaches to assessment are available, including Gordon's Functional Health Patterns (see Appendix B) and head-to-toe and body systems approaches. Regardless of the approach used, the nurse assesses the client, being alert for symptoms that will help formulate a nursing diagnosis.

Assessment information is obtained first by doing a thorough health and medical history, and listening to and observing the client. To elicit as much information as possible, the nurse should use open-ended questions, rather than questions that can be answered by a simple yes or no (Dreyer, 2006). The client should be asked questions such as the following:

"Describe what you are feeling."
"How long have you been feeling this way?"
"How did the symptoms start?"
"Describe the symptoms."
"What brought you to the hospital (clinic) today?"

These types of questions will encourage the client to give more information about his or her situation. Listen carefully for cues and record relevant information that the client shares. This information that is obtained verbally from the client is considered subjective information.

Information is also obtained by performing a physical assessment, taking vital signs, and noting diagnostic test results. This information is considered objective information.

If the client is critically ill or unable to respond verbally, much of the information will be gathered from the physical assessment and diagnostic test results, and possibly from the client's significant others.

The information from all of these sources is used to formulate a nursing diagnosis. All of this information needs to be carefully documented on the forms provided by the agency or school of nursing. When recording information, the HIPAA (Health Insurance Portability & Accountability Act; Brown, 2007) regulations need to be followed carefully. The client's name should NOT be used on the student care plan to protect client confidentiality. When the assessment is complete, proceed to the next step.

STEP 2: NURSING DIAGNOSIS (ADPIE)

Formulating a Nursing Diagnosis with Related Factors and Defining Characteristics

A working nursing diagnosis may have one, two, or three parts. One-part diagnoses are usually wellness diagnoses and contain only the NANDA-I label. For example, a beginning nursing student is trying to master nursing diagnosis and the nursing process. A label you could use might be **Readiness for enhanced Knowledge**. (The student expresses an interest in learning about the nursing process and how to make a nursing diagnosis.)

The two-part system consists of the nursing diagnosis and the "related to" (r/t) statement. "Related factors are factors that appear to show some type of patterned relationship with the nursing diagnosis: such factors may be described as antecedent to, associated with, relating to, contributing to, or abetting" (NANDA-I, 2009). The two-part system is often used when the defining characteristics, or signs and symptoms identified in the assessment, may be obvious to those caring for the client, or as in the previous example, the beginning student nurse: **Deficient Knowledge** r/t unfamiliarity with information about the nursing process and nursing diagnosis.

The three-part system consists of the nursing diagnosis, the "related to" (r/t) statement, and the defining characteristics, which are "observable cues/inferences that cluster as manifestations of an actual or wellness nursing diagnosis" (NANDA-I, 2009).

Some nurses refer to the three-part diagnostic statement as the **PES system:**

P (problem)—The nursing diagnosis label: a concise term or phrase that represents a pattern of related cues. The nursing diagnosis is taken from the official NANDA-I list.

E (etiology)—"Related to" (r/t) phrase or etiology: related cause or contributor to the problem

S (symptoms)—Defining characteristics phrase: symptoms that the nurse identified in the assessment

Using the previous example of the beginning nursing student:

> Problem: Use the nursing diagnosis label **Deficient Knowledge** from the NANDA-I list. Remember to check the definition: "Absence or deficiency of cognitive information related to a specific topic" (NANDA-I, 2009).
>
> Etiology: r/t unfamiliarity with information about the nursing process and nursing diagnosis. At this point the beginning nurse would not be familiar with available resources regarding the nursing process.
>
> Symptoms: Defining characteristics, aeb (as evidenced by) verbalization of lack of understanding. "I don't understand this, and I really don't know how to make a nursing diagnosis." When using the **PES** system, look at the **S** first, then formulate the three-part statement. (You would have gotten the **S**, signs and symptoms, which are defining characteristics, from your assessment.)

Therefore, the three-part nursing diagnosis is: **Deficient Knowledge** r/t unfamiliarity with information about the nursing process and nursing diagnosis aeb verbalization of lack of understanding.

Nursing Diagnosis Labels

There are five different kinds of nursing diagnosis labels:

Actual Nursing Diagnosis. The client has a human response to a health condition/life process. The actual nursing diagnosis is supported by defining characteristics and related factors (NANDA-I, 2009). For example: **Imbalanced Nutrition: more than body requirements** r/t excessive intake in relation to metabolic needs aeb weight 20% over ideal for height and frame, concentrating food intake at the end of the day. (Note: This is a three-part nursing diagnosis.)

Risk Nursing Diagnosis. The client/family/community is vulnerable to developing the human response to a health condition/life process. The risk diagnosis is supported by risk factors. Defining characteristics and related factors are not available because there are no problems as of yet, though they are likely to develop. For example: **Risk for imbalanced nutrition: more than body requirements:** concentrating food at the end of the day. (Note: This is a two-part nursing diagnosis.)

Health-Promotion Nursing Diagnosis. "A clinical judgment of a person's, family's, or community's motivation and desire to increase well-being and actualize human health potential as expressed by a readiness to enhance specific health behaviors such as nutrition and exercise" (NANDA-I, 2009). Both defining characteristics and related factors are found in health-promotion diagnoses. For example: **Effective Breastfeeding** r/t basic breastfeeding knowledge aeb appropriate infant weight pattern for age. (Note: This is a three-part nursing diagnosis.)

Health promotion is different than prevention in that health promotion focuses on being as healthy as possible, as opposed to preventing a disease or problem. The difference between health promotion and disease protection is that the reason for the health behavior should always be a positive one. With a health-promotion diagnosis, the outcomes and interventions should be focused on enhancing health.

Syndrome Nursing Diagnosis. A group of signs and symptoms that usually occur together. This group of symptoms is a distinct clinical picture (McCourt, 1991; NANDA-I, 2009). Syndrome diagnoses have both defining characteristics and related factors. For example:

Post-Trauma syndrome r/t physical abuse aeb alienation, anger, anxiety, and depression. (Note: This is a three-part nursing diagnosis.)

When selecting the diagnosis, consider what label is most appropriate. Ask, is this an actual problem or a risk? Do the defining characteristics suggest health promotion or a group of symptoms that occur together?

Application and Examples of Making a Nursing Diagnosis

When the assessment is complete, identify common patterns/symptoms of response *to actual or potential health problems from the assessment* and select an appropriate nursing diagnosis label using critical thinking skills. Use the steps with Case Study 1. (The same steps can be followed using an actual client assessment in the clinical setting or from a student assessment.)

> A. Highlight or underline the relevant symptoms (defining characteristics). As you review your assessment information, ask: Is this normal? Is this an ideal situation? Is this a problem for the client? You may go back and validate information with the client.
> B. Make a short list of the symptoms (underlined or highlighted information).
> C. Cluster similar symptoms.
> D. Analyze/interpret the symptoms. (What do these symptoms mean or represent when they are together?)
> E. Select a nursing diagnosis label from the NANDA-I list that fits with the appropriate defining characteristics and nursing diagnosis definition.

Case Study I—An Elderly Man with Breathing Problems

A. Underline the Symptoms (Defining Characteristics)

A 73-year-old man has been admitted to the unit with a diagnosis of chronic obstructive pulmonary disease (COPD). He states that he has "difficulty breathing when walking short distances." He also states that his "heart feels like it is racing" (heart rate is 110 beats per minute) at the same time. He states that he is "tired all the time," and while talking to you, he is continually wringing his hands and looking out the window.

B. List the Symptoms

Chronic obstructive pulmonary disease (COPD); "difficulty breathing when walking short distances"; "heart feels like it is racing"; heart rate is 110 beats per minute; "tired all the time"; continually wringing his hands and looking out the window.

C. Cluster Symptoms

Chronic obstructive pulmonary disease (COPD)

"Difficulty breathing when walking short distances"
"Heart feels like it is racing"
"Tired all the time"

Continually wringing his hands
Looking out the window

D. Analyze
**Interpret the *Subjective Symptoms*
(What the Client has Stated)**

- "Difficulty breathing when walking short distances" = exertional discomfort: a defining characteristic of **Activity intolerance**
- "Heart feels like it is racing" = abnormal heart rate response to activity: a defining characteristic of **Activity intolerance**
- "Tired all the time" = verbal report of weakness: a defining characteristic of **Activity intolerance**

Interpret the *Objective Symptoms* (Observable Information)

- Continually wringing his hands = extraneous movement, hand/arm movements: defining characteristics of **Anxiety**
- Looking out the window = poor eye contact, glancing about: defining characteristics of **Anxiety**

E. Select the Nursing Diagnosis Label

In Section II, look up *dyspnea* or *dysrhythmia (abnormal heart rate or rhythm)*, chosen because they are high priority, and you will find the nursing diagnosis **Activity intolerance** listed with these symptoms. Is this diagnosis appropriate for this client?

To validate that the diagnosis **Activity intolerance** is appropriate for the client, turn to Section III, and read the NANDA-I definition of the nursing diagnosis **Activity intolerance:** "Insufficient physiological or psychological energy to endure or complete required or desired daily activities." When reading the definition, ask, "Does this definition describe the symptoms demonstrated by the client?" "Is any more assessment information needed?" "Should I take his blood pressure or take an apical pulse rate?" If the appropriate nursing diagnosis has been selected, the definition should describe the condition that has been observed.

The client should also have defining characteristics for this particular diagnosis. Are the client symptoms that you identified in the list of defining characteristics (e.g., verbal report of fatigue, abnormal heart rate response to activity, exertional dyspnea)?

Another way to use this text and to help validate the diagnosis is to look up the client's medical diagnosis in Section

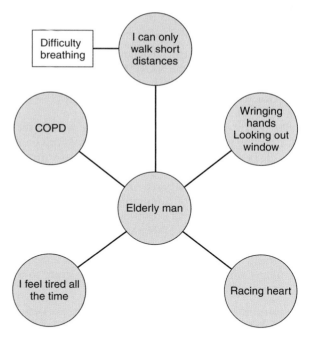

Figure I-2
Example of a concept map.

II. This client has a medical diagnosis of COPD. Is **Activity intolerance** listed with this medical diagnosis?

The process of identifying significant symptoms, clustering or grouping them into logical patterns, and then choosing an appropriate nursing diagnosis involves diagnostic reasoning (critical thinking) skills that must be learned in the process of becoming a nurse. This text serves as a tool to help the learner in this process.

A concept map may also be used to identify the nursing diagnosis: See Figure I-2 for an example.

Concept mapping diagrams the critical thinking strategy involved in using the nursing process (Abel & Freeze, 2006). Start with a blank sheet of paper; the client should be at the center of the paper. The next steps involve linking to the person via arrows the symptoms (defining characteristics) from the assessment. After the symptoms are visualized, similar ones can be put together to formulate a nursing diagnosis using another concept map (see Figure I-3).

The central theme in this concept map is the nursing diagnosis: **Activity intolerance**, with the defining characteristics/client symptoms as concepts that lead to and support the nursing diagnosis.

"Related to" Phrase or Etiology

The second part of the nursing diagnosis is the "related to" (r/t) phrase. Related factors are those that appear to show some type of patterned relationship with the nursing diagnosis. Such factors may be described as antecedent to, associated

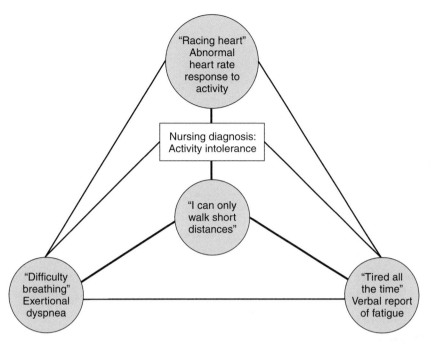

Figure I-3
Formulating a nursing diagnosis using a concept map.

with, related to, contributing to, or abetting. Only actual nursing diagnoses have related factors (NANDA-I, 2009). Pathophysiological and psychosocial changes, such as developmental age and cultural and environmental situations, may be causative or contributing factors. Exceptions to including a "related to" statement occur when the client has a "risk" or "readiness for" diagnosis. The risk diagnoses will have risk factors, and the readiness diagnoses will have defining characteristics only. This information can be found in Section III, which contains all 206 NANDA-I nursing diagnoses with definitions, defining characteristics, related factors, or risk factors.

Ideally the etiology, or cause, of the nursing diagnosis is something that can be treated by a nurse. When this is the case, the diagnosis is identified as an independent nursing diagnosis. If medical intervention is also necessary, it might be identified as a collaborative diagnosis. A carefully written, individualized r/t statement enables the nurse to plan nursing interventions that will assist the client in accomplishing goals and return to a state of optimum health.

The etiology is **not** the medical diagnosis. It may be the underlying issue contributing to the nursing diagnosis, but a medical diagnosis is **not** something the nurse can treat. In the case of the man with COPD, think about what happens when someone has COPD? How does this affect the client? What is happening to him because of this diagnosis?

For each suggested nursing diagnosis, the nurse should refer to the statements listed under the heading "Related Factors (r/t)" in Section III. These r/t factors may or may not be appropriate for the individual client. If they are not appropriate, the nurse should develop and write an r/t statement that is appropriate for the client. For the client from Case Study I, a two-part statement could be made here:

Problem = **Activity intolerance**
Etiology = r/t imbalance between oxygen supply and demand

It was already determined that the elderly man had **Activity intolerance**. With the respiratory symptoms identified from the assessment, imbalance between oxygen supply and demand is appropriate.

Defining Characteristics Phrase

The defining characteristics phrase is the third part of the three-part diagnostic system, and it consists of the signs and symptoms that have been gathered during the assessment phase. The phrase "as evidenced by" (aeb) may be used to connect the etiology (r/t) with the defining characteristics. The use of identifying defining characteristics is similar to the process the physician uses when making a medical diagnosis. For example, the physician who observes the following signs and symptoms—diminished inspiratory and expiratory capacity of the lungs, complaints of dyspnea on exertion, difficulty in inhaling and exhaling deeply, and sometimes chronic cough—may make the medical diagnosis of COPD. This same process is used to identify the nursing diagnosis of **Activity intolerance**.

Put It All Together: Writing the Three-Part Nursing Diagnosis Statement

Problem—Choose the label (nursing diagnosis) using the guidelines explained previously. A list of nursing diagnosis labels can be found in Section II and on the inside back cover.

Etiology—Write an r/t phrase (etiology). These can be found in Section II.

Symptoms—Write the defining characteristics (signs and symptoms), or the "as evidenced by" (aeb) list. A list of the signs and symptoms associated with each nursing diagnosis can be found in Section III.

Case Study 1—Elderly Man with COPD Continued

Using the information from the above case study/example, the nursing diagnostic statement would be as follows:

Problem—**Activity intolerance**
Etiology—Related to (r/t) imbalance between oxygen supply and demand
Symptoms—Verbal reports of fatigue, exertional dyspnea ("difficulty breathing when walking"), and abnormal heart rate response to activity ("racing heart")

Therefore, the nursing diagnostic statement for the elderly man with COPD is **Activity intolerance** r/t imbalance between oxygen supply and demand aeb verbal reports of fatigue, exertional dyspnea, and abnormal heart rate in response to activity.

Consider a second case study:

Case Study 2—Woman with Insomnia

As before, the nurse always begins with an assessment. To make the nursing diagnosis, the nurse follows the steps below.

A. Underline the Symptoms

A 45-year-old woman comes to the clinic and <u>asks for medication to help her sleep</u>. She states she is <u>worrying too much</u> and states, "<u>It takes me about an hour to get to sleep,</u> and <u>it is very hard to fall asleep. I feel like I can't do anything because I am so tired. My job has become very stressful because of a new boss and too much work.</u>"

B. Make a Short List of the Symptoms

Asks for medication to help her sleep; states she is worrying about too much; "It takes me about an hour to get to sleep; it is very hard to fall asleep; I feel like I can't do anything because I am so tired; My job has become very stressful because of a new boss and too much work."

C. Cluster Similar Symptoms

Asks for medication to help her sleep
"It takes me about an hour to get to sleep."
"It is very hard to fall asleep."
"I feel like I can't do anything because I am so tired."

"I am worrying too much"

"My job is stressful."
"Too much work"

D. Analyze/Interpret the Symptoms

Subjective Symptoms

- Asks for medication to help her sleep, "It takes me about an hour to get to sleep; it is very hard to fall asleep. I feel like I can't do anything because I am so tired." (all defining characteristics = verbal complaints of difficulty with sleeping)
- States she is worrying too much (anxiety)
- "My job is stressful."

Objective Symptoms

None

E. Select a Nursing Diagnosis with Related Factors and Defining Characteristics

Look up "sleep" in Section II. Listed under the heading "Sleep Pattern Disorders" in Section II is the following information:

Insomnia (nursing diagnosis) r/t anxiety and stress

This client states she is worrying too much, which may indicate anxiety; she also recently has increased job stress.

Look up **Insomnia** in Section III. Check the definition: "A disruption in amount and quality of sleep that impairs functioning." Does this describe the client in the case study? What are the related factors? What are the symptoms? Write the diagnostic statement:

Problem—**Insomnia**
Etiology—r/t anxiety, stress
Symptoms—difficulty falling asleep, "I am so tired, I can't do anything"

The nursing diagnostic statement is written in this format: **Insomnia** r/t anxiety and stress aeb (as evidenced by) difficulty falling asleep.

After the diagnostic statement is written, proceed to the next step: planning.

STEP 3: PLANNING (AD**P**IE)

This phase consists of writing **measurable client outcomes and nursing interventions** to accomplish the outcomes. Before this can be done, if the client has more than one diagnosis, the priority of the nursing diagnoses must be determined.

Nursing diagnoses should be prioritized first by immediate needs based on ABC (airway, breathing, and circulation). The highest priority nursing diagnoses should also be determined by using Maslow's hierarchy of needs. In this hierarchy, priority is generally given to immediate problems that may be life-threatening (thus ABC). For example, **Activity intolerance**, a physiological need, may be a higher priority than **Anxiety**, a love and belonging or security need. Refer to Appendix A, Nursing Diagnoses Arranged by Maslow's Hierarchy of Needs, for assistance in prioritizing nursing diagnoses.

Outcomes

After the appropriate priority of the nursing diagnoses is determined, outcomes are developed. This text includes standardized Nursing Outcomes Classification (NOC) outcomes written by a large team of University of Iowa College of Nursing faculty and students in conjunction with clinicians from a variety of settings (Moorhead et al, 2008). "Nursing-sensitive outcome (NOC) is an individual, family or community state, behavior or perception that is measured along a continuum in response to nursing interventions. The outcomes are stated as concepts that reflect a patient, caregiver, family, or community actual state, perception of behavior rather than as expected goals. . ." (Moorhead et al, 2008).

It is very important, if at all possible, for the nurse to *involve* the client in determining appropriate outcomes. The use of outcomes information creates a continuous feedback loop that is essential to ensuring evidence-based care and the best possible client outcomes, not only for individuals, but also for families, communities, and populations (Orchard et al, 2006). The minimum requirements that an outcome is rated is when the outcome is selected (i.e., the baseline measure) and when care is completed (i.e., the discharge summary). This may be sufficient in short-stay, acute-care settings. Depending on how rapid client condition changes are anticipated, some settings may evaluate once a day or once a shift. Community agencies may evaluate every visit or every other visit, for example. As measurement times are not standardized, they can be individualized for the client and the setting (Moorhead et al, 2008).

Development of appropriate outcomes can be done one of two ways: using the Nursing Outcomes Classification (NOC) list or developing an appropriate outcome statement, both of which are included in this book in Section III. There are suggested outcome statements for each nursing diagnosis in this text that can be used as written, or modified as necessary to meet the needs of the client.

When writing outcome statements, it can be helpful to use the acronym SMART, which means the outcome must be:

Specific
Measurable
Attainable
Realistic
Timed

The SMART acronym is used in business, educational, and health care settings. This method assists the nurse in identifying the client's outcomes more effectively.

The Evolve website includes a listing of additional NOC outcomes. The use of NOC outcomes can be helpful to the nurse because they contain a five-point, Likert-type rating scale that can be used to evaluate progress toward achieving the outcome. In this text the rating scale is listed, along with some of the more common indicators. As an example, the rating scale for the outcome **Sleep** is shown in Table I-2.

Because the NOC outcomes are very specific, they enhance the nursing process by helping the nurse measure and record the outcomes before and after interventions have been performed. The nurse can choose to have clients rate their own progress using the Likert-type rating scale. This involvement can help increase client motivation to progress *toward* outcomes.

After client outcomes are selected or written, and *discussed* with a client, the nurse plans nursing care and establishes a means that will help the client achieve the selected outcomes. The usual means are nursing interventions.

Interventions

Interventions are like road maps directing the best ways to provide nursing care. The more clearly a nurse writes an intervention, the easier it will be to complete the journey and arrive at the destination of successful client outcomes.

Section III supplies choices of interventions for each nursing diagnosis. The interventions are identified as independent (autonomous actions that are initiated by the nurse in response to a nursing diagnosis) or collaborative (actions that the nurse performs in collaboration with other health care professionals, and that may require a physician's order and may be in response to both medical and nursing diagnoses). The nurse may choose the interventions appropriate for the client and individualize them accordingly, or determine additional interventions.

This text also contains several suggested Nursing Interventions Classification (NIC) interventions for each nursing diagnosis to help the reader see how NIC is used along with NOC and nursing diagnoses. The NIC interventions are a comprehensive, standardized classification of treatments that nurses perform. The classification includes both physiological and psychosocial interventions and covers all nursing specialties. A listing of NIC interventions is included on the Evolve website. For more information about NIC interventions, the reader is referred to the NIC text, which is identified in the reference list (Bulechek et al, 2008).

Evidence-Based Interventions

Nursing is changing as a profession. It is essential now that each nurse develop clinical inquiry skills, which means the nurse continually questions if care is being given in the best way possible. To determine the best way of giving care, use of evidence-based practice is needed. And to make this happen, nurses need ready access to the evidence.

This text includes evidence (research)-based rationales whenever possible. The research ranges along a continuum from a case study about a single client to a systematic review performed by experts that gives quality information to guide nursing care. Every attempt has been made to supply the most current research for the nursing interventions. Some references may have earlier dates because they are classic studies that have not been replicated.

Example NOC Outcome

TABLE I-2

Sleep—0004

Domain-Functional Health (I)   Care Recipient:
Class-Energy Maintenance (A)   Data Source:
Scale(s)-Severely compromised to Not compromised (a) and Severe to None (n)
Definition: Natural periodic suspension of consciousness during which the body is restored.
Outcome Target Rating: _____ Maintain at _____ Increase to _____

Sleep Overall Rating	Severely compromised 1	Substantially compromised 2	Moderately compromised 3	Mildly compromised 4	Not compromised 5	NA
INDICATORS:						
000401 Hours of sleep	1	2	3	4	5	NA
000402 Observed hours of sleep	1	2	3	4	5	NA
000403 Sleep pattern	1	2	3	4	5	NA
000404 Sleep quality	1	2	3	4	5	NA
000405 Sleep efficiency	1	2	3	4	5	NA
000407 Sleep routine	1	2	3	4	5	NA
000418 Sleeps through the night consistently	1	2	3	4	5	NA
000408 Feelings of rejuvenation after sleep	1	2	3	4	5	NA
000410 Wakeful at appropriate times	1	2	3	4	5	NA
000419 Comfortable bed	1	2	3	4	5	NA
000420 Comfortable temperature in room	1	2	3	4	5	NA
000411 Electroencephalogram findings	1	2	3	4	5	NA
000412 Electromyogram findings	1	2	3	4	5	NA
000413 Electrooculogram findings	1	2	3	4	5	NA

	Severe 1	Substantial 2	Moderate 3	Mild 4	None 5	NA
000421 Difficulty getting to sleep	1	2	3	4	5	NA
000406 Interrupted sleep	1	2	3	4	5	NA
000409 Inappropriate napping	1	2	3	4	5	NA
000416 Sleep apnea	1	2	3	4	5	NA
000417 Dependence on sleep aids	1	2	3	4	5	NA
000422 Nightmares	1	2	3	4	5	NA
000423 Nocturia	1	2	3	4	5	NA
000424 Snoring	1	2	3	4	5	NA
000425 Pain	1	2	3	4	5	NA

From Moorhead S, Johnson M, Maas M, Swanson, E: *Nursing outcomes classification (NOC)*, ed 4, St Louis, 2008, Mosby.

Nurses in all clinical settings make hundreds of clinical decisions every day. Accurate diagnosis and selection of interventions based on searching and evaluating evidence is essential (Cruz et al, 2006; Titler, 2009). Nurses can find evidence to guide their practice in many places. Box I-1 presents several of the more common sources for information on EBN.

When using EBN, it is vitally important that the clients' concerns and individual situations be taken under consideration. The nurse must always use critical thinking when applying EBN guidelines to any particular nursing situation. Each client is unique in his or her needs and capabilities. Prescriptive guidelines can be applied inappropriately, resulting in increased problems for the client (Thompson, 2004). The goal is to provide the best care based on information from researchers, practitioners, and the recipients of care.

If you are aware of or have information on more current research, we encourage you to submit the information to customer.support@elsevier.com. We appreciate your interest in keeping this text up-to-date and current, and your support in providing the best "evidence" for state-of-the-art nursing practice.

Putting It All Together—Documenting the Care Plan

The final planning phase is documenting the actual care plan, including prioritized nursing diagnostic statements, outcomes, and interventions. This may be done electronically or by actual writing. To ensure continuity of care, the plan must be documented and shared with all health care personnel caring for the client. This text provides rationales, most of which are research based, to validate that the interventions are appropriate and workable. Because it usually takes at least 1 year from the time a manuscript is accepted for publication for it to appear in print, we have provided many websites as references for rationales and client/family teaching. In this time of rapid change in health care, we cannot wait a year for access to vital information. Websites for client/family teaching are available at the EVOLVE website.

The EVOLVE website includes also includes an electronic care plan constructor that can be easily accessed, updated, and individualized. Many agencies are using electronic records, and this is an ideal resource. See the inside front cover of this text for information regarding access to the Evolve website, or go to http://evolve.elsevier.com/Ackley/NDH.

STEP 4: IMPLEMENTATION (ADPIE)

The implementation phase of the nursing process is the actual initiation of the nursing care plan. This is the point at which you actually give nursing care. You perform the interventions that have been individualized to the client. All the hard work you put into the previous steps (ADP) is now able to be actualized to assist the client. As the interventions are performed, make sure that they are appropriate for the client. Consider that the client who was having difficulty breathing was also elderly. He may need extra time to carry

---

BOX I-1 WEBSITES FOR EVIDENCE-BASED CARE

PubMed
www.ncbi.nlm.nih.gov/entrez/query.fcgi?DB=pubmed
This site offers *free* searching of the medical and some of the nursing literature. It is provided by the National Library of Medicine and the National Institutes of Health. Information on more than 33,000 journals is found here.

CINAHL: The Cumulative Index to Nursing and Allied Health Literature
www.ebscohost.com/cinahl/
This is the best site in which to search the nursing literature. There is a cost to use this database. It is available in most school and medical/nursing libraries.

The Joanna Briggs Institute for Evidence-Based Nursing and Midwifery
www.joannabriggs.edu.au
This site identifies areas in which nurses need summarized evidence on which to base their practice; facilitates systematic reviews of international research; undertakes multisite, randomized, controlled clinical trials in areas in which research is needed; and prepares easy-to-read summaries of best practice in the form of Practice Information Sheets based on the results of systematic reviews.

The Cochrane Collaboration
www.cochrane.org
This international collaboration facilitates the creation, maintenance, and dissemination of more than 1000 systematic reviews of the effects of health care interventions in multiple conditions. More than 60 interdisciplinary working groups and collaborative review groups are composed of people from around the world who share an interest in developing and maintaining systematic reviews relevant to a particular health area.

out any activity. Check the rationale or research that is provided to see "why" the intervention is being used. The evidence should support the individualized actions that you are implementing.

Client outcomes are achieved by the performance of the nursing interventions. During this phase the nurse continues to assess the client to determine whether the interventions are effective and the desired outcomes are met.

STEP 5: EVALUATION (ADPIE)

Although evaluation is listed as the last phase of the nursing process, it is actually an integral part of each phase and something the nurse does continually. When evaluation is performed as the last phase, the nurse refers to the client's outcomes and determines whether they were met. If the outcomes were not met, the nurse begins again with assessment and determines the reason they were not met. Remember the SMART acronym? Were the outcomes **S**pecific? Were the outcomes **M**easurable? Did the client's heart rate decrease? Did the client indicate that it was easier to breathe when walking from his bed to the bathroom? Were the outcomes **A**ttainable and **R**ealistic? Did he still report, "being tired?" Did you allow adequate **T**ime for a positive outcome? Also ask yourself if you identified the correct nursing diagnosis. Should the interventions be changed? At this point the nurse can look up any new symptoms or conditions that have been identified and adjust the care plan as needed. When using EBN, it is at this point the nurse determines whether the practice that was followed was effective.

Another important part of the evaluation phase is documentation. The nurse should use the facility's tool for documentation and record the nursing activity that was performed and results of implementing nursing interventions. Many facilities use problem-oriented charting, in which the nurse is required to evaluate the care and client outcomes as part of charting. Documentation is also necessary for legal reasons because in a legal dispute, *if it wasn't charted/ recorded, it wasn't done.*

Many health care providers are using critical pathways to plan nursing care. The use of nursing diagnoses should be an integral part of any critical pathway to ensure that nursing care needs are being assessed and appropriate nursing interventions are planned and implemented.

The use of nursing diagnoses, NOC outcomes, and NIC interventions ensures that nurses are speaking a common language when providing nursing care. This system also is easily computerized for simplified documentation and analysis of patterns of care. Nursing diagnosis is the essence of nursing, used to ensure that clients receive excellent, holistic nursing care.

Just as nurses continually evaluate the interventions and outcomes of care delivered, so too must they continually evaluate the research supporting the interventions, to provide evidence-based care. The nursing process is continually evolving. In this text, our goal is to present state-of-the-art information to assist the nurse and nursing student to provide the best nursing care possible.

REFERENCES

Abel W, Freeze M: Evaluation of concept mapping in an associate degree nursing program, *J Nurs Educ* 45(9):356-364, 2006.

Bradley D, Dixon JF: Staff nurses creating safe passage with evidence-based practice, *Nurs Clin North Am* 44(1):71-81, 2009.

Brown B: Top 10 HIPAA misconceptions, *J Health Care Compliance* 9(1):41–45, 2007.

Bulechek GM, Butcher HK, McCloskey Dochterman J: *Nursing interventions classification (NIC),* ed 5, St Louis, 2008, Mosby.

Cruz D, Pimenta C, Lunney M: Teaching how to make accurate nurses' diagnoses using an evidence-based practice model. In R Levin, H Feldman (eds): *Teaching evidence-based practice in nursing,* New York, 2006, Springer.

Dreyer L: The patient interview: learn to communicate, *RDH* 26(2):46–50, 2006.

Fineout-Overholt E, Johnston L: Teaching EBP: asking searchable, answerable clinical questions, *Worldviews Evid Based Nurs* 2(3):157–160, 2005.

Hockenberry M, Wilson D, Barrera P: Implementing evidence-based nursing practice in a pediatric hospital, *Pediatr Nurs* 32(4):371–376, 2006.

Joint Commission 2009 National Patient Safety Goals: Available at www.jointcommission.org/PatientSafety/NationalPatient SafetyGoals/09_hap_npsgs.htm, retrieved July 21, 2009.

McCourt AE: Syndromes in nursing: a continuing concern. In Carroll-Johnson, editor: *Classification of nursing diagnoses: proceedings of the ninth Conference of North American Nursing Diagnosis Association,* Philadelphia, 1991, Lippincott, pp. 79–82.

Moorhead S, Johnson M, Maas M et al: *Nursing outcomes classification (NOC),* ed 4, St Louis, 2008, Mosby.

NANDA International: *Nursing diagnoses—definitions and classification 2009-2011,* Philadelphia, 2009, Wiley-Blackwell.

Orchard C, Reid-Haughian C, Vanderlee R: Health outcomes for better information and care (HOBIC): integrating patient outcome information into nursing undergraduate curricula, *Can J Nurs Leadersh* 19(3):28–33, 2006.

Spear HJ: Evidence-based nursing practice: making progress and making a difference, *Worldviews Evid Based Nurs* 3(2):52–54, 2006.

Thompson C: Fortuitous phenomena: On complexity, pragmatic randomized controlled trials, and knowledge for evidence-based practice, *Worldviews Evid Based Nurs* 1:9–17, 2004.

Titler M: The evidence for evidence-based practice implementation. In R Hughes (ed): *Patient safety and quality: an evidence-based handbook for nurses,* Rockville, MD, 2009, Agency for Healthcare Research and Quality.

Guide to Nursing Diagnoses

Section II is an alphabetical listing of client symptoms, client problems, medical diagnoses, psychiatric diagnoses, and clinical states. Each of these will have a list of possible nursing diagnoses. You may use this section to find suggestions for nursing diagnoses for your client.

- Assess the client using the format provided by the clinical setting.
- Locate the client's symptoms, problems, clinical state, diagnoses, surgeries, and diagnostic testing in the alphabetical listing contained in this section.
- Note suggestions given for appropriate nursing diagnoses.
- Evaluate the suggested nursing diagnoses to determine if they are appropriate for the client and have information that was found in the assessment.
- Use Section III (which contains an alphabetized list of all NANDA-I approved nursing diagnoses) to validate this information and check the definition, related factors, and defining characteristics. Determine if the nursing diagnosis you have selected is appropriate for the client.

A

A

Abdominal Distention

Constipation r/t decreased activity, decreased fluid intake, decreased fiber intake, pathological process

Dysfunctional gastrointestinal **Motility** r/t decreased perfusion of intestines, medication effect

Nausea r/t irritation of gastrointestinal tract

Imbalanced **Nutrition**: less than body requirements r/t nausea, vomiting

Acute **Pain** r/t retention of air, gastrointestinal secretions

Delayed **Surgical** recovery r/t retention of gas, secretions

Abdominal Hysterectomy

See Hysterectomy

Abdominal Pain

Dysfunctional gastrointestinal **Motility** r/t decreased perfusion, medication effect

Acute **Pain** r/t injury, pathological process

See cause of Abdominal Pain

Abdominal Surgery

Constipation r/t decreased activity, decreased fluid intake, anesthesia, opioids

Ineffective **Health** maintenance r/t knowledge deficit regarding self-care after surgery

Dysfunctional gastrointestinal **Motility** r/t medication effect, trauma from surgery

Imbalanced **Nutrition**: less than body requirements r/t high metabolic needs, decreased ability to ingest or digest food

Acute **Pain** r/t surgical procedure

Ineffective peripheral tissue **Perfusion** r/t immobility, abdominal surgery

Risk for **Infection**: Risk factor: invasive procedure

See Surgery, Perioperative Care; Surgery, Postoperative Care; Surgery, Preoperative Care

Abdominal Trauma

Disturbed **Body** image r/t scarring, change in body function, need for temporary colostomy

Ineffective **Breathing** pattern r/t abdominal distention, pain

Deficient **Fluid** volume r/t hemorrhage

Dysfunctional gastrointestinal **Motility** r/t decreased perfusion

Acute **Pain** r/t abdominal trauma

Risk for **Infection**: Risk factor: possible perforation of abdominal structures

Ablation, Radiofrequency Catheter

Fear r/t invasive procedure

Risk for decreased cardiac tissue **Perfusion**: Risk factor: catheterization of heart

Abortion, Induced

Compromised family **Coping** r/t unresolved feelings about decision

Ineffective **Health** maintenance r/t deficient knowledge regarding self-care after abortion

Acute **Pain** r/t surgical intervention

Chronic low **Self-Esteem** r/t feelings of guilt

Chronic **Sorrow** r/t loss of potential child

Risk for **Bleeding**: Risk factor: trauma from abortion

Risk for delayed **Development**: Risk factors: unplanned or unwanted pregnancy

Risk for **Infection**: Risk factors: open uterine blood vessels, dilated cervix

Risk for **Post-Trauma** syndrome: Risk factor: psychological trauma of abortion

Risk for **Spiritual** distress: Risk factor: perceived moral implications of decision

Abortion, Spontaneous

Disturbed **Body** image r/t perceived inability to carry pregnancy, produce child

Disabled family **Coping** r/t unresolved feelings about loss

Ineffective **Coping** r/t personal vulnerability

Interrupted **Family** processes r/t unmet expectations for pregnancy and childbirth

Fear r/t implications for future pregnancies

Grieving r/t loss of fetus

Ineffective **Health** maintenance r/t deficient knowledge regarding self-care after abortion

Acute **Pain** r/t uterine contractions, surgical intervention

Situational low **Self-Esteem** r/t feelings about loss of fetus

Chronic **Sorrow** r/t loss of potential child

Risk for **Bleeding**: Risk factor: trauma from abortion

Risk for **Infection**: Risk factors: septic or incomplete abortion of products of conception, open uterine blood vessels, dilated cervix

Risk for **Post-Trauma** syndrome: Risk factor: psychological trauma of abortion

Risk for **Spiritual** distress: Risk factor: loss of fetus

Abruptio Placentae <36 Weeks

Anxiety r/t unknown outcome, change in birth plans

Death **Anxiety** r/t unknown outcome, hemorrhage, or pain

Interrupted **Family** processes r/t unmet expectations for pregnancy and childbirth

Fear r/t threat to well-being of self and fetus

Impaired **Gas** exchange: placental r/t decreased uteroplacental area

Ineffective **Health** maintenance r/t deficient knowledge regarding self-care with disorder

Acute **Pain** r/t irritable uterus, hypertonic uterus

Impaired **Tissue** integrity: maternal r/t possible uterine rupture

Risk for **Bleeding**: Risk factor: separation of placenta from uterus causing bleeding

Risk for disproportionate **Growth**: Risk factor: uteroplacental insufficiency

Risk for **Infection**: Risk factor: partial separation of placenta

Risk for disturbed **Maternal/Fetal** dyad: Risk factors: trauma of process, lack of energy of mother

Risk for **Shock**: Risk factors: separation of placenta from uterus

Abscess Formation

Ineffective **Health** maintenance r/t deficient knowledge regarding self-care with abscess

Ineffective **Protection** r/t inadequate nutrition, abnormal blood profile, drug therapy, depressed immune function

Impaired **Tissue** integrity r/t altered circulation, nutritional deficit or excess

Abuse, Child

See Child Abuse

Abuse, Spouse, Parent, or Significant Other

Anxiety r/t threat to self-concept, situational crisis of abuse

Caregiver role strain r/t chronic illness, self-care deficits, lack of respite care, extent of caregiving required

Impaired verbal **Communication** r/t psychological barriers of fear

Compromised family **Coping** r/t abusive patterns

Defensive **Coping** r/t low self-esteem

Dysfunctional **Family** processes r/t inadequate coping skills

Insomnia r/t psychological stress

Post-Trauma syndrome r/t history of abuse

Powerlessness r/t lifestyle of helplessness

Chronic low **Self-Esteem** r/t negative family interactions

Risk for self-directed **Violence**: Risk factor: history of abuse

Accessory Muscle Use (to Breathe)

Ineffective **Breathing** pattern (See **Breathing** pattern, ineffective, Section III)

See Asthma; Bronchitis; COPD (Chronic Obstructive Pulmonary Disease); Respiratory Infections, Acute Childhood

Accident Prone

Adult **Failure** to thrive r/t fatigue

Acute **Confusion** r/t altered level of consciousness

Ineffective **Coping** r/t personal vulnerability, situational crises

Risk for **Injury**: Risk factor: history of accidents

Achalasia

Ineffective **Coping** r/t chronic disease

Acute **Pain** r/t stasis of food in esophagus

Impaired **Swallowing** r/t neuromuscular impairment

Risk for **Aspiration**: Risk factor: nocturnal regurgitation

Acid-Base Imbalances

Risk for **Electrolyte** imbalance: Risk factors: renal dysfunction, treatment-related side effects (e. g., medications, drains)

Acidosis, Metabolic

Acute **Confusion** r/t acid-base imbalance, associated electrolyte imbalance

Impaired **Memory** r/t effect of metabolic acidosis on brain function

Imbalanced **Nutrition**: less than body requirements r/t inability to ingest, absorb nutrients

Risk for **Electrolyte** imbalance: Risk factor: effect of metabolic acidosis on renal function

Risk for **Injury**: Risk factors: disorientation, weakness, stupor

Risk for decreased cardiac tissue **Perfusion**: Risk factor: dysrhythmias from hyperkalemia

Risk for **Shock**: Risk factors: abnormal metabolic state, presence of acid state impairing function

Acidosis, Respiratory

Activity intolerance r/t imbalance between oxygen supply and demand

Impaired **Gas** exchange r/t ventilation perfusion imbalance

Impaired **Memory** r/t hypoxia

Risk for decreased cardiac tissue **Perfusion**: Risk factor: dysrhythmias associated with respiratory acidosis

Acne

Disturbed **Body** image r/t biophysical changes associated with skin disorder

Ineffective self **Health** management r/t deficient knowledge (medications, personal care, cause)

Impaired **Skin** integrity r/t hormonal changes (adolescence, menstrual cycle)

ACS (Acute Coronary Syndrome)

See (MI) Myocardial Infarction

Acquired Immunodeficiency Syndrome

See AIDS (Acquired Immunodeficiency Syndrome)

Acromegaly

Activity intolerance (See **Activity** intolerance, Section III)

Ineffective **Airway** clearance r/t airway obstruction by enlarged tongue

Disturbed **Body** image r/t changes in body function and appearance

Impaired physical **Mobility** r/t joint pain

Sexual dysfunction r/t changes in hormonal secretions

Activity Intolerance, Potential to Develop

Risk for **Activity** intolerance (See **Activity** intolerance, risk for, Section III)

A

Acute Abdominal Pain

Deficient **Fluid** volume r/t air and fluids trapped in bowel, inability to drink

Acute **Pain** r/t pathological process

Risk for dysfunctional gastrointestinal **Motility**: Risk factor: ineffective gastrointestinal tissue perfusion

See cause of Abdominal Pain

Acute Alcohol Intoxication

Ineffective **Breathing** pattern r/t depression of the respiratory center

Acute **Confusion** r/t central nervous system depression

Dysfunctional **Family** processes r/t abuse of alcohol

Risk for **Aspiration**: Risk factor: depressed reflexes with acute vomiting

Risk for **Infection**: Risk factor: impaired immune system from altered nutrition

Acute Back

Anxiety r/t situational crisis, back injury

Constipation r/t decreased activity, effect of pain medication

Ineffective **Coping** r/t situational crisis, back injury

Ineffective **Health** maintenance r/t deficient knowledge regarding self-care with painful back

Impaired physical **Mobility** r/t pain

Acute **Pain** r/t back injury

Acute Confusion

See Confusion, Acute

Acute Respiratory Distress Syndrome

See ARDS (Acute Respiratory Distress Syndrome)

Acute Lymphocytic Leukemia (ALL)

See Cancer; Chemotherapy; Child with Chronic Condition; Leukemia

Adams-Stokes Syndrome

See Dysrhythmia

Addiction

See Alcoholism; Drug Abuse

Addison's Disease

Activity intolerance r/t weakness, fatigue

Disturbed **Body** image r/t increased skin pigmentation

Deficient **Fluid** volume r/t failure of regulatory mechanisms

Ineffective **Health** maintenance r/t deficient knowledge

Imbalanced **Nutrition**: less than body requirements r/t chronic illness

Risk for **Injury**: Risk factor: weakness

Adenoidectomy

Ineffective **Airway** clearance r/t hesitation or reluctance to cough as a result of pain, fear

Ineffective **Health** maintenance r/t deficient knowledge of postoperative care

Nausea r/t anesthesia effects, drainage from surgery

Acute **Pain** r/t surgical incision

Risk for **Aspiration**: Risk factors: postoperative drainage, impaired swallowing

Risk for deficient **Fluid** volume: Risk factors: decreased intake as a result of painful swallowing, effects of anesthesia

Risk for imbalanced **Nutrition**: less than body requirements: Risk factors: hesitation or reluctance to swallow

Adhesions, Lysis of

See Abdominal Surgery

Adjustment Disorder

Anxiety r/t inability to cope with psychosocial stressor

Risk-prone health **Behavior** r/t assault to self-esteem

Disturbed personal **Identity** r/t psychosocial stressor (specific to individual)

Situational low **Self-Esteem** r/t change in role function

Impaired **Social** interaction r/t absence of significant others or peers

Adjustment Impairment

Risk-prone health **Behavior** (See **Behavior**, health, risk-prone, Section III)

Adolescent, Pregnant

Anxiety r/t situational and maturational crisis, pregnancy

Disturbed **Body** image r/t pregnancy superimposed on developing body

Decisional **Conflict**: keeping child versus giving up child versus abortion r/t lack of experience with decision making, interference with decision making, multiple or divergent sources of information, lack of support system

Disabled family **Coping** r/t highly ambivalent family relationships, chronically unresolved feelings of guilt, anger, despair

Ineffective **Coping** r/t situational and maturational crisis, personal vulnerability

Ineffective **Denial** r/t fear of consequences of pregnancy becoming known

Interrupted **Family** processes r/t unmet expectations for adolescent, situational crisis

Fear r/t labor and delivery

Delayed **Growth** and development r/t pregnancy

Ineffective **Health** maintenance r/t deficient knowledge with denial of pregnancy, desire to keep pregnancy secret, fear

Deficient **Knowledge** r/t pregnancy, infant growth and development, parenting

Noncompliance r/t denial of pregnancy

Imbalanced **Nutrition**: less than body requirements r/t lack of knowledge of nutritional needs during pregnancy and as growing adolescent

Ineffective **Role** performance r/t pregnancy

Situational low **Self-Esteem** r/t feelings of shame and guilt about becoming or being pregnant

Impaired **Social** interaction r/t self-concept disturbance

Social isolation r/t absence of supportive significant others

Risk for impaired **Attachment**: Risk factor: anxiety associated with the parent role

Risk for **Constipation**: Risk factors: hormonal effects, inadequate fiber in diet, inadequate fluid in diet

Risk for delayed **Development**: Risk factor: unplanned or unwanted pregnancy

Risk for urge urinary **Incontinence**: Risk factor: pressure on bladder by growing uterus

Risk for disturbed **Maternal/Fetal** dyad: Risk factors: immaturity, substance use

Risk for impaired **Parenting**: Risk factors: adolescent parent, unplanned or unwanted pregnancy, single parent

Readiness for enhanced **Childbearing** process: reports appropriate prenatal lifestyle

Adoption, Giving Child Up For

Decisional **Conflict** r/t unclear personal values or beliefs, perceived threat to value system, support system deficit

Ineffective **Coping** r/t final decision

Interrupted **Family** processes r/t conflict within family regarding relinquishment of child

Grieving r/t loss of child, loss of role of parent

Insomnia r/t depression or trauma of relinquishment of child

Social isolation r/t making choice that goes against values of significant others

Chronic **Sorrow** r/t loss of relationship with child

Risk for **Post-Trauma** syndrome: Risk factor: psychological trauma of relinquishment of child

Risk for **Spiritual** distress: Risk factor: perceived moral implications of decision

Readiness for enhanced **Spiritual** well-being: harmony with self regarding final decision

Adrenocortical Insufficiency

Deficient **Fluid** volume r/t insufficient ability to reabsorb water

Ineffective **Protection** r/t inability to tolerate stress

Delayed **Surgical** recovery r/t inability to respond to stress

Risk for **Shock**: Risk factor: deficient fluid volume

See Addison's Disease; Shock, Hypovolemic

Advance Directives

Death **Anxiety** r/t planning for end-of-life health decisions

Decisional **Conflict** r/t unclear personal values or beliefs, perceived threat to value system, support system deficit

Grieving r/t possible loss of self, significant other

Readiness for enhanced **Spiritual** well-being: harmonious interconnectedness with self, others, higher power, God

Affective Disorders

Constipation r/t inactivity, decreased fluid intake

Ineffective **Coping** r/t complicated grieving

Adult **Failure** to thrive r/t altered mood state

Fatigue r/t psychological demands

Ineffective **Health** maintenance r/t lack of ability to make good judgments regarding ways to obtain help

Hopelessness r/t feeling of abandonment, long-term stress

Insomnia r/t inactivity

Chronic low **Self-Esteem** r/t repeated unmet expectations

Sexual dysfunction r/t loss of sexual desire

Social isolation r/t ineffective coping

Chronic **Sorrow** r/t chronic mental illness

Risk for complicated **Grieving**: Risk factor: lack of previous resolution of former grieving response

Risk for **Loneliness**: Risk factors: pattern of social isolation, feelings of low self-esteem

Risk for **Suicide**: Risk factor: panic state

See specific disorder: Depression (Major Depressive Disorder); Dysthymic Disorder; Manic Disorder, Bipolar I

Age-Related Macular Degeneration

See Macular Degeneration

Aggressive Behavior

Fear r/t real or imagined threat to own well-being

Risk for other-directed **Violence** (See **Violence**, other-directed, risk for, Section III)

Risk for self-directed **Violence** (See **Violence**, self-directed, risk for, Section III)

Aging

Death **Anxiety** r/t fear of unknown, loss of self, impact on significant others

Impaired **Dentition** r/t ineffective oral hygiene

Adult **Failure** to thrive r/t depression, apathy, fatigue

Grieving r/t multiple losses, impending death

Ineffective self **Health** management r/t deficient knowledge: medication, nutrition, exercise, coping strategies

Functional urinary **Incontinence** r/t impaired vision, impaired cognition, neuromuscular limitations, altered environmental factors

Impaired individual **Resilience** r/t aging, multiple losses

Disturbed **Sensory** perception: visual/auditory r/t aging process

Sleep deprivation r/t aging-related sleep-stage shifts

Chronic **Sorrow** r/t multiple losses

Ineffective **Thermoregulation** r/t aging

Risk for **Caregiver** role strain: Risk factor: inability to handle increasing needs of significant other

Risk for **Injury**: Risk factor: disturbed sensory perception

Risk for **Loneliness**: Risk factors: inadequate support system, role transition, health alterations, depression, fatigue

Readiness for enhanced community **Coping**: providing social support and other resources identified as needed for elderly client

Readiness for enhanced family **Coping**: ability to gratify needs, address adaptive tasks

Readiness for enhanced **Knowledge**: specify: need to improve health

Readiness for enhanced **Nutrition**: need to improve health

Readiness for enhanced **Relationship**: demonstrates understanding of partner's insufficient function

Readiness for enhanced **Self Health** management: knowledge about medication, nutrition, exercise, coping strategies

Readiness for enhanced **Sleep**: need to improve sleep

Readiness for enhanced **Spiritual** well-being: one's experience of life's meaning, harmony with self, others, higher power, God, environment

Readiness for enhanced **Urinary** elimination: need to improve health

Agitation

Acute **Confusion** r/t side effects of medication, hypoxia, decreased cerebral perfusion, alcohol abuse or withdrawal, substance abuse or withdrawal, sensory deprivation or overload

Sleep deprivation r/t sundown syndrome

See cause of Agitation

Agoraphobia

Anxiety r/t real or perceived threat to physical integrity

Ineffective **Coping** r/t inadequate support systems

Fear r/t leaving home, going out in public places

Impaired **Social** interaction r/t disturbance in self-concept

Social isolation r/t altered thought process

Agranulocytosis

Ineffective **Health** maintenance r/t deficient knowledge of protective measures to prevent infection

Delayed **Surgical** recovery r/t abnormal blood profile

Risk for **Infection**: Risk factor: abnormal blood profile

AIDS (Acquired Immunodeficiency Syndrome)

Death **Anxiety** r/t fear of premature death

Disturbed **Body** image r/t chronic contagious illness, cachexia

Caregiver role strain r/t unpredictable illness course, presence of situation stressors

Diarrhea r/t inflammatory bowel changes

Disturbed **Energy** field r/t chronic illness

Interrupted **Family** processes r/t distress about diagnosis of human immunodeficiency virus (HIV) infection

Fatigue r/t disease process, stress, poor nutritional intake

Fear r/t powerlessness, threat to well-being

Grieving: family/parental r/t potential or impending death of loved one

Grieving: individual r/t loss of physio-psychosocial well-being

Ineffective **Health** maintenance r/t deficient knowledge regarding transmission of infection, lack of exposure to information, misinterpretation of information

Hopelessness r/t deteriorating physical condition

Imbalanced **Nutrition**: less than body requirements r/t decreased ability to eat and absorb nutrients as a result of anorexia, nausea, diarrhea; oral candidiasis pathology in gastrointestinal tract

Chronic **Pain** r/t tissue inflammation and destruction

Ineffective **Protection** r/t risk for infection secondary to inadequate immune system

Impaired individual **Resilience** r/t chronic illness

Situational low **Self-Esteem** r/t crisis of chronic contagious illness

Ineffective **Sexuality** pattern r/t possible transmission of disease

Social isolation r/t self-concept disturbance, therapeutic isolation

Chronic **Sorrow** r/t living with long-term chronic illness

Spiritual distress r/t challenged beliefs or moral system

Risk for deficient **Fluid** volume: Risk factors: diarrhea, vomiting, fever, bleeding

Risk for **Infection**: Risk factor: inadequate immune system

Risk for **Loneliness**: Risk factor: social isolation

Risk for impaired **Oral** mucous membrane: Risk factor: immunological deficit

Risk for impaired **Skin** integrity: Risk factors: immunological deficit, diarrhea

Risk for **Spiritual** distress: Risk factor: physical illness

See AIDS, Child; Cancer; Pneumonia

AIDS Dementia

Chronic **Confusion** r/t viral invasion of nervous system

See Dementia

AIDS, Child

Parental role conflict r/t intimidation with invasive or restrictive modalities

Impaired **Parenting** r/t congenital acquisition of infection secondary to intravenous (IV) drug use, multiple sexual partners, history of contaminated blood transfusion

See AIDS (Acquired Immunodeficiency Syndrome); Child with Chronic Condition; Hospitalized Child; Terminally Ill Child, Adolescent; Terminally Ill Child, Infant/Toddler; Terminally Ill Child, Preschool Child; Terminally Ill Child, School-Age Child/Preadolescent; Terminally Ill Child/Death of Child, Parent

Airway Obstruction/Secretions

Ineffective **Airway** clearance (See **Airway** clearance, ineffective, Section III)

Alcohol Withdrawal

Anxiety r/t situational crisis, withdrawal

Acute **Confusion** r/t effects of alcohol withdrawal

Ineffective **Coping** r/t personal vulnerability

Dysfunctional **Family** processes r/t abuse of alcohol

Ineffective **Health** maintenance r/t deficient knowledge regarding chronic illness or effects of alcohol consumption

Insomnia r/t effect of alcohol withdrawal, anxiety

Imbalanced **Nutrition**: less than body requirements r/t poor dietary habits

Chronic low **Self-Esteem** r/t repeated unmet expectations

Disturbed **Sensory** perception: visual, auditory, kinesthetic, tactile, olfactory r/t neurochemical imbalance in brain

Risk for deficient **Fluid** volume: Risk factors: excessive diaphoresis, agitation, decreased fluid intake

Risk for other-directed **Violence**: Risk factor: substance withdrawal

Risk for self-directed **Violence**: Risk factor: substance withdrawal

Alcoholism

Anxiety r/t loss of control

Risk-prone health **Behavior** r/t lack of motivation to change behaviors, addiction

Acute **Confusion** r/t alcohol abuse

Chronic **Confusion** r/t neurological effects of chronic alcohol intake

Defensive **Coping** r/t alcoholism

Disabled family **Coping** r/t codependency issues due to alcoholism

Ineffective **Coping** r/t use of alcohol to cope with life events

Ineffective **Denial** r/t refusal to acknowledge alcoholism

Dysfunctional **Family** process r/t alcohol abuse

Impaired **Home** maintenance r/t memory deficits, fatigue

Insomnia r/t irritability, nightmares, tremors

Impaired **Memory** r/t alcohol abuse

Self **Neglect** r/t effects of alcohol abuse

Imbalanced **Nutrition**: less than body requirements r/t anorexia

Powerlessness r/t alcohol addiction

Ineffective **Protection** r/t malnutrition, sleep deprivation

Chronic low **Self-Esteem** r/t failure at life events

Social isolation r/t unacceptable social behavior, values

Risk for **Injury**: Risk factor: alteration in sensory or perceptual function

Risk for **Loneliness**: Risk factor: unacceptable social behavior

Risk for other-directed **Violence**: Risk factors: reactions to substances used, impulsive behavior, disorientation, impaired judgment

Risk for self-directed **Violence**: Risk factors: reactions to substances used, impulsive behavior, disorientation, impaired judgment

Alcoholism, Dysfunctional Family Processes

Dysfunctional **Family** processes (See **Family** processes, dysfunctional, Section III)

Alkalosis

See Metabolic Alkalosis

ALL (Acute Lymphocytic Leukemia)

See Cancer; Chemotherapy; Child with a Chronic Condition; Leukemia

Allergies

Latex **Allergy** response r/t hypersensitivity to natural rubber latex

Ineffective **Health** maintenance r/t deficient knowledge regarding allergies

Risk for latex **Allergy** response: Risk factor: repeated exposure to products containing latex

Alopecia

Disturbed **Body** image r/t loss of hair, change in appearance

Deficient **Knowledge** r/t self-care needed to promote hair growth

Altered Mental Status

See Confusion, Acute; Confusion, Chronic; Memory Deficit

ALS (Amyotrophic Lateral Sclerosis)

See Amyotrophic Lateral Sclerosis (ALS)

Alzheimer's Disease

Caregiver role strain r/t duration and extent of caregiving required

Chronic **Confusion** r/t Alzheimer's disease

Compromised family **Coping** r/t interrupted family processes

Impaired **Environmental** interpretation syndrome r/t Alzheimer's disease

Adult **Failure** to thrive r/t difficulty in reasoning, judgment, memory, concentration

Fear r/t loss of self

Ineffective **Health** maintenance r/t deficient knowledge of caregiver regarding appropriate care

Impaired **Home** maintenance r/t impaired cognitive function, inadequate support systems

Hopelessness r/t deteriorating condition

Insomnia r/t neurological impairment, daytime naps

Impaired **Memory** r/t neurological disturbance

Impaired physical **Mobility** r/t severe neurological dysfunction

Self **Neglect** r/t loss of cognitive function

Powerlessness r/t deteriorating condition

Self-Care deficit: specify r/t psychological or physiological impairment

Social isolation r/t fear of disclosure of memory loss

Wandering r/t cognitive impairment, frustration, physiological state

Risk for **Injury**: Risk factor: confusion

Risk for **Loneliness**: Risk factor: potential social isolation

Risk for **Relocation** stress syndrome: Risk factors: impaired psychosocial health, decreased health status

Risk for other-directed **Violence**: Risk factors: frustration, fear, anger

See Dementia

A

AMD (Age-Related Macular Degeneration)

See Macular Degeneration

Amenorrhea

Imbalanced **Nutrition**: less than body requirements r/t inadequate food intake

See Sexuality, Adolescent

AMI (Acute Myocardial Infarction)

See MI (Myocardial Infarction)

Amnesia

Acute **Confusion** r/t alcohol abuse, delirium, dementia, drug abuse

Dysfunctional **Family** processes r/t alcohol abuse, inadequate coping skills

Impaired **Memory** r/t excessive environmental disturbance, neurological disturbance

Post-Trauma syndrome r/t history of abuse, catastrophic illness, disaster, accident

Amniocentesis

Anxiety r/t threat to self and fetus, unknown future

Decisional **Conflict** r/t choice of treatment pending results of test

Risk for **Infection**: Risk factor: invasive procedure

Amnionitis

See Chorioamnionitis

Amniotic Membrane Rupture

See Premature Rupture of Membranes

Amputation

Disturbed **Body** image r/t negative effects of amputation, response from others

Grieving r/t loss of body part, future lifestyle changes

Ineffective **Health** maintenance r/t deficient knowledge of care of stump, rehabilitation

Impaired physical **Mobility** r/t musculoskeletal impairment, limited movement

Acute **Pain** r/t surgery, phantom limb sensation

Chronic **Pain** r/t surgery, phantom limb sensation

Ineffective peripheral tissue **Perfusion** r/t impaired arterial circulation

Impaired **Skin** integrity r/t poor healing, prosthesis rubbing

Chronic **Sorrow** r/t grief associated with loss of body part

Risk for **Bleeding**: Risk factor: vulnerable surgical site

Amyotrophic Lateral Sclerosis (ALS)

Death **Anxiety** r/t impending progressive loss of function leading to death

Ineffective **Breathing** pattern r/t compromised muscles of respiration

Impaired verbal **Communication** r/t weakness of muscles of speech, deficient knowledge of ways to compensate and alternative communication devices

Decisional **Conflict**: ventilator therapy r/t unclear personal values or beliefs, lack of relevant information

Impaired individual **Resilience** r/t chronic debilitating illness

Chronic **Sorrow** r/t chronic illness

Impaired **Swallowing** r/t weakness of muscles involved in swallowing

Impaired spontaneous **Ventilation** r/t weakness of muscles of respiration

Risk for **Aspiration**: Risk factor: impaired swallowing

Risk for **Spiritual** distress: Risk factor: chronic debilitating condition

See Neurologic Disorders

Anal Fistula

See Hemorrhoidectomy

Anaphylactic Shock

Ineffective **Airway** clearance r/t laryngeal edema, bronchospasm

Latex **Allergy** response r/t abnormal immune mechanism response

Impaired spontaneous **Ventilation** r/t acute airway obstruction

Anasarca

Excess **Fluid** volume r/t excessive fluid intake, cardiac/renal dysfunction, loss of plasma proteins

Risk for impaired **Skin** integrity: Risk factor: impaired circulation to skin

See cause of Anasarca

Anemia

Anxiety r/t cause of disease

Fatigue r/t decreased oxygen supply to the body, increased cardiac workload

Ineffective **Health** maintenance r/t deficient knowledge regarding nutritional and medical treatment of anemia

Impaired **Memory** r/t anemia

Delayed **Surgical** recovery r/t decreased oxygen supply to body, increased cardiac workload

Risk for **Bleeding** (See **Bleeding,** risk for, Section III)

Risk for **Injury**: Risk factor: alteration in peripheral sensory perception

Anemia, in Pregnancy

Anxiety r/t concerns about health of self and fetus

Fatigue r/t decreased oxygen supply to the body, increased cardiac workload

Ineffective **Health** maintenance r/t deficient knowledge regarding nutrition in pregnancy

Risk for delayed **Development**: Risk factor: reduction in the oxygen-carrying capacity of blood

Risk for **Infection**: Risk factor: reduction in oxygen-carrying capacity of blood

Risk for disturbed **Maternal/Fetal**: dyad: Risk factor: compromised oxygen transport

Anemia, Sickle Cell

See Anemia; Sickle Cell Anemia/Crisis

Anencephaly

See Neural Tube Defects

Aneurysm, Abdominal Surgery

Risk for deficient **Fluid** volume: Risk factor: hemorrhage r/t potential abnormal blood loss

Risk for **Infection**: Risk factor: invasive procedure

Risk for ineffective gastrointestinal tissue **Perfusion** (See **Perfusion,** tissue, gastrointestinal, ineffective, risk for, Section III)

Risk for ineffective renal **Perfusion**: Risk factor: prolonged ischemia of kidneys

See Abdominal Surgery

Aneurysm, Cerebral

See Craniectomy/Craniotomy; Subarachnoid Hemorrhage (if aneurysm has ruptured)

Anger

Anxiety r/t situational crisis

Risk-prone health **Behavior** r/t assault to self-esteem, disability requiring change in lifestyle, inadequate support system

Defensive **Coping** r/t inability to acknowledge responsibility for actions and results of actions

Fear r/t environmental stressor, hospitalization

Grieving r/t significant loss

Powerlessness r/t health care environment

Risk for compromised human **Dignity**: Risk factors: inadequate participation in decision making, perceived dehumanizing treatment, perceived humiliation, exposure of the body, cultural incongruity

Risk for **Post-Trauma** syndrome: Risk factor: inadequate social support

Risk for other-directed **Violence**: Risk factors: history of violence, rage reaction

Risk for self-directed **Violence**: Risk factors: history of violence, history of abuse, rage reaction

Angina

Activity intolerance r/t acute pain, dysrhythmias

Anxiety r/t situational crisis

Decreased **Cardiac** output r/t myocardial ischemia, medication effect, dysrhythmia

Ineffective **Coping** r/t personal vulnerability to situational crisis of new diagnosis, deteriorating health

Ineffective **Denial** r/t deficient knowledge of need to seek help with symptoms

Grieving r/t pain, loss of health

Ineffective **Health** maintenance r/t deficient knowledge of care of angina condition

Acute **Pain** r/t myocardial ischemia

Ineffective **Sexuality** pattern r/t disease process, medications, loss of libido

Angiocardiography (Cardiac Catheterization)

See Cardiac Catheterization

Angioplasty, Coronary

Fear r/t possible outcome of interventional procedure

Ineffective **Health** maintenance r/t deficient knowledge regarding care after procedures, measures to limit coronary artery disease

Ineffective peripheral tissue **Perfusion** r/t vasospasm, hematoma formation

Risk for **Bleeding**: Risk factors: possible damage to coronary artery, hematoma formation, hemorrhage

Risk for decreased cardiac tissue **Perfusion**: Risk factors: ventricular ischemia, dysrhythmias

Anomaly, Fetal/Newborn (Parent Dealing with)

Anxiety r/t threat to role functioning, situational crisis

Decisional **Conflict**: interventions for fetus or newborn r/t lack of relevant information, spiritual distress, threat to value system

Parental role **Conflict** r/t separation from newborn, intimidation with invasive or restrictive modalities, specialized care center policies

Disabled family **Coping** r/t chronically unresolved feelings about loss of perfect baby

Ineffective **Coping** r/t personal vulnerability in situational crisis

Interrupted **Family** processes r/t unmet expectations for perfect baby, lack of adequate support systems

Fear r/t real or imagined threat to baby, implications for future pregnancies, powerlessness

Hopelessness r/t long-term stress, deteriorating physical condition of child, lost spiritual belief

Deficient **Knowledge** r/t limited exposure to situation

Impaired **Parenting** r/t interruption of bonding process

Powerlessness r/t complication threatening fetus or newborn

Situational low **Self-Esteem** r/t perceived inability to produce a perfect child

Social isolation r/t alterations in child's physical appearance, altered state of wellness

Chronic **Sorrow** r/t loss of ideal child, inadequate bereavement support

Spiritual distress r/t test of spiritual beliefs

Risk for impaired **Attachment**: Risk factor: ill infant unable to effectively initiate parental contact as result of altered behavioral organization

Risk for complicated **Grieving**: Risk factor: loss of perfect child

Risk for disorganized **Infant** behavior: Risk factor: congenital disorder

Risk for impaired **Parenting**: Risk factors: interruption of bonding process; unrealistic expectations for self, infant, or partner; perceived threat to own emotional survival; severe stress; lack of knowledge

A

Risk for **Spiritual** distress: Risk factor: lack of normal child to raise and carry on family name

Anorectal Abscess

Disturbed **Body** image r/t odor and drainage from rectal area

Acute **Pain** r/t inflammation of perirectal area

Risk for **Constipation**: Risk factor: fear of painful elimination

Anorexia

Deficient **Fluid** volume r/t inability to drink

Imbalanced **Nutrition**: less than body requirements r/t loss of appetite, nausea, vomiting

Delayed **Surgical** recovery r/t inadequate nutritional intake

Anorexia Nervosa

Activity intolerance r/t fatigue, weakness

Disturbed **Body** image r/t misconception of actual body appearance

Constipation r/t lack of adequate food, fiber, and fluid intake

Defensive **Coping** r/t psychological impairment, eating disorder

Disabled family **Coping** r/t highly ambivalent family relationships

Ineffective **Denial** r/t fear of consequences of therapy, possible weight gain

Diarrhea r/t laxative abuse

Interrupted **Family** processes r/t situational crisis

Imbalanced **Nutrition**: less than body requirements r/t inadequate food intake, excessive exercise

Chronic low **Self-Esteem** r/t repeated unmet expectations

Ineffective **Sexuality** pattern r/t loss of libido from malnutrition

Ineffective family **Therapeutic** regimen management r/t family conflict, excessive demands on family associated with complexity of condition and treatment

Risk for **Infection**: Risk factor: malnutrition resulting in depressed immune system

Risk for **Spiritual** distress: Risk factor: low self-esteem

See Maturational Issues, Adolescent

Anosmia (Smell, Loss of Ability to)

Imbalanced **Nutrition**: less than body requirements r/t loss of appetite associated with loss of smell

Disturbed **Sensory** perception: olfactory r/t altered sensory reception, transmission, integration

Antepartum Period

See Pregnancy, Normal; Prenatal Care, Normal

Anterior Repair, Anterior Colporrhaphy

Urinary retention r/t edema of urinary structures

Risk for urge urinary **Incontinence**: Risk factor: trauma to bladder

See Vaginal Hysterectomy

Anticoagulant Therapy

Ineffective **Health** maintenance r/t deficient knowledge regarding precautions to take with anticoagulant therapy

Risk for **Bleeding**: Risk Factors: altered clotting function from anticoagulant

Risk for deficient **Fluid** volume: hemorrhage: Risk factor: altered clotting mechanism

Antisocial Personality Disorder

Defensive **Coping** r/t excessive use of projection

Ineffective **Coping** r/t frequently violating the norms and rules of society

Hopelessness r/t abandonment

Impaired **Social** interaction r/t sociocultural conflict, chemical dependence, inability to form relationships

Spiritual distress r/t separation from religious or cultural ties

Ineffective family **Therapeutic** regimen management r/t excessive demands on family

Risk for **Loneliness**: Risk factor: inability to interact appropriately with others

Risk for impaired **Parenting**: Risk factors: inability to function as parent or guardian, emotional instability

Risk for **Self-Mutilation**: Risk factors: self-hatred, depersonalization

Risk for other-directed **Violence**: Risk factor: history of violence

Anuria

See Renal Failure

Anxiety

Anxiety (See **Anxiety**, Section III)

Anxiety Disorder

Ineffective **Activity** planning r/t unrealistic perception of events

Anxiety r/t unmet security and safety needs

Death **Anxiety** r/t fears of unknown, powerlessness

Decisional **Conflict** r/t low self-esteem, fear of making a mistake

Defensive **Coping** r/t overwhelming feelings of dread

Disabled family **Coping** r/t ritualistic behavior, actions

Ineffective **Coping** r/t inability to express feelings appropriately

Ineffective **Denial** r/t overwhelming feelings of hopelessness, fear, threat to self

Disturbed **Energy** field r/t hopelessness, helplessness

Insomnia r/t psychological impairment, emotional instability

Powerlessness r/t lifestyle of helplessness

Self-Care deficit r/t ritualistic behavior, activities

Sleep deprivation r/t prolonged psychological discomfort

Risk for **Spiritual** distress: Risk factor: psychological distress

Aortic Aneurysm Repair (Abdominal Surgery)

See Abdominal Surgery; Aneurysm, Abdominal Surgery

Aortic Valvular Stenosis

See Congenital Heart Disease/Cardiac Anomalies

Aphasia

Anxiety r/t situational crisis of aphasia

Impaired verbal **Communication** r/t decrease in circulation to brain

Ineffective **Coping** r/t loss of speech

Ineffective **Health** maintenance r/t deficient knowledge regarding information on aphasia and alternative communication techniques

Aplastic Anemia

Activity intolerance r/t imbalance between oxygen supply and demand

Anxiety r/t deficient knowledge of disease process and treatment

Impaired **Protection** r/t inadequate immune function

Delayed **Surgical** recovery r/t risk for infection

Risk for **Bleeding**: Risk factor: inadequate clotting factors

Risk for **Infection**: Risk factor: inadequate immune function

Apnea in Infancy

See Premature Infant (Child); Premature Infant (Parent); SIDS (Sudden Infant Death Syndrome)

Apneustic Respirations

Ineffective **Breathing** pattern r/t perception or cognitive impairment, neurological impairment

See cause of Apneustic Respirations

Appendectomy

Deficient **Fluid** volume r/t fluid restriction, hypermetabolic state, nausea, vomiting

Ineffective **Health** maintenance r/t deficient knowledge regarding self-care after appendectomy

Acute **Pain** r/t surgical incision

Delayed **Surgical** recovery r/t rupture of appendix

Risk for **Infection**: Risk factors: perforation or rupture of appendix, surgical incision, peritonitis

See Hospitalized Child; Surgery, Postoperative

Appendicitis

Deficient **Fluid** volume r/t anorexia, nausea, vomiting

Acute **Pain** r/t inflammation

Risk for **Infection**: Risk factor: possible perforation of appendix

Apprehension

Anxiety r/t threat to self-concept, threat to health status, situational crisis

Death **Anxiety** r/t apprehension over loss of self, consequences to significant others

AMD (Age-Related Macular Degeneration)

See Macular Degeneration

ARDS (Acute Respiratory Distress Syndrome)

Ineffective **Airway** clearance r/t excessive tracheobronchial secretions

Death **Anxiety** r/t seriousness of physical disease

Impaired **Gas** exchange r/t damage to alveolar-capillary membrane, change in lung compliance

Delayed **Surgical** recovery r/t complications associated with respiratory pathology

Impaired spontaneous **Ventilation** r/t damage to alveolar capillary membrane

See Child with Chronic Condition; Ventilator Client

Arrhythmia

See Dysrhythmia

Arterial Insufficiency

Ineffective peripheral tissue **Perfusion** r/t interruption of arterial flow

Delayed **Surgical** recovery r/t ineffective tissue perfusion

Arthritis

Activity intolerance r/t chronic pain, fatigue, weakness

Disturbed **Body** image r/t ineffective coping with joint abnormalities

Ineffective **Health** maintenance r/t deficient knowledge regarding care of arthritis

Impaired physical **Mobility** r/t musculoskeletal impairment

Chronic **Pain** r/t progression of joint deterioration

Self-Care deficit: specify r/t pain, musculoskeletal impairment

See JRA (Juvenile Rheumatoid Arthritis)

Arthrocentesis

Acute **Pain** r/t invasive procedure

Arthroplasty (Total Hip Replacement)

See Total Joint Replacement (Total Knee, Total Hip, Shoulder); Surgery, Perioperative; Surgery, Postoperative; Surgery, Preoperative

Arthroscopy

Ineffective **Health** maintenance r/t deficient knowledge regarding procedure, postoperative restrictions

Ascites

Ineffective **Breathing** pattern r/t increased abdominal girth

Ineffective **Health** maintenance r/t deficient knowledge of care with condition of ascites

Imbalanced **Nutrition**: less than body requirements r/t loss of appetite

Chronic **Pain** r/t altered body function

See cause of Ascites; Cancer; Cirrhosis

Asphyxia, Birth

Ineffective **Breathing** pattern r/t depression of breathing reflex secondary to anoxia

Ineffective **Coping** r/t uncertainty of child outcome

Fear (parental) r/t concern over safety of infant

Impaired **Gas** exchange r/t poor placental perfusion, lack of initiation of breathing by newborn

Grieving r/t loss of "perfect" child, concern of loss of future abilities

A

Impaired spontaneous **Ventilation** r/t brain injury

Risk for impaired Attachment: Risk factors: ill infant who is unable to initiate parental contact, hospitalization in critical care environment

Risk for delayed Development: Risk factor: lack of oxygen to brain

Risk for disproportionate Growth: Risk factor: lack of oxygen to brain

Risk for disorganized Infant behavior: Risk factor: lack of oxygen to brain

Risk for Injury: Risk factor: lack of oxygen to brain

Risk for ineffective cerebral tissue Perfusion: Risk factor: poor placental perfusion or cord compression resulting in lack of oxygen to brain

Risk for Post-Trauma syndrome: parental: Risk factor: psychological trauma of sudden potential for loss of newborn

Aspiration, Danger of

Risk for Aspiration (See **Aspiration**, risk for, Section III)

Assault Victim

Post-Trauma syndrome r/t assault

Rape-Trauma syndrome r/t rape

Impaired individual **Resilience** r/t frightening experience, post-trauma stress response

Risk for Post-Trauma syndrome: Risk factors: perception of event, inadequate social support, unsupportive environment, diminished ego strength, duration of event

Risk for Spiritual distress: Risk factors: physical, psychological stress

Assaultive Client

Risk for Injury: Risk factors: confused thought process, impaired judgment

Risk for other-directed Violence: Risk factors: paranoid ideation, anger

Asthma

Activity intolerance r/t fatigue, energy shift to meet muscle needs for breathing to overcome airway obstruction

Ineffective **Airway** clearance r/t tracheobronchial narrowing, excessive secretions

Anxiety r/t inability to breathe effectively, fear of suffocation

Disturbed **Body** image r/t decreased participation in physical activities

Ineffective **Breathing** pattern r/t anxiety

Ineffective **Coping** r/t personal vulnerability to situational crisis

Ineffective self **Health** management (See **Health** management, self, ineffective, in Section III)

Impaired **Home** maintenance r/t deficient knowledge regarding control of environmental triggers

Sleep deprivation r/t ineffective breathing pattern, cough

Readiness for enhanced **Self Health** management (See **Self Health** management, readiness for enhanced, in Section III)

See Child with Chronic Condition; Hospitalized Child

Ataxia

Anxiety r/t change in health status

Disturbed **Body** image r/t staggering gait

Impaired physical **Mobility** r/t neuromuscular impairment

Risk for Falls: Risk factors: gait alteration, instability

Atelectasis

Ineffective **Breathing** pattern r/t loss of functional lung tissue, depression of respiratory function or hypoventilation because of pain

Impaired **Gas** exchange r/t decreased alveolar-capillary surface

Atherosclerosis

See MI (Myocardial Infarction); CVA (Cerebrovascular Accident); Peripheral Vascular Disease (PVD)

Athlete's Foot

Ineffective **Health** maintenance r/t deficient knowledge regarding treatment and prevention of athlete's foot

Impaired **Skin** integrity r/t effects of fungal agent

See Itching; Pruritus

ATN (Acute Tubular Necrosis)

See Renal Failure

Atrial Fibrillation

See Dysrhythmia

Atrial Septal Defect

See Congenital Heart Disease/Cardiac Anomalies

Attention Deficit Disorder

Risk-prone health **Behavior** r/t intense emotional state

Disabled family **Coping** r/t significant person with chronically unexpressed feelings of guilt, anxiety, hostility, and despair

Chronic low **Self-Esteem** r/t difficulty in participating in expected activities, poor school performance

Social isolation r/t unacceptable social behavior

Risk for delayed Development: Risk factor: behavior disorders

Risk for Loneliness: Risk factor: social isolation

Risk for impaired Parenting: Risk factor: lack of knowledge of factors contributing to child's behavior

Risk for Spiritual distress: Risk factor: poor relationships

Auditory Problems

See Hearing Impairment

Autism

Impaired verbal **Communication** r/t speech and language delays

Compromised family **Coping** r/t parental guilt over etiology of disease, inability to accept or adapt to child's condition, inability to help child and other family members seek treatment

Delayed **Growth** and development r/t inability to develop relations with other human beings, inability to identify own body as separate from those of other people, inability to integrate concept of self

Disturbed personal **Identity** r/t inability to distinguish between self and environment, inability to identify own body as separate from those of other people, inability to integrate concept of self

Self **Neglect** r/t impaired socialization

Impaired **Social** interaction r/t communication barriers, inability to relate to others, failure to develop peer relationships

Risk for delayed **Development**: Risk factor: autism

Risk for **Loneliness**: Risk factors: health alterations, change in cognition

Risk for **Self-Mutilation**: Risk factor: autistic state

Risk for other-directed **Violence**: Risk factors: frequent destructive rages toward others secondary to extreme response to changes in routine, fear of harmless things

Risk for self-directed **Violence**: Risk factors: frequent destructive rages toward self, secondary to extreme response to changes in routine, fear of harmless things

See Child with Chronic Condition; Mental Retardation

Autonomic Dysreflexia

Autonomic dysreflexia r/t bladder distention, bowel distention, noxious stimuli

Risk for **Autonomic** dysreflexia: Risk factors: bladder distention, bowel distention, noxious stimuli

Autonomic Hyperreflexia

See Autonomic Dysreflexia

B

Baby Care

Readiness for enhanced **Childbearing** process: demonstrates appropriate feeding and baby care techniques, along with attachment to infant and providing a safe environment

Back Pain

Anxiety r/t situational crisis, back injury

Ineffective **Coping** r/t situational crisis, back injury

Disturbed **Energy** field r/t chronic pain

Ineffective **Health** maintenance r/t deficient knowledge regarding prevention of further injury, proper body mechanics

Impaired physical **Mobility** r/t pain

Acute **Pain** r/t back injury

Chronic **Pain** r/t back injury

Risk for **Constipation**: Risk factors: decreased activity, side effect of pain medication

Risk for **Disuse** syndrome: Risk factor: severe pain

Bacteremia

Risk for **Infection**: Risk factor: compromised immune system

See Infection; Infection, Potential for

Barrel Chest

See Aging (if appropriate); COPD (Chronic Obstructive Pulmonary Disease)

Bathing/Hygiene Problems

Impaired bed **Mobility** r/t chronic physically limiting condition

Self **Neglect** (See **Neglect**, self, Section III)

Bathing **Self-Care** deficit (See **Self-Care** deficit, bathing, Section III)

Battered Child Syndrome

Dysfunctional **Family** processes r/t inadequate coping skills

Sleep deprivation r/t prolonged psychological discomfort

Chronic **Sorrow** r/t situational crises

Risk for **Aspiration**: Risk factor: propped bottle

Risk for **Post-Trauma** syndrome: Risk factors: physical abuse, incest, rape, molestation

Risk for **Self-Mutilation**: Risk factors: feelings of rejection, dysfunctional family

See Child Abuse

Battered Person

See Abuse, Spouse, Parent, or Significant Other

Bedbugs, Infestation

Impaired **Home** maintenance r/t deficient knowledge regarding prevention of bedbug infestation

Impaired **Skin** integrity r/t bites of bedbugs

See Itching; Pruritus

Bed Mobility, Impaired

Impaired bed **Mobility** (See **Mobility**, bed, impaired, Section III)

Bed Rest, Prolonged

Deficient **Diversional** activity r/t prolonged bed rest

Impaired bed **Mobility** r/t neuromuscular impairment

Social isolation r/t prolonged bed rest

Risk for **Disuse** syndrome: Risk factor: prolonged immobility

Risk for **Loneliness**: Risk factor: prolonged bed rest

Bedsores

See Pressure Ulcer

Bedwetting

See Enuresis; Toilet Training

Bell's Palsy

Disturbed **Body** image r/t loss of motor control on one side of face

Imbalanced **Nutrition**: less than body requirements r/t difficulty with chewing

Acute **Pain** r/t inflammation of facial nerve

Risk for **Injury** (eye): Risk factor: dysfunction of facial nerve

Benign Prostatic Hypertrophy

See BPH (Benign Prostatic Hypertrophy); Prostatic Hypertrophy

Bereavement

Grieving r/t loss of significant person

Insomnia r/t grief

Chronic **Sorrow** r/t death of loved one, chronic illness, disability

Risk for complicated **Grieving**: Risk factor: death of a loved one

Risk for **Spiritual** distress: Risk factor: death of a loved one

Biliary Atresia

Anxiety r/t surgical intervention, possible liver transplantation

Impaired **Comfort** r/t inflammation of skin, itching

Imbalanced **Nutrition**: less than body requirements r/t decreased absorption of fat and fat-soluble vitamins, poor feeding

Risk for **Bleeding**: Risk factors: vitamin K deficiency, altered clotting mechanisms

Risk for ineffective **Breathing** pattern: Risk factors: enlarged liver, development of ascites

Risk for impaired **Skin** integrity: Risk factor: pruritus

See Child with Chronic Condition; Cirrhosis (as complication); Hospitalized Child; Terminally Ill Child, Adolescent; Terminally Ill Child, Infant/Toddler; Terminally Ill Child, Preschool Child; Terminally Ill Child, School-Age-Child/Preadolescent; Terminally Ill Child/Death of Child, Parent

Biliary Calculus

See Cholelithiasis

Biliary Obstruction

See Jaundice

Bilirubin Elevation in Neonate

Neonatal **Jaundice** (See **Jaundice**, neonatal, Section III)

Biopsy

Fear r/t outcome of biopsy

Ineffective **Health** maintenance r/t deficient knowledge regarding biopsy site, further needed health care

Bioterrorism

Contamination r/t exposure to bioterrorism

Risk for **Infection**: Risk factor: exposure to harmful biological agent

Risk for **Post-Trauma** syndrome: Risk factor: perception of event of bioterrorism

Bipolar Disorder I (Most Recent Episode, Depressed or Manic)

Ineffective **Activity** planning r/t unrealistic perception of events

Risk-prone health **Behavior** r/t low state of optimism

Ineffective **Coping** r/t complicated grieving

Disturbed **Energy** field r/t disharmony of mind, body, spirit

Fatigue r/t psychological demands

Ineffective **Health** maintenance r/t lack of ability to make good judgments regarding ways to obtain help

Self-Care deficit: specify r/t depression, cognitive impairment

Chronic low **Self-Esteem** r/t repeated unmet expectations

Social isolation r/t ineffective coping

Risk for complicated **Grieving**: Risk factor: lack of previous resolution of former grieving response

Risk for **Loneliness**: Risk factors: stress, conflict

Risk for **Spiritual** distress: Risk factor: mental illness

See Depression (Major Depressive Disorder); Manic Disorder, Bipolar I

Birth Asphyxia

See Asphyxia, Birth

Birth Control

See Contraceptive Method

Bladder Cancer

Urinary retention r/t clots obstructing urethra

See Cancer; TURP (Transurethral Resection of the Prostate)

Bladder Distention

Urinary retention r/t high urethral pressure caused by weak detrusor, inhibition of reflex arc, blockage, strong sphincter

Bladder Training

Disturbed **Body** image r/t difficulty maintaining control of urinary elimination

Ineffective **Health** maintenance r/t deficient knowledge regarding incontinence self-care

Functional urinary **Incontinence** r/t altered environment; sensory, cognitive, mobility deficit

Stress urinary **Incontinence** r/t degenerative change in pelvic muscles and structural supports

Urge urinary **Incontinence** r/t decreased bladder capacity, increased urine concentration, overdistention of bladder

Bladder Training, Child

See Toilet Training

Bleeding Tendency

Risk for **Bleeding** (See **Bleeding**, risk for, Section III)

Risk for delayed **Surgical** recovery: Risk factor: bleeding tendency

Blepharoplasty

Disturbed **Body** image r/t effects of surgery

Ineffective **Health** maintenance r/t deficient knowledge regarding postoperative care of surgical area

Blindness

Interrupted **Family** processes r/t shift in health status of family member (change in visual acuity)

Impaired **Home** maintenance r/t decreased vision

Ineffective **Role** performance r/t alteration in health status (change in visual acuity)

Self-Care deficit: specify r/t inability to see to be able to perform activities of daily living

Disturbed **Sensory** perception: visual r/t altered sensory reception, transmission, integration

Risk for delayed **Development**: Risk factor: vision impairment

Risk for **Injury**: Risk factor: sensory dysfunction

See Vision Impairment

Blood Disorder

Ineffective **Protection** r/t abnormal blood profile

See cause of Blood Disorder

Blood Pressure Alteration

See Hypotension; HTN (Hypertension)

Blood Sugar Control

Risk for unstable blood **Glucose** level (See **Glucose** level, blood, unstable, risk for, Section III)

Blood Transfusion

Anxiety r/t possibility of harm from transfusion

See Anemia

Body Dysmorphic Disorder

Disturbed **Body** image r/t overinvolvement in physical appearance

Body Image Change

Disturbed **Body** image (See **Body** image, disturbed, Section III)

Body Temperature, Altered

Ineffective **Thermoregulation** (See **Thermoregulation**, ineffective, Section III)

Bone Marrow Biopsy

Fear r/t unknown outcome of results of biopsy

Ineffective **Health** maintenance r/t deficient knowledge of expectations after procedure, disease treatment after biopsy

Acute **Pain** r/t bone marrow aspiration

See disease necessitating bone marrow biopsy (e.g., Leukemia)

Borderline Personality Disorder

Ineffective **Activity** planning r/t unrealistic perception of events

Anxiety r/t perceived threat to self-concept

Defensive **Coping** r/t difficulty with relationships, inability to accept blame for own behavior

Ineffective **Coping** r/t use of maladjusted defense mechanisms (e.g., projection, denial)

Powerlessness r/t lifestyle of helplessness

Social isolation r/t immature interests

Ineffective family **Therapeutic** regimen management r/t manipulative behavior of client

Risk for **Caregiver** role strain: Risk factors: inability of care receiver to accept criticism, care receiver taking advantage of others to meet own needs or having unreasonable expectations

Risk for **Self-Mutilation**: Risk factors: ineffective coping, feelings of self-hatred

Risk for **Spiritual** distress: Risk factor: poor relationships associated with behaviors attributed to borderline personality disorder

Risk for self-directed **Violence**: Risk factors: feelings of need to punish self, manipulative behavior

Boredom

Deficient **Diversional** activity r/t environmental lack of diversional activity

Social isolation r/t altered state of wellness

Botulism

Deficient **Fluid** volume r/t profuse diarrhea

Ineffective **Health** maintenance r/t deficient knowledge regarding prevention of botulism, care after episode

Bowel Incontinence

Bowel incontinence r/t decreased awareness of need to defecate, loss of sphincter control, fecal impaction

Bowel Obstruction

Constipation r/t decreased motility, intestinal obstruction

Deficient **Fluid** volume r/t inadequate fluid volume intake, fluid loss in bowel

Imbalanced **Nutrition**: less than body requirements r/t nausea, vomiting

Acute **Pain** r/t pressure from distended abdomen

Bowel Resection

See Abdominal Surgery

Bowel Sounds, Absent or Diminished

Constipation r/t decreased or absent peristalsis

Deficient **Fluid** volume r/t inability to ingest fluids, loss of fluids in bowel

Delayed **Surgical** recovery r/t inability to obtain adequate nutritional status

Risk for dysfunctional gastrointestinal **Motility** (See **Motility**, gastrointestinal, dysfunctional, risk for, Section III)

Bowel Sounds, Hyperactive

Diarrhea r/t increased gastrointestinal motility

Bowel Training

Bowel incontinence r/t loss of control of rectal sphincter

Ineffective **Health** maintenance r/t deficient knowledge regarding treatment of bowel incontinence

Bowel Training, Child

See Toilet Training

BPH (Benign Prostatic Hypertrophy)

Ineffective **Health** maintenance r/t deficient knowledge regarding self-care with prostatic hypertrophy

Insomnia r/t nocturia

Urinary retention r/t obstruction

Risk for urge urinary **Incontinence**: Risk factors: detrusor muscle instability with impaired contractility, involuntary sphincter relaxation

Risk for **Infection**: Risk factors: urinary residual after voiding, bacterial invasion of bladder

See Prostatic Hypertrophy

Bradycardia

Decreased **Cardiac** output r/t slow heart rate supplying inadequate amount of blood for body function

Ineffective **Health** maintenance r/t deficient knowledge of condition, effects of cardiac medications

Risk for ineffective cerebral tissue **Perfusion**: Risk factors: decreased cardiac output secondary to bradycardia, vagal response

Bradypnea

Ineffective **Breathing** pattern r/t neuromuscular impairment, pain, musculoskeletal impairment, perception or cognitive impairment, anxiety, fatigue or decreased energy, effects of drugs

See cause of Bradypnea

Brain Injury

See Intracranial Pressure, Increased

Brain Surgery

See Craniectomy/Craniotomy

Brain Tumor

Acute **Confusion** r/t pressure from tumor

Fear r/t threat to well-being

Grieving r/t potential loss of physiosocial-psychosocial well-being

Decreased **Intracranial** adaptive capacity r/t presence of brain tumor

Acute **Pain** r/t pressure from tumor

Disturbed **Sensory** perception: specify r/t tumor growth compressing brain tissue

Risk for **Injury**: Risk factors: sensory-perceptual alterations, weakness

See Cancer; Chemotherapy; Child with Chronic Condition; Craniectomy/Craniotomy; Hospitalized Child; Radiation Therapy; Terminally Ill Child, Adolescent; Terminally Ill Child, Infant/Toddler; Terminally Ill Child, Preschool Child; Terminally Ill Child, School-Age Child/Preadolescent; Terminally Ill Child/Death of Child, Parent

Braxton Hicks Contractions

Activity intolerance r/t increased perception of contractions with increased gestation

Anxiety r/t uncertainty about beginning labor

Fatigue r/t lack of sleep

Stress urinary **Incontinence** r/t increased pressure on bladder with contractions

Insomnia r/t contractions when lying down

Ineffective **Sexuality** pattern r/t fear of contractions

Breast Biopsy

Fear r/t potential for diagnosis of cancer

Ineffective **Health** maintenance r/t deficient knowledge regarding appropriate postoperative care of breasts

Risk for **Spiritual** distress: Risk factor: fear of diagnosis of cancer

Breast Cancer

Death **Anxiety** r/t diagnosis of cancer

Ineffective **Coping** r/t treatment, prognosis

Fear r/t diagnosis of cancer

Sexual dysfunction r/t loss of body part, partner's reaction to loss

Chronic **Sorrow** r/t diagnosis of cancer, loss of body integrity

Risk for **Spiritual** distress: Risk factor: fear of diagnosis of cancer

See Cancer; Chemotherapy; Mastectomy; Radiation Therapy

Breast Examination, Self

See SBE (Self-Breast Examination)

Breast Lumps

Fear r/t potential for diagnosis of cancer

Ineffective **Health** maintenance r/t deficient knowledge regarding appropriate care of breasts

Breast Pumping

Ineffective **Health** maintenance r/t deficient knowledge regarding breast milk expression and storage

Risk for **Infection**: Risk factors: contaminated breast pump, incomplete emptying of breast

Risk for impaired **Skin** integrity: Risk factor: high suction

Breastfeeding, Effective

Effective **Breastfeeding** (See **Breastfeeding**, effective, Section III)

Breastfeeding, Ineffective

Ineffective **Breastfeeding** (See **Breastfeeding**, ineffective, Section III)

See Infant Feeding Pattern, Ineffective; Painful Breasts, Engorgement; Painful Breasts, Sore Nipples

Breastfeeding, Interrupted

Interrupted **Breastfeeding** (See **Breastfeeding**, interrupted, Section III)

Breath Sounds, Decreased or Absent

See Atelectasis; Pneumothorax

Breathing Pattern Alteration

Ineffective **Breathing** pattern r/t neuromuscular impairment, pain, musculoskeletal impairment, perception or cognitive impairment, anxiety, decreased energy or fatigue

Breech Birth

Anxiety: maternal r/t threat to self, infant

Fear: maternal r/t danger to infant, self

Impaired **Gas** exchange: fetal r/t compressed umbilical cord

Risk for **Aspiration**: fetal: Risk factor: birth of body before head

Risk for delayed **Development**: Risk factor: compressed umbilical cord

Risk for impaired **Tissue** integrity: fetal: Risk factor: difficult birth

Risk for impaired **Tissue** integrity: maternal: Risk factor: difficult birth

Bronchitis

Ineffective **Airway** clearance r/t excessive thickened mucus secretion

Anxiety r/t potential chronic condition

Ineffective **Health** maintenance r/t deficient knowledge regarding care of condition

Readiness for enhanced **Self Health** management: wishes to stop smoking

Bronchopulmonary Dysplasia

Activity intolerance r/t imbalance between oxygen supply and demand

Excess **Fluid** volume r/t sodium and water retention

Imbalanced **Nutrition**: less than body requirements r/t poor feeding, increased caloric needs as a result of increased work of breathing

See Child with Chronic Condition; Hospitalized Child; Respiratory Conditions of the Neonate

Bronchoscopy

Risk for **Aspiration**: Risk factor: temporary loss of gag reflex

Risk for **Injury**: Risk factors: complication of pneumothorax, laryngeal edema, hemorrhage (if biopsy done)

Bruits, Carotid

Risk for ineffective cerebral tissue **Perfusion**: Risk factors: interruption of carotid blood flow to brain

Bryant's Traction

See Traction and Casts

Buck's Traction

See Traction and Casts

Buerger's Disease

See Peripheral Vascular Disease (PVD)

Bulimia

Disturbed **Body** image r/t misperception about actual appearance, body weight

Compromised family **Coping** r/t chronically unresolved feelings of guilt, anger, hostility

Defensive **Coping** r/t eating disorder

Diarrhea r/t laxative abuse

Fear r/t food ingestion, weight gain

Noncompliance r/t negative feelings toward treatment regimen

Imbalanced **Nutrition**: less than body requirements r/t induced vomiting, excessive exercise

Powerlessness r/t urge to purge self after eating

Chronic low **Self-Esteem** r/t lack of positive feedback

See Maturational Issues, Adolescent

Bunion

Ineffective **Health** maintenance r/t deficient knowledge regarding appropriate care of feet

Bunionectomy

Ineffective **Health** maintenance r/t deficient knowledge regarding postoperative care of feet

Impaired physical **Mobility** r/t sore foot

Impaired **Walking** r/t pain associated with surgery

Risk for **Infection**: Risk factors: surgical incision, advanced age

Burns

Disturbed **Body** image r/t altered physical appearance

Deficient **Diversional** activity r/t long-term hospitalization

Fear r/t pain from treatments, possible permanent disfigurement

Grieving r/t loss of bodily function, loss of future hopes and plans

Hypothermia r/t impaired skin integrity

Impaired physical **Mobility** r/t pain, musculoskeletal impairment, contracture formation

Imbalanced **Nutrition**: less than body requirements r/t increased metabolic needs, anorexia, protein and fluid loss

Acute **Pain** r/t burn injury, treatments

Ineffective peripheral tissue **Perfusion** r/t circumferential burns, impaired arterial/venous circulation

Post-Trauma syndrome r/t life-threatening event

Impaired **Skin** integrity r/t injury of skin

Delayed **Surgical** recovery r/t ineffective tissue perfusion

Risk for ineffective **Airway** clearance: Risk factors: potential tracheobronchial obstruction, edema

Risk for deficient **Fluid** volume: Risk factors: loss from skin surface, fluid shift

Risk for **Infection**: Risk factors: loss of intact skin, trauma, invasive sites

Risk for **Peripheral** neurovascular dysfunction: Risk factor: eschar formation with circumferential burn

Risk for **Post-Trauma** syndrome: Risk factors: perception, duration of event that caused burns

See Hospitalized Child; Safety, Childhood

Bursitis

Impaired physical **Mobility** r/t inflammation in joint

Acute **Pain** r/t inflammation in joint

Bypass Graft

See Coronary Artery Bypass Grafting (CABG)

C

CABG (Coronary Artery Bypass Grafting)

See Coronary Artery Bypass Grafting (CABG)

C

Cachexia

Adult **Failure** to thrive r/t imbalanced nutrition: less than body requirements

Imbalanced **Nutrition**: less than body requirements r/t inability to ingest food because of biological factors

Ineffective **Protection** r/t inadequate nutrition

Calcium Alteration

See Hypercalcemia; Hypocalcemia

Cancer

Activity intolerance r/t side effects of treatment, weakness from cancer

Death **Anxiety** r/t unresolved issues regarding dying

Disturbed **Body** image r/t side effects of treatment, cachexia

Decisional **Conflict** r/t selection of treatment choices, continuation or discontinuation of treatment, "do not resuscitate" decision

Constipation r/t side effects of medication, altered nutrition, decreased activity

Compromised family **Coping** r/t prolonged disease or disability progression that exhausts supportive ability of significant others

Ineffective **Coping** r/t personal vulnerability in situational crisis, terminal illness

Ineffective **Denial** r/t complicated grieving process

Fear r/t serious threat to well-being

Grieving r/t potential loss of significant others, high risk for infertility

Ineffective **Health** maintenance r/t deficient knowledge regarding prescribed treatment

Hopelessness r/t loss of control, terminal illness

Insomnia r/t anxiety, pain

Impaired physical **Mobility** r/t weakness, neuromusculoskeletal impairment, pain

Imbalanced **Nutrition**: less than body requirements r/t loss of appetite, difficulty swallowing, side effects of chemotherapy, obstruction by tumor

Impaired **Oral** mucous membrane r/t chemotherapy, effects of radiation, oral pH changes, decreased oral secretions

Chronic **Pain** r/t metastatic cancer

Powerlessness r/t treatment, progression of disease

Ineffective **Protection** r/t cancer suppressing immune system

Ineffective **Role** performance r/t change in physical capacity, inability to resume prior role

Self-Care deficit: specify r/t pain, intolerance to activity, decreased strength

Impaired **Skin** integrity r/t immunological deficit, immobility

Social isolation r/t hospitalization, lifestyle changes

Chronic **Sorrow** r/t chronic illness of cancer

Spiritual distress r/t test of spiritual beliefs

Risk for **Bleeding**: Risk factor: bone marrow depression from chemotherapy

Risk for **Disuse** syndrome: Risk factors: immobility, fatigue

Risk for impaired **Home** maintenance: Risk factor: lack of familiarity with community resources

Risk for **Infection**: Risk factor: inadequate immune system

Risk for compromised **Resilience**: Risk factors: multiple stressors, pain, chronic illness

Risk for **Spiritual** distress: Risk factor: physical illness of cancer

Readiness for enhanced **Spiritual** well-being: desire for harmony with self, others, higher power, God, when faced with serious illness

See Chemotherapy; Child with Chronic Condition; Hospitalized Child; Leukemia; Radiation Therapy; Terminally Ill Child, Adolescent; Terminally Ill Child, Infant/Toddler; Terminally Ill Child, Preschool Child; Terminally Ill Child, School-Age Child/Preadolescent; Terminally Ill Child/Death of Child, Parent

Candidiasis, Oral

Ineffective **Health** maintenance r/t deficient knowledge regarding care of infected mouth

Impaired **Oral** mucous membrane r/t overgrowth of infectious agent, depressed immune function

Capillary Refill Time, Prolonged

Impaired **Gas** exchange r/t ventilation perfusion imbalance

Ineffective peripheral tissue **Perfusion** r/t interruption of arterial or venous flow

See Shock, Hypovolemic

Carbon Monoxide Poisoning

See Smoke Inhalation

Cardiac Arrest

Post-Trauma syndrome r/t experiencing serious life event

See cause of Cardiac Arrest

Cardiac Catheterization

Anxiety r/t invasive procedure, uncertainty of outcome of procedure

Ineffective **Health** maintenance r/t deficient knowledge regarding procedure, postprocedure care, treatment and prevention of coronary artery disease

Risk for **Injury**: hematoma: Risk factor: invasive procedure

Risk for decreased cardiac tissue **Perfusion**: Risk factors: ventricular ischemia, dysrhythmia

Risk for **Peripheral** neurovascular dysfunction: Risk factor: vascular obstruction

Cardiac Disorders

Decreased **Cardiac** output r/t cardiac disorder

Risk for decreased cardiac tissue **Perfusion** r/t cardiac disorder

See specific cardiac disorder

Cardiac Disorders in Pregnancy

Activity intolerance r/t cardiac pathophysiology, increased demand because of pregnancy, weakness, fatigue

Anxiety r/t unknown outcomes of pregnancy, family well-being

Death **Anxiety** r/t potential danger of condition

Compromised family **Coping** r/t prolonged hospitalization or maternal incapacitation that exhausts supportive capacity of significant others

Ineffective **Coping** r/t personal vulnerability

Interrupted **Family** processes r/t hospitalization, maternal incapacitation, changes in roles

Fatigue r/t metabolic, psychological, and emotional demands

Fear r/t potential maternal effects, potential poor fetal or maternal outcome

Ineffective **Health** maintenance r/t deficient knowledge regarding treatment, restrictions with cardiac disorder

Powerlessness r/t illness-related regimen

Ineffective **Role** performance r/t changes in lifestyle, expectations from disease process with superimposed pregnancy

Situational low **Self-Esteem** r/t situational crisis, pregnancy

Social isolation r/t limitations of activity, bed rest or hospitalization, separation from family and friends

Risk for delayed **Development**: Risk factor: poor maternal oxygenation

Risk for deficient **Fluid** volume: Risk factor: sudden changes in circulation after delivery of placenta

Risk for excess **Fluid** volume: Risk factors: compromised regulatory mechanism with increased afterload, preload, circulating blood volume

Risk for impaired **Gas** exchange: Risk factor: pulmonary edema

Risk for disproportionate **Growth**: Risk factor: poor maternal oxygenation

Risk for disturbed **Maternal/Fetal** dyad: Risk factor: compromised oxygen transport

Risk for decreased cardiac tissue **Perfusion**: Risk factor: strain on compromised heart from work of pregnancy, delivery

Risk for compromised **Resilience**: Risk factors: multiple stressors, fear

Risk for **Spiritual** distress: Risk factor: fear of diagnosis for self and infant

Cardiac Dysrhythmia

See Dysrhythmia

Cardiac Output, Decreased

Decreased **Cardiac** output r/t cardiac dysfunction

Cardiac Tamponade

Decreased **Cardiac** output r/t fluid in pericardial sac

See Pericarditis

Cardiogenic Shock

See Shock, Cardiogenic

Caregiver Role Strain

Caregiver role strain (See **Caregiver** role strain, Section III)

Risk for compromised **Resilience**: Risk factor: stress of prolonged caregiving

Carious Teeth

See Cavities in Teeth

Carotid Endarterectomy

Fear r/t surgery in vital area

Ineffective **Health** maintenance r/t deficient knowledge regarding postoperative care

Risk for ineffective **Airway** clearance: Risk factor: hematoma compressing trachea

Risk for **Injury**: Risk factor: possible hematoma formation

Risk for ineffective cerebral tissue **Perfusion**: Risk factors: hemorrhage, clot formation

Carpal Tunnel Syndrome

Impaired physical **Mobility** r/t neuromuscular impairment

Chronic **Pain** r/t unrelieved pressure on median nerve

Self-Care deficit: bathing, dressing, feeding r/t pain

Carpopedal Spasm

See Hypocalcemia

Casts

Deficient **Diversional** activity r/t physical limitations from cast

Ineffective **Health** maintenance r/t deficient knowledge regarding cast care, personal care with cast

Impaired physical **Mobility** r/t limb immobilization

Self-Care deficit: bathing, dressing, feeding r/t presence of cast(s) on upper extremities

Self-Care deficit: toileting r/t presence of cast(s) on lower extremities

Impaired **Walking** r/t cast(s) on lower extremities, fracture of bones

Risk for **Peripheral** neurovascular dysfunction: Risk factor: mechanical compression from cast

Risk for impaired **Skin** integrity: Risk factor: unrelieved pressure on skin

See Traction and Casts

Cataract Extraction

Anxiety r/t threat of permanent vision loss, surgical procedure

Ineffective **Health** maintenance r/t deficient knowledge regarding postoperative restrictions

Disturbed **Sensory** perception: vision r/t edema from surgery

Risk for **Injury**: Risk factors: increased intraocular pressure, accommodation to new visual field

See Vision Impairment

Cataracts

Disturbed **Sensory** perception: vision r/t altered sensory input

See Vision Impairment

Catatonic Schizophrenia

Impaired verbal **Communication** r/t muteness

Impaired **Memory** r/t cognitive impairment

Impaired physical **Mobility** r/t cognitive impairment, maintenance of rigid posture, inappropriate or bizarre postures

Imbalanced **Nutrition**: less than body requirements r/t decrease in outside stimulation, loss of perception of hunger, resistance to instructions to eat

Social isolation r/t inability to communicate, immobility

See Schizophrenia

Catheterization, Urinary

Ineffective **Health** maintenance r/t deficient knowledge of normal sensation of catheter in place, care of catheter

Risk for **Infection**: Risk factor: invasive procedure

Cavities in Teeth

Impaired **Dentition** r/t ineffective oral hygiene, barriers to self-care, economic barriers to professional care, nutritional deficits, dietary habits

Cellulitis

Ineffective **Health** maintenance r/t lack of knowledge regarding prevention of further incidences of infection

Acute **Pain** r/t inflammatory changes in tissues from infection

Ineffective peripheral tissue **Perfusion** r/t edema

Impaired **Tissue** integrity r/t inflammatory process damaging skin and underlying tissue

Risk for vascular **Trauma**: Risk factor: infusion of antibiotics

Cellulitis, Periorbital

Hyperthermia r/t infectious process

Acute **Pain** r/t edema and inflammation of skin/tissues

Disturbed **Sensory** perception: visual r/t decreased visual fields secondary to edema of eyelids

Impaired **Skin** integrity r/t inflammation or infection of skin, tissues

See Hospitalized Child

Central Line Insertion

Ineffective **Health** maintenance r/t deficient knowledge regarding precautions to take when central line is in place

Risk for **Infection**: Risk factor: invasive procedure

Risk for vascular **Trauma** (See **Trauma**, vascular, risk for, Section III)

Cerebral Aneurysm

See Craniectomy/Craniotomy; Intracranial Pressure, Increased; Subarachnoid Hemorrhage

Cerebral Palsy

Impaired verbal **Communication** r/t impaired ability to articulate or speak words because of facial muscle involvement

Deficient **Diversional** activity r/t physical impairments, limitations on ability to participate in recreational activities

Impaired physical **Mobility** r/t spasticity, neuromuscular impairment or weakness

Imbalanced **Nutrition**: less than body requirements r/t spasticity, feeding or swallowing difficulties

Self-Care deficit: specify r/t neuromuscular impairments, sensory deficits

Impaired **Social** interaction r/t impaired communication skills, limited physical activity, perceived differences from peers

Chronic **Sorrow** r/t presence of chronic disability

Risk for **Falls**: Risk factor: impaired physical mobility

Risk for **Injury**: Risk factors: muscle weakness, inability to control spasticity

Risk for impaired **Parenting**: Risk factor: caring for child with overwhelming needs resulting from chronic change in health status

Risk for **Spiritual** distress: Risk factors: psychological stress associated with chronic illness

See Child with Chronic Condition

Cerebral Perfusion

Risk for ineffective cerebral tissue **Perfusion** (See **Perfusion**, tissue, cerebral, ineffective, risk for, Section III)

Cerebrovascular Accident (CVA)

See CVA (Cerebrovascular Accident)

Cervicitis

Ineffective **Health** maintenance r/t deficient knowledge regarding care and prevention of condition

Ineffective **Sexuality** pattern r/t abstinence during acute stage

Risk for **Infection**: Risk factors: spread of infection, recurrence of infection

Cesarean Delivery

Anxiety r/t unmet expectations for childbirth, unknown outcome of surgery

Disturbed **Body** image r/t surgery, unmet expectations for childbirth

Interrupted **Family** processes r/t unmet expectations for childbirth

Fear r/t perceived threat to own well-being

Ineffective **Health** maintenance r/t deficient knowledge regarding postoperative care

Impaired physical **Mobility** r/t pain

Acute **Pain** r/t surgical incision

Ineffective **Role** performance r/t unmet expectations for childbirth

Situational low **Self-Esteem** r/t inability to deliver child vaginally

Risk for **Bleeding**: Risk factor: surgery

Risk for imbalanced **Fluid** volume: Risk factors: loss of blood, fluid shifts

Risk for **Infection**: Risk factor: surgical incision

Risk for **Urinary** retention: Risk factor: regional anesthesia

Readiness for enhanced **Childbearing** process: a pattern of preparing for, maintaining, and strengthening care of newborn

Chemical Dependence

See Alcoholism; Drug Abuse; Cocaine Abuse; Substance Abuse

Chemotherapy

Death **Anxiety** r/t chemotherapy not accomplishing desired results

Disturbed **Body** image r/t loss of weight, loss of hair

Fatigue r/t disease process, anemia, drug effects

Ineffective **Health** maintenance r/t deficient knowledge regarding action, side effects, way to integrate chemotherapy into lifestyle

Nausea r/t effects of chemotherapy

Imbalanced **Nutrition**: less than body requirements r/t side effects of chemotherapy

Impaired **Oral** mucous membrane r/t effects of chemotherapy

Ineffective **Protection** r/t suppressed immune system, decreased platelets

Delayed **Surgical** recovery r/t compromised immune system

Risk for **Bleeding**: Risk factors: vomiting, diarrhea

Risk for **Infection**: Risk factor: immunosuppression

Risk for vascular **Trauma**: Risk factor: infusion of irritating chemicals

See Cancer

Chest Pain

Fear r/t potential threat of death

Acute **Pain** r/t myocardial injury, ischemia

Risk for decreased cardiac tissue **Perfusion**: Risk factor: ventricular ischemia

See Angina; MI (Myocardial Infarction)

Chest Tubes

Ineffective **Breathing** pattern r/t asymmetrical lung expansion secondary to pain

Impaired **Gas** exchange r/t decreased functional lung tissue

Acute **Pain** r/t presence of chest tubes, injury

Risk for **Injury**: Risk factor: presence of invasive chest tube

Cheyne-Stokes Respiration

Ineffective **Breathing** pattern r/t critical illness

See cause of Cheyne-Stokes Respiration

CHF (Congestive Heart Failure)

Activity intolerance r/t weakness, fatigue

Decreased **Cardiac** output r/t impaired cardiac function

Constipation r/t activity intolerance

Fatigue r/t disease process

Fear r/t threat to one's own well-being

Excess **Fluid** volume r/t impaired excretion of sodium and water

Impaired **Gas** exchange r/t excessive fluid in interstitial space of lungs, alveoli

Ineffective self **Health** management (See **Health** management, self, ineffective, Section III)

Powerlessness r/t illness-related regimen

Risk for **Shock**: Risk factors: decreased contractility of heart, increased afterload

Readiness for enhanced **Self Health** management (See **Self Health** management, readiness for enhanced, Section III)

See Child with Chronic Condition; Congenital Heart Disease/ Cardiac Anomalies; Hospitalized Child

Chickenpox

See Communicable Diseases, Childhood

Child Abuse

Deficient **Diversional** activity r/t diminished or absent environmental or personal stimuli

Interrupted **Family** processes r/t inadequate coping skills

Fear r/t threat of punishment for perceived wrongdoing

Delayed **Growth** and development r/t inadequate caretaking, stimulation deficiencies

Insomnia r/t hypervigilance, anxiety

Imbalanced **Nutrition**: less than body requirements r/t inadequate caretaking

Acute **Pain** r/t physical injuries

Impaired **Parenting** r/t psychological impairment, physical or emotional abuse of parent, substance abuse, unrealistic expectations of child

Post-Trauma syndrome r/t physical abuse, incest, rape, molestation

Chronic low **Self-Esteem** r/t lack of positive feedback, excessive negative feedback

Impaired **Skin** integrity r/t altered nutritional state, physical abuse

Social isolation: family imposed r/t fear of disclosure of family dysfunction and abuse

Risk for delayed **Development**: Risk factors: shaken baby syndrome, abuse

Risk for disproportionate **Growth**: Risk factor: abuse

Risk for **Poisoning**: Risk factors: inadequate safeguards, lack of proper safety precautions, accessibility of illicit substances because of impaired home maintenance

Risk for **Suffocation**: Risk factors: unattended child, unsafe environment

Risk for **Trauma**: Risk factors: inadequate precautions, cognitive or emotional difficulties

Child Neglect

See Child Abuse; Failure to Thrive, Nonorganic

Child with Chronic Condition

Activity intolerance r/t fatigue associated with chronic illness

Decisional **Conflict** r/t treatment options, conflicting values

Parental role **Conflict** r/t separation from child as a result of chronic illness, home care of child with special needs, interruptions of family life resulting from home care regimen

Compromised family **Coping** r/t prolonged overconcern for child; distortion of reality regarding child's health problem, including extreme denial about its existence or severity

Disabled family **Coping** r/t prolonged disease or disability progression that exhausts supportive capacity of significant others

Ineffective **Coping**: child r/t situational or maturational crises

Deficient **Diversional** activity r/t immobility, monotonous environment, frequent or lengthy treatments, reluctance to participate, self-imposed social isolation

Interrupted **Family** processes r/t intermittent situational crisis of illness, disease, hospitalization

Delayed **Growth** and development r/t effects of physical disability, prescribed dependence, separation from significant others

Ineffective **Health** maintenance r/t exhausting family resources (finances, physical energy, support systems)

Impaired **Home** maintenance r/t overtaxed family members (e.g., exhausted, anxious)

Hopelessness: child r/t prolonged activity restriction, long-term stress, lack of involvement in or passively allowing care as a result of parental overprotection

Insomnia: child or parent r/t time-intensive treatments, exacerbation of condition, 24-hour care needs

Deficient **Knowledge** r/t knowledge or skill acquisition regarding health practices, acceptance of limitations, promotion of maximal potential of child, self-actualization of rest of family

Imbalanced **Nutrition**: less than body requirements r/t anorexia, fatigue from physical exertion

Imbalanced **Nutrition**: more than body requirements r/t effects of steroid medications on appetite

Chronic **Pain** r/t physical, biological, chemical, or psychological factors

Powerlessness: child r/t health care environment, illness-related regimen, lifestyle of learned helplessness

Chronic low **Self-Esteem** r/t actual or perceived differences; peer acceptance; decreased ability to participate in physical, school, and social activities

Ineffective **Sexuality** pattern: parental r/t disrupted relationship with sexual partner

Impaired **Social** interaction r/t developmental lag or delay, perceived differences

Social isolation: family r/t actual or perceived social stigmatization, complex care requirements

Chronic **Sorrow** r/t developmental stages and missed opportunities or milestones that bring comparisons with social or personal norms, unending caregiving as reminder of loss

Risk for delayed **Development**: Risk factor: chronic illness

Risk for disproportionate **Growth**: Risk factor: chronic illness

Risk for **Infection**: Risk factor: debilitating physical condition

Risk for impaired **Parenting**: Risk factors: impaired or disrupted bonding, caring for child with perceived overwhelming care needs

Readiness for enhanced family **Coping**: impact of crisis on family values, priorities, goals, or relationships; changes in family choices to optimize wellness

Childbirth

Readiness for enhanced **Childbearing** process (See **Childbearing** process, readiness for enhanced, Section III)

See Labor, Normal; Postpartum, Normal Care

Chills

Hyperthermia r/t infectious process

Chlamydia Infection

See STD (Sexually Transmitted Disease)

Chloasma

Disturbed **Body** image r/t change in skin color

Choking or Coughing with Feeding

Impaired **Swallowing** r/t neuromuscular impairment

Risk for **Aspiration**: Risk factors: depressed cough and gag reflexes

Cholecystectomy

Ineffective **Health** maintenance r/t deficient knowledge regarding postoperative care

Imbalanced **Nutrition**: less than body requirements r/t high metabolic needs, decreased ability to digest fatty foods

Acute **Pain** r/t trauma from surgery

Risk for deficient **Fluid** volume: Risk factors: restricted intake, nausea, vomiting

See Abdominal Surgery

Cholelithiasis

Ineffective **Health** maintenance r/t deficient knowledge regarding care of disease

Imbalanced **Nutrition**: less than body requirements r/t anorexia, nausea, vomiting

Acute **Pain** r/t obstruction of bile flow, inflammation in gallbladder

Chorioamnionitis

Anxiety r/t threat to self and infant

Grieving r/t guilt about potential loss of ideal pregnancy and birth

Hyperthermia r/t infectious process

Situational low **Self-Esteem** r/t guilt about threat to infant's health

Risk for delayed **Growth** and development: Risk factor: risk of preterm birth

Risk for **Infection**: Risk factor: infection transmission from mother to fetus; infection in fetal environment

Chronic Confusion

See Confusion, Chronic

Chronic Lymphocytic Leukemia

See Cancer; Chemotherapy; Leukemia

Chronic Obstructive Pulmonary Disease (COPD)

See COPD (Chronic Obstructive Pulmonary Disease)

Chronic Pain

See Pain, Chronic

Chronic Renal Failure

See Renal Failure

Chvostek's Sign

See Hypocalcemia

Circumcision

Ineffective **Health** maintenance r/t deficient knowledge (parental) regarding care of surgical area

Acute **Pain** r/t surgical intervention

Risk for **Bleeding**: Risk factor: surgical trauma

Risk for **Infection**: Risk factor: surgical wound

Cirrhosis

Chronic **Confusion** r/t chronic organic disorder with increased ammonia levels, substance abuse

Diarrhea r/t dietary changes, medications

Fatigue r/t malnutrition

Ineffective **Health** maintenance r/t deficient knowledge regarding correlation between lifestyle habits and disease process

Nausea r/t irritation to gastrointestinal system

Imbalanced **Nutrition**: less than body requirements r/t loss of appetite, nausea, vomiting

Chronic **Pain** r/t liver enlargement

Chronic low **Self-Esteem** r/t chronic illness

Chronic **Sorrow** r/t presence of chronic illness

Risk for **Bleeding**: Risk factors: impaired blood coagulation, bleeding from portal hypertension

Risk for **Injury**: Risk factors: substance intoxication, potential delirium tremens

Risk for impaired **Oral** mucous membranes: Risk factors: altered nutrition, inadequate oral care

Risk for impaired **Skin** integrity: Risk factors: altered nutritional state, altered metabolic state

Cleft Lip/Cleft Palate

Ineffective **Airway** clearance r/t common feeding and breathing passage, postoperative laryngeal, incisional edema

Ineffective **Breastfeeding** r/t infant anomaly

Impaired verbal **Communication** r/t inadequate palate function, possible hearing loss from infected eustachian tubes

Fear: parental r/t special care needs, surgery

Grieving r/t loss of perfect child

Ineffective **Health** maintenance r/t lack of parental knowledge regarding feeding techniques, wound care, use of elbow restraints

Ineffective **Infant** feeding pattern r/t cleft lip, cleft palate

Impaired physical **Mobility** r/t imposed restricted activity, use of elbow restraints

Impaired **Oral** mucous membrane r/t surgical correction

Acute **Pain** r/t surgical correction, elbow restraints

Impaired **Skin** integrity r/t incomplete joining of lip, palate ridges

Chronic **Sorrow** r/t birth of child with congenital defect

Risk for **Aspiration**: Risk factor: common feeding and breathing passage

Risk for disturbed **Body** image: Risk factors: disfigurement, speech impediment

Risk for delayed **Development**: Risk factor: inadequate nutrition resulting from difficulty feeding

Risk for deficient **Fluid** volume: Risk factor: inability to take liquids in usual manner

Risk for disproportionate **Growth**: Risk factor: inability to feed with normal techniques

Risk for **Infection**: Risk factors: invasive procedure, disruption of eustachian tube development, aspiration

Clotting Disorder

Fear r/t threat to well-being

Ineffective **Health** maintenance r/t deficient knowledge regarding treatment of disorder

Risk for **Bleeding**: Risk factor: impaired clotting

See Anticoagulant Therapy; DIC (Disseminated Intravascular Coagulation); Hemophilia

Cocaine Abuse

Ineffective **Breathing** pattern r/t drug effect on respiratory center

Chronic **Confusion** r/t excessive stimulation of nervous system by cocaine

Ineffective **Coping** r/t inability to deal with life stresses

See Drug Abuse; Substance Abuse

Cocaine Baby

See Crack Baby; Infant of Substance-Abusing Mother

Codependency

Caregiver role strain r/t codependency

Impaired verbal **Communication** r/t psychological barriers

Decisional **Conflict** r/t support system deficit

Ineffective **Coping** r/t inadequate support systems

Ineffective **Denial** r/t unmet self-needs

Powerlessness r/t lifestyle of helplessness

Cold, Viral

Ineffective **Health** maintenance r/t deficient knowledge regarding care of viral condition, prevention of further infections

Readiness for enhanced **Comfort** (See **Comfort**, readiness for enhanced, Section III)

Colectomy

Constipation r/t decreased activity, decreased fluid intake

C

Ineffective **Health** maintenance r/t deficient knowledge regarding procedure, postoperative care

Imbalanced **Nutrition**: less than body requirements r/t high metabolic needs, decreased ability to ingest or digest food

Acute **Pain** r/t recent surgery

Risk for **Infection**: Risk factor: invasive procedure

See Abdominal Surgery

Colitis

Diarrhea r/t inflammation in colon

Deficient **Fluid** volume r/t frequent stools

Acute **Pain** r/t inflammation in colon

See Crohn's Disease; Inflammatory Bowel Disease (Child and Adult)

Collagen Disease

See specific disease (e.g., Lupus Erythematosus; JRA [Juvenile Rheumatoid Arthritis]); Congenital Heart Disease/Cardiac Anomalies

Colostomy

Disturbed **Body** image r/t presence of stoma, daily care of fecal material

Ineffective **Health** maintenance r/t deficient knowledge regarding care of stoma, integrating colostomy care into lifestyle

Ineffective **Sexuality** pattern r/t altered body image, self-concept

Social isolation r/t anxiety about appearance of stoma and possible leakage of stool

Risk for **Constipation**: Risk factor: inappropriate diet

Risk for **Diarrhea**: Risk factor: inappropriate diet

Risk for impaired **Skin** integrity: Risk factor: irritation from bowel contents

Colporrhaphy, Anterior

See Vaginal Hysterectomy

Coma

Death **Anxiety**: significant others r/t unknown outcome of coma state

Interrupted **Family** processes r/t illness or disability of family member

Functional urinary **Incontinence** r/t neurological dysfunction

Self-Care deficit: specify r/t neuromuscular impairment

Ineffective family **Therapeutic** regimen management r/t complexity of therapeutic regimen

Risk for **Aspiration**: Risk factors: impaired swallowing, loss of cough or gag reflex

Risk for **Disuse** syndrome: Risk factor: altered level of consciousness impairing mobility

Risk for **Injury**: Risk factor: potential seizure activity

Risk for impaired **Oral** mucous membrane: Risk factor: dry mouth

Risk for impaired **Skin** integrity: Risk factor: immobility

Risk for **Spiritual** distress: significant others: Risk factors: loss of ability to relate to loved one, unknown outcome of coma

See cause of Coma

Comfort, Loss of

Impaired **Comfort** (See **Comfort**, impaired, Section III)

Readiness for enhanced **Comfort** (See **Comfort**, readiness for enhanced, Section III)

Communicable Diseases, Childhood (e.g., Measles, Mumps, Rubella, Chickenpox, Scabies, Lice, Impetigo)

Impaired **Comfort** r/t pruritus, inflammation or infection of skin, subdermal organisms

Deficient **Diversional** activity r/t imposed isolation from peers, disruption in usual play activities, fatigue, activity intolerance

Ineffective **Health** maintenance r/t nonadherence to appropriate immunization schedules, lack of prevention of transmission of infection

Acute **Pain** r/t impaired skin integrity, edema

Risk for **Infection**: transmission to others: Risk factor: contagious organisms

See Meningitis/Encephalitis; Respiratory Infections, Acute Childhood; Reye's Syndrome

Communication

Readiness for enhanced **Communication** (See **Communication**, readiness for enhanced, Section III)

Communication Problems

Impaired verbal **Communication** (See **Communication**, verbal, impaired, Section III)

Community Coping

Ineffective community **Coping** (See **Coping**, community, ineffective, Section III)

Readiness for enhanced community **Coping**: community sense of power to manage stressors, social supports available, resources available for problem solving

Compartment Syndrome

Fear r/t possible loss of limb, damage to limb

Acute **Pain** r/t pressure in compromised body part

Ineffective peripheral tissue **Perfusion** r/t increased pressure within compartment

Compulsion

See (OCD) Obsessive-Compulsive Disorder

Conduction Disorders (Cardiac)

See Dysrhythmia

Confusion, Acute

Acute **Confusion** r/t older than 70 years of age with hospitalization, alcohol abuse, delirium, dementia, drug abuse

Adult **Failure** to thrive r/t confusion

Confusion, Chronic

Chronic **Confusion** r/t Alzheimer's disease, Korsakoff's psychosis, multiinfarct dementia, cerebrovascular accident, head injury

Adult **Failure** to thrive r/t confusion

Impaired **Memory** r/t fluid and electrolyte imbalance, neurological disturbances, excessive environmental disturbances, anemia, acute or chronic hypoxia, decreased cardiac output

See Alzheimer's Disease; Dementia

Confusion, Possible

Risk for acute **Confusion** (See **Confusion**, acute, risk for, Section III)

Congenital Heart Disease/ Cardiac Anomalies

ACYANOTIC

Patent ductus arteriosus, atrial/ventricular septal defect, pulmonary stenosis, endocardial cushion defect, aortic valvular stenosis, coarctation of aorta

CYANOTIC

Tetralogy of Fallot, tricuspid atresia, transposition of great vessels, truncus arteriosus, total anomalous pulmonary venous return, hypoplastic left lung

Activity intolerance r/t fatigue, generalized weakness, lack of adequate oxygenation

Ineffective **Breathing** pattern r/t pulmonary vascular disease

Decreased **Cardiac** output r/t cardiac dysfunction

Excess **Fluid** volume r/t cardiac defect, side effects of medication

Impaired **Gas** exchange r/t cardiac defect, pulmonary congestion

Delayed **Growth** and development r/t inadequate oxygen and nutrients to tissues

Imbalanced **Nutrition**: less than body requirements r/t fatigue, generalized weakness, inability of infant to suck and feed, increased caloric requirements

Risk for delayed **Development**: Risk factor: inadequate oxygen and nutrients to tissues

Risk for deficient **Fluid** volume: Risk factor: side effects of diuretics

Risk for disproportionate **Growth**: Risk factor: inadequate oxygen and nutrients to tissues

Risk for disorganized **Infant** behavior: Risk factor: invasive procedures

Risk for **Poisoning**: Risk factor: potential toxicity of cardiac medications

Risk for ineffective **Thermoregulation**: Risk factor: neonatal age

See Child with Chronic Condition; Hospitalized Child

Congestive Heart Failure (CHF)

See CHF (Congestive Heart Failure)

Conjunctivitis

Acute **Pain** r/t inflammatory process

Disturbed **Sensory** perception r/t change in visual acuity resulting from inflammation

Consciousness, Altered Level of

Acute **Confusion** r/t alcohol abuse, delirium, dementia, drug abuse

Chronic **Confusion** r/t multiinfarct dementia, Korsakoff's psychosis, head injury, Alzheimer's disease, cerebrovascular accident

Adult **Failure** to thrive r/t altered level of consciousness

Functional urinary **Incontinence** r/t neurological dysfunction

Decreased **Intracranial** adaptive capacity r/t brain injury

Impaired **Memory** r/t neurological disturbances

Self-Care deficit: specify r/t neuromuscular impairment

Risk for **Aspiration**: Risk factors: impaired swallowing, loss of cough or gag reflex

Risk for **Disuse** syndrome: Risk factors: impaired mobility resulting from altered level of consciousness

Risk for impaired **Oral** mucous membrane: Risk factor: dry mouth

Risk for ineffective cerebral tissue **Perfusion** r/t increased intracranial pressure, altered cerebral perfusion

Risk for impaired **Skin** integrity: Risk factor: immobility

See cause of Altered Level of Consciousness

Constipation

Constipation (See **Constipation**, Section III)

Constipation, Perceived

Perceived **Constipation** (See **Constipation**, perceived, Section III)

Constipation, Risk for

Risk for **Constipation** (See **Constipation**, risk for, Section III)

Contamination

Contamination (See **Contamination**, Section III)

Risk for **Contamination** (See **Contamination**, risk for, Section III)

Continent Ileostomy (Kock Pouch)

Ineffective **Coping** r/t stress of disease, exacerbations caused by stress

Ineffective **Health** maintenance r/t deficient knowledge regarding postoperative care

Imbalanced **Nutrition**: less than body requirements r/t malabsorption

Risk for **Injury**: Risk factors: failure of valve, stomal cyanosis, intestinal obstruction

See Abdominal Surgery

Contraceptive Method

Decisional **Conflict**: method of contraception r/t unclear personal values or beliefs, lack of experience or interference with decision making, lack of relevant information, support system deficit

Ineffective **Sexuality** pattern r/t fear of pregnancy

Readiness for enhanced **Self Health** management: requesting information about available and appropriate birth control methods

Conversion Disorder

Anxiety r/t unresolved conflict

C

Risk-prone health **Behavior** r/t multiple stressors

Ineffective **Coping** r/t personal vulnerability

Hopelessness r/t long-term stress

Disturbed personal **Identity** r/t overwhelming stress

Impaired physical **Mobility** r/t physical conversion symptom

Powerlessness r/t lifestyle of helplessness

Ineffective **Role** performance r/t physical conversion system

Chronic low **Self-Esteem** r/t unsatisfactory or inadequate interpersonal relationships

Impaired **Social** interaction r/t altered thought process

Risk for **Injury**: Risk factors: physical conversion symptom

Convulsions

Anxiety r/t concern over controlling convulsions

Ineffective **Health** maintenance r/t deficient knowledge regarding need for medication and care during seizure activity

Impaired **Memory** r/t neurological disturbance

Risk for **Aspiration**: Risk factor: impaired swallowing

Risk for delayed **Development**: Risk factor: seizures

Risk for **Injury**: Risk factor: seizure activity

See Seizure Disorders, Adult; Seizure Disorders, Childhood

COPD (Chronic Obstructive Pulmonary Disease)

Activity intolerance r/t imbalance between oxygen supply and demand

Ineffective **Airway** clearance r/t bronchoconstriction, increased mucus, ineffective cough, infection

Anxiety r/t breathlessness, change in health status

Death **Anxiety** r/t seriousness of medical condition, difficulty being able to "catch breath," feeling of suffocation

Interrupted **Family** processes r/t role changes

Impaired **Gas** exchange r/t ventilation-perfusion inequality

Ineffective self **Health** management (See **Health** management, self, ineffective, Section III)

Noncompliance r/t reluctance to accept responsibility for changing detrimental health practices

Imbalanced **Nutrition**: less than body requirements r/t decreased intake because of dyspnea, unpleasant taste in mouth left by medications

Powerlessness r/t progressive nature of disease

Self-Care deficit: specify: r/t fatigue from the increased work of breathing

Chronic low **Self-Esteem** r/t chronic illness

Sleep deprivation r/t breathing difficulties when lying down

Impaired **Social** interaction r/t social isolation because of oxygen use, activity intolerance

Chronic **Sorrow** r/t presence of chronic illness

Risk for **Infection**: Risk factor: stasis of respiratory secretions

Readiness for enhanced **Self Health** management (See **Self Health** management, readiness for enhanced, Section III)

Coping

Readiness for enhanced **Coping** (See **Coping**, readiness for enhanced, Section III)

Coping Problems

Defensive **Coping** (See **Coping**, defensive, Section III)

Ineffective **Coping** (See **Coping**, ineffective, Section III)

See Community Coping; Family Problems

Corneal Reflex, Absent

Risk for **Injury**: Risk factors: accidental corneal abrasion, drying of cornea

Corneal Transplant

Risk for **Infection**: Risk factors: invasive procedure, surgery

Readiness for enhanced **Self Health** management: describes need to rest and avoid strenuous activities during healing phase

Coronary Artery Bypass Grafting (CABG)

Decreased **Cardiac** output r/t dysrhythmia, depressed cardiac function, increased systemic vascular resistance

Fear r/t outcome of surgical procedure

Deficient **Fluid** volume r/t intraoperative fluid loss, use of diuretics in surgery

Ineffective **Health** maintenance r/t deficient knowledge regarding postprocedure care, lifestyle adjustment after surgery

Acute **Pain** r/t traumatic surgery

Risk for perioperative positioning **Injury**: Risk factors: hypothermia, extended supine position

Costovertebral Angle Tenderness

See Kidney Stone; Pyelonephritis

Cough, Ineffective

Ineffective **Airway** clearance r/t decreased energy, fatigue, normal aging changes

See Bronchitis; COPD (Chronic Obstructive Pulmonary Disease); Pulmonary Edema

Crack Abuse

See Cocaine Abuse; Drug Abuse; Substance Abuse

Crack Baby

Disorganized **Infant** behavior r/t prematurity, pain, lack of attachment

Risk for impaired **Attachment**: Risk factors: parent's inability to meet infant's needs, substance abuse

See Infant of Substance-Abusing Mother

Crackles in Lungs, Coarse

Ineffective **Airway** clearance r/t excessive secretions in airways, ineffective cough

See cause of Coarse Crackles in Lungs

Crackles in Lungs, Fine

Ineffective **Breathing** pattern r/t fatigue, surgery, decreased energy

See Bronchitis or Pneumonia (if from pulmonary infection); CHF (Congestive Heart Failure) (if cardiac in origin); Infection

Craniectomy/Craniotomy

Adult **Failure** to thrive r/t altered cerebral tissue perfusion

Fear r/t threat to well-being

Decreased **Intracranial** adaptive capacity r/t brain injury, intracranial hypertension

Impaired **Memory** r/t neurological surgery

Acute **Pain** r/t recent surgery, headache

Risk for **Injury**: Risk factor: potential confusion

Risk for ineffective cerebral tissue **Perfusion**: Risk factors: cerebral edema, increased intracranial pressure

See Coma (if relevant)

Crepitation, Subcutaneous

See Pneumothorax

Crisis

Anxiety r/t threat to or change in environment, health status, interaction patterns, situation, self-concept, or role functioning; threat of death of self or significant other

Death **Anxiety** r/t feelings of hopelessness associated with crisis

Compromised family **Coping** r/t situational or developmental crisis

Ineffective **Coping** r/t situational or maturational crisis

Disturbed **Energy** field r/t disharmony caused by crisis

Fear r/t crisis situation

Grieving r/t potential significant loss

Impaired individual **Resilience** r/t onset of crisis

Situational low **Self-Esteem** r/t perception of inability to handle crisis

Spiritual distress r/t intense suffering

Risk for **Spiritual** distress: Risk factors: physical or psychological stress, natural disasters, situational losses, maturational losses

Crohn's Disease

Anxiety r/t change in health status

Ineffective **Coping** r/t repeated episodes of diarrhea

Diarrhea r/t inflammatory process

Ineffective **Health** maintenance r/t deficient knowledge regarding management of disease

Imbalanced **Nutrition**: less than body requirements r/t diarrhea, altered ability to digest and absorb food

Acute **Pain** r/t increased peristalsis

Powerlessness r/t chronic disease

Risk for deficient **Fluid** volume: Risk factor: abnormal fluid loss with diarrhea

Croup

See Respiratory Infections, Acute Childhood

Cryosurgery for Retinal Detachment

See Retinal Detachment

Cushing's Syndrome

Activity intolerance r/t fatigue, weakness

Disturbed **Body** image r/t change in appearance from disease process

Excess **Fluid** volume r/t failure of regulatory mechanisms

Ineffective **Health** maintenance r/t deficient knowledge regarding needed care

Sexual dysfunction r/t loss of libido

Impaired **Skin** integrity r/t effects of increased cortisol

Risk for **Infection**: Risk factor: suppression of immune system caused by increased cortisol levels

Risk for **Injury**: Risk factors: decreased muscle strength, osteoporosis

Cuts (Wounds)

See Lacerations

CVA (Cerebrovascular Accident)

Anxiety r/t situational crisis, change in physical or emotional condition

Disturbed **Body** image r/t chronic illness, paralysis

Caregiver role strain r/t cognitive problems of care receiver, need for significant home care

Impaired verbal **Communication** r/t pressure damage, decreased circulation to brain in speech center informational sources

Chronic **Confusion** r/t neurological changes

Constipation r/t decreased activity

Ineffective **Coping** r/t disability

Adult **Failure** to thrive r/t neurophysiological changes

Interrupted **Family** processes r/t illness, disability of family member

Grieving r/t loss of health

Ineffective **Health** maintenance r/t deficient knowledge regarding self-care after CVA

Impaired **Home** maintenance r/t neurological disease affecting ability to perform activities of daily living

Functional urinary **Incontinence** r/t neurological dysfunction

Reflex urinary **Incontinence** r/t loss of feeling to void

Impaired **Memory** r/t neurological disturbances

Impaired physical **Mobility** r/t loss of balance and coordination

Unilateral **Neglect** r/t disturbed perception from neurological damage

Self-Care deficit: specify r/t decreased strength and endurance, paralysis

Disturbed **Sensory** perception: visual, tactile, kinesthetic r/t neurologic deficit

Impaired **Social** interaction r/t limited physical mobility, limited ability to communicate

C

Impaired **Swallowing** r/t neuromuscular dysfunction

Impaired **Transfer** ability r/t limited physical mobility

Impaired **Walking** r/t loss of balance and coordination

Risk for **Aspiration**: Risk factors: impaired swallowing, loss of gag reflex

Risk for **Disuse** syndrome: Risk factor: paralysis

Risk for **Injury**: Risk factor: disturbed sensory perception

Risk for ineffective cerebral tissue **Perfusion** r/t clot, emboli, or hemorrhage from cerebral vessel

Risk for impaired **Skin** integrity: Risk factor: immobility

Cyanosis, Central with Cyanosis of Oral Mucous Membranes

Impaired **Gas** exchange r/t alveolar-capillary membrane changes

Cyanosis, Peripheral with Cyanosis of Nail Beds

Ineffective peripheral tissue **Perfusion** r/t interruption of arterial flow, severe vasoconstriction, cold temperatures

Cystic Fibrosis

Activity intolerance r/t imbalance between oxygen supply and demand

Ineffective **Airway** clearance r/t increased production of thick mucus

Anxiety r/t dyspnea, oxygen deprivation

Disturbed **Body** image r/t changes in physical appearance, treatment of chronic lung disease (clubbing, barrel chest, home oxygen therapy)

Impaired **Gas** exchange r/t ventilation-perfusion imbalance

Impaired **Home** maintenance r/t extensive daily treatment, medications necessary for health, mist or oxygen tents

Imbalanced **Nutrition**: less than body requirements r/t anorexia; decreased absorption of nutrients, fat; increased work of breathing

Chronic **Sorrow** r/t presence of chronic disease

Risk for **Caregiver** role strain: Risk factors: illness severity of care receiver, unpredictable course of illness

Risk for deficient **Fluid** volume: Risk factors: decreased fluid intake, increased work of breathing

Risk for **Infection**: Risk factors: thick, tenacious mucus; harboring of bacterial organisms; immunocompromised state

Risk for **Spiritual** distress: Risk factor: presence of chronic disease

See Child with Chronic Condition; Hospitalized Child; Terminally Ill Child, Adolescent; Terminally Ill Child, Infant/Toddler; Terminally Ill Child, Preschool Child; Terminally Ill Child, School-Age Child/Preadolescent; Terminally Ill Child/Death of Child, Parent

Cystitis

Ineffective **Health** maintenance r/t deficient knowledge regarding methods to treat and prevent urinary tract infections

Acute **Pain**: dysuria r/t inflammatory process in bladder

Impaired **Urinary** elimination: frequency r/t urinary tract infection

Risk for urge urinary **Incontinence**: Risk factor: infection in bladder

Cystocele

Ineffective **Health** maintenance r/t deficient knowledge regarding personal care, Kegel exercises to strengthen perineal muscles

Stress urinary **Incontinence** r/t prolapsed bladder

Urge urinary **Incontinence** r/t prolapsed bladder

Cystoscopy

Ineffective **Health** maintenance r/t deficient knowledge regarding postoperative care

Urinary retention r/t edema in urethra obstructing flow of urine

Risk for **Infection**: Risk factor: invasive procedure

D

Deafness

Impaired verbal **Communication** r/t impaired hearing

Disturbed **Sensory** perception: auditory r/t alteration in sensory reception, transmission, integration

Risk for delayed **Development** r/t impaired hearing

Risk for **Injury** r/t alteration in sensory perception

Death

Risk for sudden infant **Death** syndrome (SIDS) (See **Death** syndrome, infant, sudden, risk for, Section III)

Death, Oncoming

Death Anxiety r/t unresolved issues surrounding dying

Compromised family **Coping** r/t client's inability to provide support to family

Ineffective **Coping** r/t personal vulnerability

Fear r/t threat of death

Grieving r/t loss of significant other

Powerlessness r/t effects of illness, oncoming death

Social isolation r/t altered state of wellness

Spiritual distress r/t intense suffering

Readiness for enhanced **Spiritual** well-being: desire of client and family to be in harmony with each other and higher power, God

See Terminally Ill Child, Adolescent; Terminally Ill Child, Infant/Toddler; Terminally Ill Child, Preschool Child; Terminally Ill Child, School-Age Child/Preadolescent; Terminally Ill Child/Death of Child, Parent

Decisions, Difficulty Making

Decisional **Conflict** r/t support system deficit, perceived threat to value system, multiple or divergent sources of information, lack of relevant information, unclear personal values or beliefs

Readiness for enhanced **Decision-Making** (See **Decision-Making**, readiness for enhanced, Section III)

Decubitus Ulcer

See Pressure Ulcer

Deep Vein Thrombosis (DVT)

See DVT (Deep Vein Thrombosis)

Defensive Behavior

Defensive **Coping** r/t nonacceptance of blame, denial of problems or weakness

Ineffective **Denial** r/t inability to face situation realistically

Dehiscence, Abdominal

Fear r/t threat of death, severe dysfunction

Acute **Pain** r/t stretching of abdominal wall

Impaired **Skin** integrity r/t altered circulation, malnutrition, opening in incision

Delayed **Surgical** recovery r/t altered circulation, malnutrition, opening in incision

Impaired **Tissue** integrity r/t exposure of abdominal contents to external environment

Risk for deficient **Fluid** volume: Risk factor: altered circulation associated with opening of wound and exposure of abdominal contents

Risk for **Infection**: Risk factor: loss of skin integrity

Dehydration

Deficient **Fluid** volume r/t active fluid volume loss

Ineffective **Health** maintenance r/t deficient knowledge regarding treatment and prevention of dehydration

Impaired **Oral** mucous membrane r/t decreased salivation, fluid deficit

See cause of Dehydration

Delirium

Acute **Confusion** r/t effects of medication, response to hospitalization, alcohol abuse, substance abuse, sensory deprivation or overload

Adult **Failure** to thrive r/t delirium

Impaired **Memory** r/t delirium

Sleep deprivation r/t nightmares

Risk for **Injury**: Risk factor: altered level of consciousness

Delirium Tremens (DT)

See Alcohol Withdrawal

Delivery

See Labor, Normal

Delusions

Anxiety r/t content of intrusive thoughts

Impaired verbal **Communication** r/t psychological impairment, delusional thinking

Acute **Confusion** r/t alcohol abuse, delirium, dementia, drug abuse

Ineffective **Coping** r/t distortion and insecurity of life events

Adult **Failure** to thrive r/t delusional state

Risk for other-directed **Violence**: Risk factor: delusional thinking

Risk for self-directed **Violence**: Risk factor: delusional thinking

Dementia

Chronic **Confusion** r/t neurological dysfunction

Impaired **Environmental** interpretation syndrome r/t dementia

Adult **Failure** to thrive r/t depression, apathy

Interrupted **Family** processes r/t disability of family member

Impaired **Home** maintenance r/t inadequate support system

Functional urinary **Incontinence** r/t neuromuscular impairment

Insomnia r/t neurological impairment, naps during the day

Impaired physical **Mobility** r/t neuromuscular impairment

Self **Neglect** r/t cognitive impairment

Imbalanced **Nutrition**: less than body requirements r/t psychological impairment

Self-Care deficit: specify r/t psychological or neuromuscular impairment

Chronic **Sorrow** r/t loss of mental function

Risk for **Caregiver** role strain: Risk factors: number of caregiving tasks, duration of caregiving required

Risk for **Falls**: Risk factor: diminished mental status

Risk for **Injury**: Risk factors: confusion, decreased muscle coordination

Risk for impaired **Skin** integrity: Risk factors: altered nutritional status, immobility

Denial of Health Status

Ineffective **Denial** r/t lack of perception about health status effects of illness

Ineffective self **Health** management r/t denial of seriousness of health situation

Dental Caries

Impaired **Dentition** r/t ineffective oral hygiene, barriers to self-care, economic barriers to professional care, nutritional deficits, dietary habits

Ineffective self **Health** maintenance r/t lack of knowledge regarding prevention of dental disease

Dentition Problems

See Dental Caries

Depression (Major Depressive Disorder)

Death **Anxiety** r/t feelings of lack of self-worth

Constipation r/t inactivity, decreased fluid intake

Ineffective **Coping** r/t grieving

Disturbed **Energy** field r/t disharmony

Impaired **Environmental** interpretation syndrome r/t severe mental functional impairment

Adult **Failure** to thrive r/t depression

Fatigue r/t psychological demands

Ineffective **Health** maintenance r/t lack of ability to make good judgments regarding ways to obtain help

Hopelessness r/t feeling of abandonment, long-term stress

Insomnia r/t inactivity

Self **Neglect** r/t depression, cognitive impairment

D

Powerlessness r/t pattern of helplessness

Chronic low **Self-Esteem** r/t repeated unmet expectations

Sexual dysfunction r/t loss of sexual desire

Social isolation r/t ineffective coping

Chronic **Sorrow** r/t unresolved grief

Risk for complicated **Grieving**: Risk factor: lack of previous resolution of former grieving response

Risk for **Suicide**: Risk factor: panic state

Dermatitis

Anxiety r/t situational crisis imposed by illness

Impaired **Comfort** r/t itching

Ineffective **Health** maintenance r/t deficient knowledge regarding methods to decrease inflammation

Impaired **Skin** integrity r/t side effect of medication, allergic reaction

See Itching

Despondency

Hopelessness r/t long-term stress

See Depression (Major Depressive Disorder)

Destructive Behavior Toward Others

Risk-prone health **Behavior** r/t intense emotional state

Ineffective **Coping** r/t situational crises, maturational crises, personal vulnerability

Risk for other-directed **Violence** (See **Violence**, other-directed, risk for, Section III)

Developmental Concerns

Delayed **Growth** and development (See **Growth** and development, delayed, Section III)

INDIVIDUAL/ENVIRONMENTAL/CAREGIVER

Risk for delayed **Development** (See **Development**, delayed, risk for, Section III)

See Growth and Development Lag

Diabetes in Pregnancy

See Gestational Diabetes (Diabetes in Pregnancy)

Diabetes Insipidus

Deficient **Fluid** volume r/t inability to conserve fluid

Ineffective **Health** maintenance r/t deficient knowledge regarding care of disease, importance of medications

Diabetes Mellitus

Adult **Failure** to thrive r/t undetected disease process

Ineffective **Health** maintenance r/t complexity of therapeutic regimen

Ineffective self **Health** management (See **Health** management, self, ineffective, Section III)

Noncompliance r/t restrictive lifestyle; changes in diet, medication, exercise

Imbalanced **Nutrition**: less than body requirements r/t inability to use glucose (type 1 [insulin-dependent] diabetes)

Imbalanced **Nutrition**: more than body requirements r/t excessive intake of nutrients (type 2 diabetes)

Ineffective peripheral tissue **Perfusion** r/t impaired arterial circulation

Powerlessness r/t perceived lack of personal control

Disturbed **Sensory** perception r/t ineffective tissue perfusion

Sexual dysfunction r/t neuropathy associated with disease

Risk for unstable blood **Glucose** level (See **Glucose** level, blood, unstable, risk for, Section III)

Risk for **Infection**: Risk factors: hyperglycemia, impaired healing, circulatory changes

Risk for **Injury**: Risk factors: hypoglycemia or hyperglycemia from failure to consume adequate calories, failure to take insulin

Risk for dysfunctional gastrointestinal **Motility**: Risk factor: complication of diabetes

Risk for impaired **Skin** integrity: Risk factor: loss of pain perception in extremities

Readiness for enhanced **Self Health** management (See **Self Health** management, readiness for enhanced, Section III)

See Hyperglycemia; Hypoglycemia

Diabetes Mellitus, Juvenile (IDDM Type I)

Risk-prone health **Behavior** r/t inadequate comprehension, inadequate social support, low self-efficacy

Disturbed **Body** image r/t imposed deviations from biophysical and psychosocial norm, perceived differences from peers

Ineffective **Health** maintenance r/t parental/child deficient knowledge regarding dietary management, medication administration, physical activity, and interaction between the three; daily changes in diet, medications, illness, stress, activity associated with child's growth spurts and needs; need to instruct other caregivers and teachers regarding signs and symptoms of hypoglycemia or hyperglycemia and treatment

Noncompliance r/t disturbed body image, impaired adjustment attributable to adolescent maturational crises

Imbalanced **Nutrition**: less than body requirements r/t inability of body to adequately metabolize and use glucose and nutrients, increased caloric needs of child to promote growth and physical activity participation with peers

Acute **Pain** r/t insulin injections, peripheral blood glucose testing

See Diabetes Mellitus; Child with Chronic Condition; Hospitalized Child

Diabetic Coma

Acute **Confusion** r/t hyperglycemia, presence of excessive metabolic acids

Deficient **Fluid** volume r/t hyperglycemia resulting in polyuria

Ineffective self **Health** management r/t lack of understanding of preventive measures, adequate blood sugar control

Risk for unstable blood **Glucose** level (See **Glucose** level, blood, unstable, risk for, Section III)

Risk for **Infection**: Risk factors: hyperglycemia, changes in vascular system

See Diabetes Mellitus

Diabetic Ketoacidosis

See Ketoacidosis, Diabetic

Diabetic Retinopathy

Grieving r/t loss of vision

Ineffective **Health** maintenance r/t deficient knowledge regarding preserving vision with treatment if possible, use of low-vision aids

Disturbed **Sensory** perception r/t change in sensory reception

See Vision Impairment; Blindness

Dialysis

See Hemodialysis; Peritoneal Dialysis

Diaphragmatic Hernia

See Hiatal Hernia

Diarrhea

Diarrhea r/t infection, change in diet, gastrointestinal disorders, stress, medication effect, impaction

DIC (Disseminated Intravascular Coagulation)

Fear r/t threat to well-being

Deficient **Fluid** volume: hemorrhage r/t depletion of clotting factors

Risk for **Bleeding**: Risk factors: microclotting within vascular system, depleted clotting factors

Risk for ineffective gastrointestinal tissue **Perfusion** (See **Perfusion**, tissue, gastrointestinal, ineffective, risk for, Section III)

Digitalis Toxicity

Decreased **Cardiac** output r/t drug toxicity affecting cardiac rhythm, rate

Ineffective self **Health** management r/t deficient knowledge regarding action, appropriate method of administration of digitalis

Dignity, Loss of

Risk for compromised human **Dignity** (See **Dignity**, human, compromised, risk for, Section III)

Dilation and Curettage (D&C)

Ineffective **Health** maintenance r/t deficient knowledge regarding postoperative self-care

Acute **Pain** r/t uterine contractions

Risk for **Bleeding**: Risk factor: surgical procedure

Risk for **Infection**: Risk factor: surgical procedure

Risk for ineffective **Sexuality** pattern: Risk factors: painful coitus, fear associated with surgery on genital area

Dirty Body (for Prolonged Period)

Self **Neglect** r/t mental illness, substance abuse, cognitive impairment

Discharge Planning

Ineffective **Health** maintenance r/t lack of material sources

Impaired **Home** maintenance r/t family member's disease or injury interfering with home maintenance

Deficient **Knowledge** r/t lack of exposure to information for home care

Discomforts of Pregnancy

Disturbed **Body** image r/t pregnancy-induced body changes

Impaired **Comfort** r/t enlarged abdomen, swollen feet

Constipation r/t decreased gastrointestinal tract motility, pressure from enlarged uterus, supplementary iron

Fatigue r/t hormonal, metabolic, body changes

Stress urinary **Incontinence** r/t enlarged uterus, fetal movement

Insomnia r/t psychological stress, fetal movement, muscular cramping, urinary frequency, shortness of breath

Nausea r/t hormone effect

Acute **Pain**: headache r/t hormonal changes of pregnancy

Acute **Pain**: leg cramps r/t nerve compression, calcium/phosphorus/potassium imbalance

Risk for **Constipation**: Risk factors: decreased intestinal motility, inadequate fiber in diet

Risk for **Injury**: Risk factors: faintness and/or syncope caused by vasomotor lability or postural hypotension, venous stasis in lower extremities

Dislocation of Joint

Acute **Pain** r/t dislocation of a joint

Self-Care deficit: specify r/t inability to use a joint

Risk for **Injury**: Risk factor: unstable joint

Dissecting Aneurysm

Fear r/t threat to well-being

See Abdominal Surgery; Aneurysm, Abdominal Surgery

Disseminated Intravascular Coagulation (DIC)

See DIC (Disseminated Intravascular Coagulation)

Dissociative Identity Disorder (Not Otherwise Specified)

Anxiety r/t psychosocial stress

Ineffective **Coping** r/t personal vulnerability in crisis of accurate self-perception

Disturbed personal **Identity** r/t inability to distinguish self caused by multiple personality disorder, depersonalization, disturbance in memory

Impaired **Memory** r/t altered state of consciousness

Disturbed **Sensory** perception: auditory, visual r/t psychological stress

See Multiple Personality Disorder (Dissociative Identity Disorder)

Distress

Anxiety r/t situational crises, maturational crises

Death **Anxiety** r/t denial of one's own mortality or impending death

D

Disturbed **Energy** field r/t disruption in flow of energy as result of pain, depression, fatigue, anxiety, stress

Disuse Syndrome, Potential to Develop

Risk for **Disuse** syndrome: Risk factors: paralysis, mechanical immobilization, prescribed immobilization, severe pain, altered level of consciousness

Diversional Activity, Lack of

Deficient **Diversional** activity r/t environmental lack of diversional activity as in frequent hospitalizations, lengthy treatments

Diverticulitis

Constipation r/t dietary deficiency of fiber and roughage

Diarrhea r/t increased intestinal motility caused by inflammation

Deficient **Knowledge** r/t diet needed to control disease, medication regimen

Imbalanced **Nutrition**: less than body requirements r/t loss of appetite

Acute **Pain** r/t inflammation of bowel

Risk for deficient **Fluid** volume: Risk factor: diarrhea

Dizziness

Decreased **Cardiac** output r/t dysfunctional electrical conduction

Impaired physical **Mobility** r/t dizziness

Risk for **Falls**: Risk factor: difficulty maintaining balance

Risk for ineffective cerebral tissue **Perfusion**: Risk factor: interruption of cerebral arterial blood flow

Domestic Violence

Anxiety r/t threat to self-concept, situational crisis of abuse

Impaired verbal **Communication** r/t psychological barriers of fear

Compromised family **Coping** r/t abusive patterns

Defensive **Coping** r/t low self-esteem

Dysfunctional **Family** processes r/t inadequate coping skills

Insomnia r/t psychological stress

Post-trauma syndrome r/t history of abuse

Powerlessness r/t lifestyle of helplessness

Situational low **Self-Esteem** r/t negative family interactions

Risk for **Post-Trauma** syndrome: Risk factor: inadequate social support

Risk for compromised **Resilience**: Risk factor: effects of abuse

Risk for other-directed **Violence**: Risk factor: history of abuse

Down Syndrome

See Child with Chronic Condition; Mental Retardation

Dress Self (Inability to)

Dressing **Self-Care** deficit r/t intolerance to activity, decreased strength and endurance, pain, discomfort, perceptual or cognitive impairment, neuromuscular impairment, musculoskeletal impairment, depression, severe anxiety

Dribbling of Urine

Overflow urinary **Incontinence** r/t degenerative changes in pelvic muscles and urinary structures

Stress urinary **Incontinence** r/t degenerative changes in pelvic muscles and urinary structures

Drooling

Impaired **Swallowing** r/t neuromuscular impairment, mechanical obstruction

Risk for **Aspiration**: Risk factor: impaired swallowing

Dropout from School

Impaired individual **Resilience** (See **Resilience**, individual, impaired, Section III)

Drug Abuse

Anxiety r/t threat to self-concept, lack of control of drug use

Risk-prone health **Behavior** r/t addiction

Ineffective **Coping** r/t situational crisis

Insomnia r/t effects of drugs

Noncompliance r/t denial of illness

Imbalanced **Nutrition**: less than body requirements r/t poor eating habits

Powerlessness r/t feeling unable to change patterns of drug abuse

Impaired individual **Resilience** (See **Resilience**, individual, impaired, Section III)

Disturbed **Sensory** perception: specify r/t substance intoxication

Sexual dysfunction r/t actions and side effects of drug abuse

Sleep deprivation r/t prolonged psychological discomfort

Impaired **Social** interaction r/t disturbed thought processes from drug abuse

Spiritual distress r/t separation from religious, cultural ties

Risk for **Injury**: Risk factors: hallucinations, drug effects

Risk for other-directed **Violence**: Risk factor: poor impulse control

See Cocaine Abuse; Substance Abuse

Drug Withdrawal

Anxiety r/t physiological withdrawal

Acute **Confusion** r/t effects of substance withdrawal

Ineffective **Coping** r/t situational crisis, withdrawal

Insomnia r/t effects of medications

Noncompliance r/t denial of illness

Imbalanced **Nutrition**: less than body requirements r/t poor eating habits

Disturbed **Sensory** perception: specify r/t substance intoxication

Risk for other-directed **Violence**: Risk factors: poor impulse control, hallucinations

D

Risk for self-directed **Violence**: Risk factors: poor impulse control, hallucinations

See Drug Abuse

Dry Eye

Deficient **Knowledge** r/t treatment of dry eye

See Conjunctivitis; Keratoconjunctivitis Sicca

DT (Delirium Tremens)

See Alcohol Withdrawal

DVT (Deep Vein Thrombosis)

Constipation r/t inactivity, bed rest

Ineffective **Health** maintenance r/t deficient knowledge regarding self-care needs, treatment regimen, outcome

Impaired physical **Mobility** r/t pain in extremity, forced bed rest

Acute **Pain** r/t vascular inflammation, edema

Ineffective peripheral tissue **Perfusion** r/t deficient knowledge of aggravating factors

Delayed **Surgical** recovery r/t impaired physical mobility

See Anticoagulant Therapy

Dying Client

See Terminally Ill Adult; Terminally Ill Adolescent; Terminally Ill Child, Infant/Toddler; Terminally Ill Child, Preschool Child; Terminally Ill Child, School-Age Child/Preadolescent; Terminally Ill Child/Death of Child, Parent

Dysfunctional Eating Pattern

Imbalanced **Nutrition**: less than body requirements r/t psychological factors

Imbalanced **Nutrition**: more than body requirements r/t psychological factors

See Anorexia Nervosa; Bulimia; Maturational Issues, Adolescent; Obesity

Dysfunctional Family Unit

See Family Problems

Dysfunctional Ventilatory Weaning

Dysfunctional **Ventilatory** weaning response r/t physical, psychological, situational factors

Dysmenorrhea

Ineffective **Health** maintenance r/t deficient knowledge regarding prevention and treatment of painful menstruation

Nausea r/t prostaglandin effect

Acute **Pain** r/t cramping from hormonal effects

Dyspareunia

Sexual dysfunction r/t lack of lubrication during intercourse, alteration in reproductive organ function

Dyspepsia

Anxiety r/t pressures of personal role

Ineffective **Health** maintenance r/t deficient knowledge regarding treatment of disease

Acute **Pain** r/t gastrointestinal disease, consumption of irritating foods

Dysphagia

Impaired **Swallowing** r/t neuromuscular impairment

Risk for **Aspiration**: Risk factor: loss of gag or cough reflex

Dysphasia

Impaired verbal **Communication** r/t decrease in circulation to brain

Impaired **Social** interaction r/t difficulty in communicating

Dyspnea

Activity intolerance r/t imbalance between oxygen supply and demand

Anxiety r/t ineffective breathing pattern

Ineffective **Breathing** pattern r/t compromised cardiac or pulmonary function, decreased lung expansion, neurological impairment affecting respiratory center, extreme anxiety

Fear r/t threat to state of well-being, potential death

Impaired **Gas** exchange r/t alveolar-capillary damage

Insomnia r/t difficulty breathing, positioning required for effective breathing

Sleep deprivation r/t ineffective breathing pattern

Dysrhythmia

Activity intolerance r/t decreased cardiac output

Decreased **Cardiac** output r/t altered electrical conduction

Fear r/t threat of death, change in health status

Ineffective **Health** maintenance r/t deficient knowledge regarding self-care with disease

Risk for ineffective cerebral tissue **Perfusion**: Risk factor: decreased cardiac output from dysrhythmia

Dysthymic Disorder

Ineffective **Coping** r/t impaired social interaction

Ineffective **Health** maintenance r/t inability to make good judgments regarding ways to obtain help

Insomnia r/t anxious thoughts

Chronic low **Self-Esteem** r/t repeated unmet expectations

Ineffective **Sexuality** pattern r/t loss of sexual desire

Social isolation r/t ineffective coping

See Depression (Major Depressive Disorder)

Dystocia

Anxiety r/t difficult labor, deficient knowledge regarding normal labor pattern

Ineffective **Coping** r/t situational crisis

Fatigue r/t prolonged labor

Grieving r/t loss of ideal labor experience

Acute **Pain** r/t difficult labor, medical interventions

Powerlessness r/t perceived inability to control outcome of labor

Risk for delayed Development: Risk factor: difficult labor and birth

Risk for deficient Fluid volume: Risk factor: hemorrhage secondary to uterine atony

Risk for disproportionate Growth: Risk factor: difficult labor and birth

Risk for Infection: Risk factor: prolonged rupture of membranes

Risk for ineffective cerebral tissue Perfusion: fetal: Risk factor: difficult labor and birth

Risk for impaired Tissue integrity: maternal and fetal: Risk factor: difficult labor

Dysuria

Impaired Urinary elimination r/t urinary tract infection

Risk for urge urinary Incontinence: Risk factors: detrusor hyperreflexia from cystitis, urethritis

E

ECMO (Extracorporeal Membrane Oxygenator)

Death Anxiety r/t emergency condition, hemorrhage

Decreased Cardiac output r/t ineffective function of the heart

Impaired Gas exchange (See **Gas** exchange, impaired, Section III)

E. Coli Infection

Fear r/t serious illness, unknown outcome

Deficient Knowledge r/t how to prevent disease; care of self with serious illness

See Gastroenteritis; Gastroenteritis, Child; Hospitalized Child

Ear Surgery

Ineffective Health maintenance r/t deficient knowledge regarding postoperative restrictions, expectations, care

Acute Pain r/t edema in ears from surgery

Disturbed Sensory perception: hearing r/t invasive surgery of ears, dressings

Risk for delayed Development: Risk factor: hearing impairment

Risk for Falls: Risk factor: dizziness from excessive stimuli to vestibular apparatus

See Hospitalized Child

Earache

Acute Pain r/t trauma, edema, infection

Disturbed Sensory perception: auditory r/t altered sensory reception, transmission, integration

Eclampsia

Interrupted Family processes r/t unmet expectations for pregnancy and childbirth

Fear r/t threat of well-being to self and fetus

Risk for Aspiration: Risk factor: seizure activity

Risk for delayed Development: Risk factor: uteroplacental insufficiency

Risk for excess Fluid volume: Risk factor: decreased urine output as a result of renal dysfunction

Risk for disproportionate Growth: Risk factor: uteroplacental insufficiency

Risk for ineffective cerebral tissue Perfusion: fetal: Risk factor: uteroplacental insufficiency

ECT (Electroconvulsive Therapy)

Decisional Conflict r/t lack of relevant information

Fear r/t real or imagined threat to well-being

Impaired Memory r/t effects of treatment

See Depression (Major Depressive Disorder)

Ectopic Pregnancy

Death Anxiety r/t emergency condition, hemorrhage

Disturbed Body image r/t negative feelings about body and reproductive functioning

Fear r/t threat to self, surgery, implications for future pregnancy

Deficient Fluid volume r/t loss of blood

Acute Pain r/t stretching or rupture of implantation site

Ineffective Role performance r/t loss of pregnancy

Situational low Self-Esteem r/t loss of pregnancy, inability to carry pregnancy to term

Chronic Sorrow r/t loss of pregnancy, potential loss of fertility

Risk for ineffective Coping: Risk factor: loss of pregnancy

Risk for interrupted Family processes: Risk factor: situational crisis

Risk for Infection: Risk factors: traumatized tissue, blood loss

Risk for Spiritual distress: Risk factor: grief process

Eczema

Disturbed Body image r/t change in appearance from inflamed skin

Impaired Comfort: pruritus r/t inflammation of skin

Ineffective Health maintenance r/t deficient knowledge regarding how to decrease inflammation and prevent further outbreaks

Impaired Skin integrity r/t side effect of medication, allergic reaction

ED (Erectile Dysfunction)

See Erectile Dysfunction (ED); Impotence

Edema

Excess Fluid volume r/t excessive fluid intake, cardiac dysfunction, renal dysfunction, loss of plasma proteins

Ineffective Health maintenance r/t deficient knowledge regarding treatment of edema

Risk for impaired Skin integrity: Risk factors: impaired circulation, fragility of skin

See cause of Edema

Elder Abuse

See Abuse, Spouse, Parent, or Significant Other

Elderly

See Aging

Electroconvulsive Therapy

See ECT (Electroconvulsive Therapy)

Electrolyte Imbalance

Risk for **Electrolyte** imbalance (See **Electrolyte** imbalance, risk for, Section III)

Emaciated Person

Adult **Failure** to thrive r/t imbalanced nutrition: less than body requirements

Imbalanced **Nutrition**: less than body requirements r/t inability to ingest food, digest food, absorb nutrients because of biological, psychological, economic factors

Embolectomy

Fear r/t threat of great bodily harm from embolus

Ineffective peripheral tissue **Perfusion** r/t presence of embolus

Risk for **Bleeding**: Risk factors: postoperative complication, surgical area

See Surgery, Postoperative Care

Emboli

See Pulmonary Embolism

Embolism in Leg or Arm

Ineffective peripheral tissue **Perfusion** r/t arterial obstruction from clot

Emesis

Nausea (See **Nausea**, Section III)

See Vomiting

Emotional Problems

See Coping Problems

Empathy

Readiness for enhanced community **Coping**: social supports, being available for problem solving

Readiness for enhanced family **Coping**: basic needs met, desire to move to higher level of health

Readiness for enhanced **Spiritual** well-being: desire to establish interconnectedness through spirituality

Emphysema

See COPD (Chronic Obstructive Pulmonary Disease)

Emptiness

Social isolation r/t inability to engage in satisfying personal relationships

Chronic **Sorrow** r/t unresolved grief

Spiritual distress r/t separation from religious or cultural ties

Encephalitis

See Meningitis/Encephalitis

Endocardial Cushion Defect

See Congenital Heart Disease/Cardiac Anomalies

Endocarditis

Activity intolerance r/t reduced cardiac reserve, prescribed bed rest

Decreased **Cardiac** output r/t inflammation of lining of heart and change in structure of valve leaflets, increased myocardial workload

Ineffective **Health** maintenance r/t deficient knowledge regarding treatment of disease, preventive measures against further incidence of disease

Acute **Pain** r/t biological injury, inflammation

Risk for imbalanced **Nutrition**: less than body requirements: Risk factors: fever, hypermetabolic state associated with fever

Risk for ineffective cerebral tissue **Perfusion**: Risk factor: possible presence of emboli in cerebral circulation

Risk for ineffective peripheral tissue **Perfusion**: Risk factor: possible presence of emboli in peripheral circulation

Endometriosis

Grieving r/t possible infertility

Ineffective **Health** maintenance r/t deficient knowledge about disease condition, medications, other treatments

Nausea r/t prostaglandin effect

Acute **Pain** r/t onset of menses with distention of endometrial tissue

Sexual dysfunction r/t painful intercourse

Endometritis

Anxiety r/t prolonged hospitalization, fear of unknown

Ineffective **Health** maintenance r/t deficient knowledge regarding condition, treatment, antibiotic regimen

Hyperthermia r/t infectious process

Acute **Pain** r/t infectious process in reproductive tract

Enuresis

Ineffective **Health** maintenance r/t unachieved developmental task, neuromuscular immaturity, diseases of urinary system

See Toilet Training

Environmental Interpretation Problems

Chronic **Confusion** r/t impaired environmental interpretation syndrome

Impaired **Environmental** interpretation syndrome r/t dementia, chronic neurological disease, depression, alcoholism

Adult **Failure** to thrive r/t impaired environmental interpretation syndrome

Impaired **Memory** r/t environmental disturbances

Risk for **Injury**: Risk factor: lack of orientation to person, place, time, circumstances

See cause of Environmental Interpretation Problem

Epididymitis

Anxiety r/t situational crisis, pain, threat to future fertility

E

Ineffective **Health** maintenance r/t deficient knowledge regarding treatment for pain and infection

Acute **Pain** r/t inflammation in scrotal sac

Ineffective **Sexuality** pattern r/t edema of epididymis and testes

Epiglottitis

See Respiratory Infections, Acute Childhood (Croup, Epiglottis, Pertussis, Pneumonia, Respiratory Syncytial Virus)

Epilepsy

Anxiety r/t threat to role functioning

Ineffective **Health** maintenance r/t deficient knowledge regarding seizures and seizure control

Ineffective self **Health** management r/t deficient knowledge regarding seizure control

Impaired **Memory** r/t seizure activity

Risk for **Aspiration**: Risk factors: impaired swallowing, excessive secretions

Risk for delayed **Development**: Risk factor: seizure disorder

Risk for **Injury**: Risk factor: environmental factors during seizure

See Seizure Disorders, Adult; Seizure Disorders, Childhood

Episiotomy

Anxiety r/t fear of pain

Disturbed **Body** image r/t fear of resuming sexual relations

Impaired physical **Mobility** r/t pain, swelling, tissue trauma

Acute **Pain** r/t tissue trauma

Sexual dysfunction r/t altered body structure, tissue trauma

Impaired **Skin** integrity r/t perineal incision

Risk for **Infection**: Risk factor: tissue trauma

Epistaxis

Fear r/t large amount of blood loss

Risk for deficient **Fluid** volume: Risk factor: excessive fluid loss

Epstein-Barr Virus

See Mononucleosis

Erectile Dysfunction (ED)

Situational low **Self-esteem** r/t physiological crisis, inability to practice usual sexual activity

Sexual dysfunction r/t altered body function

Readiness for enhanced **Knowledge**: information regarding treatment for erectile dysfunction

See Impotence

Esophageal Varices

Fear r/t threat of death

Risk for **Bleeding**: Risk factor: portal hypertension, distended variceal vessels that can easily rupture

See Cirrhosis

Esophagitis

Ineffective **Health** maintenance r/t deficient knowledge regarding treatment of disease

Acute **Pain** r/t inflammation of esophagus

ETOH Withdrawal

See Alcohol Withdrawal

Evisceration

See Dehiscence, Abdominal

Exhaustion

Impaired individual **Resilience** (See **Resilience**, individual, impaired, Section III)

Disturbed **Sleep** pattern (See **Sleep** pattern, disturbed, Section III)

Exposure to Hot or Cold Environment

Risk for imbalanced **Body** temperature: Risk factor: exposure

External Fixation

Disturbed **Body** image r/t trauma, change to affected part

Risk for **Infection**: Risk factor: presence of pins inserted into bone

See Fracture

Eye Surgery

Anxiety r/t possible loss of vision

Ineffective **Health** maintenance r/t deficient knowledge regarding postoperative activity, medications, eye care

Self-Care deficit r/t impaired vision

Disturbed **Sensory** perception: visual r/t surgical procedure

Risk for **Injury**: Risk factor: impaired vision

See Hospitalized Child; Vision Impairment

Extracorporeal Membrane Oxygenator (ECMO)

See ECMO (Extracorporeal Membrane Oxygenator)

F

Failure to Thrive, Adult

Adult **Failure** to thrive r/t depression, apathy, fatigue

Failure to Thrive, Nonorganic

Delayed **Growth** and development r/t parental deficient knowledge, lack of stimulation, nutritional deficit, long-term hospitalization

Disorganized **Infant** behavior (See **Infant** behavior, disorganized, Section III)

Insomnia r/t inconsistency of caretaker; lack of quiet, consistent environment

Imbalanced **Nutrition**: less than body requirements r/t inadequate type or amounts of food for infant, inappropriate feeding techniques

Impaired **Parenting** r/t lack of parenting skills, inadequate role modeling

Chronic low **Self-Esteem**: parental r/t feelings of inadequacy, support system deficiencies, inadequate role model

Social isolation r/t limited support systems, self-imposed situation

Risk for impaired **Attachment**: Risk factor: inability of parents to meet infant's needs

Risk for delayed **Development** (See **Development**, delayed, risk for, Section III)

Risk for disproportionate **Growth** (See **Growth**, disproportionate, risk for, Section III)

Falls, Risk for

Risk for **Falls** (See **Falls**, risk for, Section III)

Family Problems

Compromised family **Coping** (See **Coping**, family, compromised, Section III)

Disabled family **Coping** (See **Coping**, family, disabled, Section III)

Interrupted **Family** processes r/t situation transition and/or crises, developmental transition and/or crises

Ineffective family **Therapeutic** regimen management r/t complexity of health care system, complexity of therapeutic regimen, decisional conflicts, economic difficulties, excessive demands made on individual or family, family conflict

Readiness for enhanced family **Coping**: needs sufficiently gratified, adaptive tasks effectively addressed to enable goals of self-actualization to surface

Family Process

Readiness for enhanced **Family** processes (See **Family** processes, readiness for enhanced, Section III)

Readiness for enhanced **Relationship** (See **Relationship**, readiness for enhanced, Section III)

Fatigue

Disturbed **Energy** field r/t disharmony

Fatigue (See **Fatigue**, Section III)

Fear

Death **Anxiety** r/t fear of death

Fear r/t identifiable physical or psychological threat to person

Febrile Seizures

See Seizure Disorders, Childhood

Fecal Impaction

See Impaction of Stool

Fecal Incontinence

Bowel incontinence r/t neurological impairment, gastrointestinal disorders, anorectal trauma

Feeding Problems, Newborn

Ineffective **Breastfeeding** (See **Breastfeeding**, ineffective, Section III)

Interrupted **Breastfeeding** r/t maternal or infant illness, prematurity, maternal employment, contraindications to breastfeeding, need to abruptly wean infant

Disorganized **Infant** behavior r/t prematurity, immature neurological system

Ineffective **Infant** feeding pattern r/t prematurity, neurological impairment or delay, oral hypersensitivity, prolonged nothing-by-mouth status

Impaired **Swallowing** r/t prematurity

Risk for delayed **Development**: Risk factor: inadequate nutrition

Risk for deficient **Fluid** volume: Risk factor: inability to take in adequate amount of fluids

Risk for disproportionate **Growth**: Risk factor: feeding problems

Femoral Popliteal Bypass

Anxiety r/t threat to or change in health status

Acute **Pain** r/t surgical trauma, edema in surgical area

Ineffective peripheral tissue **Perfusion** r/t impaired arterial circulation

Risk for **Bleeding**: Risk factor: surgery on arteries

Risk for **Infection**: Risk factor: invasive procedure

Fetal Alcohol Syndrome

See Infant of Substance-Abusing Mother

Fetal Distress/Nonreassuring Fetal Heart Rate Pattern

Fear r/t threat to fetus

Ineffective peripheral tissue **Perfusion**: fetal r/t interruption of umbilical cord blood flow

Fever

Hyperthermia r/t infectious process, damage to hypothalamus, exposure to hot environment, medications, anesthesia, inability or decreased ability to perspire

Fibrocystic Breast Disease

See Breast Lumps

Filthy Home Environment

Impaired **Home** maintenance (See **Home** maintenance, impaired, Section III)

Self **Neglect** r/t mental illness, substance abuse, cognitive impairment

Financial Crisis in the Home Environment

Impaired **Home** maintenance r/t insufficient finances

Fistulectomy

See Hemorrhoidectomy

Flail Chest

Ineffective **Breathing** pattern r/t chest trauma

Fear r/t difficulty breathing

Impaired **Gas** exchange r/t loss of effective lung function

Impaired spontaneous **Ventilation** r/t paradoxical respirations

Flashbacks

Post-Trauma syndrome r/t catastrophic event

Flat Affect

Adult **Failure** to thrive r/t apathy

F

Hopelessness r/t prolonged activity restriction creating isolation, failing or deteriorating physiological condition, long-term stress, abandonment, lost belief in transcendent values or higher power or God

Risk for Loneliness: Risk factors: social isolation, lack of interest in surroundings

See Depression (Major Depressive Disorder); Dysthymic Disorder

Flesh-Eating Bacteria (Necrotizing Fasciitis)

See Necrotizing Fasciitis (Flesh-Eating Bacteria)

Fluid Balance

Readiness for enhanced **Fluid** balance (See **Fluid** balance, readiness for enhanced, Section III)

Fluid Volume Deficit

Deficient **Fluid** volume r/t active fluid loss, failure of regulatory mechanisms

Risk for Shock: Risk factor: hypovolemia

Fluid Volume Excess

Excess **Fluid** volume r/t compromised regulatory mechanism, excess sodium intake

Fluid Volume Imbalance, Risk for

Risk for imbalanced **Fluid** volume: Risk factor: major invasive surgeries

Foodborne Illness

Diarrhea r/t infectious material in gastrointestinal tract

Deficient **Fluid** volume r/t active fluid loss

Deficient **Knowledge** r/t care of self with serious illness, prevention of further incidences of foodborne illness

Nausea r/t contamination irritating stomach

Risk for dysfunctional gastrointestinal **Motility**: Risk factor: contaminated food

See Gastroenteritis; Gastroenteritis, Child; Hospitalized Child; E. coli Infection

Food Intolerance

Risk for dysfunctional gastrointestinal **Motility**: Risk factor: food intolerance

Foreign Body Aspiration

Ineffective **Airway** clearance r/t obstruction of airway

Ineffective **Health** maintenance r/t parental deficient knowledge regarding high-risk items

Impaired **Home** maintenance r/t inability to maintain orderly and clean surroundings

Risk for Suffocation: Risk factor: inhalation of small objects

See Safety, Childhood

Formula Feeding

Grieving: maternal r/t loss of desired breastfeeding experience

Ineffective **Health** maintenance r/t maternal deficient knowledge regarding formula feeding

Risk for Constipation: infant: Risk factor: iron-fortified formula

Risk for Infection: infant: Risk factors: lack of passive maternal immunity, supine feeding position

Fracture

Deficient **Diversional** activity r/t immobility

Ineffective **Health** maintenance r/t deficient knowledge regarding care of fracture

Impaired physical **Mobility** r/t limb immobilization

Acute **Pain** r/t muscle spasm, edema, trauma

Impaired **Walking** r/t limb immobility

Risk for ineffective peripheral tissue **Perfusion**: Risk factors: immobility, presence of cast

Risk for **Peripheral** neurovascular dysfunction: Risk factors: mechanical compression, treatment of fracture

Risk for impaired **Skin** integrity: Risk factors: immobility, presence of cast

Fractured Hip

See Hip Fracture

Frequency of Urination

Stress urinary **Incontinence** r/t degenerative change in pelvic muscles and structural support

Urge urinary **Incontinence** r/t decreased bladder capacity, irritation of bladder stretch receptors causing spasm, alcohol, caffeine, increased fluids, increased urine concentration, over-distended bladder

Urinary retention r/t high urethral pressure caused by weak detrusor, inhibition of reflex arc, strong sphincter, blockage

Impaired **Urinary** elimination r/t anatomical obstruction, sensory-motor impairment, urinary tract infection

Friendship

Readiness for enhanced **Relationship**: express desire to enhance communication between partners

Frostbite

Acute **Pain** r/t decreased circulation from prolonged exposure to cold

Ineffective peripheral tissue **Perfusion** r/t damage to extremities from prolonged exposure to cold

Impaired **Tissue** integrity r/t freezing of skin and tissues

See Hypothermia

Frothy Sputum

See CHF (Congestive Heart Failure); Pulmonary Edema; Seizure Disorders, Adult; Seizure Disorders, Childhood

Fusion, Lumbar

Anxiety r/t fear of surgical procedure, possible recurring problems

Ineffective **Health** maintenance r/t deficient knowledge regarding postoperative mobility restrictions, body mechanics

Impaired physical **Mobility** r/t limitations from surgical procedure, presence of brace

Acute **Pain** r/t discomfort at bone donor site, surgical operation

Risk for **Injury**: Risk factor: improper body mechanics

Risk for perioperative positioning **Injury**: Risk factor: immobilization during surgery

G

Gag Reflex, Depressed or Absent

Impaired **Swallowing** r/t neuromuscular impairment

Risk for **Aspiration**: Risk factors: depressed cough or gag reflex

Gallop Rhythm

Decreased **Cardiac** output r/t decreased contractility of heart

Gallstones

See Cholelithiasis

Gang Member

Impaired individual **Resilience** (See **Resilience**, individual, impaired, Section III)

Gangrene

Fear r/t possible loss of extremity

Ineffective peripheral tissue **Perfusion** r/t obstruction of arterial flow

Gas Exchange, Impaired

Impaired **Gas** exchange r/t ventilation-perfusion imbalance

Gastric Ulcer

See GI Bleed (Gastrointestinal Bleeding); Ulcer, Peptic (Duodenal or Gastric)

Gastritis

Imbalanced **Nutrition**: less than body requirements r/t vomiting, inadequate intestinal absorption of nutrients, restricted dietary regimen

Acute **Pain** r/t inflammation of gastric mucosa

Risk for deficient **Fluid** volume: Risk factors: excessive loss from gastrointestinal tract as a result of vomiting, decreased intake

Gastroenteritis

Diarrhea r/t infectious process involving intestinal tract

Deficient **Fluid** volume r/t excessive loss from gastrointestinal tract from diarrhea, vomiting

Ineffective **Health** maintenance r/t deficient knowledge regarding treatment of disease

Nausea r/t irritation to gastrointestinal system

Imbalanced **Nutrition**: less than body requirements r/t vomiting, inadequate intestinal absorption of nutrients, restricted dietary intake

Acute **Pain** r/t increased peristalsis causing cramping

See Gastroenteritis, Child

Gastroenteritis, Child

Ineffective **Health** maintenance r/t lack of parental knowledge regarding fluid and dietary changes

Impaired **Skin** integrity: diaper rash r/t acidic excretions on perineal tissues

See Gastroenteritis; Hospitalized Child

Gastroesophageal Reflux

Ineffective **Airway** clearance r/t reflux of gastric contents into esophagus and tracheal or bronchial tree

Ineffective **Health** maintenance r/t deficient knowledge regarding antireflux regimen (e.g., positioning, change in diet)

Acute **Pain** r/t irritation of esophagus from gastric acids

Risk for **Aspiration**: Risk factor: entry of gastric contents in tracheal or bronchial tree

Gastroesophageal Reflux: Child

Ineffective **Airway** clearance r/t reflux of gastric contents into esophagus and tracheal or bronchial tree

Anxiety: parental r/t possible need for surgical intervention

Deficient **Fluid** volume r/t persistent vomiting

Ineffective **Health** maintenance r/t deficient knowledge regarding antireflux regimen (e.g., positioning, oral or enteral feeding techniques, medications), possible home apnea monitoring

Imbalanced **Nutrition**: less than body requirements r/t poor feeding, vomiting

Risk for **Aspiration**: Risk factor: entry of gastric contents in tracheal or bronchial tree

Risk for impaired **Parenting**: Risk factors: disruption in bonding as a result of irritable or inconsolable infant; lack of sleep for parents

See Child with Chronic Condition; Hospitalized Child

Gastrointestinal Bleeding (GI Bleed)

See GI Bleed (Gastrointestinal Bleeding)

Gastrointestinal Hemorrhage

See GI Bleed (Gastrointestinal Bleeding)

Gastrointestinal Surgery

Risk for **Injury**: Risk factor: inadvertent insertion of nasogastric tube through gastric incision line

Risk for ineffective gastrointestinal tissue **Perfusion** (See **Perfusion**, tissue, gastrointestinal, ineffective, risk for, Section III)

See Abdominal Surgery

Gastroschisis/Omphalocele

Ineffective **Airway** clearance r/t complications of anesthetic effects

Impaired **Gas** exchange r/t effects of anesthesia, subsequent atelectasis

Grieving r/t threatened loss of infant, loss of perfect birth or infant because of serious medical condition

Risk for deficient **Fluid** volume: Risk factors: inability to feed because of condition, subsequent electrolyte imbalance

Risk for **Infection**: Risk factor: disrupted skin integrity with exposure of abdominal contents

Risk for **Injury**: Risk factors: disrupted skin integrity, ineffective protection

Gastrostomy

Risk for impaired **Skin** integrity: Risk factor: presence of gastric contents on skin

See Tube Feeding

Genital Herpes

See Herpes Simplex II

Genital Warts

See STD (Sexually Transmitted Disease)

Gestational Diabetes (Diabetes in Pregnancy)

Anxiety r/t threat to self and/or fetus

Ineffective **Health** maintenance: maternal r/t deficient knowledge regarding care of diabetic condition in pregnancy

Impaired **Nutrition**: less than body requirements r/t decreased insulin production and glucose uptake in cells

Impaired **Nutrition**: more than body requirements: fetal r/t excessive glucose uptake

Powerlessness r/t lack of control over outcome of pregnancy

Risk for delayed **Development**: fetal: Risk factor: endocrine disorder of mother

Risk for disproportionate **Growth**: fetal: Risk factor: endocrine disorder of mother

Risk for disturbed **Maternal/Fetal** dyad: Risk factor: impaired glucose metabolism

Risk for impaired **Tissue** integrity: fetal: Risk factors: macrosomia, congenital defects, birth injury

Risk for impaired **Tissue** integrity: maternal: Risk factor: delivery of large infant

See Diabetes Mellitus

GI Bleed (Gastrointestinal Bleeding)

Fatigue r/t loss of circulating blood volume, decreased ability to transport oxygen

Fear r/t threat to well-being, potential death

Deficient **Fluid** volume r/t gastrointestinal bleeding

Imbalanced **Nutrition**: less than body requirements r/t nausea, vomiting

Acute **Pain** r/t irritated mucosa from acid secretion

Risk for ineffective **Coping**: Risk factors: personal vulnerability in crisis, bleeding, hospitalization

Gingivitis

Impaired **Dentition** r/t ineffective oral hygiene, barriers to self-care

Impaired **Oral** mucous membrane r/t ineffective oral hygiene

Glaucoma

Deficient **Knowledge** r/t treatment and self-care for disease

Disturbed **Sensory** perception: visual r/t increased intraocular pressure

See Vision Impairment

Glomerulonephritis

Excess **Fluid** volume r/t renal impairment

Ineffective **Health** maintenance r/t deficient knowledge regarding care of disease

Imbalanced **Nutrition**: less than body requirements r/t anorexia, restrictive diet

Acute **Pain** r/t edema of kidney

Gonorrhea

Ineffective **Health** maintenance r/t deficient knowledge regarding treatment and prevention of disease

Acute **Pain** r/t inflammation of reproductive organs

Risk for **Infection**: Risk factor: spread of organism throughout reproductive organs

See STD (Sexually Transmitted Disease)

Gout

Ineffective **Health** maintenance r/t deficient knowledge regarding medications and home care

Impaired physical **Mobility** r/t musculoskeletal impairment

Chronic **Pain** r/t inflammation of affected joint

Grand Mal Seizure

See Seizure Disorders, Adult; Seizure Disorders, Childhood

Grandiosity

Defensive **Coping** r/t inaccurate perception of self and abilities

Grandparents Raising Grandchildren

Anxiety r/t change in role status

Decisional **Conflict** r/t support system deficit

Parental role **Conflict** r/t change in parental role

Compromised family **Coping** r/t family role changes

Interrupted **Family** processes r/t family roles shift

Ineffective **Role** performance r/t role transition

Ineffective family **Therapeutic** regimen management r/t excessive demands on individual or family

Risk for impaired **Parenting**: Risk factor: role strain

Risk for **Powerlessness**: Risk factors: role strain, situational crisis, aging

Risk for **Spiritual** distress: Risk factor: life change

Readiness for enhanced **Parenting**: physical and emotional needs of children are met

Graves' Disease

See Hyperthyroidism

Grieving

Grieving r/t anticipated or actual significant loss, change in life status, style, or function

Grieving, Complicated

Complicated **Grieving** r/t expected or sudden death of a significant other, emotional instability, lack of social support

Risk for complicated **Grieving**: Risk factors: death of a significant other, emotional instability, lack of social support

Groom Self (Inability to)

Dressing **Self-Care** deficit (See **Self-Care** deficit, dressing, Section III)

Growth and Development Lag

Delayed **Growth** and development (See **Growth** and development, delayed, Section III)

Risk for disproportionate **Growth** (See **Growth**, disproportionate, risk for, Section III)

See Developmental Concerns

Guillain-Barré Syndrome

Impaired spontaneous **Ventilation** r/t weak respiratory muscles

See Neurologic Disorders

Guilt

Grieving r/t potential loss of significant person, animal, prized material possession, change in life role

Impaired individual **Resilience** (See **Resilience**, individual, impaired, Section III)

Situational low **Self-Esteem** r/t unmet expectations of self

Chronic **Sorrow** r/t unresolved grieving

Risk for complicated **Grieving**: Risk factors: actual loss of significant person, animal, prized material possession, change in life role

Risk for **Post-Trauma** syndrome: Risk factor: exaggerated sense of responsibility for traumatic event

Readiness for enhanced **Spiritual** well-being: desire to be in harmony with self, others, higher power or God

H

H1N1

See Influenza

Hair Loss

Disturbed **Body** image r/t psychological reaction to loss of hair

Imbalanced **Nutrition**: less than body requirements r/t inability to ingest food because of biological, psychological, economic factors

Halitosis

Impaired **Dentition** r/t ineffective oral hygiene

Impaired **Oral** mucous membrane r/t ineffective oral hygiene

Hallucinations

Anxiety r/t threat to self-concept

Acute **Confusion** r/t alcohol abuse, delirium, dementia, mental illness, drug abuse

Ineffective **Coping** r/t distortion and insecurity of life events

Adult **Failure** to thrive r/t altered mental status

Risk for **Self-Mutilation**: Risk factor: command hallucinations

Risk for other-directed **Violence**: Risk factors: catatonic excitement, manic excitement, rage or panic reactions, response to violent internal stimuli

Risk for self-directed **Violence**: Risk factors: catatonic excitement, manic excitement, rage or panic reactions, response to violent internal stimuli

Head Injury

Ineffective **Breathing** pattern r/t pressure damage to breathing center in brainstem

Acute **Confusion** r/t brain injury

Decreased **Intracranial** adaptive capacity r/t brain injury

Disturbed **Sensory** perception: specify r/t pressure damage to sensory centers in brain

Risk for ineffective cerebral tissue **Perfusion**: Risk factors: effects of increased intracranial pressure, trauma to brain

See Neurologic Disorders

Headache

Disturbed **Energy** field r/t disharmony

Acute **Pain** r/t lack of knowledge of pain control techniques or methods to prevent headaches

Ineffective self **Health** management r/t lack of knowledge, identification, elimination of aggravating factors

Health Maintenance Problems

Ineffective **Health** maintenance (See **Health** maintenance, ineffective, Section III)

Health-Seeking Person

Readiness for enhanced **Self Health** management (See **Self Health** management, readiness for enhanced, Section III)

Hearing Impairment

Impaired verbal **Communication** r/t inability to hear own voice

Disturbed **Sensory** perception: auditory r/t altered state of auditory system

Social isolation r/t difficulty with communication

Heart Attack

See MI (Myocardial Infarction)

Heart Failure

See CHF (Congestive Heart Failure)

Heart Surgery

See Coronary Artery Bypass Grafting (CABG)

Heartburn

Ineffective **Health** maintenance r/t deficient knowledge regarding information about factors that cause esophageal reflex

Nausea r/t gastrointestinal irritation

Acute **Pain**: heartburn r/t gastroesophageal reflux

Risk for imbalanced **Nutrition**: less than body requirements: Risk factor: pain after eating

Heat Stroke

Deficient **Fluid** volume r/t profuse diaphoresis

Hyperthermia r/t vigorous activity, hot environment

H

Hematemesis

See GI Bleed (Gastrointestinal Bleeding)

Hematuria

See Kidney Stone; UTI (Urinary Tract Infection)

Hemianopia

Anxiety r/t change in vision

Unilateral **Neglect** r/t effects of disturbed perceptual abilities

Disturbed **Sensory** perception: visual r/t altered sensory reception, transmission, integration

Risk for **Injury**: Risk factor: disturbed sensory perception

Hemiplegia

Anxiety r/t change in health status

Disturbed **Body** image r/t functional loss of one side of body

Impaired physical **Mobility** r/t loss of neurological control of involved extremities

Unilateral **Neglect** r/t effects of disturbed perceptual abilities

Self-Care deficit: specify: r/t neuromuscular impairment

Impaired **Transfer** ability r/t partial paralysis

Impaired **Walking** r/t loss of neurological control of involved extremities

Risk for **Injury**: Risk factor: impaired mobility

Risk for impaired **Skin** integrity: Risk factors: alteration in sensation, immobility

See CVA (Cerebrovascular Accident)

Hemodialysis

Ineffective **Coping** r/t situational crisis

Interrupted **Family** processes r/t changes in role responsibilities as a result of therapy regimen

Excess **Fluid** volume r/t renal disease with minimal urine output

Ineffective **Health** maintenance r/t deficient knowledge regarding hemodialysis procedure, restrictions, blood access care

Noncompliance: dietary restrictions r/t denial of chronic illness

Powerlessness r/t treatment regimen

Risk for **Caregiver** role strain: Risk factor: complexity of care receiver treatment

Risk for deficient **Fluid** volume: Risk factor: excessive removal of fluid during dialysis

Risk for **Infection**: Risk factors: exposure to blood products, risk for developing hepatitis B or C

Risk for **Injury**: clotting of blood access: Risk factor: abnormal surface for blood flow

See Renal Failure; Renal Failure, Acute/Chronic, Child

Hemodynamic Monitoring

Risk for **Infection**: Risk factor: invasive procedure

Risk for **Injury**: Risk factors: inadvertent wedging of catheter, dislodgement of catheter, disconnection of catheter with embolism

Hemolytic Uremic Syndrome

Deficient **Fluid** volume r/t vomiting, diarrhea

Nausea r/t effects of uremia

Risk for **Injury**: Risk factors: decreased platelet count, seizure activity

Risk for impaired **Skin** integrity: Risk factor: diarrhea

See Hospitalized Child; Renal Failure, Acute/Chronic, Child

Hemophilia

Fear r/t high risk for AIDS infection from contaminated blood products

Ineffective **Health** maintenance r/t knowledge and skill acquisition regarding home administration of intravenous clotting factors, protection from injury

Impaired physical **Mobility** r/t pain from acute bleeds, imposed activity restrictions

Acute **Pain** r/t bleeding into body tissues

Risk for **Bleeding**: Risk factors: deficient clotting factors, child's developmental level, age-appropriate play, inappropriate use of toys or sports equipment

See Child with Chronic Condition; Hospitalized Child; Maturational Issues, Adolescent

Hemoptysis

Fear r/t serious threat to well-being

Risk for ineffective **Airway** clearance: Risk factor: obstruction of airway with blood and mucus

Risk for deficient **Fluid** volume: Risk factor: excessive loss of blood

Hemorrhage

Fear r/t threat to well-being

Deficient **Fluid** volume r/t massive blood loss

See cause of Hemorrhage; Hypovolemic Shock

Hemorrhoidectomy

Anxiety r/t embarrassment, need for privacy

Constipation r/t fear of pain with defecation

Ineffective **Health** maintenance r/t deficient knowledge regarding pain relief, use of stool softeners, dietary changes

Acute **Pain** r/t surgical procedure

Urinary retention r/t pain, anesthetic effect

Risk for **Bleeding**: Risk factors: inadequate clotting, trauma from surgery

Hemorrhoids

Impaired **Comfort** r/t itching in rectal area

Constipation r/t painful defecation, poor bowel habits

Ineffective **Health** maintenance r/t deficient knowledge regarding care of condition

Hemothorax

Deficient **Fluid** volume r/t blood in pleural space

See Pneumothorax

Hepatitis

Activity intolerance r/t weakness or fatigue caused by infection

Deficient **Diversional** activity r/t isolation

Fatigue r/t infectious process, altered body chemistry

Ineffective **Health** maintenance r/t deficient knowledge regarding disease process and home management

Imbalanced **Nutrition**: less than body requirements r/t anorexia, impaired use of proteins and carbohydrates

Acute **Pain** r/t edema of liver, bile irritating skin

Social isolation r/t treatment-imposed isolation

Risk for deficient **Fluid** volume: Risk factor: excessive loss of fluids from vomiting and diarrhea

Hernia

See Hiatal Hernia; Inguinal Hernia Repair

Herniated Disk

See Low Back Pain

Herniorrhaphy

See Inguinal Hernia Repair

Herpes in Pregnancy

Fear r/t threat to fetus, impending surgery

Situational low **Self-Esteem** r/t threat to fetus as a result of disease process

Risk for **Infection**: Risk factors: transplacental transfer during primary herpes, exposure to active herpes during birth process

See Herpes Simplex II

Herpes Simplex I

Impaired **Oral** mucous membrane r/t inflammatory changes in mouth

Herpes Simplex II

Ineffective **Health** maintenance r/t deficient knowledge regarding treatment, prevention, spread of disease

Acute **Pain** r/t active herpes lesion

Situational low **Self-Esteem** r/t expressions of shame or guilt

Sexual dysfunction r/t disease process

Impaired **Tissue** integrity r/t active herpes lesion

Impaired **Urinary** elimination r/t pain with urination

Herpes Zoster

See Shingles

HHNC (Hyperosmolar Hyperglycemic Nonketotic Coma)

See Hyperosmolar Hyperglycemic Nonketotic Coma (HHNC)

Hiatal Hernia

Ineffective **Health** maintenance r/t deficient knowledge regarding care of disease

Nausea r/t effects of gastric contents in esophagus

Imbalanced **Nutrition**: less than body requirements r/t pain after eating

Acute **Pain** r/t gastroesophageal reflux

Hip Fracture

Acute **Confusion** r/t sensory overload, sensory deprivation, medication side effects

Constipation r/t immobility, opioids, anesthesia

Fear r/t outcome of treatment, future mobility, present helplessness

Impaired physical **Mobility** r/t surgical incision, temporary absence of weight bearing

Acute **Pain** r/t injury, surgical procedure

Powerlessness r/t health care environment

Self-Care deficit: specify r/t musculoskeletal impairment

Impaired **Transfer** ability r/t immobilization of hip

Impaired **Walking** r/t temporary absence of weight bearing

Risk for **Bleeding**: Risk factors: postoperative complication, surgical blood loss

Risk for **Infection**: Risk factor: invasive procedure

Risk for **Injury**: Risk factors: dislodged prosthesis, unsteadiness when ambulating

Risk for perioperative positioning **Injury**: Risk factors: immobilization, muscle weakness, emaciation

Risk for impaired **Skin** integrity: Risk factor: immobility

Hip Replacement

See Total Joint Replacement (Total Hip/Total Knee/Shoulder)

Hirschsprung's Disease

Constipation: bowel obstruction r/t inhibited peristalsis as a result of congenital absence of parasympathetic ganglion cells in distal colon

Grieving r/t loss of perfect child, birth of child with congenital defect even though child expected to be normal within 2 years

Ineffective **Health** maintenance r/t parental deficient knowledge regarding temporary stoma care, dietary management, treatment for constipation or diarrhea

Imbalanced **Nutrition**: less than body requirements r/t anorexia, pain from distended colon

Acute **Pain** r/t distended colon, incisional postoperative pain

Impaired **Skin** integrity r/t stoma, potential skin care problems associated with stoma

See Hospitalized Child

Hirsutism

Disturbed **Body** image r/t excessive hair

Hitting Behavior

Acute **Confusion** r/t dementia, alcohol abuse, drug abuse, delirium

Risk for other-directed **Violence** (See **Violence**, other-directed, risk for, Section III)

HIV (Human Immunodeficiency Virus)

Fear r/t possible death

Ineffective **Protection** r/t depressed immune system

See AIDS (Acquired Immune Deficiency Syndrome)

Hodgkin's Disease

See Anemia; Cancer; Chemotherapy

Home Maintenance Problems

Impaired **Home** maintenance (See **Home** maintenance, impaired, Section III)

Homelessness

Impaired **Home** maintenance r/t impaired cognitive or emotional functioning, inadequate support system, insufficient finances

Self **Neglect** r/t mental illness, substance abuse, cognitive impairment

Powerlessness r/t interpersonal interactions

Risk for **Trauma**: Risk factor: being in high-crime neighborhood

Hope

Readiness for enhanced **Hope** (See **Hope**, readiness for enhanced, Section III)

Hopelessness

Hopelessness (See **Hopelessness**, Section III)

Hospitalized Child

Activity intolerance r/t fatigue associated with acute illness

Anxiety: separation (child) r/t familiar surroundings and separation from family and friends

Compromised family **Coping** r/t possible prolonged hospitalization that exhausts supportive capacity of significant people

Ineffective **Coping**: parent r/t possible guilt regarding hospitalization of child, parental inadequacies

Deficient **Diversional** activity r/t immobility, monotonous environment, frequent or lengthy treatments, reluctance to participate, therapeutic isolation, separation from peers

Interrupted **Family** processes r/t situational crisis of illness, disease, hospitalization

Fear r/t deficient knowledge or maturational level with fear of unknown, mutilation, painful procedures, surgery

Delayed **Growth** and development r/t regression or lack of progression toward developmental milestones as a result of frequent or prolonged hospitalization, inadequate or inappropriate stimulation, cerebral insult, chronic illness, effects of physical disability, prescribed dependence

Hopelessness: child r/t prolonged activity restriction, uncertain prognosis

Insomnia: child or parent r/t 24-hour care needs of hospitalization

Acute **Pain** r/t treatments, diagnostic or therapeutic procedures

Powerlessness: child r/t health care environment, illness-related regimen

Risk for impaired **Attachment**: Risk factor: separation

Risk for delayed **Growth** and development: regression: Risk factors: disruption of normal routine, unfamiliar environment or caregivers, developmental vulnerability of young children

Risk for **Injury**: Risk factors: unfamiliar environment, developmental age, lack of parental knowledge regarding safety (e.g., side rails, IV site/pole)

Risk for imbalanced **Nutrition**: less than body requirements: Risk factors: anorexia, absence of familiar foods, cultural preferences

Readiness for enhanced family **Coping**: impact of crisis on family values, priorities, goals, relationships in family

See Child with Chronic Condition

Hostile Behavior

Risk for other-directed **Violence**: Risk factor: antisocial personality disorder

HTN (Hypertension)

Ineffective self **Health** management (See **Health** management, self, ineffective, Section III)

Noncompliance r/t side effects of treatments, lack of understanding regarding importance of controlling hypertension

Imbalanced **Nutrition**: more than body requirements r/t lack of knowledge of relationship between diet and disease process

Readiness for enhanced **Self Health** management (See **Self Health** management, readiness for enhanced, Section III)

Human Immunodeficiency Virus (HIV)

See AIDS (Acquired Immune Deficiency Syndrome); HIV (Human Immunodeficiency Virus)

Humiliating Experience

Risk for compromised human **Dignity** (See **Dignity**, human, compromised, risk for, Section III)

Huntington's Disease

Decisional **Conflict** r/t whether to have children

See Neurologic Disorders

Hydrocele

Acute **Pain** r/t severely enlarged hydrocele

Ineffective **Sexuality** pattern r/t recent surgery on area of scrotum

Hydrocephalus

Decisional **Conflict** r/t unclear or conflicting values regarding selection of treatment modality

Interrupted **Family** processes r/t situational crisis

Delayed **Growth** and development r/t sequelae of increased intracranial pressure

Imbalanced **Nutrition**: less than body requirements r/t inadequate intake as a result of anorexia, nausea, vomiting, feeding difficulties

Impaired **Skin** integrity r/t impaired physical mobility, mechanical irritation

Risk for delayed **Development**: Risk factor: sequelae of increased intracranial pressure

Risk for disproportionate **Growth**: Risk factor: sequelae of increased intracranial pressure

Risk for **Infection**: Risk factor: sequelae of invasive procedure (shunt placement)

Risk for ineffective cerebral tissue **Perfusion**: Risk factors: interrupted flow, hypervolemia of cerebral ventricles

See Normal Pressure Hydrocephalous (NPH); Child with Chronic Condition; Hospitalized Child; Mental Retardation (if appropriate); Premature Infant (Child); Premature Infant (Parent)

Hygiene, Inability to Provide Own

Adult **Failure** to thrive r/t depression, apathy as evidenced by inability to perform self-care

Self **Neglect** (See **Neglect**, self, Section III)

Self-Care deficit: **bathing** (See **Self-care** deficit, bathing, Section III)

Hyperactive Syndrome

Decisional **Conflict** r/t multiple or divergent sources of information regarding education, nutrition, medication regimens; willingness to change own food habits; limited resources

Parental role **Conflict**: when siblings present r/t increased attention toward hyperactive child

Compromised family **Coping** r/t unsuccessful strategies to control excessive activity, behaviors, frustration, anger

Ineffective **Role** performance: parent r/t stressors associated with dealing with hyperactive child, perceived or projected blame for causes of child's behavior, unmet needs for support or care, lack of energy to provide for those needs

Chronic low **Self-Esteem** r/t inability to achieve socially acceptable behaviors; frustration; frequent reprimands, punishment, or scolding for uncontrolled activity and behaviors; mood fluctuations and restlessness; inability to succeed academically; lack of peer support

Impaired **Social** interaction r/t impulsive and overactive behaviors, concomitant emotional difficulties, distractibility and excitability

Risk for delayed **Development**: Risk factor: behavior disorders

Risk for impaired **Parenting**: Risk factor: disruptive or uncontrollable behaviors of child

Risk for other-directed **Violence**: parent or child: Risk factors: frustration with disruptive behavior, anger, unsuccessful relationships

Hyperalimentation

See TPN (Total Parenteral Nutrition)

Hyperbilirubinemia

Anxiety: parent r/t threat to infant, unknown future

Parental role **Conflict** r/t interruption of family life because of care regimen

Neonatal **Jaundice** r/t abnormal breakdown of red blood cells following birth

Imbalanced **Nutrition**: less than body requirements (infant) r/t disinterest in feeding because of jaundice-related lethargy

Disturbed **Sensory** perception: visual (infant) r/t use of eye patches for protection of eyes during phototherapy

Risk for disproportionate **Growth**: infant: Risk factor: disinterest in feeding because of jaundice-related lethargy

Risk for **Imbalanced** body temperature: infant: Risk factor: phototherapy

Risk for **Injury**: infant: Risk factors: kernicterus, phototherapy lights

Hypercalcemia

Decreased **Cardiac** output r/t bradydysrhythmia

Impaired physical **Mobility** r/t decreased tone in smooth and striated muscle

Imbalanced **Nutrition**: less than body requirements r/t gastrointestinal manifestations of hypercalcemia (nausea, anorexia, ileus)

Risk for **Disuse** syndrome: Risk factor: comatose state impairing mobility

Hypercapnia

Fear r/t difficulty breathing

Impaired **Gas** exchange r/t ventilation perfusion imbalance

Hyperemesis Gravidarum

Anxiety r/t threat to self and infant, hospitalization

Deficient **Fluid** volume r/t vomiting

Impaired **Home** maintenance r/t chronic nausea, inability to function

Nausea r/t hormonal changes of pregnancy

Imbalanced **Nutrition**: less than body requirements r/t vomiting

Powerlessness r/t health care regimen

Social isolation r/t hospitalization

Hyperglycemia

Ineffective self **Health** management r/t complexity of therapeutic regimen, decisional conflicts, economic difficulties, unsupportive family, insufficient cues to action, deficient knowledge, mistrust, lack of acknowledgment of seriousness of condition

Risk for unstable blood **Glucose** level (See **Glucose** level, blood, unstable, risk for, Section III)

See Diabetes Mellitus

Hyperkalemia

Risk for **Activity** intolerance: Risk factor: muscle weakness

Risk for excess **Fluid** volume: Risk factor: untreated renal failure

Risk for decreased cardiac tissue **Perfusion**: Risk factor: abnormal electrolyte level affecting heart electrical conduction

Hypernatremia

Risk for deficient **Fluid** volume: Risk factors: abnormal water loss, inadequate water intake

Hyperosmolar Hyperglycemic Nonketotic Coma (HHNC)

Acute **Confusion** r/t dehydration, electrolyte imbalance

Deficient **Fluid** volume r/t polyuria, inadequate fluid intake

Risk for **Electrolyte** imbalance r/t effect of metabolic state on kidney function

Risk for **Injury**: seizures: Risk factors: hyperosmolar state, electrolyte imbalance

See Diabetes Mellitus; Diabetes Mellitus, Juvenile

Hyperphosphatemia

Deficient **Knowledge** r/t dietary changes needed to control phosphate levels

See Renal Failure

Hypersensitivity to Slight Criticism

Defensive **Coping** r/t situational crisis, psychological impairment, substance abuse

Hypertension (HTN)

See HTN (Hypertension)

Hyperthermia

Hyperthermia (See **Hyperthermia**, Section III)

Hyperthyroidism

Activity intolerance r/t increased oxygen demands from increased metabolic rate

Anxiety r/t increased stimulation, loss of control

Diarrhea r/t increased gastric motility

Ineffective **Health** maintenance r/t deficient knowledge regarding medications, methods of coping with stress

Insomnia r/t anxiety, excessive sympathetic discharge

Imbalanced **Nutrition**: less than body requirements r/t increased metabolic rate, increased gastrointestinal activity

Risk for **Injury**: eye damage: Risk factor: protruding eyes without sufficient lubrications

Hyperventilation

Ineffective **Breathing** pattern r/t anxiety, acid-base imbalance

Hypocalcemia

Activity intolerance r/t neuromuscular irritability

Ineffective **Breathing** pattern r/t laryngospasm

Imbalanced **Nutrition**: less than body requirements r/t effects of vitamin D deficiency, renal failure, malabsorption, laxative use

Hypoglycemia

Acute **Confusion** r/t insufficient blood glucose to brain

Ineffective self **Health** management r/t deficient knowledge regarding disease process, self-care

Imbalanced **Nutrition**: less than body requirements r/t imbalance of glucose and insulin level

Risk for unstable blood **Glucose** level (See **Glucose** level, blood, unstable, risk for, Section III)

See Diabetes Mellitus; Diabetes Mellitus, Juvenile

Hypokalemia

Activity intolerance r/t muscle weakness

Risk for decreased cardiac tissue **Perfusion**: Risk factor: possible dysrhythmia from electrolyte imbalance

Hypomagnesemia

Imbalanced **Nutrition**: **less than body requirements** r/t deficient knowledge of nutrition, alcoholism

See Alcoholism

Hypomania

Insomnia r/t psychological stimulus

See Manic Disorder, Bipolar I

Hyponatremia

Acute **Confusion** r/t electrolyte imbalance

Excess **Fluid** volume r/t excessive intake of hypotonic fluids

Risk for **Injury**: Risk factors: seizures, new onset of confusion

Hypoplastic Left Lung

See Congenital Heart Disease/Cardiac Anomalies

Hypotension

Decreased **Cardiac** output r/t decreased preload, decreased contractility

Risk for deficient **Fluid** volume: Risk factor: excessive fluid loss

Risk for ineffective cerebral tissue **Perfusion**: Risk factors: hypovolemia, decreased contractility, decreased afterload

Risk for ineffective gastrointestinal tissue **Perfusion** (See **Perfusion**, tissue, gastrointestinal, ineffective, risk for, Section III)

Risk for ineffective renal **Perfusion**: Risk factor: prolonged ischemia of kidneys

Risk for **Shock** (See **Shock**, risk for, Section III)

See cause of Hypotension

Hypothermia

Hypothermia (See **Hypothermia**, Section III)

Hypothyroidism

Activity intolerance r/t muscular stiffness, shortness of breath on exertion

Constipation r/t decreased gastric motility

Impaired **Gas** exchange r/t possible respiratory depression

Ineffective **Health** maintenance r/t deficient knowledge regarding disease process and self-care

Imbalanced **Nutrition**: more than body requirements r/t decreased metabolic process

Impaired **Skin** integrity r/t edema, dry or scaly skin

Hypovolemic Shock

See Shock, Hypovolemic

Hypoxia

Acute **Confusion** rv/t decreased oxygen supply to brain

Fear r/t breathlessness

Impaired **Gas** exchange r/t altered oxygen supply, inability to transport oxygen

Risk for **Shock** (See **Shock**, risk for, Section III)

Hysterectomy

Constipation r/t opioids, anesthesia, bowel manipulation during surgery

Ineffective **Coping** r/t situational crisis of surgery

Grieving r/t change in body image, loss of reproductive status

Ineffective **Health** maintenance r/t deficient knowledge regarding precautions and self-care after surgery

Acute **Pain** r/t surgical injury

Ineffective peripheral tissue **Perfusion** r/t deficient knowledge of aggravating factors (immobility)

Sexual dysfunction r/t disturbance in self-concept

Urinary retention r/t edema in area, anesthesia, opioids, pain

Risk for **Bleeding**: Risk factor: surgical procedure

Risk for **Constipation**: Risk factors: opioids, anesthesia, bowel manipulation during surgery

Risk for urge urinary **Incontinence**: Risk factors: edema in area, anesthesia, opioids, pain

See Surgery, Perioperative; Surgery, Preoperative; Surgery, Postoperative

---

I

IBS (Irritable Bowel Syndrome)

Constipation r/t low-residue diet, stress

Diarrhea r/t increased motility of intestines associated with stress

Ineffective **Health** maintenance r/t deficient knowledge regarding self-care with IBS

Ineffective self **Health** management r/t deficient knowledge, powerlessness

Chronic **Pain** r/t spasms, increased motility of bowel

Readiness for enhanced **Self Health** management: expressed desire to manage illness and prevent onset of symptoms

ICD (Implantable Cardioverter/Defibrillator)

Decreased **Cardiac** output r/t possible dysrhythmia

Ineffective **Health** maintenance r/t deficient knowledge regarding self-care, action of internal cardiac defibrillator

IDDM (Insulin-Dependent Diabetes)

See Diabetes Mellitus

Identity Disturbance/Problems

Disturbed personal **Identity** r/t situational crisis, psychological impairment, chronic illness, pain

Idiopathic Thrombocytopenic Purpura (ITP)

See ITP (Idiopathic Thrombocytopenic Purpura)

Ileal Conduit

Disturbed **Body** image r/t presence of stoma

Ineffective self **Health** management r/t new skills required to care for appliance and self

Deficient **Knowledge** r/t care of stoma

Ineffective **Sexuality** pattern r/t altered body function and structure

Social isolation r/t alteration in physical appearance, fear of accidental spill of ostomy contents

Risk for latex **Allergy** response: Risk factor: repeated exposures to latex associated with treatment and management of disease

Risk for impaired **Skin** integrity: Risk factor: difficulty obtaining tight seal of appliance

Ileostomy

Disturbed **Body** image r/t presence of stoma

Diarrhea r/t dietary changes, alteration in intestinal motility

Ineffective self **Health** management r/t new skills required to care for appliance and self

Deficient **Knowledge** r/t limited practice of stoma care, dietary modifications

Ineffective **Sexuality** pattern r/t altered body function and structure

Social isolation r/t alteration in physical appearance, fear of accidental spill of ostomy contents

Risk for impaired **Skin** integrity: Risk factors: difficulty obtaining tight seal of appliance, caustic drainage

Ileus

Deficient **Fluid** volume r/t loss of fluids from vomiting, fluids trapped in bowel

Dysfunctional gastrointestinal **Motility** r/t effects of surgery, decreased perfusion of intestines, medication effect

Nausea r/t gastrointestinal irritation

Acute **Pain** r/t pressure, abdominal distention

Immobility

Ineffective **Breathing** pattern r/t inability to deep breathe in supine position

Acute **Confusion**: elderly r/t sensory deprivation from immobility

Constipation r/t immobility

Adult **Failure** to thrive r/t limited physical mobility

Impaired physical **Mobility** r/t medically imposed bed rest

Ineffective peripheral tissue **Perfusion** r/t interruption of venous flow

Powerlessness r/t forced immobility from health care environment

Impaired **Walking** r/t limited physical mobility

Risk for **Disuse** syndrome: Risk factor: immobilization

Risk for impaired **Skin** integrity: Risk factors: pressure on immobile parts, shearing forces when moved

Immunization

Readiness for enhanced **Immunization** status (See **Immunization** status, readiness for enhanced, Section III)

Immunosuppression

Risk for **Infection**: Risk factor: immunosuppression

Impaction of Stool

Constipation r/t decreased fluid intake, less than adequate amounts of fiber and bulk-forming foods in diet, medication effect, or immobility

Imperforate Anus

Anxiety r/t ability to care for newborn

Deficient **Knowledge** r/t home care for newborn

Impaired **Skin** integrity r/t pruritus

Impetigo

Ineffective **Health** maintenance r/t parental deficient knowledge regarding care of impetigo

See Communicable Diseases, Childhood

Implantable Cardioverter/ Defibrillator (ICD)

See ICD (Implantable Cardioverter/Defibrillator)

Impotence

Situational low **Self-Esteem** r/t physiological crisis, inability to practice usual sexual activity

Sexual dysfunction r/t altered body function

Readiness for enhanced **Knowledge**: treatment information for erectile dysfunction

See Erectile Dysfunction (ED)

Inactivity

Activity intolerance r/t imbalance between oxygen supply and demand, sedentary lifestyle, weakness, immobility

Impaired physical **Mobility** r/t intolerance to activity, decreased strength and endurance, depression, severe anxiety, musculoskeletal impairment, perceptual or cognitive impairment, neuromuscular impairment, pain, discomfort

Risk for **Constipation**: Risk factor: insufficient physical activity

Incompetent Cervix

See Premature Dilation of the Cervix (Incompetent Cervix)

Incontinence of Stool

Disturbed **Body** image r/t inability to control elimination of stool

Bowel incontinence r/t decreased awareness of need to defecate, loss of sphincter control

Toileting **Self-Care** deficit r/t toileting needs

Situational low **Self-Esteem** r/t inability to control elimination of stool

Risk for impaired **Skin** integrity: Risk factor: presence of stool

Incontinence of Urine

Functional urinary **Incontinence** r/t altered environment; sensory, cognitive, or mobility deficits

Overflow urinary **Incontinence** r/t relaxation of pelvic muscles and changes in urinary structures

Reflex urinary **Incontinence** r/t neurological impairment

Stress urinary **Incontinence** (See **Incontinence**, urinary, stress, Section III)

Urge urinary **Incontinence** (See **Incontinence**, urinary, urge, Section III)

Toileting **Self-Care** deficit r/t neuromuscular dysfunction

Situational low **Self-Esteem** r/t inability to control passage of urine

Risk for impaired **Skin** integrity: Risk factor: presence of urine

Indigestion

Nausea r/t gastrointestinal irritation

Imbalanced **Nutrition**: less than body requirements r/t discomfort when eating

Induction of Labor

Anxiety r/t medical interventions

Decisional **Conflict** r/t perceived threat to idealized birth

Ineffective **Coping** r/t situational crisis of medical intervention in birthing process

Acute **Pain** r/t contractions

Situational low **Self-Esteem** r/t inability to carry out normal labor

Risk for **Injury**: maternal and fetal: Risk factors: hypertonic uterus, potential prematurity of newborn

Readiness for enhanced **Family** processes: family support during induction of labor

Infant Apnea

See Premature Infant (Child); Respiratory Conditions of the Neonate; SIDS (Sudden Infant Death Syndrome)

Infant Behavior

Disorganized **Infant** behavior r/t pain, oral/motor problems, feeding intolerance, environmental overstimulation, lack of containment or boundaries, prematurity, invasive or painful procedures

Risk for disorganized **Infant** behavior: Risk factors: pain, oral/motor problems, environmental overstimulation, lack of containment or boundaries

Readiness for enhanced organized **Infant** behavior: stable physiologic measures, use of some self-regulatory measures

Infant Care

Readiness for enhanced **Childbearing** process: a pattern of preparing for, maintaining, and strengthening care of newborn infant

Infant Feeding Pattern, Ineffective

Ineffective infant **Feeding** pattern r/t prematurity, neurological impairment or delay, oral hypersensitivity, prolonged nothing-by-mouth order

Infant of Diabetic Mother

Decreased **Cardiac** output r/t cardiomegaly

Deficient **Fluid** volume r/t increased urinary excretion and osmotic diuresis

Delayed **Growth** and development r/t prolonged and severe postnatal hypoglycemia

Imbalanced **Nutrition**: less than body requirements r/t hypotonia, lethargy, poor sucking, postnatal metabolic changes from hyperglycemia to hypoglycemia and hyperinsulinism

Risk for delayed **Development**: Risk factors: prolonged and severe postnatal hypoglycemia

Risk for impaired **Gas** exchange: Risk factors: increased incidence of cardiomegaly, prematurity

Risk for disproportionate **Growth**: Risk factors: prolonged and severe postnatal hypoglycemia

See Premature Infant (Child); Respiratory Conditions of the Neonate

Infant of Substance-Abusing Mother (Fetal Alcohol Syndrome, Crack Baby, Other Drug Withdrawal Infants)

Ineffective **Airway** clearance r/t pooling of secretions from the lack of adequate cough reflex, effects of viral or bacterial lower airway infection as a result of altered protective state

Interrupted **Breastfeeding** r/t use of drugs or alcohol by mother

Diarrhea r/t effects of withdrawal, increased peristalsis from hyperirritability

Ineffective infant **Feeding** pattern r/t uncoordinated or ineffective sucking reflex

Delayed **Growth** and development r/t effects of maternal use of drugs, effects of neurological impairment, decreased attentiveness to environmental stimuli or inadequate stimuli

Insomnia r/t hyperirritability or hypersensitivity to environmental stimuli

Imbalanced **Nutrition**: less than body requirements r/t feeding problems; uncoordinated or ineffective suck and swallow; effects of diarrhea, vomiting, or colic associated with maternal substance abuse

Impaired **Parenting** r/t impaired or absent attachment behaviors, inadequate support systems

Disturbed **Sensory** perception r/t hypersensitivity to environmental stimuli

Risk for delayed **Development**: Risk factor: substance abuse

Risk for disproportionate **Growth**: Risk factor: substance abuse

Risk for **Infection**: skin, meningeal, respiratory: Risk factor: effects of withdrawal

See Cerebral Palsy; Child with Chronic Condition; Crack Baby; Failure to Thrive, Nonorganic; Hospitalized Child; Hyperactive Syndrome; Premature Infant (Child); SIDS (Sudden Infant Death Syndrome)

Infantile Polyarteritis

See Kawasaki Disease

Infantile Spasms

See Seizure Disorders, Childhood

Infection

Hyperthermia r/t increased metabolic rate

Ineffective **Protection** r/t inadequate nutrition, abnormal blood profiles, drug therapies, treatments

Risk for vascular **Trauma**: Risk factors: infusion of antibiotics

Infection, Potential for

Risk for **Infection** (See **Infection**, risk for, Section III)

Infertility

Ineffective self **Health** management r/t deficient knowledge about infertility

Powerlessness r/t infertility

Chronic **Sorrow** r/t inability to conceive a child

Spiritual distress r/t inability to conceive a child

Inflammatory Bowel Disease (Child and Adult)

Ineffective **Coping** r/t repeated episodes of diarrhea

Diarrhea r/t effects of inflammatory changes of the bowel

Deficient **Fluid** volume r/t frequent and loose stools

Imbalanced **Nutrition**: less than body requirements r/t anorexia, decreased absorption of nutrients from gastrointestinal tract

Acute **Pain** r/t abdominal cramping and anal irritation

Impaired **Skin** integrity r/t frequent stools, development of anal fissures

Social isolation r/t diarrhea

See Child with Chronic Condition; Crohn's Disease; Hospitalized Child; Maturational Issues, Adolescent

Influenza

Deficient **Fluid** volume r/t inadequate fluid intake

Ineffective **Health** maintenance r/t deficient knowledge regarding self-care

Ineffective self **Health** management r/t lack of knowledge regarding preventive immunizations

Hyperthermia r/t infectious process

Acute **Pain** r/t inflammatory changes in joints

Readiness for enhanced **Knowledge**: about information to prevent or treat influenza

Inguinal Hernia Repair

Impaired physical **Mobility** r/t pain at surgical site and fear of causing hernia to rupture

Acute **Pain** r/t surgical procedure

Urinary retention r/t possible edema at surgical site

Risk for **Infection**: Risk factor: surgical procedure

Injury

Risk for **Falls**: Risk factors: orthostatic hypotension, impaired physical mobility, diminished mental status

Risk for **Injury**: Risk factor: environmental conditions interacting with client's adaptive and defensive resources

Insomnia

Insomnia (See **Insomnia**, Section III)

I

Insulin Shock

See Hypoglycemia

Intermittent Claudication

Deficient **Knowledge** r/t lack of knowledge of cause and treatment of peripheral vascular diseases

Acute **Pain** r/t decreased circulation to extremities with activity

Ineffective peripheral tissue **Perfusion** r/t interruption of arterial flow

Risk for **Injury**: Risk factor: tissue hypoxia

Readiness for enhanced **Knowledge**: prevention of pain and impaired circulation

See Peripheral Vascular Disease (PVD)

Internal Cardioverter/Defibrillator (ICD)

See ICD (Implantable Cardioverter/Defibrillator)

Internal Fixation

Impaired **Walking** r/t repair of fracture

Risk for **Infection**: Risk factors: traumatized tissue, broken skin

See Fracture

Interstitial Cystitis

Acute **Pain** r/t inflammatory process

Impaired **Urinary** elimination r/t inflammation of bladder

Risk for **Infection**: Risk factor: suppressed inflammatory response

Intervertebral Disk Excision

See Laminectomy

Intestinal Obstruction

See Ileus

Intoxication

Anxiety r/t loss of control of actions

Acute **Confusion** r/t alcohol abuse

Ineffective **Coping** r/t use of mind-altering substances as a means of coping

Impaired **Memory** r/t effects of alcohol on mind

Disturbed **Sensory** perception r/t neurochemical imbalance in brain from substance

Risk for **Aspiration**: Risk factors: diminished mental status, vomiting

Risk for **Falls**: Risk factor: diminished mental status

Risk for other-directed **Violence**: Risk factor: inability to control thoughts and actions

Intraaortic Balloon Counterpulsation

Anxiety r/t device providing cardiovascular assistance

Decreased **Cardiac** output r/t failing heart needing counterpulsation

Compromised family **Coping** r/t seriousness of significant other's medical condition

Impaired physical **Mobility** r/t restriction of movement because of mechanical device

Risk for **Peripheral** neurovascular dysfunction: Risk factors: vascular obstruction of balloon catheter, thrombus formation, emboli, edema

Intracranial Pressure, Increased

Ineffective **Breathing** pattern r/t pressure damage to breathing center in brainstem

Acute **Confusion** r/t increased intracranial pressure

Adult **Failure** to thrive r/t undetected changes from increased intracranial pressure

Decreased **Intracranial** adaptive capacity r/t sustained increase in intracranial pressure

Impaired **Memory** r/t neurological disturbance

Disturbed **Sensory** perception r/t pressure damage to sensory centers in brain

Risk for ineffective cerebral tissue **Perfusion**: Risk factors: body position, cerebral vessel circulation deficits

See cause of Increased Intracranial Pressure

Intrauterine Growth Retardation

Anxiety: maternal r/t threat to fetus

Ineffective **Coping**: maternal r/t situational crisis, threat to fetus

Impaired **Gas** exchange r/t insufficient placental perfusion

Delayed **Growth** and development r/t insufficient supply of oxygen and nutrients

Imbalanced **Nutrition**: less than body requirements r/t insufficient placenta

Situational low **Self-Esteem**: maternal r/t guilt about threat to fetus

Spiritual distress r/t unknown outcome of fetus

Risk for **Powerlessness**: Risk factor: unknown outcome of fetus

Intravenous Therapy

Risk for vascular **Trauma**: Risk factor: infusion of irritating chemicals

Intubation, Endotracheal or Nasogastric

Disturbed **Body** image r/t altered appearance with mechanical devices

Impaired verbal **Communication** r/t endotracheal tube

Imbalanced **Nutrition**: less than body requirements r/t inability to ingest food because of the presence of tubes

Impaired **Oral** mucous membrane r/t presence of tubes

Acute **Pain** r/t presence of tube

Irregular Pulse

See Dysrhythmia

Irritable Bowel Syndrome (IBS)

See IBS (Irritable Bowel Syndrome)

Isolation

Impaired individual **Resilience** (See **Resilience**, individual, impaired, Section III)

Social isolation (See **Social** isolation, Section III)

Itching

Impaired **Comfort** r/t inflammation of skin causing itching

Risk for impaired **Skin** integrity: Risk factor: scratching

ITP (Idiopathic Thrombocytopenic Purpura)

Deficient **Diversional** activity r/t activity restrictions, safety precautions

Ineffective **Protection** r/t decreased platelet count

Risk for **Bleeding**: Risk factors: decreased platelet count, developmental level, age-appropriate play

See Hospitalized Child

J

Jaundice

Neonatal **Jaundice** (See **Jaundice**, neonatal, Section III)

Risk for **Bleeding**: Risk factor: impaired liver function

Risk for impaired **Liver** function: Risk factors: possible viral infection, medication effect

Risk for impaired **Skin** integrity: Risk factors: pruritus, itching

See Cirrhosis; Hepatitis

Jaundice, Neonatal

Neonatal **Jaundice** (See **Jaundice**, neonatal, Section III)

Risk for ineffective gastrointestinal tissue **Perfusion**: Risk factor: liver dysfunction

Readiness for enhanced **Self Health** management: expresses desire to manage treatment: assessment of jaundice when infant is discharged from the hospital, when to call the physician, and possible preventive measures such as frequent breastfeeding

See Hyperbilirubinemia

Jaw Pain and Heart Attacks

See Angina; Chest Pain; MI (Myocardial Infarction)

Jaw Surgery

Deficient **Knowledge** r/t emergency care for wired jaws (e.g., cutting bands and wires), oral care

Imbalanced **Nutrition**: less than body requirements r/t jaws wired closed

Acute **Pain** r/t surgical procedure

Impaired **Swallowing** r/t edema from surgery

Risk for **Aspiration**: Risk factor: wired jaws

Jittery

Anxiety r/t unconscious conflict about essential values and goals, threat to or change in health status

Death **Anxiety** r/t unresolved issues relating to end of life

Risk for **Post-Trauma** syndrome: Risk factors: occupation, survivor's role in event, inadequate social support

Jock Itch

Ineffective self **Health** management r/t prevention and treatment

Impaired **Skin** integrity r/t moisture and irritating or tight-fitting clothing

See Itching

Joint Dislocation

See Dislocation of Joint

Joint Pain

See Arthritis; Bursitis; JRA (Juvenile Rheumatoid Arthritis); Osteoarthritis; Rheumatoid Arthritis

Joint Replacement

Risk for **Peripheral** neurovascular dysfunction: Risk factor: orthopedic surgery

See Total Joint Replacement (Total Hip/Total Knee/Shoulder)

JRA (Juvenile Rheumatoid Arthritis)

Impaired **Comfort** r/t altered health status

Fatigue r/t chronic inflammatory disease

Delayed **Growth** and development r/t effects of physical disability, chronic illness

Impaired physical **Mobility** r/t pain, restricted joint movement

Acute **Pain** r/t swollen or inflamed joints, restricted movement, physical therapy

Self-Care deficit: feeding, bathing, dressing, toileting r/t restricted joint movement, pain

Risk for compromised human **Dignity**: Risk factors: perceived intrusion by clinicians, invasion of privacy

Risk for **Injury**: Risk factors: impaired physical mobility, splints, adaptive devices, increased bleeding potential from antiinflammatory medications

Risk for complicated **Resilience**: Risk factor: chronic condition

Risk for situational low **Self-Esteem**: Risk factor: disturbed body image

Risk for impaired **Skin** integrity: Risk factors: splints, adaptive devices

See Child with Chronic Condition; Hospitalized Child

Juvenile Onset Diabetes

See Diabetes Mellitus, Juvenile

K

Kaposi's Sarcoma

Risk for compromised human **Dignity**: Risk factor: use of undefined medical terms

Risk for complicated **Grieving**: Risk factor: loss of social support

Risk for impaired **Religiosity**: Risk factors: illness/hospitalization, ineffective coping

Risk for compromised **Resilience**: Risk factor: serious illness

See AIDS (Acquired Immune Deficiency Syndrome)

Kawasaki Disease

Anxiety: parental r/t progression of disease, complications of arthritis, and cardiac involvement

Impaired **Comfort** r/t altered health status

Hyperthermia r/t inflammatory disease process

Imbalanced **Nutrition**: less than body requirements r/t impaired oral mucous membranes

Impaired **Oral** mucous membrane r/t inflamed mouth and pharynx; swollen lips that become dry, cracked, fissured

Acute **Pain** r/t enlarged lymph nodes; erythematous skin rash that progresses to desquamation, peeling, denuding of skin

Impaired **Skin** integrity r/t inflammatory skin changes

Risk for imbalanced **Fluid** volume: Risk factor: hypovolemia

Risk for decreased cardiac tissue **Perfusion**: Risk factor: cardiac involvement

See Hospitalized Child

Kegel Exercise

Stress urinary **Incontinence** r/t degenerative change in pelvic muscles

Urge urinary **Incontinence** r/t inflammation of bladder

Risk for urge urinary **Incontinence**: Risk factors: overactive bladder dysfunction; urinary tract infection; dietary risk factors: consumption of caffeine

Readiness for enhanced **Self Health** management: desires information to relieve incontinence

Keloids

Disturbed **Body** image r/t presence of scar tissue at site of a healed skin injury

Readiness for enhanced **Self Health** management: desire to have information to manage condition

Keratoconjunctivitis Sicca (Dry Eye Syndrome)

Risk for **Infection** r/t dry eyes

See Conjunctivitis

Keratoplasty

See Corneal Transplant

Ketoacidosis, Diabetic

Deficient **Fluid** volume r/t excess excretion of urine, nausea, vomiting, increased respiration

Impaired **Memory** r/t fluid and electrolyte imbalance

Noncompliance: diabetic regimen r/t ineffective coping with chronic disease

Imbalanced **Nutrition**: less than body requirements r/t body's inability to use nutrients

Risk for unstable blood **Glucose** level: Risk factor: deficient knowledge of diabetes management (e.g., action plan)

Risk for **Powerlessness**: Risk factor: illness-related regimen

Risk for compromised **Resilience**: Risk factor: complications of disease

See Diabetes Mellitus

Ketoacidosis: Alcoholic

See Alcohol Withdrawal; Alcoholism

Keyhole Heart Surgery

See MIDCAB (Minimally Invasive Direct Coronary Artery Bypass)

Kidney Disease Screening

Readiness for enhanced **Self Health** management: seeks information for screening

Kidney Failure

See Renal Failure

Kidney Stone

Deficient **Knowledge** r/t fluid requirements and dietary restrictions

Overflow urinary **Incontinence** r/t bladder outlet obstruction

Acute **Pain** r/t obstruction from renal calculi

Impaired **Urinary** elimination: urgency and frequency r/t anatomical obstruction, irritation caused by stone

Risk for imbalanced **Fluid** volume: Risk factor: hypovolemia

Risk for **Infection**: Risk factor: obstruction of urinary tract with stasis of urine

Kidney Transplant

Decisional **Conflict** r/t acceptance of donor kidney

Ineffective **Protection** r/t immunosuppressive therapy

Risk for ineffective renal **Perfusion**: Risk factor: complications from transplant procedure

Readiness for enhanced **Decision-Making**: expresses desire to enhance understanding of choices

Readiness for enhanced **Family** processes: adapting to life without dialysis

Readiness for enhanced **Self Health** management: desire to manage the treatment and prevention of complications post transplant

Readiness for enhanced **Spiritual** well-being: heightened coping, living without dialysis

See Nephrectomy; Renal Failure; Renal Transplantation, Donor; Renal Transplantation, Recipient; Surgery, Perioperative Care; Surgery, Postoperative Care; Surgery, Preoperative Care

Kidney Tumor

See Wilms' Tumor

Kissing Disease

See Mononucleosis

Knee Replacement

See Total Joint Replacement (Total Hip/Total Knee/Shoulder)

Knowledge

Readiness for enhanced **Knowledge** (See **Knowledge**, readiness for enhanced, Section III)

Knowledge, Deficient

Ineffective **Health** maintenance r/t lack of or significant alteration in communication skills (written, verbal, and/or gestural)

Deficient **Knowledge** (See **Knowledge**, deficient, Section III)

Kock Pouch

See Continent Ileostomy (Kock Pouch)

Korsakoff's Syndrome

Acute **Confusion** r/t alcohol abuse

Dysfunctional **Family** processes r/t alcoholism as possible cause of syndrome

Impaired **Memory** r/t neurological changes

Self **Neglect** r/t cognitive impairment

Risk for **Falls**: Risk factor: cognitive impairment

Risk for **Injury**: Risk factors: sensory dysfunction, lack of coordination when ambulating

Risk for impaired **Liver** function: Risk factor: substance abuse (alcohol)

Risk for imbalanced **Nutrition**: less than body requirements: Risk factor: lack of adequate balanced intake

L

Labor, Induction of

See Induction of Labor

Labor, Normal

Anxiety r/t fear of the unknown, situational crisis

Impaired **Comfort** r/t labor

Fatigue r/t childbirth

Deficient **Knowledge** r/t lack of preparation for labor

Acute **Pain** r/t uterine contractions, stretching of cervix and birth canal

Impaired **Tissue** integrity r/t passage of infant through birth canal, episiotomy

Risk for deficient **Fluid** volume: Risk factor: excessive loss of blood

Risk for **Infection**: Risk factors: multiple vaginal examinations, tissue trauma, prolonged rupture of membranes

Risk for **Injury**: fetal: Risk factor: hypoxia

Risk for **Post-Trauma** syndrome: Risk factors: trauma or violence associated with labor pains, medical or surgical interventions, history of sexual abuse

Risk for **Powerlessness**: Risk factor: labor process

Readiness for enhanced **Childbearing** process: responds appropriately, is proactive, bonds with infant and uses support systems

Readiness for enhanced family **Coping**: significant other providing support during labor

Readiness for enhanced **Power**: expresses readiness to enhance participation in choices regarding treatment during labor

Readiness for enhanced **Self Health** management: prenatal care and childbirth education birth process, posttrauma

Labyrinthitis

Ineffective self **Health** management r/t delay in seeking treatment for respiratory and ear infections

Risk for **Injury** r/t dizziness

Readiness for enhanced **Self Health** management: management of episodes

See Ménière's Disease

Lacerations

Risk for **Infection**: Risk factor: broken skin

Risk for **Trauma**: Risk factor: children playing with dangerous objects

Readiness for enhanced **Self Health** management: proper care of injury

Lactation

See Breastfeeding, Effective; Breastfeeding, Ineffective; Breastfeeding, Interrupted

Lactic Acidosis

Decreased **Cardiac** output r/t altered heart rate/rhythm, preload, and contractility

Risk for **Electrolyte** imbalance: Risk factor: impaired regulatory mechanism

Risk for decreased cardiac tissue **Perfusion**: Risk factor: hypoxia

See Ketoacidosis, Diabetic

Lactose Intolerance

Readiness for enhanced **Knowledge**: interest in identifying lactose intolerance, treatment, and substitutes for milk products

See Abdominal Distention; Diarrhea

Laminectomy

Anxiety r/t change in health status, surgical procedure

Impaired **Comfort** r/t surgical procedure

Deficient **Knowledge** r/t appropriate postoperative and postdischarge activities

Impaired physical **Mobility** r/t neuromuscular impairment

Acute **Pain** r/t localized inflammation and edema

Disturbed **Sensory** perception: tactile r/t possible edema or nerve injury

Urinary retention r/t competing sensory impulses, effects of opioids or anesthesia

Risk for **Bleeding**: Risk factor: surgery

Risk for **Infection**: Risk factor: invasive procedure

Risk for perioperative positioning **Injury**: Risk factor: prone position

Risk for ineffective cardiac, cerebral, peripheral tissue **Perfusion**: Risk factors: edema, hemorrhage, embolism

See Scoliosis; Surgery, Perioperative; Surgery, Postoperative; Surgery, Preoperative

Language Impairment

See Speech Disorders

Laparoscopic Laser Cholecystectomy

See Cholecystectomy; Laser Surgery

Laparoscopy

Urge urinary **Incontinence** r/t pressure on the bladder from gas

Acute **Pain**: shoulder r/t gas irritating the diaphragm

Risk for ineffective gastrointestinal tissue **Perfusion**: Risk factor: complications from procedure

Laparotomy

See Abdominal Surgery

Large Bowel Resection

See Abdominal Surgery

Laryngectomy

Ineffective **Airway** clearance r/t surgical removal of glottis, decreased humidification of air

Death **Anxiety** r/t unknown results of surgery

Disturbed **Body** image r/t change in body structure and function

Impaired **Comfort** r/t surgery

Impaired verbal **Communication** r/t removal of larynx

Interrupted **Family** processes r/t surgery, serious condition of family member, difficulty communicating

Grieving r/t loss of voice, fear of death

Ineffective self **Health** management r/t deficient knowledge regarding self-care with laryngectomy

Imbalanced **Nutrition**: less than body requirements r/t absence of oral feeding, difficulty swallowing, increased need for fluids

Impaired **Oral** mucous membrane r/t absence of oral feeding

Chronic **Sorrow** r/t change in body image

Impaired **Swallowing** r/t edema, laryngectomy tube

Risk for compromised human **Dignity**: Risk factor: loss of control of body function

Risk for **Electrolyte** imbalance: Risk factor: fluid imbalance

Risk for complicated **Grieving**: Risk factors: loss, major life event

Risk for **Infection**: Risk factors: invasive procedure, surgery

Risk for **Powerlessness**: Risk factors: chronic illness, change in communication

Risk for compromised **Resilience**: Risk factor: change in health status

Risk for situational low **Self-Esteem**: Risk factor: disturbed body image

Laser Surgery

Impaired **Comfort** r/t surgery

Constipation r/t laser intervention in vulval and perianal areas

Deficient **Knowledge** r/t preoperative and postoperative care associated with laser procedure

Acute **Pain** r/t heat from laser

Risk for **Bleeding**: Risk factor: surgery

Risk for **Infection**: Risk factor: delayed heating reaction of tissue exposed to laser

Risk for **Injury**: Risk factor: accidental exposure to laser beam

LASIK Eye Surgery (Laser-Assisted in Situ Keratomileusis)

Impaired **Comfort** r/t surgery

Decisional **Conflict** r/t decision to have the surgery

Risk for **Infection** r/t surgery

Readiness for enhanced **Self Health** management: surgical procedure pre- and postoperative teaching and expectations

Latex Allergy

Latex **Allergy** response (See **Allergy** response, latex, Section III)

Risk for latex **Allergy** response (See **Allergy** response, latex, risk for, Section III)

Readiness for enhanced **Knowledge**: prevention and treatment of exposure to latex products

Laxative Abuse

Perceived **Constipation** r/t health belief, faulty appraisal, impaired thought processes

Lead Poisoning

Contamination r/t flaking, peeling paint in presence of young children

Impaired **Home** maintenance r/t presence of lead paint

Risk for delayed **Development**: Risk factor: lead poisoning

Left Heart Catheterization

See Cardiac Catheterization

Legionnaires' Disease

Contamination r/t contaminated water in air-conditioning systems

See Pneumonia

Lens Implant

See Cataract Extraction; Vision Impairment

Lethargy/Listlessness

Adult **Failure** to thrive r/t apathy

Fatigue r/t decreased metabolic energy production

Insomnia r/t internal or external stressors

Risk for ineffective cerebral tissue **Perfusion**: Risk factor: lack of oxygen supply to brain

See cause of Lethargy/Listlessness

Leukemia

Ineffective **Protection** r/t abnormal blood profile

Risk for imbalanced **Fluid** volume: Risk factors: nausea, vomiting, bleeding, side effects of treatment

Risk for **Infection**: Risk factor: ineffective immune system

Risk for compromised **Resilience**: Risk factor: serious illness

See Cancer; Chemotherapy

Leukopenia

Ineffective **Protection** r/t leukopenia

Risk for **Infection**: Risk factor: low white blood cell count

L

Level of Consciousness, Decreased

See Confusion, Acute; Confusion, Chronic

Lice

Impaired **Comfort** r/t inflammation, pruritus

Impaired **Home** maintenance r/t close unsanitary, overcrowded conditions

Self **Neglect** r/t lifestyle

Readiness for enhanced **Self Health** management: preventing and treating infestation

See Communicable Diseases, Childhood

Lifestyle, Sedentary

Sedentary **Lifestyle** (See **Lifestyle**, sedentary, Section III)

Lightheadedness

See Dizziness; Vertigo

Limb Reattachment Procedures

Anxiety r/t unknown outcome of reattachment procedure, use and appearance of limb

Disturbed **Body** image r/t unpredictability of function and appearance of reattached body part

Grieving r/t unknown outcome of reattachment procedure

Spiritual distress r/t anxiety about condition

Stress overload r/t multiple coexisting stressors, physical demands

Risk for **Bleeding**: Risk factor: severed vessels

Risk for perioperative positioning **Injury**: Risk factor: immobilization

Risk for **Peripheral** neurovascular dysfunction: Risk factors: trauma, orthopedic and neurovascular surgery, compression of nerves and blood vessels

Risk for **Powerlessness**: Risk factor: unknown outcome of procedure

Risk for impaired **Religiosity**: Risk factors: suffering, hospitalization

See Surgery, Postoperative Care

Liposuction

Disturbed **Body** image r/t dissatisfaction with unwanted fat deposits in body

Risk for compromised **Resilience**: Risk factor: body image disturbance

Readiness for enhanced **Decision-Making**: expressed desire to make decision regarding liposuction

Readiness for enhanced **Self-Concept**: satisfaction with new body image

See Surgery, Perioperative Care; Surgery, Postoperative Care; Surgery, Preoperative Care

Lithotripsy

Readiness for enhanced **Self Health** management: expresses desire for information related to procedure and after care and prevention of stones

See Kidney Stone

Liver Biopsy

Anxiety r/t procedure and results

Risk for deficient **Fluid** volume: Risk factor: hemorrhage from biopsy site

Risk for **Powerlessness**: Risk factor: inability to control outcome of procedure

Liver Cancer

Risk for impaired **Liver** function: Risk factor: disease process

Risk for ineffective gastrointestinal tissue **Perfusion**: Risk factor: liver dysfunction

Risk for compromised **Resilience**: Risk factor: serious illness

See Cancer; Chemotherapy; Radiation Therapy

Liver Disease

See Cirrhosis; Hepatitis

Liver Function

Risk for impaired **Liver** function (See **Liver** function, impaired, risk for, Section III)

Liver Transplant

Impaired **Comfort** r/t surgical pain

Decisional **Conflict** r/t acceptance of donor liver

Ineffective **Protection** r/t immunosuppressive therapy

Risk for impaired **Liver** function: Risk factors: possible rejection, infection

Readiness for enhanced **Family** processes: change in physical needs of family member

Readiness for enhanced **Self Health** management: desire to manage the treatment and prevention of complications posttransplant

Readiness for enhanced **Spiritual** well-being: heightened coping

See Surgery, Perioperative Care; Surgery, Postoperative Care; Surgery, Preoperative Care

Living Will

Moral **Distress** r/t end-of-life decisions

Readiness for enhanced **Decision-Making**: expresses desire to enhance understanding of choices for decision making

Readiness for enhanced **Relationship**: shares information with others

Readiness for enhanced **Religiosity**: request to meet with religious leaders or facilitators

Readiness for enhanced **Resilience**: uses effective communication

Readiness for enhanced **Spiritual** well-being: acceptance of and preparation for end of life

See Advance Directives

Lobectomy

See Thoracotomy

Loneliness

Spiritual distress r/t loneliness, social alienation

Risk for **Loneliness** (See **Loneliness**, risk for, Section III)

L

Risk for impaired **Religiosity**: Risk factor: lack of social interaction

Risk for situational low **Self-Esteem**: Risk factors: failure, rejection

Readiness for enhanced **Hope**: expresses desire to enhance interconnectedness with others

Readiness for enhanced **Relationship**: expresses satisfaction with complementary relation between partners

Loose Stools (Bowel Movements)

Diarrhea r/t increased gastric motility

Risk for dysfunctional gastrointestinal **Motility**: Risk factor: diarrhea

See cause of Loose Stools; Diarrhea

Loss of Bladder Control

See Incontinence of Urine

Loss of Bowel Control

See Incontinence of Stool

Lou Gehrig's Disease

See Amyotrophic Lateral Sclerosis (ALS)

Low Back Pain

Impaired **Comfort** r/t back pain

Ineffective **Health** maintenance r/t deficient knowledge regarding self-care with back pain

Impaired physical **Mobility** r/t back pain

Chronic **Pain** r/t degenerative processes, musculotendinous strain, injury, inflammation, congenital deformities

Urinary retention r/t possible spinal cord compression

Risk for **Powerlessness**: Risk factor: living with chronic pain

Readiness for enhanced **Self Health** management: expressed desire for information to manage pain

Low Blood Pressure

See Hypotension

Low Blood Sugar

See Hypoglycemia

Lower GI Bleeding

See GI Bleed (Gastrointestinal Bleeding)

Lumbar Puncture

Anxiety r/t invasive procedure and unknown results

Deficient **Knowledge** r/t information about procedure

Acute **Pain** r/t possible loss of cerebrospinal fluid

Risk for **Infection**: Risk factor: invasive procedure

Risk for ineffective cerebral tissue **Perfusion**: Risk factor: treatment-related side effects

Lumpectomy

Decisional **Conflict** r/t treatment choices

Readiness for enhanced **Knowledge**: preoperative and postoperative care

Readiness for enhanced **Spiritual** well-being: hope of benign diagnosis

See Cancer

Lung Cancer

See Cancer; Chemotherapy; Radiation Therapy; Thoracotomy

Lung surgery

See Thoracotomy

Lupus Erythematosus

Disturbed **Body** image r/t change in skin, rash, lesions, ulcers, mottled erythema

Fatigue r/t increased metabolic requirements

Ineffective **Health** maintenance r/t deficient knowledge regarding medication, diet, activity

Acute **Pain** r/t inflammatory process

Powerlessness r/t unpredictability of course of disease

Impaired **Religiosity** r/t ineffective coping with disease

Chronic **Sorrow** r/t presence of chronic illness

Spiritual distress r/t chronicity of disease, unknown etiology

Risk for decreased cardiac tissue **Perfusion**: Risk factor: altered circulation

Risk for compromised **Resilience**: Risk factor: chronic disease

Risk for impaired **Skin** integrity: Risk factors: chronic inflammation, edema, altered circulation

Lyme Disease

Impaired **Comfort** r/t inflammation

Fatigue r/t increased energy requirements

Deficient **Knowledge** r/t lack of information concerning disease, prevention, treatment

Acute **Pain** r/t inflammation of joints, urticaria, rash

Risk for decreased **Cardiac** output: Risk factor: dysrhythmia

Risk for **Powerlessness**: Risk factor: possible chronic condition

Lymphedema

Disturbed **Body** image r/t change in appearance of body part with edema

Excess **Fluid** volume r/t compromised regulatory system; inflammation, obstruction, or removal of lymph glands

Deficient **Knowledge** r/t management of condition

Risk for situational low **Self-Esteem** r/t disturbed body image

Lymphoma

See Cancer

Macular Degeneration

Risk-prone health **Behavior** r/t deteriorating vision

Ineffective **Coping** r/t visual loss

Compromised **Family** coping r/t deteriorating vision of family member

Hopelessness r/t deteriorating vision

Sedentary **Lifestyle** r/t visual loss

Self **Neglect** r/t change in vision

Disturbed **Sensory** perception: visual r/t blurred, distorted, dim, or absent central vision

Social isolation r/t inability to drive because of visual changes

Risk for **Falls**: Risk factor: visual difficulties

Risk for **Injury**: Risk factor: inability to distinguish traffic lights

Risk for **Powerlessness**: Risk factor: deteriorating vision

Risk for impaired **Religiosity**: Risk factor: possible lack of transportation

Risk for compromised **Resilience**: Risk factor: changing vision

Readiness for enhanced **Self Health** management: appropriate choices of daily activities for meeting the goals of a treatment program

Magnetic Resonance Imaging (MRI)

See MRI (Magnetic Resonance Imaging)

Major Depressive Disorder

Interrupted **Family** processes r/t change in health status of family member

Self **Neglect** r/t psychological disorder

Risk for **Loneliness**: Risk factors: social isolation associated with feelings of sadness, hopelessness

Risk for compromised **Resilience**: Risk factor: psychological disorder

See Depression (Major Depressive Disorder)

Malabsorption Syndrome

Diarrhea r/t lactose intolerance, gluten sensitivity, resection of small bowel

Deficient **Knowledge** r/t lack of information about diet and nutrition

Dysfunctional gastrointestinal **Motility** r/t disease state

Imbalanced **Nutrition**: less than body requirements r/t inability of body to absorb nutrients because of biological factors

Risk for **Electrolyte** imbalance: Risk factor: hypovolemia

Risk for imbalanced **Fluid** volume: Risk factor: diarrhea

Risk for disproportionate **Growth**: Risk factor: malnutrition from malabsorption

See Abdominal Distention

Maladaptive Behavior

See Crisis; Post-Trauma Syndrome; Suicide Attempt

Malaise

See Fatigue

Malaria

Contamination r/t geographic area

Risk for **Contamination**: Risk factors: increased environmental exposure (not wearing protective clothing, not using insecticide or repellant on skin and in room in areas where infected mosquitoes are present); inadequate defense mechanisms (inappropriate use of prophylactic regimen)

Risk for impaired **Liver** function: Risk factor: complications of disease

Readiness for enhanced community **Coping**: uses resources available for problem solving

Readiness for enhanced **Immunization** status: expresses desire to enhance immunization status and knowledge of immunization standards

Readiness for enhanced **Resilience**: immunization status

See Anemia

Male Infertility

See Erectile Dysfunction (ED); Infertility

Malignancy

See Cancer

Malignant Hypertension (Arteriolar Nephrosclerosis)

Decreased **Cardiac** output r/t altered afterload, altered contractility

Fatigue r/t disease state, increased blood pressure

Excess **Fluid** volume r/t decreased renal function

Disturbed **Sensory** perception: visual r/t altered sensory reception from papilledema

Risk for acute **Confusion**: Risk factors: increased blood urea nitrogen or creatine levels

Risk for imbalanced **Fluid** volume: Risk factors: hypertension, altered renal function

Risk for ineffective cerebral tissue **Perfusion**: Risk factor: hypertension

Risk for ineffective renal **Perfusion**: Risk factor: hypertension

Readiness for enhanced **Self Health** management: expresses desire to manage the illness, high blood pressure

Malignant Hyperthermia

Hyperthermia r/t anesthesia reaction associated with inherited condition

Risk for ineffective renal **Perfusion**: Risk factor: hyperthermia

Readiness for enhanced **Self Health** management: knowledge of risk factors

Malnutrition

Adult **Failure** to thrive r/t undetected malnutrition

Ineffective self **Health** management r/t inadequate nutrition

Deficient **Knowledge** r/t misinformation about normal nutrition, social isolation, lack of food preparation facilities

Self **Neglect** r/t inadequate nutrition

Imbalanced **Nutrition**: less than body requirements r/t inability to ingest food, digest food, or absorb nutrients because of biological, psychological, or economic factors; institutionalization (i.e., lack of menu choices)

Ineffective **Protection** r/t inadequate nutrition

Risk for disproportionate **Growth**: Risk factor: malnutrition

M

Risk for **Powerlessness**: Risk factor: possible inability to provide adequate nutrition

Mammography

Readiness for enhanced **Resilience**: responsibility for self-care

Readiness for enhanced **Self Health** management: follows guidelines for screening

Manic Disorder, Bipolar I

Anxiety r/t change in role function

Risk-prone health **Behavior** r/t low self-efficacy

Ineffective **Coping** r/t situational crisis

Ineffective **Denial** r/t fear of inability to control behavior

Interrupted **Family** processes r/t family member's illness

Ineffective self **Health** management r/t unpredictability of client, excessive demands on family, chronic illness, social support deficit

Impaired **Home** maintenance r/t altered psychological state, inability to concentrate

Disturbed personal **Identity** r/t manic state

Insomnia r/t constant anxious thoughts

Self **Neglect** r/t manic state

Noncompliance r/t denial of illness

Imbalanced **Nutrition**: less than body requirements r/t lack of time and motivation to eat, constant movement

Impaired individual **Resilience** r/t psychological disorder

Ineffective **Role** performance r/t impaired social interactions

Sleep deprivation r/t hyperagitated state

Risk for **Caregiver** role strain: Risk factor: unpredictability of condition

Risk for imbalanced **Fluid** volume: Risk factor: hypovolemia

Risk for **Powerlessness**: Risk factor: inability to control changes in mood

Risk for impaired **Religiosity**: Risk factor: depression

Risk for **Spiritual** distress: Risk factor: depression

Risk for **Suicide**: Risk factor: bipolar disorder

Risk for self- or other-directed **Violence**: Risk factors: hallucinations, delusions

Readiness for enhanced **Hope**: expresses desire to enhance problem-solving goals

Manipulation of Organs, Surgical Incision

Impaired **Comfort** r/t incision; surgery

Deficient **Knowledge** r/t lack of exposure to information regarding care after surgery and at home

Urinary retention r/t swelling of urinary meatus

Risk for **Infection**: Risk factor: presence of urinary catheter

Manipulative Behavior

Defensive **Coping** r/t superior attitude toward others

Ineffective **Coping** r/t inappropriate use of defense mechanisms

Self **Neglect** r/t maintaining control

Self-Mutilation r/t use of manipulation to obtain nurturing relationship with others

Impaired **Social** interaction r/t self-concept disturbance

Risk for **Loneliness**: Risk factor: inability to interact appropriately with others

Risk for situational low **Self-Esteem**: Risk factor: history of learned helplessness

Risk for **Self-Mutilation**: Risk factor: inability to cope with increased psychological or physiological tension in healthy manner

Marasmus

See Failure to Thrive, Nonorganic

Marfan Syndrome

Decreased **Cardiac** output r/t dilation of the aortic root, dissection or rupture of the aorta

Disturbed **Sensory** perception: visual r/t myopia associated with Marfan syndrome

Risk for decreased cardiac tissue **Perfusion**: Risk factor: heart-related complications from Marfan syndrome

Readiness for enhanced **Self Health** management: describes reduction of risk factors

See Mitral Valve Prolapse; Scoliosis

Marshall-Marchetti-Krantz Operation

PREOPERATIVE

Stress urinary **Incontinence** r/t weak pelvic muscles and pelvic supports

POSTOPERATIVE

Impaired **Comfort** r/t surgical procedure

Deficient **Knowledge** r/t lack of exposure to information regarding care after surgery and at home

Acute **Pain** r/t manipulation of organs, surgical incision

Urinary retention r/t swelling of urinary meatus

Risk for **Bleeding**: Risk factor: surgical procedure

Risk for **Infection**: Risk factor: presence of urinary catheter

Mastectomy

Death **Anxiety** r/t threat of mortality associated with breast cancer

Disturbed **Body** image r/t loss of sexually significant body part

Impaired **Comfort** r/t altered body image; difficult diagnosis

Fear r/t change in body image, prognosis

Deficient **Knowledge** r/t self-care activities

Nausea r/t chemotherapy

Acute **Pain** r/t surgical procedure

Sexual dysfunction r/t change in body image, fear of loss of femininity

Chronic **Sorrow** r/t disturbed body image, unknown long-term health status

Spiritual distress r/t change in body image

Risk for **Infection**: Risk factors: surgical procedure; broken skin

M

Risk for impaired physical **Mobility**: Risk factors: nerve or muscle damage, pain

Risk for **Post-Trauma** syndrome: Risk factors: loss of body part, surgical wounds

Risk for **Powerlessness**: Risk factor: fear of unknown outcome of procedure

Risk for compromised **Resilience**: Risk factor: altered body image

See Cancer; Modified Radical Mastectomy; Surgery, Perioperative; Surgery, Postoperative; Surgery, Preoperative

Mastitis

Anxiety r/t threat to self, concern over safety of milk for infant

Ineffective **Breastfeeding** r/t breast pain, conflicting advice from health care providers

Deficient **Knowledge** r/t antibiotic regimen, comfort measures

Acute **Pain** r/t infectious disease process, swelling of breast tissue

Ineffective **Role** performance r/t change in capacity to function in expected role

Risk for disturbed **Maternal/Fetal** dyad: Risk factors: interrupted/ineffective breastfeeding

Maternal Infection

Ineffective **Protection** r/t invasive procedures, traumatized tissue

See Postpartum, Normal Care

Maturational Issues, Adolescent

Risk-prone health **Behavior** r/t inadequate comprehension, negative attitude toward health care

Ineffective **Coping** r/t maturational crises

Interrupted **Family** processes r/t developmental crises of adolescence resulting from challenge of parental authority and values, situational crises from change in parental marital status

Deficient **Knowledge**: potential for enhanced health maintenance r/t information misinterpretation, lack of education regarding age-related factors

Impaired **Social** interaction r/t ineffective, unsuccessful, or dysfunctional interaction with peers

Social isolation r/t perceived alteration in physical appearance, social values not accepted by dominant peer group

Risk for **Injury/Trauma**: Risk factor: thrill-seeking behaviors

Risk for situational low **Self-Esteem**: Risk factor: developmental changes

Readiness for enhanced **Communication**: expressing willingness to communicate with parental figures

Readiness for enhanced **Relationship**: expresses desire to enhance communication with parental figures

See Sexuality, Adolescent; Substance Abuse (if relevant)

Maze III Procedure

See Dysrhythmia; Open Heart Surgery

MD (Muscular Dystrophy)

See Muscular Dystrophy (MD)

Measles (Rubeola)

See Communicable Diseases, Childhood

Meconium Aspiration

See Respiratory Conditions of the Neonate

Melanoma

Disturbed **Body** image r/t altered pigmentation, surgical incision

Fear r/t threat to well-being

Ineffective **Health** maintenance r/t deficient knowledge regarding self-care and treatment of melanoma

Acute **Pain** r/t surgical incision

Readiness for enhanced **Self Health** management: describes reduction of risk factors; protection from sunlight's ultraviolet rays

See Cancer

Melena

Fear r/t presence of blood in feces

Risk for imbalanced **Fluid** volume: Risk factor: hemorrhage

See GI Bleed (Gastrointestinal Bleeding)

Memory Deficit

Impaired **Memory** (See **Memory**, impaired, Section III)

Ménière's Disease

Risk for **Injury**: Risk factor: symptoms from disease

Readiness for enhanced **Self Health** management: expresses desire to manage illness

See Dizziness; Nausea; Vertigo

Meningitis/Encephalitis

Ineffective **Airway** clearance r/t seizure activity

Impaired **Comfort** r/t altered health status

Excess **Fluid** volume r/t increased intracranial pressure, syndrome of inappropriate secretion of antidiuretic hormone

Delayed **Growth** and development r/t effects of physical disability

Decreased **Intracranial** adaptive capacity r/t sustained increase in intracranial pressure of 10 to 15 mm Hg

Impaired **Mobility** r/t neuromuscular or central nervous system insult

Acute **Pain** r/t biological injury

Disturbed **Sensory** perception: hearing r/t central nervous system infection, ear infection

Disturbed **Sensory** perception: kinesthetic r/t central nervous system infection

Disturbed **Sensory** perception: visual r/t photophobia attributable to central nervous system infection

Risk for **Aspiration**: Risk factor: seizure activity

Risk for acute **Confusion**: Risk factor: infection of brain

Risk for **Falls**: Risk factor: neuromuscular dysfunction

Risk for **Injury**: Risk factor: seizure activity

M

Risk for ineffective cerebral tissue **Perfusion**: Risk factors: inflamed cerebral tissues and meninges, increased intracranial pressure; infection

Risk for compromised **Resilience**: Risk factor: illness

Risk for **Shock**: Risk factor: infection

Readiness for enhanced **Immunization** status: expresses desire to enhance immunization status and knowledge of immunization standards

See Hospitalized Child

Meningocele

See Neural Tube Defects

Menopause

Impaired **Comfort** r/t symptoms associated with menopause

Insomnia r/t hormonal shifts

Impaired **Memory** r/t change in hormonal levels

Sexual dysfunction r/t menopausal changes

Ineffective **Sexuality** pattern r/t altered body structure, lack of physiological lubrication, lack of knowledge of artificial lubrication

Ineffective **Thermoregulation** r/t changes in hormonal levels

Risk for urge urinary **Incontinence**: Risk factor: changes in hormonal levels affecting bladder function

Risk for imbalanced **Nutrition**: more than body requirements: Risk factor: change in metabolic rate caused by fluctuating hormone levels

Risk for **Powerlessness**: Risk factor: changes associated with menopause

Risk for compromised **Resilience**: Risk factor: menopause

Risk for situational low **Self-Esteem**: Risk factors: developmental changes, menopause

Readiness for enhanced **Self-Care**: expresses satisfaction with body image

Readiness for enhanced **Self Health** management: verbalized desire to manage menopause

Readiness for enhanced **Spiritual** well-being: desire for harmony of mind, body, and spirit

Menorrhagia

Fear r/t loss of large amounts of blood

Risk for deficient **Fluid** volume: Risk factor: excessive loss of menstrual blood

Mental Illness

Risk-prone health **Behavior** r/t low self-efficacy

Compromised family **Coping** r/t lack of available support from client

Defensive **Coping** r/t psychological impairment, substance abuse

Disabled family **Coping** r/t chronically unexpressed feelings of guilt, anxiety, hostility, or despair

Ineffective **Coping** r/t situational crisis, coping with mental illness

Ineffective **Denial** r/t refusal to acknowledge abuse problem, fear of the social stigma of disease

Disturbed personal **Identity** r/t psychoses

Chronic **Sorrow** r/t presence of mental illness

Stress overload r/t multiple coexisting stressors

Ineffective family **Therapeutic** regimen management r/t chronicity of condition, unpredictability of client, unknown prognosis

Risk for **Loneliness**: Risk factor: social isolation

Risk for **Powerlessness**: Risk factor: lifestyle of helplessness

Risk for compromised **Resilience**: Risk factor: chronic illness

Mental Retardation

Impaired verbal **Communication** r/t developmental delay

Interrupted **Family** processes r/t crisis of diagnosis and situational transition

Grieving r/t loss of perfect child, birth of child with congenital defect or subsequent head injury

Delayed **Growth** and development r/t cognitive or perceptual impairment, developmental delay

Impaired **Home** maintenance r/t insufficient support systems

Self **Neglect** r/t learning disability

Self-Care deficit: bathing, dressing, feeding, toileting r/t perceptual or cognitive impairment

Self-Mutilation r/t inability to express tension verbally

Social isolation r/t delay in accomplishing developmental tasks

Spiritual distress r/t chronic condition of child with special needs

Stress overload r/t intense, repeated stressor (chronic condition)

Impaired **Swallowing** r/t neuromuscular impairment

Risk for delayed **Development**: Risk factor: cognitive or perceptual impairment

Risk for disproportionate **Growth**: Risk factor: mental retardation

Risk for impaired **Religiosity**: Risk factor: social isolation

Risk for **Self-Mutilation**: Risk factors: separation anxiety, depersonalization

Readiness for enhanced family **Coping**: adaptation and acceptance of child's condition and needs

See Child with Chronic Condition; Safety, Childhood

Metabolic Acidosis

See Ketoacidosis, Alcoholic; Ketoacidosis, Diabetic

Metabolic Alkalosis

Deficient **Fluid** volume r/t fluid volume loss, vomiting, gastric suctioning, failure of regulatory mechanisms

Metastasis

See Cancer

Methicillin-Resistant Staphylococcus Aureus (MRSA)

See MRSA (Methicillin-Resistant Staphylococcus aureus)

MI (Myocardial Infarction)

Anxiety r/t threat of death, possible change in role status

Death **Anxiety** r/t seriousness of medical condition

Decreased **Cardiac** output r/t ventricular damage, ischemia, dysrhythmias

Constipation r/t decreased peristalsis from decreased physical activity, medication effect, change in diet

Ineffective family **Coping** r/t spouse or significant other's fear of partner loss

Ineffective **Denial** r/t fear, deficient knowledge about heart disease

Interrupted **Family** processes r/t crisis, role change

Fear r/t threat to well-being

Ineffective **Health** maintenance r/t deficient knowledge regarding self-care and treatment

Acute **Pain** r/t myocardial tissue damage from inadequate blood supply

Situational low **Self-Esteem** r/t crisis of MI

Ineffective **Sexuality** pattern r/t fear of chest pain, possibility of heart damage

Risk for decreased cardiac tissue **Perfusion**: Risk factors: coronary artery spasm, hypertension, hypoxia

Risk for **Powerlessness**: Risk factor: acute illness

Risk for **Shock**: Risk factors: hypotension, hypoxia

Risk for **Spiritual** distress: Risk factors: physical illness: MI

Readiness for enhanced **Knowledge**: expresses an interest in learning about condition

See Angioplasty (Coronary); Coronary Artery Bypass Grafting (CABG)

MIDCAB (Minimally Invasive Direct Coronary Artery Bypass)

Risk for **Bleeding**: Risk factor: surgery

Risk for **Infection**: Risk factor: large breasts on incision line

Readiness for enhanced **Self Health** management: pre- and postoperative care associated with the surgery

See Angioplasty, Coronary; Coronary Artery Bypass Grafting (CABG)

Midlife Crisis

Ineffective **Coping** r/t inability to deal with changes associated with aging

Powerlessness r/t lack of control over life situation

Spiritual distress r/t questioning beliefs or value system

Readiness for enhanced **Relationship**: meets goals for lifestyle change

Readiness for enhanced **Spiritual** well-being: desire to find purpose and meaning to life

Migraine Headache

Disturbed **Energy** field r/t pain, disruption of normal flow of energy

Impaired **Comfort** r/t altered health status

Ineffective **Health** maintenance r/t deficient knowledge regarding prevention and treatment of headaches

Acute **Pain**: headache r/t vasodilation of cerebral and extracerebral vessels

Risk for compromised **Resilience**: Risk factors: chronic illness, impaired comfort

Readiness for enhanced **Self Health** management: expressed desire to manage the illness

Milk Intolerance

See Lactose Intolerance

Minimally Invasive Direct Coronary Bypass (MIDCAB)

See MIDCAB (Minimally Invasive Direct Coronary Artery Bypass)

Miscarriage

See Pregnancy Loss

Mitral Stenosis

Activity intolerance r/t imbalance between oxygen supply and demand

Anxiety r/t possible worsening of symptoms, activity intolerance, fatigue

Decreased **Cardiac** output r/t incompetent heart valves, abnormal forward or backward blood flow, flow into a dilated chamber, flow through an abnormal passage between chambers

Fatigue r/t reduced cardiac output

Ineffective **Health** maintenance r/t deficient knowledge regarding self-care with disorder

Risk for **Infection**: Risk factors: invasive procedure, risk for endocarditis

Risk for decreased cardiac tissue **Perfusion**: Risk factor: incompetent heart valve

Mitral Valve Prolapse

Anxiety r/t symptoms of condition: palpitations, chest pain

Fatigue r/t abnormal catecholamine regulation, decreased intravascular volume

Fear r/t lack of knowledge about mitral valve prolapse, feelings of having a heart attack

Ineffective **Health** maintenance r/t deficient knowledge regarding methods to relieve pain and treat dysrhythmia and shortness of breath, need for prophylactic antibiotics before invasive procedures

Acute **Pain** r/t mitral valve regurgitation

Risk for **Infection**: Risk factor: invasive procedures

Risk for ineffective cerebral tissue **Perfusion**: Risk factor: postural hypotension

Risk for **Powerlessness**: Risk factor: unpredictability of onset of symptoms

Readiness for enhanced **Knowledge**: expresses an interest in learning about condition

Mobility, Impaired Bed

Impaired bed **Mobility** (See **Mobility**, bed, impaired, Section III)

M

Mobility, Impaired Physical

Impaired physical **Mobility** (See **Mobility**, physical, impaired, Section III)

Risk for **Falls**: Risk factor: impaired physical mobility

Mobility, Impaired Wheelchair

Impaired wheelchair **Mobility** (See **Mobility**, wheelchair, impaired, Section III)

Modified Radical Mastectomy

Decisional **Conflict** r/t treatment of choice

Readiness for enhanced **Communication**: willingness to enhance communication

See Mastectomy

Motion Sickness

See Labyrinthitis

Mononucleosis

Activity intolerance r/t generalized weakness

Impaired **Comfort** r/t sore throat, muscle aches

Fatigue r/t disease state, stress

Ineffective **Health** maintenance r/t deficient knowledge concerning transmission and treatment of disease

Hyperthermia r/t infectious process

Acute **Pain** r/t enlargement of lymph nodes, oropharyngeal edema

Impaired **Swallowing** r/t enlargement of lymph nodes, oropharyngeal edema

Risk for **Injury**: Risk factor: possible rupture of spleen

Risk for **Loneliness**: Risk factor: social isolation

Mood Disorders

Risk-prone health **Behavior** r/t hopelessness, altered locus of control

Caregiver role strain r/t symptoms associated with disorder of care receiver

Self **Neglect** r/t depression

Social isolation r/t alterations in mental status

Risk for situational low **Self-Esteem**: Risk factor: unpredictable changes in mood

Readiness for enhanced **Communication**: expresses feelings

See specific disorder: Depression (Major Depressive Disorder); Dysthymic Disorder; Hypomania; Manic Disorder, Bipolar I

Moon Face

Disturbed **Body** image r/t change in appearance from disease and medication

Risk for situational low **Self-Esteem**: Risk factor: change in body image

See Cushing's Syndrome

Moral/Ethical Dilemmas

Decisional **Conflict** r/t questioning personal values and belief, which alter decision

Moral **Distress** r/t conflicting information guiding moral or ethical decision making

Risk for **Powerlessness**: Risk factor: lack of knowledge to make a decision

Risk for **Spiritual** distress: Risk factor: moral or ethical crisis

Readiness for enhanced **Decision-Making**: expresses desire to enhance congruency of decisions with personal values and goals

Readiness for enhanced **Religiosity**: requests assistance in expanding religious options

Readiness for enhanced **Resilience**: vulnerable state

Readiness for enhanced **Spiritual** well-being: request for interaction with others regarding difficult decisions

Morning Sickness

See Hyperemesis Gravidarum; Pregnancy, Normal

Mottling of Peripheral Skin

Ineffective peripheral tissue **Perfusion** r/t interruption of arterial flow, decreased circulating blood volume

Risk for vascular **Trauma**: Risk factor: nature of solution

Mourning

See Grieving

Mouth Lesions

See Mucous Membranes, Impaired Oral

MRI (Magnetic Resonance Imaging)

Anxiety r/t fear of being in closed spaces

Deficient **Knowledge** r/t unfamiliarity with information resources; exam information

Readiness for enhanced **Knowledge**: expresses interest in learning about exam

Readiness for enhanced **Self Health** management: describes reduction of risk factors associated with exam

MRSA (Methicillin-Resistant Staphylococcus Aureus)

Hyperthermia r/t infection

Impaired **Skin** integrity r/t infection

Delayed **Surgical** recovery r/t infection

Impaired **Tissue** integrity r/t wound, infection

Risk for **Loneliness**: Risk factor: physical isolation

Risk for compromised **Resilience**: Risk factor: illness

Risk for **Shock**: Risk factor: sepsis

Mucocutaneous Lymph Node Syndrome

See Kawasaki Disease

Mucous Membrane, Impaired Oral

Impaired **Oral** mucous membrane (See **Oral** mucous membrane, impaired, Section III)

Multiinfarct Dementia

See Dementia

Multiple Gestation

Anxiety r/t uncertain outcome of pregnancy

Death **Anxiety** r/t maternal complications associated with multiple gestation

Fatigue r/t physiological demands of a multifetal pregnancy and/or care of more than one infant

Impaired **Home** maintenance r/t fatigue

Stress urinary **Incontinence** r/t increased pelvic pressure

Insomnia r/t impairment of normal sleep pattern; parental responsibilities

Neonatal **Jaundice** r/t feeding pattern not well established

Deficient **Knowledge** r/t caring for more than one infant

Impaired physical **Mobility** r/t increased uterine size

Imbalanced **Nutrition**: less than body requirements r/t physiological demands of a multifetal pregnancy

Stress overload r/t multiple coexisting stressors, family demands

Impaired **Transfer** ability r/t enlarged uterus

Risk for ineffective **Breastfeeding**: Risk factors: lack of support, physical demands of feeding more than one infant

Risk for **Constipation**: Risk factor: enlarged uterus

Risk for delayed **Development**: fetus: Risk factor: multiple gestation

Risk for disproportionate **Growth**: fetus: Risk factor: multiple gestation

Readiness for enhanced **Childbearing** process: demonstrates appropriate care for infant and mother

Readiness for enhanced **Family** processes: family adapting to change with more than one infant

Multiple Personality Disorder (Dissociative Identity Disorder)

Anxiety r/t loss of control of behavior and feelings

Disturbed **Body** image r/t psychosocial changes

Defensive **Coping** r/t unresolved past traumatic events, severe anxiety

Ineffective **Coping** r/t history of abuse

Hopelessness r/t long-term stress

Disturbed personal **Identity** r/t severe child abuse

Chronic low **Self-Esteem** r/t rejection, failure

Risk for **Self-Mutilation**: Risk factor: need to act out to relieve stress

Readiness for enhanced **Communication**: willingness to discuss problems associated with condition

See Dissociative Identity Disorder (Not Otherwise Specified)

Multiple Sclerosis (MS)

Ineffective **Activity** planning r/t unrealistic perception of personal competence

Ineffective **Airway** clearance r/t decreased energy or fatigue

Disturbed **Energy** field r/t disruption in energy flow resulting from disharmony between mind and body

Impaired physical **Mobility** r/t neuromuscular impairment

Self **Neglect** r/t functional impairment

Powerlessness r/t progressive nature of disease

Self-Care deficit: specify r/t neuromuscular impairment

Disturbed **Sensory** perception: specify r/t pathology in sensory tracts

Sexual dysfunction r/t biopsychosocial alteration of sexuality

Chronic **Sorrow** r/t loss of physical ability

Spiritual distress r/t perceived hopelessness of diagnosis

Urinary retention r/t inhibition of the reflex arc

Risk for latex **Allergy** response: Risk factor: possible repeated exposures to latex associated with intermittent catheterizations

Risk for **Disuse** syndrome: Risk factor: physical immobility

Risk for **Injury**: Risk factors: altered mobility, sensory dysfunction

Risk for imbalanced **Nutrition**: less than body requirements: Risk factors: impaired swallowing, depression

Risk for **Powerlessness**: Risk factor: chronic illness

Risk for impaired **Religiosity**: Risk factor: illness

Readiness for enhanced **Self-Care**: expresses desire to enhance knowledge of strategies and responsibility for self-care

Readiness for enhanced **Self Health** management: expresses a desire to manage condition

Readiness for enhanced **Spiritual** well-being: struggling with chronic debilitating condition

See Neurologic Disorders

Mumps

See Communicable Diseases, Childhood

Murmurs

Decreased **Cardiac** output r/t altered preload/afterload

Risk for decreased cardiac tissue **Perfusion**: Risk factor: incompetent valve

Muscular Atrophy/Weakness

Risk for **Disuse** syndrome: Risk factor: impaired physical mobility

Risk for **Falls**: Risk factor: impaired physical mobility

Muscular Dystrophy (MD)

Activity intolerance r/t fatigue

Ineffective **Activity** planning r/t unrealistic perception of personal competence

Ineffective **Airway** clearance r/t muscle weakness and decreased ability to cough

Constipation r/t immobility

Disturbed **Energy** field r/t illness

Fatigue r/t increased energy requirements to perform activities of daily living

Impaired **Mobility** r/t muscle weakness and development of contractures

Self **Neglect** r/t functional impairment

Imbalanced **Nutrition**: less than body requirements r/t impaired swallowing or chewing

Imbalanced **Nutrition**: more than body requirements r/t inactivity

Self-Care deficit: feeding, bathing, dressing, toileting r/t muscle weakness and fatigue

Impaired **Transfer** ability r/t muscle weakness

Impaired **Walking** r/t muscle weakness

Risk for **Aspiration**: Risk factor: impaired swallowing

Risk for ineffective **Breathing** pattern: Risk factor: muscle weakness

Risk for **Disuse** syndrome: Risk factor: complications of immobility

Risk for **Falls**: Risk factor: muscle weakness

Risk for impaired **Gas** exchange: Risk factors: ineffective airway clearance and ineffective breathing pattern caused by muscle weakness

Risk for **Infection**: Risk factor: pooling of pulmonary secretions as a result of immobility and muscle weakness

Risk for **Injury**: Risk factors: muscle weakness and unsteady gait

Risk for decreased cardiac tissue **Perfusion**: Risk factor: hypoxia associated with cardiomyopathy

Risk for **Powerlessness**: Risk factor: chronic condition

Risk for impaired **Religiosity**: Risk factor: illness

Risk for compromised **Resilience**: Risk factor: chronic illness

Risk for impaired **Skin** integrity: Risk factors: immobility, braces, or adaptive devices

Risk for situational low **Self-Esteem**: Risk factor: presence of chronic condition

Readiness for enhanced **Self-Concept**: acceptance of strength and abilities

See Child with Chronic Condition; Hospitalized Child

MVA (Motor Vehicle Accident)

See Fracture; Head Injury; Injury; Pneumothorax

Myasthenia Gravis

Ineffective **Airway** clearance r/t decreased ability to cough and swallow

Interrupted **Family** processes r/t crisis of dealing with diagnosis

Fatigue r/t paresthesia, aching muscles

Impaired physical **Mobility** r/t defective transmission of nerve impulses at the neuromuscular junction

Imbalanced **Nutrition**: less than body requirements r/t difficulty eating and swallowing

Impaired **Swallowing** r/t neuromuscular impairment

Risk for **Caregiver** role strain: Risk factor: severity of illness of client

Risk for impaired **Religiosity**: Risk factor: illness

Risk for compromised **Resilience**: Risk factor: new diagnosis of chronic, serious illness

Readiness for enhanced **Spiritual** well-being: heightened coping with serious illness

See Neurologic Disorders

Mycoplasma Pneumonia

See Pneumonia

Myelocele

See Neural Tube Defects

Myelogram, Contrast

Acute **Pain** r/t irritation of nerve roots

Urinary retention r/t pressure on spinal nerve roots

Risk for deficient **Fluid** volume: Risk factor: possible dehydration

Risk for ineffective cerebral tissue **Perfusion**: Risk factors: hypotension, loss of cerebrospinal fluid

Myelomeningocele

See Neural Tube Defects

Myocardial Infarction (MI)

See MI (Myocardial Infarction)

Myocarditis

Activity intolerance r/t reduced cardiac reserve and prescribed bed rest

Decreased **Cardiac** output r/t altered preload/afterload

Deficient **Knowledge** r/t treatment of disease

Risk for decreased cardiac tissue **Perfusion**: Risk factors: hypoxia, hypovolemia, cardiac tamponade

Readiness for enhanced **Knowledge**: treatment of disease

See CHF (Congestive Heart Failure), if appropriate

Myringotomy

Fear r/t hospitalization, surgical procedure

Ineffective **Health** maintenance r/t deficient knowledge regarding care after surgery

Acute **Pain** r/t surgical procedure

Disturbed **Sensory** perception r/t possible hearing impairment

Risk for **Infection**: Risk factor: invasive procedure

See Ear Surgery

Myxedema

See Hypothyroidism

N

Narcissistic Personality Disorder

Risk-prone health **Behavior** r/t low self-efficacy

Decisional **Conflict** r/t lack of realistic problem-solving skills

Defensive **Coping** r/t grandiose sense of self

Interrupted **Family** processes r/t taking advantage of others to achieve own goals

Disturbed **Personal** identity r/t psychological impairment

Impaired individual **Resilience** r/t psychological disorders

Impaired **Social** interaction r/t self-concept disturbance

Risk for **Loneliness** r/t inability to interact appropriately with others

Risk for **Self-Mutilation**: Risk factor: inadequate coping

Narcolepsy

Anxiety r/t fear of lack of control over falling asleep

Disturbed **Sleep** pattern r/t uncontrollable desire to sleep

Risk for **Trauma**: Risk factor: falling asleep during potentially dangerous activity

Readiness for enhanced **Sleep**: expression of willingness to enhance sleep

Narcotic Use

Risk for **Constipation**: Risk factor: effects of opioids on peristalsis

See Substance Abuse (if relevant)

Nasogastric Suction

Impaired **Oral** mucous membrane r/t presence of nasogastric tube

Risk for imbalanced **Fluid** volume: Risk factor: loss of gastrointestinal fluids without adequate replacement

Risk for dysfunctional gastrointestinal **Motility**: Risk factor: blockage in the intestines

Nausea

Nausea: biophysical, situational, treatment-related (See **Nausea**, Section III)

Near-Drowning

Ineffective **Airway** clearance r/t aspiration, impaired gas exchange

Aspiration r/t aspiration of fluid into the lungs

Fear: parental r/t possible death of child, possible permanent and debilitating sequelae

Impaired **Gas** exchange r/t laryngospasm, holding breath, aspiration

Grieving r/t potential death of child, unknown sequelae, guilt about accident

Ineffective **Health** maintenance r/t parental deficient knowledge regarding safety measures appropriate for age

Hypothermia r/t central nervous system injury, prolonged submersion in cold water

Risk for delayed **Development**/disproportionate **Growth**: Risk factors: hypoxemia, cerebral anoxia

Risk for complicated **Grieving**: Risk factors: potential death of child, unknown sequelae, guilt about accident

Risk for **Infection**: Risk factors: aspiration, invasive monitoring

Risk for ineffective cerebral tissue **Perfusion**: Risk factor: hypoxia

Readiness for enhanced **Spiritual** well-being: struggle with survival of life-threatening situation

See Child with Chronic Condition; Hospitalized Child; Safety, Childhood; Terminally Ill Child/Death of Child, Parent

Nearsightedness

Readiness for enhanced **Self Health** management: early diagnosis and appropriate referral for eyeglasses or contact lenses when nearsightedness is suspected; signs that may indicate a vision problem, including sitting close to television, holding books very close when reading, or having difficulty reading the blackboard in school or signs on a wall

Nearsightedness; Corneal Surgery

See LASIK Eye Surgery (Laser-Assisted in Situ Keratomileusis)

Neck Vein Distention

Decreased **Cardiac** output r/t decreased contractility of heart resulting increased preload

Excess **Fluid** volume r/t excess fluid intake, compromised regulatory mechanisms

See CHF (Congestive Heart Failure)

Necrosis, Renal Tubular; ATN (Acute Tubular Necrosis); Necrosis, Acute Tubular

See Renal Failure

Necrotizing Enterocolitis (NEC)

Ineffective **Breathing** pattern r/t abdominal distention, hypoxia

Diarrhea r/t infection

Disturbed **Energy** field r/t illness

Deficient **Fluid** volume r/t vomiting, gastrointestinal bleeding

Neonatal **Jaundice** r/t feeding pattern not well established

Imbalanced **Nutrition**: less than body requirements r/t decreased ability to absorb nutrients, decreased perfusion to gastrointestinal tract

Risk for **Infection**: Risk factors: bacterial invasion of gastrointestinal tract, invasive procedures

Risk for dysfunctional gastrointestinal **Motility**: Risk factor: infection

Risk for ineffective gastrointestinal **Perfusion**: Risk factors: shunting of blood away from mesenteric circulation and toward vital organs as a result of perinatal stress, hypoxia

See Hospitalized Child; Premature Infant (Child)

Necrotizing Fasciitis (Flesh-Eating Bacteria)

Decreased **Cardiac** output r/t tachycardia and hypotension

Fear r/t possible fatal outcome of disease

Grieving r/t poor prognosis associated with disease

Hyperthermia r/t presence of infection

Acute **Pain** r/t toxins interfering with blood flow

Ineffective peripheral tissue **Perfusion** r/t thrombosis of the subcutaneous blood vessels, leading to necrosis of nerve fibers

Ineffective **Protection** r/t cellulites resistant to treatment

Risk for **Shock**: Risk factors: infection; sepsis

See Renal Failure; Septicemia; Shock, Septic

N

Negative Feelings About Self

Self **Neglect** r/t negative feelings

Chronic low **Self-esteem** r/t longstanding negative self-evaluation

Situational low **Self-esteem** r/t inappropriate learned negative feelings about self

Readiness for enhanced **Self-Concept** expresses willingness to enhance self-concept

Neglect, Unilateral

Unilateral **Neglect** (See **Neglect**, unilateral, Section III)

Neglectful Care of Family Member

Caregiver role strain r/t care demands of family member, lack of social or financial support

Disabled family **Coping** r/t highly ambivalent family relationships, lack of respite care

Interrupted **Family** processes r/t situational transition or crisis

Deficient **Knowledge** r/t care needs

Impaired individual **Resilience** r/t vulnerability from neglect

Risk for compromised human **Dignity**: Risk factor: inadequate participation in decision making

Neonatal Jaundice

Neonatal **Jaundice** (See **Jaundice**, neonatal, Section III)

Neonate

Readiness for enhanced **Childbearing** process: appropriate care of newborn

See Newborn, Normal; Newborn, Postmature; Newborn, Small for Gestational Age (SGA)

Neoplasm

Fear r/t possible malignancy

See Cancer

Nephrectomy

Anxiety r/t surgical recovery, prognosis

Ineffective **Breathing** pattern r/t location of surgical incision

Constipation r/t lack of return of peristalsis

Acute **Pain** r/t incisional discomfort

Spiritual distress r/t chronic illness

Impaired **Urinary** elimination r/t loss of kidney

Risk for **Bleeding**: Risk factor: surgery

Risk for **Electrolyte** imbalance: Risk factor: renal dysfunction

Risk for imbalanced **Fluid** volume: Risk factors: vascular losses, decreased intake

Risk for **Infection**: Risk factors: invasive procedure, lack of deep breathing because of location of surgical incision

Risk for ineffective renal **Perfusion**: Risk factor: renal disease

Nephrostomy, Percutaneous

Acute **Pain** r/t invasive procedure

Impaired **Urinary** elimination r/t nephrostomy tube

Risk for **Infection**: Risk factor: invasive procedure

Nephrotic Syndrome

Activity intolerance r/t generalized edema

Disturbed **Body** image r/t edematous appearance and side effects of steroid therapy

Excess **Fluid** volume r/t edema resulting from oncotic fluid shift caused by serum protein loss and renal retention of salt and water

Imbalanced **Nutrition**: less than body requirements r/t anorexia, protein loss

Imbalanced **Nutrition**: more than body requirements r/t increased appetite attributable to steroid therapy

Social isolation r/t edematous appearance

Risk for **Infection**: Risk factor: altered immune mechanisms caused by disease and effects of steroids

Risk for ineffective renal **Perfusion**: Risk factor: renal disease

Risk for impaired **Skin** integrity: Risk factor: edema

See Child with Chronic Condition; Hospitalized Child

Nerve Entrapment

See Carpal Tunnel Syndrome

Neural Tube Defects (Meningocele, Myelomeningocele, Spina Bifida, Anencephaly)

Constipation r/t immobility or less than adequate mobility

Grieving r/t loss of perfect child, birth of child with congenital defect

Delayed **Growth** and development r/t physical impairments, possible cognitive impairment

Reflex urinary **Incontinence** r/t neurogenic impairment

Total urinary **Incontinence** r/t neurogenic impairment

Urge urinary **Incontinence** r/t neurogenic impairment

Impaired **Mobility** r/t neuromuscular impairment

Chronic low **Self-Esteem** r/t perceived differences, decreased ability to participate in physical and social activities at school

Disturbed **Sensory** perception: visual r/t altered reception caused by strabismus

Impaired **Skin** integrity r/t incontinence

Risk for latex **Allergy** response: Risk factor: multiple exposures to latex products

Risk for imbalanced **Nutrition**: more than body requirements: Risk factors: diminished, limited, or impaired physical activity

Risk for **Powerlessness**: Risk factor: debilitating disease

Risk for impaired **Skin** integrity: lower extremities: Risk factor: decreased sensory perception

Readiness for enhanced family **Coping**: effective adaptive response by family members

Readiness for enhanced **Family** processes: family supports each other

See Child with Chronic Condition; Premature Infant (Child)

Neuralgia

See Trigeminal Neuralgia

N

Neuritis (Peripheral Neuropathy)

Activity intolerance r/t pain with movement

Ineffective **Health** maintenance r/t deficient knowledge regarding self-care with neuritis

Acute **Pain** r/t stimulation of affected nerve endings, inflammation of sensory nerves

See Neuropathy, Peripheral

Neurofibromatosis

Disturbed **Energy** field r/t disease

Compromised **Family** coping r/t cost and emotional needs of disease

Disturbed **Sensory** perception r/t optic nerve gliomas associated with disease

Impaired **Skin** integrity r/t café-au-lait spots

Risk for delayed **Development**: learning disorders including attention deficit–hyperactivity disorder, low intelligent quotient scores, and developmental delay: Risk factor: genetic disorder

Risk for disproportionate **Growth**: short stature, precocious puberty, delayed maturation, thyroid disorders: Risk factor: genetic disorder

Risk for **Injury**: Risk factor: possible problems with balance

Risk for decreased cardiac tissue **Perfusion**: Risk factor: hypertension

Risk for compromised **Resilience**: Risk factor: presence of chronic disease

Risk for **Spiritual** distress: Risk factor: possible severity of disease

Readiness for enhanced **Decision-Making**: expresses desire to enhance understanding of choices and meaning of choices, genetic counseling

Readiness for enhanced **Self Health** management: seeks cancer screening, education and genetic counseling

See Abdominal Distension; Surgery, Perioperative; Surgery, Postoperative; Surgery, Preoperative

Neurogenic Bladder

Overflow urinary **Incontinence** r/t detrusor external sphincter dyssynergia

Reflex urinary **Incontinence** r/t neurological impairment

Urinary retention r/t interruption in the lateral spinal tracts

Risk for latex **Allergy** response: Risk factors: repeated exposures to latex associated with possible repeated catheterizations

Neurologic Disorders

Ineffective **Airway** clearance r/t perceptual or cognitive impairment, decreased energy, fatigue

Acute **Confusion** r/t dementia, alcohol abuse, drug abuse, delirium

Ineffective **Coping** r/t disability requiring change in lifestyle

Disturbed **Energy** field r/t illness

Interrupted **Family** processes r/t situational crisis, illness, or disability of family member

Grieving r/t loss of usual body functioning

Impaired **Home** maintenance r/t client's or family member's disease

Impaired **Memory** r/t neurological disturbance

Impaired physical **Mobility** r/t neuromuscular impairment

Imbalanced **Nutrition**: less than body requirements r/t impaired swallowing, depression, difficulty feeding self

Powerlessness r/t progressive nature of disease

Self-Care deficit: specify r/t neuromuscular dysfunction

Sexual dysfunction r/t biopsychosocial alteration of sexuality

Social isolation r/t altered state of wellness

Impaired **Swallowing** r/t neuromuscular dysfunction

Wandering r/t cognitive impairment

Risk for **Disuse** syndrome: Risk factors: physical immobility, neuromuscular dysfunction

Risk for **Injury**: Risk factors: altered mobility, sensory dysfunction, cognitive impairment

Risk for ineffective cerebral tissue **Perfusion**: Risk factor: cerebral disease/injury

Risk for impaired **Religiosity**: Risk factor: life transition

Risk for impaired **Skin** integrity: Risk factors: altered sensation, altered mental status, paralysis

See specific condition: Alcohol Withdrawal; Amyotrophic Lateral Sclerosis (ALS); CVA (Cerebrovascular Accident); Delirium; Dementia; Guillain-Barré Syndrome; Head Injury; Huntington's Disease; Multiple Sclerosis (MS); Myasthenia Gravis; Muscular Dystrophy' Parkinson's Disease

Neuropathy, Peripheral

Chronic **Pain** r/t damage to nerves in the peripheral nervous system as a result of medication side effects, vitamin deficiency, or diabetes

Ineffective **Thermoregulation** r/t decreased ability to regulate body temperature

Risk for **Injury**: Risk factors: lack of muscle control, decreased sensation

See Peripheral Vascular Disease (PVD)

Neurosurgery

See Craniectomy/Craniotomy

Newborn, Normal

Effective **Breastfeeding** r/t normal oral structure and gestational age greater than 34 weeks

Ineffective **Protection** r/t immature immune system

Ineffective **Thermoregulation** r/t immaturity of neuroendocrine system

Risk for sudden infant **Death** syndrome: Risk factors: lack of knowledge regarding infant sleeping in prone or side-lying position, prenatal or postnatal infant smoke exposure, infant overheating or overwrapping, loose articles in the sleep environment

Risk for **Infection**: Risk factor: open umbilical stump

Risk for **Injury**: Risk factors: immaturity, need for caretaking

Readiness for enhanced **Childbearing** process: appropriate care of newborn

N

Readiness for enhanced organized **Infant** behavior: demonstrates adaptive response to pain

Readiness for enhanced **Parenting**: providing emotional and physical needs of infant

Newborn, Postmature

Hypothermia r/t depleted stores of subcutaneous fat

Impaired **Skin** integrity r/t cracked and peeling skin as a result of decreased vernix

Risk for ineffective **Airway** clearance: Risk factor: meconium aspiration

Risk for unstable **Glucose** level: Risk factor: depleted glycogen stores

Risk for **Injury**: Risk factor: hypoglycemia caused by depleted glycogen stores

Newborn, Small for Gestational Age (SGA)

Neonatal **Jaundice** r/t neonate age and difficulty feeding

Imbalanced **Nutrition**: less than body requirements r/t history of placental insufficiency

Ineffective **Thermoregulation** r/t decreased brown fat, subcutaneous fat

Risk for sudden infant **Death** syndrome: Risk factor: low birth weight

Risk for delayed **Development**: Risk factor: history of placental insufficiency

Risk for disproportionate **Growth**: Risk factor: history of placental insufficiency

Risk for **Injury**: Risk factors: hypoglycemia, perinatal asphyxia, meconium aspiration

Nicotine Addiction

Risk-prone health **Behavior** r/t smoking

Ineffective **Health** maintenance r/t lack of ability to make a judgment about smoking cessation

Powerlessness r/t perceived lack of control over ability to give up nicotine

Readiness for enhanced **Decision-Making**: expresses desire to enhance understanding and meaning of choices

Readiness for enhanced **Self Health** management: expresses desire to learn measures to stop smoking

NIDDM (Non–Insulin-Dependent Diabetes Mellitus)

Readiness for enhanced **Self Health** management: expresses desire for information on exercise and diet to manage diabetes

See Diabetes Mellitus

Nightmares

Disturbed **Energy** field r/t disharmony of body and mind

Post-Trauma syndrome r/t disaster, war, epidemic, rape, assault, torture, catastrophic illness, or accident

Nipple Soreness

Impaired **Comfort** r/t physical condition

See Painful Breasts, Sore Nipples

Nocturia

Urge urinary **Incontinence** r/t decreased bladder capacity, irritation of bladder stretch receptors causing spasm, alcohol, caffeine, increased fluids, increased urine concentration, overdistention of bladder

Impaired **Urinary** elimination r/t sensory motor impairment, urinary tract infection

Risk for **Powerlessness**: Risk factor: inability to control nighttime voiding

Nocturnal Myoclonus

See Restless Leg Syndrome; Stress

Nocturnal Paroxysmal Dyspnea

See PND (Paroxysmal Nocturnal Dyspnea)

Noncompliance

Noncompliance (See **Noncompliance**, Section III)

Non–Insulin-Dependent Diabetes Mellitus (NIDDM)

See Diabetes Mellitus

Normal Pressure Hydrocephalus (NPH)

Impaired verbal **Communication** r/t obstruction of flow of cerebrospinal fluid

Acute **Confusion** r/t dementia caused by obstruction to flow of cerebrospinal fluid

Impaired **Memory** r/t neurological disturbance

Risk for **Falls**: Risk factor: unsteady gait as a result of obstruction of cerebrospinal fluid

Risk for ineffective cerebral tissue **Perfusion**: Risk factor: fluid pressing on the brain

Norwalk Virus

See Viral Gastroenteritis

NSTEMI (non–ST-elevation myocardial infarction)

See MI (Myocardial Infarction)

Nursing

See Breastfeeding, Effective; Breastfeeding, Ineffective; Breastfeeding, Interrupted

Nutrition

Readiness for enhanced **Nutrition** (See **Nutrition**, readiness for enhanced, Section III)

Nutrition, Imbalanced

Imbalanced **Nutrition**: less than body requirements (See **Nutrition**: less than body requirements, imbalanced, Section III)

Imbalanced **Nutrition**: more than body requirements (See **Nutrition**: more than body requirements, imbalanced, Section III)

Risk for imbalanced **Nutrition**: more than body requirements (See **Nutrition**: more than body requirements, imbalanced, risk for, Section III)

O

Obesity

Risk-prone health **Behavior**: r/t negative attitude toward health care

Disturbed **Body** image r/t eating disorder, excess weight

Imbalanced **Nutrition**: more than body requirements r/t caloric intake exceeding energy expenditure

Chronic low **Self-Esteem** r/t ineffective coping, overeating

Readiness for enhanced **Nutrition**: expresses willingness to enhance nutrition

OBS (Organic Brain Syndrome)

See Organic Mental Disorders

Obsessive-Compulsive Disorder (OCD)

See OCD (Obsessive-Compulsive Disorder)

Obstruction, Bowel

See Bowel Obstruction

Obstructive Sleep Apnea

Insomnia r/t blocked airway

Imbalanced **Nutrition**: more than body requirements r/t excessive intake related to metabolic need

See PND (Paroxysmal Nocturnal Dyspnea)

OCD (Obsessive-Compulsive Disorder)

Ineffective **Activity** planning r/t unrealistic perception of events

Anxiety r/t threat to self-concept, unmet needs

Risk-prone health **Behavior** r/t inadequate comprehension associated with repetitive thoughts

Decisional **Conflict** r/t inability to make a decision for fear of reprisal

Disabled family **Coping** r/t family process being disrupted by client's ritualistic activities

Ineffective **Coping** r/t expression of feelings in an unacceptable way, ritualistic behavior

Powerlessness r/t unrelenting repetitive thoughts to perform irrational activities

Impaired individual **Resilience** r/t psychological disorder

Risk for situational low **Self-Esteem**: Risk factor: inability to control repetitive thoughts and actions

ODD (Oppositional Defiant Disorder)

Anxiety r/t feelings of anger and hostility toward authority figures

Risk-prone health **Behavior** r/t multiple stressors associated with condition

Ineffective **Coping** r/t lack of self-control or perceived lack of self-control

Disabled **Family** coping r/t feelings of anger, hostility; defiant behavior toward authority figures

Chronic or situational low **Self-Esteem** r/t poor self-control and disruptive behaviors

Impaired **Social** interaction r/t being touchy or easily annoyed, blaming others for own mistakes, constant trouble in school

Social isolation r/t unaccepted social behavior

Ineffective family **Therapeutic** regimen management r/t difficulty in limit setting and managing oppositional behaviors

Risk for impaired **Parenting**: Risk factors: children's difficult behaviors and inability to set limits

Risk for **Powerlessness**: Risk factor: inability to deal with difficulty behaviors

Risk for **Spiritual** distress: Risk factors: anxiety and stress in dealing with difficulty behaviors

Risk for other-directed **Violence**: Risk factors: history of violence, threats of violence against others; history of antisocial behavior; history of indirect violence

Older Adult

See Aging

Oliguria

Deficient **Fluid** volume r/t active fluid loss, failure of regulatory mechanism

See Cardiac Output, Decreased; Renal Failure; Shock, Hypovolemic

Omphalocele

See Gastroschisis/Omphalocele

Oophorectomy

Risk for ineffective **Sexuality** pattern: Risk factor: altered body function

See Surgery, Perioperative; Surgery, Postoperative; Surgery, Preoperative

OPCAB (Off-Pump Coronary Artery Bypass)

See Angioplasty, Coronary; Coronary Artery Bypass Grafting (CABG)

Open Heart Surgery

Risk for decreased cardiac tissue **Perfusion**: Risk factor: cardiac surgery

See Coronary Artery Bypass Grafting (CABG); Dysrhythmia

Open Reduction of Fracture with Internal Fixation (Femur)

Anxiety r/t outcome of corrective procedure

Impaired physical **Mobility** r/t postoperative position, abduction of leg, avoidance of acute flexion

Powerlessness r/t loss of control, unanticipated change in lifestyle

Risk for perioperative positioning **Injury**: Risk factor: immobilization

Risk for **Peripheral** neurovascular dysfunction: Risk factors: mechanical compression, orthopedic surgery, immobilization

See Surgery, Postoperative Care

O

Opiate Use

Risk for **Constipation**: Risk factor: effects of opiates on peristalsis

See Drug Abuse; Drug Withdrawal

Opportunistic Infection

Delayed **Surgical** recovery r/t abnormal blood profiles, impaired healing

Risk for **Infection**: Risk factor: abnormal blood profiles

See AIDS (Acquired Immunodeficiency Syndrome); HIV (Human Immunodeficiency Virus)

Oppositional Defiant Disorder (ODD)

See ODD (Oppositional Defiant Disorder)

Oral Mucous Membrane, Impaired

Impaired **Oral** mucous membrane (See **Oral** mucous membrane, impaired, Section III)

Oral Thrush

See Candidiasis, Oral

Orchitis

Readiness for enhanced **Self Health** management: follows recommendations for mumps vaccination

See Epididymitis

Organic Mental Disorders

Adult **Failure** to thrive r/t undetected organic mental disorder

Impaired **Social** interaction r/t disturbed thought processes

Risk for **Injury**: Risk factors: disorientation to time, place, person

See Dementia

Orthopedic Traction

Ineffective **Role** performance r/t limited physical mobility

Impaired **Social** interaction r/t limited physical mobility

Impaired **Transfer** ability r/t limited physical mobility

Risk for impaired **Religiosity**: Risk factor: immobility

See Traction and Casts

Orthopnea

Ineffective **Breathing** pattern r/t inability to breathe with head of bed flat

Decreased **Cardiac** output r/t inability of heart to meet demands of body

Orthostatic Hypotension

See Dizziness

Osteoarthritis

Activity intolerance r/t pain after exercise or use of joint

Acute **Pain** r/t movement

Impaired **Transfer** ability r/t pain

See Arthritis

Osteomyelitis

Deficient **Diversional** activity r/t prolonged immobilization, hospitalization

Fear: parental r/t concern regarding possible growth plate damage caused by infection, concern that infection may become chronic

Ineffective **Health** maintenance r/t continued immobility at home, possible extensive casts, continued antibiotics

Hyperthermia r/t infectious process

Impaired physical **Mobility** r/t imposed immobility as a result of infected area

Acute **Pain** r/t inflammation in affected extremity

Risk for **Constipation**: Risk factor: immobility

Risk for **Infection**: Risk factor: inadequate primary and secondary defenses

Risk for impaired **Skin** integrity: Risk factor: irritation from splint or cast

See Hospitalized Child

Osteoporosis

Deficient **Knowledge** r/t diet, exercise, need to abstain from alcohol and nicotine

Impaired physical **Mobility** r/t pain, skeletal changes

Imbalanced **Nutrition**: less than body requirements r/t inadequate intake of calcium and vitamin D

Acute **Pain** r/t fracture, muscle spasms

Risk for **Injury**: fracture: Risk factors: lack of activity, risk of falling resulting from environmental hazards, neuromuscular disorders, diminished senses, cardiovascular responses, responses to drugs

Risk for **Powerlessness**: Risk factor: debilitating disease

Readiness for enhanced **Self Health** management: expresses desire to manage the treatment of illness and prevent complications

Ostomy

See Child with Chronic Condition; Colostomy; Ileal Conduit; Ileostomy

Otitis Media

Acute **Pain** r/t inflammation, infectious process

Disturbed **Sensory** perception: auditory r/t incomplete resolution of otitis media, presence of excess drainage in middle ear

Risk for delayed **Development**: speech and language: Risk factor: frequent otitis media

Risk for **Infection**: Risk factors: eustachian tube obstruction, traumatic eardrum perforation, infectious disease process

Readiness for enhanced **Knowledge**: information on treatment and prevention of disease

Ovarian Carcinoma

Death **Anxiety** r/t unknown outcome, possible poor prognosis

Fear r/t unknown outcome, possible poor prognosis

Ineffective **Health** maintenance r/t deficient knowledge regarding self-care, treatment of condition

Readiness for enhanced **Family** processes: family functioning meets needs of client

O

Readiness for enhanced **Resilience**: participates in support groups

See Chemotherapy; Hysterectomy; Radiation Therapy

P

Pacemaker

Anxiety r/t change in health status, presence of pacemaker

Death **Anxiety** r/t worry over possible malfunction of pacemaker

Deficient **Knowledge** r/t self-care program, when to seek medical attention

Acute **Pain** r/t surgical procedure

Risk for **Bleeding**: Risk factor: surgery

Risk for **Infection**: Risk factors: invasive procedure, presence of foreign body (catheter and generator)

Risk for decreased cardiac tissue **Perfusion**: Risk factor: pacemaker malfunction

Risk for **Powerlessness**: Risk factor: presence of electronic device to stimulate heart

Readiness for enhanced **Self Health** management: appropriate health care management of pacemaker

Paget's Disease

Disturbed **Body** image r/t possible enlarged head, bowed tibias, kyphosis

Deficient **Knowledge** r/t appropriate diet high in protein and calcium, mild exercise

Chronic **Sorrow** r/t chronic condition with altered body image

Risk for **Trauma**: fracture: Risk factor: excessive bone destruction

Pain, Acute

Disturbed **Energy** field r/t unbalanced energy field

Acute **Pain** (See **Pain**, acute, Section III)

Pain, Chronic

Impaired **Comfort** r/t altered health status

Disturbed **Energy** field r/t unbalanced energy field

Chronic **Pain** (See **Pain**, chronic, Section III)

Painful Breasts, Engorgement

Impaired **Comfort** r/t physical condition

Acute **Pain** r/t distention of breast tissue

Ineffective **Role** performance r/t change in physical capacity to assume role of breastfeeding mother

Impaired **Tissue** integrity r/t excessive fluid in breast tissues

Risk for ineffective **Breastfeeding**: Risk factors: pain, infant's inability to latch on to engorged breast

Risk for **Infection**: Risk factor: milk stasis

Risk for disturbed **Maternal/Fetal** dyad: Risk factor: discomfort

Painful Breasts, Sore Nipples

Ineffective **Breastfeeding** r/t pain

Impaired **Comfort** r/t physical condition

Acute **Pain** r/t cracked nipples

Ineffective **Role** performance r/t change in physical capacity to assume role of breastfeeding mother

Impaired **Skin** integrity r/t mechanical factors involved in suckling, breastfeeding management

Risk for **Infection**: Risk factor: break in skin

Pallor of Extremities

Ineffective peripheral tissue **Perfusion** r/t interruption of vascular flow

Palpitations (Heart Palpitations)

See Dysrhythmia

Pancreatic Cancer

Death **Anxiety** r/t possible poor prognosis of disease process

Ineffective family **Coping** r/t poor prognosis

Fear r/t poor prognosis of the disease

Grieving r/t shortened life span

Deficient **Knowledge** r/t disease-induced diabetes, home management

Spiritual distress r/t poor prognosis

Risk for impaired **Liver** function: Risk factor: complications from underlying disease

See Cancer; Chemotherapy; Radiation Therapy; Surgery, Perioperative; Surgery, Postoperative; Surgery, Preoperative

Pancreatitis

Ineffective **Breathing** pattern r/t splinting from severe pain

Ineffective **Denial** r/t ineffective coping, alcohol use

Diarrhea r/t decrease in pancreatic secretions resulting in steatorrhea

Adult **Failure** to thrive r/t pain

Deficient **Fluid** volume r/t vomiting, decreased fluid intake, fever, diaphoresis, fluid shifts

Ineffective **Health** maintenance r/t deficient knowledge concerning diet, alcohol use, medication

Nausea r/t irritation of gastrointestinal system

Imbalanced **Nutrition**: less than body requirements r/t inadequate dietary intake, increased nutritional needs as a result of acute illness, increased metabolic needs caused by increased body temperature

Acute **Pain** r/t irritation and edema of the inflamed pancreas

Chronic **Sorrow** r/t chronic illness

Readiness for enhanced **Comfort**: expresses desire to enhance comfort

Panic Disorder (Panic Attacks)

Ineffective **Activity** planning r/t unrealistic perception of events

Anxiety r/t situational crisis

P

Risk-prone health **Behavior** r/t low self-efficacy

Ineffective **Coping** r/t personal vulnerability

Disturbed personal **Identity** r/t situational crisis

Post-Trauma syndrome r/t previous catastrophic event

Social isolation r/t fear of lack of control

Risk for **Loneliness**: Risk factor: inability to socially interact because of fear of losing control

Risk for **Post-Trauma** syndrome: Risk factors: perception of the event, diminished ego strength

Risk for **Powerlessness**: Risk factor: ineffective coping skills

Readiness for enhanced **Coping**: seeks problem-oriented and emotion-oriented strategies to manage condition

See Anxiety; Anxiety Disorder

Paralysis

Disturbed **Body** image r/t biophysical changes, loss of movement, immobility

Impaired **Comfort** r/t prolonged immobility

Constipation r/t effects of spinal cord disruption, inadequate fiber in diet

Ineffective **Health** maintenance r/t deficient knowledge regarding self-care with paralysis

Impaired **Home** maintenance r/t physical disability

Reflex urinary **Incontinence** r/t neurological impairment

Impaired physical **Mobility** r/t neuromuscular impairment

Impaired wheelchair **Mobility** r/t neuromuscular impairment

Self **Neglect** r/t functional impairment

Powerlessness r/t illness-related regimen

Self-Care deficit: specify r/t neuromuscular impairment

Sexual dysfunction r/t loss of sensation, biopsychosocial alteration

Chronic **Sorrow** r/t loss of physical mobility

Impaired **Transfer** ability r/t paralysis

Risk for latex **Allergy** response: Risk factor: possible repeated urinary catheterizations

Risk for **Disuse** syndrome: Risk factor: paralysis

Risk for **Falls**: Risk factor: paralysis

Risk for **Injury**: Risk factors: altered mobility, sensory dysfunction

Risk for **Post-Trauma** syndrome: Risk factor: event causing paralysis

Risk for impaired **Religiosity**: Risk factors: immobility, possible lack of transportation

Risk for compromised **Resilience**: Risk factor: chronic disability

Risk for situational low **Self-Esteem**: Risk factor: change in body image and function

Risk for impaired **Skin** integrity: Risk factors: altered circulation, altered sensation, immobility

Readiness for enhanced **Self-Care**: expresses desire to enhance knowledge and responsibility for strategies for self-care

See Child with Chronic Condition; Hemiplegia; Hospitalized Child; Neural Tube Defects; Spinal Cord Injury

Paralytic Ileus

Constipation r/t decreased gastric motility

Deficient **Fluid** volume r/t loss of fluids from vomiting, retention of fluid in bowel

Dysfunctional **Gastrointestinal** motility r/t bowel obstruction

Nausea r/t gastrointestinal irritation

Impaired **Oral** mucous membrane r/t presence of nasogastric tube

Acute **Pain** r/t pressure, abdominal distention

See Bowel Obstruction

Paranoid Personality Disorder

Ineffective **Activity** planning r/t unrealistic perception of events

Anxiety r/t uncontrollable intrusive, suspicious thoughts

Risk-prone health **Behavior** r/t intense emotional state

Disturbed personal **Identity** r/t difficulty with reality testing

Impaired individual **Resilience** r/t psychological disorder

Chronic low **Self-Esteem** r/t inability to trust others

Disturbed **Sensory** perception: specify r/t psychological dysfunction, suspicious thoughts

Social isolation r/t inappropriate social skills

Risk for **Loneliness**: Risk factor: social isolation

Risk for **Post-Trauma** syndrome: Risk factor: exaggerated sense of responsibility

Risk for **Suicide**: Risk factor: psychiatric illness

Risk for other-directed **Violence**: Risk factor: being suspicious of others and others' actions

Paraplegia

See Spinal Cord Injury

Parathyroidectomy

Anxiety r/t surgery

Risk for ineffective **Airway** clearance: Risk factors: edema or hematoma formation, airway obstruction

Risk for **Bleeding**: Risk factor: surgery

Risk for impaired verbal **Communication**: Risk factors: possible laryngeal damage, edema

Risk for **Infection**: Risk factor: surgical procedure

See Hypocalcemia

Parent Attachment

Risk for impaired **Attachment** (See **Attachment**, impaired, risk for, Section III)

Readiness for enhanced **Childbearing** process: demonstrates appropriate care of newborn

See Parental Role Conflict

Parental Role Conflict

Parental role **Conflict** (See **Conflict**, parental role, Section III)

Chronic **Sorrow** r/t difficult parent-child relationship

Risk for **Spiritual** distress: Risk factor: altered relationships

Readiness for enhanced **Parenting**: willingness to enhance parenting

P

Parenting

Readiness for enhanced **Parenting** (See **Parenting**, readiness for enhanced, Section III)

Parenting, Impaired

Impaired **Parenting** (See **Parenting**, impaired, Section III)

Chronic **Sorrow** r/t difficult parent-child relationship

Risk for **Spiritual** distress: Risk factor: altered relationships

Parenting, Risk for Impaired

Risk for impaired **Parenting** (See **Parenting**, impaired, risk for, Section III)

See Parenting, Impaired

Paresthesia

Disturbed **Sensory** perception: tactile r/t altered sensory reception, transmission, integration

Risk for **Injury** r/t inability to feel temperature changes, pain

Parkinson's Disease

Impaired verbal **Communication** r/t decreased speech volume, slowness of speech, impaired facial muscles

Constipation r/t weakness of defecation muscles, lack of exercise, inadequate fluid intake, decreased autonomic nervous system activity

Adult **Failure** to thrive r/t depression associated with chronic progressive disease

Imbalanced **Nutrition**: less than body requirements r/t tremor, slowness in eating, difficulty in chewing and swallowing

Chronic **Sorrow** r/t loss of physical capacity

Risk for **Injury**: Risk factors: tremors, slow reactions, altered gait

See Neurologic Disorders

Paroxysmal Nocturnal Dyspnea (PND)

See PND (Paroxysmal Nocturnal Dyspnea)

Patent Ductus Arteriosus (PDA)

See Congenital Heart Disease/Cardiac Anomalies

Patient-Controlled Analgesia (PCA)

See PCA (Patient-Controlled Analgesia)

Patient Education

Deficient **Knowledge** r/t lack of exposure to information, information misinterpretation, unfamiliarity with information resources to manage illness

Readiness for enhanced **Decision-Making**: expresses desire to enhance understanding of choices for decision making

Readiness for enhanced **Knowledge** (specify): interest in learning

Readiness for enhanced **Self Health** management: expresses desire for information to manage the illness

Readiness for enhanced **Spiritual** well-being: desires to reach harmony with self, others, higher power/God

PCA (Patient-Controlled Analgesia)

Impaired **Comfort** r/t condition requiring PCA, pruritus from medication side effects

Deficient **Knowledge** r/t self-care of pain control

Nausea r/t side effects of medication

Risk for **Injury**: Risk factors: possible complications associated with PCA

Risk for vascular **Trauma**: Risk factor: insertion site and length of insertion time

Readiness for enhanced **Knowledge**: appropriate management of PCA

Pectus Excavatum

See Marfan Syndrome

Pediculosis

See Lice

PEG (Percutaneous Endoscopic Gastrostomy)

See Tube Feeding

Pelvic Inflammatory Disease (PID)

See PID (Pelvic Inflammatory Disease)

Penile Prosthesis

Ineffective **Sexuality** pattern r/t use of penile prosthesis

Risk for **Infection**: Risk factor: invasive surgical procedure

Risk for situational low **Self-Esteem**: Risk factors: ineffective sexuality pattern

Readiness for enhanced **Self Health** management: seeks information regarding care and use of prosthesis

See Erectile Dysfunction (ED); Impotence

Peptic Ulcer

See Ulcer, Peptic (Duodenal or Gastric)

Percutaneous Transluminal Coronary Angioplasty (PTCA)

See Angioplasty, Coronary

Pericardial Friction Rub

Acute **Pain** r/t inflammation, effusion

Delayed **Surgical** recovery r/t complications associated with cardiac problems

Risk for decreased cardiac tissue **Perfusion**: Risk factors: inflammation in pericardial sac, fluid accumulation compressing heart

Pericarditis

Activity intolerance r/t reduced cardiac reserve, prescribed bed rest

Deficient **Knowledge** r/t unfamiliarity with information sources

Acute **Pain** r/t biological injury, inflammation

Delayed **Surgical** recovery r/t complications associated with cardiac problems

Risk for imbalanced **Nutrition**: less than body requirements r/t fever, hypermetabolic state associated with fever

Risk for decreased cardiac tissue **Perfusion**: Risk factor: inflammation in pericardial sac

P

Risk for ineffective renal **Perfusion**: Risk factor: decreased cardiac tissue perfusion

Perioperative Positioning

Risk for perioperative positioning **Injury** (See **Injury**, positioning, perioperative, risk for, Section III)

Peripheral Neuropathy

See Neuropathy, Peripheral

Peripheral Neurovascular Dysfunction

Risk for **Peripheral** neurovascular dysfunction (See **Peripheral** neurovascular dysfunction, risk for, Section III)

See Neuropathy, Peripheral; Peripheral Vascular Disease (PVD)

Peripheral Vascular Disease (PVD)

Activity intolerance r/t imbalance between peripheral oxygen supply and demand

Ineffective **Health** maintenance r/t deficient knowledge regarding self-care and treatment of disease

Chronic **Pain**: intermittent claudication r/t ischemia

Ineffective peripheral tissue **Perfusion** r/t disease process

Risk for **Falls**: Risk factor: altered mobility

Risk for **Injury**: Risk factors: tissue hypoxia, altered mobility, altered sensation

Risk for **Peripheral** neurovascular dysfunction: Risk factor: possible vascular obstruction

Risk for impaired **Skin** integrity: Risk factor: altered circulation or sensation

Readiness for enhanced **Self Health** management: self-care and treatment of disease

See Neuropathy, Peripheral; Peripheral Neurovascular Dysfunction

Peritoneal Dialysis

Ineffective **Breathing** pattern r/t pressure from dialysate

Impaired **Home** maintenance r/t complex home treatment of client

Deficient **Knowledge** r/t treatment procedure, self-care with peritoneal dialysis

Acute **Pain** r/t instillation of dialysate, temperature of dialysate

Chronic **Sorrow** r/t chronic disability

Risk for ineffective **Coping**: Risk factor: disability requiring change in lifestyle

Risk for imbalanced **Fluid** volume: Risk factor: medical procedure

Risk for **Infection**: peritoneal: Risk factor: invasive procedure, presence of catheter, dialysate

Risk for **Powerlessness**: Risk factor: chronic condition and care involved

See Child with Chronic Condition; Hemodialysis; Hospitalized Child; Renal Failure; Renal Failure, Acute/Chronic, Child

Peritonitis

Ineffective **Breathing** pattern r/t pain, increased abdominal pressure

Constipation r/t decreased oral intake, decrease of peristalsis

Deficient **Fluid** volume r/t retention of fluid in bowel with loss of circulating blood volume

Nausea r/t gastrointestinal irritation

Imbalanced **Nutrition**: less than body requirements r/t nausea, vomiting

Acute **Pain** r/t inflammation, stimulation of somatic nerves

Risk for dysfunctional gastrointestinal **Motility**: Risk factor: gastrointestinal disease

Pernicious Anemia

Diarrhea r/t malabsorption of nutrients

Fatigue r/t imbalanced nutrition: less than body requirements

Impaired **Memory** r/t anemia; lack of adequate red blood cells

Nausea r/t altered oral mucous membrane; sore tongue, bleeding gums

Imbalanced **Nutrition**: less than body requirements r/t lack of appetite associated with nausea and altered oral mucous membrane

Impaired **Oral** mucous membrane r/t vitamin deficiency; inability to absorb vitamin B_{12} associated with lack of intrinsic factor

Risk for **Falls**: Risk factors: dizziness, lightheadedness

Risk for **Peripheral** neurovascular dysfunction: Risk factor: anemia

Persistent Fetal Circulation

See Congenital Heart Disease/Cardiac Anomalies

Personal Identity Problems

Disturbed personal **Identity** (See **Identity**, personal, disturbed, Section III)

Personality Disorder

Ineffective **Activity** planning r/t unrealistic perception of events

Impaired individual **Resilience** r/t psychological disorder

See specific disorder: Antisocial Personality Disorder; Borderline Personality Disorder; OCD (Obsessive-Compulsive Disorder); Paranoid Personality Disorder

Pertussis (Whooping Cough)

See Respiratory Infections, Acute Childhood

Pesticide Contamination

Contamination r/t use of environmental contaminants; pesticides

Risk for disproportionate **Growth**: Risk factor: environmental contamination

Petechiae

See Anticoagulant Therapy; Clotting Disorder; DIC (Disseminated Intravascular Coagulation); Hemophilia

Petit Mal Seizure

Readiness for enhanced **Self Health** management: wears medical alert bracelet; limits hazardous activities such as driving, swimming, working at heights, operating equipment

See Epilepsy

Pharyngitis

See Sore Throat

Phenylketonuria (PKU)

See PKU (Phenylketonuria)

Pheochromocytoma

Anxiety r/t symptoms from increased catecholamines—headache, palpitations, sweating, nervousness, nausea, vomiting, syncope

Ineffective **Health** maintenance r/t deficient knowledge regarding treatment and self-care

Insomnia r/t high levels of catecholamines

Nausea r/t increased catecholamines

Risk for decreased cardiac tissue **Perfusion**: Risk factor: hypertension

See Surgery, Perioperative; Surgery, Postoperative; Surgery, Preoperative

Phlebitis

See Thrombophlebitis

Phobia (Specific)

Fear r/t presence or anticipation of specific object or situation

Powerlessness r/t anxiety about encountering unknown or known entity

Impaired individual **Resilience** r/t psychological disorder

Readiness for enhanced **Power**: expresses readiness to enhance identification of choices that can be made for change

See Anxiety; Anxiety Disorder; Panic Disorder (Panic Attacks)

Photosensitivity

Ineffective **Health** maintenance r/t deficient knowledge regarding medications inducing photosensitivity

Risk for impaired **Skin** integrity: Risk factor: exposure to sun

Physical Abuse

See Abuse, Child; Abuse, Spouse, Parent, or Significant Other

Pica

Anxiety r/t stress from urge to eat nonnutritive substances

Imbalanced **Nutrition**: less than body requirements r/t eating nonnutritive substances

Impaired **Parenting** r/t lack of supervision, food deprivation

Risk for **Constipation**: Risk factor: presence of undigestible materials in gastrointestinal tract

Risk for **Infection**: Risk factor: ingestion of infectious agents via contaminated substances

Risk for gastrointestinal **Motility**: Risk factor: abnormal eating behavior

Risk for **Poisoning**: Risk factor: ingestion of substances containing lead

See Anemia

PID (Pelvic Inflammatory Disease)

Ineffective **Health** maintenance r/t deficient knowledge regarding self-care, treatment of disease

Acute **Pain** r/t biological injury; inflammation, edema, congestion of pelvic tissues

Ineffective **Sexuality** pattern r/t medically imposed abstinence from sexual activities until acute infection subsides, change in reproductive potential

Risk for urge urinary **Incontinence**: Risk factors: inflammation, edema, congestion of pelvic tissues

Risk for **Infection**: Risk factors: insufficient knowledge to avoid exposure to pathogens; proper hygiene, nutrition, other health habits

See Maturational Issues, Adolescent; STD (Sexually Transmitted Disease)

PIH (Pregnancy-Induced Hypertension/Preeclampsia)

Anxiety r/t fear of the unknown, threat to self and infant, change in role functioning

Death **Anxiety** r/t threat of preeclampsia

Deficient **Diversional** activity r/t bed rest

Interrupted **Family** processes r/t situational crisis

Impaired **Home** maintenance r/t bed rest

Deficient **Knowledge** r/t lack of experience with situation

Impaired physical **Mobility** r/t medically prescribed limitations

Impaired **Parenting** r/t bed rest

Powerlessness r/t complication threatening pregnancy, medically prescribed limitations

Ineffective **Role** performance r/t change in physical capacity to assume role of pregnant woman or resume other roles

Situational low **Self-Esteem** r/t loss of idealized pregnancy

Impaired **Social** interaction r/t imposed bed rest

Risk for imbalanced **Fluid** volume: Risk factors: hypertension, altered renal function

Risk for **Injury**: fetal: Risk factors: decreased uteroplacental perfusion, seizures

Risk for **Injury**: maternal: Risk factors: vasospasm, high blood pressure

Readiness for enhanced **Knowledge**: desire for information on managing condition

See Malignant Hypertension (Arteriolar Nephrosclerosis)

Piloerection

Hypothermia r/t exposure to cold environment

Pimples

See Acne

Pink Eye

See Conjunctivitis

Pinworms

Impaired **Comfort** r/t itching

Impaired **Home** maintenance r/t inadequate cleaning of bed linen and toilet seats

Insomnia r/t discomfort

Readiness for enhanced **Self Health** management: proper handwashing; short, clean fingernails; avoiding hand, mouth, nose contact with unwashed hands; appropriate cleaning of bed linen and toilet seats

Pituitary Cushing's

See Cushing's Syndrome

PKU (Phenylketonuria)

Risk for delayed **Development**: Risk factors: not following strict dietary program; eating foods extremely low in phenylalanine; avoiding eggs, milk, any foods containing aspartame (NutraSweet)

Readiness for enhanced **Self Health** management: testing for PKU and following prescribed dietary regimen

Placenta Abruptio

Death **Anxiety** r/t threat of mortality associated with bleeding

Fear r/t threat to self and fetus

Ineffective **Health** maintenance r/t deficient knowledge regarding treatment and control of hypertension associated with placenta abruptio

Acute **Pain**: abdominal/back r/t premature separation of placenta before delivery

Risk for **Bleeding**: Risk factor: placenta abruptio

Risk for deficient **Fluid** volume: Risk factor: maternal blood loss

Risk for disturbed **Maternal/Fetal** dyad: Risk factor: complication of pregnancy

Risk for **Powerlessness**: Risk factors: complications of pregnancy and unknown outcome

Risk for **Shock**: Risk factor: hypovolemia

Risk for **Spiritual** distress: Risk factor: fear from unknown outcome of pregnancy

Placenta Previa

Death **Anxiety** r/t threat of mortality associated with bleeding

Disturbed **Body** image r/t negative feelings about body and reproductive ability, feelings of helplessness

Ineffective **Coping** r/t threat to self and fetus

Deficient **Diversional** activity r/t long-term hospitalization

Interrupted **Family** processes r/t maternal bed rest, hospitalization

Fear r/t threat to self and fetus, unknown future

Impaired **Home** maintenance r/t maternal bed rest, hospitalization

Impaired physical **Mobility** r/t medical protocol, maternal bed rest

Ineffective **Role** performance r/t maternal bed rest, hospitalization

Situational low **Self-Esteem** r/t situational crisis

Spiritual distress r/t inability to participate in usual religious rituals, situational crisis

Risk for **Bleeding**: Risk factor: placenta previa

Risk for **Constipation**: Risk factor: bed rest, pregnancy

Risk for deficient **Fluid** volume: Risk factor: maternal blood loss

Risk for imbalanced **Fluid** volume: Risk factor: maternal blood loss

Risk for **Injury**: fetal and maternal: Risk factors: threat to uteroplacental perfusion, hemorrhage

Risk for disturbed **Maternal/Fetal** dyad: Risk factor: complication of pregnancy

Risk for impaired **Parenting**: Risk factors: maternal bed rest, hospitalization

Risk for ineffective peripheral tissue **Perfusion**: placental: Risk factors: dilation of cervix, loss of placental implantation site

Risk for **Powerlessness**: Risk factors: complications of pregnancy and unknown outcome

Risk for **Shock**: Risk factor: hypovolemia

Plantar Fasciitis

Impaired **Comfort** r/t pain

Impaired physical **Mobility** r/t discomfort

Acute **Pain** r/t inflammation

Chronic **Pain** r/t inflammation

Pleural Effusion

Ineffective **Breathing** pattern r/t pain

Excess **Fluid** volume r/t compromised regulatory mechanisms; heart, liver, or kidney failure

Hyperthermia r/t increased metabolic rate secondary to infection

Acute **Pain** r/t inflammation, fluid accumulation

Pleural Friction Rub

Ineffective **Breathing** pattern r/t pain

Acute **Pain** r/t inflammation, fluid accumulation

See cause of Pleural Friction Rub

Pleural Tap

See Pleural Effusion

Pleurisy

Ineffective **Breathing** pattern r/t pain

Impaired **Gas** exchange r/t ventilation perfusion imbalance

Acute **Pain** r/t pressure on pleural nerve endings associated with fluid accumulation or inflammation

Risk for ineffective **Airway** clearance: Risk factors: increased secretions, ineffective cough because of pain

Risk for **Infection**: Risk factor: exposure to pathogens

Risk for impaired physical **Mobility**: Risk factors: activity intolerance, inability to "catch breath"

PMS (Premenstrual Tension Syndrome)

Fatigue r/t hormonal changes

Excess **Fluid** volume r/t alterations of hormonal levels inducing fluid retention

Deficient **Knowledge** r/t methods to deal with and prevent syndrome

Acute **Pain** r/t hormonal stimulation of gastrointestinal structures

Risk for **Powerlessness**: Risk factors: lack of knowledge and ability to deal with symptoms

Risk for compromised **Resilience**: Risk factor: PMS symptoms

Readiness for enhanced **Communication**: willingness to express thoughts and feelings about PMS

Readiness for enhanced **Self Health** management: desire for information to manage and prevent symptoms

PND (Paroxysmal Nocturnal Dyspnea)

Anxiety r/t inability to breathe during sleep

Ineffective **Breathing** pattern r/t increase in carbon dioxide levels, decrease in oxygen levels

Insomnia r/t suffocating feeling from fluid in lungs on awakening from sleep

Sleep deprivation r/t inability to breathe during sleep

Risk for decreased cardiac tissue **Perfusion**: Risk factor: hypoxia

Risk for **Powerlessness**: Risk factor: inability to control nocturnal dyspnea

Readiness for enhanced **Sleep**: expresses willingness to learn measures to enhance sleep

Pneumonectomy

See Thoracotomy

Pneumonia

Activity intolerance r/t imbalance between oxygen supply and demand

Ineffective **Airway** clearance r/t inflammation and presence of secretions

Impaired **Gas** exchange r/t decreased functional lung tissue

Ineffective self **Health** management r/t deficient knowledge regarding self-care and treatment of disease

Hyperthermia r/t dehydration, increased metabolic rate, illness

Deficient **Knowledge** r/t risk factors predisposing person to pneumonia, treatment

Imbalanced **Nutrition**: less than body requirements r/t loss of appetite

Impaired **Oral** mucous membrane r/t dry mouth from mouth breathing, decreased fluid intake

Risk for acute **Confusion**: Risk factor: underlying illness

Risk for deficient **Fluid** volume: Risk factor: inadequate intake of fluids

Risk for vascular **Trauma**: Risk factor: irritation from IV antibiotics

Readiness for enhanced **Immunization** status: expresses desire to increase immunization status

See Respiratory Infections, Acute Childhood

Pneumothorax

Fear r/t threat to own well-being, difficulty breathing

Impaired **Gas** exchange r/t ventilation-perfusion imbalance

Acute **Pain** r/t recent injury, coughing, deep breathing

Risk for **Injury**: Risk factor: possible complications associated with closed chest drainage system

See Chest Tubes

Poliomyelitis

Readiness for enhanced **Immunization** status: expresses desire to increase immunization status

See Paralysis

Poisoning, Risk for

Risk for **Poisoning** (See **Poisoning**, risk for, Section III)

Polydipsia

Readiness for enhanced **Fluid** balance: no excessive thirst when diabetes is controlled

See Diabetes Mellitus

Polyphagia

Readiness for enhanced **Nutrition**: knowledge of appropriate diet for diabetes

See Diabetes Mellitus

Polyuria

Readiness for enhanced **Urinary** elimination: willingness to learn measures to enhance urinary elimination

See Diabetes Mellitus

Postoperative Care

See Surgery, Postoperative

Postpartum Depression

Anxiety r/t new responsibilities of parenting

Risk-prone health **Behavior** r/t lack of support systems

Disturbed **Body** image r/t normal postpartum recovery

Ineffective **Coping** r/t hormonal changes, maturational crisis

Fatigue r/t childbirth, postpartum state

Impaired **Home** maintenance r/t fatigue, care of newborn

Deficient **Knowledge** r/t lifestyle changes

Impaired **Parenting** r/t hormone-induced depression

Ineffective **Role** performance r/t new responsibilities of parenting

Sexual dysfunction r/t fear of another pregnancy, postpartum pain, lochia flow

Sleep deprivation r/t environmental stimulation of newborn

Impaired **Social** interaction r/t change in role functioning

Risk for **Post-Trauma** syndrome: Risk factors: trauma or violence associated with labor and birth process, medical/surgical interventions, history of sexual abuse

Risk for situational low **Self-Esteem**: Risk factor: decreased power over feelings of sadness

Risk for **Spiritual** distress: Risk factors: altered relationships, social isolation

Readiness for enhanced **Hope**: expresses desire to enhance hope and interconnectedness with others

See Depression (Major Depressive Disorder)

P

Postpartum Hemorrhage

Activity intolerance r/t anemia from loss of blood

Death **Anxiety** r/t threat of mortality associated with bleeding

Disturbed **Body** image r/t loss of ideal childbirth

Interrupted **Breastfeeding** r/t separation from infant for medical treatment

Decreased **Cardiac** output r/t hypovolemia

Fear r/t threat to self, unknown future

Deficient **Fluid** volume r/t uterine atony, loss of blood

Impaired **Home** maintenance r/t lack of stamina

Deficient **Knowledge** r/t lack of exposure to situation

Acute **Pain** r/t nursing and medical interventions to control bleeding

Ineffective peripheral tissue **Perfusion** r/t hypovolemia

Risk for **Bleeding**: Risk factor: postpartum complications

Risk for imbalanced **Fluid** volume: Risk factor: maternal blood loss

Risk for **Infection**: Risk factors: loss of blood, depressed immunity

Risk for disturbed **Maternal/Fetal** dyad: Risk factor: complication of pregnancy

Risk for impaired **Parenting**: Risk factor: weakened maternal condition

Risk for **Powerlessness**: Risk factor: acute illness

Risk for **Shock**: Risk factor: hypovolemia

Postpartum, Normal Care

Anxiety r/t change in role functioning, parenting

Effective **Breastfeeding** r/t basic breastfeeding knowledge, support of partner and health care provider

Constipation r/t hormonal effects on smooth muscles, fear of straining with defecation, effects of anesthesia

Fatigue r/t childbirth, new responsibilities of parenting, body changes

Acute **Pain** r/t episiotomy, lacerations, bruising, breast engorgement, headache, sore nipples, epidural or intravenous (IV) site, hemorrhoids

Sexual dysfunction r/t recent childbirth

Impaired **Skin** integrity r/t episiotomy, lacerations

Sleep deprivation r/t care of infant

Impaired **Urinary** elimination r/t effects of anesthesia, tissue trauma

Risk for **Constipation**: Risk factors: hormonal effects on smooth muscles, fear of straining with defecation, effects of anesthesia

Risk for imbalanced **Fluid** volume: Risk factors: shift in blood volume, edema

Risk for urge urinary **Incontinence**: Risk factors: effects of anesthesia or tissue trauma

Risk for **Infection**: Risk factors: tissue trauma, blood loss

Readiness for enhanced family **Coping**: adaptation to new family member

Readiness for enhanced **Hope**: desire to increase hope

Readiness for enhanced **Parenting**: expressing willingness to enhance parenting skills

Post-Trauma Syndrome

Post-Trauma syndrome (See **Post-Trauma** syndrome, Section III)

Post-Trauma Syndrome, Risk for

Risk for **Post-Trauma** syndrome (See **Post-Trauma** syndrome, risk for, Section III)

Post-Traumatic Stress Disorder (PTSD)

See PTSD (Post-Traumatic Stress Disorder)

Potassium, Increase/Decrease

See Hyperkalemia; Hypokalemia

Power/Powerlessness

Powerlessness (See **Powerlessness**, Section III)

Risk for **Powerlessness** (See **Powerlessness**, risk for, Section III)

Readiness for enhanced **Power** (See **Power**, readiness for enhanced, Section III)

Preeclampsia

See PIH (Pregnancy-Induced Hypertension/Preeclampsia)

Pregnancy, Cardiac Disorders

See Cardiac Disorders in Pregnancy

Pregnancy-Induced Hypertension/ Preeclampsia (PIH)

See PIH (Pregnancy-Induced Hypertension/Preeclampsia)

Pregnancy Loss

Anxiety r/t threat to role functioning, health status, situational crisis

Compromised family **Coping** r/t lack of support by significant other because of personal suffering

Ineffective **Coping** r/t situational crisis

Grieving r/t loss of pregnancy, fetus, or child

Complicated **Grieving** r/t sudden loss of pregnancy, fetus, or child

Acute **Pain** r/t surgical intervention

Ineffective **Role** performance r/t inability to assume parenting role

Ineffective **Sexuality** pattern r/t self-esteem disturbance resulting from pregnancy loss and anxiety about future pregnancies

Chronic **Sorrow** r/t loss of a fetus or child

Spiritual distress r/t intense suffering

Risk for **Bleeding**: Risk factor: pregnancy complication

Risk for deficient **Fluid** volume: Risk factor: blood loss

Risk for complicated **Grieving**: Risk factor: loss of pregnancy

Risk for **Infection**: Risk factor: retained products of conception

Risk for **Powerlessness**: Risk factor: situational crisis

Risk for **Spiritual** distress: Risk factor: intense suffering

Readiness for enhanced **Communication**: willingness to express feelings and thoughts about loss

Readiness for enhanced **Hope**: expresses desire to enhance hope

Readiness for enhanced **Spiritual** well-being: desire for acceptance of loss

Pregnancy, Normal

Anxiety r/t unknown future, threat to self secondary to pain of labor

Disturbed **Body** image r/t altered body function and appearance

Interrupted **Family** processes r/t developmental transition of pregnancy

Fatigue r/t increased energy demands

Fear r/t labor and delivery

Deficient **Knowledge** r/t primiparity

Nausea r/t hormonal changes of pregnancy

Imbalanced **Nutrition**: less than body requirements r/t growing fetus, nausea

Imbalanced **Nutrition**: more than body requirements r/t deficient knowledge regarding nutritional needs of pregnancy

Sleep deprivation r/t uncomfortable pregnancy state

Impaired **Urinary** elimination r/t frequency caused by increased pelvic pressure and hormonal stimulation

Risk for **Constipation**: Risk factor: pregnancy

Risk for **Sexual** dysfunction: Risk factors: altered body function, self-concept, body image with pregnancy

Readiness for enhanced **Childbearing** process: appropriate prenatal care

Readiness for enhanced family **Coping**: satisfying partner relationship, attention to gratification of needs, effective adaptation to developmental tasks of pregnancy

Readiness for enhanced **Family** processes: family adapts to change

Readiness for enhanced **Nutrition**: desire for knowledge of appropriate nutrition during pregnancy

Readiness for enhanced **Parenting**: expresses willingness to enhance parenting skills

Readiness for enhanced **Relationship**: meeting developmental goals associated with pregnancy

Readiness for enhanced **Self Health** management: seeks information for prenatal self care

Readiness for enhanced **Spiritual** well-being: new role as parent

See Discomforts of Pregnancy

Premature Dilation of the Cervix (Incompetent Cervix)

Ineffective **Activity** planning r/t unrealistic perception of events

Ineffective **Coping** r/t bed rest, threat to fetus

Deficient **Diversional** activity r/t bed rest

Fear r/t potential loss of infant

Grieving r/t potential loss of infant

Deficient **Knowledge** r/t treatment regimen, prognosis for pregnancy

Impaired physical **Mobility** r/t imposed bed rest to prevent preterm birth

Powerlessness r/t inability to control outcome of pregnancy

Ineffective **Role** performance r/t inability to continue usual patterns of responsibility

Situational low **Self-Esteem** r/t inability to complete normal pregnancy

Sexual dysfunction r/t fear of harm to fetus

Impaired **Social** interaction r/t bed rest

Risk for **Infection**: Risk factors: invasive procedures to prevent preterm birth

Risk for **Injury**: fetal: Risk factors: preterm birth, use of anesthetics

Risk for **Injury**: maternal: Risk factors: surgical procedures to prevent preterm birth (e.g., cerclage)

Risk for compromised **Resilience**: Risk factor: complication of pregnancy

Risk for **Spiritual** distress: Risk factors: physical/psychological stress

Premature Infant (Child)

Impaired **Gas** exchange r/t effects of cardiopulmonary insufficiency

Delayed **Growth** and development: developmental lag r/t prematurity, environmental and stimulation deficiencies, multiple caretakers

Disorganized **Infant** behavior r/t prematurity

Insomnia r/t noisy and noxious intensive care environment

Neonatal **Jaundice** r/t infant experiences difficulty making transition to extrauterine life

Imbalanced **Nutrition**: less than body requirements r/t delayed or understimulated rooting reflex, easy fatigue during feeding, diminished endurance

Disturbed **Sensory** perception r/t noxious stimuli, noisy environment

Impaired **Swallowing** r/t decreased or absent gag reflex, fatigue

Ineffective **Thermoregulation** r/t large body surface/weight ratio, immaturity of thermal regulation, state of prematurity

Risk for delayed **Development**: Risk factor: prematurity

Risk for disproportionate **Growth**: Risk factor: prematurity

Risk for **Infection**: Risk factors: inadequate, immature, or undeveloped acquired immune response

Risk for **Injury**: Risk factor: prolonged mechanical ventilation, retinopathy of prematurely (ROP) secondary to 100% oxygen environment

Readiness for enhanced organized **Infant** behavior: use of some self-regulatory measures

P

Premature Infant (Parent)

Ineffective **Breastfeeding** r/t disrupted establishment of effective pattern secondary to prematurity or insufficient opportunities

Decisional **Conflict** r/t support system deficit, multiple sources of information

Parental role **Conflict** r/t expressed concerns, expressed inability to care for child's physical, emotional, or developmental needs

Compromised family **Coping** r/t disrupted family roles and disorganization, prolonged condition exhausting supportive capacity of significant persons

Grieving r/t loss of perfect child possibly leading to complicated grieving

Complicated **Grieving** (prolonged) r/t unresolved conflicts

Chronic **Sorrow** r/t threat of loss of a child, prolonged hospitalization

Spiritual distress r/t challenged belief or value systems regarding moral or ethical implications of treatment plans

Risk for impaired **Attachment**: Risk factors: separation, physical barriers, lack of privacy

Risk for disturbed **Maternal/Fetal** dyad: Risk factor: complication of pregnancy

Risk for **Powerlessness**: Risk factor: inability to control situation

Risk for compromised **Resilience**: Risk factor: premature infant

Risk for **Spiritual** distress: Risk factors: challenged belief or value systems regarding moral or ethical implications of treatment plans

Readiness for enhanced **Family** process: adaptation to change associated with premature infant

See Child with Chronic Condition; Hospitalized Child

Premature Rupture of Membranes

Anxiety r/t threat to infant's health status

Disturbed **Body** image r/t inability to carry pregnancy to term

Ineffective **Coping** r/t situational crisis

Grieving r/t potential loss of infant

Situational low **Self-Esteem** r/t inability to carry pregnancy to term

Risk for **Infection**: Risk factor: rupture of membranes

Risk for **Injury**: fetal: Risk factor: risk of premature birth

Risk for disturbed **Maternal/Fetal** dyad: Risk factor: complication of pregnancy

Premenstrual Tension Syndrome (PMS)

See PMS (Premenstrual Tension Syndrome)

Prenatal Care, Normal

Readiness for enhanced **Childbearing** process: appropriate prenatal lifestyle

Readiness for enhanced **Knowledge**: appropriate prenatal care

Readiness for enhanced **Spiritual** well-being: new role as parent

See Pregnancy, Normal

Prenatal Testing

Anxiety r/t unknown outcome, delayed test results

Acute **Pain** r/t invasive procedures

Risk for **Infection** r/t invasive procedures during amniocentesis or chorionic villus sampling

Risk for **Injury**: fetal r/t invasive procedures

Preoperative Teaching

See Surgery, Preoperative Care

Pressure Ulcer

Impaired **Comfort** r/t pressure ulcer

Impaired bed **Mobility** r/t intolerance to activity, pain, cognitive impairment, depression, severe anxiety

Imbalanced **Nutrition**: less than body requirements r/t limited access to food, inability to absorb nutrients because of biological factors, anorexia

Acute **Pain** r/t tissue destruction, exposure of nerves

Impaired **Skin** integrity: stage I or II pressure ulcer r/t physical immobility, mechanical factors, altered circulation, skin irritants

Impaired **Tissue** integrity: stage III or IV pressure ulcer r/t altered circulation, impaired physical mobility

Risk for **Infection**: Risk factors: physical immobility, mechanical factors (shearing forces, pressure, restraint, altered circulation, skin irritants)

Preterm Labor

Anxiety r/t threat to fetus, change in role functioning, change in environment and interaction patterns, use of tocolytic drugs

Ineffective **Coping** r/t situational crisis, preterm labor

Deficient **Diversional** activity r/t long-term hospitalization

Grieving r/t loss of idealized pregnancy, potential loss of fetus

Impaired **Home** maintenance r/t medical restrictions

Impaired physical **Mobility** r/t medically imposed restrictions

Ineffective **Role** performance r/t inability to carry out normal roles secondary to bed rest or hospitalization, change in expected course of pregnancy

Situational low **Self-Esteem** r/t threatened ability to carry pregnancy to term

Sexual dysfunction r/t actual or perceived limitation imposed by preterm labor and/or prescribed treatment, separation from partner because of hospitalization

Sleep deprivation r/t change in usual pattern secondary to contractions, hospitalization, treatment regimen

Impaired **Social** interaction r/t prolonged bed rest or hospitalization

Risk for **Injury**: fetal: Risk factors: premature birth, immature body systems

Risk for **Injury**: maternal: Risk factor: use of tocolytic drugs

Risk for **Powerlessness**: Risk factor: lack of control over preterm labor

Risk for vascular **Trauma**: Risk factor: IV medication

P

Readiness for enhanced **Childbearing** process: appropriate prenatal lifestyle

Readiness for enhanced **Comfort**: expresses desire to enhance relaxation

Readiness for enhanced **Communication**: willingness to discuss thoughts and feelings about situation

Problem-Solving Ability

Defensive **Coping** r/t situational crisis

Readiness for enhanced **Communication**: willing to share ideas with others

Readiness for enhanced **Relationship**: shares information and ideas between partners

Readiness for enhanced **Resilience**: identifies available resources

Readiness for enhanced **Spiritual** well-being: desires to draw on inner strength and find meaning and purpose to life

Projection

Anxiety r/t threat to self-concept

Defensive **Coping** r/t inability to acknowledge that own behavior may be a problem, blaming others

Chronic low **Self-Esteem** r/t failure

Impaired **Social** interaction r/t self-concept disturbance, confrontational communication style

Risk for **Loneliness**: Risk factor: blaming others for problems

Risk for **Post-Trauma** syndrome: Risk factor: diminished ego strength

See Paranoid Personality Disorder

Prolapsed Umbilical Cord

Fear r/t threat to fetus, impending surgery

Ineffective peripheral tissue **Perfusion**: fetal r/t interruption in umbilical blood flow

Risk for **Injury**: fetal: Risk factors: cord compression, ineffective tissue perfusion

Risk for **Injury**: maternal: Risk factor: emergency surgery

Prostatectomy

See TURP (Transurethral Resection of the Prostate)

Prostatic Hypertrophy

Ineffective **Health** maintenance r/t deficient knowledge regarding self-care and prevention of complications

Insomnia r/t nocturia

Urinary retention r/t obstruction

Risk for urge urinary **Incontinence**: Risk factor: small bladder capacity

Risk for **Infection**: Risk factors: urinary residual after voiding, bacterial invasion of bladder

See BPH (Benign Prostatic Hypertrophy)

Prostatitis

Impaired **Comfort** r/t inflammation

Ineffective **Health** maintenance r/t deficient knowledge regarding treatment

Urge urinary **Incontinence** r/t irritation of bladder

Ineffective **Protection** r/t depressed immune system

Protection, Altered

Ineffective **Protection** (See **Protection**, ineffective, Section III)

Pruritus

Impaired **Comfort** r/t itching

Deficient **Knowledge** r/t methods to treat and prevent itching

Risk for impaired **Skin** integrity: Risk factor: scratching from pruritus

Psoriasis

Disturbed **Body** image r/t lesions on body

Impaired **Comfort** r/t irritated skin

Ineffective **Health** maintenance r/t deficient knowledge regarding treatment modalities

Powerlessness r/t lack of control over condition with frequent exacerbations and remissions

Impaired **Skin** integrity r/t lesions on body

Psychosis

Ineffective **Activity** planning r/t compromised ability to process information

Ineffective **Health** maintenance r/t cognitive impairment, ineffective individual and family coping

Self **Neglect** r/t mental disorder

Impaired individual **Resilience** r/t psychological disorder

Situational low **Self-Esteem** r/t excessive use of defense mechanisms (e.g., projection, denial, rationalization)

Risk for **Post-Trauma** syndrome: Risk factor: diminished ego strength

See Schizophrenia

PTCA (Percutaneous Transluminal Coronary Angioplasty)

See Angioplasty, Coronary

PTSD (Posttraumatic Stress Disorder)

Anxiety r/t exposure to internal or external cues that symbolize or resemble an aspect of the traumatic event

Death **Anxiety** r/t psychological stress associated with traumatic event

Ineffective **Breathing** pattern r/t hyperventilation associated with anxiety

Ineffective **Coping** r/t extreme anxiety

Disturbed **Energy** field r/t disharmony of mind, body, spirit

Insomnia r/t recurring nightmares

Post-Trauma syndrome r/t exposure to a traumatic event

Disturbed **Sensory** perception r/t psychological stress

Sleep deprivation r/t nightmares associated with traumatic event

Spiritual distress r/t feelings of detachment or estrangement from others

P

Risk for **Powerlessness**: Risk factors: flashbacks, reliving event

Risk for self- or other-directed **Violence**: Risk factors: fear of self or others

Readiness for enhanced **Comfort**: expresses desire to enhance relaxation

Readiness for enhanced **Communication**: willingness to express feelings and thoughts

Readiness for enhanced **Spiritual** well-being: desire for harmony after stressful event

Pulmonary Edema

Anxiety r/t fear of suffocation

Ineffective **Breathing** pattern r/t presence of tracheobronchial secretions

Impaired **Gas** exchange r/t extravasation of extravascular fluid in lung tissues and alveoli

Ineffective **Health** maintenance r/t deficient knowledge regarding treatment regimen

Sleep deprivation r/t inability to breathe

Risk for decreased cardiac tissue **Perfusion**: Risk factor: heart failure

See CHF (Congestive Heart Failure)

Pulmonary Embolism

Decreased **Cardiac** output r/t right ventricular failure secondary to obstructed pulmonary artery

Fear r/t severe pain, possible death

Impaired **Gas** exchange r/t altered blood flow to alveoli secondary to lodged embolus

Deficient **Knowledge** r/t activities to prevent embolism, self-care after diagnosis of embolism

Acute **Pain** r/t biological injury, lack of oxygen to cells

Ineffective peripheral tissue **Perfusion**: r/t deep vein thrombus formation

Delayed **Surgical** recovery r/t complications associated with respiratory difficulty

See Anticoagulant Therapy

Pulmonary Stenosis

See Congenital Heart Disease/Cardiac Anomalies

Pulse Deficit

Decreased **Cardiac** output r/t dysrhythmia

See Dysrhythmia

Pulse Oximetry

Readiness for enhanced **Knowledge**: information associated with treatment regimen

See Hypoxia

Pulse Pressure, Increased

See Intracranial Pressure, Increased

Pulse Pressure, Narrowed

See Shock, Hypovolemic

Pulses, Absent or Diminished Peripheral

Ineffective peripheral tissue **Perfusion** r/t interruption of arterial flow

Risk for **Peripheral** neurovascular dysfunction: Risk factors: fractures, mechanical compression, orthopedic surgery trauma, immobilization, burns, vascular obstruction

See cause of Absent or Diminished Peripheral Pulses

Purpura

See Clotting Disorder

Pyelonephritis

Ineffective **Health** maintenance r/t deficient knowledge regarding self-care, treatment of disease, prevention of further urinary tract infections

Insomnia r/t urinary frequency

Acute **Pain** r/t inflammation and irritation of urinary tract

Impaired **Urinary** elimination r/t irritation of urinary tract

Risk for urge urinary **Incontinence**: Risk factor: irritation of urinary tract

Risk for ineffective renal **Perfusion**: Risk factor: infection

Pyloric Stenosis

Imbalanced **Nutrition**: less than body requirements r/t vomiting secondary to pyloric sphincter obstruction

Acute **Pain** r/t abdominal fullness

Risk for imbalanced **Fluid** volume: Risk factors: vomiting, dehydration

See Hospitalized Child

Pyloromyotomy (Pyloric Stenosis Repair)

See Surgery Preoperative, Perioperative, Postoperative

R

RA (Rheumatoid Arthritis)

See Rheumatoid Arthritis (RA)

Rabies

Ineffective **Health** maintenance r/t deficient knowledge regarding care of wound, isolation, and observation of infected animal

Acute **Pain** r/t multiple immunization injections

Risk for ineffective cerebral tissue **Perfusion**: Risk factor: rabies virus

Readiness for enhanced **Immunization** status: desires to enhance immunization status

Radial Nerve Dysfunction

Acute **Pain** r/t trauma to hand or arm

See Neuropathy, Peripheral

Radiation Therapy

Activity intolerance r/t fatigue from possible anemia

Disturbed **Body** image r/t change in appearance, hair loss

Diarrhea r/t irradiation effects

Fatigue r/t malnutrition from lack of appetite, nausea, and vomiting

Deficient **Knowledge** r/t what to expect with radiation therapy

Nausea r/t side effects of radiation

Imbalanced **Nutrition**: less than body requirements r/t anorexia, nausea, vomiting, irradiation of areas of pharynx and esophagus

Impaired **Oral** mucous membrane r/t irradiation effects

Ineffective **Protection** r/t suppression of bone marrow

Risk for **Powerlessness**: Risk factors: medical treatment and possible side effects

Risk for compromised **Resilience**: Risk factor: radiation treatment

Risk for impaired **Skin** integrity: Risk factor: irradiation effects

Risk for **Spiritual** distress: Risk factors: radiation treatment, prognosis

Radical Neck Dissection

See Laryngectomy

Rage

Risk-prone health **Behavior** r/t multiple stressors

Impaired individual **Resilience** r/t poor impulse control

Stress overload r/t multiple coexisting stressors

Risk for **Self-Mutilation**: Risk factor: command hallucinations

Risk for **Suicide**: Risk factor: desire to kill self

Risk for other-directed **Violence**: Risk factors: panic state, manic excitement, organic brain syndrome

Rape-Trauma Syndrome

Rape-Trauma syndrome (See **Rape-Trauma** syndrome, Section III)

Chronic **Sorrow** r/t forced loss of virginity

Risk for **Post-Trauma** syndrome: Risk factors: trauma or violence associated with rape

Risk for **Powerlessness**: Risk factor: inability to control thoughts about incident

Risk for **Spiritual** distress: Risk factor: forced loss of virginity

Rash

Impaired **Comfort** r/t pruritus

Impaired **Skin** integrity r/t mechanical trauma

Risk for latex **Allergy** response: Risk factor: allergy to products associated with latex

Risk for **Infection**: Risk factors: traumatized tissue, broken skin

Readiness for enhanced **Immunization** status: desire to prevent infectious disease

Rationalization

Defensive **Coping** r/t situational crisis, inability to accept blame for consequences of own behavior

Ineffective **Denial** r/t fear of consequences, actual or perceived loss

Impaired individual **Resilience** r/t psychological disturbance

Risk for **Post-Trauma** syndrome: Risk factor: survivor's role in event

Readiness for enhanced **Communication**: expressing desire to share thoughts and feelings

Readiness for enhanced **Spiritual** well-being: possibility of seeking harmony with self, others, higher power, God

Rats, Rodents in the Home

Impaired **Home** maintenance r/t lack of knowledge, insufficient finances

See Filthy Home Environment

Raynaud's Disease

Deficient **Knowledge** r/t lack of information about disease process, possible complications, self-care needs regarding disease process and medication

Ineffective peripheral tissue **Perfusion** r/t transient reduction of blood flow

RDS (Respiratory Distress Syndrome)

See Respiratory Conditions of the Neonate

Rectal Fullness

Constipation r/t decreased activity level, decreased fluid intake, inadequate fiber in diet, decreased peristalsis, side effects from antidepressant or antipsychotic therapy

Risk for **Constipation**: Risk factor: habitual denial or ignoring of urge to defecate

Rectal Lump

See Hemorrhoids

Rectal Pain/Bleeding

Constipation r/t pain on defecation

Deficient **Knowledge** r/t possible causes of rectal bleeding, pain, treatment modalities

Acute **Pain** r/t pressure of defecation

Risk for **Bleeding**: Risk factor: rectal disease

Rectal Surgery

See Hemorrhoidectomy

Rectocele Repair

Constipation r/t painful defecation

Ineffective **Health** maintenance r/t deficient knowledge of postoperative care of surgical site, dietary measures, exercise to prevent constipation

Acute **Pain** r/t surgical procedure

Urinary retention r/t edema from surgery

R

Risk for **Bleeding**: Risk factor: surgery

Risk for urge urinary **Incontinence**: Risk factor: edema from surgery

Risk for **Infection**: Risk factors: surgical procedure, possible contamination of site with feces

Reflex Incontinence

Reflex urinary **Incontinence** (See **Incontinence**, urinary, reflex, Section III)

Regression

Anxiety r/t threat to or change in health status

Defensive **Coping** r/t denial of obvious problems, weaknesses

Self **Neglect** r/t functional impairment

Powerlessness r/t health care environment

Impaired individual **Resilience** r/t psychological disturbance

Ineffective **Role** performance r/t powerlessness over health status

See Hospitalized Child; Separation Anxiety

Regretful

Anxiety r/t situational or maturational crises

Death **Anxiety** r/t feelings of not having accomplished goals in life

Risk for **Spiritual** distress: Risk factor: inability to forgive

Rehabilitation

Ineffective **Coping** r/t loss of normal function

Impaired physical **Mobility** r/t injury, surgery, psychosocial condition warranting rehabilitation

Self-Care deficit: specify r/t impaired physical mobility

Readiness for enhanced **Comfort**: expresses desire to enhance feeling of comfort

Readiness for enhanced **Self-Concept**: accepts strengths and limitations

Readiness for enhanced **Self Health** management: expression of desire to manage rehabilitation

Relaxation Techniques

Anxiety r/t disturbed energy field

Readiness for enhanced **Comfort**: expresses desire to enhance relaxation

Readiness for enhanced **Religiosity**: requests religious materials or experiences

Readiness for enhanced **Resilience**: desire to enhance resilience

Readiness for enhanced **Self-Concept**: willingness to enhance self-concept

Readiness for enhanced **Self Health** management: desire to manage illness

Readiness for enhanced **Spiritual** well-being: seeking comfort from higher power

Religiosity

Impaired **Religiosity** (See **Religiosity**, impaired, Section III)

Risk for impaired **Religiosity** (See **Religiosity**, impaired, risk for, Section III)

Readiness for enhanced **Religiosity** (See **Religiosity**, readiness for enhanced, Section III)

Religious Concerns

Spiritual distress r/t separation from religious or cultural ties

Risk for impaired **Religiosity**: Risk factors: ineffective support, coping, caregiving

Risk for **Spiritual** distress: Risk factors: physical or psychological stress

Readiness for enhanced **Spiritual** well-being: desire for increased spirituality

Relocation Stress Syndrome

Relocation stress syndrome (See **Relocation** stress syndrome, Section III)

Risk for **Relocation** stress syndrome (See **Relocation** stress syndrome, risk for, Section III)

Renal Failure

Activity intolerance r/t effects of anemia, congestive heart failure

Death **Anxiety** r/t unknown outcome of disease

Decreased **Cardiac** output r/t effects of congestive heart failure, elevated potassium levels interfering with conduction system

Impaired **Comfort** r/t pruritus

Ineffective **Coping** r/t depression resulting from chronic disease

Fatigue r/t effects of chronic uremia and anemia

Excess **Fluid** volume r/t decreased urine output, sodium retention, inappropriate fluid intake

Noncompliance r/t complex medical therapy

Imbalanced **Nutrition**: less than body requirements r/t anorexia, nausea, vomiting, altered taste sensation, dietary restrictions

Impaired **Oral** mucous membrane r/t irritation from nitrogenous waste products

Chronic **Sorrow** r/t chronic illness

Spiritual distress r/t dealing with chronic illness

Impaired **Urinary** elimination r/t effects of disease, need for dialysis

Risk for **Electrolyte** imbalance: Risk factor: renal dysfunction

Risk for **Infection**: Risk factor: altered immune functioning

Risk for **Injury**: Risk factors: bone changes, neuropathy, muscle weakness

Risk for impaired **Oral** mucous membrane: Risk factors: dehydration, effects of uremia

Risk for ineffective renal **Perfusion**: Risk factor: renal disease

Risk for **Powerlessness**: Risk factor: chronic illness

Risk for **Shock**: Risk factor: infection

R

Renal Failure, Acute/Chronic, Child

Disturbed **Body** image r/t growth retardation, bone changes, visibility of dialysis access devices (shunt, fistula), edema

Deficient **Diversional** activity r/t immobility during dialysis

See Child with Chronic Condition; Hospitalized Child; Renal Failure

Renal Failure, Nonoliguric

Anxiety r/t change in health status

Risk for deficient **Fluid** volume: Risk factor: loss of large volumes of urine

See Renal Failure

Renal Transplantation, Donor

Decisional **Conflict** r/t harvesting of kidney from traumatized donor

Moral **Distress** r/t conflict among decision makers, end-of-life decisions, time constraints for decision making

Spiritual distress r/t grieving from loss of significant person

Readiness for enhanced **Communication**: expressing thoughts and feelings about situation

Readiness for enhanced family **Coping**: decision to allow organ donation

Readiness for enhanced **Decision-Making**: expresses desire to enhance understanding and meaning of choices

Readiness for enhanced **Resilience**: decision to donate organs

Readiness for enhanced **Spirituality**: inner peace resulting from allowance of organ donation

See Nephrectomy

Renal Transplantation, Recipient

Anxiety r/t possible rejection, procedure

Impaired **Health** maintenance r/t long-term home treatment after transplantation, diet, signs of rejection, use of medications

Deficient **Knowledge** r/t specific nutritional needs, possible paralytic ileus, fluid or sodium restrictions

Ineffective **Protection** r/t immunosuppression therapy

Impaired **Urinary** elimination r/t possible impaired renal function

Risk for **Bleeding**: Risk factor: surgical procedure

Risk for **Infection**: Risk factor: use of immunosuppressive therapy to control rejection

Risk for ineffective renal **Perfusion**: Risk factor: transplanted kidney

Risk for **Shock**: Risk factor: possible hypovolemia

Risk for **Spiritual** distress: Risk factor: obtaining transplanted kidney from someone's traumatic loss

Readiness for enhanced **Spiritual** well-being: acceptance of situation

See Kidney Transplant

Respiratory Acidosis

See Acidosis, Respiratory

Respiratory Conditions of the Neonate (Respiratory Distress Syndrome [RDS], Meconium Aspiration, Diaphragmatic Hernia)

Ineffective **Airway** clearance r/t sequelae of attempts to breathe in utero resulting in meconium aspiration

Ineffective **Breathing** pattern r/t prolonged ventilator dependence

Fatigue r/t increased energy requirements and metabolic demands

Impaired **Gas** exchange r/t decreased surfactant, immature lung tissue

Risk for **Infection**: Risk factors: tissue destruction or irritation as a result of aspiration of meconium fluid

See Bronchopulmonary Dysplasia; Hospitalized Child; Premature Infant, Child

Respiratory Distress

See Dyspnea

Respiratory Distress Syndrome (RDS)

See Respiratory Conditions of the Neonate

Respiratory Infections, Acute Childhood (Croup, Epiglottitis, Pertussis, Pneumonia, Respiratory Syncytial Virus)

Activity intolerance r/t generalized weakness, dyspnea, fatigue, poor oxygenation

Ineffective **Airway** clearance r/t excess tracheobronchial secretions

Anxiety/Fear r/t oxygen deprivation, difficulty breathing

Ineffective **Breathing** pattern r/t inflamed bronchial passages, coughing

Deficient **Fluid** volume r/t insensible losses (fever, diaphoresis), inadequate oral fluid intake

Impaired **Gas** exchange r/t insufficient oxygenation as a result of inflammation or edema of epiglottis, larynx, bronchial passages

Hyperthermia r/t infectious process

Imbalanced **Nutrition**: less than body requirements r/t anorexia, fatigue, generalized weakness, poor sucking and breathing coordination, dyspnea

Risk for **Aspiration**: Risk factors: inability to coordinate breathing, coughing, sucking

Risk for **Infection**: transmission to others: Risk factor: virulent infectious organisms

Risk for **Injury** (to pregnant others): Risk factors: exposure to aerosolized medications (e.g., ribavirin, pentamidine), resultant potential fetal toxicity

Risk for **Suffocation**: Risk factors: inflammation of larynx, epiglottis

See Hospitalized Child

Respiratory Syncytial Virus

See Respiratory Infections, Acute Childhood

Restless Leg Syndrome

Insomnia r/t leg discomfort during sleep relieved by frequent leg movement

Sleep deprivation r/t frequent leg movements

See Stress

Retarded Growth and Development

See Growth and Development Lag

Retching

Nausea r/t chemotherapy, postsurgical anesthesia, irritation to gastrointestinal system, stimulation of neuropharmacological mechanisms

Imbalanced Nutrition: less than body requirements r/t inability to ingest food

Retinal Detachment

Anxiety r/t change in vision, threat of loss of vision

Deficient Knowledge r/t symptoms, need for early intervention to prevent permanent damage

Disturbed Sensory perception: visual r/t changes in vision, sudden flashes of light, floating spots, blurring of vision

Risk for impaired Home maintenance: Risk factors: postoperative care, activity limitations, care of affected eye

Risk for compromised Resilience: Risk factor: possible loss of vision

See Vision Impairment

Retinopathy, Diabetic

See Diabetic Retinopathy

Retinopathy of Prematurity (ROP)

Risk for Injury: Risk factors: prolonged mechanical ventilation, ROP secondary to 100% oxygen environment

See Retinal Detachment

Reye's Syndrome

Ineffective Breathing pattern r/t neuromuscular impairment

Compromised family Coping r/t acute situational crisis

Deficient Fluid volume r/t vomiting, hyperventilation

Excess Fluid volume: cerebral r/t cerebral edema

Impaired Gas exchange r/t hyperventilation, sequelae of increased intracranial pressure

Grieving r/t uncertain prognosis and sequelae

Ineffective Health maintenance r/t deficient knowledge regarding use of salicylates during viral illness of child

Imbalanced Nutrition: less than body requirements r/t effects of liver dysfunction, vomiting

Situational low Self-Esteem: family r/t negative perceptions of self, perceived inability to manage family situation, expressions of guilt

Disturbed Sensory perception r/t cerebral edema

Impaired Skin integrity r/t effects of decorticate or decerebrate posturing, seizure activity

Risk for Injury: Risk factors: combative behavior, seizure activity

Risk for impaired Liver function: Risk factor: infection

Risk for ineffective cerebral tissue Perfusion: Risk factor: infection

See Hospitalized Child

Rh Factor Incompatibility

Anxiety r/t unknown outcome of pregnancy

Neonatal **Jaundice** r/t Rh factor incompatibility

Deficient Knowledge r/t treatment regimen from lack of experience with situation

Powerlessness r/t perceived lack of control over outcome of pregnancy

Risk for Injury: fetal: Risk factors: intrauterine destruction of red blood cells, transfusions

Readiness for enhanced Self Health management: prenatal care, compliance with diagnostic and treatment regimen

Rhabdomyolysis

Ineffective Coping r/t seriousness of condition

Impaired physical Mobility r/t myalgia and muscle weakness

Impaired Urinary elimination r/t presence of myoglobin in the kidneys

Risk for deficient Fluid volume: Risk factor: reduced blood flow to kidneys

Risk for ineffective renal Perfusion: Risk factor: possible renal failure

Risk for Shock: Risk factor: hypovolemia

Readiness for enhanced Self Health management: seeks information to avoid condition

See Renal Failure

Rheumatic Fever

See Endocarditis

Rheumatoid Arthritis (RA)

Imbalanced Nutrition: less than body requirements r/t loss of appetite

Risk for compromised Resilience: Risk factor: chronic, painful, progressive disease

See Arthritis; JRA (Juvenile Rheumatoid Arthritis)

Rib Fracture

Ineffective Breathing pattern r/t fractured ribs

Acute Pain r/t movement, deep breathing

See Ventilator Client (if relevant)

Ridicule of Others

Defensive Coping r/t situational crisis, psychological impairment, substance abuse

Risk for Post-Trauma syndrome: Risk factor: perception of the event

Ringworm of Body

Impaired Comfort r/t pruritus

Impaired Skin integrity r/t presence of macules associated with fungus

See Itching; Pruritus

Ringworm of Nails

Disturbed **Body** image r/t appearance of nails, removed nails

Ringworm of Scalp

Disturbed **Body** image r/t possible hair loss (alopecia)

See Itching; Pruritus

Risk for Relocation Stress Syndrome

Risk for **Relocation** stress syndrome (See **Relocation** stress syndrome, risk for, Section III)

Roaches, Invasion of Home with

Impaired **Home** maintenance r/t lack of knowledge, insufficient finances

See Filthy Home Environment

Role Performance, Altered

Ineffective **Role** performance (See **Role** performance, ineffective, Section III)

ROP (Retinopathy of Prematurity)

See Retinopathy of Prematurity (ROP)

RSV (Respiratory Syncytial Virus)

See Respiratory Infection, Acute Childhood

Rubella

See Communicable Diseases, Childhood

Rubor of Extremities

Ineffective peripheral tissue **Perfusion** r/t interruption of arterial flow

See Peripheral Vascular Disease (PVD)

Ruptured Disk

See Low Back Pain

S

SAD (Seasonal Affective Disorder)

Readiness for enhanced **Resilience**: uses SAD lights during winter months

See Depression (Major Depressive Disorder)

Sadness

Complicated **Grieving** r/t actual or perceived loss

Spiritual distress r/t intense suffering

Risk for **Powerlessness**: Risk factor: actual or perceived loss

Risk for **Spiritual** distress: Risk factor: loss of loved one

Readiness for enhanced **Communication**: willingness to share feelings and thoughts

Readiness for enhanced **Spiritual** well-being: desire for harmony after actual or perceived loss

See Depression (Major Depressive Disorder); Major Depressive Disorder

Safe Sex

Readiness for enhanced **Self Health** management: taking appropriate precautions during sexual activity to keep from contacting a sexually transmitted disease

See Sexuality, Adolescent; STD (Sexually Transmitted Disease)

Safety, Childhood

Deficient **Knowledge**: potential for enhanced health maintenance r/t parental knowledge and skill acquisition regarding appropriate safety measures

Risk for **Aspiration** (See **Aspiration**, risk for, Section III)

Risk for **Injury/Trauma**: Risk factors: developmental age, altered home maintenance

Risk for impaired **Parenting**: Risk factors: lack of available and effective role model, lack of knowledge, misinformation from other family members (old wives' tales)

Risk for **Poisoning**: Risk factors: use of lead-based paint; presence of asbestos or radon gas; drugs not locked in cabinet; household products left in accessible area (bleach, detergent, drain cleaners, household cleaners); alcohol and perfume within reach of child; presence of poisonous plants; atmospheric pollutants

Readiness for enhanced **Childbearing** process: appropriate knowledge for care of child

Readiness for enhanced **Immunization** status: expresses desire to enhance immunization status

Salmonella

Impaired **Home** maintenance r/t improper preparation or storage of food, lack of safety measures when caring for pet reptile

Risk for **Electrolyte** imbalance: Risk factor: diarrhea

Readiness for enhanced **Self Health** management: avoiding improperly prepared or stored food, wearing gloves when handling pet reptiles or their feces

See Gastroenteritis; Gastroenteritis, Child

Salpingectomy

Decisional **Conflict** r/t sterilization procedure

Grieving r/t possible loss from tubal pregnancy

Risk for impaired **Urinary** elimination: Risk factor: trauma to ureter during surgery

See Hysterectomy; Surgery, Perioperative Care; Surgery, Postoperative Care; Surgery, Preoperative Care

Sarcoidosis

Anxiety r/t change in health status

Impaired **Gas** exchange r/t ventilation-perfusion imbalance

Ineffective **Health** maintenance r/t deficient knowledge regarding home care and medication regimen

Acute **Pain** r/t possible disease affecting joints

Ineffective **Protection** r/t immune disorder

Risk for decreased cardiac tissue **Perfusion**: Risk factor: dysrhythmias

Risk for impaired **Skin** integrity: Risk factor: immunological disorder

SARS (Severe Acute Respiratory Syndrome)

Risk for **Infection**: Risk factor: increased environmental exposure (travelers in close proximity to infected persons, traveling when a fever is present)

Readiness for enhanced **Knowledge**: information regarding travel and precautions to avoid exposure to SARS

See Pneumonia

SBE (Self-Breast Examination)

Readiness for enhanced **Knowledge**: self-breast examination

Readiness for enhanced **Self Health** management: desires to have information about SBE

Scabies

See Communicable Diseases, Childhood

Scared

Anxiety r/t threat of death, threat to or change in health status

Death **Anxiety** r/t unresolved issues surrounding end-of-life decisions

Fear r/t hospitalization, real or imagined threat to own well-being

Impaired individual **Resilience** r/t violence

Readiness for enhanced **Communication**: willingness to share thoughts and feelings

Schizophrenia

Ineffective **Activity** planning r/t compromised ability to process information

Anxiety r/t unconscious conflict with reality

Impaired verbal **Communication** r/t psychosis, disorientation, inaccurate perception, hallucinations, delusions

Ineffective **Coping** r/t inadequate support systems, unrealistic perceptions, inadequate coping skills, disturbed thought processes, impaired communication

Deficient **Diversional** activity r/t social isolation, possible regression

Interrupted **Family** processes r/t inability to express feelings, impaired communication

Fear r/t altered contact with reality

Ineffective **Health** maintenance r/t cognitive impairment, ineffective individual and family coping, lack of material resources

Impaired **Home** maintenance r/t impaired cognitive or emotional functioning, insufficient finances, inadequate support systems

Hopelessness r/t long-term stress from chronic mental illness

Disturbed personal **Identity** r/t psychiatric disorder

Insomnia r/t sensory alterations contributing to fear and anxiety

Impaired **Memory** r/t psychosocial condition

Self **Neglect** r/t psychosis

Imbalanced **Nutrition**: less than body requirements r/t fear of eating, lack of awareness of hunger, disinterest toward food

Impaired individual **Resilience** r/t psychological disorder

Self-Care deficit: specify r/t loss of contact with reality, impairment of perception

Disturbed **Sensory** perception r/t biochemical imbalances for sensory distortion (illusions, hallucinations)

Sleep deprivation r/t intrusive thoughts, nightmares

Impaired **Social** interaction r/t impaired communication patterns, self-concept disturbance, disturbed thought processes

Social isolation r/t lack of trust, regression, delusional thinking, repressed fears

Chronic **Sorrow** r/t chronic mental illness

Spiritual distress r/t loneliness, social alienation

Ineffective family **Therapeutic** regimen management r/t chronicity and unpredictability of condition

Risk for **Caregiver** role strain: Risk factors: bizarre behavior of client, chronicity of condition

Risk for compromised human **Dignity**: Risk factor: stigmatizing label

Risk for **Loneliness**: Risk factor: inability to interact socially

Risk for **Post-Trauma** syndrome: Risk factor: diminished ego strength

Risk for **Powerlessness**: Risk factor: intrusive, distorted thinking

Risk for impaired **Religiosity**: Risk factors: ineffective coping, lack of security

Risk for **Suicide**: Risk factor: psychiatric illness

Risk for self- and other-directed **Violence**: Risk factors: lack of trust, panic, hallucinations, delusional thinking

Readiness for enhanced **Hope**: expresses desire to enhance interconnectedness with others and problem-solve to meet goals

Readiness for enhanced **Power**: expresses willingness to enhance participation in choices for daily living and health and enhance knowledge for participation in change

Sciatica

See Neuropathy, Peripheral

Scoliosis

Risk-prone health **Behavior** r/t lack of developmental maturity to comprehend long-term consequences of noncompliance with treatment procedures

Disturbed **Body** image r/t use of therapeutic braces, postsurgery scars, restricted physical activity

Ineffective **Breathing** pattern r/t restricted lung expansion caused by severe curvature of spine

Impaired **Comfort** r/t altered health status and body image

Impaired **Gas** exchange r/t restricted lung expansion as a result of severe presurgery curvature of spine, immobilization

Impaired physical **Mobility** r/t restricted movement, dyspnea caused by severe curvature of spine

Acute **Pain** r/t musculoskeletal restrictions, surgery, reambulation with cast or spinal rod

Impaired **Skin** integrity r/t braces, casts, surgical correction

Chronic **Sorrow** r/t chronic disability

S

Ineffective **Health** maintenance r/t deficient knowledge regarding treatment modalities, restrictions, home care, postoperative activities

Risk for **Infection**: Risk factor: surgical incision

Risk for perioperative positioning **Injury**: Risk factor: prone position

Risk for compromised **Resilience**: Risk factor: chronic condition

Readiness for enhanced **Self Health** management: desires knowledge regarding treatment for condition

See Hospitalized Child; Maturational Issues, Adolescent

Sedentary Lifestyle

Activity intolerance r/t sedentary lifestyle

Sedentary **Lifestyle** (See **Lifestyle**, sedentary, Section III)

Readiness for enhanced **Coping**: seeking knowledge of new strategies to adjust to sedentary lifestyle

Self-Health Management, Ineffective

Ineffective self **Health** management (See **Health** management, self, ineffective, Section III)

Self-Health Management, Readiness for Enhanced

Readiness for enhanced **Self Health** management (See **Self Health** management, readiness for enhanced, Section III)

Seizure Disorders, Adult

Acute **Confusion** r/t postseizure state

Social isolation r/t unpredictability of seizures, community-imposed stigma

Risk for ineffective **Airway** clearance: Risk factor: accumulation of secretions during seizure

Risk for **Falls**: Risk factor: uncontrolled seizure activity

Risk for **Powerlessness**: Risk factor: possible seizure

Risk for compromised **Resilience**: Risk factor: chronic illness

Readiness for enhanced **Knowledge**: anticonvulsive therapy

Readiness for enhanced **Self-Care**: expresses desire to enhance knowledge and responsibility for self-care

See Epilepsy

Seizure Disorders, Childhood (Epilepsy, Febrile Seizures, Infantile Spasms)

Ineffective **Health** maintenance r/t lack of knowledge regarding anticonvulsive therapy, fever reduction (febrile seizures)

Social isolation r/t unpredictability of seizures, community-imposed stigma

Risk for ineffective **Airway** clearance: Risk factor: accumulation of secretions during seizure

Risk for delayed **Development** and disproportionate growth: Risk factors: effects of seizure disorder, parental overprotection

Risk for **Falls**: Risk factor: possible seizure

Risk for **Injury**: Risk factors: uncontrolled movements during seizure, falls, drowsiness caused by anticonvulsants

See Epilepsy

Self-Breast Examination (SBE)

See SBE (Self-Breast Examination)

Self-Care

Readiness for enhanced **Self-Care** (See **Self-Care**, readiness for enhanced, Section III)

Self-Care Deficit, Bathing

Bathing **Self-Care** deficit (See **Self-Care** deficit, bathing, Section III)

Self-Care Deficit, Dressing

Dressing **Self-Care** deficit (See **Self-Care** deficit, dressing, Section III)

Self-Care Deficit, Feeding

Feeding **Self-Care** deficit (See **Self-Care** deficit, feeding, Section III)

Self-Care Deficit, Toileting

Toileting **Self-Care** deficit (See **Self-Care** deficit, toileting, Section III)

Self-Concept

Readiness for enhanced **Self-Concept** (See **Self-Concept**, readiness for enhanced, Section III)

Self-Destructive Behavior

Post-Trauma syndrome r/t unresolved feelings from traumatic event

Risk for **Self-Mutilation**: Risk factors: feelings of depression, rejection, self-hatred, depersonalization; command hallucinations

Risk for **Suicide**: Risk factor: history of self-destructive behavior

Risk for self-directed **Violence**: Risk factors: panic state, history of child abuse, toxic reaction to medication

Self-Esteem, Chronic Low

Chronic low **Self-esteem** (See **Self-esteem**, low, chronic, Section III)

Self-Esteem, Situational Low

Situational low **Self-Esteem** (See **Self-Esteem**, low, situational, Section III)

Risk for situational low **Self-Esteem** (See **Self-Esteem**, low, situational, risk for, Section III)

Self-Mutilation, Risk for

Self-Mutilation (See **Self-Mutilation**, Section III)

Risk for **Self-Mutilation** (See **Self-Mutilation**, risk for, Section III)

Senile Dementia

Sedentary **Lifestyle** r/t lack of interest

See Dementia

Sensory/Perceptual Alterations

Disturbed **Sensory** perception (See **Sensory** perception, disturbed, Section III)

S

Separation Anxiety

Ineffective **Coping** r/t maturational and situational crises, vulnerability related to developmental age, hospitalization, separation from family and familiar surroundings, multiple caregivers

Insomnia r/t separation for significant others

Risk for impaired **Attachment**: Risk factor: separation

See Hospitalized Child

Sepsis, Child

Imbalanced **Nutrition**: less than body requirements r/t anorexia, generalized weakness, poor sucking reflex

Ineffective peripheral tissue **Perfusion**: r/t arterial or venous blood flow exchange problems, septic shock

Delayed **Surgical** recovery r/t presence of infection

Ineffective **Thermoregulation** r/t infectious process, septic shock

Risk for impaired **Skin** integrity: Risk factors: desquamation caused by disseminated intravascular coagulation

See Hospitalized Child; Premature Infant, Child

Septicemia

Imbalanced **Nutrition**: less than body requirements r/t anorexia, generalized weakness

Ineffective peripheral tissue **Perfusion** r/t decreased systemic vascular resistance

Risk for imbalanced **Fluid** volume r/t vasodilation of peripheral vessels, leaking of capillaries

Risk for **Shock**: Risk factors: hypotension, hypovolemia

See Sepsis, Child; Shock, Septic

Severe Acute Respiratory Syndrome (SARS)

See SARS (Severe Acute Respiratory Syndrome); Pneumonia

Sexual Dysfunction

Sexual dysfunction (See **Sexual** dysfunction, Section III)

Chronic **Sorrow** r/t loss of ideal sexual experience, altered relationships

See Erectile Dysfunction (ED)

Sexuality, Adolescent

Disturbed **Body** image r/t anxiety caused by unachieved developmental milestone (puberty) or deficient knowledge regarding reproductive maturation as manifested by amenorrhea or expressed concerns regarding lack of growth of secondary sex characteristics

Decisional **Conflict**: sexual activity r/t undefined personal values or beliefs, multiple or divergent sources of information, lack of relevant information

Deficient **Knowledge**: potential for enhanced health maintenance r/t multiple or divergent sources of information or lack of relevant information regarding sexual transmission of disease, contraception, prevention of toxic shock syndrome

See Maturational Issues, Adolescent

Sexuality Pattern, Ineffective

Ineffective **Sexuality** pattern (See **Sexuality** pattern, ineffective, Section III)

Sexually Transmitted Disease (STD)

See STD (Sexually Transmitted Disease)

Shaken Baby Syndrome

Decreased **Intracranial** adaptive capacity r/t brain injury

Impaired **Parenting** r/t stress, history of being abusive

Impaired individual **Resilience** r/t poor impulse control

Stress overload r/t intense repeated family stressors, family violence

Risk for other-directed **Violence**: Risk factors: history of violence against others, perinatal complications

See Child Abuse; Suspected Child Abuse and Neglect (SCAN), Child; Suspected Child Abuse and Neglect (SCAN), Parent

Shakiness

Anxiety r/t situational or maturational crisis, threat of death

Shame

Situational low **Self-Esteem** r/t inability to deal with past traumatic events, blaming of self for events not under one's control

Shingles

Impaired **Comfort** r/t inflammation

Acute **Pain** r/t vesicular eruption along the nerves

Ineffective **Protection** r/t abnormal blood profiles

Social isolation r/t altered state of wellness, contagiousness of disease

Risk for **Infection**: Risk factor: tissue destruction

Readiness for enhanced **Immunization** status: expresses desire to enhance immunization status

See Itching

Shivering

Impaired **Comfort** r/t altered health status

Fear r/t serious threat to health status

Hypothermia r/t exposure to cool environment

Risk for **Injury**: Risk factor: prolonged shock resulting in multiple organ failure or death

Risk for decreased cardiac tissue **Perfusion**: Risk factor: hypotension, hypovolemia

Risk for ineffective renal **Perfusion**: Risk factor: hypovolemia

Risk for **Shock** (See **Shock**, risk for, Section III)

See Shock, Cardiogenic; Shock, Hypovolemic; Shock, Septic

Shock, Cardiogenic

Decreased **Cardiac** output r/t decreased myocardial contractility, dysrhythmia

Shock, Hypovolemic

Deficient **Fluid** volume r/t abnormal loss of fluid, trauma, third spacing

S

Shock, Septic

Deficient **Fluid** volume r/t abnormal loss of fluid through capillaries, pooling of blood in peripheral circulation

Ineffective **Protection** r/t inadequately functioning immune system

See Sepsis, Child; Septicemia

Shoulder Repair

Self-Care deficit: bathing, dressing, feeding r/t immobilization of affected shoulder

Risk for perioperative positioning **Injury**: Risk factor: immobility

See Surgery, Preoperative; Surgery, Perioperative; Surgery, Postoperative; Total Joint Replacement (Total Hip/Total Knee/Shoulder)

Sickle Cell Anemia/Crisis

Activity intolerance r/t fatigue, effects of chronic anemia

Impaired **Comfort** r/t altered health status

Deficient **Fluid** volume r/t decreased intake, increased fluid requirements during sickle cell crisis, decreased ability of kidneys to concentrate urine

Impaired physical **Mobility** r/t pain, fatigue

Acute **Pain** r/t viscous blood, tissue hypoxia

Ineffective peripheral tissue **Perfusion** r/t effects of red cell sickling, infarction of tissues

Risk for disproportionate **Growth**: Risk factor: chronic illness

Risk for **Infection**: Risk factor: alterations in splenic function

Risk for decreased cardiac tissue **Perfusion**: Risk factors: effects of red cell sickling, infarction of tissues

Risk for ineffective cerebral, gastrointestinal, renal tissue **Perfusion**: Risk factors: effects of red cell sickling, infarction of tissues

Risk for compromised **Resilience**: Risk factor: chronic illness

Readiness for enhanced **Immunization** status: receives appropriate immunizations to prevent disease

See Child with Chronic Condition; Hospitalized Child

SIDS (Sudden Infant Death Syndrome)

Anxiety/Fear: parental r/t life-threatening event

Interrupted **Family** processes r/t stress as a result of special care needs of infant with apnea

Grieving r/t potential loss of infant

Insomnia: parental/infant r/t home apnea monitoring

Deficient **Knowledge**: potential for enhanced health maintenance r/t knowledge or skill acquisition of cardiopulmonary resuscitation and home apnea monitoring

Impaired **Resilience** r/t sudden loss

Risk for sudden infant **Death** syndrome (See **Death** syndrome, infant, sudden, risk for, Section III)

Risk for **Powerlessness**: Risk factor: unanticipated life-threatening event

See Terminally Ill Child/Death of Child, Parent

Situational Crisis

Ineffective **Coping** r/t situational crisis

Interrupted **Family** processes r/t situational crisis

Readiness for enhanced **Communication**: willingness to share feelings and thoughts

Readiness for enhanced **Religiosity**: requests religious material and/or experiences

Readiness for enhanced **Resilience**: desire to enhance resilience

Readiness for enhanced **Spiritual** well-being: desire for harmony following crisis

SJS (Stevens-Johnson Syndrome)

See Stevens-Johnson Syndrome (SJS)

Skin Cancer

Ineffective **Health** maintenance r/t deficient knowledge regarding self-care with skin cancer

Ineffective **Protection** r/t weakened immune system

Impaired **Skin** integrity r/t abnormal cell growth in skin, treatment of skin cancer

Readiness for enhanced **Knowledge**: self-care to prevent and treat skin cancer

Readiness for enhanced **Self Health** management: follows preventive measures

Skin Disorders

Impaired **Skin** integrity (See **Skin** integrity, impaired, Section III)

Skin Integrity, Risk for Impaired

Risk for impaired **Skin** integrity (See **Skin** integrity, impaired, risk for, Section III)

Skin Turgor, Change in Elasticity

Deficient **Fluid** volume r/t active fluid loss

Sleep

Readiness for enhanced **Sleep** (See **Sleep**, readiness for enhanced, Section III)

Sleep Apnea

See PND (Paroxysmal Nocturnal Dyspnea)

Sleep Deprivation

Fatigue r/t lack of sleep

Disturbed **Sensory** perception r/t lack of sleep

Sleep deprivation (See **Sleep** deprivation, Section III)

Sleep Pattern Disorders

Insomnia (See **Insomnia**, Section III)

Sleep Pattern, Disturbed, Parent/Child

Insomnia: child r/t anxiety or fear

Insomnia: parent r/t parental responsibilities, stress

See Suspected Child Abuse and Neglect (SCAN), Child and Parent

S

Slurring of Speech

Impaired verbal **Communication** r/t decrease in circulation to brain, brain tumor, anatomical defect, cleft palate

Situational low **Self-Esteem** r/t speech impairment

See Communication Problems

Small Bowel Resection

See Abdominal Surgery

Smell, Loss of Ability to

Risk for **Injury**: Risk factors: inability to detect gas fumes, smoke smells

See Anosmia

Smoke Inhalation

Ineffective **Airway** clearance r/t smoke inhalation

Impaired **Gas** exchange r/t ventilation perfusion imbalance

Risk for acute **Confusion**: Risk factor: decreased oxygen supply

Risk for **Poisoning**: Risk factor: exposure to carbon monoxide

Readiness for enhanced **Self Health** management: functioning smoke detectors and carbon monoxide detectors in home and work, plan for escape route worked out and reviewed

See Atelectasis; Burns; Pneumonia

Smoking Behavior

Risk-prone health **Behavior** r/t smoking

Altered **Health** maintenance r/t denial of effects of smoking, lack of effective support for smoking withdrawal

Readiness for enhanced **Knowledge**: expresses interest in smoking cessation

Social Interaction, Impaired

Impaired **Social** interaction (See **Social** interaction, impaired, Section III)

Social Isolation

Social isolation (See **Social** isolation, Section III)

Sociopathic Personality

See Antisocial Personality Disorder

Sodium, Decrease/Increase

See Hyponatremia; Hypernatremia

Somatization Disorder

Anxiety r/t unresolved conflicts channeled into physical complaints or conditions

Ineffective **Coping** r/t lack of insight into underlying conflicts

Ineffective **Denial** r/t displaces psychological stress to physical symptoms

Nausea r/t anxiety

Chronic **Pain** r/t unexpressed anger, multiple physical disorders, depression

Impaired individual **Resilience** r/t possible psychological disorders

Sore Nipples, Breastfeeding

Ineffective **Breastfeeding** r/t deficient knowledge regarding correct feeding procedure

See Painful Breasts, Sore Nipples

Sore Throat

Impaired **Comfort** r/t sore throat

Deficient **Knowledge** r/t treatment, relief of discomfort

Impaired **Oral** mucous membrane r/t inflammation or infection of oral cavity

Impaired **Swallowing** r/t irritation of oropharyngeal cavity

Sorrow

Grieving r/t loss of significant person, object, or role

Chronic **Sorrow** (See **Sorrow**, chronic, Section III)

Readiness for enhanced **Communication**: expresses thoughts and feelings

Readiness for enhanced **Spiritual** well-being: desire to find purpose and meaning of loss

Spastic Colon

See IBS (Irritable Bowel Syndrome)

Speech Disorders

Anxiety r/t difficulty with communication

Impaired verbal **Communication** r/t anatomical defect, cleft palate, psychological barriers, decrease in circulation to brain

Delayed **Growth** and development r/t effects of physical or mental disability

Disturbed **Sensory** perception (auditory) r/t altered sensory reception, transmission, and/or integration

Spina Bifida

See Neural Tube Defects

Spinal Cord Injury

Deficient **Diversional** activity r/t long-term hospitalization, frequent lengthy treatments

Fear r/t powerlessness over loss of body function

Complicated **Grieving** r/t loss of usual body function

Sedentary **Lifestyle** r/t lack of resources or interest

Impaired wheelchair **Mobility** r/t neuromuscular impairment

Urinary retention r/t inhibition of reflex arc

Risk for latex **Allergy** response: Risk factor: continuous or intermittent catheterization

Risk for **Autonomic** dysreflexia: Risk factors: bladder or bowel distention, skin irritation, deficient knowledge of patient and caregiver

Risk for ineffective **Breathing** pattern: Risk factor: neuromuscular impairment

Risk for **Infection**: Risk factors: chronic disease, stasis of body fluids

Risk for **Loneliness**: Risk factor: physical immobility

Risk for **Powerlessness**: Risk factor: loss of function

See Child with Chronic Condition; Hospitalized Child; Neural Tube Defects; Paralysis

Spinal Fusion

Impaired bed **Mobility** r/t impaired ability to turn side to side while keeping spine in proper alignment

Impaired physical **Mobility** r/t musculoskeletal impairment associated with surgery, possible back brace

Readiness for enhanced **Knowledge**: expresses interest in information associated with surgery

See Acute Back; Back Pain; Scoliosis; Surgery, Preoperative Care; Surgery, Perioperative Care; Surgery, Postoperative Care

Spiritual Distress

Spiritual distress (See **Spiritual** distress, Section III)

Risk for **Spiritual** distress (See **Spiritual** distress, risk for, Section III)

Spiritual Well-Being

Readiness for enhanced **Spiritual** well-being (See **Spiritual** well-being, readiness for enhanced, Section III)

Splenectomy

See Abdominal Surgery

Sprains

Impaired physical **Mobility** r/t injury

Acute **Pain** r/t physical injury

Stapedectomy

Acute **Pain** r/t headache

Disturbed **Sensory** perception: auditory r/t hearing loss caused by edema from surgery

Risk for **Falls**: Risk factor: dizziness

Risk for **Infection**: Risk factor: invasive procedure

Stasis Ulcer

Impaired **Tissue** integrity r/t chronic venous congestion

See CHF (Congestive Heart Failure); Varicose Veins

STD (Sexually Transmitted Disease)

Impaired **Comfort** r/t infection

Fear r/t altered body function, risk for social isolation, fear of incurable illness

Ineffective **Health** maintenance r/t deficient knowledge regarding transmission, symptoms, treatment of STD

Ineffective **Sexuality** pattern r/t illness, altered body function

Social isolation r/t fear of contracting or spreading disease

Risk for **Infection**: spread of infection: Risk factor: lack of knowledge concerning transmission of disease

Readiness for enhanced **Knowledge**: seeks information regarding prevention and treatment of STDs

See Maturational Issues, Adolescent; PID (Pelvic Inflammatory Disease)

STEMI (ST-Elevation Myocardial Infarction)

See MI (Myocardial Infarction)

Stent (Coronary Artery Stent)

Risk for **Injury**: Risk factor: complications associated with stent placement

Risk for decreased cardiac tissue **Perfusion**: Risk factor: possible restenosis

Risk for vascular **Trauma**: Risk factor: insertion site, catheter width

Readiness for enhanced **Decision-Making**: expresses desire to enhance risk benefit analysis, understanding and meaning of choices, and decisions regarding treatment

See Angioplasty, Coronary; Cardiac Catheterization

Sterilization Surgery

Decisional **Conflict** r/t multiple or divergent sources of information, unclear personal values or beliefs

See Surgery, Preoperative Care; Surgery, Perioperative Care; Surgery, Postoperative Care; Tubal Ligation; Vasectomy

Stertorous Respirations

Ineffective **Airway** clearance r/t pharyngeal obstruction

Stevens-Johnson Syndrome (SJS)

Impaired **Oral** mucous membrane r/t immunocompromised condition associated with allergic medication reaction

Acute **Pain** r/t painful skin lesions and painful oral mucosa lesions

Impaired **Skin** integrity r/t allergic medication reaction

Risk for acute **Confusion**: Risk factors: dehydration, electrolyte disturbances

Risk for imbalanced **Fluid** volume: Risk factors: factors affecting fluid needs (hypermetabolic state, hyperthermia), excessive losses through normal routes (vomiting and diarrhea)

Risk for **Infection**: Risk factor: broken skin

Risk for impaired **Liver** function: Risk factor: infection

Stillbirth

See Pregnancy Loss

Stoma

See Colostomy; Ileostomy

Stomatitis

Impaired **Oral** mucous membrane r/t pathological conditions of oral cavity

Stone, Kidney

See Kidney Stone

Stool, Hard/Dry

Constipation r/t inadequate fluid intake, inadequate fiber intake, decreased activity level, decreased gastric motility

S

Straining with Defecation

Decreased **Cardiac** output r/t vagal stimulation with dysrhythmia resulting from Valsalva maneuver

Constipation r/t less than adequate fluid intake, less than adequate dietary intake

Strep Throat

Risk for **Infection**: Risk factor: exposure to pathogen

See Sore Throat

Stress

Anxiety r/t feelings of helplessness, feelings of being threatened

Ineffective **Coping** r/t ineffective use of problem-solving process, feelings of apprehension or helplessness

Disturbed **Energy** field r/t low energy level, feelings of hopelessness

Fear r/t powerlessness over feelings

Stress overload r/t intense or multiple stressors

Risk for **Post-Trauma** syndrome: Risk factors: perception of event, survivor's role in event

Readiness for enhanced **Communication**: shows willingness to share thoughts and feelings

Readiness for enhanced **Spiritual** well-being: expresses desire for harmony and peace in stressful situation

See Anxiety

Stress Overload

Stress overload (See **Stress** overload, Section III)

Stress Urinary Incontinence

Stress urinary **Incontinence** r/t degenerative change in pelvic muscles

Risk for urge urinary **Incontinence**: Risk factor: involuntary sphincter relaxation

See Incontinence of Urine

Stridor

Ineffective **Airway** clearance r/t obstruction, tracheobronchial infection, trauma

Stroke

See CVA (Cerebrovascular Accident)

Stuttering

Anxiety r/t impaired verbal communication

Impaired verbal **Communication** r/t anxiety, psychological problems

Subarachnoid Hemorrhage

Acute **Pain**: headache r/t irritation of meninges from blood, increased intracranial pressure

Risk for ineffective cerebral tissue **Perfusion**: Risk factor: bleeding from cerebral vessel

See Intracranial Pressure, Increased

Substance Abuse

Compromised/disabled family **Coping** r/t codependency issues

Defensive **Coping** r/t substance abuse

Ineffective **Coping** r/t use of substances to cope with life events

Ineffective **Denial** r/t refusal to acknowledge substance abuse problem

Dysfunctional **Family** processes r/t substance abuse

Insomnia r/t irritability, nightmares, tremors

Risk for impaired **Attachment**: Risk factor: substance abuse

Risk for **Suicide**: Risk factor: substance abuse

Risk for vascular **Trauma**: Risk factor: chemical irritant

Risk for self- or other-directed **Violence**: Risk factors: reactions to substances used, impulsive behavior, disorientation, impaired judgment

Readiness for enhanced **Coping**: seeking social support and knowledge of new strategies

Readiness for enhanced **Self-Concept**: accepting strengths and limitations

See Alcoholism; Drug Abuse; Maturational Issues, Adolescent

Substance Abuse, Adolescent

See Alcohol Withdrawal; Maturational Issues, Adolescent; Substance Abuse

Substance Abuse in Pregnancy

Defensive **Coping** r/t denial of situation, differing value system

Ineffective **Health** maintenance r/t addiction

Deficient **Knowledge** r/t lack of exposure to information regarding effects of substance abuse in pregnancy

Noncompliance r/t differing value system, cultural influences, addiction

Risk for impaired **Attachment**: Risk factors: substance abuse, inability of parent to meet infant's or own personal needs

Risk for **Infection**: Risk factors: intravenous drug use, lifestyle

Risk for **Injury**: fetal: Risk factor: effects of drugs on fetal growth and development

Risk for **Injury**: maternal: Risk factor: drug use

Risk for impaired **Parenting**: Risk factor: lack of ability to meet infant's needs

See Alcoholism; Drug Abuse; Substance Abuse

Sucking Reflex

Effective **Breastfeeding** r/t regular and sustained sucking and swallowing at breast

Sudden Infant Death Syndrome (SIDS)

See SIDS (Sudden Infant Death Syndrome)

Suffocation, Risk for

Risk for **Suffocation** (See **Suffocation**, risk for, Section III)

Suicide Attempt

Risk-prone health **Behavior** r/t low self-efficacy

Ineffective **Coping** r/t anger, complicated grieving

Hopelessness r/t perceived or actual loss, substance abuse, low self-concept, inadequate support systems

S

Post-Trauma response r/t history of traumatic events, abuse, rape, incest, war, torture

Impaired individual **Resilience** r/t poor impulse control

Situational low **Self-Esteem** r/t guilt, inability to trust, feelings of worthlessness or rejection

Social isolation r/t inability to engage in satisfying personal relationships

Spiritual distress r/t hopelessness, despair

Risk for **Post-Trauma** syndrome: Risk factor: survivor's role in suicide attempt

Risk for **Suicide** (See **Suicide**, risk for, Section III)

Readiness for enhanced **Communication**: willingness to share thoughts and feelings

Readiness for enhanced **Spiritual** well-being: desire for harmony and inner strength to help redefine purpose for life

See Violent Behavior

Support System

Readiness for enhanced family **Coping**: ability to adapt to tasks associated with care, support of significant other during health crisis

Readiness for enhanced **Family** processes: activities support the growth of family members

Readiness for enhanced **Parenting**: children or other dependent person(s) expressing satisfaction with home environment

Suppression of Labor

See Preterm Labor; Tocolytic Therapy

Surgery, Perioperative Care

Risk for imbalanced **Fluid** volume: Risk factor: surgery

Risk for perioperative positioning **Injury**: Risk factors: predisposing condition, prolonged surgery

Surgery, Postoperative Care

Activity intolerance r/t pain, surgical procedure

Anxiety r/t change in health status, hospital environment

Deficient **Knowledge** r/t postoperative expectations, lifestyle changes

Nausea r/t manipulation of gastrointestinal tract, postsurgical anesthesia

Imbalanced **Nutrition**: less than body requirements r/t anorexia, nausea, vomiting, decreased peristalsis

Ineffective peripheral tissue **Perfusion** r/t hypovolemia, circulatory stasis, obesity, prolonged immobility, decreased coughing, decreased deep breathing

Acute **Pain** r/t inflammation or injury in surgical area

Delayed **Surgical** recovery r/t extensive surgical procedure, postoperative surgical infection

Urinary retention r/t anesthesia, pain, fear, unfamiliar surroundings, client's position

Risk for **Bleeding**: Risk factor: surgical procedure

Risk for ineffective **Breathing** pattern: Risk factors: pain, location of incision, effects of anesthesia or opioids

Risk for **Constipation**: Risk factors: decreased activity, decreased food or fluid intake, anesthesia, pain medication

Risk for imbalanced **Fluid** volume: Risk factors: hypermetabolic state, fluid loss during surgery, presence of indwelling tubes

Risk for **Infection**: Risk factors: invasive procedure, pain, anesthesia, location of incision, weakened cough as a result of aging

Surgery, Preoperative Care

Anxiety r/t threat to or change in health status, situational crisis, fear of the unknown

Insomnia r/t anxiety about upcoming surgery

Deficient **Knowledge** r/t preoperative procedures, postoperative expectations

Readiness for enhanced **Knowledge**: shows understanding of preoperative and postoperative expectations for self-care

Surgical Recovery, Delayed

Delayed **Surgical** recovery (See **Surgical** recovery, delayed, Section III)

Suspected Child Abuse and Neglect (SCAN), Child

Ineffective **Activity** planning r/t lack of family support

Anxiety/Fear: child r/t threat of punishment for perceived wrongdoing

Disturbed personal **Identity** r/t dysfunctional family processes

Rape-Trauma syndrome r/t altered lifestyle because of abuse, changes in residence

Risk for compromised **Resilience**: Risk factor: adverse situation

Readiness for enhanced community **Coping**: obtaining resources to prevent child abuse, neglect

See Child Abuse; Hospitalized Child; Maturational Issues, Adolescent

Suspected Child Abuse and Neglect (SCAN), Parent

Disabled family **Coping** r/t dysfunctional family, underdeveloped nurturing parental role, lack of parental support systems or role models

Dysfunctional **Family** processes r/t inadequate coping skills

Ineffective **Health** maintenance r/t deficient knowledge of parenting skills as a result of unachieved developmental tasks

Impaired **Home** maintenance r/t disorganization, parental dysfunction, neglect of safe and nurturing environment

Impaired **Parenting** r/t unrealistic expectations of child; lack of effective role model; unmet social, emotional, or maturational needs of parents; interruption in bonding process

Powerlessness r/t inability to perform parental role responsibilities

Impaired individual **Resilience** r/t poor impulse control

Chronic low **Self-Esteem** r/t lack of successful parenting experiences

Risk for other-directed **Violence**: parent to child: Risk factors: inadequate coping mechanisms, unresolved stressors, unachieved maturational level by parent

S

Suspicion

Disturbed personal **Identity** r/t psychiatric disorder

Powerlessness r/t repetitive paranoid thinking

Impaired **Social** interaction r/t disturbed thought processes, paranoid delusions, hallucinations

Risk for self- or other-directed **Violence**: Risk factor: inability to trust

Swallowing Difficulties

Impaired **Swallowing** (See **Swallowing**, impaired, Section III)

Swine Flu (H1N1)

See Influenza

Syncope

Anxiety r/t fear of falling

Decreased **Cardiac** output r/t dysrhythmia

Impaired physical **Mobility** r/t fear of falling

Social isolation r/t fear of falling

Risk for **Falls**: Risk factor: syncope

Risk for **Injury**: Risk factors: altered sensory perception, transient loss of consciousness, risk for falls

Risk for ineffective cerebral tissue **Perfusion**: Risk factor: interruption of blood flow

Syphilis

See STD (Sexually Transmitted Disease)

Systemic Lupus Erythematosus

See Lupus Erythematosus

T

T & A (Tonsillectomy and Adenoidectomy)

Ineffective **Airway** clearance r/t hesitation or reluctance to cough because of pain

Deficient **Knowledge**: potential for enhanced health maintenance r/t insufficient knowledge regarding postoperative nutritional and rest requirements, signs and symptoms of complications, positioning

Nausea r/t gastric irritation, pharmaceuticals, anesthesia

Acute **Pain** r/t surgical incision

Risk for **Aspiration/Suffocation**: Risk factors: postoperative drainage and impaired swallowing

Risk for deficient **Fluid** volume: Risk factors: decreased intake because of painful swallowing, effects of anesthesia (nausea, vomiting), hemorrhage

Risk for imbalanced **Nutrition**: less than body requirements: Risk factors: hesitation or reluctance to swallow

Tachycardia

See Dysrhythmia

Tachypnea

Ineffective **Breathing** pattern r/t pain, anxiety

See cause of Tachypnea

Tardive Dyskinesia

Ineffective self **Health** management r/t complexity of therapeutic regimen or medication

Deficient **Knowledge** r/t cognitive limitation in assimilating information relating to side effects associated with neuroleptic medications

Disturbed **Sensory** perception r/t tardive dyskinesia

Risk for **Injury**: Risk factor: drug-induced abnormal body movements

Taste Abnormality

Adult **Failure** to thrive r/t imbalanced nutrition: less than body requirements associated with taste abnormality

Disturbed **Sensory** perception: gustatory r/t medication side effects; altered sensory reception, transmission, integration; aging changes

TB (Pulmonary Tuberculosis)

Ineffective **Airway** clearance r/t increased secretions, excessive mucus

Ineffective **Breathing** pattern r/t decreased energy, fatigue

Fatigue r/t disease state

Impaired **Gas** exchange r/t disease process

Ineffective self **Health** management r/t deficient knowledge of prevention and treatment regimen

Impaired **Home** maintenance management r/t client or family member with disease

Hyperthermia r/t infection

Risk for **Infection**: Risk factors: insufficient knowledge regarding avoidance of exposure to pathogens

Readiness for enhanced **Self Health** management: takes medications according to prescribed protocol for prevention and treatment

TBI (Traumatic Brain Injury)

Interrupted **Family** processes r/t traumatic injury to family member

Chronic **Sorrow** r/t change in health status and functional ability

Risk for **Post-Trauma** syndrome: Risk factor: perception of event causing TBI

Risk for impaired **Religiosity**: Risk factor: impaired physical mobility

Risk for compromised **Resilience**: Risk factor: crisis of injury

See Head Injury; Neurologic Disorders

TD (Traveler's Diarrhea)

Diarrhea r/t travel

Risk for deficient **Fluid** volume: Risk factors: excessive loss of fluids, diarrhea

Risk for **Infection**: Risk factors: insufficient knowledge regarding avoidance of exposure to pathogens (water supply, iced drinks, local cheeses, ice cream, undercooked meat, fish and shellfish, uncooked vegetables, unclean eating utensils, improper handwashing)

Temperature, Decreased

Hypothermia r/t exposure to cold environment

Temperature, Increased

Hyperthermia r/t dehydration, illness, trauma

Temperature Regulation, Impaired

Ineffective **Thermoregulation** r/t trauma, illness

TEN (Toxic Epidermal Necrolysis)

See Toxic Epidermal Necrolysis (TEN)

Tension

Anxiety r/t threat to or change in health status, situational crisis

Disturbed **Energy** field r/t change in health status, discouragement, pain

Readiness for enhanced **Communication**: expresses willingness to share feelings and thoughts

See Stress

Terminally Ill Adult

Death **Anxiety** r/t unresolved issues relating to death and dying

Disturbed **Energy** field r/t impending disharmony of mind, body, spirit

Risk for **Spiritual** distress: Risk factor: impending death

Readiness for enhanced **Religiosity**: requests religious material and/or experiences

Readiness for enhanced **Spiritual** well-being: desire to achieve harmony of mind, body, spirit

See Terminally Ill Child/Death of Child, Parent

Terminally Ill Child, Adolescent

Disturbed **Body** image r/t effects of terminal disease, already critical feelings of group identity and self-image

Ineffective **Coping** r/t inability to establish personal and peer identity because of the threat of being different or not being healthy, inability to achieve maturational tasks

Impaired **Social** interaction/**Social** isolation r/t forced separation from peers

See Child with Chronic Condition; Hospitalized Child, Terminally Ill Child/Death of Child, Parent

Terminally Ill Child, Infant/Toddler

Ineffective **Coping** r/t separation from parents and familiar environment attributable to inability to understand dying process

See Child with Chronic Condition, Terminally Ill Child/Death of Child, Parent

Terminally Ill Child, Preschool Child

Fear r/t perceived punishment, bodily harm, feelings of guilt caused by magical thinking (i.e., believing that thoughts cause events)

See Child with Chronic Condition, Terminally Ill Child/Death of Child, Parent

Terminally Ill Child, School-Age Child/Preadolescent

Fear r/t perceived punishment, body mutilation, feelings of guilt

See Child with Chronic Condition, Terminally Ill Child/Death of Child, Parent

Terminally Ill Child/Death of Child, Parent

Decisional **Conflict** r/t continuation or discontinuation of treatment, do-not-resuscitate decision, ethical issues regarding organ donation

Compromised family **Coping** r/t inability or unwillingness to discuss impending death and feelings with child or support child through terminal stages of illness

Ineffective **Denial** r/t complicated grieving

Interrupted **Family** processes r/t situational crisis

Grieving r/t death of child

Hopelessness r/t overwhelming stresses caused by terminal illness

Insomnia r/t grieving process

Impaired **Parenting** r/t risk for overprotection of surviving siblings

Powerlessness r/t inability to alter course of events

Impaired **Social** interaction r/t complicated grieving

Social isolation: imposed by others r/t feelings of inadequacy in providing support to grieving parents

Social isolation: self-imposed r/t unresolved grief, perceived inadequate parenting skills

Spiritual distress r/t sudden and unexpected death, prolonged suffering before death, questioning the death of youth, questioning the meaning of one's own existence

Risk for complicated **Grieving**: Risk factors: prolonged, unresolved, obstructed progression through stages of grief and mourning

Risk for compromised **Resilience**: Risk factor: impending death

Readiness for enhanced family **Coping**: impact of crisis on family values, priorities, goals, or relationships; expressed interest or desire to attach meaning to child's life and death

Tetralogy of Fallot

See Congenital Heart Disease/Cardiac Anomalies

Therapeutic Regimen Management, Ineffective: Family

Ineffective family **Therapeutic** regimen management (See **Therapeutic** regimen management, family, ineffective, Section III)

T

Therapeutic Touch

Disturbed **Energy** field r/t low energy levels, disturbance in energy fields, pain, depression, fatigue

Thermoregulation, Ineffective

Ineffective **Thermoregulation** (See **Thermoregulation**, ineffective, Section III)

Thoracentesis

See Pleural Effusion

Thoracotomy

Activity intolerance r/t pain, imbalance between oxygen supply and demand, presence of chest tubes

Ineffective **Airway** clearance r/t drowsiness, pain with breathing and coughing

Ineffective **Breathing** pattern r/t decreased energy, fatigue, pain

Deficient **Knowledge** r/t self-care, effective breathing exercises, pain relief

Acute **Pain** r/t surgical procedure, coughing, deep breathing

Risk for **Bleeding**: Risk factor: surgery

Risk for **Infection**: Risk factor: invasive procedure

Risk for **Injury**: Risk factor: disruption of closed-chest drainage system

Risk for perioperative positioning **Injury**: Risk factor: lateral positioning, immobility

Risk for vascular **Trauma**: Risk factor: chemical irritant; antibiotics

Thought Disorders

See Schizophrenia

Thrombocytopenic Purpura

See ITP (Idiopathic Thrombocytopenic Purpura)

Thrombophlebitis

Constipation r/t inactivity, bed rest

Deficient **Diversional** activity r/t bed rest

Deficient **Knowledge** r/t pathophysiology of condition, self-care needs, treatment regimen and outcome

Sedentary **Lifestyle** r/t deficient knowledge of benefits of physical exercise

Impaired physical **Mobility** r/t pain in extremity, forced bed rest

Acute **Pain** r/t vascular inflammation, edema

Ineffective peripheral tissue **Perfusion** r/t interruption of venous blood flow

Delayed **Surgical** recovery r/t complication associated with inactivity

Risk for **Bleeding**: Risk factors: treatment; anticoagulants

Risk for **Injury**: Risk factor: possible embolus

Risk for vascular **Trauma**: Risk factor: anticoagulant therapy

See Anticoagulant Therapy

Thyroidectomy

Risk for ineffective **Airway** clearance r/t edema or hematoma formation, airway obstruction

Risk for impaired verbal **Communication**: Risk factors: edema, pain, vocal cord of laryngeal nerve damage

Risk for **Injury**: Risk factor: possible parathyroid damage or removal

See Surgery, Preoperative Care; Surgery, Perioperative Care; Surgery, Postoperative Care

TIA (Transient Ischemic Attack)

Acute **Confusion** r/t hypoxia

Readiness for enhanced **Self Health** management: obtains knowledge regarding treatment prevention of inadequate oxygenation

See Syncope

Tic Disorder

See Tourette's Syndrome (TS)

Tinea Capitis

Impaired **Comfort** r/t inflammation from pruritus

See Ringworm of Scalp

Tinea Corporis

See Ringworm of Body

Tinea Cruris

See Jock Itch; Itching; Pruritus

Tinea Pedis

See Athlete's Foot; Itching; Pruritus

Tinea Unguium (Onychomycosis)

See Ringworm of Nails

Tinnitus

Ineffective **Health** maintenance r/t deficient knowledge regarding self-care with tinnitus

Disturbed **Sensory** perception: auditory r/t altered sensory reception, transmission, integration

Tissue Damage, Corneal, Integumentary, or Subcutaneous

Impaired **Tissue** integrity (See **Tissue** integrity, impaired, Section III)

Tissue Perfusion, Ineffective Peripheral

Ineffective peripheral tissue **Perfusion** (See **Perfusion**, tissue, peripheral, ineffective, Section III)

Toilet Training

Deficient **Knowledge**: parent r/t signs of child's readiness for training

Risk for **Constipation**: Risk factor: withholding stool

Risk for **Infection**: Risk factor: withholding urination

Toileting Problems

Toileting **Self-Care** deficit r/t impaired transfer ability, impaired mobility status, intolerance of activity, neuromuscular impairment, cognitive impairment

Impaired **Transfer** ability r/t neuromuscular deficits

T

Tonsillectomy and Adenoidectomy (T & A)

See T & A (Tonsillectomy and Adenoidectomy)

Toothache

Impaired **Dentition** r/t ineffective oral hygiene, barriers to self-care, economic barriers to professional care, nutritional deficits, lack of knowledge regarding dental health

Acute **Pain** r/t inflammation, infection

Total Anomalous Pulmonary Venous Return

See Congenital Heart Disease/Cardiac Anomalies

Total Joint Replacement (Total Hip/Total Knee/Shoulder)

Disturbed **Body** image r/t large scar, presence of prosthesis

Impaired physical **Mobility** r/t musculoskeletal impairment, surgery, prosthesis

Risk for **Injury**: neurovascular: Risk factors: altered peripheral tissue perfusion, altered mobility, prosthesis

See Surgery, Preoperative Care; Surgery, Perioperative Care; Surgery, Postoperative Care

Total Parenteral Nutrition (TPN)

See TPN (Total Parenteral Nutrition)

Tourette's Syndrome (TS)

Hopelessness r/t inability to control behavior

Impaired individual **Resilience** r/t uncontrollable behavior

Risk for situational low **Self-Esteem**: Risk factors: uncontrollable behavior, motor and phonic tics

See Attention Deficit Disorder

Toxemia

See PIH (Pregnancy-Induced Hypertension/Preeclampsia)

Toxic Epidermal Necrolysis (TEN) (Erythema multiforme)

Death **Anxiety** r/t uncertainty of prognosis

Disturbed **Sensory** perception (visual) r/t altered sensory reception associated with visual changes from conjunctival inflammation and scarring

See Stevens-Johnson Syndrome (SJS)

TPN (Total Parenteral Nutrition)

Imbalanced **Nutrition**: less than body requirements r/t inability to ingest or digest food or absorb nutrients as a result of biological or psychological factors

Risk for **Fluid** volume excess: Risk factor: rapid administration of TPN

Risk for **Infection**: Risk factors: concentrated glucose solution, invasive administration of fluids

Risk for vascular **Trauma**: Risk factors: insertion site, length of treatment time

Tracheoesophageal Fistula

Ineffective **Airway** clearance r/t aspiration of feeding because of inability to swallow

Imbalanced **Nutrition**: less than body requirements r/t difficulties in swallowing

Risk for **Aspiration**: Risk factors: common passage of air and food

Risk for vascular **Trauma**: Risk factors: venous medications and site

See Respiratory Conditions of the Neonate; Hospitalized Child

Tracheostomy

Ineffective **Airway** clearance r/t increased secretions, mucous plugs

Anxiety r/t impaired verbal communication, ineffective airway clearance

Disturbed **Body** image r/t abnormal opening in neck

Impaired verbal **Communication** r/t presence of mechanical airway

Deficient **Knowledge** r/t self-care, home maintenance management

Acute **Pain** r/t edema, surgical procedure

Risk for **Aspiration**: Risk factor: presence of tracheostomy

Risk for **Bleeding**: Risk factor: surgical incision

Risk for **Infection**: Risk factors: invasive procedure, pooling of secretions

Traction and Casts

Constipation r/t immobility

Deficient **Diversional** activity r/t immobility

Impaired physical **Mobility** r/t imposed restrictions on activity because of bone or joint disease injury

Acute **Pain** r/t immobility, injury, or disease

Self-Care deficit: feeding, dressing, bathing, toileting r/t degree of impaired physical mobility, body area affected by traction or cast

Impaired **Transfer** ability r/t presence of traction, casts

Risk for **Disuse** syndrome: Risk factor: mechanical immobilization

See Casts

Transfer Ability

Impaired **Transfer** ability (See **Transfer** ability, impaired, Section III)

Transient Ischemic Attack (TIA)

See TIA (Transient Ischemic Attack)

Transposition of Great Vessels

See Congenital Heart Disease/Cardiac Anomalies

Transurethral Resection of the Prostate (TURP)

See TURP (Transurethral Resection of the Prostate)

Trauma in Pregnancy

Anxiety r/t threat to self or fetus, unknown outcome

Deficient **Knowledge** r/t lack of exposure to situation

Acute **Pain** r/t trauma

Impaired **Skin** integrity r/t trauma

Risk for **Bleeding**: Risk factor: trauma

T

Risk for imbalanced **Fluid** volume: Risk factor: fluid loss

Risk for **Infection**: Risk factor: traumatized tissue

Risk for **Injury**: fetal: Risk factor: premature separation of placenta

Risk for disturbed **Maternal/Fetal** dyad: Risk factor: complication of pregnancy

Trauma, Risk for

Risk for **Trauma** (See **Trauma**, risk for, Section III)

Traumatic Brain Injury (TBI)

See TBI (Traumatic Brain Injury); Intracranial Pressure, Increased

Traumatic Event

Post-Trauma syndrome r/t previously experienced trauma

Traveler's Diarrhea (TD)

See TD (Traveler's Diarrhea)

Trembling of Hands

Anxiety/Fear r/t threat to or change in health status, threat of death, situational crisis

Tricuspid Atresia

See Congenital Heart Disease/Cardiac Anomalies

Trigeminal Neuralgia

Ineffective self **Health** management r/t deficient knowledge regarding prevention of stimuli that trigger pain

Imbalanced **Nutrition**: less than body requirements r/t pain when chewing

Acute **Pain** r/t irritation of trigeminal nerve

Risk for **Injury** (eye): Risk factor: possible decreased corneal sensation

Truncus Arteriosus

See Congenital Heart Disease/Cardiac Anomalies

TS (Tourette's Syndrome)

See Tourette's Syndrome (TS)

TSE (Testicular Self-Examination)

Readiness for enhanced **Self Health** management: seeks information regarding self-examination

Tubal Ligation

Decisional **Conflict** r/t tubal sterilization

See Laparoscopy

Tube Feeding

Risk for **Aspiration**: Risk factors: improperly administered feeding, improper placement of tube, improper positioning of client during and after feeding, excessive residual feeding or lack of digestion, altered gag reflex

Risk for imbalanced **Fluid** volume: Risk factor: inadequate water administration with concentrated feeding

Risk for imbalanced **Nutrition**: less than body requirements: Risk factors: intolerance to tube feeding, inadequate calorie replacement to meet metabolic needs

Tuberculosis (TB)

See TB (Pulmonary Tuberculosis)

TURP (Transurethral Resection of the Prostate)

Deficient **Knowledge** r/t postoperative self-care, home maintenance management

Acute **Pain** r/t incision, irritation from catheter, bladder spasms, kidney infection

Urinary retention r/t obstruction of urethra or catheter with clots

Risk for **Bleeding**: Risk factor: surgery

Risk for deficient **Fluid** volume: Risk factors: fluid loss, possible bleeding

Risk for urge urinary **Incontinence**: Risk factor: edema from surgical procedure

Risk for **Infection**: Risk factors: invasive procedure, route for bacteria entry

Risk for ineffective renal **Perfusion**: Risk factor: hypovolemia

Ulcer, Peptic (Duodenal or Gastric)

Fatigue r/t loss of blood, chronic illness

Ineffective **Health** maintenance r/t lack of knowledge regarding health practices to prevent ulcer formation

Nausea r/t gastrointestinal irritation

Acute **Pain** r/t irritated mucosa from acid secretion

Risk for ineffective gastrointestinal tissue **Perfusion**: Risk factor: ulcer

See GI Bleed (Gastrointestinal Bleeding)

Ulcerative Colitis

See Inflammatory Bowel Disease (Child and Adult)

Ulcers, Stasis

See Stasis Ulcer

Unilateral Neglect of One Side of Body

Unilateral **Neglect** (See **Neglect**, unilateral, Section III)

Unsanitary Living Conditions

Impaired **Home** maintenance r/t impaired cognitive or emotional functioning, lack of knowledge, insufficient finances

Urgency to Urinate

Urge urinary **Incontinence** (See **Incontinence**, urinary, urge, Section III)

Risk for urge urinary **Incontinence** (See **Incontinence**, urinary, urge, risk for, Section III)

Urinary Diversion

See Ileal Conduit

Urinary Elimination, Impaired

Impaired **Urinary** elimination (See **Urinary** elimination, impaired, Section III)

Urinary Incontinence

See Incontinence of Urine

Urinary Readiness

Readiness for enhanced **Urinary** elimination (See **Urinary** elimination, readiness for enhanced, Section III)

Urinary Retention

Urinary retention (See **Urinary** retention, Section III)

Urinary Tract Infection (UTI)

See UTI (Urinary Tract Infection)

Urolithiasis

See Kidney Stone

Uterine Atony in Labor

See Dystocia

Uterine Atony in Postpartum

See Postpartum Hemorrhage

Uterine Bleeding

See Hemorrhage; Postpartum Hemorrhage; Shock, Hypovolemic

UTI (Urinary Tract Infection)

Ineffective **Health** maintenance r/t deficient knowledge regarding methods to treat and prevent UTIs

Acute **Pain**: dysuria r/t inflammatory process in bladder

Impaired **Urinary** elimination: frequency r/t urinary tract infection

Risk for urge urinary **Incontinence**: Risk factor: hyperreflexia from cystitis

Risk for ineffective renal **Perfusion**: Risk factor: infection

V

VAD (Ventricular Assist Device)

See Ventricular Assist Device (VAD)

Vaginal Hysterectomy

Urinary retention r/t edema at surgical site

Risk for urge urinary **Incontinence**: Risk factors: edema, congestion of pelvic tissues

Risk for **Infection**: Risk factor: surgical site

Risk for perioperative-positioning **Injury**: Risk factor: lithotomy position

See Postpartum Hemorrhage

Vaginitis

Impaired **Comfort** r/t pruritus, itching

Ineffective **Health** maintenance r/t deficient knowledge regarding self-care with vaginitis

Ineffective **Sexuality** pattern r/t abstinence during acute stage, pain

Vagotomy

See Abdominal Surgery

Value System Conflict

Decisional **Conflict** r/t unclear personal values or beliefs

Spiritual distress r/t challenged value system

Readiness for enhanced **Spiritual** well-being: desire for harmony with self, others, higher power, God

Varicose Veins

Ineffective **Health** maintenance r/t deficient knowledge regarding health care practices, prevention, treatment regimen

Chronic **Pain** r/t impaired circulation

Ineffective peripheral tissue **Perfusion** r/t venous stasis

Risk for impaired **Skin** integrity: Risk factor: altered peripheral tissue perfusion

Vascular Dementia (Formerly Called Multiinfarct Dementia)

See Dementia

Vascular Obstruction, Peripheral

Anxiety r/t lack of circulation to body part

Acute **Pain** r/t vascular obstruction

Ineffective peripheral tissue **Perfusion** r/t interruption of circulatory flow

Risk for **Peripheral** neurovascular dysfunction: Risk factor: vascular obstruction

Vasectomy

Decisional **Conflict** r/t surgery as method of permanent sterilization

Vasocognopathy

See Alzheimer's Disease; Dementia

Venereal Disease

See STD (Sexually Transmitted Disease)

Ventilation, Impaired Spontaneous

Impaired spontaneous **Ventilation** (See **Ventilation**, spontaneous, impaired, Section III)

Ventilator Client

Ineffective **Airway** clearance r/t increased secretions, decreased cough and gag reflex

Ineffective **Breathing** pattern r/t decreased energy and fatigue as a result of possible altered nutrition: less than body requirements

Impaired verbal **Communication** r/t presence of endotracheal tube, decreased mentation

Fear r/t inability to breathe on own, difficulty communicating

Impaired **Gas** exchange r/t ventilation-perfusion imbalance

Powerlessness r/t health treatment regimen

Social isolation r/t impaired mobility, ventilator dependence

Impaired spontaneous **Ventilation** r/t metabolic factors, respiratory muscle fatigue

Dysfunctional **Ventilatory** weaning response r/t psychological, situational, physiological factors

Risk for latex **Allergy** response: Risk factor: repeated exposure to latex products

Risk for **Infection**: Risk factors: presence of endotracheal tube, pooled secretions

Risk for compromised **Resilience**: Risk factor: illness

See Child with Chronic Condition; Hospitalized Child; Respiratory Conditions of the Neonate

Ventilatory Weaning Response, Dysfunctional (DVWR)

Dysfunctional **Ventilatory** weaning response (See **Ventilatory** weaning response, dysfunctional, Section III)

Ventricular Assist Device (VAD)

Risk for vascular **Trauma**: Risk factor: insertion site

Readiness for enhanced **Decision-Making**: expresses desire to enhance the understanding of the meaning of choices regarding implanting a ventricular assist device

See Open Heart Surgery

Ventricular Fibrillation

See Dysrhythmia

Vertigo

Disturbed **Sensory** perception: kinesthetic r/t altered sensory reception, transmission, integration; medications

See Syncope

Violent Behavior

Risk for other-directed **Violence** (See **Violence**, other-directed, risk for, Section III)

Risk for self-directed **Violence** (See **Violence**, self-directed, risk for, Section III)

Viral Gastroenteritis

Diarrhea r/t infectious process, rotavirus, Norwalk virus

Ineffective self **Health** management r/t inadequate handwashing

Risk for dysfunctional gastrointestinal **Motility**: Risk factor: infection

See Gastroenteritis, Child

Vision Impairment

Fear r/t loss of sight

Disturbed **Sensory** perception r/t altered sensory reception associated with impaired vision

Social isolation r/t altered state of wellness, inability to see

Risk for compromised **Resilience**: Risk factor: presence of new crisis

See Blindness; Cataracts; Glaucoma

Vomiting

Nausea r/t chemotherapy, postsurgical anesthesia, irritation to the gastrointestinal system, stimulation of neuropharmacological mechanisms

Risk for **Electrolyte** imbalance: Risk factor: vomiting

Risk for imbalanced **Fluid** volume: Risk factors: decreased intake, loss of fluids with vomiting

Risk for imbalanced **Nutrition**: less than body requirements: Risk factor: inability to ingest food

von Recklinghausen's Disease

See Neurofibromatosis

Walking Impairment

Impaired **Walking** (See **Walking**, impaired, Section III)

Wandering

Wandering (See **Wandering**, Section III)

Weakness

Fatigue r/t decreased or increased metabolic energy production

Risk for **Falls**: Risk factor: weakness

Weight Gain

Imbalanced **Nutrition**: more than body requirements r/t excessive intake in relation to metabolic need

Weight Loss

Imbalanced **Nutrition**: less than body requirements r/t inability to ingest food because of biological, psychological, economic factors

Wellness-Seeking Behavior

Readiness for enhanced **Self Health** management: expresses desire for increased control of health practice

Wernicke-Korsakoff Syndrome

See Korsakoff's Syndrome

West Nile Virus

See Meningitis/Encephalitis

Wheelchair Use Problems

Impaired wheelchair **Mobility** (See **Mobility**, wheelchair, impaired, Section III)

Wheezing

Ineffective **Airway** clearance r/t tracheobronchial obstructions, secretions

Wilms' Tumor

Constipation r/t obstruction associated with presence of tumor

Acute **Pain** r/t pressure from tumor

See Chemotherapy; Hospitalized Child; Radiation Therapy; Surgery, Preoperative Care; Surgery, Perioperative Care; Surgery, Postoperative Care

Withdrawal from Alcohol

See Alcohol Withdrawal

Withdrawal from Drugs

See Drug Withdrawal

Wounds (open)

See Lacerations

Wound Debridement

Acute **Pain** r/t debridement of wound

Impaired **Tissue** integrity r/t debridement, open wound

Risk for **Infection**: Risk factors: open wound, presence of bacteria

Wound Dehiscence, Evisceration

Fear r/t client fear of body parts "falling out," surgical procedure not going as planned

Imbalanced **Nutrition**: less than body requirements r/t inability to digest nutrients, need for increased protein for healing

Risk for deficient **Fluid** volume: Risk factors: inability to ingest nutrients, obstruction, fluid loss

Risk for **Injury**: Risk factor: exposed abdominal contents

Risk for delayed **Surgical** recovery: Risk factors: separation of wound, exposure of abdominal contents

Wound Infection

Disturbed **Body** image r/t dysfunctional open wound

Hyperthermia r/t increased metabolic rate, illness, infection

Imbalanced **Nutrition**: less than body requirements r/t biological factors, infection, hyperthermia

Impaired **Tissue** integrity r/t wound, presence of infection

Risk for imbalanced **Fluid** volume: Risk factor: increased metabolic rate

Risk for **Infection**: spread of: Risk factor: imbalanced nutrition: less than body requirements

Risk for delayed **Surgical** recovery: Risk factor: presence of infection

W

Section III is a listing of nursing diagnosis care plans according to NANDA-I. The care plans are arranged alphabetically by diagnostic concept.

MAKING AN ACCURATE NURSING DIAGNOSIS

Verify the accuracy of the previously suggested nursing diagnoses (from Section II) for the client. To do this:

- Read the definition for the suggested nursing diagnosis and determine if it sounds appropriate.
- Compare the Defining Characteristics with the symptoms that were identified from the client data collected.
- Compare the Risk Factors with the symptoms that were identified from the client data collected (if it is a "Risk for" Nursing Diagnosis; they do not have defining characteristics).

WRITING OUTCOMES, STATEMENTS, AND NURSING INTERVENTIONS

After selecting the appropriate nursing diagnosis, use this section to write outcomes and interventions:

- Use the NOC/NIC outcomes and interventions with the associated rating scales.
- Use the Client Outcomes/Nursing Interventions as written by the authors and contributors.
- Read the rationales; the majority of rationales are based on nursing or clinical research that validates the efficacy of the interventions.

Following these steps, you will be able to write a nursing care plan:

- Follow this care plan to administer nursing care to the client.
- Document all steps and evaluate and update the care plan as needed.

Activity intolerance   *Betty J. Ackley, MSN, EdS, RN*   A

NANDA-I

Definition

Insufficient physiological or psychological energy to endure or complete required or desired daily activities

Defining Characteristics

Abnormal blood pressure response to activity; abnormal heart rate response to activity; EKG changes reflecting arrhythmias; EKG changes reflecting ischemia; exertional discomfort; exertional dyspnea; verbal report of fatigue; verbal report of weakness

Related Factors (r/t)

Bed rest; generalized weakness; imbalance between oxygen supply/demand; immobility; sedentary lifestyle

NOC   (Nursing Outcomes Classification)

Suggested NOC Outcomes

Activity Tolerance, Endurance, Energy Conservation, Self-Care: Instrumental Activities of Daily Living (IADLs)

Example NOC Outcome with Indicators
Endurance as evidenced by the following indicators: Performance of usual routine/Activity/Concentration/Muscle endurance/Eating pattern/Libido/Energy restored after rest/Blood oxygen level (Rate the outcome and indicators of **Endurance:** 1 = severely compromised, 2 = substantially compromised, 3 = moderately compromised, 4 = mildly compromised, 5 = not compromised [see Section I].)

Client Outcomes

Client Will (Specify Time Frame):

- Participate in prescribed physical activity with appropriate changes in heart rate, blood pressure, and breathing rate; maintain monitor patterns (rhythm and ST segment) within normal limits
- State symptoms of adverse effects of exercise and report onset of symptoms immediately
- Maintain normal skin color, and skin is warm and dry with activity
- Verbalize an understanding of the need to gradually increase activity based on testing, tolerance, and symptoms
- Demonstrate increased tolerance to activity

NIC   (Nursing Interventions Classification)

Suggested NIC Interventions

Activity Therapy, Energy Management

Example NIC Activities—Energy Management
Monitor cardiorespiratory response to activity; Monitor location and nature of discomfort or pain during movement/activity

Nursing Interventions and *Rationales*

- Determine cause of activity intolerance (see Related Factors) and determine whether cause is physical, psychological, or motivational. *Determining the cause of a problem can help direct appropriate interventions.*
- If mainly on bed rest, minimize cardiovascular deconditioning by positioning the client in an upright position several times daily if possible. *Deconditioning of the cardiovascular system occurs*

• = Independent   ▲ = Collaborative   **EBN** = Evidence-Based Nursing   **EB** = Evidence-Based

within days and involves fluid shifts, fluid loss, decreased cardiac output, decreased peak oxygen uptake, and increased resting heart rate (Fletcher, 2005; Fauci et al, 2008). A study found that diabetic clients developed orthostatic hypotension after 48 hours of bed rest, possibly from altered cardiovascular reflexes (Schneider et al, 2009).

- Assess the client daily for appropriateness of activity and bed rest orders. Mobilize the client as soon as it is possible. *With bed rest there is a shift of fluids from the extremities to the thoracic cavity from the loss of gravitational stress. Positioning in an upright position helps maintain optimal fluid distribution and maintain orthostatic tolerance (Perme & Chandrashekar, 2009).* **EB:** *A study utilizing tomography demonstrated significant decreased strength in the hip, thigh, and calf muscles in elderly orthopedic clients, as well as bone mineral loss with immobility (Berg et al, 2007).*
- If client is mostly immobile, consider use of a transfer chair: a chair that becomes a stretcher. *Using a transfer chair where the client is pulled onto a flat surface and then seated upright in the chair can help previously immobile clients get out of bed (Nelson et al, 2003; Perme & Chandrashekar, 2009).*
- When appropriate, gradually increase activity, allowing the client to assist with positioning, transferring, and self-care as possible. Progress from sitting in bed to dangling, to standing, to ambulation. Always have the client dangle at the bedside before trying standing to evaluate for postural hypotension. *Postural hypotension is very common in the elderly (Krecinic et al, 2009).*
- When getting a client up, observe for symptoms of intolerance such as nausea, pallor, dizziness, visual dimming, and impaired consciousness, as well as changes in vital signs. *When an adult rises to the standing position, 300 to 800 mL of blood pools in the lower extremities. As a result, symptoms of central nervous system hypoperfusion may occur, including feelings of weakness, nausea, headache, lightheadedness, dizziness, blurred vision, fatigue, tremulousness, palpitations, and impaired cognition (Bradley & Davis, 2003).*
- ▲ If the client experiences symptoms of postural hypotension as outlined above, take precautions when getting the client out of bed. Put graduated compression stockings on client or use lower limb compression bandaging if ordered to return blood to the heart and brain. Have the client dangle at the side of the bed with legs hanging over the edge of the bed, flex and extend feet several times after sitting up, then stand up slowly with someone holding the client. If client becomes light headed or dizzy, return them to bed immediately. *Postural hypotension is common and can occur with both younger and older clients from immobility and deconditioning. Use of compression stockings or leg bandaging can help return fluid from the lower extremities back where it collects from immobility to the heart and brain (Gorelik et al, 2009; Platts et al, 2009).*
- Perform range-of-motion (ROM) exercises if the client is unable to tolerate activity or is mostly immobile. See care plan for **Risk for Disuse syndrome**.
- Monitor and record the client's ability to tolerate activity: note pulse rate, blood pressure, monitor pattern, dyspnea, use of accessory muscles, and skin color before, during and after the activity. If the following signs and symptoms of cardiac decompensation develop, activity should be stopped immediately:
  - Onset of chest discomfort
  - Dyspnea
  - Palpitations
  - Excessive fatigue
  - Lightheadedness, confusion, ataxia, pallor, cyanosis, nausea, or any peripheral circulatory insufficiency
  - Dysrhythmia
  - Exercise hypotension (drop in systolic blood pressure of 10 mm Hg from baseline blood pressure despite an increase in workload)
  - Excessive rise in blood pressure (systolic >180 mm Hg or diastolic >110 mm Hg) NOTE: These are upper limits; activity may be stopped before reaching these values
  - Inappropriate bradycardia (drop in heart rate >10 beats/min or <50 beats/min)
  - Increased heart rate above 100 beats/min
- ▲ Instruct the client to stop the activity immediately and report to the physician if the client is experiencing the following symptoms: new or worsened intensity or increased frequency of discomfort; tightness or pressure in chest, back, neck, jaw, shoulders, and/or arms; palpitations; dizziness; weakness; unusual and extreme fatigue; excessive air hunger. *These are common symptoms of angina and are caused by a temporary insufficiency of coronary blood supply. Symptoms typically last for*

• = Independent ▲ = Collaborative **EBN** = Evidence-Based Nursing **EB** = Evidence-Based

minutes as opposed to momentary twinges. If symptoms last longer than 5 to 10 minutes, the client should be evaluated by a physician. Pulse rate and arterial blood oxygenation indicate cardiac/exercise tolerance; pulse oximetry identifies hypoxia (Grimes, 2007; Schmitz, 2007).

- Observe and document skin integrity several times a day. **Activity intolerance,** *if resulting in immobility, may lead to pressure ulcers. Mechanical pressure, moisture, friction, and shearing forces all predispose to their development (Fauci et al, 2008).* Refer to the care plan **Risk for impaired Skin integrity.**

- Assess for constipation. If present, refer to care plan for **Constipation. Activity intolerance** is associated with increased risk of constipation.

▲ Refer the client to physical therapy to help increase activity levels and strength.

▲ Consider a dietitian referral to assess nutritional needs related to activity intolerance, provide nutrition as needed. If client is unable to eat food, use enteral or parenteral feedings as needed.

- Recognize that malnutrition causes significant morbidity due to the loss of lean body mass. *Providing nutrition early helps maintain muscle and immune system function, and reduce hospital length of stay (McClave et al, 2009; Racco, 2009).*

- Provide emotional support and encouragement to the client to gradually increase activity. Work with the client to set mutual goals that increase activity levels. *Fear of breathlessness, pain, or falling may decrease willingness to increase activity.*

▲ Observe for pain before activity. If possible, treat pain before activity and ensure that the client is not heavily sedated. *Pain restricts the client from achieving a maximal activity level and is often exacerbated by movement.*

▲ Obtain any necessary assistive devices or equipment needed before ambulating the client (e.g., walkers, canes, crutches, portable oxygen). *Assistive devices can help increase mobility (Yeom, Keller, & Fleury, 2009).*

▲ Use a gait walking belt when ambulating the client. *Gait belts improve the caregiver's grasp, reducing the incidence of injuries (Nelson et al, 2003).*

Activity Intolerance Due to Respiratory Disease

- If the client is able to walk and has chronic obstructive pulmonary disease (COPD), use the traditional 6–minute walk distance to evaluate ability to walk. **EB:** *The 6–minute walk test predicted mortality in COPD clients (Pinto-Plata et al, 2004).*

▲ Ensure that the chronic pulmonary client has oxygen saturation testing with exercise. Use supplemental oxygen to keep oxygen saturation 90% or above or as prescribed with activity. *Clients with COPD may suffer from inadequate gas exchange. Oxygen therapy can improve exercise ability and ability to think in hypoxemic clients (Celli, MacNee, & ATS/ERS Task Force, 2004).*

- Monitor a respiratory client's response to activity by observing for symptoms of respiratory intolerance such as increased dyspnea, loss of ability to control breathing rhythmically, use of accessory muscles, nasal flaring, appearance of facial distress, and skin tone changes such as pallor and cyanosis (Perme & Chandrashekar, 2009).

- Instruct and assist a COPD client in using conscious, controlled breathing techniques during exercise, including pursed-lip breathing, and inspiratory muscle use. **EBN:** *A systematic review found pursed-lip breathing effective in decreasing dyspnea (Carrieri-Kohlman et al, 2008).* **EB:** *A systematic review found that inspiratory muscle training was effective in increasing endurance of the client and decreasing dyspnea (Langer et al, 2009).*

▲ Evaluate the client's nutritional status. Refer to a dietitian if needed. Use nutritional supplements to increase nutritional level if needed. *Improved nutrition may help increase inspiratory muscle function and decrease dyspnea.* **EBN:** *A study found that almost half of a group of clients with COPD were malnourished, which can lead to an exacerbation of the disease (Odencrants, Ehnfors, & Ehrenbert, 2008).*

▲ For the client in the intensive care unit, consider mobilizing the client in a four-phase method if there is sufficient knowledgeable staff available to protect the client from harm. *Even intensive care unit clients receiving mechanical ventilation can be mobilized safely if a multidisciplinary team is present to support, protect, and monitor the client for intolerance to activity (Perme & Chandrashekar, 2009).*

▲ Refer the COPD client to a pulmonary rehabilitation program. **EB:** *A Cochrane review found that pulmonary rehabilitation has been shown to relieve dyspnea and fatigue (Lacasse et al, 2006). Another*

● = Independent ▲ = Collaborative **EBN** = Evidence-Based Nursing **EB** = Evidence-Based

Cochrane review found pulmonary rehabilitation effective to decrease mortality and rate of readmission for the client who was recently discharged after treatment for an exacerbation of COPD (Puhan et al, 2009).

Activity Intolerance Due to Cardiovascular Disease

- If the client is able to walk and has heart failure, consider use of the 6–minute walk test to determine physical ability. **EB:** *The 6–minute walk test is a simple, safe, and inexpensive exercise test to predict functional capacity (Du et al, 2009).*
- Allow for periods of rest before and after planned exertion periods such as meals, baths, treatments, and physical activity. *Both physical and emotional rest help lower arterial pressure and reduce the workload of the myocardium (Fauci et al, 2008).*
- ▲ Refer to heart failure program or cardiac rehabilitation program for education, evaluation, and guided support to increase activity and rebuild life. **EB:** *Exercise can help many clients with heart failure. A carefully monitored exercise program can improve both exercise capacity and quality of life in mild to moderate heart failure clients (Rees et al, 2004).*
- See care plan for **Decreased Cardiac output** for further interventions.

 ### Geriatric

- Slow the pace of care. Allow the client extra time to carry out physical activities. *Slow gait in the elderly may be related to fear of falling; decreased strength in muscles, reduced balance or visual acuity, knee flexion contractures, and foot pain.*
- Encourage families to help/allow an elderly client to be independent in whatever activities possible. *Sometimes families believe they are assisting by allowing clients to be sedentary. Encouraging activity not only enhances good functioning of the body's systems but also promotes a sense of worth (Fauci et al, 2008).*
- ▲ Assess for swaying, poor balance, weakness, and fear of falling while elders stand/walk. If present, refer to physical therapy. *Fear of falling and repeat falling is common in the elderly population. Balance rehabilitation provides individualized treatment for persons with various deficits associated with balance (Studer, 2008).* Refer to the care plan for **Risk for Falls** and **Impaired Walking**.
- ▲ Evaluate medications the client is taking to see if they could be causing activity intolerance. Medications such as beta-blockers; lipid lowering agents, which can damage muscle; some antihypertensives; and lowering the blood pressure to normal in the elderly can result in decreased functioning. *Elderly may need a blood pressure of 140/80 or higher in order to walk without dizziness. It is important that medications be reviewed to ensure they are not resulting in less function of the elderly client (Haque, 2007). Many of the medications found on the Beers List of medications that are inappropriate to prescribe for elderly clients can result in decreased function from dizziness and delirium (Molony, 2009).* **EB:** *A study found that cases of orthostatic hypotension with syncope in the elderly were commonly associated with use of vasoactive medications (Mussi et al, 2009).*
- ▲ If the client has heart disease causing activity intolerance, refer for cardiac rehabilitation. **EB:** *A study found that elderly clients with coronary heart disease who participate in cardiac rehabilitation programs had significantly lower mortality rates (Suaya et al, 2009).*
- ▲ Refer the disabled elderly client to physical therapy for functional training including gait training, stepping, and sit-to-stand exercises, or for strength training. **EB:** *Functional decline from hospital-associated deconditioning is common in the elderly, and acute inpatient rehabilitation can be effective in preventing this condition (Kortebein, 2009). A study found that intensive functional training improved balance and coordination more than strength training (Krebs, Scarborough & McGibbon, 2007).* **EB:** *A Cochrane review found that progressive resistance strength training is effective in elderly clients to improve function (Liu & Latham, 2009).*
- When mobilizing the elderly client, watch for orthostatic hypotension accompanied by dizziness and fainting. *Postural hypotension can be detected in up to 30% of elderly clients. These methods can help prevent falls (Tinetti, 2003).*
- Teach compensatory strategies for orthostatic (postural) hypotension. *Older adults develop arterial stiffness and reduced autonomic nervous system functioning. Their baroreceptors respond slowly so they are less able to maintain blood pressure when standing (Sclater & Alagiakrishnan, 2006).*

● = Independent   ▲ = Collaborative   **EBN** = Evidence-Based Nursing   **EB** = Evidence-Based

Home Care

▲ Begin discharge planning as soon as possible with case manager or social worker to assess need for home support systems and the need for community or home health services.

▲ Assess the home environment for factors that contribute to decreased activity tolerance such as stairs or distance to the bathroom. Refer to occupational therapy, if needed, to assist the client in restructuring the home and ADL patterns. *During hospitalization, clients and families often estimate energy requirements at home inaccurately because the hospital's availability of staff support distorts the level of care that will be needed.*

▲ Refer to physical therapy for strength training and possible weight training, to regain strength, increase endurance, and improve balance. If the client is homebound, the physical therapist can also initiate cardiac rehabilitation.

● Normalize the client's activity intolerance; encourage progress with positive feedback. The client's experience should be validated as within expected norms. Recognition of progress enhances motivation. **EBN:** *In qualitative studies, fatigued women reported that they felt distressed when health care providers invalidated their experiences of fatigue (Patusky, 2002; Asbring & Narvanen, 2004).*

● Teach the client/family the importance of and methods for setting priorities for activities, especially those having a high energy demand (e.g., home/family events). Instruct in realistic expectations. **EBN:** *Unrealistic expectations provoke guilt feelings in the client, leading to efforts that can exceed the client's energy capacity (Patusky, 2002).*

● Provide the client/family with resources such as senior centers, exercise classes, educational and recreational programs, and volunteer opportunities that can aid in promoting socialization and appropriate activity. *Social isolation can be an outcome of and contribute to activity intolerance.*

● Discuss the importance of sexual activity as part of daily living. Instruct the client in adaptive techniques to conserve energy during sexual interactions.

● Instruct the client and family in the importance of maintaining proper nutrition.

● Instruct in use of dietary supplements as indicated. *Illness may suppress appetite, leading to inadequate nutrition.*

▲ Refer to medical social services as necessary to assist the family in adjusting to major changes in patterns of living because of activity intolerance.

● Assess the need for long-term supports for optimal activity tolerance of priority activities (e.g., assistive devices, oxygen, medication, catheters, massage), especially for a hospice client. Evaluate intermittently.

▲ Refer to home health aide services to support the client and family through changing levels of activity tolerance. Introduce aide support early. Instruct the aide to promote independence in activity as tolerated.

● Allow terminally ill clients and their families to guide care. *Control by the client or family respects their autonomy and promotes effective coping.*

● Provide increased attention to comfort and dignity of the terminally ill client in care planning. *Interventions should be provided as much for psychological effect as for physiological support. For example, oxygen may be more valuable as a support to the client's psychological comfort than as a booster of oxygen saturation.*

▲ Institute case management of frail elderly to support continued independent living.

Client/Family Teaching and Discharge Planning

● Instruct the client on techniques to utilize for avoiding activity intolerance.

● Teach the client to use controlled breathing techniques with activity.

● Teach the client techniques to decrease dizziness from postural hypotension when standing up.

● Help client with energy conservation and work simplification techniques in ADLs.

● Describe to the client the symptoms of activity intolerance, including which symptoms to report to the physician.

● Explain to the client how to use assistive devices, oxygen, or medications before or during activity.

● Help client set up an activity log to record exercise and exercise tolerance.

ⓔvolve   See the EVOLVE website for Weblinks for client education resources.

● = Independent   ▲ = Collaborative   **EBN** = Evidence-Based Nursing   **EB** = Evidence-Based

REFERENCES

Asbring P, Narvanen A: Patient power and control: a study of women with uncertain illness trajectories, *Qual Health Res* 14(2): 226, 2004.

Berg HE, Eiken O, Miklavcic L et al: Hip, thigh and calf muscle atrophy and bone loss after 5-week bedrest inactivity, *Eur J Appl Physiol* 99(3):283–289, 2007.

Bradley JG, Davis KA: Orthostatic hypertension, *Am Fam Physician* 68(12):2393–2398, 2003.

Carrieri-Kohlman V, Donesky-Cuenco D: Dyspnea management. An EBP guideline. In Ackley B, Ladwig G, Swann BA et al, editors: *Evidence-based nursing care guidelines: medical-surgical interventions,* Philadelphia, 2008, Mosby.

Celli BR, MacNee W, ATS/ERS Task Force: Standards for the diagnosis and treatment of patients with COPD: a summary of the ATS/ERS position paper, *Eur Respir J* 23(6):932, 2004.

Du H, Newton PJ, Salamonson Y et al: A review of the six-minute walk test: its implication as a self-administered assessment tool, *Eur J Cardiovasc Nurs* 8(1):2–8, 2009.

Fauci A, Braunwald E, Kasper DL et al: *Harrison's principles of internal medicine,* ed 17, New York, 2008, McGraw-Hill.

Fletcher K: Immobility: geriatric self-learning module, *Medsurg Nurs* 14(1):35, 2005.

Gorelik O, Almozzino-Sarafian D, Litvinov V et al: Seating-induced postural hypotension is common in older patients with decompensated heart failure and may be prevented by lower limb compression bandaging. *Gerontology,* 55(2):138–144, 2009.

Grimes K: Heart disease. In O'Sullivan SB & Schmitz JT, editors: *Physical rehabilitation,* ed 5, Philadelphia, 2007, F.A. Davis.

Haque R: *Polypharmacy in the elderly—cardiovascular component.* Presentation at conference: new directions in cardiovascular disease, March 10, 2007, Jackson, MI.

Kortebein P: Rehabilitation for hospital-associated deconditioning, *Am J Phys Med Rehabil* 88(1):66–77, 2009.

Krebs DE, Scarborough DM, McGibbon CA: Functional vs. strength training in disabled elderly outpatients, *Am J Phys Med Rehabil* 86(2):93–103, 2007.

Krecinic T, Mattace-Raso F, Van Der Velde N et al: Orthostatic hypotension in older persons: a diagnostic algorithm, *J Nutr Health Aging* 13(6):572–575, 2009.

Lacasse Y, Goldstein R, Lasserson T et al: Pulmonary rehabilitation for chronic obstructive pulmonary disease, *Cochrane Database Syst Rev* (3):CD003793, 2006.

Langer D, Hendriks E, Burtin C et al: A clinical practice guideline for physiotherapists treating patients with chronic obstructive pulmonary disease based on a systematic review of available evidence, *Clin Rehabil* 23(5):445–462, 2009.

Liu CJ, Latham NK: Progressive resistance strength training for improving physical function in older adults, *Cochrane Database Syst Rev* (3): CD002759, 2009.

McClave S, Martindale R, Vanek V et al: Guidelines for the provision and assessment of nutrition support therapy in the adult critically ill patient: Society of Critical Care Medicine (SCCM) and American Society for Parenteral and Enteral Nutrition (A.S.P.E.N.), *JPEN J Parenter Enteral Nutr* 33(3):277–316, 2009.

Molony SL: Monitoring medication use in older adults, *Am J Nurs* 109(1):68–78, 2009.

Mussi C, Ungar A, Salvioli G et al: Orthostatic hypotension as cause of syncope in patients older than 65 years admitted to emergency departments for transient loss of consciousness, *J Gerontol A Biol Sci Med Sci* 64(7):801–806, 2009.

Nelson A, Owen B, Lloyd JD et al: Safe patient handling and movement, *Am J Nurs* 103(3):32, 2003.

Odencrants S, Ehnfors M, Ehrenbert A: Nutritional status and patient characteristics for hospitalized older patients with chronic obstructive pulmonary disease, *J Clin Nurs* 17(13):1771–1778, 2008.

Patusky KL: Relatedness theory as a framework for the treatment of fatigued women, *Arch Psychiatr Nurs* 5:224, 2002.

Perme C, Chandrashekar R: Early mobility and walking program for patients in intensive care units: creating a standard of care, *Am J Crit Care,* 18(3):212–221, 2009.

Pinto-Plata VM, Cote C, Cabral H et al: The 6-min walk distance: change over time and value as a predictor of survival in severe COPD, *Eur Respir J* 23(1):23, 2004.

Platts SH, Tushorn JA, Riberiro LC et al: Compression garments as countermeasures to orthostatic intolerance, *Aviat Spac Environ Med* 80(5):437–442, 2009.

Puhan M, Scharplatz M, Troosters T et al: Pulmonary rehabilitation following exacerbations of chronic obstructive pulmonary disease, *Cochrane Database Syst Rev* (1):CD005305, 2009.

Racco M: Nutrition in the ICU, *RN* 72(1):26–30, 2009.

Rees K, Taylor RS, Singh et al: Exercise based rehabilitation for heart failure, *Cochrane Database Syst Rev* (3):CD003331, 2004

Schmitz TJ: Vital signs. In O'Sullivan SB & Schmitz TJ, editors: *Physical rehabilitation,* ed 5, Philadelphia, 2007, F.A. Davis.

Schneider SM, Roberts RA, Amorim F et al. Impaired orthostatic response in patients with type 2 diabetes mellitus after 48 hours of bedrest, *Endocr Pract* 15(2):104–110, 2009.

Sclater A, Alagiakrishnan K: Orthostatic hypotension: a primary care primer for assessment and treatment, *Geriatrics* 59(8):22, 2006.

Studer M: Keep it moving: advances in gait training techniques help clients reduce balance issues, *Rehabil Manag* 21(5):10–15, 2008.

Suaya JA, Stason WB, Ades PA et al: Cardiac rehabilitation and survival in older coronary patients, *J Am Coll Cardiol* 54(1):25–33, 2009.

Tinetti ME: Preventing falls in elderly persons, *N Engl J Med* 348(1):421, 2003.

Yeom HA, Keller C, Fleury J: Interventions for promoting mobility in community-dwelling older adults, *J Am Acad Nurse Pract* 21(2):95–100, 2009.

Risk for Activity intolerance   *Betty J. Ackley, MSN, EdS, RN*

NANDA-I

Definition

At risk for experiencing insufficient physiological or psychological energy to endure or complete required or desired daily activities

● = Independent   ▲ = Collaborative   **EBN** = Evidence-Based Nursing   **EB** = Evidence-Based

Risk Factors

Deconditioned status; history of previous intolerance; inexperience with the activity; presence of circulatory problems; presence of respiratory problems

NOC, NIC, Client Outcomes, Nursing Interventions, Client/Family Teaching and Discharge Planning, *Rationales,* and References

Refer to care plan for **Activity intolerance.**

Ineffective Activity planning   *France Maltais, BSc, MEd, and Gail B. Ladwig, MSN, RN, CHTP*

Definition

Inability to prepare for a set of actions fixed in time and under certain conditions

Defining Characteristics

Verbalization of fear toward a task to be undertaken; verbalization of worries toward a task to be undertaken; excessive anxieties toward a task to be undertaken; pattern of failure of behavior; lack of plan; lack of resources; lack of sequential organization; procrastination; unmet goals for chosen activity

Related Factors (r/t)

Compromised ability to process information; defensive flight behavior when faced with proposed solution; hedonism; lack of family support; lack of friend support; unrealistic perception of events; unrealistic perception of personal competence

 (Nursing Outcomes Classification)

Suggested NOC Outcomes

Cognition; Cognition Orientation; Concentration; Decision-Making; Information Processing; Memory

Example NOC Outcome with Indicators
Cognition as evidenced by the following indicators: Communication clear and appropriate for age/Comprehension of the meaning of situations/Information processing/Alternatives weighed when making decisions (Rate the outcome and indicators of **Cognition:** 1 = severely compromised, 2 = substantially compromised, 3 = moderately compromised, 4 = mildly compromised, 5 = not compromised [see Section I].)

Client Outcomes

Client Will (Specify Time Frame):

- State fear(s) and worry of task to be undertaken
- Identify and verbalize symptoms of anxiety toward task to be undertaken
- State a plan/resources/goal/organization and time frame for task to be undertaken

NIC **(Nursing Interventions Classification)**

Suggested NIC Interventions

Anxiety Reduction, Behavior Management, Behavior Modification, Calming Technique, Coping Enhancement, Memory Training, Planning Assistance, Sequence Guidance

Example NIC Activities—Coping Enhancement
Assist client in developing an objective appraisal of the event; Explore with client previous methods of dealing with life problems

● = Independent   ▲ = Collaborative   **EBN** = Evidence-Based Nursing   **EB** = Evidence-Based

Nursing Interventions and *Rationales*

- Establish a contract (McFarland et al, 1996, 1999).
  - Before the first conference/meeting with the client, begin by establishing an agenda and get the assurance that the client will participate. Record the information. Give precise information on the upcoming session. At each session identify precisely the tasks to be accomplished for each session and the upcoming tasks for subsequent session. *It is important that the client use a sequential organizational model with the nurse/health care provider (Debray et al, 2005).*
  - Identify the people who will be involved in the attainment of the objective or the person in charge. *The role and the rules are definite (e.g., The nurse will hold the interview of the day for the verbalization of feelings; the social worker will meet with the client two times a week, the priest [pastor] etc.).*
  - Ask the client how they perceive the situation in order to gather their personal vision of the problem and how they envisage their self-involvement. Specify the goals. *"It is the client's own thoughts and goals that are of prime importance" (Greenberg & Padesky, 2004).*
  - Assess the client's actual level of function (functionality) (at work, in school, at the hospital) by identifying actual dysfunctional behaviors.
  - ▲ Refer the client for cognitive behavioral therapy. The work for the client begins with the understanding that their thoughts affect their emotions and reactions and therefore the success of meeting their objectives. Explain the EPEC* system in order to have a realistic concept of the situation. Suggest that the client change their self-concept, for example, "Stop thinking of yourself as powerless." *The planning of the project (event) will depend in large part on the vision of the person with the problem and on their abilities (perception). Changing this perception may lead to self-confidence and a sense of accomplishment (emotions), which will translate into appropriate actions leading to successful behaviors (Cottraux et al, 2001; Fortinash, Holoday-Worret, & Boissonneault, 2002; Auger, 2006).*
  - Confront and restructure the following unrealistic idea "Running away is a better reaction when confronted with a dangerous object." The true syllogism is "running away is the reaction when confronted with an object that is 'imagined' to be dangerous." Instruct the client to practice and repeat the following statement: "I have the power to change by changing my ideas." *Determine with accuracy the real nature of the danger and the probability that the danger will manifest itself. It is in experimentation that a person will be able to measure their abilities. This is the nature of the contract (Debray et al, 2005).*
- Lower the anxiety level tied to the client's fear of not succeeding (Auger, 2006). **EB:** *This review of randomized placebo-controlled trials indicates that CBT is efficacious for adult anxiety disorders (Hofmann & Smits, 2008).*
  - Research the client's rising anxiety behaviors and show evidence of "the client's catastrophic" thoughts by repeating what negative thoughts the client has expressed, for example, "It would be dreadful if I would not succeed" "I can never do..." *With the confrontation, work to consider the consequences of the dangers of not succeeding such as boredom, or regrettable or disagreeable outcomes that are not as catastrophic as the client suggests. Work to change the dramatic interpretation of the situation by the client by using correct words, appropriate to the actual seriousness of the consequences (Ladouceur, Marchand, & Boivert, 1999; Wilson & Branch, 2006).*
  - Verify if the lack of success of the project would lower the client's self-image. *Reinforce the idea that making an effort is better than no action (Auger, 2006).*
  - Work on excessive generalization in regards to a unique event of all possible situations. It is often necessary to go back over premature experiences of loss of control of the environment. *The gravity of the situation and inability to succeed are always exaggerated when anxiety is dysfunctional (Cottraux et al, 2001).*
  - Encourage the person to look into a problem and at the same time make a list of priorities. Have the client drill and repeat the following statements: "I have the ability to take on more than one challenge at the same time"; and "It is in action that I measure myself, thought will never demonstrate any proof of my abilities."
- Evaluate in a fair way the client's ability to do a job, study, end the task, and participate in a program (identify the problem) (Filion, 1989).
  - Distinguish the "dream" of the project. The dream is blurred (vague) as much as the plan is detailed, clear, precise, and verifiable.

• = Independent   ▲ = Collaborative   **EBN** = Evidence-Based Nursing   **EB** = Evidence-Based

- Work on the project at the same time.
- Determine as fairly as possible the success factors needed for the planning and success of the project: financial resources; the family situation; prior medical, psychiatric and psychosocial conditions; material resources; and the ability to manage stress (Ladouceur, Marchand, & Boivert, 1999).
- Identify the informational needs of the person: understanding of their state of health, supervision of their treatment if they are receiving treatment, diet, and important telephone numbers (McFarland, Wasli, & Gerety, 1999).
- Identify and reinforce the elements of the client's personality which may help them to succeed with their plan. Have the client drill and repeat: "I can change my goals (dreams) with a plan." (McFarland, Wasli, & Gerety, 1999).

- Assist the client to plan in a realistic way for work, studies, or the choice not to continue a project *(determination des objectifs)* (Auger, 2006).
  - Determine the general objective, which consists of the final goal after multiple divided approaches during a prolonged time (3 months, 1 year or 3 years).
  - Carry out the general objective by using secondary objectives in successive stages and in a logical progression. Remember that the attainment of these objectives may imply a modification of the schedule. Use a schedule, calendar, or agenda to write down the dates. For realistic planning: choose simple tasks, limit long hours of work, protect bio-psycho-social well-being, improve techniques (of relaxation, of study, of concentration, of memory, aptitude of reading, writing, the way of taking notes).
  - Each secondary objective will be followed by detailed mini-objectives, those to be attained in a specific time period (1 month to 1 week). It will be a question of precise movements.
- Finally, determine the micro-objectives; they will be determined by a series of questions that the person can ask immediately or over the course of several hours. Drill and repeat: "I have the advantage to clearly attain my objectives and take the necessary steps to attain them, otherwise I risk turning round and round like a traveler without a compass." *Repetition leads successively to the attainment of micro-objectives, secondary objectives, and the overall general objective. These first steps are of capital importance. In effect, we only control (and yet imperfectly) the micro-objectives. If the micro-objectives are not attained, then the whole pyramid will collapse (Filion, 1989).*
- Anticipate the obstacles the client may encounter. *This helps the client to increase their motivation and their responsibility to obtain their objectives and develop a plan of action. (Auger, 2006).*
  - Help the person to make a contract with themselves, independently. *The discipline is in the rigor of their choices.*
  - Establish a safeguard that will be helpful in pursuing the goal. It should be nonpunitive, but help the client to remember the importance of the instrument's use to attain the micro-objectives, the base of success. It could be written down like this: "Each evening I will work on my books for 30 minutes. If I do it I will prepare myself a good snack, otherwise I don't merit this snack"; "I am going to take a 30–minute walk for 2 days. If I do it I will let myself watch TV for 1 hour, otherwise I will take a 1 hour walk for the next 2 days." Drill and repeat: "I will realize my goals no matter what."
- Correctly orient the individual towards things that can help him or her attain the objectives (evaluation of the work in progress).
  - Ask yourself the following questions: is the person alone, are they capable of attaining their objective in a day or would it be better to get something going with a support team? What is the proof that this person can realistically attain their objectives?
  - Discuss the resources that the person has already used in order to verify if the changes assert themselves. Identify the potentially pivotal helping people (McFarland, Wasli, & Gerety, 1999).
  - ▲ Clarify and coordinate the project in collaboration with a multidisciplinary team in the field and with other specialists (doctor, employment center, teacher, technician, etc.).
  - Redefine the project's needs. Specify the steps that should be accomplished to attain the objectives of the project. It is often necessary to redo each step in the course of the project.
  - If necessary, coordinate the orientation of the person towards other structures or treatments that have not been used, for example: individual or group therapy, an educational support person, a financial aid person.

• = Independent   ▲ = Collaborative   **EBN** = Evidence-Based Nursing   **EB** = Evidence-Based

- Tackle the fears and worries and make a cognitive reconstruction. Drill and Repeat: "I can change false ideas which make me believe that I am unable to carry out (achieve) my plan" (Ladouceur, Marchand, & Boivert, 1999).

Note: The above interventions may be adapted for the geriatric and multicultural client, and for home care and client/family teaching and discharge planning.

Refer to care plans **Anxiety, Readiness for enhanced family Coping, Readiness for enhanced Decision-Making, Fear, Readiness for enhanced Hope, Readiness for enhanced Power, Readiness for enhanced Spiritual well-being, Readiness for enhanced Self Health management** for additional interventions.

⊖volve   See the EVOLVE website for Weblinks for client education resources.

REFERENCES

Auger L: *Vivre avec sa tête ou avec son cœur (Live with your head or with your heart)*, Centre la Pensée Réaliste, republication par Pierre Bovo, 2006.

Cottraux J, Note I, Yao SN et al: A randomized controlled trial of cognitive therapy versus intensive behavior therapy in obsessive compulsive disorder, *Psychother Psychosom* 70(6):288–297, 2001.

Debray Q, Kindynis S, Leclère M et al: *The protocols of treatment of pathological personalities. Cognitive behavioral approach*, Paris, 2005, Masson.

Filion F: *J'améliore mes plans d'action*, Québec, 1989, C.A.E.R. Ed.

Fortinash K, Holoday-Worret, P, Boissonneault H: *Soins infirmiers, santé mentale et psychiatrie*, Laval, Quebec, 2003, Beauchemin.

Greenberg D, Padesky C: *Grief and anxiety: understand and overcome by the cognitive approach*, Québec, 2004, Décarie Éditeur.

Hofmann SG, Smits JA: Cognitive-behavioral therapy for adult anxiety disorders: a meta-analysis of randomized placebo-controlled trials, *J Clin Psychiatry* 69(4):621–632, 2008.

Ladouceur R, Marchand A, Boivert JM: *Anxiety disorder. Cognitive and behavioral approach*, Montreal, 1999, Gaétan Morin E.

McFarland GK, Wasli EL, Gerety EK: *Santé mentale, démarche de soins et diagnostics infirmiers*, ed 2, Paris, l996, l999, Masson.

Wilson R, Branch R: *Cognitive behavioural therapy for dummies*, Philadelphia, 2006, John Wiley & Sons. *EPEC

*(E) **event**; (P) everybody has a/his own **perception**; (E) source/origin of their own **emotions**; (C [for comportement in French]) specific **behavior**

Ineffective Airway clearance   *Betty J. Ackley, MSN, EdS, RN*   ⊖volve

NANDA-I

Definition

Inability to clear secretions or obstructions from the respiratory tract to maintain a clear airway

Defining Characteristics

Absent cough; adventitious breath sounds (rales, crackles, rhonchi, wheezes); changes in respiratory rate and rhythm; cyanosis; difficulty vocalizing; diminished breath sounds; dyspnea; excessive sputum; orthopnea; restlessness; wide-eyed

Related Factors (r/t)

Environmental

Second-hand smoke; smoke inhalation; smoking

Obstructed Airway

Airway spasm; excessive mucus; exudate in the alveoli; foreign body in airway; presence of artificial airway; retained secretions; secretions in the bronchi

Physiological

Allergic airways; asthma; COPD; hyperplasia of the bronchial walls; infection; neuromuscular dysfunction

NOC   (Nursing Outcomes Classification)

Suggested NOC Outcomes

Aspiration Prevention; Respiratory Status: Airway Patency, Gas Exchange, Ventilation

• = Independent   ▲ = Collaborative   **EBN** = Evidence-Based Nursing   **EB** = Evidence-Based

---

Example NOC Outcome with Indicators

Respiratory Status: Ventilation as evidenced by the following indicators: Respiratory rate/Moves sputum out of airway/Adventitious breath sounds not present/Shortness of breath not present/Auscultated breath sounds/Auscultated vocalization/Chest x-ray findings IER (Rate each indicator of **Respiratory Status: Ventilation:** 1 = severe deviation from normal range, 2 = substantial deviation from normal range, 3 = moderate deviation from normal range, 4 = mild deviation from normal range, 5 = no deviation from normal range [see Section I].)

Client Outcomes

Client Will (Specify Time Frame):

- Demonstrate effective coughing and clear breath sounds
- Maintain a patent airway at all times
- Explain methods useful to enhance secretion removal
- Explain the significance of changes in sputum to include color, character, amount, and odor
- Identify and avoid specific factors that inhibit effective airway clearance

NIC (Nursing Interventions Classification)

Suggested NIC Interventions

Airway Management, Airway Suctioning, Cough Enhancement

Example NIC Activities—Airway Management

Instruct how to cough effectively; auscultate breath sounds, noting areas of decreased or absent ventilation and presence of adventitious sounds

Nursing Interventions and *Rationales*

- Auscultate breath sounds q 1 to 4 hours. *Breath sounds are normally clear or scattered fine crackles at bases, which clear with deep breathing. The presence of coarse crackles during late inspiration indicates fluid in the airway; wheezing indicates an airway obstruction (Fauci et al, 2008).*
- Monitor respiratory patterns, including rate, depth, and effort. *A normal respiratory rate for an adult without dyspnea is 12 to 16 (Bickley & Szilagyi, 2009). With secretions in the airway, the respiratory rate will increase.*
- Monitor blood gas values and pulse oxygen saturation levels as available. *An oxygen saturation of less than 90% (normal: 95% to 100%) or a partial pressure of oxygen of less than 80 (normal: 80 to 100) indicates significant oxygenation problems (Clark, Giuliano, & Chen, 2006).*
- ▲ Administer oxygen as ordered. *Oxygen administration has been shown to correct hypoxemia (Wong & Elliott, 2009).*
- Position the client to optimize respiration (e.g., head of bed elevated 30–45 degrees and repositioned at least every 2 hours). *An upright position allows for maximal lung expansion; lying flat causes abdominal organs to shift toward the chest, which crowds the lungs and makes it more difficult to breathe.* **EB:** *In a mechanically ventilated client, there is a decreased incidence of pneumonia if the client is positioned at a 45–degree semirecumbent position as opposed to a supine position (Seckel, 2006).*
- Help the client deep breathe and perform controlled coughing. Have the client inhale deeply, hold breath for several seconds, and cough two or three times with mouth open while tightening the upper abdominal muscles. *This technique can help increase sputum clearance and decrease cough spasms (Donahue, 2002). Controlled coughing uses the diaphragmatic muscles, making the cough more forceful and effective.*
- If the client has obstructive lung disease, such as COPD, cystic fibrosis, or bronchiectasis, consider helping the client use the forced expiratory technique, the "huff cough." The client does a series of coughs while saying the word "huff." *This technique prevents the glottis from closing during the cough and is effective in clearing secretions (van der Schans, 2007; Bhowmik et al, 2009).*
- ▲ Encourage the client to use an incentive spirometer if ordered. Recognize that controlled coughing and deep breathing may be just as effective. **EB:** *A study of postoperative abdominal surgery clients demonstrated that coughing and deep breathing clients versus use of an incentive spirometer resulted*

● = Independent ▲ = Collaborative **EBN** = Evidence-Based Nursing **EB** = Evidence-Based

in no significant difference in oxygenation (Genc, Yildirim, & Gnerli, 2004). A Cochrane review found that use of incentive spirometry was not more effective than positive pressure breathing techniques (Freitas et al, 2007).

- Encourage activity and ambulation as tolerated. If unable to ambulate the client, turn the client from side to side at least every 2 hours. *Body movement helps mobilize secretions.* **EB:** *Changes of postoperative position from sitting to standing are very important to improve outcomes, and the supine position should be avoided (Nielsen, Holte, & Kehlet, 2003).* See interventions for **Impaired Gas exchange** for further information on positioning a respiratory client.
- Encourage fluid intake of up to 2500 mL/day within cardiac or renal reserve. *Fluids help minimize mucosal drying and maximize ciliary action to move secretions.*
▲ Administer medications such as bronchodilators or inhaled steroids as ordered. Watch for side effects such as tachycardia or anxiety with bronchodilators, or inflamed pharynx with inhaled steroids. *Bronchodilators decrease airway resistance, improve the efficiency of respiratory movements, improve exercise tolerance, and can reduce symptoms of dyspnea on exertion (Barnett, 2008).*
▲ Provide postural drainage, percussion, and vibration as ordered. **EB:** *A Cochrane review of studies demonstrated that there is no advantage of chest physiotherapy over other airway clearance techniques for cystic fibrosis clients (Main, Prasad, & Schans, 2005).*
- Observe sputum, noting color, odor, and volume. *Normal sputum is clear or gray and minimal; abnormal sputum is green, yellow, or bloody; malodorous; and often copious.*

Critical Care

▲ If the client is intubated and is stable, consider getting the client up to sit at the edge of the bed, transfer to a chair, or walk as appropriate, if an effective interdisciplinary team is developed to keep the client safe. *For every week of bed rest, muscle strength can decrease 20%; early ambulation helped clients develop a positive outlook (Perme & Chandrashekar, 2009).*
▲ If the client is intubated, consider use of kinetic therapy, using a kinetic bed that slowly moves the client with 40–degree turns. **EBN:** *A study demonstrated that use of the kinetic bed versus turning clients every 2 hours resulted in decreased ventilator-associated pneumonia and atelectasis (Ahrens et al, 2004). Rotational therapy decreases the incidence of pneumonia, but had little effect on mortality rates, number of days on ventilator, or number of days in the ICU (Goldhill et al, 2007).*
- When suctioning an endotracheal tube or tracheostomy tube for a client on a ventilator, do the following:
  - Explain the process of suctioning beforehand and ensure the client is not in pain or overly anxious. *Suctioning can be a frightening experience; an explanation along with adequate pain relief or needed sedation can reduce stress, anxiety, and pain.*
  - Hyperoxygenate before and between endotracheal suction sessions. *Studies have demonstrated that hyperoxygenation helps prevent oxygen desaturation in a suctioned client (Pedersen et al, 2009).*
  - Suction for less than 15 seconds. *Studies demonstrated that because of a drop in the partial pressure of oxygen with suctioning, that preferably no more than 10 seconds be used actually suctioning, with the entire procedure taking 15 seconds (Pedersen et al, 2009).*
  - Use a closed, in-line suction system. Closed in-line suctioning has minimal effects on heart rate, respiratory rate, tidal volume, and oxygen saturation (Seymour et al, 2009). **EB:** *A study demonstrated that endotracheal suctioning using a closed system resulted in less deoxygenation of the client than when disconnecting the tubing for suctioning (Maggiore et al, 2003).*
  - Avoid saline instillation during suctioning. **EBN:** *Repeated studies have demonstrated that saline instillation before suctioning has an adverse effect on oxygen saturation in both adults and children (Rauen et al, 2008; Pederson et al, 2009).*
  - Document results of coughing and suctioning, particularly client tolerance and secretion characteristics such as color, odor, and volume.

Pediatric

- Educate parents about the risk factors for ineffective airway clearance such as foreign body ingestion and passive smoke exposure. **EB:** *Studies indicate the most common types of pediatric foreign bodies include vegetables, nuts, small toys, and other pieces of food (Midulla, Guidi, & Barbato, 2005).*

• = Independent   ▲ = Collaborative   **EBN** = Evidence-Based Nursing   **EB** = Evidence-Based

- See the care plan **Risk for Suffocation** for more interventions on choking. **EB:** *Passive smoke exposure significantly increases the risk of respiratory infections in children (Chatzimicael et al, 2008).*
- Educate children and parents on the importance of adherence to peak expiratory flow (PEF) monitoring for asthma self-management. **EBN:** *Children adherent to at least once-daily PEF monitoring were less likely to have an asthma episode than those who were less adherent (Burkhart, Rayens, & Revelette, 2007).*
- Educate parents and other caregivers that cough and cold medication bought over the counter are not safe for a child under 2 unless specifically ordered by a health care provider. *Over the counter cold and cough medications are no longer recommended for children under the age of 2 unless recommended by a health care provider. Minimal data exist to support their effectiveness, and overuse can cause harm (Ky et al, 2006; Woo, 2008).*

Geriatric

- Encourage ambulation as tolerated without causing exhaustion. *Immobility is often harmful to the elderly because it decreases ventilation and increases stasis of secretions, leading to atelectasis or pneumonia (Fletcher, 2005).*
- Actively encourage the elderly to deep breathe and cough. *Cough reflexes are blunted, and coughing is decreased in the elderly (Miller, 2004).*
- Ensure adequate hydration within cardiac and renal reserves. *The elderly are prone to dehydration, and therefore more viscous secretions, because they frequently use diuretics or laxatives and forget to drink adequate amounts of water (Miller, 2004).*

Home Care

- Some of the above interventions may be adapted for home care use.
- ▲ Begin discharge planning as soon as possible with case manager or social worker to assess need for home support systems, assistive devices, and community or home health services.
- Assess home environment for factors that exacerbate airway clearance problems (e.g., presence of allergens, lack of adequate humidity in air, poor air flow, stressful family relationships). **EBN:** *Home environmental triggers of asthma have been found to include dust/dust mites, animal dander, mold, perfumes/detergents, and cigarette smoke. Psychosocial triggers included family tensions, physical activity, anxiety/stress, and friends/peer pressure (Navaie-Waliser et al, 2004).*
- Assess affective climate within family and family support system. *Problems with respiratory function and resulting anxiety can provoke anger and frustration in the client. Feelings may be displaced onto caregiver and require intervention to ensure continued caregiver support.* Refer to care plan for **Caregiver role strain.**
- Refer to GOLD and ACP-ASIM/ACCP guidelines for management of home care and indications of hospital admission criteria (Chojnowski, 2003).
- When respiratory procedures are being implemented, explain equipment and procedures to family members, and provide needed emotional support. *Family members assuming responsibility for respiratory monitoring often find this stressful. They may not have been able to assimilate fully any instructions provided by hospital staff.*
- When electrically based equipment for respiratory support is being implemented, evaluate home environment for electrical safety, proper grounding, and so on. Ensure that notification is sent to the local utility company, the emergency medical team, and police and fire departments.
- Provide family with support for care of a client with chronic or terminal illness. *Breathing difficulty can provoke extreme anxiety, which can interfere with the client's ability or willingness to adhere to the treatment plan.*
- Refer to care plan for **Anxiety.** *Witnessing breathing difficulties and facing concerns of dealing with chronic or terminal illness can create fear in caregiver. Fear inhibits effective coping.* **EBN:** *Parents of a child with cystic fibrosis particularly benefit from nursing support. Parents deal with devastation upon receiving the diagnosis, a sense of fear and isolation, an overwhelming sense of guilt and powerlessness, vigilance, and returning to normalcy (Carpenter & Narsavage, 2004).* Refer to care plan for **Powerlessness.**

• = Independent   ▲ = Collaborative   **EBN** = Evidence-Based Nursing   **EB** = Evidence-Based

- Instruct the client to avoid exposure to persons with upper respiratory infections, to avoid crowds of people, and wash hands after each exposure to groups of people, or public places.
▲ Determine client adherence to medical regimen. Instruct the client and family in importance of reporting effectiveness of current medications to physician. *Inappropriate use of medications (too much or too little) can influence amount of respiratory secretions.*
- Teach the client when and how to use inhalant or nebulizer treatments at home.
- Teach the client/family importance of maintaining regimen and having PRN drugs easily accessible at all times. *Success in avoiding emergency or institutional care may rest solely on medication compliance or availability.* **EBN:** *Parents/family have been found to have inadequate knowledge about recognition of asthma attacks, triggers, and management (Navaie-Waliser et al, 2004).*
- Instruct the client and family in the importance of maintaining proper nutrition, adequate fluids, rest, and behavioral pacing for energy conservation and rehabilitation.
- Instruct in use of dietary supplements as indicated. *Illness may suppress appetite, leading to inadequate nutrition. Supplements will allow clients to eat with minimal energy consumption.*
- Identify an emergency plan, including criteria for use. *Ineffective airway clearance can be life-threatening.*
▲ Refer for home health aide services for assistance with ADLs. *Clients with decreased oxygenation and copious respiratory secretions are often unable to maintain energy for ADLs.*
▲ Assess family for role changes and coping skills. Refer to medical social services as necessary. *Clients with decreased oxygenation are unable to maintain role activities and therefore experience frustration and anger, which may pose a threat to family integrity. Family counseling to adapt to role changes may be needed.*
▲ For the client dying at home with a terminal illness, if the death rattle is present with gurgling, rattling, or crackling sounds in the airway with each breath, recognize that anticholinergic medications can often help control symptoms, if given early in the process. *Anticholinergic medications can help decrease the accumulation of secretions, but do not decrease existing secretions. This medication must be administered early in the process to be effective (Hipp & Letizia, 2009).*
▲ For the client with a death rattle, nursing care includes turning to mobilize secretions, keeping the head of the bed elevated for postural drainage of secretions, and avoiding suctioning. *Suctioning is a distressing and painful event for clients and families, and is rarely effective in decreasing the death rattle (Hipp & Letizia, 2009).*

Client/Family Teaching and Discharge Planning

▲ Teach the importance of not smoking. Refer to a smoking cessation program, and encourage clients who relapse to keep trying to quit. Ensure that client receives appropriate medications to support smoking cessation from the primary health care provider. **EB:** *A systemic review of research demonstrated that the combination of medications and an intensive, prolonged counseling program supporting smoking cessation were effective in promoting long-term abstinence from smoking (Fiore et al, 2008). A Cochrane review found that use of the medication varenicline (Chantix) increased the rate of smoking withdrawal two to three times more than smoking withdrawal without use of medications (Cahill, Stead, & Lancaster, 2008).*
▲ Teach the client how to use a flutter clearance device if ordered, which vibrates to loosen mucus and gives positive pressure to keep airways open (Bhowmik et al, 2009). **EB:** *A study demonstrated that use of the mucus clearance device had improved exercise performance compared with COPD clients who use a sham device (Wolkove et al, 2004). A Cochrane review found that there was no clear evidence that oscillation was more or less effective than other forms of physiotherapy for airway clearance in cystic fibrosis (Morrison & Agnew, 2009).*
▲ Teach the client how to use peak expiratory flow rate (PEFR) meter if ordered and when to seek medical attention if PEFR reading drops. Also teach how to use metered dose inhalers and self-administer inhaled corticosteroids as ordered following precautions to decrease side effects.
- Teach the client how to deep breathe and cough effectively. **EB:** *Controlled coughing uses the diaphragmatic muscles, making the cough more forceful and effective (Bellone et al, 2000).*
- Teach the client/family to identify and avoid specific factors that exacerbate ineffective airway clearance, including known allergens and especially smoking (if relevant) or exposure to secondhand smoke.

• = Independent   ▲ = Collaborative   **EBN** = Evidence-Based Nursing   **EB** = Evidence-Based

- Educate the client and family about the significance of changes in sputum characteristics, including color, character, amount, and odor. *With this knowledge, the client and family can identify early the signs of infection and seek treatment before acute illness occurs.*
- Teach the client/family need to take ordered antibiotics until the prescription has run out. *Taking the entire course of antibiotics helps to eradicate bacterial infection, which decreases lingering, chronic infection.*
- Teach the family of the dying client in hospice with a death rattle, that rarely are clients aware of the fluid that has accumulated, and help them find evidence of comfort in the client's nonverbal behavior (Hipp & Letizia, 2009).

⊘volve   See the EVOLVE website for Weblinks for client education.

REFERENCES

Ahrens T, Kollef M, Stewart J et al: Effect of kinetic therapy on pulmonary complications, *Am J Crit Care* 13(5):376, 2004.

Barnett M: Nursing management of chronic obstructive pulmonary disease, *Br J Nurs* 17(21):1314–1318, 2008.

Bellone A, Lascioli R, Raschi S et al: Chest physical therapy in patients with acute exacerbation of chronic bronchitis: effectiveness of three modes, *Arch Phys Med Rehabil* 81(5):558, 2000.

Bhowmik A, Chahal K, Austin G et al: Improving mucociliary clearance in chronic obstructive pulmonary disease, *Respir Med* 103(4):496–502, 2009.

Bickley LS, Szilagyi P: *Guide to physical examination,* ed 10, Philadelphia, 2009, Lippincott, Williams and Wilkins.

Burkhart PV, Rayens MK, Revelette WR: Improved health outcomes with peak flow monitoring for children with asthma, *J Asthma* 44(2):137–142, 2007.

Cahill K, Stead LF, Lancaster T: Nicotine receptor partial agonists for smoking cessation, *Cochrane Database Syst Rev* 16(3):CD006103, 2008.

Carpenter DR, Narsavage GL: One breath at a time: living with cystic fibrosis, *J Pediatr Nurs* 19(1):25, 2004.

Chatzimicael A, Tsalkidis A, Cassimos D et al: Effect of passive smoking on lung function and respiratory infection, *Indian J Pediatr* 75(4):335–340, 2008.

Chojnowski D: "GOLD" standards for acute exacerbation in COPD, *Nurs Pract* 28(5):26, 2003.

Clark AP, Giuliano K, Chen HM: Pulse oximetry revised, *Clin Nurse Spec* 20(6):268–272, 2006.

Donahue M: "Spare the cough, spoil the airway": back to the basics in airway clearance, *Pediatr Nurs* 28(2):119, 2002.

Fauci A, Braunwald E, Kasper DL et al: *Harrison's principles of internal medicine,* ed 17, New York, 2008, McGraw-Hill.

Fiore MC, Jaen CR, Baker TB et al: Treating tobacco use and dependence clinical practice guideline, 2008 update. Rockville MD, 2008, U.S. Department of Health and Human Services, Public Health Service.

Fletcher K: Immobility: geriatric self-learning module, *Medsurg Nurs* 14(1):35, 2005.

Freitas ER, Soares BG, Cardoso JR et al: Incentive spirometry for preventing pulmonary complications after coronary artery bypass graft, *Cochrane Database Syst Rev* (3):CD004466, 2007.

Genc A, Yildirim Y, Gnerli A: Researching of the effectiveness of deep breathing and incentive spirometry in postoperative early stage, *Fizyoterapi Rehabil* 15(1), 2004.

Goldhill DR, Imhoff M, McLean B et al: Rotational bed therapy to prevent and treat respiratory complications: a review and meta-analysis. *Am J Crit Care* 16(1):50–61, 2007.

Hipp B, Letizia MJ: Understanding and responding to the death rattle in dying patients. *Medsurg Nurs* 18(1):17–21, 2009.

Ky, Krawcdzyk J, Gharahbaghian L et al: (Updated July 14, 2006). *Toxicity, cough and cold preparation,* available at: http://emedicine.medscape.com/article/1010513–print. Accessed March 28, 2009.

Maggiore SM, Lellouche F, Pigeot J et al: Prevention of endotracheal suctioning-induced alveolar decruitement in acute lung injury, *Am J Respir Crit Care Med* 167(9):1215, 2003.

Main E, Prasad A, Schans C: Conventional chest physiotherapy compared to other airway clearance techniques for cystic fibrosis, *Cochrane Database Syst Rev,* (1):CD002011, 2005.

Midulla F, Guidi R, Barbato A: Foreign body aspiration in children, *Pediatr Int* 47(6):663–668, 2005.

Miller CA: *Nursing for wellness in older adults,* ed 4, Philadelphia, 2004, Lippincott.

Morrison L, Agnew J: Oscillating devices for airway clearance in people with cystic fibrosis, *Cochrane Database Syst Rev* (1):CD006842, 2009.

Navaie-Waliser M, Misener M, Mersman C et al: Evaluating the needs of children with asthma in home care: the vital role of nurses as caregivers and educators, *Public Health Nurs* 21(4):306, 2004.

Nielsen KG, Holte K, Kehlet H: Effects of posture on postoperative pulmonary function, *Acta Anaesthesiol Scand* 47(10):1270, 2003.

Pedersen CM, Rosendahl-Nielsen M, Hjermind J et al: Endotracheal suctioning of the adult intubated patient—what is the evidence? *Intensive Crit Care Nurs* 25(1):21–30, 2009.

Perme C, Chandrashekar R: Early mobility and walking program for patients in intensive care units: creating a standard of care, *Am J Crit Care* 18(3):212–220, 2009.

Rauen CA, Chulay M, Bridges E et al: Seven evidence-based practice habits: putting some sacred cows out to pasture, *Crit Care Nurs* 28(2):98–123, 2008.

Seckel M: Implementing evidence-based practice guidelines to minimize ventilator-associated pneumonia, *AACN News* 24(1):8–10, 2006.

Seymour C, Cross B, Cooke C et al: Physiologic impact of closed-system endotracheal suctioning in spontaneously breathing patients receiving mechanical ventilation, *Respir Care* 54(3):367–374, 2009.

van der Schans CP: Conventional chest physical therapy for obstructive lung disease, *Respir Care* 52(9):1198–1206, 2007.

Wolkove N, Baltzan MA Jr, Kamel H et al: A randomized trial to evaluate the sustained efficacy of a mucus clearance device in ambulatory patients with chronic obstructive pulmonary disease, *Can Respir J* 11(8):567, 2004.

Wong M, Elliott M: The use of medical orders in acute care oxygen therapy, *Br J Nurs* 18(8):462–464, 2009.

Woo T: Pharmacology of cough and cold medicines, *J Pediatr Health Care* 22(2):73–79, 2008.

• = Independent   ▲ = Collaborative   **EBN** = Evidence-Based Nursing   **EB** = Evidence-Based

Latex Allergy response   *Leslie H. Nicoll, PhD, MBA, RN, BC, and DeLancey Nicoll, SN*

 NANDA-I

Definition

A hypersensitive reaction to natural latex rubber products

Defining Characteristics

Life-threatening reactions occurring <1 hour after exposure to latex protein: Bronchospasm; cardiac arrest; contact urticaria progressing to generalized symptoms; dyspnea; edema of the lips; edema of the throat; edema of the tongue; edema of the uvula; hypotension; respiratory arrest; syncope; tightness in chest; wheezing

Orofacial characteristics: Edema of eyelids; edema of sclera; erythema of the eyes; facial erythema; facial itching; itching of the eyes; oral itching; nasal congestion; nasal erythema; nasal itching; rhinorrhea; tearing of the eyes

Gastrointestinal characteristics: Abdominal pain; nausea

Generalized characteristics: Flushing; generalized discomfort; generalized edema; increasing complaint of total body warmth; restlessness

Type IV reactions occurring >1 hour after exposure to latex protein: Discomfort reaction to additives such as thiurams and carbamates; eczema; irritation; redness

Related Factors (r/t)

Hypersensitivity to natural latex rubber protein

 NOC   **(Nursing Outcomes Classification)**

Suggested NOC Outcomes

Allergic Response: Localized, Systemic; Immune Hypersensitivity Response; Symptom Severity; Tissue Integrity: Skin and Mucous Membranes

Example NOC Outcome with Indicators
Immune Hypersensitivity Response as evidenced by the following indicators: Respiratory, cardiac, gastrointestinal, renal, and neurological function status IER/Free of allergic reactions (Rate each indicator of **Immune Hypersensitivity Response:** 1 = Severely compromised 2 = Substantially compromised, 3 = Moderately compromised, 4 = Mildly compromised, 5 = Not compromised [see Section I].) IER, In expected range.

Client Outcomes

Client Will (Specify Time Frame):

- Identify presence of NRL allergy
- List history of risk factors
- Identify type of reaction
- State reasons not to use or to have anyone use latex products
- Experience a latex-safe environment for all health care procedures
- Avoid areas where there is powder from NRL gloves
- State the importance of wearing a MedicAlert bracelet and wear one
- State the importance of carrying an emergency kit with a supply of nonlatex gloves, antihistamines, and an autoinjectable epinephrine syringe (EpiPen), and carry one

NIC   **(Nursing Interventions Classification)**

Suggested NIC Interventions

Allergy Management, Latex Precautions

● = Independent   ▲ = Collaborative   **EBN** = Evidence-Based Nursing   **EB** = Evidence-Based

Example NIC Activities—Latex Precautions
Question client or appropriate other about history of systemic reaction or sensitization to NRL (e.g., facial or scleral edema, tearing eyes, urticaria, rhinitis, and wheezing); Place an allergy band on client.

Nursing Interventions and *Rationales*

- Identify clients at risk: those persons who are most likely to exhibit a sensitivity to NRL that may result in varying degrees of reactivity. Consider the following client groups:
  - Persons with neural tube defects including spina bifida, myelomeningocele/meningocele. **EB:** *Spina bifida clients are known to be a high-risk group for latex allergy and sensitization due numerous operations beginning soon after birth (Cremer et al, 2007).* **EB:** *Spina bifida clients are high risk for NRL (Rolland & O'Hehir, 2008).*
  - Children who have experienced three or more surgeries, particularly as a neonate. **EB:** *A significant correlation between the total number of surgeries, particularly during the first year of life, and degree of sensitization has been established (Sparta et al, 2004).* **EB:** *The frequency of latex allergy in children requiring multiple surgery ranges from 16.7% to 65% (Nucera, Schiavino, & Sabato, 2006).*
  - Children with chronic renal failure. **EB:** *Children with chronic renal failure are at risk because of their intense exposure to latex through catheters, gloves, and anesthetic equipment during frequent hospitalizations from early life on (Dehlink et al, 2004).*
  - Atopic individuals (persons with a tendency to have multiple allergic conditions) including allergies to food products. Particular allergies to fruits and vegetables including bananas, avocado, celery, fig, chestnut, papaya, potato, tomato, melon, and passion fruit are significant. **EB:** *The existence of other forms of atopy are related to increased risk of latex sensitization (Wan & Lue, 2007).* **EB:** *Based on a study of food allergies, Hev b UDP glucose pyrophosphorylase has been identified as a novel allergen in NRL able to cause latex-fruit allergy syndrome and as a potential panallergen in vegetable foods (Conti et al, 2007).*
  - Persons who possess a known or suspected NRL allergy by having exhibited an allergic or anaphylactic reaction, positive skin testing, or positive IgE antibodies against latex. **EB:** *Persons who are sensitized or have demonstrated an NRL allergy are at risk, even when a latex-free environment is adopted (Taylor & Erkek, 2004).* **EB:** *The use of skin-prick testing with latex extracts and specific IgE detection for the diagnosis of NRL allergy in suspected clients is directed to identification of risk factors (Mari et al 2007).*
  - Persons who have had an ongoing occupational exposure to NRL, including health care workers (HCWs), rubber industry workers, bakers, laboratory personnel, food handlers, hairdressers, janitors, policemen, and firefighters. **EB:** *Occupational exposure is different from that among children with spina bifida; it has been suggested that occupational exposure is from NRL glove proteins inhaled through powders as opposed to particle-bound latex proteins in urinary catheters (Barbara et al, 2004).* **EB:** *HCWs have an increased risk of sensitization and allergic symptoms to latex (Bousquet et al, 2006).* **EB:** *In health care workers, approximately 2.8% to 18% are reportedly sensitized (Wan & Lue, 2007).* **EB:** *The prevalence of a type I allergy to NRL in dental hygienists appears similar to that reported for other oral health care professionals and is greater than the general population (Hamann, Rodgers, & Sullivan, 2005).* **EB:** *While many argue that the implementation of universal precautions is a driving factor behind the increase of latex allergy in health care workers, researchers at the University of Minnesota dispute that claim (McCall, Horwitz, & Kammeyer-Mueller, 2003).*
- Take a thorough history of the client at risk. **EB:** *A complete and thorough history remains as the most reliable screening test to predict the likelihood of an anaphylactic reaction (Hepner & Castells, 2003).* **EB:** *The vast majority of the clients diagnosed with latex allergy informed of their diagnosis when seeking medical care during which they would be exposed (Garcia, 2007).*
- Question the client about associated symptoms of itching, swelling, and redness after contact with rubber products such as rubber gloves, balloons, and barrier contraceptives, or swelling of the tongue and lips after dental examinations. **EB:** *Latex allergy is an IgE-mediated hypersensitivity to NRL, presenting a wide range of clinical symptoms such as, angioedema, swelling, cough, asthma, and anaphylactic reactions (Deval et al, 2008).*

● = Independent   ▲ = Collaborative   **EBN** = Evidence-Based Nursing   **EB** = Evidence-Based

- Consider a skin prick test with NRL extracts to identify IgE-mediated immunity. **EB:** *Skin prick tests with well-characterized latex extracts are highly sensitive and specific predictors of latex-specific IgE antibodies (Ownby, 2003).* **EB:** *Ammoniated latex extract shows a higher sensitivity in comparison with nonammoniated products (Bernardini et al, 2008).*

- Consider the use of a provocation test (cutaneous, sublingual, mucous, conjictival) for latex allergy diagnosis confirmation. **EB:** *Latex allergy diagnosis was confirmed by specific provocation tests (Nucera, Schiavino, & Sabato, 2006).* **EB:** *Nasal provocation test is a more sensitive testing method as compared to the glove use test (Unsel et al, 2009).*

- All latex-sensitive clients are treated as if they have NRL allergy. **EB:** *Even if a person has not experienced an NRL reaction, if it can be documented that he or she has been sensitized, then he or she should be treated as if he or she has an NRL allergy. Every hospital and scientific research facility should institute a comprehensive emergency treatment program for NRL allergic clients and workers; latex-safe areas in their facilities; and a prevention program that includes the wide use of latex-free gloves and absence of powdered gloves throughout these facilities (Edlich et al, 2003).* **EB:** *Reducing exposure to latex is a safe and more economical alternative to complete removal of the individual from the place of employment (Ranta & Ownby, 2004).*

- Clients with spina bifida and others with a positive history of NRL sensitivity or NRL allergy should have all medical/surgical/dental procedures performed in a latex-controlled environment. **EB:** *Allergen avoidance and substitution and the use of latex-safe devices including synthetic gloves are essential for the affected client (Lukesova, Krcmova, & Kopecky, 2005).* **EB:** *A latex-controlled environment is defined as one in which no latex gloves are used in the room or surgical suite and no latex accessories (catheters, adhesives, tourniquet, and anesthesia equipment) come in contact with the client (Joint Task Force on Practice Parameters, 1998).* **EB:** *Clients who are latex allergic should have a surgical procedure performed as the first case in the morning, when the levels of latex aeroallergens are the smallest (Cleveland Clinic Foundation, 2009).*

- In select high risk atopic individuals, a specific immunotherapy regimen should be discussed with their health care provider. **EB:** *Current subcutaneous and sublingual immunotherapy schedules have been tested for treatment of latex allergy with evidence of efficacy but the risks of adverse events are high (Rolland & O'Hehir, 2008).* **EB:** *Sublingual immunotherapy represents an efficient therapeutic tool for the management of latex allergic clients (Nucera et al, 2008).*

- The most effective approach to preventing NRL anaphylaxis is complete latex avoidance. **EB:** *Prevention is the cornerstone in the management of latex sensitization (Hepner & Castells, 2003).* **EB:** *The use of no-latex gloves has to be the best choice from the preventative point of view (Filon & Cerchi, 2008).*

- Materials and items that contain NRL must be identified, and latex-free alternatives must be found. **EB:** *The development of a guide listing latex-containing drugs is essential for the primary prevention of allergic reactions to this substance in hospital. (Navarrete et al 2006).* **EB:** *Effective September 1998, all medical devices must be labeled regarding their latex content (Hubbard, 1997).* **EB:** *Substitution of powdered latex gloves with low-protein, powder-free NRL gloves or latex-free gloves promises benefits to both workers' health and cost and human resource savings for employers (LaMontagne et al, 2006).*

- In health care settings, general use of latex gloves having negligible allergen content, powder-free latex gloves, and nonlatex gloves and medical articles should be considered in an effort to minimize exposure to latex allergen. **EB:** *Simple measures such as the avoidance of unnecessary glove use, the use of nonpowdered latex gloves by all workers, and use of nonlatex gloves by sensitized subjects can stop the progression of latex symptoms and can avoid new cases of sensitization (Filon & Radman, 2006).* **EB:** *Surgical powdered latex gloves were the major predisposing factor for latex sensitization measured by latex-specific IgE among anesthesiologists (Tatsumi et al, 2005).*

- If latex gloves are chosen for protection from blood or body fluids, a reduced-protein, powder-free glove should be selected. **EB:** *Until well-accepted, standardized tests are available, total protein serves as a useful indicator of the exposure of concern. Protein levels below 50 mg/g are considered the least allergenic (Muller, 2003).*

- See Box III-1 for examples of products that may contain NRL and safe alternatives that are available. **EB:** *Anaphylaxis from NRL allergy is a medical emergency and must be treated as such. Latex is a potent allergen, and a type I anaphylactic reaction may be immediate in sensitized individuals. Acute treatment must be carried out in a latex-free environment (Hepner & Castells, 2003).*

• = Independent   ▲ = Collaborative   **EBN** = Evidence-Based Nursing   **EB** = Evidence-Based

BOX III-1 PRODUCTS THAT MAY CONTAIN LATEX AND LATEX-FREE ALTERNATIVES USED IN HEALTH CARE SETTINGS

Frequently Contain Latex	Latex-Free Alternative
Ace wraps	Teds, pneumatic boots
Airways	Hudson airways, oxygen masks
Ambu (bag-valve) masks (black or blue reusable)	Clear, disposable ambu-bags
Band-Aids	Sterile dressing with plastic tape or tegaderm
Blood pressure cuffs	Dura-Cuf Critikon Vital Answers or use over gown or stockinetter
Catheter, indwelling	Silicone foley (Kendall, Argyle, Baxter)
Catheter, straight	Plastic (Mentor, Bard)
	Double, triple lumen (Bard, Rusch)
Chux	Disposable underpads
Disposable gloves, latex, non-sterile	Sensicare gloves
Dressings—Moleskin, Micropore, Coban (3M)	Tegaderm (3M), Steri-strips
Electrode pads	3M, Baxter electrocardiogram pads
	Dantec surface electrocardiogram pads
Endotracheal tubes	Mallinckrodt, Sheridan, Portex tube styletes
	Laryngeal mask airway
Gloves, sterile and exam, surgical and medical	Vinyl, neoprene gloves (Neolon, Tachylon, Tru-touch, Elastryn)
Heplock-PRN adapter	Use stopcock to inject medications
IV solutions and tubing systems	Baxter, Abbott, Walrus tubing
	Walrus anesthesia sets are latex-free
	Abbott IV fluid
Medication syringes	Becton Dickinson angiocaths and syringes
	Concord Portex, Bard syringes
Medication vials	Remove latex stopper
Oral and nasal airways	Hudson airways, oxygen masks
OR caps with elastic (bouffant)	Caps with ties
Oxygen tubing	Nasal, face mask
Stethoscope tubing	Do not let tubing touch client, cover with web roll
Suction tubing	Mallinckrodt, Yankauer, Davol suction catheters
Tape—cloth, adhesive, paper	Plastic, silk, 3M Microfoam Blenderm, Durapore
Tourniquets	Latex-free tourniquet (blue)

Home Care

- Assess the home environment for presence of NRL products (e.g., balloons, condoms, gloves, and products of related allergies, such as bananas, avocados, and poinsettia plants). **EB:** *Strict compliance with latex avoidance instructions is essential both inside and outside the hospital. Greater emphasis should be placed on reducing latex exposure in the home and school environments, as such contact could maintain positive IgE-antibody levels (Dieguez et al, 2006).*
- At onset of care, assess client history and current status of NRL allergy response. **EBN:** *A complete and thorough history remains as the most reliable screening test to predict the likelihood of an anaphylactic reaction (American Association of Nurse Anesthetists, 1998).*
- ▲ Seek medical care as necessary.
- Do not use NRL products in caregiving.
- Assist the client in identifying and obtaining alternatives to NRL products. **EBN:** *Preventing exposure to latex is the key to managing and preventing this allergy. Providing a safe environment for clients with NRL allergy is the responsibility of all health care professionals (American Association of Nurse*

• = Independent   ▲ = Collaborative   **EBN** = Evidence-Based Nursing   **EB** = Evidence-Based

BOX III-2 LATEX PRODUCTS AND SAFE ALTERNATIVES OUTSIDE OF THE HEALTH-CARE SETTING

Containing Latex	Latex-Free Alternative
Balloons	Mylar balloons
Balls, Koosh ball	Vinyl, Thornton sport ball
Belt for clothing	Leather or cloth belts
Beach shoes	Cotton socks
Bungee cords	Rope or twine
Cleaning/kitchen gloves	Vinyl gloves
Condoms	Polyurethane Avanti for males
	Polyurethane Reality for females
Crib mattress pads	Heavy cotton pads
Elastic bands	Paper clips, staples, twine
Elastic on legs, waist of clothing, disposable diapers, rubber pants	Velcro closures
	Cloth diapers
Halloween rubber masks	Plastic mask or water-based paints
Pacifiers	Plastic pacifier "The First Years"
	Silicone—Pur, Gerber, Soft-Flex
Racquet handles	Leather handles
Raincoats/slickers	Nylon or synthetic waterproof coats
Swim fins	Clear plastic fins
Telephone cords	Clear cords

Data in boxes 1 and 2 from: American Association of Nurse Anesthetists: *AANA latex protocol,* Park Ridge, Il, 1998, The Association, pp 1–9; National Institute for Occupational Safety and Health: *Preventing allergic reactions to natural rubber latex in the workplace,* Cincinnati, July 1998, The Institute; Hepner DL, Castells MC: Latex allergy: an update, *Anesth Analg* 96(4):1219–1229, 2003.

Anesthetists, 1998). **EB:** *Avoidance management should be individualized, taking into consideration factors such as age, activity, occupation, hobbies, residential conditions, and the client's level of personal anxiety (Joint Task Force on Practice Parameters, 1998).*

Client/Family Teaching and Discharge Planning

- Provide written information about NRL allergy and sensitivity. **EB:** *Client education is the most important preventive strategy. Client should be carefully instructed about "hidden" latex, cross reactions (particularly foods) and unforeseen risks during medical procedures (Joint Task Force on Practice Parameters, 1998; American College of Allergy, Asthma & Immunology, 2009).*
- ▲ Instruct the client to inform health care professionals if he or she has an NRL allergy, particularly if he or she is scheduled for surgery. **EB:** *It is essential to recognize which clients and colleagues are sensitized to latex to provide appropriate treatment and to establish adequate prevention (Hepner & Castells, 2003).*
- Teach the client what products contain NRL and to avoid direct contact with all latex products and foods that trigger allergic reactions. **EBN:** *Once an individual becomes allergic to latex, special precautions are needed to prevent exposures. Teaching is an effective strategy (Society for Gastroenterology Nurses and Associates, Inc., 2004).*
- See Box III-2 for examples of products found in the community that may contain NRL and safe alternatives that are available.
- Teach the client to avoid areas where powdered latex gloves are used, as well as where latex balloons are inflated or deflated. **EB:** *Powder from gloves acts as a carrier for latex protein (Hepner & Castells, 2003).*
- Instruct the client with NRL allergy to wear a medical identification bracelet and/or carry a medical identification card. **EB:** *Identification of the client with NRL allergy is critical for preventing problems and for early intervention with appropriate treatment if an exposure occurs (Joint Task Force on Practice Parameters, 1998; Hepner & Castells, 2003).*

• = Independent   ▲ = Collaborative   **EBN** = Evidence-Based Nursing   **EB** = Evidence-Based

- Instruct the client to carry an emergency kit with a supply of nonlatex gloves, antihistamines, and an autoinjectable epinephrine syringe (EpiPen). **EB:** *An autoinjectable epinephrine syringe should be prescribed to sensitized clients who are at risk for an anaphylactic episode with accidental latex exposure (Joint Task Force on Practice Parameters, 1998; National Institute for Occupational Safety and Health, 1998; American College of Allergy, Asthma & Immunology, 2009).*

ⓔvolve   See the EVOLVE website for World Wide Web resources for client education.

REFERENCES

American Association of Nurse Anesthetists: *AANA latex protocol,* Park Ridge, Il, 1998, The Association.

American College of Allergy, Asthma & Immunology: *Anaphylaxis*: www.acaai.org/public/advice/anaph.htm, accessed April 17, 2009.

Barbara J, Santais MC, Levy DA et al: Inhaled cornstarch glove powder increases latex-induced airway hyper-sensitivity in guinea pigs, *Clin Exp Allergy* 34(6):978–983, 2004.

Bernardini R, Pucci N, Azzari C et al: Sensitivity and specificity of different skin prick tests with latex extracts in pediatric patients with suspected natural rubber latex allergy—a cohort study, *Pediatr Allergy Immunol* 19(4):315–318, 2008.

Bousquet J, Flahault A, Vandenplas O et al: Natural rubber latex allergy among health care workers: a systematic review of the evidence, *J Allergy Clin Immunol* 118(2):447–454, 2006.

Cleveland Clinic Foundation: *How to Manage a Latex-Allergic Patient*: www.uam.es/departamentos/medicina/anesnet/gtoa/latex/manage .htm. Accessed April 16, 2009.

Conti A, Giuffrida MG, Hoffmann-Sommergruber K et al: Identification of latex UDP glucose pyrophosphorylase (Hev b UDPGP) as a novel cause of latex fruit allergy syndrome, *Eur Ann Allergy Clin Immunol* 39(4):116–118, 2007.

Cremer R, Lorbacher M, Hering F et al: Natural rubber latex sensitization and allergy in patient with spina bifida, urogenital disorders and oesophageal atresia compared with a normal pediatric population, *Eur J Pediatr Surg* 17(3):194–198, 2007.

Dehlink E, Prandstetter C, Eiwegger T et al: Increased prevalence of latex-sensitization among children with chronic renal failure, *Allergy* 59(7):734–738, 2004.

Deval R, Ramesh V, Prasad GB et al: Natural rubber latex allergy, *Indian J Dermatol Venereol Leprolo.* 74(4):304–310, 2008.

Dieguez Pastor MC, Anton Girones M, Blanco R et al: Latex allergy in children: a follow-up study, *Allergol Immunopathol (Madr)* 34(1):17–22, 2006.

Edlich RF, Woodard CR, Hill LG et al: Latex allergy: a life-threatening epidemic for scientists, healthcare personnel, and their patients, *J Long Term Eff Med Implants* 13(1):11–19, 2003.

Filon FL, Radman G: Latex allergy: a follow up study of 1040 healthcare workers, *Occup Environ Med* 63(2):121–125, 2006.

Filon FL Cerchi R: Epidemiology of latex allergy in healthcare workers, *Med Lav* 99(2):108–112, 2008.

Garcia JA: Type I latex allergy: a follow-up study, *J Investig Allergol Clin Immunol.* 17(3):164–167, 2007.

Hamann CP, Rodgers PA, Sullivan KM: Prevalence of type I natural rubber latex allergy among dental hygienists, *J Dent Hyg* 79(2):7, 2005.

Hepner DL, Castells MC: Latex allergy: an update, *Anesth Analg* 96(4):1219–1229, 2003.

Hubbard WK: Department of Health and Human Services. Food and Drug Administration: natural rubber-containing medical devices–user labeling, *Federal Register* 62:189, 1997.

Joint Task Force on Practice Parameters; American Academy of Allergy, Asthma and Immunology; American College of Allergy, Asthma and Immunology; and the Joint Council of Allergy, Asthma and Immu-nology: The diagnosis and management of anaphylaxis, *J Allergy Clin Immunol* 101(6 Pt 2):S465, 1998.

LaMontagne AD, Radi S, Elder DS et al: Primary prevention of latex related sensitization and occupational asthma: a systematic review, *Occup Environ Med* 63(5):359–364, 2006.

Lukesova S, Krcmova I, Kopecky O: Latex allergy—report on two cases, *Cas Lek Cesk* 144(9):641–643, 2005.

Mari A, Scala E, D'Ambrosio C et al: Latex allergy within a cohort of not-at-risk subjects with respiratory symptoms: prevalence of latex sensitization and assessment of diagnostic tools, *Int Arch Allergy Immunol* 143(2):135–143, 2007.

McCall BP, Horwitz IB, Kammeyer-Mueller JD: Have health conditions associated with latex increased since the issuance of universal precautions? *Am J Public Health* 93(4):599–604, 2003.

Muller BA: Minimizing latex exposure and allergy: how to avoid or reduce sensitization in the healthcare setting, *Postgrad Med* 113(4):91–96, 2003.

National Institute for Occupational Safety and Health: *Preventing allergic reactions to natural rubber latex in the workplace,* Cincinnati, 1998, The Institute.

Navarrete MA, Salas A, Palacios L et al: Latex allergy, *Farm Hosp.* 30(3):177–186, 2006.

Nucera E, Schiavino D, Pollastrini E: Sublingual desensitization in children with congenital malformations and latex allergy, *Pediatr Allergy Immunol* 17(8):606–612, 2006.

Nucera E, Schiavino D, Sabato V et al: Sublingual immunotherapy for latex allergy: tolerability and safety profile of rush build-up phase, *Curr Med Res Opin* 24(4):1147–1154, 2008.

Ownby DR: Strategies for distinguishing asymptomatic latex sensitization from true occupational allergy or asthma, *Ann Allergy Asthma Immunol* 90(5 Suppl 2):42–46, 2003.

Ranta PM, Ownby DR: A review of natural-rubber latex allergy in healthcare workers, *Clin Infect Dis* 38(2):252–256, 2004.

Rolland JM, O'Hehir RE: Latex allergy: a model for therapy, *Clin Exp Allergy* 38(6):898–912, 2008.

Society for Gastroenterology Nurses and Associates, Inc: SGNA Guidelines for preventing sensitivity and allergic reactions to natural rubber latex in the workplace, *Gastroenterol Nurs* 27(4):191–197, 2004.

Sparta G, Kemper MJ, Gerber AC et al: Latex allergy in children with urological malformation and chronic renal failure, *J Urol* 171(4):1647–1649, 2004.

Tatsumi K, Ide T, Kitaguchi K et al: Prevalence and risk factors for latex sensitization among anesthesiologists, *Masui* 54(2):195–201, 2005.

Taylor JS, Erkek E: Latex allergy: diagnosis and management, *Dermatol Ther* 17 (4): 289–301, 2004.

Unsel M, Mete N, Ardeniz O et al: The importance of nasal provocation test in the diagnosis of natural rubber latex allergy, *Allergy* 64(6):862–867, 2009.

Wan KS, Lue HC: Latex allergy in health care workers in Taiwan: prevalence, clinical features, *Int Arch Occup Environ Health* 80(5):455–457, 2007.

● = Independent   ▲ = Collaborative   **EBN** = Evidence-Based Nursing   **EB** = Evidence-Based

Risk for latex Allergy response   *Leslie H. Nicoll, PhD, MBA, RN, BC, and DeLancey Nicoll, SN*

NANDA-I

Definition

Risk of hypersensitivity to natural latex rubber products

Risk Factors

Allergies to avocados, bananas, chestnuts, kiwis, poinsettia plants, and tropical fruits; history of allergies; history of asthma; history of reaction to latex; multiple surgical procedures, especially from infancy; professions with daily exposure to latex

NOC   (Nursing Outcomes Classification)

Suggested NOC Outcomes

Allergic Response: Systemic; Immune Hypersensitivity Response; Knowledge: Health Behavior; Risk Control; Risk Detection; Tissue Integrity: Skin and Mucous Membranes

Example **NOC** Outcome with Indicators
Immune Hypersensitivity Response as evidenced by the following indicators: Respiratory, cardiac, gastrointestinal, renal, and neurological function status (Rate each indicator of **Immune Hypersensitivity Response:** 1 = severely compromised, 2 = substantially compromised, 3 = moderately compromised, 4 = mildly compromised, 5 = not compromised [see Section I].)

Client Outcomes

Client Will (Specify Time Frame):
- State risk factors for NRL allergy
- Request latex-free environment
- Demonstrate knowledge of plan to treat NRL allergic reaction

NIC   (Nursing Interventions Classification)

Suggested NIC Interventions

Allergy Management, Latex Precautions, Environmental Risk Protection

Example **NIC** Activities—Latex Precautions
Question patient or appropriate other about history of systemic reaction to NRL (e.g., facial or scleral edema, tearing eyes, urticaria, rhinitis, and wheezing); Place allergy band on client

Nursing Interventions and *Rationales*

- Clients at high risk need to be identified, such as those with frequent bladder catheterizations, occupational exposure to latex, past history of atopy (hay fever, asthma, dermatitis, or food allergy to fruits such as bananas, avocados, papaya, chestnut, or kiwi); those with a history of anaphylaxis of uncertain etiology, especially if associated with surgery; health care workers; and females exposed to barrier contraceptives and routine examinations during gynecological and obstetric procedures. **EB:** *Although latex allergy is a limited phenomenon, it is nevertheless quite frequent within risk groups. Most clients have simultaneously many risk factors for the development of such an allergy, and the occurrence of several risk factors increases severity of the allergy (Gentili et al, 2006).* **EB:** *Latex allergy is an increasingly common condition because the use of latex products is widespread (Eustachio et al, 2003).* **EB:** *Health care professionals, hospital clients, and rubber industry workers have noted a marked increase in allergic reactions to NRL in the past 10 years (Ranta & Ownby, 2004).* **EB:** *Recent studies have shown that allergy to NRL is significantly associated with hypersensitivity to certain foods, including avocados, chestnuts, papayas, kiwis, potatoes, tomatoes,*

• = Independent   ▲ = Collaborative   **EBN** = Evidence-Based Nursing   **EB** = Evidence-Based

and bananas (Isola et al, 2003). **EB:** *A latex-directed history is the primary method of identifying latex sensitivity, although both skin and serum testing are available and are increasingly accurate (Hepner & Castells, 2003; Society of Gastroenterology Nurses and Associates, Inc., 2004).*

- Clients with spina bifida are a high-risk group for NRL allergy and should remain latex-free from the first day of life. **EB:** *The SB population bears a disease-associated propensity for latex sensitization. This effect cannot be explained exclusively by a higher number of operations and differences related to atopy, age, or gender (Eiwegger et al, 2006).* **EB:** *Latex allergy in spina bifida children is a multifactoral situation related with a disease-associated propensity for latex sensitization, early exposure, and number of surgical procedures. Prophylactic measures to avoid the exposure, not only in the sanitary environment, through the institution of latex-safe routes and every day, prevent potentially serious allergic reactions (Ausili et al, 2007).* **EB:** *Latex-free precautions from birth in children with spina bifida are more effective in preventing latex sensitization than the same precautions instituted in later life (Nieto et al, 2002).*
- Children who are on home ventilation should be assessed for NRL allergy. **EB:** *This study showed a high incidence of NRL allergy in children on home ventilation. All children on home ventilation should be screened for NRL allergy to prevent untoward reactions from exposure to latex (Nakamura et al, 2000).*
- Children with chronic renal failure should be assessed for NRL allergy. **EB:** *This study demonstrated a high incidence of NRL in children with chronic renal failure. Children with chronic renal failure are at risk because of their intense exposure to latex through catheters, gloves, and anesthetic equipment during frequent hospitalizations from early life on (Dehlink et al, 2004).*
- Assess for NRL allergy in clients who are exposed to "hidden" latex. **EB:** *Case studies have reported on serious complications in clients exposed to latex through hair glue (Cogen & Beezhold, 2002) and microdermabrasion (Farris & Rietschel, 2002). Workers are at high risk of becoming sensitized to latex allergens when exposed to excessive dust produced by loom tuning machines (Lopata et al 2007).*
- See care plan for **Latex Allergy response**.

Home Care

▲ Ensure that the client has a medical plan if a response develops. *Prompt treatment decreases potential severity of response.*
- See care plan for **Latex Allergy response**. Note client history and environmental assessment.

Client/Family Teaching and Discharge Planning

▲ A client who has had symptoms of NRL allergy or who suspects he or she is allergic to latex should tell his or her employer and contact his or her institution's occupational health services. **EB:** *Occupational health services can arrange testing by an allergist. If an allergy is present, measures to protect the client's well-being in the workplace should be instituted (National Institute for Occupational Safety and Health, 1998).*
- Provide written information about latex allergy and sensitivity. **EB:** *Client education is the most important preventive strategy. Client should be carefully instructed about "hidden" latex; cross reactions, particularly foods; and unforeseen risks during medical procedures (Joint Task Force on Practice Parameters, 1998).*
- Health care workers should avoid the use of latex gloves and seek alternatives such as gloves made from nitrile. **EB:** *The risk of NRL allergy appears to be largely linked to occupational exposure and NRL-associated occupational asthma is due almost solely to powdered glove use. Airborne NRL is dependent on the use of powdered NRL gloves; conversion to non-NRL or nonpowdered NRL substitutes results in predictable rapid disappearance of detectable levels of aeroallergen (Brown et al, 2004).* **EB:** *A case study report of two nurses indicated worsening symptoms when they worked in an environment with powdered gloves, even though they avoided direct skin contact with latex (Amr & Suk, 2004).* **EB:** *The level of dexterity provided by latex and nitrile SafeSkin gloves for tasks on a gross dexterity level are comparable and health workers will benefit from the nonallergenic properties of nitrile (Sawyer & Bennett 2006).*
- Health care institutions should develop prevention programs for the use of latex-free gloves and the absence of powdered gloves; they should also establish latex-safe areas in their facilities. **EB:** *Latex allergy has become a global epidemic, affecting clients, health care workers, and scientific personnel (Edlich et al, 2003). The use of powder-free, low-protein latex gloves as an alternative to powdered*

● = Independent   ▲ = Collaborative   **EBN** = Evidence-Based Nursing   **EB** = Evidence-Based

latex gloves significantly reduces the incidence of latex allergy and latex-induced asthma, as well as the prevalence of latex-related symptoms (Occupational Health, 2008).
- See **Latex Allergy response**.

Ⓔvolve See the EVOLVE website for Weblinks for client education resources.

REFERENCES

Amr S, Suk WA: Latex allergy and occupational asthma in healthcare workers: adverse outcomes, *Environ Health Perspect* 112(3):378–381, 2004.

Ausili E, Tabacco F, Focarelli B et al: Prevalence of latex allergy in spina bifida: genetic and environmental risk factors, *Eur Rev Med Pharmacol Sci* 11(3):149–153, 2007.

Brown RH, Taenkhum K, Buckley TJ et al: Different latex aeroallergen size distributions between powdered surgical and examination gloves: significance for environmental avoidance, *J Allergy Clin Immunol* 114(2):358–363, 2004.

Cogen FC, Beezhold DH: Hair glue anaphylaxis: a hidden latex allergy, *Ann Allergy Asthma Immunol* 88(1):61–63, 2002.

Dehlink E, Prandstetter C, Eiwegger T et al: Increased prevalence of latex-sensitization among children with chronic renal failure, *Allergy* 59(7):734–738, 2004.

Edlich RF, Woodard CR, Hill LG et al: Latex allergy: a life-threatening epidemic for scientists, healthcare personnel, and their patients, *J Long Term Eff Med Implants* 13(1):11–19, 2003.

Eiwegger T, Dehlink E, Schwindt J et al: Early exposure to latex products mediates latex sensitization in spina bifida but not in other diseases with comparable latex exposure rates, *Clin Exp Allergy* 36(10):1242–1246, 2006.

Eustachio N, Cristina CM, Antonio F et al: A discussion of natural rubber latex allergy with special reference to children: clinical considerations, *Curr Drug Targets Immune Endocr Metabol Disord* 3(3):171–180, 2003.

Farris PK, Rietschel RL: An unusual acute urticarial response following microdermabrasion, *Dermatol Surg* 28(7):606–608, 2002.

Gentili A, Lima M, Ricci G et al: Secondary prevention of latex allergy in children: analysis of results, *Pediatr Med Chir*, 28(4–6):83–90, 2006.

Hepner DL, Castells MC: Latex allergy: an update, *Anesth Analg* 96(4):1219–1229, 2003.

Isola S, Ricciardi L, Saitta S et al: Latex allergy and fruit cross-reaction in subjects who are nonatopic, *Allergy Asthma Proc* 24(3):193–197, 2003.

Joint Task Force on Practice Parameters; American Academy of Allergy, Asthma and Immunology; American College of Allergy, Asthma and Immunology; and the Joint Council of Allergy, Asthma and Immunology: The diagnosis and management of anaphylaxis, *J Allergy Clin Immunol* 101(6 Pt 2):S465, 1998.

Lopata AL, Adams S, Kirstein F et al: Occupational allergy to latex among loom turners in a textile factory, *Int Arch Allergy Immunol* 144(1):64–68, 2007.

Nakamura CT, Ferdman RM, Keens TG et al: Latex allergy in children on home mechanical ventilation, *Chest* 118(4):1000–1003, 2000.

National Institute for Occupational Safety and Health: *Preventing allergic reactions to natural rubber latex in the workplace,* Cincinnati, 1998, The Institute.

Nieto A, Mazon A, Pamies R et al: Efficacy of latex avoidance for primary prevention of latex sensitization in children with spina bifida, *J Pediatr* 140(3):370–372, 2002.

Occupational Health, *First national guideline on latex allergy*, Jun; 60(6): 37, 2008: www.personneltoday.com/articles/2008/09/01/46035/first-national-guideline-on-latex-allergy.html. Accessed on August 17, 2009.

Ranta PM, Ownby DR: A review of natural-rubber latex allergy in healthcare workers, *Clin Infect Dis* 38(2):252–256, 2004.

Sawyer J, Bennett A: Comparing the level of dexterity offered by latex and nitrile SafeSkin gloves, *Ann Occup Hyg* 50(3):289–296, 2006.

Society of Gastroenterology Nurses and Associates, Inc: SGNA Guidelines for preventing sensitivity and allergic reactions to natural rubber latex in the workplace, *Gastroenterol Nurs* 27(4):191–197, 2004.

Anxiety   *Ruth McCaffrey, DNP, ARNP*   Ⓔvolve

NANDA-I

Definition

A vague uneasy feeling of discomfort or dread accompanied by an autonomic response (the source often nonspecific or unknown to the individual); a feeling of apprehension caused by anticipation of danger. It is an alerting signal that warns of impending danger and enables the individual to take measures to deal with threat

Defining Characteristics

Behavioral

Diminished productivity; expressed concerns due to change in life events; extraneous movement; fidgeting; glancing about; insomnia; poor eye contact; restlessness; scanning; vigilance

Affective

Apprehensive; anguish; distressed; fearful; feelings of inadequacy; focus on self; increased wariness; irritability; jittery; overexcited; painful increased helplessness; persistent increased helplessness; rattled; regretful; uncertainty; worried

• = Independent   ▲ = Collaborative   **EBN** = Evidence-Based Nursing   **EB** = Evidence-Based

Physiological

Facial tension; hand tremors; increased perspiration; increased tension; shakiness; trembling; voice quivering

Sympathetic

Anorexia; cardiovascular excitation; diarrhea; dry mouth; facial flushing; heart pounding; increased blood pressure; increased pulse; increased reflexes; increased respiration; pupil dilation; respiratory difficulties; superficial vasoconstriction; twitching; weakness

Parasympathetic

Abdominal pain; decreased blood pressure; decreased pulse; diarrhea; faintness; fatigue; nausea; sleep disturbance; tingling in extremities; urinary frequency; urinary hesitancy; urinary urgency

Cognitive

Awareness of physiologic symptoms; blocking of thought; confusion; decreased perceptual field; difficulty concentrating; diminished ability to learn; diminished ability to problem solve; fear of unspecified consequences; forgetfulness; impaired attention; preoccupation; rumination; tendency to blame others

Related Factors (r/t)

Change in: economic status, environment, health status, interaction patterns, role function, role status; exposure to toxins; familial association; heredity; interpersonal contagion; interpersonal transmission; maturational crises; situational crises; stress; substance abuse; threat of death; threat to: economic status, environment, health status, interaction patterns, role function, role status; self-concept; unconscious conflict about essential goals of life; unconscious conflict about essential values; unmet needs

NOC   (Nursing Outcomes Classification)

Suggested NOC Outcomes

Aggression Self-Control, Anxiety Level, Anxiety Self-Control, Coping, Impulse Self-Control

Example NOC Outcome with Indicators
Anxiety Self-Control as evidenced by the following indicators: Eliminates precursors of anxiety/Monitors physical manifestations of anxiety/Controls anxiety response (Rate the outcome and indicators of **Anxiety Self-Control:** 1 = never demonstrated, 2 = rarely demonstrated, 3 = sometimes demonstrated, 4 = often demonstrated, 5 = consistently demonstrated [see Section I].)

Client Outcomes

Client Will (Specify Time Frame):

- Identify and verbalize symptoms of anxiety
- Identify, verbalize, and demonstrate techniques to control anxiety
- Verbalize absence of or decrease in subjective distress
- Have vital signs that reflect baseline or decreased sympathetic stimulation
- Have posture, facial expressions, gestures, and activity levels that reflect decreased distress
- Demonstrate improved concentration and accuracy of thoughts
- Identify and verbalize anxiety precipitants, conflicts, and threats
- Demonstrate return of basic problem-solving skills
- Demonstrate increased external focus
- Demonstrate some ability to reassure self

• = Independent   ▲ = Collaborative   **EBN** = Evidence-Based Nursing   **EB** = Evidence-Based

NIC   (Nursing Interventions Classification)

Suggested NIC Intervention

Anxiety Reduction

Example NIC Activities—Anxiety Reduction
Use a calm, reassuring approach; explain all procedures, including sensations likely to be experienced during the procedure

Nursing Interventions and *Rationales*

- Assess the client's level of anxiety and physical reactions to anxiety (e.g., tachycardia, tachypnea, nonverbal expressions of anxiety). Consider using the Hamilton Anxiety Scale, which grades 14 symptoms on a scale of 0 (not present) to 4 (very severe). Symptoms evaluated are mood, tension, fear, insomnia, concentration, worry, depressed mood, somatic complaints, and cardiovascular, respiratory, gastrointestinal, genitourinary, autonomic, and behavioral symptoms. **EBN:** *Reliability and validity of the Hamilton anxiety scale have been supported by research (Flood & Buckwalter, 2009).* **EBN:** *Anxiety is a risk factor for major adverse cardiac risk events in persons with stable coronary artery disease (Frasure-Smith & Lesperance, 2008).*
- Rule out withdrawal from alcohol, sedatives, or smoking as the cause of anxiety. **EB:** *One third of respondents in this study with an alcohol use disorder (abuse or dependence) were three times more likely to have an anxiety disorder (Hasin, 2006).*
- Identify and limit, discontinue, or be aware of the use of any stimulants such as caffeine, nicotine, theophylline, terbutaline sulfate, amphetamines, and cocaine. **EB:** *Many substances cause or potentially cause anxiety symptoms (Bolton et al, 2006).*
- If the situational response is rational, use empathy to encourage the client to interpret the anxiety symptoms as normal. **EBN:** *The way a nurse interacts with a client influences his/her quality of life. Providing psychological and social support can reduce the symptoms and problems associated with anxiety (Wagner & Bear, 2009).*
- If irrational thoughts or fears are present, offer the client accurate information and encourage him or her to talk about the meaning of the events contributing to the anxiety. **EBN:** *During the diagnosis and management of cancer, highlighting the importance of the meaning of events to an individual is an important factor in helping clients to identify what makes them anxious. Acknowledgment of this meaning may help to reduce anxiety (Antoni, 2006).*
- Encourage the client to use positive self-talk such as, "Anxiety won't kill me," "I can do this one step at a time," "Right now I need to breathe and stretch," "I don't have to be perfect." **EBN:** *Cognitive therapies focus on changing behaviors and feelings by changing thoughts. Replacing negative self-statements with positive self-statements helps to decrease anxiety (Roemer & Orsillo, 2006).*
- Intervene when possible to remove sources of anxiety. **EBN:** *Anxiety has a negative effect on quality of life that persists over time (Sareen et al, 2006).*
- Explain all activities, procedures, and issues that involve the client; use nonmedical terms and calm, slow speech. Do this in advance of procedures when possible, and validate the client's understanding. **EBN:** *Effective nurse-client communication is critical to efficient care provision (Finke, Light, & Kitko, 2008).*
- Ascertain client preferences about the desire to be distracted before and during noxious medical procedures. **EBN:** *Clients have individual preferences for the use of distraction during anxiety-provoking procedures. This is especially true when the client is a child (Cohen, 2008).* **EB:** *The uses of music, storytelling, and distraction have been shown to reduce preoperative anxiety (Gilmartin & Wright, 2007).*
- Provide backrubs/massage for the client to decrease anxiety. **EBN:** *Massage and aromatherapy significantly decreased anxiety or perception of tension (Mansky & Wallerstedt, 2006).*
- Use therapeutic touch and healing touch techniques. **EBN:** *Various techniques that involve intention to heal, laying on of hands, clearing the energy field surrounding the body, and transfer of healing energy from the environment through the healer to the subject can reduce anxiety (Mansky & Wallerstedt, 2006).* **EBN:** *Anxiety was significantly reduced in a therapeutic touch placebo condition. Healing touch*

• = Independent   ▲ = Collaborative   **EBN** = Evidence-Based Nursing   **EB** = Evidence-Based

may be one of the most useful nursing interventions available to reduce anxiety (Maville, Bowen & Benham, 2008).

- Guided imagery can be used to decrease anxiety. **EBN:** *Anxiety was decreased with the use of guided imagery during an intervention for postoperative pain (Gonzales et al, 2008).*
- Suggest yoga to the client **EB:** *Studies have supported the benefits of yoga as an effective modality for reducing anxiety (Mansky & Wallerstedt, 2006).*
- Provide clients with a means to listen to music of their choice or audiotapes. Provide a quiet place and encourage clients to listen for 20 minutes. **EBN:** *Music listening reduces anxiety and pain (McCaffrey & Locsin, 2006).* **EBN:** *Chemotherapy clients who used audiotapes had lower anxiety than a control group (Mansky & Wallerstedt, 2006).*

Pediatric

- The above interventions may be adapted for the pediatric client.

Geriatric

- ▲ Monitor the client for depression. Use appropriate interventions and referrals. **EB:** *Anxiety often accompanies or masks depression in elderly adults. Clients who have depression and anxiety, are socially isolated, or are severely ill should be asked whether they've been thinking about ending their life or wanting to die (Conner et al, 2006).* **EB:** *Anxiety and depression are associated with overall health status, emotional and cognitive functioning, and fatigue (Beaudreau & O'Hara, 2008). The sociological and psychological aspects of depression are also associated with culture and the meaning attached to one's culture (Giger & Davidhizar, 2008).*
- Older adults report less worry than younger adults. **EB:** *There were no age differences in the report of somatic and affective symptoms. Thus, worry appears to play a less prominent role in the presentation of anxiety in older adults. These findings suggest that older adults do experience anxiety differently than younger adults (Brenes, 2006).*
- Observe for adverse changes if antianxiety drugs are taken. *Age renders clients more sensitive to both the clinical and toxic effects of many antianxiety agents (Belcher et al, 2006).*
- Provide a quiet environment with diversion. *Excessive noise increases anxiety; involvement in a quiet activity can be soothing to the elderly (Chaudhury, 2006).*
- Provide alternative interventions such as massage therapy, guided imagery, aroma therapy to complement traditional medical regimens. *Effective nursing practice for reducing anxiety in elderly clients provides a challenge and an opportunity for nurses and family caregivers to blend alternative therapies with technology to provide more individualized and holistic client care.* **EBN:** *Massage intervention significantly reduced pain and anxiety in elderly clients (Manskey & Wallerstedt, 2006; Carrington et al, 2008).*

Multicultural

- Assess for the presence of culture-bound anxiety states. **EBN:** *The context in which anxiety is experienced and the response to anxiety are culturally mediated (Emery, 2006). African American women and men have historically been through heartbreaking experiences as they have fought to maintain their family and survive the subjugation and horror of the slavery experience. However, because of the way in which the African American family has been forced into structured a matrifocal system, African American women in particular have suffered from cultural-bound anxiety more often than their male counterparts. Even for those African American women who were not personally involved, the anxiety lives on in family stories and by association with the culture (Cherry & Giger, 2008; Giger et al, 2008; Giger & Davidhizar, 2008).*
- Identify how anxiety is manifested in the culturally diverse client. **EBN:** *Anxiety is manifested differently from culture to culture through cognitive to somatic symptoms (Kisely & Simon, 2006).*
- Acknowledge that value conflicts from acculturation stresses may contribute to increased anxiety. **EBN:** *Challenges to traditional beliefs and values are anxiety provoking (Halbreich et al, 2007).*
- For the diverse client experiencing preoperative anxiety, provide music of their choice. **EBN:** *Music intervention was found to have cross-cultural validity in the reduction of preoperative anxiety in Chinese male clients (Twiss, Seaver, & McCaffrey, 2006).*

• = Independent   ▲ = Collaborative   **EBN** = Evidence-Based Nursing   **EB** = Evidence-Based

Home Care

- The above interventions may be adapted for home care use.
- ▲ Assess for suicidal ideation. Implement emergency plan as indicated. *Suicidal ideation may occur in response to co-occurring depression or a sense of hopelessness over severe anxiety symptoms or once antidepressant medications have been started (Mitchell et al, 2009).* See care plan for **Risk for Suicide.**
- Assess for influence of anxiety on medical regimen. **EBN:** *The ability to direct attention is necessary for self-care and independence and was reduced for several months after surgery in older women newly diagnosed with breast cancer (Larsson et al, 2008).*
- Assess for presence of depression. *Depression and anxiety co-occur frequently (Schoevers et al, 2008).*
- Assist family to be supportive of the client in the face of anxiety symptoms. **EBN:** *Social support, self-esteem, and optimism were all positively related to positive health practices, and social support was positively related to self-esteem and optimism (Cooper et al, 2006).*
- ▲ Consider referral for the prescription of antianxiety or antidepressant medications for clients who have panic disorder (PD) or other anxiety-related psychiatric disorders. **EBN:** *The use of antidepressants, especially SSRI medications, is effective in many cases of anxiety (Katzman, 2009).*
- ▲ Assist the client/family to institute medication regimen appropriately. Instruct in side effects, importance of taking medications as ordered, and effects to report immediately to nurse or physician. *Antianxiety and antidepressant medications have side effects that may prompt the client to discontinue use, sometimes with additional uncomfortable effects. Some medications may be used to overdose. Antidepressant medications can take up to several weeks for full effect, and the client may discontinue use prematurely if there is little effect or if the medication is effective and the client considers it no longer necessary (Antai-Otong, 2006).*
- ▲ Refer for psychiatric home health care services for client reassurance and implementation of a therapeutic regimen. **EBN:** *Psychiatric home care nurses can address issues relating to the client's anxiety, including agoraphobia, with or without coexisting depression. Behavioral interventions in the home can assist the client to participate more effectively in the treatment plan (Brown et al, 2006).*

Client/Family Teaching and Discharge Planning

- ▲ Teach use of appropriate community resources in emergency situations (e.g., suicidal thoughts), such as hotlines, emergency departments, law enforcement, and judicial systems. **EB:** *The method of suicide prevention found to be most effective is a systematic, direct-screening procedure that has a high potential for institutionalization (Simon et al, 2007).*
- Teach the client/family the symptoms of anxiety. **EBN:** *Information is empowering and reduces anxiety (Godfrey, Parten, & Buchner, 2006).*
- Help client to define anxiety levels (from "easily tolerated" to "intolerable") and select appropriate interventions. **EBN:** *Mild anxiety enhances learning and adaptation, but moderate to severe anxiety may impede or immobilize progress (Kolcaba, Tilton, & Drouin, 2006).*
- Teach the client techniques to self-manage anxiety. **EBN:** *Teaching clients anxiety reduction techniques can help them manage side effects with self-care behaviors (Lu & Wykle, 2007).*
- Teach progressive muscle relaxation techniques. **EBN:** *A significant reduction in anxiety level was obtained by using progressive muscle relaxation interventions (Lolak et al, 2008).*
- Teach relaxation breathing for occasional use: client should breathe in through nose, fill slowly from abdomen upward while thinking "re," and then breathe out through mouth, from chest downward, and think "lax." **EBN:** *Anxiety management training effectively treats both specific and generalized anxiety (Janeway, 2009).*
- Teach the client about the benefits of listening to music to self-manage anxiety. **EBN:** *Findings support the use of music as an independent nursing intervention for preoperative anxiety in clients having day surgery (Cook et al, 2005).*
- Teach the client to visualize or fantasize about the absence of anxiety or pain, successful experience of the situation, resolution of conflict, or outcome of procedure. **EBN:** *Use of guided imagery has been useful for reducing anxiety (Tyron & McKay, 2009).*
- Teach relationship between a healthy physical and emotional lifestyle and a realistic mental attitude. **EBN:** *Exercise is an excellent means of decreasing anxiety (DeMoor et al, 2006).*

• = Independent ▲ = Collaborative **EBN** = Evidence-Based Nursing **EB** = Evidence-Based

- Provide family members with information to help them to distinguish between a panic attack and serious physical illness symptoms. Instruct family members to consult a health care professional if they have questions. **EBN:** *Education on managing anxiety disorders must include family members because they are the ones usually called on to take the client for emergency care. Family members can be expert informants because of their familiarity with the client's history and symptoms (Carr, 2009).*

⊝volve   See the EVOLVE website for Weblinks for client education resources.

REFERENCES

Antai-Otong D: The art of prescribing antidepressants in late-life depression: prescribing principals, *Perspect Psychiatr Care* 42(2):149–153, 2006.

Antoni M: Reduction of cancer-specific thought intrusions and anxiety symptoms with a stress management intervention among women undergoing treatment for breast cancer, *Am J Psychiatr* 163(10):1791–1797, 2006.

Beaudreau S, O'Hara R: Late-life anxiety and cognitive impairment: a review, *Am J Geriatr Psychiatry* 16(10):790–803, 2008.

Belcher V, Fried T, Agostini J et al: Views of older adults on patient participation in medication-related decision making, *J Gen Intern Med* 21(4):298–303, 2006.

Bolton J, Cox B, Clara I et al: Use of alcohol and drugs to self-medicate anxiety disorders in a nationally representative sample, *J Nerv Men Dis* 194(11):818–825, 2006.

Brenes G: Age differences in the presentation of anxiety, *Aging Men Health* 19(3):298–302, 2006.

Brown E, Raue P, Schulberg H et al: Clinical competencies: caring for late-life depression in home care patients, *J Gerontol Nurs* 32(9):10–14, 2006.

Carr A: The effectiveness of family therapy and systemic interventions for adult-focused problems, *J Fam Ther* 31(1):46–74, 2009.

Carrington R, Papaleontiou M, Ong A et al: Self-management strategies to reduce pain and improve function among older adults in community settings: a review of the evidence, *Pain Med* 9(4):409–424, 2008.

Chaudhury H: Nurses' perception of single-occupancy versus multi-occupancy rooms in acute care environments: an exploratory comparative assessment, *Appl Nurs Res* 19(3):118–125, 2006.

Cherry B, Giger J: African-Americans. In Giger J, Davidhizar R, editors: *Transcultural nursing: assessment and intervention,* ed 5, St Louis, 2008, Mosby.

Cohen LL: Behavioral approaches to anxiety and pain management for pediatric venous access, *Pediatrics* 122(3):134–139, 2008.

Conner K, Duberstein P, Beckman A et al: Planning of suicide attempts among depressed inpatients ages 50 and over, *J Affect Disord* 96(1–2):212–220, 2006.

Cook M, Chaboyer W, Schluter P et al: The effect of music on preoperative anxiety in day surgery, *J Adv Nurs* 52(1):47–55, 2005.

Cooper C, Katona C, Orrell M et al: Coping strategies and anxiety in caregivers of people with Alzheimer's disease: the LASER-AD study, *J Affect Disord* 90(1):15–20, 2006.

DeMoor MHM, Beem AL, Stubbe D et al: Regular exercise, anxiety, depression and personality: a population-based study, *Prev Med* 42(4):273–279, 2006.

Emery P: Building a new culture of aging: revolutionizing long-term care, *J Christ Nurs* 23(1):16–24, 2006.

Finke E, Light J, Kitko L: A systematic review of the effectiveness of nurse communication with patients with complex communication needs with a focus on the use of augmentative and alternative communication, *J Clin Nurs* 17(16):2102–2115, 2008.

Flood M, Buckwalter KC: Recommendations for mental health care of older adults: Part 1—an overview of depression and anxiety, *J Gerontol Nurs* 35(2):26–34, 2009.

Flood M, Buckwalter KC: Recommendations for mental health care: an overview of depression and anxiety. *J Gerontol Nurs* 35(2):26–34, 2009.

Frasure-Smith N, Lesperance F: Depression and anxiety as predictors of 2–year cardiac events in patients with stable coronary artery disease, *Arch Gen Psychiatry* 65(1):62–71, 2008.

Giger J, Davidhizar R: *Transcultural nursing: assessment and intervention,* ed 5, St Louis, 2008, Mosby, 190–238.

Giger J, Appel S, Davidhizar R et al: Church and spirituality in the lives of the African American community, *J Transcult Nurs* 19(4):375–383, 2008.

Gilmartin J, Wright K: The nurses' role in day surgery: a literature review, *Int Nurs Rev* 54(2):183–190, 2007.

Godfrey B, Parten C, Buckner E: Identification of special care needs: the comparison of the cardiothoracic intensive care unit patient and nurse, *Dimens Crit Care Nurs* 25(6):275–282, 2006.

Gonzales EA, Ledesma RJA, McAllister DJ et al: The effect of guided imagery on postoperative outcomes in patients undergoing same-day surgical procedures, *AANA J* 76(5):374–375, 2008.

Halbreich Y, Alarcon RD, Calil H et al: Culturally-sensitive complaints of depressions and anxieties in women, *J Affect Disord* 102(1–3):159–176, 2007.

Hasin D: Diagnosis of comorbid psychiatric disorders in substance users assessed with the psychiatric research interview for substance and mental disorders for DSM-IV, *Am J Psychiatry* 163(4):689–696, 2006.

Janeway D: An integrated approach to the diagnosis and treatment of anxiety within the practice of cardiology, *Cardiol Rev* 17(1):36–43, 2009.

Katzman M: Current considerations in the treatment of generalized anxiety disorder, *CNS Drugs* 23(2):103–120, 2009.

Kisely S, Simon G: An international study comparing the effect of medically explained and unexplained somatic symptoms on psychosocial outcome, *J Psychosom Res* 60(2):125–130, 2006.

Kolcaba K, Tilton C, Drouin C: Comfort theory: a unifying framework to enhance the practice environment, *J Nurs Admin* 36(11):538–544, 2006.

Larsson I, Jonsson C, Olsson A et al: Women's experience of physical activity following breast cancer treatment, *Scand J Caring Sci* 22(3):422–429, 2008.

Lolak S, Connors G, Sheridan M et al: Effects of progressive muscle relaxation training on anxiety and depression in patients enrolled in an outpatient pulmonary rehabilitation program, *Psychother Psychosom* 77(2):119–125, 2008.

Lu Y, Wykle M: Relationships between caregiver stress and self-care behaviors in response to symptoms, *Clin Nurs Res* 16(1):29–43, 2007.

Mansky PJ, Wallerstedt DB: Complementary medicine in palliative care and cancer symptom management, *Cancer J* 12(5):425–431, 2006.

Maville J, Bowen J, Benham G: Effect of healing touch on stress perception and biological correlates, *Holist Nurs Pract* 22(2):103–110, 2008.

McCaffrey R, Locsin R: The effect of music on pain and acute confusion in older adults undergoing hip and knee surgery, *Holist Nurs Pract,* 20(5):218–224, 2006.

• = Independent   ▲ = Collaborative   **EBN** = Evidence-Based Nursing   **EB** = Evidence-Based

Mitchell A, Skraida TJ, Kim Y et al: Depression, anxiety and quality of life in suicide survivors, *Arch Psychiatr Nurs* 23(1):2–10, 2009.

Roemer L, Orsillo SM: An open trial of acceptance-based behavior therapy for generalized anxiety disorder, *Behav Ther* 38(1):72–85, 2006.

Sareen J, Jacobi F, Cox BJ et al: Disability and poor quality of life associated with comorbid anxiety disorders and physical conditions, *Arch Intern Med* 166(19):2109–2116, 2006.

Schoevers R, Van HL, Koppelmans V et al: Managing the patient with co-morbid depression and an anxiety disorder, *Drugs* 68(12):1621–1634, 2008.

Simon N, Zalta A, Otto M et al: The association of comorbid anxiety disorders with suicide attempts and suicidal ideation in outpatients with bipolar disorder, *J Psychiatr Res* 41(3–4):255–264, 2007.

Twiss E, Seaver J, McCaffrey R: The effect of music listening on anxiety and postoperative ventilation in older adults undergoing cardiovascular surgery, *Nurs Crit Care* 23(5):245–251, 2006.

Tyron W, McKay D: Memory modification as an outcome variable in anxiety disorder treatment, *J Anxiety Disord* 23(4):546–556, 2009.

Wagner D, Bear M: Patient satisfaction with nursing care: a concept analysis within a nursing framework, *J Adv Nurs* 65(3):692–701, 2009.

Death Anxiety   *Ruth McCaffrey, DNP, ARNP*

 NANDA-I

Definition

Vague uneasy feeling of discomfort or dread generated by perceptions of a real or imagined threat to one's existence

Defining Characteristics

Reports concerns of overworking the caregiver; reports deep sadness; reports fear of developing terminal illness; reports fear of loss of mental abilities when dying; reports fear of pain related to dying; reports fear of premature death; reports fear of the process of dying; reports fear of prolonged dying; reports fear of suffering related to dying; reports feeling powerless over dying; reports negative thoughts related to death and dying; reports worry about the impact on one's own death on significant others

Related Factors (r/t)

Anticipating adverse consequences of general anesthesia; anticipating impact of death on others; anticipating pain; anticipating suffering; confronting reality of terminal disease; discussions on topic of death; experiencing dying process; near-death experience; nonacceptance of own mortality; observations related to death; perceived proximity of death; uncertainty about an encounter with a higher power; uncertainty about the existence of a higher power; uncertainty about life after death; uncertainty of prognosis

NOC   (Nursing Outcomes Classification)

Suggested NOC Outcomes

Dignified Life Closure, Fear, Self-Control, Health Beliefs: Perceived Threat

Example NOC Outcome with Indicators
Dignified Life Closure as evidenced by the following indicators: Expresses readiness for death/Resolves important issues/Shares feelings about dying/Discusses spiritual concerns (Rate the outcome and indicators of **Dignified Life Closure:** 1 = never demonstrated, 2 = rarely demonstrated, 3 = sometimes demonstrated, 4 = often demonstrated, 5 = consistently demonstrated [see Section I].)

Client Outcomes

Client Will (Specify Time Frame):

- State concerns about impact of death on others
- Express feelings associated with dying
- Seek help in dealing with feelings
- Discuss concerns about God or higher being
- Discuss realistic goals
- Use prayer or other religious practice for comfort

• = Independent   ▲ = Collaborative   **EBN** = Evidence-Based Nursing   **EB** = Evidence-Based

(Nursing Interventions Classification)

Suggested NIC Interventions

Dying Care, Grief Work Facilitation, Spiritual Support

Example NIC Activities—Dying Care
Communicate willingness to discuss death; Support patient and family through stages of grief

Nursing Interventions and *Rationales*

- Assess the psychosocial maturity of the individual. **EB:** *As psychosocial maturity and age increase, death anxiety decreases. Findings have shown that psychosocial maturity is a better predictor of death anxiety than is age (Halliday & Boughton, 2008).*
- ▲ Assess clients for pain and provide pain relief measures. **EBN:** *Managing pain takes a multidisciplinary approach in palliative care of the dying client (Ferrell, Levy, & Paice, 2008).*
- Assess client for fears related to death. **EBN:** *Acknowledging and responding to these fears is the core of end-of-life palliative care (Nadworny, 2007).*
- Assist clients with life planning: consider and redefine main life goals, focus on areas of strength and/or goals that will provide satisfaction, adopt realistic goals and recognize those that are impossible to achieve. **EB:** *Life planning processes affect self-esteem and self-concept by changing unrealistic goals (Ferrell, Levy, & Paice, 2008).* **EB:** *Increased levels of death anxiety may block future thoughts (Ferrell, Levy, & Paice, 2008).*
- Assist clients with life review and reminiscence. **EB:** *Life reviewing can foster the integration of past conflicts. It can improve ego integrity and life satisfaction, lower depression, and reduce stress (Heyland et al, 2006).*
- Provide music of a client's choosing. **EBN:** *Music therapy is a nonpharmacological nursing intervention that may be used to promote relaxation (McCaffrey & Locsin, 2006).* **EB:** *Music may be beneficial in easing emotional, physical, and spiritual distress as death approaches (Cox, 2006).*
- Provide social support for families, understanding what is most important to families who are caring for clients at the end of life. **EBN:** *The elements rated as extremely important at the end of life of a family member were (1) to have trust and confidence in the doctors, (2) to be honestly told about the prognosis of the family member, and (3) resolving conflicts with the dying family member and saying goodbye (Heyland et al, 2006).*
- Encourage clients to pray. **EBN:** *Prayer, scripture reading, and clergy visits were found to comfort some hospice clients, but sometimes specific religious tenets may be troubling and need to be resolved before the client can find peace (Gilbert, 2008).*

 ### Geriatric

- Carefully assess older adults for issues regarding death anxiety. **EBN:** *Elders differ in their readiness for death. Some still have goals that they want to reach. These goals may not always be realistic (Bente et al, 2006). As client advocate, nurses can be confident the decisions made by older adults are accurate and reflect a lifelong set of values that were important to the decision-making process (Martin & Roberto, 2006).* **EB:** *Old age raises questions for many adults, such as whether we face a painful death, what happens after death, and if our lives had meaning (Goldsteen et al, 2006).*
- Provide back massage for clients who have anxiety regarding issues such as death. **EBN:** *Massage significantly decreased anxiety or perception of tension (Frenkel & Shah, 2008).*
- Refer to care plan for **Grieving.**

 ### Multicultural

- Assist clients to identify with their culture and its values. **EB:** *The process of identification with one's culture is identified as a coping mechanism that may protect the individual from increased death anxiety (Lobar, Youngblut, & Brooten, 2006).* **EBN:** *Practices related to life support, DNR, advanced*

directives, and routines and rituals at the end of life are related to cultural orientation. Depending on the cultural orientation, specific members are responsible for communication related to death and dying (Fordham, Giger, & Davidhizar, 2006). Findings from one study suggest that faith and Christianity may also be better predictors of death anxiety as a cultural indicator than other variables. Christians scored significantly lower for death anxiety than both nonreligious and Muslim groups, and Muslims scored significantly higher than the nonreligious group (Gareth & McAdie, 2009).

- Refer to care plans for **Anxiety** and **Grieving.**

Home Care

- The above interventions may be adapted for home care.
- Identify times and places when anxiety is greatest. Provide for psychological support at those times, using such strategies as personal contact, telephone contact, diversionary activities, or therapeutic self. *Anxiety may be related to earlier events associated with home setting or daily patterns that created pain and now serve as triggers (Jakobsson et al, 2006).*
- Support religious beliefs; encourage client to participate in services and activities of choice. *Belief in a supreme being/higher power provides a feeling of ever-present help (Gilbert, 2008).*
- ▲ Refer to medical social services or mental health services, including support groups as appropriate (e.g., anticipatory grieving groups from hospice, visiting volunteers of hospice). *Referral to specialty groups may be a key part of the nursing plan (Jakobsson et al, 2006).*
- Encourage the client to verbalize feelings to family/caregivers, counselors, and self. *Expression of feelings relieves fear burden and allows examination and validation of feelings (Bluck et al, 2008).*
- Identify client's preferences for end-of-life care; provide assistance in honoring preferences as much as practicable. **EB:** *Many changes occur in the final hours of life. Family members of those dying at home need to be prepared for these changes, both to understand what is happening and to provide care (Kehl et al, 2008).*
- ▲ Assist the client in making contact with death-related planning organizations, if appropriate: such as the Cremation Society and funeral homes. *Planning and direct action (contracting for after-death care) often relieve anxiety and provide the client with a measure of control (Bente et al, 2006).*
- With client, create a memento book reflecting life achievements. Leave in the home for regular review by client. If family will be the recipient, a memento book serves as both an opportunity for life review and a means of proactively leaving something behind for survivors. *Memento books and written life goals are tangible milestones related to life and death. They provide comfort, reassurance, hope, and direction for the client and more definition for client/caregiver expectations. It gives client a sense of focus, decreasing feelings of powerlessness over death (Eliott & Olver, 2007).*
- ▲ Refer for psychiatric home health care services for client reassurance and implementation of a therapeutic regimen. Psychiatric home care nurses can address issues relating to client's death anxiety, including family relationships. *Behavioral interventions in the home can assist client to participate more effectively in the treatment plan (Jakobsson et al, 2006).*
- Refer to care plan for **Powerlessness.**

Client/Family Teaching and Discharge Planning

- Promote more effective communication to family members engaged in the caregiving role. Encourage them to talk to their loved one about areas of concern. Both caregivers and care receivers avoid discussing. **EBN:** *Increasing the knowledge of and access to palliative care decreases suffering before death (Jakobsson et al, 2006).*
- Allow family members to be physically close to their dying loved one, giving them permission, instruction, and opportunities to touch. Keep family members informed. **EBN:** *Tertiary care centers are criticized for not providing a peaceful death experience (Nelson et al, 2006).*
- To increase clients' knowledge about end-of-life issues, teach them and their family members about options for care, such as advance directives. **EBN:** *Educating clients and families about end-of-life options will provide security and reduce anxiety (Kehl et al, 2008).*

⊖volve   See the EVOLVE website for Weblinks for client education resources.

● = Independent   ▲ = Collaborative   **EBN** = Evidence-Based Nursing   **EB** = Evidence-Based

REFERENCES

Bente A, Swane C, Halberg I et al: Being given a cancer diagnosis in old age: a phenomenological study, *Int J Nurs Stud* 43(8):1101–1109, 2006.

Bluck S, Dirk J, MacKay M et al: Life experience with death; related to death attitudes and to the use of death related memories, *Death Stud* 32(6):524–549, 2008.

Cox R: Music thanatology: reconstructing end-of-life care, *J Hum Caring* 10(2):1091–1099, 2006.

Eliott J, Olver I: Hope and hoping in the talk of dying cancer patients, *Soc Sci Med* 64(1):138–149, 2007.

Ferrell B, Levy MH, Paice J: Managing pain from advanced cancer in the palliative care setting, *Clin J Oncol Nurs* 12(4):575–581, 2008.

Fordham P, Giger J, Davidhizar R: Multi-cultural and multi-ethnic considerations and advanced directives: developing cultural competency, *J Cult Divers* 13(1):3–9, 2006.

Frenkel M, Shah V: Complementary medicine can benefit palliative care—part 2, *J Palliat Care* 15(6):288–293, 2008.

Gareth JM, McAdie T: Are personality, well-being and death anxiety related to religious affiliation? *Ment Health Relig Cult* 12(2):115–120, 2009.

Gilbert RB: More than a parting prayer: lessons in care-giving for the dying, *Crisis Loss* 16(3):261–263, 2008.

Goldsteen M, Houtepen R, Proot I et al: What is a good death? Terminally ill patients dealing with normative expectations around death and dying, *Patient Educ Couns* 64(1–3):378–386, 2006.

Halliday L, Boughton M: The moderating effect of death experience on death anxiety: implications for nursing education, *J Hosp Palliat Nurs* 10(2):76–82, 2008.

Healing Touch International, Inc: www.healingtouchinternational.org. Accessed Nov. 3, 2009.

Heyland D, Dodek P, Groll D et al: What matters most in end-of-life care: perceptions of seriously ill patients and their family members *CMAJ* 174(5):627–633, 2006.

Jakobsson E, Bergh I, Ohlen J et al: Utilization of health-care services at the end-of-life, *Health Policy* 80(2):245–250, 2006.

Kehl KA, Kirchhoff KT, Finster MP et al: Materials to prepare families for dying at home, *J Palliat Med* 11(7):969–972, 2008.

Lobar S, Youngblut J, Brooten D: Cross-cultural beliefs, ceremonies, and rituals surrounding death of a loved one, *Pediatr Nurs* 32(1):44–50, 2006.

Martin V, Roberto K: Assessing the stability of values and health care preferences of older adults: a long term comparison study, *J Gerontol Nurs* 32(11):23–31, 2006.

McCaffrey R, Locsin R: The effect of music on pain and acute confusion in older adults undergoing hip and knee surgery, *Holist Nurs Pract*, 20(5):218–224, 2006

Nadworny SW: The hospital vigil, fulfilling a patient's wish not to die alone, *Caring* 26(11):52–54, 2007.

Nelson J, Angus D, Weissfeld L et al: End-of-life care for the critically ill: a national intensive care unit survey, *Crit Care Med* 34(10):2547–2553, 2006.

Risk for Aspiration *Betty J. Ackley, MSN, EdS, RN* ⊖volve

NANDA-I

Definition

At risk for entry of gastrointestinal secretions, oropharyngeal secretions, solids, or fluids into the tracheobronchial passages

Risk Factors

Decreased gastrointestinal motility; delayed gastric emptying; depressed cough; depressed gag reflex; facial surgery; facial trauma; gastrointestinal tubes; incompetent lower esophageal sphincter; increased gastric residual; increased intragastric pressure; impaired swallowing; medication administration; neck trauma; neck surgery; oral surgery; oral trauma; presence of endotracheal tube; presence of tracheostomy tube; reduced level of consciousness; situations hindering elevation of upper body; tube feedings; wired jaws

NOC (Nursing Outcomes Classification)

Suggested NOC Outcomes

Aspiration Prevention, Respiratory Status: Ventilation, Swallowing Status

Example NOC Outcome with Indicators
Respiratory Status: Ventilation as evidenced by the following indicators: Adventitious breath sounds/Dyspnea at rest/Dyspnea with exertion/Tactile fremitus/Accumulation of sputum/Accessory muscle use (Rate the outcome and indicators of **Respiratory Status: Ventilation:** 1 = severe, 2 = substantial, 3 = moderate, 4 = mild, 5 = none [see Section I].)

 = Independent   ▲ = Collaborative   **EBN** = Evidence-Based Nursing   **EB** = Evidence-Based

Client Outcomes

Client Will (Specify Time Frame):

- Maintain patent airway and clear lung sounds
- Swallow and digest oral, nasogastric, or gastric feeding without aspiration

NIC   (Nursing Interventions Classification)

Suggested NIC Intervention

Aspiration Precautions

Example NIC Activities—Aspiration Precautions
Monitor level of consciousness, cough reflex, gag reflex, and swallowing ability; Check NG or gastrostomy residual before feeding

Nursing Interventions and *Rationales*

- Monitor respiratory rate, depth, and effort. Note any signs of aspiration such as dyspnea, cough, cyanosis, wheezing, hoarseness, or fever. *Signs of aspiration should be detected as soon as possible to prevent further aspiration and to initiate treatment that can be lifesaving. Because of laryngeal pooling and residue in clients with dysphagia, silent aspiration (i.e., not manifested by choking or coughing) may occur (Ramsey, Smithard, & Kalra, 2005; Guy & Smith, 2009).*
- Auscultate lung sounds frequently and before and after feedings; note any new onset of crackles or wheezing. **EB:** *Bronchial auscultation of lung sounds was shown to be specific in identifying clients at risk for aspirating (Shaw et al, 2004).*
- Take vital signs frequently, noting onset of a temperature, increased respiratory rate.
- Before initiating oral feeding, check client's gag reflex and ability to swallow by feeling the laryngeal prominence as the client attempts to swallow. *A client can aspirate even with an intact gag reflex (Wieseke, Bantz, & Siktberg, 2008).* If client is having problems swallowing, see nursing interventions for **Impaired Swallowing**.
- If client needs to be fed, feed slowly and allow adequate time for chewing and swallowing. **EB:** *Multiple studies have found that it takes 35 minutes or more to feed a client who wants to eat. (Simmons, Osterweil, & Schnelle, 2001; Simmons & Schnelle, 2004; Simmons, 2008).*
- When feeding client, watch for signs of impaired swallowing or aspiration, including coughing, choking, and spitting food.
- Have suction machine available when feeding high-risk clients. If aspiration does occur, suction immediately. *A client with aspiration needs immediate suctioning and may need further lifesaving interventions such as intubation.*
- Keep head of bed elevated at 30 to 45 degrees, preferably sitting up in a chair at 90 degrees when feeding. Keep head elevated for an hour afterward. *Maintaining a sitting position with and after meals can help decrease aspiration pneumonia (Guy & Smith, 2009).* **EB:** *A study demonstrated that the number of clients developing a fever was significantly reduced when kept sitting upright after eating (Matsui et al, 2002).*
- ▲ Note presence of any nausea, vomiting, or diarrhea. Treat nausea promptly with antiemetics.
- If the client shows symptoms of nausea and vomiting, position on side. *The side-lying position can help the client expel the vomitus, and decrease possible aspiration.*
- Listen to bowel sounds frequently, noting if they are decreased, absent, or hyperactive. *Decreased or absent bowel sounds can indicate an ileus with possible vomiting and aspiration; increased high-pitched bowel sounds can indicate a mechanical bowel obstruction with possible vomiting and aspiration (Fauci et al, 2008).*
- Note new onset of abdominal distention or increased rigidity of abdomen. *Abdominal distention or rigidity can be associated with paralytic or mechanical obstruction and an increased likelihood of vomiting and aspiration (Fauci et al, 2008).*
- ▲ If client has a tracheostomy, ask for referral to speech pathologist for swallowing studies before attempting to feed. After the evaluation, the decision should be made to have cuff either inflated or deflated when client eats. **EB:** *Studies have shown that use of speaking valves for the client with a tracheostomy may reduce risk of aspiration when the client eats (Baumgartner, Bewyer, & Bruner,*

● = Independent   ▲ = Collaborative   **EBN** = Evidence-Based Nursing   **EB** = Evidence-Based

2008). **EB:** *A study found that a tracheostomy was not associated with increased aspiration (Sharma et al, 2007).*

- Provide meticulous oral care including brushing of teeth at least two times per day. Good oral care can prevent contamination of the mouth, which can be aspirated. **EB:** *Research has shown that excellent dental care/oral care can be effective in preventing hospital-acquired (or extended care–acquired) pneumonia (Garcia, 2005; Ishikawa et al 2008; Sarin et al, 2008; Arpin, 2009).*

Enteral Feedings

- Insert nasogastric feeding tube using the internal nares to distal-lower esophageal-sphincter distance, an updated version of the Hanson method. The ear-to-nose-to-xiphoid-process is often inaccurate. **EBN:** *A study demonstrated that the revised Hanson's method was more accurate in predicting the correct distance than the traditional method (Ellet et al, 2005).*
- ▲ Check to make sure the initial nasogastric feeding tube placement was confirmed by x-ray, with the openings of the tube in the stomach, not the esophagus. This is especially important if a small-bore feeding tube is used, although larger tubes used for feedings or medication administration should be verified by x-ray also. *X-ray verification of placement remains the gold standard for determining safe placement of feeding tubes (Bankhead et al, 2009).*
- Keep the nasogastric tube securely taped.
- Measure and record the length of the tube that is outside of the body at defined intervals to help ensure correct placement. *As part of maintaining correct placement, it is helpful to note the length of the tube outside of the body; it is possible for a tube to slide out and be in the esophagus, without obvious disruption of the tape (Metheny, 2006; Bankhead et al, 2009).*
- Note the placement of the tube on any x-rays that are done on the client. *Acutely ill clients receive frequent x-rays. These are available for the nurse to determine continued correct placement of the NG tube (Ackerman & Mick, 2006; Metheny, 2006).*
- Check the pH of the aspirate. If the pH reading is 4 or less, the tube is probably in the stomach. *Recognize that the pH may not indicate correct placement if the client is receiving continuous tube feedings, is receiving a hydrogen ion blocker, has blood in the aspirate, or is receiving antacids (Ackerman & Mick, 2006; Bankhead et al, 2009).*
- Determine placement of feeding tube before each feeding or every 4 hours if client is on continuous feeding. Note length of tube outside of body, any recent x-ray results, pH of aspirate if relevant, and characteristic appearance of aspirate; do not rely on air insufflation method. **EBN:** *The auscultatory air insufflation method is not reliable for differentiating between gastric or respiratory placement (Metheny et al, 2006; Bankhead et al, 2009).*
- ▲ Check for gastric residual volume during continuous feedings or before feedings; if residual is greater than 200 mL, hold feedings following institutional protocol (Guy & Smith, 2009). **EBN:** *Monitoring gastric residual as evidence of risk for aspiration may or may not be effective (Metheny et al, 2006; Metheny et al, 2008); however, it still should be done at intervals (Bankhead et al, 2009) especially if there is a question of tube feeding intolerance. The practice of holding tube feedings if there is increased residual reduces the amount of calories given to the client. If the client has a small-bore feeding tube, it is difficult to check gastric residual volume and may be inaccurate. It may be prudent to use large-bore multiple port tubes during the first few days of tube feedings (Metheny et al, 2005; Metheny et al, 2008).* **EBN:** *A study of the effectiveness of either returning gastric residual volumes to the client, or discarding them resulted in inconclusive findings with complications when either action was taken, and more research is needed in the area (Booker, Niedringhaus, & Eden, 2000).*
- Test for the presence of pepsin in tracheobronchial secretions to detect aspiration of enteral feedings. Avoid use of glucose testing. **EB:** *Glucose was found in tracheal secretions of clients who were not receiving enteral feedings (Bankhead et al, 2009). The detection of pepsin in tracheal secretions is considered an indicator of aspiration of gastric contents; a flat position is strongly associated with the presence of pepsin in secretions (Metheny et al, 2002; Metheny et al, 2008).*
- Do not use blue dye to tint enteral feedings. *The presence of blue and green skin and urine and serum discoloration from use of blue dye has been associated with the death of clients, (Lucarelli et al, 2004). The FDA has reported at least 12 deaths from the use of blue dye in enteral feedings (USFDA, 2003). In a study performed on rabbits, use of the blue dye was not consistently effective in identifying tracheal aspiration (Metheny et al, 2002). A study found neurotoxicity in the central nervous system from use*

of methylene blue dye in rats using methylene blue as a marker in parathyroid surgery (Vutskits et al, 2008).

- During enteral feedings, position client with head of bed elevated 30 to 45 degrees (Bankhead et al, 2009). **EBN and EB:** *A study of mechanically ventilated clients receiving tube feedings demonstrated there was an increase of the presence of pepsin (from gastric contents) in pulmonary secretions if the client was in a flat position versus being positioned with head elevated (Metheny et al, 2006). A review of aspiration in ventilator clients who were being tube-fed found support for elevating the head of the bed at least 30 degrees (Bowman et al, 2005).*

 Geriatric

- Carefully check elderly client's gag reflex and ability to swallow before feeding. *Laryngeal nerve endings are reduced in the elderly, which diminishes the gag reflex (Miller, 2004).*
- Watch for signs of aspiration pneumonia in the elderly with cerebrovascular accidents, even if there are no apparent signs of difficulty swallowing or of aspiration. *Bedside evaluation for swallowing and aspiration can be inaccurate.* **EB:** *Silent aspiration can occur in the elderly population (Butler et al, 2009).*
- ▲ Recognize that the elderly with aspiration pneumonia have fewer symptoms than younger people. *Aspiration pneumonia can be undiagnosed in the elderly population because of decreased symptoms; sometimes the only obvious symptom may be new onset of delirium (Metheny, 2007).*
- ▲ Use central nervous system depressants cautiously; elderly clients may have an increased incidence of aspiration with altered levels of consciousness. *Elderly clients have altered metabolism, distribution, and excretion of drugs. Many medications can interfere with the swallowing reflex (Wieseke, Bantz, & Siktberg, 2008; Gallagher & Naidoo, 2009).*
- Keep an elderly, mostly bedridden client sitting upright for 45 minutes to 1 hour following meals. **EB:** *A study demonstrated that the number of clients developing a fever was significantly reduced when kept sitting upright after eating (Matsui et al, 2002).*
- Recommend to families that enteral feedings may or may not be indicated for clients with dementia. Instead use hand-feeding assistance, modified food consistency as needed, or environmental alterations (Easterling & Robbins, 2008). **EBN:** *Research has demonstrated that tube feedings in this population do not prevent malnutrition or aspiration, improve survival, or reduce infections. Instead there is an increased risk for aspiration pneumonia (Keithley & Swanson, 2004).*

 Home Care

- The above interventions may be adapted for home care use.
- For clients at high risk for aspiration, obtain complete information from the discharging institution regarding institutional management.
- Assess the client and family for willingness and cognitive ability to learn and cope with swallowing, feeding, and related disorders.
- Assess caregiver understanding and reinforce teaching regarding positioning and assessment of the client for possible aspiration.
- Provide the client with emotional support in dealing with fears of aspiration. *Fear of choking can provoke extreme anxiety, which can interfere with the client's ability or willingness to adhere to the treatment plan.* Refer to care plan for **Anxiety.**
- Establish emergency and contingency plans for care of client. *Clinical safety of client between visits is a primary goal of home care nursing.*
- ▲ Have a speech and occupational therapist assess client's swallowing ability and other physiological factors and recommend strategies for working with client in the home (e.g., pureeing foods served to client; providing adaptive equipment for independence in eating). *Successful strategies allow the client to remain part of the family.*
- Obtain suction equipment for the home as necessary.
- Teach caregivers safe, effective use of suctioning devices. Inform client and family that only individuals instructed in suctioning should perform the procedure.
- ▲ Institute case management of frail elderly to support continued independent living.

• = Independent ▲ = Collaborative **EBN** = Evidence-Based Nursing **EB** = Evidence-Based

Client/Family Teaching and Discharge Planning

- Teach the client and family signs of aspiration and precautions to prevent aspiration.
- Teach the client and family how to safely administer tube feeding.

eVolve   See the EVOLVE website for Weblinks for client education resources.

REFERENCES

Ackerman MH, Mick DJ: Technologic approaches to determining proper placement of enteral feeding tubes, *AACN Adv Crit Care* 17(3):246–249, 2006.

Arpin S: Oral hygiene in elderly people in hospitals and nursing homes, *Evid Based Dent* 10(2):46, 2009.

Bankhead R, Boullata J, Brantley S et al: Aspen enteral nutrition practice recommendations, *J Parenteral Enteral Nutr* 33(2):122–167, 2009.

Baumgratner CA, Bewyer E, Bruner D: Management of communication and swallowing in intensive care: the role of the speech pathologist, *AACN Adv Crit Care* 19(4):433–443, 2008.

Booker KJ, Niedringhaus L, Eden B: Comparison of 2 methods of managing gastric residual volumes from feeding tubes, *Am J Crit Care* 9(5):318, 2000.

Bowman A, Greiner JE, Doerschug KC et al: Implementation of an evidenced-based feeding protocol and aspiration risk reduction algorithm, *Crit Care Nurs Q* 28(4):324–33, 2005.

Butler SG, Stuart A, Markley L et al: Penetration and aspiration in healthy older adults as assessed during endoscopic evaluation of swallowing, *Ann Otol Rhinol Laryngol* 118(3):190–198, 2009.

Easterling CS, Robbins E: Dementia and dysphagia, *Geriatr Nurs* 29(4):275–285, 2008.

Ellett ML, Beckstrand J, Flueckiger J et al: Predicting the insertion distance for placing gastric tubes, *Clin Nurs Res* 14(1):11, 2005.

Fauci A, Braunwald E, Kasper DL et al: *Harrison's principles of internal medicine,* ed 17, New York, 2008, McGraw-Hill.

Gallagher L, Naidoo P: Prescription drugs and their effects on swallowing, *Dysphagia* 24(2):159–166, 2009.

Garcia R: A review of the possible role of oral and dental colonization on the occurrence of health care-associated pneumonia: underappreciated risk and a call for interventions, *Am J Infect Control* 33(9):527–541, 2005.

Guy JL, Smith LH: Preventing aspiration: a common and dangerous problem for patients with cancer, *Clin J Oncol Nurs* 13(1):105–108, 2009.

Ishikawa A, Yoneyama T, Hirota K et al: Professional oral health care reduces the number of oropharyngeal bacteria, *J Dent Res* 87(6):594–598, 2008.

Keithley JK, Swanson B: Enteral nutrition: an update on practice recommendations, *Medsurg Nurs* 13(2):131, 2004.

Lucarelli MR, Shirk MB, Julian MW et al: Toxicity of food drug and cosmetic blue No. 1 dye in critically ill patients, *Chest* 125(2):793, 2004.

Matsui T, Yamaya M, Ohrui T et al: Sitting position to prevent aspiration in bed-bound patients, *Gerontology* 48(3):194, 2002.

Metheny NA: Preventing respiratory complications of tube feedings: evidence-based practice, *Am J Crit Care* 15(4):360–369, 2006.

Metheny NA: Try this: best practices in nursing care to older adults. Preventing aspiration in older adults with dysphagia, *Medsurg Nurs* 16(4):271–272, 2007.

Metheny NA, Dahms TE, Stewart BJ et al: Efficacy of dye-stained enteral formula in detecting pulmonary aspiration, *Chest* 122(1):276–81, 2002.

Metheny NA, Stewart J, Nuetzel G, et al: Effect of feeding-tube properties on residual volume measurements in tube-fed patients, *J Parenter Enteral Nutr* 29(3):192–7, 2005.

Metheny NA, Clouse RE, Chang YH et al: Tracheobronchial aspiration of gastric contents in critically ill tube-fed patients: frequency, outcomes, and risk factors, *Crit Care Med* 34(4):1007–1015, 2006.

Metheny NA, Schallom L, Oliver DA, et al: Gastric residual volume and aspiration in critically ill patients receiving gastric feedings, *Am J Crit Care* 17(6):512–520, 2008.

Miller CA: *Nursing for wellness in older adults,* ed 4, Philadelphia, 2004, Lippincott.

Ramsey D, Smithard D, Kalra L: Silent aspiration: what do we know? *Dysphagia* 20(3):218–225, 2005.

Sarin J, Balasubramaniam R, Corcoran A et al: Reducing the risk of aspiration pneumonia among elderly patients in long-term care facilities through oral health interventions, *J Am Med Dir Assoc* 9(2):128–135, 2008.

Sharma OP, Oswanski MF, Singer D et al: Swallowing disorders in trauma patients: impact of tracheostomy, *Am Surg* 73(11):1117–1121, 2007.

Shaw JL, Sharpe S, Dyson SE et al: Bronchial auscultation: an effective adjunct to speech and language therapy bedside assessment when detecting dysphagia and aspiration? *Dysphagia* 19(4):211, 2004.

Simmons SF: Feeding. In Ackley B, Ladwig G, Swan BA et al: *Evidence-based nursing care guidelines,* Philadelphia, 2008, Mosby.

Simmons SF, Schnelle JF: Individualized feeding assistance care for nursing home residents: staffing requirements to implement two interventions, *J Gerontol A Biol Sci Med Sci* 59(9):M966–973, 2004.

Simmons SF, Osterweil D, Schnelle JF: Improving food intake in nursing home residents with feeding assistance: a staffing analysis, *J Gerontol A Biol Sci Med Sci* 56(12):M790–M794, 2001.

U.S. Food and Drug Administration (USFDA). Reports of blue discoloration and death in patients receiving enteral feedings tinted with the dye, FD&C Blue no. 1. *FDA Public Health Advisory, 2003:* www.fda.gov/ForIndustry/ColorAdditives/ColorAdditivesinSpecificProducts/InMedicalDevices/ucm142395.htm. Accessed July 13, 2009.

Vutskits L, Briner A, Klauser P et al: Adverse effects of methylene blue on the central nervous system, *Anesthesiology* 108(4):684–692, 2008.

Wieseke A, Bantz D, Siktberg L: Assessment and early diagnosis of dysphagia, *Geriatr Nurs* 29(6):376–383, 2008.

Risk for impaired Attachment   *Mary A. DeWys, BS, RN, and Peg Padnos, AB, BSN, RN*

NANDA-I

Definition

Disruption of the interactive process between parent/significant other and child/infant that fosters the development of a protective and nurturing reciprocal relationship

 • = Independent   ▲ = Collaborative   EBN = Evidence-Based Nursing   EB = Evidence-Based

Risk Factors

Anxiety associated with the parent role; ill child who is unable effectively to initiate parental contact as a result of altered behavioral organization; inability of parents to meet personal needs; lack of privacy; parental conflict resulting from altered behavioral organization; physical barriers; premature infant who is unable to effectively initiate parental contact due to altered behavioral organization; separation; substance abuse

 (Nursing Outcomes Classification)

Suggested NOC Outcomes

Caregiver Adaptation to Patient Institutionalization, Child Development, Coping, Parent-Infant Attachment, Parenting Performance

Example NOC Outcomes with Indicators
Demonstrates appropriate **Child Development: 2 Months** as evidenced by the following indicators: Coos and vocalizes/Shows interest in visual stimuli/Shows interest in auditory stimuli/Smiles/Shows pleasure in interactions, especially with primary caregivers. **4 Months:** Looks at and becomes excited by mobile/Recognizes parents' voices/Smiles, laughs, and squeals. **6 months:** Smiles, laughs, squeals, imitates noise/Shows beginning signs of stranger anxiety. **12 Months:** Plays social games/Imitates vocalizations/Pulls to stand (Rate the outcome and indicators of appropriate **Child Development:** 1 = never demonstrated, 2 = rarely demonstrated, 3 = sometimes demonstrated, 4 = often demonstrated, 5 = consistently demonstrated [see Section I].)

Client Outcomes

Parent(s)/Caregiver(s) Will (Specify Time Frame):

- Be willing to consider pumping breast milk (and storing appropriately) or breastfeeding, if feasible
- Demonstrate behaviors that indicate secure attachment to infant/child
- Provide a safe environment, free of physical hazard
- Provide nurturing environment sensitive to infant/child's need for nutrition/feeding, sleeping, comfort, and social play
- Read and respond contingently to infant/child's behavior cues that signal approach/engagement or avoidance/disengagement
- Be able to calm and relieve infant/child's distress
- Support infant's self-regulation capabilities, intervening when needed
- Engage in mutually satisfying interactions that provide opportunities for attachment
- Give infant nurturing sensory experiences (e.g., holding, cuddling, stroking, rocking)
- Demonstrate an awareness of developmentally appropriate activities that are pleasurable, emotionally supportive, and growth fostering
- Avoid physical and emotional abuse and/or neglect as retribution for parent's perception of infant/child's misbehavior
- Be knowledgeable of appropriate community resources and support services

 (Nursing Interventions Classification)

Suggested NIC Interventions

Anticipatory Guidance, Attachment Process, Attachment Promotion, Coping Enhancement, Developmental Care, Attachment Process, Parent Education: Infant

Example NIC Activities—Anticipatory Guidance
Instruct about normal development and behavior, as appropriate; Provide information on realistic expectations related to the patient's behavior; Use case examples to enhance the patient's problem-solving skills, as appropriate

• = Independent   ▲ = Collaborative   **EBN** = Evidence-Based Nursing   **EB** = Evidence-Based

Nursing Interventions and *Rationales*

- Establish a trusting relationship with parent/caregiver. *Interventions must address both the infant's needs for a stimulating, responsive, and secure environment and meet the parent's developmental and emotional challenges (Barnard, 1998).* **EBN:** *An understanding of parental needs is essential to the development of effective, caring nurse-parent relationships and to help minimize parental stress in the NICU (Lam, Spence, & Halliday, 2007).*
- Encourage mothers to breastfeed their infants, and provide support. *Mothers who choose to breast-feed display enhanced sensitivity during early infancy that, in turn, may foster secure attachment (Britton, Britton, & Gronwaldt, 2006). The Baby Friendly Initiative urges that support is there for the very first breastfeeding, and that all mothers should have the opportunity to hold their babies with skin-to-skin contact for an unlimited period as soon as possible after delivery (Warren, 2008).*
- ▲ Identify factors related to postpartum depression (PPD) and major depression and offer appropriate interventions and referrals. **EB:** *The "Postpartum Bonding Questionnaire" (PBQ) is an effective instrument for identifying mothers with PPD (Brockington, Fraser, & Wilson, 2006). Toddler-parent psychotherapy increases secure attachment between toddlers and mothers who have experienced major depressive disorder since the birth of their child (Dawe, 2007).* **EBN:** *Depressive symptoms in low-income mothers have been shown to affect infant development negatively. Treatment in the home by masters-prepared psychiatric nurses was helpful in reducing depressive symptoms (Beeber et al, 2004).*
- Nurture parents so that they in turn can nurture their infant/child. **EBN:** *Provide relationship-based caregiving; when working with parents, the nurse is nurturing the developing mother-infant relationship (Lawhon, 2002). "Minding the Baby" is an interdisciplinary, relationship-based home-visiting program that addresses the relationship disruptions stemming from mothers' early trauma and history of derailed attachment (Slade et al, 2005).*
- Offer parents opportunities to verbalize their childhood fears associated with attachment. *Treatment of caregivers' own attachment difficulties and current psychopathology may also be indicated (Hardy, 2007).*
- Suggest journaling as a way for parents of hospitalized infants to cope with their stress and emotional reactions. **EBN:** *A study of parents of preterm infants, who kept journals as a means to cope with the most stressful aspects of the NICU experience, reported that the practice promoted their willingness to involve themselves in their infants' care (MacNab et al, 1998).*
- Offer parent-to-parent support to parents of NICU hospitalized and newborn infants. **EBN:** *The research found that parenting a young infant is stressful and the parents are not prepared for the complexities of caring for a newborn. Parents found support from their peer group extremely beneficial and looked to maternal and child health nurses for information and reassurance. The role of maternal and child health nurses is to facilitate access to peer groups, listen to the concerns of parents, affirm parenting skills and provide parenting information (Eronen, Pincombe, & Calabretto, 2007).*
- Encourage parents of hospitalized infants to "personalize the baby" by bringing in clothing, pictures of themselves, toys, and tapes of their voices. **EBN:** *These actions help parents claim the infant as their own. Neonatal nurses are in a unique position to support families' competence and confidence in caring for their infants at their own pace and to encourage the developing mother-infant relationship (Lawhon, 2002).*
- Encourage physical closeness using skin-to-skin experiences for parents and infants as appropriate. **EBN:** *"Kangaroo care" is one of several effective bonding and attachment strategies; others include swaddling, offering pacifier, listening to heartbeat sounds and sounds of mother's voice, rhythmic movement, and decreasing external stimuli (Ludington-Hoe, Cong, & Hashemi, 2002). Placing the newborn skin-to-skin on the mother's chest immediately after delivery until the infant latches on for the first feeding, encouraging continued breastfeeding, and keeping the mother and infant always together in the first hours and days after delivery helps to establish a bond between mother and infant (Kennell & McGrath, 2005).*
- Assist parents in developing new caregiving competencies and/or revising and extending old ones. **EBN:** *Five caregiving domains have been identified: (1) being with the infant, (2) knowing the infant as a person, (3) giving care to the infant, (4) communicating and engaging with others about needs (both infant and parental), and (5) problem-solving/decision-making/learning (Pridham et al, 1998).*
- Plan ways for parents to interact/assist with caregiving for their hospitalized/institutionalized infant/child. **EBN:** *Seeing the infant in the delivery room prior to admission to the NICU may decrease parental stress, which can be a significant barrier to attachment (Shields-Poe & Pinelli, 1997).*

• = Independent   ▲ = Collaborative   **EBN** = Evidence-Based Nursing   **EB** = Evidence-Based

Involving parents in decision making and empowering parents in their infant's care can help to alleviate parental stress (Lam, Spence, & Halliday, 2007).

- Educate parents about reading and responding sensitively to their infant's unique "body language" (behavior cues) that communicate approach ("I'm ready to play"), avoidance/stress ("I'm unhappy. I need a change."), and self-calming ("I'm helping myself"). *Providing knowledge of how infants communicate their feelings and needs offers parents guidelines for choosing their own behavioral responses (Boris, Aoki, & Zeanah, 1999).*

- Educate and support parent's ability to relieve infant/child's stress/distress. **EB:** *The more that the infant of a nonresponsive mother cries at 2 months of age, the more likely is the establishment of a negative feedback cycle that can impair attachment and feelings of security at 18 months of age (Gunnar, Brodersen, & Nachmias, 1996).*

- Guide parents in adapting their behaviors and activities with infant/child cues and changing needs. **EBN:** *Assisting parents to be responsive to infant/child cues and helping parents to be sensitive to their responsiveness to those cues are growth-fostering activities that nurses can encourage (Barnard, 1994). Model calming interventions to provide parents with tools for positive interactions with their infant/child (Karl, 1999).*

- Attend to both the parent and infant/child in an effort to strengthen high-quality parent-infant interactions. **EBN:** *The environment provided by the child's primary caregivers has tremendous impact on all aspects of child's early development as well as his or her later life (Malekpour, 2007).*

- Assist parents with providing pleasurable sensory learning experiences (i.e., sight, sound, movement, touch, and body awareness). **EBN:** *Various studies of hospitalized preterm infants who received gentle human touch (GHT) and massage showed similar positive findings: lower morbidity, shorter length of stay, fewer days on supplemental oxygen, lower neurobiologic risk scores, and higher average daily weight gain than control counterparts (Harrison, 2001).*

- Encourage parents and caregivers to massage their infants and children. *Infant massage enhances attachment through stimulation of mature sensory systems (tactile/kinesthetic) and has been shown to be an effective "low-tech" means of providing developmentally appropriate care for premature infants (Field, 2002; Beachy, 2003).*

Pediatric/Infant

- Recognize and support infant/child's capacity for self-regulation and intervene when appropriate. *Infants must learn to take in sensory information while simultaneously managing not to become overaroused and overwhelmed by stimuli (Greenspan, 1992; DeGangi & Breinbauer, 1997).*

- Provide lyrical, soothing music in the nursery and home that is appropriate for age (i.e., corrected, in the case of premature infants) and contingent with state and behavioral cues. **EBN:** *Overall beneficial effects of music therapy have been observed in preterm infants (Standley, 2002).*

- Recognize and support infant/child's attention capabilities. *"The ability to take an interest in the sights, sounds, and sensations of the world" is a significant developmental milestone (Greenspan & Wieder, 1998).*

- Encourage opportunities for mutually satisfying interactions between infant and parent. *The process of attachment involves communication and patterns of interactions between parent and infant that are synchronous and rhythmic (Rossetti, 1999). Opportunities should be provided for infants to be with their parents and hear their voices naturally (Graven, 2000).*

- Encourage opportunities for physical closeness. **EB:** *The neurodevelopmental profile was more mature for infants receiving kangaroo care. Results underscore the role of early skin-to-skin contact in the maturation of the autonomic and circadian systems in preterm infants (Feldman & Eidelman, 2003).*

Multicultural

- Discuss cultural norms with families to provide care that is appropriate for enhancing attachment with the infant/child. **EB:** *Attachment investigators provide evidence that security takes similar forms and has similar antecedents and consequences in diverse cultures. There is also evidence that security differs across culture, and the nature of the similarities and differences are not well understood (Rothbaum et al, 2007).*

• = Independent   ▲ = Collaborative   **EBN** = Evidence-Based Nursing   **EB** = Evidence-Based

- Promote the attachment process in women who have abused substances by providing a treatment environment that is culturally based and women-centered. **EBN:** *Pregnant and postpartum Asian/Pacific Islander women in substance abuse treatment identified provisions for the newborn, infant health care, parent education, and infant mother bonding as conducive to their treatment (Morelli, Fong & Oliveria, 2001).*
- Empower family members to draw on personal strengths in which multiple worldviews and values of individual members are recognized, incorporated, and negotiated. **EB:** *A respectful intervention process can reiterate a parallel process in the family in which multiple worldviews among different members are explored, accepted, appreciated, and negotiated for the benefit of the family (Lee & Mjelde-Mossey, 2004).*
- Encourage positive involvement and relationship development between children and noncustodial fathers to enhance health and development. **EB:** *Research with low-income African American fathers has shown that these fathers are strongly committed to their children, but there is a need for outside facilitation to overcome barriers that interfere with their positive involvement (Dubowitz et al, 2004).*

 Home Care

- The above interventions may be adapted for home care use.
- Assess quality of interaction between parent and infant/child. **EB:** *Parent-child relationships underpin the emotional health and well-being of infants. Difficulties within this relationship can have far-reaching consequences for both parents and children. Health visitors within public health teams have a unique opportunity to support this relationship at an early stage (Bailey, 2009).*
- Use "interaction coaching" (i.e., teaching mother to let the infant lead) so that the mother will match her style of interaction to the baby's cues. **EBN:** *Mothers with postpartum depressive symptoms who received interaction coaching demonstrated significantly greater responsiveness to their infants (Horowitz et al, 2001).*
- ▲ Provide home visitation for infants with depressed mothers and for highly stressed parents of preterm infants. **EB:** *Several studies identified home visitation as an effective intervention for depressed and stressed parents/caregivers. Such programs offered support, counseling, and developmental guidance to facilitate early attachment and bonding (Barnard, 1997; NCAST, 1994). NSTEP-P was developed to assist parents in understanding preterm infant behavior and caregiving practices for families (Barnard, 1994).*
- ▲ Identify community resources and supportive network systems for mothers showing depressive symptoms. **EBN:** *Identifying maternal depressive symptoms leading to early intervention and treatment of women at risk for depression can decrease the negative effects on infant development (Mew et al, 2003).*
- Provide supportive care for infants and children whose parents have been deployed during wartime. **EB:** *There is an interdependent nature of infants and their parents who are experiencing wartime deployment and reunion. Family roles change throughout the cycle of deployment; and parental absence has a detrimental impact on infant attachment relationships. Parents, professionals, and communities should work together to ensure the youngest family members are afforded optimal development within the context of their parent's wartime deployment (Gorman & Fitzgerald, 2007).*

ⓔvolve   See the EVOLVE website for Weblinks for client education resources.

REFERENCES

Bailey B : Parent-child relationships: developing a brief attachment-screening tool, *Community Pract* 82(3):22–26, 2009.

Barnard KE: *Caregiver/parent-child interaction feeding and teaching manual,* Seattle, 1994, NCAST.

Barnard KE: Influencing parent-child interactions. In Guralnick MJ, editor: *The effectiveness of early intervention,* Baltimore, 1997, Brooks, pp 249–268.

Barnard KE, editor: Developing, implementing, and documenting interventions with parents and young children, *Zero to Three,* February and March, 23–29, 1998.

Beachy JM: Premature infant massage in the NICU, *Neonatal Netw* 22(3):39–45, 2003.

Beeber LS, Holditch-Davis D, Belyea MJ et al: In-home intervention for depressive symptoms with low-income mothers of infants and toddlers in the United States, *Health Care Women Int* 25(6):561–580, 2004.

Boris NW, Aoki Y, Zeanah CH: The development of infant-parent attachment: considerations for assessment, *Infants Young Child* 11(4):1, 1999.

Britton JR, Britton HL, Gronwaldt V: Breastfeeding, sensitivity, and attachment, *Pediatrics* 118(5):e1436–1443, 2006.

● = Independent   ▲ = Collaborative   **EBN** = Evidence-Based Nursing   **EB** = Evidence-Based

Brockington IF, Fraser C, Wilson D: The postpartum bonding questionnaire: a validation, *Arch Womens Ment Health* 9:233–242, 2006.

Dawe S: Toddler-parent psychotherapy increases secure attachment between toddlers and mothers who have experienced major depressive disorder, *Evid Based Ment Health* 10(4):123, 2007.

DeGangi GA, Breinbauer C: The symptomatology of infants and toddlers with regulatory disorders, *J Development Learning Dis* 1(1):183–215, 1997.

Dubowitz H, Lane W, Ross K et al: The involvement of low-income African American fathers in their children's lives, and the barriers they face, *Ambul Pediatr* 4(6):505–508, 2004.

Eronen R, Pincombe J, Calabretto H: Support for stressed parents of young infants, *Neonatal Paediatr Child Health Nurs* 10(2):20–27, 2007.

Feldman R, Eidelman A: Skin-to-skin contact (kangaroo care) accelerates autonomic and neurobehavioural maturation in preterm infants, *Dev Med Child Neurol* 45(4):274, 2003.

Field T: Massage, *Med Clin North Am* 86(1):163–167, 2002.

Gorman LA, Fitzgerald HE: Ambiguous loss, family stress, and infant attachment during times of war, *Zero to Three*, 27(6):20–26, 2007.

Graven S: Sound and the developing infant in the NICU: conclusions and recommendations for care, *J Perinatol* 20(8)(Pt2):S88–S93, 2000.

Greenspan SI: *Infancy and early childhood: the practice of clinical assessment and intervention with emotional and developmental challenges.* Madison, CT, 1992, International Universities.

Greenspan SI, Wieder S: *The child with special needs: encouraging intellectual and emotional growth*, Reading, MA, 1998, Perseus.

Gunnar MR, Brodersen L, Nachmias M et al: Stress reactivity and attachment security, *Dev Psychobiol* 29(3):191–204, 1996.

Hardy LT; Attachment theory and reactive attachment disorder: theoretical perspectives and treatment implications, *J Child Adolesc Psychiatr Nurs* (1):27–39, 2007.

Harrison LL: The use of comforting touch and massage to reduce stress for preterm infants in the neonatal intensive care unit, *Newborn Infant Nurs Rev* 1:235–241, 2001.

Horowitz JA, Bell M, Trybulski J et al: Promoting responsiveness between mothers with depressive symptoms and their infants, *J Nurs Schol* 33(4):323–329, 2001.

Karl D: The interactive newborn bath, *MCN Am J Matern Child Nurs* 24(6):280–286, 1999.

Kennell J, McGrath S: Starting the process of mother-infant bonding, *Acta Paediatr* 94(6):775–777, 2005.

Lam J, Spence K, Halliday R: Parents' perception of nursing support in the neonatal intensive care unit (NICU), *Neonatal Paediatr Child Health Nurs* 10(3):19–25, 2007.

Lawhon G: Integrated nursing care: vital issues important in the humane care of the newborn, *Semin Neonatol* 7:441–446, 2002.

Lee MY, Mjelde-Mossey L: Cultural dissonance among generations: a olution-focused approach with East Asian elders and their families, *J Marital Fam Ther* 30(4):497–513, 2004.

Ludington-Hoe SM, Cong X, Hashemi F: Infant crying: nature, physiologic consequences, and select interventions, *Neonatal Netw* 21(2):29–36, 2002.

Macnab AJ, Beckett LY, Park CC et al: Journal writing as a social support strategy for parents of premature infants: a pilot study, *Patient Educ Couns* 33:149–159, 1998.

Malekpour M: Effects of attachment on early and later development, *Br J Dev Disabil* 53 part 2(105): 81–95, 2007.

Mew AM, Holditch-Davis D, Belyea M et al: Correlates of depressive symptoms in mothers of preterm infants, *Neonatal Netw* 22(5):51–60, 2003.

Morelli PT, Fong R, Oliveria J: Culturally competent substance abuse treatment for Asian/Pacific Islander women, *J Hum Behav Soc Environ* 3(3/4):263, 2001.

NCAST: *Keys to caregiving: a video program*, Seattle, 1994, NCAST.

Pridham KF: Guided participation and development of care-giving competencies for families of low birth-weight infants, *J Adv Nurs* 28(5):948–958, 1998.

Rossetti LM: *Infant-toddler assessment*, Boston, 1999, Little-Brown and Company.

Rothbaum F, Kakinuma M, Nagaoka R, et al: Attachment and amae: parent-child closeness in the United States and Japan, *J Cross Cult Psychol* (4):465–486, 2007.

Shields-Poe D, Pinelli J: Variables associated with parental stress in neonatal intensive care units, *Neonat Netw* 16(1):29, 1997.

Slade A, Sadler L, De Dios-Kenn C et al: Minding the baby: a reflective parenting program, *Psychoanal Study Child*, 60:74–100, 2005.

Standley JM: A meta-analysis of the efficacy of music for premature infants, *Pediatr Nurs* 17(2):107–113, 2002.

Warren R: Breastfeeding in the delivery room, *Br J Midwifery* 16(2):119–20, 2008.

Autonomic dysreflexia   Paula Reiss Sherwood, RN, CNRN, PhD, and Elizabeth A. Crago, RN, MSN

NANDA-I

Definition

Life-threatening, uninhibited sympathetic response of the nervous system to a noxious stimulus after a spinal cord injury at T7 or above

Defining Characteristics

Blurred vision; bradycardia; chest pain; chilling; conjunctival congestion; diaphoresis (above the injury); headache (a diffuse pain in different portions of the head and not confined to any nerve distribution area); Horner's syndrome; metallic taste in mouth; nasal congestion; pallor (below the injury); paresthesia; paroxysmal hypertension; pilomotor reflex; red splotches on skin (above the injury); tachycardia

Related Factors (r/t)

Bladder distention; bowel distention; deficient caregiver knowledge; deficient client knowledge; skin irritation

• = Independent   ▲ = Collaborative   **EBN** = Evidence-Based Nursing   **EB** = Evidence-Based

(Nursing Outcomes Classification)

Suggested NOC Outcomes

Neurological Status, Neurological Status: Autonomic, Vital Signs

Example NOC Outcome with Indicators
Neurological Status: Autonomic as evidenced by the following indicators: Systolic blood pressure/Diastolic blood pressure/Apical heart rate/Perspiration response pattern/Goose bumps response pattern/Pupil reactivity/Peripheral tissue perfusion (Rate each indicator of **Neurological Status: Autonomic:** 1 = severely compromised, 2 = substantially compromised, 3 = moderately compromised, 4 = mildly compromised, 5 = not compromised [see Section I].)

Client Outcomes/Goals

Client Will (Specify Time Frame):

- Maintain normal vital signs
- Remain free of dysreflexia symptoms
- Explain symptoms, prevention, and treatment of dysreflexia

 (Nursing Interventions Classification)

Suggested NIC Intervention

Dysreflexia Management

Example NIC Activities—Dysreflexia Management
Identify and minimize stimuli that may precipitate dysreflexia; Monitor for signs and symptoms of autonomic dysreflexia

Nursing Interventions and *Rationales*

- Monitor the client for symptoms of dysreflexia, particularly those with high-level and more extensive spinal cord injuries. See Defining Characteristics. **EB:** *Because some clients are asymptomatic, it is important to recognize risk factors for autonomic dysreflexia (AD), such as higher and more complete injuries and injuries related to trauma (Frisbie, 2006; Rabchevsky, 2006; Schottler et al, 2009). AD has also been associated with lower age groups and less time since injury (Hitzig et al, 2008).*
- ▲ Collaborate with health care practitioners to identify the cause of dysreflexia (e.g., distended bladder, impaction, pressure ulcer, urinary calculi, bladder infection, acute condition in the abdomen, penile pressure, ingrown toenail, or other source of noxious stimuli). *Noxious stimuli cause an uncontrolled sympathetic nervous system response (Widerstrom-Noga, Cruz Almeida, & Krassioukov, 2004).*
- ▲ If symptoms of dysreflexia are present, place client in high Fowler's position, remove all support hoses or binders, and immediately determine the noxious stimuli causing the response. If blood pressure cannot be decreased within 1 minute, notify the physician STAT. **EB:** *These steps promote venous pooling, decrease venous return, and decrease blood pressure. The client should be rapidly evaluated by both the physician and nurse to find the possible cause (Krassioukov et al, 2009).*
- ▲ To determine the stimulus for dysreflexia:
  - First, assess bladder function. Check for distention, and if present catheterize using an anesthetic jelly as a lubricant. Do not use Valsalva maneuver or Crede's method to empty the bladder. Ensure existing catheter patency. Also note signs of urinary tract infection. **EB:** *AD may be associated with bladder care for 30% of persons with a spinal cord injury (Anderson et al, 2006).*
  - Second, assess bowel function. Numb the bowel area with a topical anesthetic as ordered, and once agent is effective (5 minutes), check for impaction. **EB:** *AD may be associated with bowel care for 23% of persons with a spinal cord injury (Anderson et al, 2006). In particular, insertion of rectal medication and manual removal of stool have both been shown to increase systolic blood pressure (Furusawa et al, 2007).*
  - Third, assess the skin looking for any points of pressure.

• = Independent   ▲ = Collaborative   **EBN** = Evidence-Based Nursing   **EB** = Evidence-Based

▲ Initiate antihypertensive therapy as soon as ordered. **EB:** *A severely elevated blood pressure must be decreased for client safety, particularly given the client with AD's increased susceptibility to ventricular arrhythmias (Collins, Rodenbaugh, & DiCarlo, 2006).*

▲ Be careful not to increase noxious sensory stimuli. If numbing agent is ordered, use it on anus and 1 inch of rectum before attempting to remove a fecal impaction. Also spray pressure ulcer with it. If necessary to replace an obstructed catheter, use an anesthetic jelly as ordered. *Increased noxious sensory stimuli can exacerbate the abnormal response and worsen the client's prognosis.* **EB:** *In one study the use of topical lidocaine did not limit the development of autonomic dysreflexia during anorectal procedures in spinal cord injury clients (Cosman, Vu, & Plowman, 2002). AD may be associated with bladder and bowel care for persons with a spinal cord injury (Anderson et al, 2006).*

• Monitor vital signs every 3 to 5 minutes during acute event; continue to monitor vital signs after event is resolved (symptoms resolve and vital signs return to baseline). **EB:** *It is possible for the client to develop rebound hypotension after the acute event because of the use of antihypertensive medications, or symptoms of dysreflexia may reoccur (Krassioukov et al, 2009).*

• Watch for complications of dysreflexia, including signs of cerebral hemorrhage, seizures, MI, or intraocular hemorrhage. **EB:** *Extremely high blood pressure can cause intracranial hemorrhage and death (Krassioukov et al, 2009).*

• Accurately and completely record any incidences of dysreflexia; especially note the precipitating stimuli. **EB:** *It is imperative to determine both the causes of the condition and whether the condition is persistent, requiring the client to take medications routinely to prevent repeat incidences (Krassioukov et al, 2009).*

• Use the following interventions to prevent dysreflexia:
  ▪ Ensure that drainage from Foley catheter is good and that bladder is not distended.
  ▪ Ensure a regular pattern of defecation to prevent fecal impaction. **EB:** *Bladder distention and bowel impaction are common causes of dysreflexia (Furusawa et al, 2007).*
  ▪ Frequently change position of client to relieve pressure and prevent the formation of pressure ulcers.

▲ If ordered, apply an anesthetic agent to any wound below level of injury before performing wound care. **EB:** *Stimuli that would result in pain if the spinal cord were not dysfunctional can lead to AD (Krassioukov et al, 2009).*

▲ Because episodes can reoccur, notify all health care team members of the possibility of a dysreflexia episode. **EB:** *All health care personnel working with the client should be aware of the condition because symptoms could begin while the client is away from the nursing unit (Karlsson, 2006).*

▲ For female clients with spinal cord injury who become pregnant, collaborate with obstetrical health care practitioners to monitor for signs and symptoms of dysreflexia. **EB:** *Autonomic dysreflexia may signal the onset of labor or be a sign of preterm labor and obstetrical health care personnel should monitor potential cardiovascular complications (Osgood & Kuczkowski, 2006).*

 Home Care

• The above interventions may be adapted for home care use.

• Instruct the client with any known proclivity toward dysreflexia to wear a medical alert bracelet and carry a medical alert wallet card when not in a safe environment (i.e., not with someone who knows client has the condition and can respond appropriately). **EB:** *Autonomic dysreflexia is life-threatening response (Karlsson, 2006).*

▲ Establish an emergency plan: obtain physician orders for medications to be used in situations in which first aid does not work and plans to identify potential stimuli. **EB:** *Medication administered immediately can reverse early stage dysreflexia (Krassioukov et al, 2009). Dysreflexia that is not recognized and treated can result in death (Kasper, Braunwald, & Fauci, 2005).*

▲ If orders have not been obtained or client does not have medications, use emergency medical services.

• When episode of dysreflexia is resolved, monitor blood pressure every 30 to 60 minutes for next 5 hours or admit to institution for observation. **EB:** *After an episode of autonomic dysreflexia, it is not uncommon for a second episode or rebound to occur (Kasper, Braunwald, & Fauci, 2005).*

• = Independent   ▲ = Collaborative   **EBN** = Evidence-Based Nursing   **EB** = Evidence-Based

Client/Family Teaching and Discharge Planning

- Teach recognition of the earliest symptoms of dysreflexia, the actions that should be taken when they occur, and the need to summon help immediately. Give client a written card that contains this information. **EB:** *Clients and families at risk for not understanding the key elements of AD occurrence and management are clients with nontraumatic etiologies, those with T5 or lower injuries, those in the youngest age group at injury, and those who had a shorter duration of injury (Schottler et al, 2009). Risk for AD has also been linked to genetic predisposition (Brown & Jacob, 2006).*
- Teach steps to prevent dysreflexia episodes: care of bladder, bowel, and skin and prevention of other forms of noxious stimuli (i.e., not wearing clothing that is too tight). **EB:** *Data have suggested that despite having symptoms consistent with a diagnosis of AD, there are gaps in clients' understanding of treatment for the condition, particularly when the spinal cord injury is not a result of trauma (McGillivray et al, 2009).*
- Discuss the potential impact of sexual intercourse and pregnancy on autonomic dysreflexia. **EB:** *Autonomic dysreflexia has been shown to be triggered by pre- and full-term labor for women (Osgood & Kuczkowski, 2006) and by ejaculation and sperm retrieval for men (Elliott & Krassioukov, 2006; Ekland et al, 2008). Clients who develop AD during bowel and bladder care may be at higher risk for developing AD during sexual activity (Anderson et al, 2006).*

    See the EVOLVE website for Weblinks for client education resources.

REFERENCES

Anderson KD, Borisoff JF, Johnson RD et al: The impact of spinal cord injury on sexual function: Concerns of the general population, *Spinal Cord* 10:1–10, 2006.

Brown A, Jacob JE: Genetic approaches to autonomic dysreflexia, *Prog Brain Res*, 152, 299–313, 2006.

Collins HL, Rodenbaugh DW, DiCarlo SE: Spinal cord injury alters cardiac electrophysiology and increases the susceptibility to ventricular arrhythmias, *Prog Brain Res* 152:275–288, 2006.

Cosman BC, Vu TT, Plowman BK: Topical lidocaine does not limit autonomic dysreflexia during anorectal procedures in spinal cord injury: a prospective, double-blind study, *Int J Colorectal Dis* 17(2):104, 2002.

Ekland MB, Krassioukov AV, McBride KE et al: Incidence of autonomic dysreflexia and silent autonomic dysreflexia in men with spinal cord injury undergoing sperm retrieval: implications for clinical practice, *J Spinal Cord Med*, 31(1):33–9, 2008.

Elliot S, Krassioukov A: Malignant autonomic dysreflexia in spinal cord injured men, *Spinal Cord* 44:386–392, 2006.

Frisbie JH: Unstable baseline blood pressure in chronic tetraplegia, *Spinal Cord* Mar 28:1–4, 2006.

Furusawa K, Sugiyama H, Ikeda A et al: Autonomic dysreflexia during a bowel program in patients with cervical spinal cord injury, *Acta Med Okayama* 61(4): 221–227, 2007.

Hitzig SL, Tonack M, Campbell KA et al: Secondary health complications in an aging Canadian spinal cord injury sample, *Am J Phys Med Rehabil*, 87(7):545–555, 2008.

Karlsson AK: Autonomic dysfunction in spinal cord injury: clinical presentation of symptoms and signs, *Prog Brain Res*, 152:1–8, 2006.

Kasper L, Braunwald E, Fauci AS: *Harrison's principles of internal medicine,* ed 16, New York, 2005, McGraw-Hill.

Krassioukov A, Warburton DE, Teasell R et al: A systematic review of the management of autonomic dysreflexia after spinal cord injury, *Arch Phys Med Rehabil* 90(4):682–695, 2009.

McGillivray CF, Hitzig SL, Craven BC et al: Evaluating knowledge of autonomic dysreflexia among individuals with spinal cord injury and their families, *J Spinal Cord Med*, 32(1):54–62, 2009.

Osgood SL, Kuczkowski KM: Autonomic dysreflexia in a patient with spinal cord injury, *Acta Anaesthesiol Belg* 57(2):161–162, 2006.

Rabchevsky AG: Segmental organization of spinal reflexes mediating autonomic dysreflexia after spinal cord injury, *Prog Brain Res* 152:265–274, 2006.

Schottler J, Vogel L, Chafetz R et al: Patient and caregiver knowledge of autonomic dysreflexia among youth with spinal cord injury, *Spinal Cord* 47(9):681–686, 2009.

Widerstrom-Noga E, Cruz Almeida Y, Krassioukov A: Is there a relationship between chronic pain and autonomic dysreflexia in persons with cervical spinal cord injury? *J Neurotrauma* 21(2):195–204, 2004.

Risk for Autonomic dysreflexia   Betty J. Ackley, MSN, EdS, RN

NANDA-I

Definition

At risk for life-threatening, uninhibited response of the sympathetic nervous system, postspinal shock, in an individual with spinal cord injury or lesion at T6 or above (has been demonstrated in clients with injuries at T7 and T8)

Risk Factors

An injury/lesion at T6 or above AND at least one of the following noxious stimuli

• = Independent   ▲ = Collaborative   **EBN** = Evidence-Based Nursing   **EB** = Evidence-Based

B

Cardiopulmonary Stimuli

Deep vein thrombosis; pulmonary emboli

Gastrointestinal Stimuli

Bowel distention; constipation; difficult passage of feces; digital stimulation; enemas; esophageal reflux; fecal impaction; gallstones; gastric ulcers; gastrointestinal system pathology; hemorrhoids; suppositories

Musculoskeletal-Integumentary Stimuli

Cutaneous stimulation (e.g., pressure ulcer, ingrown toenail, dressings, burns, rash); fractures, heterotrophic bone; pressure over bony prominences; range-of-motion exercises, spasm; sunburns; wounds

Neurologic Stimuli

Irritating stimuli below the level of injury; painful stimuli below the level of injury

Regulatory Stimuli

Extreme environmental temperatures; temperature fluctuations

Reproductive Stimuli

Ejaculation; labor and delivery; menstruation; ovarian cyst; pregnancy sexual intercourse

Situational Stimuli

Constrictive clothing (e.g., straps, stockings, shoes); drug reactions (e.g., decongestants, sympathomimetics, vasoconstrictors); narcotic/opiod withdrawal; positioning; surgical procedures

Urological Stimuli

Bladder distention; bladder spasm; calculi; catheterization; cystitis; detrusor sphincter dyssynergia; epididymitis; instrumentation, surgery; urethritis; urinary tract infection

NOC, NIC, Client Outcomes, Nursing Interventions, Client/Family Teaching and Discharge Planning, *Rationales*, and References

Refer to care plan for **Autonomic dysreflexia**.

Risk-prone health Behavior   *Gail B. Ladwig, MSN, RN, CHTP*

 NANDA-I

Definition

Impaired ability to modify lifestyle/behaviors in a manner that improves health status

Defining Characteristics

Demonstrates nonacceptance of health status change; failure to achieve optimal sense of control; failure to take action that prevents health problems; minimizes health status change

Related Factors (r/t)

Excessive alcohol; inadequate comprehension; inadequate social support; low self-efficacy; low socioeconomic status; multiple stressors; negative attitude toward health care; smoking

 NOC   **(Nursing Outcomes Classification)**

Suggested NOC Outcomes

Participation in Health Care Decisions, Psychosocial Adjustment: Life Change, Risk Detection

---

• = Independent   ▲ = Collaborative   **EBN** = Evidence-Based Nursing   **EB** = Evidence-Based

Example NOC Outcome with Indicators
Risk Detection: as evidenced by the following indicators: Recognizes signs and symptoms that indicate risks/identifies potential health risks/participates in screening at recommended intervals/obtains information about changes in health recommendations (Rate the outcome and indicators of **Risk Detection:** 1 = never demonstrated, 2 = rarely demonstrated, 3 = sometimes demonstrated, 4 = often demonstrated, 5 = consistently demonstrated [see Section I].)

Client Outcomes

Client Will (Specify Time Frame):

- State acceptance of change in health status
- Request assistance in altering behaviors to adapt to change
- State personal goals for dealing with change in health status and means to prevent further health problems
- State experience of a period of grief that is proportional to the actual or perceived effect of the loss
- Report and/or demonstrate behavior changes mutually agreed upon with nurse as evidence of positive adaptation

(Nursing Interventions Classification)

Suggested NIC Intervention

Self-Efficacy Enhancement

Example NIC Activities—Self-Efficacy Enhancement
Explore individual's perception of his/her capability to perform the desired behavior; reinforce confidence in making behavior changes and taking action

Nursing Interventions and *Rationales*

- Assess the client's definitions of health and wellness and major barriers to health and wellness. **EBN:** *Each person has unique, individual perceptions of well-being and illness (Kiefer, 2008).*
- Allow the client adequate time to express feelings about the change in health status. **EBN:** *Important intervention for the client with a serious illness such as a malignant brain tumor (Khalili, 2007).*
- Use open-ended questions to allow the client free expression (e.g., "Tell me about your last hospitalization" or "How does this time compare?"). **EBN:** *Effective questioning facilitates a better understanding of the client and enables the development of a deeper nurse-client relationship (Jasmine, 2009).*
- Help the client work through the stages of grief. Denial is usually the initial response and may be an adaptive coping mechanism. Acknowledge that grief takes time, and give the client permission to grieve; accept crying. *The process of grieving is integral to adaptation to a disruption of health status. Denial is the initial phase of the grieving response and would be expected when a client is told of a significant change in health status (Norris & Spelic, 2002).*
- Encourage visitation and communication with family/close relatives of critically ill clients. **EBN:** *The presence of close relatives is of great importance for the ill person and must be facilitated by staff. Close relatives can help with the change brought about by critical illness (Engström & Söderberg, 2007).*
- Discuss the client's current goals. If appropriate, have the client list goals so that they can be referred to and steps can be taken to accomplish them. Support hope that the goals will be accomplished. **EBN:** *Clarification of the client/family goals and expectations will allow the nurse to clarify what is possible and to identify measures that can facilitate achievement of the goals (Northouse et al, 2002). "Hope theory" may facilitate recovery and clearer and more sustainable goals (Snyder et al, 2006).*
- Allow the client choices in daily care, particularly choices that result from the change in health status. **EBN:** *A client will demonstrate a more positive adaptation if the resources and interventions offered by the nurse are adapted to the client's perceived circumstances and needs (LeClere et al, 2002).*

• = Independent   ▲ = Collaborative   **EBN** = Evidence-Based Nursing   **EB** = Evidence-Based

- Provide assistance with activities as needed. **EBN:** *Clients' feelings of personal control increased when assistance was available to help them do things they could not do by themselves; they felt insecure and experienced emotional discomfort when assistance was lacking (Lauck, 2009).*
- Give the client positive feedback for accomplishments, no matter how small. Support the client and family and promote their strengths and coping skills. **EB:** *Support is necessary to help the client and family throughout the illness (Khalili, 2007).*
- Manipulate the environment to decrease stress; allow the client to display personal items that have meaning. **EBN:** *Appraisal uncertainty is a risk factor for a negative adaptation to health change (Dudley-Brown, 2002).*
- Maintain consistency and continuity in daily schedule. When possible, provide the same caregiver. **EBN:** *The predictability of interaction with the same nurses as a part of treatment facilitates trust, confidence, and positive adaptation (Richer & Ezer, 2002).*
- Promote use of positive spiritual influences. *Spirituality is an innate aspect of being human, and every client has the potential for spiritual growth through suffering from an illness (Tu, 2006).*
- ▲ Refer to community resources. Provide general and contact information for ease of use. **EB:** *Participating with a group of peers in a relevant activity appears to be an important factor in effectively changing behavior" (Boldy & Silfo, 2006).*

Pediatric

- Encourage visitation of children when family members are in intensive care. *Visitation of children should be supported to facilitate expression of feelings associated with major health changes in family members (Knutsson et al, 2008).*
- Involve significant others in planning and teaching. **EBN:** *Parents of critically ill children demonstrated fewer complications following their participation in a structured, hospital-based intervention (Melnyk et al, 2004).*
- Use visualization and distraction during chest physiotherapy for children with cystic fibrosis. *Although chest physiotherapy is central to the management of cystic fibrosis (CF), adherence among children is problematic. Visualization and distraction may improve compliance (Williams et al, 2007).*

Geriatric

- ▲ Assess for signs of depression resulting from illness-associated changes and make appropriate referrals. **EBN:** *Depression is a common consequence of aging. Assessments of the spouse's perception as well as of the client's factual situation may identify risk factors that are leading to a depressed state (Franzen-Dahlin, 2008).*
- Support activities that promote usefulness of older adults. **EB:** *Older adults with persistently low perceived usefulness or feelings of uselessness may be a vulnerable group with increased risk for poor health outcomes in later life (Gruenewald et al, 2009).*
- Monitor the client for agitation associated with health problems. Support family caring for elders with agitation. **EB:** *The findings in this study suggest that some symptoms, such as agitation/aggression and irritability/lability, may affect the caregivers significantly, although the symptoms' frequency and severity are low (Matsumoto et al, 2007).*

Multicultural

- Assess for the influence of cultural beliefs, norms, and values on the client's ability to modify health behavior. **EBN:** *What the client considers normal and abnormal health behavior may be based on cultural perceptions (Leininger & McFarland, 2002; Richardson, 2004; Van Bruggen, 2008).*
- Assess the role of fatalism on the client's ability to modify health behavior. **EB:** *Fatalistic perspectives, which involve the belief that you cannot control your own fate, may influence health behaviors in some African American, Asian, and Latino populations (Lerman et al, 2002; Powe & Finnie, 2003).*
- ▲ Assess for signs of depression and level of social support and make appropriate referrals. **EB:** *Increased depressed feelings and lower levels of available social support were reported by minorities in this study who had mild to moderate traumatic brain injury (Brown et al, 2004) and in other studies regardless of diagnoses (Plant & Sachs-Ericsson, 2004).*

• = Independent ▲ = Collaborative **EBN** = Evidence-Based Nursing **EB** = Evidence-Based

- Identify which family members the client can rely on for support. **EBN:** *A variety of different cultures rely on family members to cope with stress (White et al, 2002).*
- Encourage spirituality as a source of support for coping. **EBN:** *Many African Americans and Latinos identify spirituality, religiousness, prayer, and church-based approaches as coping resources (Samuel-Hodge et al, 2000; Giger et al, 2008).*
- Negotiate with the client regarding the aspects of health behavior that will need to be modified. **EBN:** *Give-and-take with the client will lead to culturally congruent care (Leininger & McFarland, 2002).*

 Home Care

- The above interventions may be adapted for home care use.
- Take the client's perspective into consideration, and use a holistic approach in assessing and responding to client planning for the future. **EBN:** *Clients with newly diagnosed diabetes do not want to become their illness (Johansson, Dahlberg, & Ekebergh, 2009).*
- Assist the client to adapt to their diagnosis and to live with the disease. **EBN:** *Despite being diagnosed with diabetes, clients still want to continue the same life and be the same persons as before—although they now carry a disease (Johansson, Dahlberg, & Ekebergh, 2009).*
- ▲ Refer the client to counselor or therapist for follow-up care. Initiate community referrals as needed (e.g., grief counseling, self-help groups). **EBN:** *Families need assistance and support in coping with health change and caregiving (Honea et al, 2008).*
- Refer to care plan for **Powerlessness.**

 Client/Family Teaching and Discharge Planning

- Assess family/caregivers for coping and teaching/learning styles. **EBN:** *The degree of optimism and pessimism influences the coping and health outcomes of caregivers of clients with Parkinson's disease (Lyons et al, 2004).*
- Foster communication between the client/family and medical staff. **EBN:** *Family members of individuals undergoing cardiopulmonary resuscitation expressed a need to be involved and present or informed at all times during the process (Wagner, 2004).* **EB:** *Psychotherapeutic interventions should not only address the clients' problems but also the support-givers' questions, needs, and psychosocial burdens (Frick et al, 2005).*
- Educate and prepare families regarding the appearance of the client and the environment before initial exposure. **EBN:** *Families indicated that knowing what to expect was helpful (Clukey, 2008).*
- Teach the client to maintain a positive outlook by listing current strengths. **EBN:** *Successful adaptation requires a coordination of efforts to fit the nursing interventions to the client's perception of the threat, personal values and beliefs, and recognition of personal strengths (Norris & Spelic, 2002).*
- Teach a client and his or her family relaxation techniques (controlled breathing, guided imagery) and help them practice. **EBN:** *Guided imagery with relaxation may be an easy-to-use self-management intervention to improve the quality of life of older adults with osteoarthritis (Baird & Sands, 2006).*
- Allow the client to proceed at own pace in learning; provide time for return demonstrations (e.g., self-injection of insulin). **EBN:** *Use clear and distinct language free of medical jargon and meaningless values (Wagner, 2004).*
- If long-term deficits are expected, inform the family as soon as possible. **EBN:** *An honest assessment shared by the nurse of a particular situation is important to the family's sense of what is expected of them in adapting to a health care change (Weiss & Chen, 2002).*
- Provide clients with information on how to access and evaluate available health information via the internet. *Client access to health information and personal health records is becoming increasingly important in today's health care society. MedlinePlus, NIH Senior Health, and ClinicalTrials.gov are designed to get medical information directly into the hands of clients (Koonce et al, 2007).*

ⓔvolve   See the EVOLVE website for Weblinks for client education resources.

• = Independent   ▲ = Collaborative   **EBN** = Evidence-Based Nursing   **EB** = Evidence-Based

REFERENCES

Baird CL, Sands LP: Effect of guided imagery with relaxation on health-related quality of life in older women with osteoarthritis, *Res Nurs Health* 29(5):442–451, 2006.

Boldy D, Silfo E: Chronic disease self-management by people from lower socio-economic backgrounds: action planning and impact, *J Integr Care* 4(4):19–25, 2006.

Brown SA, McCauley SR, Levin HS et al: Perception of health and quality of life in minorities after mild-to-moderate traumatic brain injury, *Appl Neuropsychol* 11(1):54–64, 2004.

Clukey L: Anticipatory mourning: processes of expected loss in palliative care, *Int J Palliat Nurs* 14(7):316, 318–25, 2008.

Dudley-Brown S: Prevention of psychological distress in persons with inflammatory bowel disease, *Issues Ment Health Nurs* 23:403, 2002.

Engström A, Söderberg S: Receiving power through confirmation: the meaning of close relatives for people who have been critically ill, *J Adv Nurs* 59(6):569–576, 2007.

Franzen-Dahlin A: Predictors of life situation among significant others of depressed or aphasic stroke patients, *J Clin Nurs* 17(12):1574–1580, 2008.

Frick E, Rieg-Appleson C, Tyroller M et al: Social support, affectivity, and the quality of life of patients and their support-givers prior to stem cell transplantation, *J Psychosoc Oncol* 23(4):15–34, 2005.

Giger J, Appel S, Davidhizar R et al: Church and spirituality in the lives of the African American community, *J Transcult Nurs* 19(4):375–383, 2008.

Gruenewald TL, Karlamangla AS, Greendale GA et al: Increased mortality risk in older adults with persistently low or declining feelings of usefulness to others, *J Aging Health* 21(2):398–425, 2009.

Honea NJ, Brintnall R, Given B et al: Putting evidence into practice: nursing assessment and interventions to reduce family caregiver strain and burden, *Clin J Oncol Nurs* 12(3):507–516, 2008.

Jasmine TJX: The use of effective therapeutic communication skills in nursing practice, *Singapore Nurs J* 36(1):35–38, 40, 2009.

Johansson A, Dahlberg K, Ekebergh M: A lifeworld phenomenological study of the experience of falling ill with diabetes, *Int J Nurs Stud* 46(2):197–203, 2009.

Kiefer RA: An integrative review of the concept of well-being, *Holist Nurs Pract* 22(5):244–252, 2008.

Khalili Y: Ongoing transitions: the impact of a malignant brain tumour on patient and family, *Axone* 28(3):5–13, 2007.

Knutsson S, Samuelsson IP, Hellström A et al: Children's experiences of visiting a seriously ill/injured relative on an adult intensive care unit, *J Adv Nurs* 61(2):154–162, 2008.

Koonce T, Giuse D, Beauregard J et al: Toward a more informed patient: bridging health care information through an interactive communication portal, *J Med Libr Assoc* 95(1):77, 2007.

Lauck S: Patients felt greater personal control and emotional comfort in hospital when they felt secure, informed, and valued, *Evid Based Nurs* 12(1):29, 2009.

LeClere CM, Wells DL, Craig D et al: Falling short of the mark, *Clin Nurs Res* 11(3):242–263, 2002.

Leininger MM, McFarland MR: *Transcultural nursing: concepts, theories, research and practices,* ed 3, New York, 2002, McGraw-Hill.

Lerman C, Croyle, R. Tercyak, K et al: Genetic testing: psychological aspects and implications, *J Consult Clin Psychol* 70(3):784–797, 2002.

Lyons KS, Stewart BJ, Archbold PG et al: Pessimism and optimism as early warning signs for compromised health for caregivers of patients with Parkinson's disease, *Nurs Res* 53(6):354–362, 2004.

Matsumoto N, Ikeda M, Fukuhara R et al: Caregiver burden associated with behavioral and psychological symptoms of dementia in elderly people in the local community, *Dement Geriatr Cogn Disord,* 23(4): e219–224, 2007.

Melnyk BM, Alpert-Gillis L, Feinstein NF et al: Creating opportunities for parent empowerment: program effects on the mental health/coping outcomes of critically ill young children and their mothers, *Pediatrics* 113(6):e597–607, 2004.

Norris J, Spelic SS: Supporting adaption to body image disruption, *Rehabil Nurs* 27(1):8–12, 2002.

Northouse L, Walker J, Schafenacker A et al: A family-based program of care for women with recurrent breast cancer and their family members, *Oncol Nurs Forum* 29(10):1411–1419,

Plant E, Sachs-Ericsson N: Racial and ethnic differences in depression: the roles of social support and meeting basic needs, *Consult Clin Psychol* 72(1):41–52, 2004.

Powe BD, Finnie R: Cancer fatalism: the state of the science, *Cancer Nurs* 26(6):454–465, 2003.

Richardson P: How cultural ideas help shape the conceptualization of mental illness and mental health, *Occup Ther* 9(1):5–8, 2004.

Richer MC, Ezer H: Living in it, living with it, and moving on: dimensions of meaning during chemotherapy, *Oncol Nurs Forum* 29(1):113–119, 2002.

Samuel-Hodge CD, Headen SW, Skelly AH et al: Influences on day-to-day self-management of type 2 diabetes among African-American women: spirituality, the multi-caregiver role, and other social context factors, *Diabetes Care* 23(7):928–933, 2000.

Snyder CR, Lehman KA, Kluck B et al: Hope for rehabilitation and vice versa, *Rehab Psychol* 51(2):89–112, 2006.

Tu M: Illness: an opportunity for spiritual growth, *J Altern Complement Med* 12(10):1029–1033, 2006.

Van Bruggen H: Mental health as social construct. In Creek J, Lougher L: *Occupational health and mental health,* ed 4, London, 2008, Churchill Livingstone.

Wagner JM: Lived experience of critically ill patients' family members during cardiopulmonary resuscitation, *Am J Crit Care* 13(5):416–420, 2004.

Weiss SJ, Chen JL: Factors influencing maternal mental health and family functioning during the low birthweight infant's first year of life, *J Pediatr Nurs* 17(2):114–125, 2002.

White N, Bichter J, Koeckeritz J et al: A cross-cultural comparison of family resiliency in hemodialysis patients, *J Transcult Nurs* 13(3):218–227, 2002.

Williams B, Mukhopadhyay S, Dowell J et al: Problems and solutions: accounts by parents and children of adhering to chest physiotherapy for cystic fibrosis, *Disabil Rehabil* 29(14):1097–1105, 2007.

Risk for Bleeding   *Sheri Holmes, RNC, MSN, CNS-C*   ⊝volve

NANDA-I

Definition

At risk for a decrease in blood volume that may compromise health

• = Independent   ▲ = Collaborative   **EBN** = Evidence-Based Nursing   **EB** = Evidence-Based

Risk Factors

Aneurysm; circumcision; deficient knowledge; disseminated intravascular coagulopathy; history of falls; gastrointestinal disorders (e.g., gastric ulcer disease, polyps, varices); impaired liver function (e.g., cirrhosis, hepatitis); inherent coagulopathies (e.g., thrombocytopenia); postpartum complications (e.g., uterine atony, retained placenta); pregnancy-related complications (e.g., placenta previa, molar pregnancy, abruption placenta); trauma, treatment-related side effects (e.g., surgery, medications, administration of platelet-deficient blood products, chemotherapy)

NOC   (Nursing Outcomes Classification)

Suggested NOC Outcomes

Blood Loss Severity; Blood Coagulation; Circulation Status; Knowledge: Cancer Management; Fetal Status: Antepartum, Intrapartum; Maternal Status: Antepartum, Intrapartum, Postpartum; Post-Procedure Recovery; Physical Injury Severity; Tissue Perfusion: Cellular; Vital Signs

Example NOC Outcomes with Indicators

Blood Loss Severity as evidenced by visible blood loss/Hematuria/Postsurgical bleeding/Decreased systolic blood pressure/Decreased diastolic blood pressure/Anxiety/Increased apical heart rate (Rate each indicator of **Blood Loss Severity**: 1 = severe, 2 = substantial, 3 = moderate, 4 = mild, 5 = none [see Section 1].)
Maternal Status: Postpartum as evidenced by the following indicators: Blood pressure/Apical heart rate/Uterine fundal height/Lochia amount/Lochia color/Hemoglobin (Rate each indicator of **Maternal Status: Postpartum**: 1 = severe deviation from normal range, 2 = substantial deviation from normal range, 3 = moderate deviation from normal range, 4 = mild deviation from normal range, 5 = no deviation from normal range [see Section 1].)

Client Outcomes

Client Will (Specify Time Frame):

- Maintain stable vital signs with minimal blood loss
- Explain actions can take if bleeding occurs

NIC   (Nursing Interventions Classification)

Suggested NIC Interventions

Bleeding Precautions: Post-Anesthesia Care, Bleeding Reduction: Postpartum Uterus, Bleeding Reduction: Antepartum Uterus, Hemorrhage Control, Hypovolemia Management

Example NIC Activities—Post-Anesthesia Care

Monitor oxygenation; Monitor vital signs; Monitor surgical site

Example NIC Activities—Bleeding Reduction: Postpartum Uterus

Review obstetrical history for risk factors for postpartum hemorrhage; Increase fundal massage; Evaluate for bladder distention

Nursing Interventions and *Rationales*

- Review client history for increased bleeding risk. **EB:** *Anticipate an increased risk for bleeding if client has a personal or family history of bleeding, posttrauma or postoperative bleeding, or personally used antithrombolytics in the past 5 days. Routine INR/PT preoperatively is not recommended. Clients with von Willebrand's disease (1% to 2% of population), will need a short-term or long-term course of VWD/FVIII prior to undergoing a surgical procedure to decrease the risk of bleeding. Clients with or without a history of gastrointestinal bleeding may be at increased risk for bleeding if they take selective serotonin reuptake inhibitors (SSRIs) such as fluoxetine, paroxetine, and sertraline (Mansour et al, 2006; Chee, Crawford & Watson, 2008; Franchini, 2008; Barbui et al, 2009; Korte et al, 2009).*
- Monitor signs of bleeding in the urine, stool, sputum, vomitus. Watch for nosebleeds, any petechiae, purpura, or abnormal bruising. *Disseminated intravascular coagulation (DIC) is a critical disease state that requires prompt action to avert death. It often results from a systemic infection. Spe-*

• = Independent   ▲ = Collaborative   **EBN** = Evidence-Based Nursing   **EB** = Evidence-Based

cific signs include petechiae, cyanosis of fingers and nose, and oozing of blood from three unrelated sites. The underlying cause must be treated quickly, along with maintaining homeostasis (Armola, 2007).

▲ Monitor laboratory tests that evaluate bleeding, including hemoglobin, hematocrit, INR, protime (also known as prothrombin time). **EB:** *Hemoglobin and hematocrit levels are late determinants of bleeding or hemorrhage, however they provide more objective than visual assessment of blood loss. International normalized ratio (INR) and prothrombin time measure the effects of medication on the coagulation cascade and should be drawn at least 16 hours after the dose is administered (ICSI, 2007).*

● Implement safety precautions, such as a falls prevention protocol for a client who has identified falls risk (i.e., history of falls). **EBN:** *On admission and as indicated, nurses should assess for falls risk factors that could increase the incidence of bleeding (Balas, Casey, & Happ, 2008).*

● Check vital signs at frequent intervals. *Watch for changes associated with bleeding including increased heart rate, respiratory rate, and eventually decreased blood pressure. Take orthostatic blood pressure readings lying, sitting, and standing, watching for characteristic pattern of hypotension associated with fluid loss (Lahrmann et al, 2006).*

● Watch for tachycardia and recognize that it may indicate hypovolemia. *Tachycardia in the Post-Anesthesia Care Unit (PACU) may indicate dehydration, hypovolemia, anxiety, or inadequate pain management. Even though hemorrhage is not a common problem in PACU, the presence of occult bleeding should always be considered (Noble, 2008).*

● Monitor medications for effects on increasing bleeding including aspirin, NSAIDs, and SSRIs. **EB:** *These medications have an antiplatelet effect that can increase the risk of bleeding, particularly in a client who is at risk due to illness or medications (Berger et al, 2006; ICSI, 2007; Schalekamp, Klungel, & Souverein, 2008).*

● **Safety Guidelines for Anticoagulant Administration**. Follow the approved protocol for anticoagulant administration including the time of administration; use of prepackaged medications and prefilled, or premixed parenteral therapy as ordered; laboratory tests to check before administration; and symptoms to notice before administering. *Anticoagulation therapy is complex and too frequently leads to adverse dry events (Joint Commission, 2009). Defined protocols can decrease errors in administration.*

▲ Before administering warfarin, check the INR. Hold the medication and notify the physician if the INR is outside of the recommended paremeters. **EB:** *The target INR for warfarin should be between 2.0 and 3.0 for nonvalvular atrial fibrillation; between 2.5 and 3.5 for valvular atrial fibrillation. The risk for bleeding increases substantially when the INR is greater than 4.0, and risk for thromboembolism increases when the INR is below 1.7. Even in the therapeutic ranges, clients have a 2% to 4% risk for bleeding that requires transfusion. A 15% adjustment in the dosage usually changes the level by 1.0 INR (ICSI, 2007).*

● Use a programmable infusion pump only for administration of an intravenous continuous heparin infusion (Joint Commission, 2009).

▲ Notify the dietary department when the client is receiving warfarin. *This is to ensure consistency in the amount of vitamin K in the diet (Joint Commission, 2009).*

▲ Give vitamin K orally or intravenously if needed as ordered. **EB:** *When the client's INR is greater than 5.0, it is recommended to give vitamin K, rather than just holding the warfarin. Avoid giving IM or SubQ to decrease chance of irregular absorption that can lead to warfarin resistance (DeZee et al, 2006; ICSI, 2007).*

 Client/Family Teaching and Discharge Planning

▲ **Safety Standards**. Educate clients and families about the anticoagulant medications including when to take, how often to have lab tests, and precautions that should be followed. Give the client both verbal and written instructions (Joint Commission, 2009).

▲ Educate clients about when and how they can restart their anticoagulants following surgery. **EB:** *Clients with a moderate to high risk of thromboembolism are treated to prevent thromboembolism, rather than prevent bleeding. Clients with a low risk of thromboembolism are treated to prevent bleeding rather than to prevent thromboembolism. Generally warfarin is resumed 12 to 24 hours after surgery at the previous dose. Therapeutic levels should be achieved in 6 to 12 days, with older (>70) or obese clients taking a little longer (ICSI, 2007; Douketis et al, 2008).*

● = Independent ▲ = Collaborative **EBN** = Evidence-Based Nursing **EB** = Evidence-Based

- Provide clients with education, both oral and written, that meets the standards of client education health literacy. **EB:** *Clients with low health literacy skills need to be empowered through "teach back" and "show back" techniques to assure their self-care safety (Joint Commission, 2007; Wilson, 2009; Hughes & Messerly, 2009).*
- Advise client to adopt safety practices about self-care activities. **EB:** *Shave with an electric razor. Brush teeth with a soft toothbrush. Wipe with wet wipes after stooling. Carry bandages with you at all times. Avoid sports and activities that could increase your risk for falling. Wear a medical alert bracelet or necklace (AHRQ, 2008).*
- ▲ Teach client who is taking an antithrombolytic medication to monitor the intake of foods, herbs, and dietary supplements. **EB:** *Foods high in vitamin K (e.g., spinach, broccoli, cauliflower, cabbage) can decrease the effect of the medication. Consistent intake of these foods, rather than avoidance is preferred. Increased activity will decrease the effect of warfarin. Illness, including fever, diarrhea, poor nutrition, large amounts of alcohol, and herbal supplements, such as gingko, garlic, ginseng, and omega-3 fatty acids, will increase the effect of warfarin (AHRQ, 2008).*

Postpartum Risk for Bleeding

- ▲ Based on prenatal and past medical history, determine need for IV fluids, sites, blood products, additional uterotonics prior to delivery. *Uterine atony due to prolonged labor, multiparty, general anesthesia, tocolytics, multiple gestation, abnormal placental implantation, and uterine fibroids increase the risk of bleeding during the postpartum period. Coagulopathies such as thrombocytopenia, von Willebrand's disease, need to be identified prior to delivery whenever possible. Portal hypertension resulting in esophageal varices is a rare but dangerous risk (Hoffman, 2009; Rosenfeld, Hochner-Celnikier & Ackerman, 2009).*
- Assess fundal height and lochia amount every 15 minutes for the first hour after delivery, every 30 minutes in the second hour and every 4 hours after that as needed. Support the uterus at the symphysis pubis and massage the fundus of the uterus until it is firm. Vigorous massage and downward pressure should be avoided (Chichester, 2008).
- Frequently assess for clinical signs and symptoms of blood loss, such as dizziness, fatigue, tachycardia, and hypotension. *Blood loss is frequently underestimated (500 mL for vaginal and 1000 mL for cesarean deliveries). Postpartum hemorrhage (PPH) complicates up to 5% of live births in the United States. Early PPH occurs in the first 24 hours. Late PPH occurs 24 hours to 6 weeks postpartum and complicates 1% to 2% of all live births in the United States (Hoffman, 2009).*
- ▲ Establish an emergency response process for PPH. **EBN:** *Based on outcomes from a multi-hospital study, postpartum hemorrhage occurred more frequently on the weekend than during the weekdays (Bendavid et al, 2007).*
- ▲ Administer uterotonic agent (e.g., oxytocin) at the birth of the anterior shoulder as ordered. **EB and EBN:** *Active management of the third stage of labor (early cord clamping, uterotonic agent with birth of shoulder, and controlled traction of the umbilical cord) significantly decreases the risk of postpartum hemorrhage (McDonald, 2007).*
- Educate women about the increased risk of having abnormal placental implantation with cesarean delivery and the increased risk of antepartum or postpartum bleeding. **EB:** *The placenta tends to implant over a previous uterine scar (Chichester, 2008).*

℮volve   See the EVOLVE website for Weblinks for client education resources.

REFERENCES

Agency for Healthcare Research and Quality (AHRQ): *Your guide to coumadin/warfarin therapy*: www.ahrq.gov/consumer/coumadin.htm. Accessed April 14, 2009.

Armola RR: Monitor patients for disseminated intravascular coagulation, *Nurs Crit Care* 2(5)9–15, 2007.

Balas MC, Casey CM, Happ MB: Comprehensive assessment and management of the critically ill. In Capezuti E, Zwicker D, Mezey M et al, editors: *Evidence-based geriatric nursing protocols for best practice*, ed 3, New York, 2008, Springer.

Barbui C, Andretta M, De Vitis G et al: Antidepressant drug prescription and risk of abnormal bleeding: a case-control study, *J Clin Psychopharmacol* 29(1):33–38, 2009.

Bendavid E, Kaganova Y, Needleman J et al: Complication rates on weekends and weekdays in U.S. hospitals, *Am J Med* 120(5):422–428, 2007.

Berger JS, Roncaglioni MC, Avanzini F et al: Aspirin for the primary prevention of cardiovascular events in women and men: a sex-specific meta-analysis of randomized controlled trials, *JAMA* 295(3):306–313, 2006.

Chee YL, Crawford JC, Watson HG: Guidelines on the assessment of bleeding risk prior to surgery or invasive procedures, *Br J Haematol* 140:496–504, 2008.

Chichester M: Cesarean delivery is rising: implications for care for the perianesthesia nurse, *J Perianesth Nurs* 23(5):321–334, 2008.

DeZee KJ, Shimeall WT, Douglas KM et al: Treatment of excessive anticoagulation with phytonadione (vitamin K): a meta-analysis, *Arch Intern Med* 166(4):391–397, 2006.

Douketis JD, Berger PB, Dunn AS et al: The perioperative management of antithrombotic therapy: American College of Chest Physicians Evidence-Based Clinical Practice Guidelines (8th Edition), *Chest* 133(6 Suppl):299S-339S, 2008.

Franchini M: Surgical prophylaxis in von Willebrand's disease: a difficult balance to manage, *Blood Transfus* 6(s2):s33–s38, 2008.

Hoffman C: Postpartum hemorrhage, *Postgrad Obstet Gynecol* 29(2):1–6, 2009.

Hughes S, Messerly S: Patient education: a critical component in caring for patients on warfarin, *J Cardiovasc Nurs* 24(2):171–173, 2009.

Institute for Clinical Systems Improvement (ICSI): *Antithrombotic therapy supplement,* Bloomington, Minn, 2007, Author, p. 64.

Joint Commission: *What did the doctor say? Improving health literacy to protect patient safety,* Oakbrook Terrace, IL, 2007, Author.

Joint Commission: *Accreditation Program: Critical Access Hospital National Patient Safety Goals. The Joint Commission on Accreditation of Health Care Organizations:* www.jointcommission.org/PatientSafety/NationalPatientSafetyGoals/09_cah_npsgs.htm. Accessed August 9, 2009.

Korte WC, Szadkowski C, Gahler A et al: Factor XIII substitution in surgical cancer patients at high risk for intraoperative bleeding, *Anesthesiol* 110(2)239–245, 2009.

Lahrmann H, Cortelli P, Hilz M et al: EFNS guidelines on the diagnosis and management of orthostatic hypotension, *Eur J Neurol* 13(9)930–936, 2006.

Mansour A, Pearce M, Johnson B et al: Which patients taking SSRIs are at greatest risk for bleeding? *J Fam Pract* 55(3):206–208, 2006.

McDonald S: Management of the third stage of labor, *J Midwifery Womens Health* 52(3):254–261, 2007.

Noble KA: The obesity epidemic: the impact of obesity on the perianesthesia patient, *J Perianesth Nurs* 23(6):418–425, 2008.

Rosenfeld H, Hochner-Celnikier D, Ackerman Z: Massive bleeding from ectopic varices in the postpartum period: rare but serious complication in women with portal hypertension, *Eur J Gastroenterol Hepatol* 21(9):1086–1091, 2009.

Schalekamp T, Klungel JH, Souverein PC: Increased bleeding risk with concurrent use of selective serotonin reuptake inhibitors and coumarins, *Arch Intern Med* 168(2):180–185, 2008.

Wilson M: Readability and patient education materials used for low-income populations, *Clin Nurse Spec* 23(1):33–40, 2009.

Disturbed Body image   *Gail B. Ladwig, MSN, RN, CHTP*   ⊝volve

NANDA-I

Definition

Confusion in mental picture of one's physical self

Defining Characteristics

Behaviors of acknowledgment of one's body; behaviors of avoidance on one's body; behaviors of monitoring one's body; nonverbal response to actual change in body (e.g., appearance, structure, function); nonverbal response to perceived change in body (e.g., appearance, structure, function); verbalization of feelings that reflect an altered view of one's body (e.g., appearance, structure, function); verbalization of perceptions that reflect an altered view of one's body appearance

Objective

Actual change in function; actual change in structure; behaviors of acknowledging one's body; behaviors of monitoring one's body; change in ability to estimate spatial relationship of body to environment; change in social involvement; extension of body boundary to incorporate environmental objects; intentional hiding of body part; intentional overexposure of body part; missing body part; not looking at body part; not touching body part; trauma to nonfunctioning part; unintentional hiding of body part; unintentional overexposing of body part

Subjective

Depersonalization of loss by impersonal pronouns; depersonalization of part by impersonal pronouns; emphasis on remaining strengths; fear of reaction by others; fear of rejection by others; focus on past appearance; focus on past function; focus on past strength; heightened achievement; negative feelings about body (e.g., feeling of helplessness, hopelessness, powerlessness); personalization of loss by name; personalization of part by name; preoccupation with change; preoccupation with loss; refusal to verify actual change; verbalization of change in lifestyle

Related Factors (r/t)

Biophysical; cognitive; cultural; developmental changes; illness; illness treatment; injury; perceptual; psychosocial; spiritual; surgery; trauma

• = Independent   ▲ = Collaborative   **EBN** = Evidence-Based Nursing   **EB** = Evidence-Based

(Nursing Outcomes Classification)

Suggested NOC Outcomes

Body Image, Self-Esteem, Acceptance health status: coping; Identity

Example NOC Outcome with Indicators
Body Image as evidenced by the following indicators: Congruence between body reality, body ideal, and body presentation/Satisfaction with body appearance/Adjustment to changes in physical appearance (Rate the outcome and indicators of **Body Image:** 1 = never positive, 2 = rarely positive, 3 = sometimes positive, 4 = often positive, 5 = consistently positive [see Section I].)

Client Outcomes

Client Will (Specify Time Frame):

- Demonstrate adaptation to changes in physical appearance or body function as evidenced by adjustment to lifestyle change
- Identify and change irrational beliefs and expectations regarding body size or function
- Verbalize congruence between body reality and body perception
- Describe, touch, or observe affected body part
- Demonstrate social involvement rather than avoidance and utilize adaptive coping and/or social skills
- Utilize cognitive strategies or other coping skills to improve perception of body image and enhance functioning
- Utilize strategies to enhance appearance (e.g., wig, clothing)

  (Nursing Interventions Classification)

Suggested NIC Intervention

Body Image Enhancement

Example NIC Activities—Body Image Enhancement
Determine patient's body image expectations based on developmental stage; Assist patient to identify actions that will enhance appearance

Nursing Interventions and *Rationales*

- Incorporate psychosocial questions related to body image as part of nursing assessment to identify clients at risk for body image disturbance (e.g., body builders; cancer survivors; clients with eating disorders, burns, skin disorders, polycystic ovary disease; or those with stomas/ostomies/colostomies or other disfiguring conditions). **EB:** *Assessment of psychosocial issues can help to identify clients at risk for body image concerns as a result of a disfiguring condition (Rumsey et al, 2004; Borwell, 2009).*
- If client is at risk for body image disturbance, consider using a tool such as the Body Image Quality of Life Inventory (BIQLI), or Body Areas Satisfaction Scale (Bass) which quantify both the positive and negative effects of body image on one's psychosocial quality of life. **EB:** *A favorable body image quality of life was related to higher self-esteem, optimism, and social support in both sexes and less eating disturbance among women (Cash, Jakatdar, & Williams, 2003).* **EBN:** *Using a body image scale can help nurses to identify possible body image disturbances and to plan individual nursing interventions (Giovannelli et al, 2008).*
- ▲ Assess for body dysmorphic disorder (BDD) and refer to psychiatry or other appropriate provider. **EB:** *Body dysmorphic disorder (BDD) is a prevalent and disabling preoccupation with a slight or imagined defect in appearance. Results from the small number of available randomized controlled trials (RCTs) suggest that SRIs serotonin reuptake inhibitors and CBT (cognitive behavioral therapy) may be useful in treating clients with BDD (Ipser, Sander, & Stein, 2009).*
- ▲ Assess for the possibility of muscle dysmorphia (pathological preoccupation with muscularity and leanness; occurs more often in males than in females) and make appropriate referrals. **EB:** *This*

● = Independent   ▲ = Collaborative   **EBN** = Evidence-Based Nursing   **EB** = Evidence-Based

condition is often seen among body builders or those in sports that emphasize size and bulk (e.g., wrestling) and will likely continue to increase with the societal focus on body image. Fluoxetine alone or in combination with CBT may be an effective treatment (Leone, Sedory, & Gray, 2005).

• Assess client and family response to surgery that results in a change in body and offer support. **EBN:** *A qualitative study by Notter and Burnard (2006) revealed that although many clients and family members received education before surgery, most felt the reality of it differed significantly from their expectations.*

• If nursing assessment reveals body image concerns related to a disfiguring condition, assist client in voicing his/her concerns and if appropriate, coaching the client in how to respond to questions from others in social situations. If within the nurse's level of expertise, may assist client in graded practice in social situations (e.g., going to hairdresser, swimming pool). **EB:** *Many clients with disfiguring conditions are concerned about and may avoid exposing the disfigurement to others' gaze and displays of ignorance and negative comments by others (Rumsey et al, 2004).*

▲ Refer clients with body image disturbance for CBT and/or social skills training if indicated. **EB:** *CBT and social skills training help clients learn new mental scripts for interacting with others, challenge negative thoughts and replacing these with new thoughts, and applying new behaviors and thoughts in social situations (Jarry & Ip, 2005).*

• Acknowledge denial, anger, or depression as normal feelings when adjusting to changes in body and lifestyle. However, allow client to share emotions when they are ready, rather than rushing them. **EB:** *The influence of emotion-focused coping (venting emotions and mental disengagement) on distress following disfiguring injury was associated with less body image disturbance (Fauerbach et al, 2002).*

• Encourage the client to discuss interpersonal and social conflicts that may arise. **EB:** *Changes in physical appearance and function associated with disease processes (and sometimes treatment) need to be integrated into the interaction that occurs between clients and lay caregivers (Price, 2000).*

• Explore opportunities to assist the client to develop a realistic perception of his or her body image. **EB:** *Actual body size may not be consistent with the client's perceived body size. Inaccurate perception by the client can be unhealthy (Townsend, 2003).*

• Help client describe ideal self, identify self-criticisms, and suggestions to support acceptance of self. **EBN:** *Head and neck tumor clients after tumor excision and micro-reconstructive surgery reported that they were least satisfied with their face, and 35.8% changed job because of their appearance. Job rehabilitation and body image should be incorporated into the daily care of head and neck cancer clients. For example, participants could learn how to use cosmetic strategies to improve their facial appearance during otopalatodigital (OPD) syndrome follow-up. Thus, the negative impact might be reduced (Liu, 2008).*

• Encourage clients to verbalize treatment preferences and play a role in treatment decisions. **EB:** *Women who received the treatment they preferred for stage 1 or 2 breast cancer had better body image (and mental health) than women who did not. Good communication between physicians and women improved outcomes (Figueiredo et al, 2004).*

• Encourage the clients to write a narrative description of their changes. *Expressive writing has therapeutic benefits with feelings of greater psychological well-being and fewer posttraumatic intrusion and avoidance symptoms (Atkinson et al, 2009).*

• Take cues from clients regarding readiness to look at wound (may ask if client has seen wound yet) and utilize clients' questions or comments as way to teach about wound care and healing. **EB:** *Clients with disfiguring conditions, in this case burns, respond in a variety of ways, and the severity of the disfigurement does not always predict impact on body image. Tailoring interventions to individual clients and reading their nonverbal cues likely contributes to clients' ability to heal emotionally from impact of wound on body image (Birdsall & Weinberg, 2001).*

• Encourage the client to purchase clothes that are attractive and that deemphasize their disability. **EB:** *Individuals with osteoporosis are not usually disabled but may perceive themselves as unattractive and experience social isolation as a result of ill-fitting clothes that accentuate the physical changes (Sedlak & Doheny, 2000).*

• Encourage client to participate in regular aerobic exercise when feasible. **EB:** *A systematic review of exercise during and after cancer treatment found that exercise may be an effective intervention to improve body image but depends on many factors (e.g., stage of treatment, client lifestyle) (Knols, Aaronson, & Uebelhart, 2005).* **EB:** *A meta-analysis examined research regarding the impact of exercise on*

• = Independent   ▲ = Collaborative   **EBN** = Evidence-Based Nursing   **EB** = Evidence-Based

body image and concluded that exercise was associated with improved body image (Hausenblas & Fallon, 2006).

▲ Provide client with a list of appropriate community resources (e.g., Reach to Recovery, Ostomy Association). **EB:** *Motivation, sharing of experiences, camaraderie with and support from peers, and knowledge of not being alone have been identified as advantages of group learning (Payne, 1993).*

Geriatric

- Focus on remaining abilities. Have client make a list of strengths. **EB:** *Results from unstructured interviews with women aged 61 to 92 years regarding their perceptions and feelings about their aging bodies suggest that women exhibit the internalization of ageist beauty norms, even as they assert that health is more important to them than physical attractiveness and comment on the "naturalness" of the aging process (Hurd, 2000).*
- Encourage regular exercise for the elderly. **EB:** *Researchers in this study conclude that regular exercise had positive effects on the self-esteem and body image of elderly women (Anonymous, 2001).*

Multicultural

- Assess for the influence of cultural beliefs, norms, and values on the client's body image. **EBN:** *The client's body image may be based on cultural perceptions, as well as influences from the larger social context. Use of pan-ethnic status such as Asian or Hispanic may obscure important ethnic group differences (Yates, Edman, & Aruguete, 2004).* **EBN:** *Body image is affected by relationships between tactile space and visual space, special behavior, and proximity to others (Giger & Davidhizar, 2008). Each client should be assessed for body image based on the phenomenon of communication, time, space, social organization, environmental control, and biological variations (Giger & Davidhizar, 2008). With body and increased BMI, there is a direct correlation among race, socioeconomic status, community socioeconomic disadvantaged status, and individual health behaviors; each of these factors are known to be independent predictors of body image and increased BMI in ethnically/racially diverse populations (Robert & Reither, 2004).*
- Assess for the presence of conflicting cultural demands. **EBN:** *Poor peer socialization and family rigidity were found to be related to the preoccupation with body size and slimness in a young female Mexican American population (Kuba & Harris, 2001).*
- Assess for the presence of depressive symptoms. **EBN:** *Body image attitudes were significantly related to depressive symptoms in a study of diverse postpartum women (Walker et al, 2002).*
- Acknowledge that body image disturbances can affect all individuals regardless of culture, race, or ethnicity. **EBN:** *Body image disturbances are pervasive across Western cultures and appear to increase in other cultures with acculturation to Western ideals (Hebl, King, & Lin, 2004).* **EB:** *Non-Caucasian girls were found to report higher internalization of the thin ideal than their Caucasian peers (Hermes & Keele, 2003).*

Home Care

- The above interventions may be adapted for home care use.
- Assess client's level of social support as it is one of the determinants of client's recovery and emotional health. **EBN:** *Females who perceived they have good social support were found to adapt better to changes in body image after stoma surgery (Brown & Randle, 2005).*
- Assess family/caregiver level of acceptance of client's body changes. **EB:** *Family members' expressions and reactions were found to impact women's coping, and negative reactions in particular increased the women's level of anxiety. Negative feedback from family/caregiver can influence client's reactions and ability to adjust to body changes negatively (Brown & Randle, 2005).*
- Recognize that older women may continue their younger preoccupation with weight and recurrent dieting, despite being at normal weight. Assess source of low weight or weight loss with this in mind. **EB:** *Reports suggest that elderly women continue to be preoccupied with being thin. Increased awareness of eating habits and weight preoccupation in elderly women has been recommended (Fallaz et al, 1999).*
- Encourage client to discuss concerns related to sexuality and provide support or information as indicated. Many conditions that affect body image also affect sexuality. **EB:** *Brown & Randle (2005)*

• = Independent   ▲ = Collaborative   **EBN** = Evidence-Based Nursing   **EB** = Evidence-Based

found that clients (particularly females) with stomas often believe they are less sexually attractive after surgery, though their sexual partner may not share that view. However, clients who underwent urostomy surgery often experienced a decrease in sexual functioning.

- Teach all aspects of care. Involve client and caregivers in self-care as soon as possible. Do this in stages if client still has difficulty looking at or touching changed body part. **EB:** *Prostate cancer clients need interventions that assist them to manage the effects of their disease. Programs need to include spouses because they also are negatively affected by the disease and can influence client outcomes (Kershaw et al, 2008).*

▲ Refer for prosthetic device if appropriate. **EB:** *Swanson, Stube, and Edman (2005) found that use of the C-Leg for lower-limb amputees improved body image due to feeling more secure in public (stability of device) and ability to walk with a more natural gait.*

Client/Family Teaching and Discharge Planning

- Teach appropriate care of surgical site (e.g., mastectomy site, amputation site, ostomy site, etc.). **EBN:** *Integration of a cosmetic program into the routine nursing care for oral cancer clients is highly recommended. This study confirmed that cosmetic rehabilitation had positive effects on the body image of oral cancer clients (Huang & Liu, 2008).*

- Inform client of available community support groups; such as Internet discussion boards. **EB:** *Many people living with long-term conditions would like to be in contact with their peers, and Internet discussion boards represent a cost-effective and interactive way of achieving this (Armstrong & Powell, 2009).*

- Encourage significant others to offer support. **EB:** *Clients in this study with heart failure managed depressive symptoms that affect health-related quality of life by engaging in activities such as exercise and reading, and by using positive thinking, spirituality, and social support. Helping clients find enhanced social support is important (Dekker et al, 2009).*

▲ Refer clients who are having difficulty with personal acceptance, personal and social body image disruption, sexual concerns, reduced self-care skills, and the management of surgical complications to an interdisciplinary team or specialist (e.g., ostomy nurse) if available. **EBN:** *There is sufficient research-based evidence to conclude that intestinal ostomy surgery exerts a clinically relevant impact on health-related quality of life (HRQOL), and that nursing interventions can ameliorate this effect (Pittman, Kozell & Gray, 2009).* **EB:** *Clients who had a stoma had problems with body image (Ross et al, 2006).*

 See the EVOLVE website for Weblinks for client education resources.

REFERENCES

Anonymous: Active seniors less susceptible to depression, *J Phys Educ Recreat Dance* 72(1):9–11, 2001.

Armstrong N, Powell J: Patient perspectives on health advice posted on internet discussion boards: a qualitative study, *Health Expect* 12(3):313–20, 2009.

Atkinson R, Hare T, Merriman M et al: Therapeutic benefits of expressive writing in an electronic format, *Nurs Adm Q* 33(3):212–215, 2009.

Birdsall C, Weinberg K: Adult clients looking at their burn injuries for the first time, *J Burn Care Rehabal* 22(5):360–364, 2001.

Borwell B: Rehabilitation and stoma care: addressing the psychological needs, *Br J Nurs* 18(4):S20–2–S24–5, 2009.

Brown H, Randle J: Living with a stoma: a review of the literature, *J Clin Nurs* 14(1):74–81, 2005.

Cash TF, Jakatdar TA, Williams EF: The body image quality of life inventory: further validation with college men and women, *Body Image* 11(4):279–287, 2003.

Dekker RL, Peden AR, Lennie TA et al: Living with depressive symptoms: patients with heart failure, *Am J Crit Care* 18(4):310–318, 2009.

Fallaz AF, Bernstein M, Van Nes MC et al: Weight loss preoccupation in aging women: a review, *J Nutr Health Aging* 3:177–181, 1999.

Fauerbach JA, Heinberg LJ, Lawrence JW et al: Coping with body image changes following a disfiguring burn injury, *Health Psychol* 21(2):115–121, 2002.

Figueiredo MI, Cullen J, Yi-Ting H et al: Breast cancer treatment in older women: does getting what you want improve your long-term body image and mental health? *J Clin Oncol* 22(19):4002–4009, 2004.

Giger J, Davidhizar R: *Transcultural nursing: assessment and intervention*, ed 4, St Louis, 2008, Mosby.

Giovannelli TS, Cash TF, Henson JM, et al: The measurement of body-image dissatisfaction-satisfaction: is rating importance important? *Body Image* 5(2):216–223, 2008.

Hausenblas HA, Fallon E: Exercise and body image: a meta-analysis, *Psychol Health* 21(1):33–47, 2006.

Hebl MR, King EB, Lin J: The swimsuit becomes us all: ethnicity, gender, and vulnerability to self-objectification, *Pers Soc Psychol Bull* 30(10):1322–1331, 2004.

Hermes SF, Keel PK: The influence of puberty and ethnicity on awareness and internalization of the thin ideal, *Int J Eat Disord* 33(4):465–467, 2003.

● = Independent   ▲ = Collaborative   **EBN** = Evidence-Based Nursing   **EB** = Evidence-Based

Huang S, Liu HE: Effectiveness of cosmetic rehabilitation on the body image of oral cancer patients in Taiwan, *Support Care Cancer* 16(9):981–986, 2008.

Hurd LC: Older women's body image and embodied experience: an exploration, *J Women Aging* 12(3–4):77–97, 2000.

Ipser JC, Sander C, Stein DJ: Pharmacotherapy and psychotherapy for body dysmorphic disorder, *Cochrane Database Syst Rev* (1): CD005332, 2009.

Jarry JL, Ip K: The effectiveness of stand-alone cognitive-behavioural therapy for body image: a meta-analysis, *Body Image* 2(4):317–331, 2005.

Kershaw TS, Mood DW, Newth G et al: Longitudinal analysis of a model to predict quality of life in prostate cancer patients and their spouses, *Ann Behav Med* 36(2):117–128, 2008.

Knols R, Aaronson NK, Uebelhart D: Physical exercise in cancer clients during and after medical treatment: a systematic review of randomized and controlled clinical trials, *J Clin Oncol* 23(19):3830–3842, 2005.

Kuba SA, Harris DJ: Eating disturbances in women of color: an exploratory study of contextual factors in the development of disordered eating in Mexican American women, *Health Care Women Int* 22(3):281–298, 2001.

Leone JE, Sedory EJ, Gray, KA: Recognition and treatment of muscle dysmorphia and related body image disorders, *J Athl Train* 40(4):352–359, 2005.

Liu HE: Changes of satisfaction with appearance and working status for head and neck tumor patients, *J Clin Nurs* 17(14):1930–1938, 2008.

Notter J, Burnard P: Preparing for loop ileostomy surgery: women's accounts from a qualitative study, *Int J Nurs Studies* 43(2):147–159, 2006.

Payne J: The contribution of group learning to the rehabilitation of spinal cord injured adults, *Rehabil Nurs* 18:375–379, 1993.

Pittman J, Kozell K, Gray M: Should WOC nurses measure health-related quality of life in patients undergoing intestinal ostomy surgery? *J Wound Ostomy Continence Nurs* 36(3):254–65, 2009.

Price B: Altered body image: managing social encounters, *Int J Palliat Nurs* 6(4):179–185, 2000.

Robert SA, Reither EN: A multilevel analysis of race, community disadvantage, and body mass index among adults in the U.S., *Soc Sci Med* 59(12):2421–2434, 2004.

Ross L, Abild-Nielsen AG, Thomsen BL et al: Quality of life of Danish colorectal cancer patients with and without a stoma, *Support Care Cancer* 15(5):505–13, 2006.

Rumsey N, Clarke A, White P et al: Altered body image: appearance related concerns of people with visible disfigurement, *J Adv Nursing* 48(5):443–453, 2004.

Sedlak CA, Doheny MO: Fashion tips for women with osteoporosis, *Orthop Nurs* 19(5):31–35, 2000.

Swanson E, Stube J, Edman, P: Function and body image levels in individuals with transfemoral amputation using the C-Leg, *JPO* 17(3):80–84, 2005.

Townsend MC: *Psychiatric mental health nursing: concepts of care,* Saddle River, NJ, 2003, F.A. Davis.

Walker L, Timmerman GM, Kim M et al: Relationships between body image and depressive symptoms during postpartum in ethnically diverse, low income women, *Women Health* 36(3):101–121, 2002.

Yates A, Edman J, Aruguete M: Ethnic differences in BMI and body/self-dissatisfaction among Whites, Asian subgroups, Pacific Islanders, and African-Americans, *J Adolesc Health* 34(4):300–307, 2004.

Risk for imbalanced Body temperature   *Betty J. Ackley, MSN, EdS, RN*

NANDA-I

Definition

At risk for failure to maintain body temperature within a normal range

Risk Factors

Altered metabolic rate; dehydration, exposure to extremes of environmental temperature; extremes of age or weight, illness affecting temperature regulation, inactivity, inappropriate clothing for environmental temperature, medications causing vasoconstriction, medications causing vasodilation, sedation, trauma affecting temperature regulation, vigorous activity

NOC, NIC, Client Outcomes, Nursing Interventions, Client/Family Teaching and Discharge Planning, *Rationales*, and References

Refer to care plans for **Ineffective Thermoregulation**, **Hyperthermia**, or **Hypothermia**.

Bowel incontinence   *Mikel Gray, PhD, CUNP, CCCN, FAANP, FAAN*   ⊝volve

NANDA-I

Definition

Change in normal bowel elimination habits characterized by involuntary passage of stool

Defining Characteristics

Constant dribbling of soft stool, fecal odor; inability to delay defecation; fecal staining of bedding; fecal staining of clothing; inability to delay defecation; inability to recognize urge to defecate; inatten-

• = Independent   ▲ = Collaborative   **EBN** = Evidence-Based Nursing   **EB** = Evidence-Based

tion to urge to defecate; recognizes rectal fullness but reports inability to expel formed stool; red perianal skin; self-report of inability to recognize rectal fullness; urgency

Related Factors (r/t)

Abnormally high abdominal pressure; abnormally high intestinal pressure; chronic diarrhea; colorectal lesions; dietary habits; environmental factors (e.g., inaccessible bathroom); general decline in muscle tone; immobility; impaired cognition; impaired reservoir capacity; incomplete emptying of bowel; laxative abuse; loss of rectal sphincter control; lower motor nerve damage; medications; rectal sphincter abnormality; impaction; stress; toileting self-care deficit; upper motor nerve damage

 (Nursing Outcomes Classification)

Suggested NOC Outcomes

Bowel Continence, Bowel Elimination

Example NOC Outcome with Indicators
Bowel Continence as evidenced by the following indicators: Maintains predictable pattern of stool evacuation/Maintains control of stool passage/Evacuates stool at least every 3 days (Rate the outcome and indicators of **Bowel Continence:** 1 = never demonstrated, 2 = rarely demonstrated, 3 = sometimes demonstrated, 4 = often demonstrated, 5 = consistently demonstrated [see Section I].)

Client Outcomes

Client Will (Specify Time Frame):

- Have regular, complete evacuation of fecal contents from the rectal vault (pattern may vary from every day to every 3 days)
- Have regulation of stool consistency (soft, formed stools)
- Reduce or eliminate frequency of incontinent episodes
- Demonstrate intact skin in the perianal/perineal area
- Demonstrate the ability to isolate, contract, and relax pelvic muscles (when incontinence related to sphincter incompetence or high-tone pelvic floor dysfunction)
- Increase pelvic muscle strength (when incontinence related to sphincter incompetence)

 (Nursing Interventions Classification)

Suggested NIC Interventions

Bowel Incontinence Care, Bowel Incontinence Care: Encopresis, Bowel Training

Example NIC Interventions—Bowel Incontinence Care
Determine physical or psychological cause of fecal incontinence; Instruct patient/family to record fecal output, as appropriate

Nursing Interventions and *Rationales*

- In a private setting, directly question any client at risk about the presence of fecal incontinence. If the client reports altered bowel elimination patterns, problems with bowel control, or "uncontrollable diarrhea," complete a focused nursing history including previous and present bowel elimination routines, dietary history, frequency and volume of uncontrolled stool loss, and aggravating and alleviating factors. *Unless questioned directly, clients are often hesitant to report the presence of fecal incontinence (Fisher, Bliss, & Savik, 2008). The nursing history determines the patterns of stool elimination, to characterize involuntary stool loss, and the likely etiology of the incontinence (Norton & Chelvanayagam, 2000).*
- Women who have been pregnant and have delivered one or more children vaginally should be routinely screened for fecal incontinence. **EB:** *A study of women during a routine gynecologic exam revealed a 26.8% prevalence of anal and urinary incontinence symptoms, and the majority stated a desire to receive professional advice and assistance with these symptoms. However, 67% were not asked about their condition (Griffiths, Makam, & Edwards, 2006).*

• = Independent　▲ = Collaborative　**EBN** = Evidence-Based Nursing　**EB** = Evidence-Based

▲ In close consultation with a physician or advanced practice nurse, consider routine use of a validated tool that focuses on bowel elimination patterns. *More than 23 validated symptom questionnaires have been developed and validated for the evaluation of urinary and fecal incontinence (Avery et al, 2007).*

▲ Complete a focused physical assessment including inspection of perineal skin, pelvic muscle strength assessment, digital examination of the rectum for presence of impaction and anal sphincter strength, and evaluation of functional status (mobility, dexterity, visual acuity). *A focused physical examination (including a vaginal examination to determine coexisting pelvic organ prolapse) assists in determining the severity of fecal leakage and its likely etiology; it should be completed prior to functional testing such as anorectal manometry or anal sphincter electromyography (Rao, 2006).*

● Complete an assessment of cognitive function. *Dementia, acute confusion, and mental retardation are risk factors for fecal incontinence (Norton & Chelvanaygam, 2000; Quander et al, 2006).*

● Document patterns of stool elimination and incontinent episodes through a bowel record, including frequency of bowel movements, stool consistency, frequency and severity of incontinent episodes, precipitating factors, and dietary and fluid intake. *This document, used to confirm the verbal history, assists in determining the likely etiology of stool incontinence and serves as a baseline to evaluate treatment efficacy (Norton & Chelvanayagam, 2000).*

● Assess associated bowel elimination symptoms including rectal urgency, constipation, and feelings of incomplete bowel elimination despite defecation. *Rectal urgency, constipation, and feelings of incomplete bowel evacuation have been associated with an increased likelihood of fecal incontinence episodes in women (Bharucha et al, 2008; Schnelle et al, 2009).*

● Assess stool consistency and its influence on risk for stool loss. *Several classification systems for stool have been promulgated (Bliss et al, 2001b). They assist the nurse and client to differentiate between normal soft, formed stool, hardened stools associated with constipation, and liquid stools associated with diarrhea.* **EBN:** *A study of stool consistency found good reliability when evaluated by professional nurses, student nurses, and clients. Word-only descriptors yielded equivocal consistency when assessed by subjects as did tools that combined words with illustrations of various stool consistencies (Bliss et al, 2001b). Less well-formed (loose or liquid) stool is associated with an increased and severity and frequency of fecal incontinence episodes (Bliss et al, 2004; Bharucha et al, 2008).*

● Identify conditions contributing to or causing fecal incontinence. *Fecal incontinence is frequently multifactorial. Accurate assessment of the probable etiology of fecal incontinence is necessary to select a treatment plan likely to control or eliminate the condition (Lazarescu, Turnbull, & Vanner, 2009).*

● Improve access to toileting:
  ■ Identify usual toileting patterns among persons in the acute care or long-term care facility and plan opportunities for toileting accordingly.
  ■ Provide assistance with toileting for clients with limited access or impaired functional status (mobility, dexterity, access).
  ■ Institute a prompted toileting program for persons with impaired cognitive status (retardation, dementia).
  ■ Provide adequate privacy for toileting.
  ■ Respond promptly to requests for assistance with toileting.
  Acute or transient fecal incontinence frequently occurs in the acute care or long-term care facility because of inadequate access to toileting facilities, insufficient assistance with toileting, or inadequate privacy when attempting to toilet (Bliss et al, 2000).

● Counsel clients with fecal incontinence associated with liquid stools (diarrhea) about methods to normalize stool consistency via dietary fiber or fiber supplements. *A liquid stool is associated with an increased likelihood of fecal incontinence (Bliss et al, 2000).* **EBN:** *Daily supplementation of dietary fiber using a product containing psyllium improved stool consistency and reduced frequency of incontinent stools (Bliss et al, 2001a).*

● For the client with intermittent episodes of fecal incontinence related to acute changes in stool consistency, begin a bowel reeducation program consisting of:
  ■ Cleansing the bowel of impacted stool if indicated
  ■ Normalizing stool consistency by adequate intake of fluids (30 mL/kg of body weight/day) and dietary or supplemental fiber
  ■ Establishing a regular routine of fecal elimination based on established patterns of bowel elimination (patterns established prior to onset of incontinence)

● = Independent ▲ = Collaborative **EBN** = Evidence-Based Nursing **EB** = Evidence-Based

Bowel reeducation is designed to reestablish normal defecation patterns and to normalize stool consistency in order to reduce or eliminate the risk of recurring fecal incontinence associated with changes in stool consistency (Doughty & Jensen, 2006).

▲ Begin a prompted defecation program for the adult with dementia, mental retardation, or related learning disabilities. Prompted urine and fecal elimination programs have been shown to reduce or eliminate incontinence in the long-term care facility and in community settings (Doughty & Jensen, 2006).

▲ Begin a scheduled stimulation defecation program for persons with neurological conditions causing fecal incontinence including the following steps:
  ■ Cleanse the bowel of impacted fecal material before beginning the program.
  ■ Implement strategies to normalize stool consistency including adequate intake of fluid and fiber and avoidance of foods associated with diarrhea.
  ■ Determine a regular schedule for bowel elimination (typically every day or every other day) based on prior patterns of bowel elimination whenever feasible.
  ■ Provide a stimulus before assisting the client to a position on the toilet; digital stimulation, a stimulating suppository, "mini-enema," or pulsed evacuation enema may be used for stimulation.

The scheduled, stimulated program relies on consistency of stool, and a mechanical or chemical stimulus to produce a bolus contraction of the rectum with evacuation of fecal material (Doughty & Jensen, 2006).

▲ Begin a reeducation or pelvic floor muscle exercise program for the person with sphincter incompetence or high-tone pelvic floor muscle dysfunction of the pelvic muscles, or refer persons with fecal incontinence related to sphincter dysfunction to a nurse specialist or other therapist with clinical expertise in these techniques of care. **EB:** *There is insufficient evidence to conclude that bowel reeducation or pelvic floor muscle exercise programs are effective for the management of fecal incontinence in adults, but the existing evidence does provide adequate support to consider implementing this intervention in selected clients, particularly given the potential for benefit in the absence of harmful side effects (Norton, Hosker, & Brazzelli, 2006). A nonrandomized cohort study of 281 clients with fecal incontinence revealed modest improvement in most clients undergoing pelvic floor muscle rehabilitation and profound improvement in a minority of subjects (Terra et al, 2006).*

▲ Consider a pelvic muscle training program or electrical stimulation program in clients with urgency to defecate and fecal incontinence related to recurrent diarrhea or fecal incontinence associated with myogenic disorders affecting the pelvic floor muscles. *Mixed data suggest that while pelvic floor muscle training improves anorectal squeeze and related factors, its effect on fecal incontinence may be modest. Clients undergoing pelvic floor muscle training tend to have perceptions of control over bowel function (Naimy et al, 2007; Sun et al, 2008).*

● Institute a structured skin care regimen that incorporates three essential steps: cleanse, moisturize, and protect. Select a cleanser with a pH range comparable to that of normal skin (usually labeled "pH balanced"), moisturize with an emollient to replace lipids removed with cleansing, and protect with a skin protectant containing a petrolatum, dimethicone, or zinc oxide base, or a no-sting skin barrier. Skin that is exposed to urine and/or stool should be cleansed daily and following major incontinence episodes. When feasible, select a product that combined two or all three of these processes into a single step. Ensure that products are available at the bedside when caring for a client with total incontinence in an inpatient facility. *Urinary incontinence, particularly when combined with fecal incontinence or use of absorptive pads or adult containment briefs, increases the risk of incontinence-associated dermatitis.* **EBN:** *A structured skin care regimen based on a three-step process (cleanse, moisturize, and protect) is effective for the prevention of incontinence-associated dermatitis (Gray et al, 2007).*

● Cleanse the perineal and perianal skin following each episode of fecal incontinence. *Frequent cleaning with soap and water may compromise perianal skin integrity and enhance the irritation produced by fecal leakage (Gray et al, 2007).*

● Apply a moisture barrier containing dimethicone or zinc oxide to clients with severe urinary incontinence or those with double urinary and fecal incontinence. *Clients with very severe incontinence and those with double fecal and urinary incontinence (particularly when the stool is liquefied) typically require a product with vigorous moisture barrier qualities. Petrolatum-based products containing dimethicone or zinc oxide are preferred (Gray et al, 2007).*

● = Independent   ▲ = Collaborative   **EBN** = Evidence-Based Nursing   **EB** = Evidence-Based

▲ Consult the physician or advanced practice nurse concerning use of a skin protectant. Apply protectant and teach care providers how to apply to affected areas. *A petrolatum-, dimethicone-, or zinc oxide–based skin protectant should be applied to skin exposed to fecal incontinence to prevent incontinence-associated dermatitis, or to promote healing in affected skin (Gray, 2008). A thin layer of an antifungal powder may be layered beneath the ointment, but excessive application may paradoxically retain moisture and diminish its effectiveness (Evans & Gray, 2003; Gray, 2008).*

• Assist the client to select and apply a containment device for occasional episodes of fecal incontinence. *A fecal containment device will prevent soiling of clothing and reduce odors in the client with uncontrolled stool loss (Brazzelli, Shirran, & Vale, 2003). Counsel clients, and especially male clients who may be hesitant to use pads, who have low volume fecal soiling that an absorbent dressing may be used to absorb fecal soiling.* **EBN:** *A study of 75 community persons with fecal incontinence who used an absorptive dressing used to contain mucus and stool leakage after surgery revealed that the device was preferred over traditional pads in 92% (Bliss & Savik, 2008).*

• Teach the caregiver of the client with frequent episodes of fecal incontinence and limited mobility to regularly monitor the sacrum and perineal area for pressure ulcerations. *Limited mobility, particularly when combined with fecal incontinence, increases the risk of pressure ulceration. Routine cleansing, pressure reduction techniques, and management of fecal and urinary incontinence reduce this risk (Johanson, Irizarry & Doughty, 1997; Schnelle et al, 1997).*

▲ Teach the client with more frequent stool loss to apply an anal continence plug in consultation with the physician. *The anal continence plug is a device that can reduce or eliminate persistent liquid or solid stool incontinence in selected clients (Doherty, 2004).*

• Apply a fecal pouch to the critically ill client with frequent stool loss, particularly when fecal incontinence produces altered perianal skin integrity. *Fecal pouches contain stool loss, reduce odor, and protect the perianal skin from chemical irritation related to contact with stool (Fiers & Thayer, 2000; Waldrop & Doughty, 2000).*

▲ Consult a physician or advanced practice nurse about insertion of a bowel management system in the critically ill client with frequent stool loss, particularly when fecal incontinence produces altered perianal skin integrity. *Three systems are commercially available; each allows drainage of liquid stool from the bowel, and one system enables irrigation of the bowel in cases where the stool is formed but contact with the skin contraindicated, such as clients with severe burns affecting the perianal and perineal area. A quality improvement project demonstrated that incontinence-associated dermatitis, lower stage pressure ulcers, and the severity of fecal incontinence were reduced after introduction of a bowel management system (Benoit & Watts, 2007).*

Geriatric

• Evaluate all elderly clients for established or acute fecal incontinence when the elderly client enters the acute or long-term care facility and intervene as indicated. *The prevalence of fecal incontinence, which often coexists with urinary incontinence, is approximately 50% in long-term care and 20% in acute care facilities (Hunskaar et al, 2005; Junkin & Selekof, 2007).*

• Determine the client's cognitive level using a screening tool such as the Mini-Mental State Exam (MMSE) or Mini-Cog. **EB:** *Use of a standard evaluation tool such as the MMSE can help determine the client's abilities and assist in planning appropriate nursing interventions. Acute or established dementias increase the risk of fecal incontinence among the elderly (Borson et al, 2005; Wilber et al, 2005; Borson et al, 2006).*

Home Care

• The above interventions may be adapted for home care use.

• Assess and teach a bowel management program to support continence. Address timing, diet, fluids, and actions taken independently to deal with bowel incontinence. *Identifying factors that change level of incontinence may guide interventions. If client has been taking over-the-counter medications or home remedies, it is important to consider their influence.*

• Instruct caregiver to provide clothing that is nonrestrictive, can be manipulated easily for toileting, and can be changed with ease. *Avoidance of complicated maneuvers increases the chance of success in toileting programs and decreases the client's risk for embarrassing incontinent episodes.*

• = Independent ▲ = Collaborative **EBN** = Evidence-Based Nursing **EB** = Evidence-Based

- Evaluate self-care strategies of community-dwelling elders; strengthen adaptive behaviors and counsel elders about altering strategies that compromise general health. **EBN:** *A survey of 242 community-dwelling elders reveals multiple self-care strategies designed to alleviate or prevent intermittent episodes of fecal incontinence. The most common included use of containment or protective devices and dietary alterations designed to normalize stool consistency. However, elders also reported reductions in physical activity and exercise, potentially compromising overall mobility and health (Bliss, Fischer, & Savik, 2005).*
- Assist the family in arranging care in a way that allows the client to participate in family or favorite activities without embarrassment. *Careful planning can both help client retain dignity and maintain integrity of family patterns.*
- ▲ If the client is limited to bed (or bed and chair), provide a commode or bedpan that can be easily accessed. If necessary, refer the client to physical therapy services to learn side transfers and to build strength for transfers.
- ▲ If the client is frequently incontinent, refer for home health aide services to assist with hygiene and skin care.
- Teach the client and family to perform a bowel reeducation program; scheduled, stimulated program; or other strategies to manage fecal incontinence.
- Teach the client and family about common dietary sources for fiber, as well as supplemental fiber or bulking agents as indicated.
- ▲ Refer the family to support services to assist with in-home management of fecal incontinence as indicated.
- Teach nursing colleagues and nonprofessional care providers the importance of providing toileting opportunities and adequate privacy for the client in an acute or long-term care facility.

NOTE: Refer to nursing diagnoses **Diarrhea** and **Constipation** for detailed management of these related conditions.

evolve   See the EVOLVE website for Weblinks for client education resources.

REFERENCES

Avery KN, Bosch JL, Gotoh M et al: Questionnaires to assess urinary and anal incontinence: review and recommendations, *J Urol* 177(1):39–49, 2007.

Benoit RA, Watts CY: The effect of a pressure ulcer prevention program and a bowel management program (BMS) in reducing pressure ulcer prevalence in an ICU setting, *J Wound Ostomy* 34(2):163–175, 2007.

Bharucha AE, Seide BM, Zinsmeister AR et al: Relation of bowel habits to fecal incontinence in women, *Am J Gastroenterol* 103(6):1470–5, 2008.

Bliss DZ, Savik K: Use of an absorbent dressing specifically for fecal incontinence, *J Wound Ostomy Continence Nurs* 35(2):221–8, 2008.

Bliss DZ, Fischer LR, Savik K: Managing fecal incontinence: self-care practices of older adults. *J Gerontol Nurs* 31(7):35–44, 2005.

Bliss DZ, Johnson S, Savik K et al: Fecal incontinence in hospitalized patients who are acutely ill, *Nurs Res* 49(2):101–108, 2000.

Bliss DZ, Larson SJ, Burr JK et al: Reliability of a stool consistency classification system, *J Wound Ostomy Cont Nurs* 28(6):305–313, 2001a.

Bliss DZ, Jung HJ, Savik K et al: Supplementation with dietary fiber improves fecal incontinence, *Nurs Res* 50(4):203–213, 2001b.

Bliss DZ, Fischer LR, Savik K et al: Severity of fecal incontinence in community-living elderly in a health maintenance organization, *Res Nurs Health* 27(3):162–73, 2004.

Borson S, Scanlan JM, Watanabe J et al: Simplifying detection of cognitive impairment: comparison of the Mini-Cog and Mini-Mental State Examination in a multiethnic sample, *J Am Geriatr Soc* 53(5):871–874, 2005.

Borson S, Scanlan J, Watanabe J et al: Improving identification of cognitive impairment in primary care, *Int J Geriatr Psychiatry* 21(4):349–355, 2006.

Brazzelli M, Shirran E, Vale L: Absorbent products for containing urinary and/or fecal incontinence in adults, *Cochrane Database Syst Rev* 3:CD001406, 2003.

Doherty W: Managing fecal incontinence or leakage: the Peristeen Anal Plug, *Br J Nurs* 13(21):1293–1297, 2004.

Doughty DB, Jensen LL: Assessment and management of the patient with fecal incontinence and related bowel dysfunction. In Doughty DB, editor: *Urinary and fecal incontinence: current management concepts,* ed 2, St Louis, 2006, Elsevier.

Evans EC, Gray M: What interventions are effective for the prevention and treatment of cutaneous candidiasis? *J Wound Ostomy Continence Nurs* 30(1):11–16, 2003.

Fiers S, Thayer D: Management of intractable incontinence. In: Doughty DB, editor: *Urinary and fecal incontinence: nursing management,* ed 2, St Louis, 2000, Mosby.

Fisher K, Bliss DZ, Savik K: Comparison of recall and daily self-report of fecal incontinence severity, *J Wound Ostomy Continence Nurs* 35(5):515–520, 2008.

Gray M: Perineal skin care for the continence professional, *Continence UK J* 2(2):29–39; 2008.

Gray M, Bliss DZ, Doughty DB et al: Incontinence-associated dermatitis: a consensus, *J Wound Ostomy Continence Nurs* 34(1):45–54, 2007.

Griffiths AN, Makam A, Edwards GJ: Should we actively screen for urinary and anal incontinence in the general gynecology outpatients setting? A prospective observational study, *J Obstet Gynecol* 26(5):442–444, 2006.

Hunskaar S, Burgio K, Clark A et al: Epidemiology of urinary (UI) and fecal (FI) incontinence and pelvic organ prolapse (POP) 3rd *International Consultation on Incontinence,* ed 3, Plymouth, England, 2005, Health Publication, Plymbridge Distributors.

Johanson JF, Irizarry F, Doughty A: Risk factors for fecal incontinence in a nursing home population, *J Clin Gastroenterol* 24:156, 1997.

Junkin J, Selekof J: Prevalence of incontinence and associated skin injury in an acute care population, *J Wound Ostomy Continence Nurs* 34(3):260–269, 2007.

Lazarescu A, Turnbull GK, Vanner S: Investigating and treating fecal incontinence: when and how, *Can J Gastroenterol* 23(4):301–308, 2009.

Naimy N, Lindam AT, Bakka A et al: Biofeedback vs. electrostimulation in the treatment of postdelivery anal incontinence: a randomized, clinical trial, *Dis Colon Rectum* 50(12):2040–2046, 2007.

Norton C, Chelvanayagam S: A nursing assessment tool for adult with fecal incontinence, *J Wound Ostomy Cont Nurs* 27(5):279–291, 2000.

Norton C, Hosker G, Brazzelli M: Biofeedback and/or sphincter exercises for the treatment of faecal incontinence in adults, *Cochrane Database Syst Rev* 2:CD002111, 2006.

Quander CR, Morris MC, Mendes de Leon CF et al: Association of fecal incontinence with physical disability and impaired cognitive function, *Am J Gastroenterol* 101(11):2588–2593, 2006.

Rao SS: A balancing view: fecal incontinence: test or treat empirically: which strategy is best? *Am J Gastroenterol* 101(12):2683–2684, 2006.

Schnelle JF, Adamson GM, Cruise PA et al: Skin disorders and moisture in incontinent nursing home residents: intervention implications, *J Am Geriatr Soc* 45(10):1182–1188, 1997.

Schnelle JF, Simmons SF, Beuscher L et al: Prevalence of constipation symptoms in fecally incontinent nursing home residents, *J Am Geriatr Soc* 57(4):647–652, 2009.

Sun D, Zhao P, Jia H et al: Results of biofeedback therapy together with electrical stimulation in faecal incontinence with myogenic lesions, *Acta Chirurgica Belgica* 108(3):313–317, 2008.

Terra MP, Dobben AC, Berghmans B et al: Electrical stimulation and pelvic floor muscle training with biofeedback in patients with fecal incontinence: a cohort study of 281 patients, *Dis Colon Rectum* 49(8):1149–1159, 2006.

Waldrop J, Doughty DB: Pathophysiology of bowel dysfunction and fecal incontinence. In Doughty DB, editor: *Urinary and fecal incontinence: nursing management,* ed 2, St Louis, 2000, Mosby.

Wilber S, Lofgren S, Mager T et al: An evaluation of two screening tools for cognitive impairment in older emergency department patients, *Acad Emerg Med* 12(7):612–616, 2005.

Effective Breastfeeding   *Teresa Howell, MSN, RN, CNE*    ⊖volve

NANDA-I

Definition

Mother-infant dyad/family exhibits adequate proficiency and satisfaction with breastfeeding process

Defining Characteristics

Adequate infant elimination patterns for age; appropriate infant weight pattern for age; eagerness of infant to nurse; effective mother-infant communication patterns; infant content after feeding; maternal verbalization of satisfaction with the breastfeeding process; mother able to position infant at breast to promote a successful latching-on response; regular suckling at the breast; regular swallowing at the breast; signs of oxytocin release; sustained suckling at the breast; sustained swallowing at the breast; symptoms of oxytocin release

Related Factors (r/t)

Basic breastfeeding knowledge; infant gestational age >34 weeks; maternal confidence; normal breast structure; normal infant oral structure; support source

NOC   (Nursing Outcomes Classification)

Suggested NOC Outcomes

Breastfeeding Establishment: Infant, Maternal, Breastfeeding Maintenance

Example NOC Outcome with Indicators
Breastfeeding Establishment: Infant as evidenced by the following indicators: Proper alignment and latch-on/Proper areolar grasp/Proper areolar compression/Correct suck and tongue placement/Audible swallow/Nursing a minimum of 5 to 10 minutes per breast/Minimum 8 feedings per day/Urinations per day appropriate for age/Weight gain appropriate for age (Rate the outcome and indicators of **Breastfeeding Establishment: Infant:** 1 = not adequate, 2 = slightly adequate, 3 = moderately adequate, 4 = substantially adequate, 5 = totally adequate [see Section I].)

Client Outcomes

Client Will (Specify Time Frame):

• Maintain effective breastfeeding

 • = Independent   ▲ = Collaborative   **EBN** = Evidence-Based Nursing   **EB** = Evidence-Based

- Maintain normal growth patterns (infant)
- Verbalize satisfaction with breastfeeding process (mother)

NIC (Nursing Interventions Classification)

Suggested NIC Interventions

Breastfeeding Assistance, Lactation Counseling

Example NIC Activities—Breastfeeding Assistance
Discuss with parents an estimate of effort and length of time they would like to put toward breastfeeding; Provide early mother/infant contact opportunity to breastfeed within 2 hours after birth

Nursing Interventions and *Rationales*

- Encourage and facilitate early skin-to-skin contact (SSC) (position includes contact of the naked baby with the mother's bare chest within 2 hours after birth). **EBN:** *Benefits of SSC (early initiation of breastfeeding, increased ability of newborns to distinguish their mother's milk, increased breastfeeding duration and breastfeeding success) have been supported in the literature (Dabrowski, 2007).*
- Encourage rooming-in and breastfeeding on demand. **EBN:** *Successful breastfeeding and duration of breastfeeding is improved by keeping mothers and newborns together during their hospital stay (Dabrowski, 2007). **EB:** Breastfeeding can be influenced by ensuring skin-to-skin contact, keeping mothers and newborns together, and avoiding supplemental feeding unless medically indicated (CDC, 2007). Newborns should breastfeed within the first hour of life and then as indicated by hunger cues (Shannon, O'Donnell, & Skinner, 2007). Infant behavioral cues can be identified by the mother if she and her newborn are kept together in the hospital (Shannon, O'Donnell, & Skinner, 2007).*
- Monitor the breastfeeding process. **EBN:** *Breastfeeding should be observed by nurses and lactation consultants while the woman is hospitalized to identify ineffective breastfeeding patterns prior to discharge (Lewallen et al, 2006).*
- Identify opportunities to enhance knowledge and experience regarding breastfeeding. Support and teaching must be individualized to the client's level of understanding. **EBN:** *Professional support to breastfeeding mothers has demonstrated a positive effect but mothers have also identified that inconsistencies among professionals can impose a negative impact on breastfeeding (Nelson, 2007).*
- Give encouragement/positive feedback related to breastfeeding mother-infant interactions. **EBN:** *Effective breastfeeding is influenced by maternal state and the mother's knowledge of breastfeeding (Mulder, 2006). **EBN:** A precursor to effective breastfeeding is a comfortable and relaxed maternal state (Mulder, 2006). **EBN:** Support and encouragement by the nurse is indicated for successful breastfeeding (Shannon, O'Donnell, & Skinner, 2007).*
- Monitor for signs and symptoms of nipple pain and/or trauma. *These factors have been identified as impacting the continuation of breastfeeding in the first weeks of motherhood (Lewallen et al, 2006).* **EBN:** *Ensuring proper latch-on is a key intervention to decrease sore nipples (Lewallen et al, 2006).*
- Discuss prevention and treatment of common breastfeeding problems. **EBN:** *Evidence-based practice guidelines support the need to evaluate breastfeeding women's knowledge regarding the prevention and management of common problems (e.g., sore nipples, breast engorgement) associated with breastfeeding (Registered Nurses Association of Ontario, 2003).*
- Monitor infant responses to breastfeeding. **EBN:** *Monitor and assess the mom and baby for several breastfeeding sessions to evaluate maternal and infant cues, latch, nipple condition, and response to breastfeeding (Ladewig, London, & Davidson, 2010).*
- Identify current support-person network and opportunities for continued breastfeeding support. **EB:** *Education and support to breastfeeding mothers increases the length of breastfeeding and helps to promote exclusive breastfeeding (Anonymous, 2008).*
- Avoid supplemental bottle feedings and do not provide samples of formula on discharge. **EBN:** *Supplemental feedings can contribute to decreased milk supply (Lewallen et al, 2006).*
- ▲ Provide follow-up contact; as available provide home visits and/or peer counseling. **EB:** *Evidence suggests that practitioners providing extra support and attention to mothers are the key to breastfeeding success (Winterburn, 2005).*

• = Independent   ▲ = Collaborative   **EBN** = Evidence-Based Nursing   **EB** = Evidence-Based

Multicultural

- Assess for the influence of cultural beliefs, norms, and values on current breastfeeding practices. *The client's knowledge of breastfeeding may be based on cultural perceptions, as well as influences from the larger social context (Cricco-Lizza, 2004; Gill et al, 2004; Kong & Lee, 2004).* **EBN:** *A study of African American women revealed formula-feeding experiences were the norm and infant-feeding beliefs reflected responses to life experiences (Cricco-Lizza, 2004).* **EBN:** *The Hispanic mother may believe stress and anger makes bad milk, which makes a breastfeeding infant ill. Some Hispanic women neutralize the bowel when weaning from breast to bottle by feeding only anise tea for 24 hours (Gonzalez, Owens, & Esperat, 2008).* **EBN:** *Each client should be assessed for ability to breastfeed based on a culturally competent assessment of the phenomenon of communication, time, space, social organization, environmental control, and biological variations (Giger & Davidhizar, 2008).*
- Assess mothers' timing preference to begin breastfeeding. *Women from different cultures may have different beliefs about the best time to begin breastfeeding (Purnell & Paulanka, 2008).* **EBN:** *Although usual hospital practice is to begin breastfeeding immediately, some cultures (e.g., Arab heritage) do not regard colostrum as appropriate for newborns and may prefer to wait until milk is present at about 3 days of age (Purnell & Paulanka, 2008).*
- Validate the client's concerns about the amount of milk taken. **EBN:** *Provide information about physical signs that baby is getting enough milk (Lewallen et al, 2006).*

Home Care

- The above interventions may be adapted for home care use.

Client/Family Teaching and Discharge Planning

- Include the father and other family members in education about breastfeeding. *Teach the parents the signs of effective breastfeeding so they can recognize problems and know when to contact their care provider (Lowdermilk & Perry, 2007).* **EB:** *Researchers conducting a randomized controlled trial with a 2–hour intervention class on infant care and breastfeeding promotion found that the fathers in the intervention group were influential advocates for breastfeeding (Wolfberg et al, 2004).*
- Teach the client the importance of maternal nutrition. **EB:** *Consumption or avoidance of specific foods or drinks are generally not necessary. Breastfeeding mothers should consume 500 calories more than a nonpregnant, nonnursing women (Lowdermilk & Perry, 2007).*
- Reinforce the infant's subtle hunger cues (e.g., quiet-alert state, rooting, sucking, mouthing, hand-to-mouth, hand-to-hand activity) and encourage the client to nurse whenever signs are apparent. *Parents should be taught feeding cues that suggest it is a good time to breastfeed their infant.* **EBN:** *Evidence-based practice guidelines support the teaching/reinforcement of these skills as important to effective breastfeeding (Association of Women's Health Obstetric and Neonatal Nurses, 2000).*
- Review guidelines for frequency (every 2 to 3 hours, or 8 to 12 feedings per 24 hours) and duration (until suckling and swallowing slow down and satiety is reached) of feeding times. *In the first few days, frequent and regular stimulation of the breasts is important to establish an adequate milk supply; after breastfeeding is established, feeding lasts until the breasts are drained (Association of Women's Health Obstetric and Neonatal Nurses, 2000; Neifert, 2004).* **EBN:** *Evidence-based guidelines recommend assessment of infant satisfaction/satiety including infant cues and patterns of weight (Association of Women's Health Obstetric and Neonatal Nurses, 2000).*
- Provide anticipatory guidance about common infant behaviors. *Being able to anticipate and manage behaviors and problems promotes parental confidence (Association of Women's Health Obstetric and Neonatal Nurses, 2000; Milligan et al, 2000).*
- Provide information about additional breastfeeding resources. **EBN:** *Evidence-based clinical practice guidelines suggest that breastfeeding books, materials, websites, and breastfeeding support groups, which provide current and accurate information, can enhance maternal success and satisfaction with the breastfeeding process (Association of Women's Health Obstetric and Neonatal Nurses, 2000).*

ⓔvolve See the EVOLVE website for Weblinks for client education resources.

• = Independent   ▲ = Collaborative   **EBN** = Evidence-Based Nursing   **EB** = Evidence-Based

REFERENCES

Anonymous: Breastfeeding support helps reduce child mortality, *Aust Nurs J* 16(3):16, 2008.

Association of Women's Health Obstetric and Neonatal Nurses: *Evidence-based clinical practice guideline: breastfeeding support: pre-natal care through the first year (practice guideline)*, Washington DC, 2000, The Association.

Centers for Disease Control and Prevention (CDC): Breastfeeding-related maternity practices at hospitals and birth centers—United States, *MMWR Morb Mortal Wkly Rep* 57(23):621–625, 2007.

Cricco-Lizza R: Infant-feeding beliefs and experiences of black women enrolled in WIC in the New York metropolitan area, *Qual Health Res* 14(9):1197–1210, 2004.

Dabrowski GA: Skin to skin contact: giving birth back to mothers and babies, *Nurs Womens Health* 11(1):64–71, 2007.

Giger J, Davidhizar R: *Transcultural nursing: assessment and intervention*, St Louis, 2008, Mosby.

Gill SL, Reifsnider E, Mann AR et al: Assessing infant breastfeeding belief among low-income Mexican Americans, *J Perinat Educ* 13:29, 2004.

Gonzalez E, Owens D, Esperat C: Mexican Americans. In Giger J, Davidhizar R, editors: *Transcultural nursing: assessment and intervention*. St Louis, 2008, Mosby.

Kong SK, Lee DT: Factors influencing decision to breastfeed, *J Adv Nurs* 46(4):369–379, 2004.

Ladewig AW, London ML, Davidson MR: Newborn nutrition. In *Contemporary maternal-newborn nursing care*, ed 7, Upper Saddle River, NJ, 2010, Pearson.

Lewallen LP, Dick MJ, Flowers J et al: Breastfeeding support and early cessation, *J Obstet Gynecol Neonatal Nurs* 35(2):166–172, 2006.

Lowdermilk DL, Perry SE: Newborn nutrition and feeding. In Lowdermilk DL, Perry SE: *Maternity and women's healthcare*, St Louis, 2007, Mosby.

Milligan RA, Pugh LC, Bronner YL et al: Breastfeeding duration among low income women, *J Midwif Womens Health* 45(3);246–252, 2000.

Mulder PJ: A concept analysis of effective breastfeeding, *J Obstet Gynecol Neonatal Nurs* 35(3):332–339, 2006.

Neifert MR: Breastmilk transfer: positioning, latch-on, and screening for problems in milk transfer, *Clin Obstet Gynecol* 47(3):656–675, 2004.

Nelson AM: Maternal-newborn nurses' experience of inconsistent professional breastfeeding support, *J Adv Nurs* 60(1):29–38, 2007.

Purnell LD, Paulanka BJ: *Transcultural health care: a culturally competent approach*, ed 4, Philadelphia, 2008, F.A. Davis.

Registered Nurses Association of Ontario (RNAO): *Breastfeeding best practice guidelines for nurses*, Toronto, 2003, The Association.

Shannon T, O'Donnell MJ, Skinner K: Breastfeeding in the 21st century: overcoming barriers to help women and infants, *Nurs Womens Health* 11(6):569–575, 2007.

Winterburn SA: Breastfeeding support plans: an evidenced-based approach, *Prim Health Care* 15(4):36–39, 2005.

Wolfberg AJ, Michels KB, Shields W et al: Dads as breastfeeding advocates: results from a randomized controlled trial of an educational intervention, *Am J Obstet Gynecol* 191(3):708–712, 2004.

Ineffective Breastfeeding   *Teresa Howell, MSN, RN, CNE*

NANDA-I

Definition

Dissatisfaction or difficulty a mother, infant, or child experiences with the breastfeeding process

Defining Characteristics

Inadequate milk supply; infant arching at the breast; infant crying at the breast; infant inability to latch on to maternal breast correctly; infant exhibiting crying within the first hour after breastfeeding; infant exhibiting fussiness within the first hour after breastfeeding; insufficient emptying of each breast per feeding; insufficient opportunity for suckling at the breast; no observable signs of oxytocin release; nonsustained suckling at the breast; observable signs of inadequate infant intake; perceived inadequate milk supply, persistence of sore nipples beyond first week of breastfeeding; resisting latching on; unresponsive to other comfort measures; unsatisfactory breastfeeding process

Related Factors (r/t)

Infant anomaly; infant receiving supplemental feedings with artificial nipple; interruption in breastfeeding; knowledge deficit; maternal ambivalence; maternal anxiety; maternal breast anomaly; nonsupportive family; nonsupportive partner; poor infant sucking reflex; prematurity; previous breast surgery; previous history of breastfeeding failure

NOC   (Nursing Outcomes Classification)

Suggested NOC Outcomes and Example

Refer to care plan for **Effective Breastfeeding**.

Client Outcomes

Client Will (Specify Time Frame):

- Achieve effective breastfeeding (dyad)
- Verbalize/demonstrate techniques to manage breastfeeding problems (mother)
- Manifest signs of adequate intake at the breast (infant)
- Manifest positive self-esteem in relation to the infant feeding process (mother)
- Explain alternative method of infant feeding if unable to continue exclusive breastfeeding (mother)

NIC (Nursing Interventions Classification)

Suggested NIC Interventions and Example

Refer to care plan **Effective Breastfeeding**.

Nursing Interventions and *Rationales*

- Identify women with risk factors for lower breastfeeding initiation and continuation rates (age <20 years, low socioeconomic status) as well as factors contributing to ineffective breastfeeding as early as possible in the perinatal experience. **EBN:** *Prenatal breastfeeding education is a way to increase the initiation and length of breastfeeding (Gill, Reifsnider, & Lucke, 2007).*
- Provide time for clients to express expectations and concerns and give emotional support. **EBN:** *Lactation consultants and nurses play a key role in the establishment of breastfeeding (Lewallen et al, 2006).*
- Use valid and reliable tools to measure breastfeeding performance and to predict early discontinuance of breastfeeding whenever possible/feasible. **EB:** *Breastfeeding Assessment Score (BAS) has been used to identify infants at risk for early cessation of breastfeeding and may predict exclusive breastfeeding failure (Gianni et al, 2004).*
- Provide evidence-based teaching and breastfeeding assistance appropriate to the client's individualized needs (see Client/Family Teaching and Discharge Planning).
- Promote comfort and relaxation to reduce pain and anxiety. *Discomfort and increased tension are factors associated with reduced let-down reflex and premature discontinuance of breastfeeding. Anxiety and fear are associated with decreased milk production (Mezzacappa & Katkin, 2002).*
- Avoid supplemental feedings. **EBN:** *Supplementation with formula feedings has been associated with early weaning of the infant (Araujo et al, 2007). If indicated during the first few days of life, supplements ideally should be limited to 0.5 to 1 oz. of the mother's own milk after a breastfeeding attempt (Shannon, O'Donnell, & Skinner, 2007).*
- Monitor infant behavioral cues and responses to breastfeeding. **EBN:** *Infant behaviors contribute to oxytocin release and let-down, contribute to effective feeding, indicate effective breastfeeding, manifest satiety, and indicate adequacy of the feeding while contributing to positive maternal-infant attachment (White, Simon, & Bryan, 2002). Keeping the mother and newborn together in the hospital can help the mother learn to respond to her infant's behavioral cues (Shannon, O'Donnell, & Skinner, 2007).*
- Provide necessary equipment/instruction/assistance for milk expression as needed. **EBN:** *Breast massage using the Oketani method (first reported in Japan) was associated with improved quality of milk and growth and development patterns (Foda et al, 2004).*
- ▲ Provide referrals and resources: lactation consultants, nurse and peer support programs, community organizations, and written and electronic sources of information. **EBN:** *Evidenced-based guidelines and systematic reviews support the use of professionals with special skills in breastfeeding and other support programs to promote continued breastfeeding (Association of Women's Health Obstetric and Neonatal Nurses, 2000b). If a newborn is having difficulty breastfeeding beyond 24 hours a lactation consultant should be contacted (Shannon, O'Donnell, & Skinner, 2007).*
- See care plan for **Effective Breastfeeding**.

Multicultural

- Assess whether the client's concerns about the amount of milk taken during breastfeeding is contributing to dissatisfaction with the breastfeeding process. **EBN:** *Some cultures may add semisolid* *food within the first month of life as a result of concerns that the infant is not getting enough to eat and the perception that "big is healthy" (Higgins, 2000).*

- Assess the influence of family support on the decision to continue or discontinue breastfeeding. **EB:** *In one Italian study, a description of mother's characteristics that may indicate the need for more support included mothers that smoke and have had their first newborn (Bertini et al, 2003).* **EBN:** *Recent research has found that the mother's partner and family are most influential in the choice of infant feeding method and, thus, should be included in breastfeeding promotion programs for ethnically diverse women (Rose et al, 2004).*
- Assess for the influence of mother's weight on attempts to initiate and sustain breastfeeding. **EB:** *Prepregnant overweight and obesity have been associated with failure to initiate and to sustain breastfeeding among Caucasian and Hispanic women (Kugyelka, Rasmussen, & Frongillo, 2004).*
- Provide traditional ethnic foods for breastfeeding mothers. **EBN:** *Cambodians had the lowest breastfeeding initiation rate of any racial/ethnic group in Massachusetts. One barrier to breastfeeding is a lack of hospital foods that allow women to follow a traditional diet postpartum. After a staff training program on breastfeeding, and the creation of a Cambodian menu, initiation rates increased significantly more in Cambodians than in non-Cambodians. Postintervention, there was no significant difference between breastfeeding initiation rates among Cambodian women (66.7%) compared to non-Cambodians (68.9%) (Galvin et al, 2008).*
- See care plan for **Effective Breastfeeding**.

Home Care

- The above interventions may be adapted for home care use.
- Provide anticipatory guidance in relation to home management of breastfeeding. **EBN:** *Since many women maintain a career after having children, nurses should initiate teaching about pumping, maintaining milk supply, and feeding the infant while the mother is at work. Women can continue to breastfeed while working if provided education and support (Lewallen et al, 2006).*
- Investigate availability/refer to public health department, hospital home follow-up breastfeeding program, or other postdischarge support. **EBN:** *Some hospitals and public health departments have follow-up breastfeeding programs, particularly for high-risk mothers (e.g., older mothers, past history substance use, risk of physical abuse) (McNaughton, 2004).*
- Monitor for specific difficulties contributing to bonding difficulties between mother and infant.
- Refer to care plan for **Risk for impaired Attachment.**

Client/Family Teaching and Discharge Planning

- Review maternal and infant benefits of breastfeeding. **EBN:** *Information about benefits of breastfeeding can assist women/families to make informed decisions about breastfeeding (Association of Women's Health Obstetric and Neonatal Nurses, 2000a, 2000b; U.S. Department of Health and Human Services, 2000).*
- Instruct the client on maternal breastfeeding behaviors/techniques (preparation for, positioning, initiation of/promoting latch-on, burping, completion of session, and frequency of feeding). Consider use of a video. **EBN:** *Breastfeeding mothers should be evaluated to determine knowledge deficits, provide teaching, assist with breastfeeding and address any concerns the mother might have (Ladewig, London, & Davidson, 2010).*
- Teach the client self-care measures for the breastfeeding woman (e.g., breast care, management of breast/nipple discomfort, nutrition/fluid, rest/activity). **EBN:** *Painful nipples, mastitis, adequate hydration and fatigue are some of the problems a breastfeeding woman may experience (Ladewig, London, & Davidson, 2010).*
- Provide information regarding infant cues and behaviors related to breastfeeding and appropriate maternal responses (e.g., cues that infant is ready to feed, behaviors during feeding that contribute to effective breastfeeding, measures of infant feeding adequacy). *Teach the mother signs of infant readiness to feed (lusty cry, rooting and sucking behaviors when nipple is placed near baby's lips) (Ladewig, London, & Davidson, 2010).*

- Provide education to father/family/significant others as needed. *Informed support people may be needed to assist mothers with breastfeeding management issues (e.g., fatigue and sleep pattern disturbances) (Quillin & Glenn, 2004; Wolfberg et al, 2004).* **EB:** *An educational intervention demonstrated the critical role of dads in encouraging women to breastfeed her newborn (Wolfberg et al, 2004). Women who lack social support for breastfeeding can be empowered by connecting with other mothers who have chosen to breastfeed (Shannon et al, 2007).*

ⓔvolve   See the EVOLVE website for Weblinks for client education resources.

REFERENCES

See **Effective Breastfeeding** for additional references.

Araujo EC, Lopes ND, Vasconcelos MGL et al: Risk for ineffective breastfeeding: an ethnographic report, *Internet J Adv Nurs Pract* 7(2), 2007. www.ispub.com/journal/the_internet_journal_of_advanced_nursing_practice/volume_7_number_2_1/article/risk_for_ineffective_breastfeeding_an_ethnographic_report.html

Association of Women's Health Obstetric and Neonatal Nurses: *Evidence-based clinical practice guideline: breastfeeding support: prenatal care through the first year (practice guideline)*, Washington, DC, 2000a, The Association.

Association of Women's Health Obstetric and Neonatal Nurses: Evidence-based clinical practice guideline: breastfeeding support: pre-natal care through the first year (monograph), Washington, DC, 2000b, The Association.

Bertini G, Perugi S, Dani C et al: Maternal education and the incidence and duration of breast feeding: a prospective study, *J Pediatr Gastroenterol Nutr* 37(4):447–452, 2003.

Foda MI, Kawashima T, Nakamura S et al: Composition of milk obtained from unmassaged versus massaged breasts of lactating mothers, *J Pediatr Gastroenterol Nutr* 38(5):484–487, 2004.

Galvin S, Grossman X, Feldman-Winter L et al: A practical intervention to increase breastfeeding initiation among Cambodian women in the U.S., *Matern Child Health J* 12(4):545–547, 2008.

Gianni ML, Vegni C, Ferraris G et al: 96 usefulness of an early breastfeeding assessment score to predict exclusive breastfeeding failure, *Pediatr Res* 56:480, 2004.

Gill SL, Reifsnider E, Lucke JF: Effects of support on the initiation and duration of breastfeeding, *West J Nurs Res* 29(6):708–723, 2007.

Higgins B: Puerto Rican cultural beliefs: influence on infant feeding practices in western New York, *J Transcult Nurs* 11(1):19–30, 2000.

Kugyelka JG, Rasmussen KM, Frongillo EA: Maternal obesity is negatively associated with breastfeeding success among Hispanic but not Black women, *J Nutr* 134(7):1746–1753, 2004.

Ladewig AW, London ML, Davidson MR: *Contemporary maternal-newborn nursing care*, ed 7, Upper Saddle River, NJ, 2010, Pearson.

Lewallen LP, Dick MJ, Flowers J et al: Breastfeeding support and early cessation, *J Obstet Gynecol Neonatal Nurs* 35(2):166–172, 2006.

McNaughton DB: Nurse home visits to maternal-child clients: a review of intervention research, *Public Health Nurs* 21(3):207–219, 2004.

Mezzacappa ES, Katkin ES: Breast-feeding is associated with reduced perceived stress and negative mood in mothers, *Health Psychol* 21(2):187–193, 2002.

Quillin SI, Glenn LL: Interaction between feeding method and co-sleeping on maternal-newborn sleep, *J Obstet Gynecol Neonatal Nurs* 33(5):580–8, 2004.

Rose VA, Warrington VO, Linder R et al: Factors influencing infant feeding method in an urban community, *J Natl Med Assoc* 96(3):325–331, 2004.

Shannon T, O'Donnell MJ, Skinner K: Breastfeeding in the 21st century: Overcoming barriers to help women and infants, *Nursing for Women's Health* 11(6):569–575, 2007.

U.S. Department of Health and Human Services: *HHS blueprint for action on breastfeeding*, Washington DC, 2000, U.S. Department of Health and Human Services, Office on Women's Health.

White C, Simon M, Bryan A: Using evidence to education birthing center nursing staff: about infant states, cues, and behaviors, *MCN Am J Matern Child Nurs* 27(5):294–298, 2002.

Wolfberg AJ, Michels KB, Shields W et al: Dads as breastfeeding advocates: results from a randomized controlled trial of an educational intervention, *Am J Obstet Gynecol* 191(3):708–712, 2004.

Interrupted Breastfeeding   *Teresa Howell, MSN, RN, CNE*

NANDA-I

Definition

Break in the continuity of the breastfeeding process as a result of inability or inadvisability to put baby to breast for feeding

Defining Characteristics

Infant receives no nourishment at the breast for some or all feedings; lack of knowledge about expression of breast milk; lack of knowledge about storage of breast milk; maternal desire to eventually provide breast milk for child's nutritional needs; maternal desire to maintain breastfeeding for child's nutritional needs; maternal desire to provide breast milk for child's nutritional needs; separation of mother and child

• = Independent   ▲ = Collaborative   **EBN** = Evidence-Based Nursing   **EB** = Evidence-Based

Related Factors (r/t)

Contraindications to breastfeeding; infant illness; maternal employment; maternal illness; need to abruptly wean infant; prematurity

NOC   (Nursing Outcomes Classification)

Suggested NOC Outcomes

Breastfeeding Maintenance, Knowledge: Breastfeeding, Parent-Infant Attachment

> ### Example NOC Outcome with Indicators
>
> **Breastfeeding Maintenance** as evidenced by the following indicators: Infant's growth and development in normal range/ability to safely collect and store breastmilk/awareness that breastfeeding can continue beyond infancy/knowledge of benefits from continued breastfeeding (Rate the outcome and indicators of **Breastfeeding Establishment: Infant:** 1 = not adequate, 2 = slightly adequate, 3 = moderately adequate, 4 = substantially adequate, 5 = totally adequate [see Section I].)

Client Outcomes

Client Will (Specify Time Frame):

Infant

- Receive mother's breast milk if not contraindicated by maternal conditions (e.g., certain drugs, infections) or infant conditions (e.g., true breast milk jaundice)

Maternal

- Maintain lactation
- Achieve effective breastfeeding or satisfaction with the breastfeeding experience
- Demonstrate effective methods of breast milk collection and storage

NIC   (Nursing Interventions Classification)

Suggested NIC Interventions

Bottle Feeding, Emotional Support, Lactation Counseling

> ### Example NIC Activities—Lactation Counseling
>
> Instruct parents on how to differentiate between perceived and actual insufficient milk supply; Encourage employers to provide opportunities for and private facilities for lactating mothers to pump and store breast milk during the work day

Nursing Interventions and *Rationales*

- Discuss mother's desire/intention to begin or resume breastfeeding. **EBN:** *It is very important that key personnel in the hospital (lactation consultants and nurses) assist mothers with getting breastfeeding off to a good start, especially with first-time breastfeeders who have no experience to rely on (Lewallen et al, 2006). Interventions to enhance a mother's confidence in breastfeeding should be initiated by health care providers (Dunn et al, 2006).*
- Provide anticipatory guidance to the mother/family regarding potential duration of the interruption when possible/feasible. *When conditions require a temporary interruption of breastfeeding, every opportunity should be taken to address the primary reason and provide nursing intervention (Lewallen et al, 2006).* **EBN:** *The likelihood of continuing/resuming breastfeeding decreases the longer feeding is delayed and formula supplements are used (Lewallen et al, 2006).*
- Reassure mother/family that early measures to sustain lactation and promote parent-infant attachment can make it possible to resume breastfeeding when the condition/situation requiring interruption is resolved. **EBN:** *Dunn et al (2006) suggest that a predictor of early cessation of breastfeeding is a low level of confidence by the mother.*

• = Independent   ▲ = Collaborative   **EBN** = Evidence-Based Nursing   **EB** = Evidence-Based

- Reassure the mother/family that the infant will benefit from any amount of breast milk provided. **EBN:** *The perception of insufficient milk supply is a common reason women discontinue breastfeeding (Lewallen et al, 2006).*
▲ Collaborate with the mother/family/health care providers/employers (as needed) to develop a plan for expression of breast milk/infant feeding/kangaroo care/SSC. *Nurses should collaborate with the mother to determine her individual preference of techniques to express breast milk (Lowdermilk & Perry, 2007).*
- Monitor for signs indicating infants' ability to and interest in breastfeeding. **EBN:** *An infant's contentedness and ability to be soothed (aspects of responsiveness) contribute to mothers' evaluation of self in relation to confidence and competence (Pridham, Lin, & Brown, 2001).*
- Observe mother performing psychomotor skill (expression, storage, alternative feeding, kangaroo care, and/or breastfeeding) and assist as needed. *The nurse's presence and involvement allow for identification of those areas for which assistance, clarification, and/or support are needed and promote maternal confidence (Hong et al, 2003).*
▲ Provide and/or assist with arrangements and/or necessary equipment. **EBN:** *Working women and those with chronic illness have specific needs including assistance with arrangement of space and time for milk expression (hand or pump) and anticipatory guidance for planning for pumping schedules, using alternative feeding positions/approaches to promote successful breastfeeding (Ortiz, McGilligan, & Kelly, 2004; Rojjanasrirat, 2004; Schaefer, 2004).*
▲ Use supplementation only as medically indicated. **EBN:** *Supplementation with formula feedings has been associated with early weaning of the infant (Araujo et al, 2007).*
- Provide anticipatory guidance for common problems associated with interrupted breastfeeding (e.g., incomplete emptying of milk glands, diminishing milk supply, infant difficulty with resuming breastfeeding, or infant refusal of alternative feeding method). **EBN:** *The most common reason for discontinuation of breastfeeding was the perception of insufficient milk supply (Lewallen et al, 2006).* **EBN:** *One measure to decrease interruption of breastfeeding due to perceived inadequate milk supply (PIM) is teaching by the clinician because many women perceive crying, fussiness, and wakeful as signs that their baby is not receiving enough milk (Gatti, 2008).*
▲ Initiate follow-up and make appropriate referrals. **EBN:** *Breastfeeding women receiving nurse and peer counselor support had longer duration of breastfeeding, and infants had fewer sick visits and reported use of fewer medications than those receiving usual care (Pugh et al, 2002).*
- Assist the client to accept and learn an alternative method of infant feeding if effective breastfeeding is not achieved. **EBN:** *If it is clear that breastfeeding cannot be achieved after the interruption and an alternative feeding method must be instituted, the mother needs support and education (Mozingo et al, 2000).*
- See care plans for **Effective Breastfeeding** and **Ineffective Breastfeeding**.

Multicultural

- Assess for the influence of cultural beliefs, norms, and values on current decision to stop breastfeeding. **EBN:** *The client's decision to halt breastfeeding may be based on cultural perceptions, as well as influences from the larger social context (Cricco-Lizza, 2004; Newton, 2004). A study of Thai nurses suggests that beliefs about breastfeeding and postpartum practices of the nurse care provider may also have implications for clients' breastfeeding experiences (Kaewsarn, Moyle, & Creedy, 2003). The Hispanic mother may believe stress and anger makes bad milk, which makes a breastfeeding infant ill (Gonzalez, Owens, & Esperat, 2008). Some Hispanic women neutralize the bowel when weaning from breast to bottle by feeding only anise tea for 24 hours (Gonzalez, Owens, & Esperat, 2008).*
- Teach culturally appropriate techniques for maintaining lactation. **EBN:** *The Oketani method of breast massage is used by Japanese and other Asian women. Oketani breast massage improved quality of human milk by increasing total solids, lipids, casein concentration, and gross energy (Foda et al, 2004).*
- Validate the client's feelings with regard to the difficulty of or her dissatisfaction with breastfeeding. **EBN:** *In a Scandinavian study the first 5 weeks was a vulnerable period and found factors associated with continuing to breastfeed. They concluded that interventions should be aimed at improving self-efficacy and resources available to those at risk (Kronborg & Vaeth, 2004).*
- See care plans for **Effective Breastfeeding** and **Ineffective Breastfeeding**.

• = Independent   ▲ = Collaborative   **EBN** = Evidence-Based Nursing   **EB** = Evidence-Based

Home Care

- The above interventions may be adapted for home care use.

Client/Family Teaching and Discharge Planning

- Teach mother effective methods to express breast milk. **EBN:** *Expressing breast milk by hand may be more effective in the removal of colostrum in the immediate postpartum period than the use of electric pumps (Ladewig, London & Davidson, 2010). Mother's should be taught the technique of hand expressing breast milk so engorgement can be addressed when electrical pumps are not available (Ladewig, London & Davidson, 2010).*
- Teach mother/parents about kangaroo care. **EBN:** *Parents can use skin-to-skin care to promote attachment and provide closeness to their infant (Ladewig, London & Davidson, 2010).* **EBN:** *Prefeeding behavior can be facilitated by the father through skin-to-skin contact (Erlandsson et al, 2007).*
- Instruct mother on safe breast milk handling techniques. **EBN:** *Storage and handling practices can optimize the nutritional value and provide protection against contaminants (Philipp, 2003).*
- See care plans for **Effective Breastfeeding** and **Ineffective Breastfeeding**.

⊖volve   See the EVOLVE website for Weblinks for client education resources.

REFERENCES

See **Effective Breastfeeding** for additional references.

Araujo EC, Lopes ND, Vasconcelos MGL et al: Risk for ineffective breastfeeding: an ethnographic report, *Int J Adv Nurs Pract* 7(2). Available at www.ispub.com/ostia/index.php?xmlFilePath5journals/ijanp/vol7n2/breast.xml. Accessed on March 5, 2007.

Cricco-Lizza R: Infant-feeding beliefs and experiences of black women enrolled in WIC in the New York metropolitan area, *Qual Health Res* 14(9):1197–1210, 2004.

Dunn S, Davies B, McCleary L et al: The relationship between vulnerability factors and breastfeeding outcomes, *J Obstet Gynecol Neonat Nurs* 35(1):87–97, 2006.

Erlandsson K, Dsilna A, Fagerberg I et al: Skin-to-skin care with the father after cesarean birth and its effect on newborn crying and prefeeding behavior, *Birth* 34(2):105–113, 2007.

Foda MI, Kawashima T, Nakamura S et al: Composition of milk obtained from unmassaged versus massaged breasts of lactating mothers, *J Pediatr Gastroenterol Nutr* 38(5): 484–487, 2004.

Gatti L: Maternal perceptions of insufficient milk supply in breastfeeding, *J Nurs Scholarsh* 40(4):355–363, 2008.

Gonzalez E, Owens D, Esperat C: Mexican Americans. In Giger J, Davidhizar R, editors: *Transcultural nursing: assessment and intervention*, St Louis, 2008, Mosby.

Hong TM, Callister LC, Schwartz R: First-time mothers' views of breastfeeding support from nurses, *MCN Am J Matern Child Nurs* 28:10, 2003.

Kaewsarn P, Moyle W, Creedy D: Thai nurses' beliefs about breastfeeding and postpartum practices, *J Clin Nurs* 12:467, 2003.

Kronborg H, Vaeth M: The influence of psychosocial factors on the duration of breastfeeding, *Scand J Public Health* 32:210, 2004.

Ladewig LP, London ML, Davidson MR: *Contemporary maternal-newborn nursing care*, ed 7, Upper Saddle River, NJ, 2010, Pearson.

Lewallen LP, Dick MJ, Flowers J et al: Breastfeeding support and early cessation, *J Obstet Gynecol Neonatal Nurs* 35(2):166–172, 2006.

Lowdermilk DL, Perry SE: *Maternity and Women's Healthcare*, St Louis, 2007, Mosby.

Mozingo JN, Davis MW, Droppleman PG et al: "It wasn't working." Women's experiences with short-term breastfeeding, *MCN Am J Matern Child Nurs* 25(3):120–126, 2000.

Newton ER: The epidemiology of breastfeeding, *Clin Obstet Gynecol* 47:613, 2004.

Ortiz J, McGilligan K, Kelly P: Duration of breast milk expression among working mothers enrolled in an employer-sponsored lactation program, *Pediatric Nurs* 30:111, 2004.

Philipp B: Encouraging patients to use a breast pump, *Contemp Ob Gyn* 1:88–100, 2003.

Pridham K, Lin CY, Brown R: Mothers' evaluation of their caregiving for premature and full-term infants through the first year: contributing factors, *Res Nurs Health* 24(3):157–169, 2001.

Pugh LC, Milligan RA, Frick KD et al: Breastfeeding duration, costs, and benefits of a support program for low-income breast-feeding women, *Birth* 29(2):95–100, 2002.

Rojjansrirat W: Working women's breastfeeding experiences, *MCN Am J Matern Child Nurs* 29:248, 2004.

Schaefer KM: Breastfeeding in chronic illness: the voices of women with fibromyalgia, *MCN Am J Matern Child Nurs* 29:248, 2004.

Ineffective Breathing pattern   *Betty J. Ackley, MSN, EdS, RN*   ⊖volve

NANDA-I

Definition

Inspiration and/or expiration that does not provide adequate ventilation

● = Independent ▲ = Collaborative **EBN** = Evidence-Based Nursing **EB** = Evidence-Based

Defining Characteristics

Alterations in depth of breathing; altered chest excursion; assumption of three-point position; bradypnea; decreased expiratory pressure; decreased inspiratory pressure; decreased minute ventilation; decreased vital capacity; dyspnea; increased anterior-posterior diameter; nasal flaring; orthopnea; prolonged expiration phase; pursed-lip breathing; tachypnea; use of accessory muscles to breathe

Related Factors (r/t)

Anxiety; body position; bony deformity; chest wall deformity; cognitive impairment; fatigue; hyperventilation; hypoventilation syndrome; musculoskeletal impairment; neurological immaturity; neuromuscular dysfunction; obesity; pain; perception impairment; respiratory muscle fatigue; spinal cord injury

 (Nursing Outcomes Classification)

Suggested NOC Outcomes

Respiratory Status: Airway Patency, Ventilation; Vital Signs

Example NOC Outcome with Indicators
Respiratory Status: Ventilation as evidenced by the following indicators: Respiratory rate/ Respiratory rhythm/ Depth of inspiration/Chest expansion symmetrical/Ease of breathing/Tidal volume/Vital capacity (Rate each indicator of **Respiratory Status: Ventilation:** 1 = severe deviation from normal range, 2 = substantial deviation from normal range, 3 = moderate deviation from normal range, 4 = mild deviation from normal range, 5 = no deviation from normal range [see Section I].)

Client Outcomes

Client Will (Specify Time Frame):

- Demonstrate a breathing pattern that supports blood gas results within the client's normal parameters
- Report ability to breathe comfortably
- Demonstrate ability to perform pursed-lip breathing and controlled breathing
- Identify and avoid specific factors that exacerbate episodes of ineffective breathing patterns

NIC   **(Nursing Interventions Classification)**

Suggested NIC Interventions

Airway Management, Respiratory Monitoring

Example NIC Activities—Airway Management
Encourage slow, deep breathing; turning; and coughing; Monitor respiratory and oxygenation status as appropriate

Nursing Interventions and *Rationales*

- Monitor respiratory rate, depth, and ease of respiration. Normal respiratory rate is 14 to 16 breaths/min in the adult (Bickley & Szilagyi, 2009). **EBN:** *When the respiratory rate exceeds 30 breaths/min, along with other physiological measures, a study demonstrated that a significant physiological alteration existed (Considine, 2005; Hagle, 2008).*
- Note pattern of respiration. If client is dyspneic, note what seems to cause the dyspnea, the way in which the client deals with the condition, and how the dyspnea resolves or gets worse.
- Note amount of anxiety associated with the dyspnea. *A normal respiratory pattern is regular in a healthy adult. To assess dyspnea, it is important to consider all of its dimensions, including antecedents, mediators, reactions, and outcomes.* **EBN:** *A qualitative study demonstrated that experienced nurses working with COPD clients frequently used the degree of anxiety as an indicator of an acute exacerbation of COPD (Bailey, Colella, & Mossey, 2004).*
- Attempt to determine if client's dyspnea is physiological or psychological in cause. **EB:** *A study found that when the cause was psychological (medically unexplained dyspnea), there was affective*

• = Independent   ▲ = Collaborative   **EBN** = Evidence-Based Nursing   **EB** = Evidence-Based

dyspnea, anxiety, and tingling in the extremities. Whereas when the dyspnea was physiological, there was associated wheezing, cough, sputum, and palpitations (Han et al, 2008).

Psychological Dyspnea—Hyperventilation

- Monitor for symptoms of hyperventilation including rapid respiratory rate, sighing breaths, light-headedness, numbness and tingling of hands and feet, palpitations, and sometimes chest pain (Bickley & Szilagyi, 2009).
- Assess cause of hyperventilation by asking client about current emotions and psychological state. **EB:** *A study demonstrated that clients with idiopathic hyperventilation were more anxious and had a higher depression score than control subjects (Jack et al, 2004).*
- Ask the client to breathe with you to slow down respiratory rate. *Maintain eye contact and give reassurance. By making the client aware of respirations and giving support, the client may gain control of the breathing rate.*
- ▲ Consider having the client breathe in and out of a paper bag as tolerated. *This simple treatment helps associated symptoms of hypervention including help retain carbon dioxide which will decrease associated symptoms of hyperventilation (Bickley & Szilagyi, 2009).*
- ▲ If client has chronic problems with hyperventilation, numbness and tingling in extremities, dizziness, and other signs of panic attacks, refer for counseling. **EB:** *Cognitive behavioral therapy can be helpful for panic attacks, as can also respiratory feedback utilizing measurement of CO_2 levels using a capnometry device to give the client feedback on rate and depth of breathing (Meuret, Wilhelm, & Roth, 2004).*

Physiological Dyspnea

- ▲ Ensure that client in acute dyspneic state has received any ordered medications, oxygen, and any other treatment needed.
- Determine severity of dyspnea using a rating scale such as the modified Borg scale, rating dyspnea 0 (best) to 10 (worst) in severity. An alternative scale is the Visual Analogue Scale (VAS) with dyspnea rated as 0 (best) to 100 (worst). **EBN and EB:** *In an emergency room study, the modified Borg scale correlated well with clinical measurements of respiratory function and was found helpful by both clients and nurses (Kendrick, Baxi, & Smith, 2000).*
- Note use of accessory muscles, nasal flaring, retractions, irritability, confusion, or lethargy. *These symptoms signal increasing respiratory difficulty and increasing hypoxia.*
- Observe color of tongue, oral mucosa, and skin for signs of cyanosis. *Cyanosis of the tongue and oral mucosa is central cyanosis and generally represents a medical emergency. Peripheral cyanosis of nail beds or lips may or may not be serious (Fauci et al, 2008; Bickley & Szilagyi, 2009).*
- Auscultate breath sounds, noting decreased or absent sounds, crackles, or wheezes. *These abnormal lung sounds can indicate a respiratory pathology associated with an altered breathing pattern.*
- ▲ Monitor oxygen saturation continuously using pulse oximetry. Note blood gas results as available. *An oxygen saturation of less than 90% (normal: 95% to 100%) or a partial pressure of oxygen of less than 80 mm Hg (normal: 80 to 100 mm Hg) indicates significant oxygenation problems (Clark, Giuliano, & Chen, 2006).*
- Using touch on the shoulder, coach the client to slow respiratory rate, demonstrating slower respirations; making eye contact with the client; and communicating in a calm, supportive fashion. *The nurse's presence, reassurance, and help in controlling the client's breathing can be beneficial in decreasing anxiety.* **EBN:** *A study demonstrated that anxiety is an important indicator of severity of client's disease with COPD (Bailey, 2004).*
- Support the client in using pursed-lip and controlled breathing techniques. *Pursed-lip breathing results in increased use of intercostal muscles, decreased respiratory rate, increased tidal volume, and improved oxygen saturation levels (Dechman & Wilson, 2004; Faager, Stahle, & Larsen, 2008).* **EBN:** *A systematic review found pursed-lip breathing effective in decreasing dyspnea (Carrieri-Kohlman & Donesky-Cuenco, 2008).*
- If the client is acutely dyspneic, consider having the client lean forward over a bedside table, resting elbows on the table if tolerated. *Leaning forward can help decrease dyspnea, possibly because gastric pressure allows better contraction of the diaphragm (Langer et al, 2009). This is called the tripod position and is used during times of distress, including when walking.*

• = Independent   ▲ = Collaborative   **EBN** = Evidence-Based Nursing   **EB** = Evidence-Based

- Position the client in an upright or semi-Fowler's position. *An upright position facilitates lung expansion.* See Nursing Interventions and Rationales for **Impaired Gas exchange** for further information on positioning.
▲ Administer oxygen as ordered. *Oxygen administration has been shown to correct hypoxemia which causes dyspnea (Wong & Elliott, 2009).*
- Increase client's activity to walking three times per day as tolerated. Assist the client to use oxygen during activity as needed. See Nursing Interventions and Rationales for **Activity intolerance**. *Supervised exercise has been shown to decrease dyspnea and increase tolerance to activity (Fauci et al, 2008).*
- Schedule rest periods before and after activity. *Respiratory clients with dyspnea are easily exhausted and need additional rest.*
▲ Evaluate the client's nutritional status. Refer to a dietitian if needed. Use nutritional supplements to increase nutritional level if needed. *Improved nutrition may help increase inspiratory muscle function and decrease dyspnea.* **EBN:** *a study found that almost half of a group of client with COPD were malnourished, which can lead to an exacerbation of the disease (Odencrants, Ehnfors, & Ehrenbert, 2008).*
- Provide small, frequent feedings. *Small feedings are given to avoid compromising ventilatory effort and to conserve energy. Clients with dyspnea often do not eat sufficient amounts of food because their priority is breathing.*
- Offer a fan to move the air in the environment. **EBN:** *A systematic review found that the movement of cool air on the face can be effective in relieving dyspnea in pulmonary clients (Carrieri-Kohlman & Donesky-Cuenco, 2008).*
- Encourage the client to take deep breaths at prescribed intervals and do controlled coughing.
- Help the client with chronic respiratory disease to evaluate dyspnea experience to determine if similar to previous incidences of dyspnea and to recognize that he or she made it through those incidences. Encourage the client to be self-reliant if possible, use problem-solving skills, and maximize use of social support. *The focus of attention on sensations of breathlessness has an impact on judgment used to determine the intensity of the sensation.* **EBN:** *A study demonstrated that the most frequently used coping styles for clients with COPD were being optimistic and self-reliant, using problem-solving skills, and receiving social support (Baker & Scholz, 2002).*
- See **Ineffective Airway clearance** if client has a problem with increased respiratory secretions.
▲ Refer the COPD client for pulmonary rehabilitation. **EB:** *A Cochrane study found pulmonary rehabilitation programs highly effective and safe for a client who has an exacerbation of COPD (Puhan et al, 2009).*

Geriatric

- Encourage ambulation as tolerated. *Immobility is harmful to the elderly because it decreases ventilation and increases stasis of secretions (Fletcher, 2005).*
- Encourage elderly clients to sit upright or stand and to avoid lying down for prolonged periods during the day. *Thoracic aging results in decreased lung expansion; an erect position fosters maximal lung expansion (Fletcher, 2005).*

Home Care

- The above interventions may be adapted for home care use.
- Work with the client to determine what strategies are most helpful during times of dypsnea. Educate and empower the client to self-manage the disease associated with impaired gas exchange. **EBN and EB:** *A study found that use of oxygen, self use of medication and getting some fresh air were most helpful in dealing with dyspnea (Thomas, 2009). Evidence-based reviews have found that self-management offers COPD clients effective options for managing the illness, leading to more positive outcomes (Kaptein et al, 2008).*
- Assist the client and family with identifying other factors that precipitate or exacerbate episodes of ineffective breathing patterns (i.e., stress, allergens, stairs, activities that have high energy requirements). *Awareness of precipitating factors helps clients avoid them and decreases risk of ineffective breathing episodes.*

• = Independent   ▲ = Collaborative   **EBN** = Evidence-Based Nursing   **EB** = Evidence-Based

- Assess client knowledge of and compliance with medication regimen. *Client/family may need repetition of instructions received at hospital discharge, and may require reiteration as fear of a recent crisis decreases. Fear interferes with the ability to assimilate new information.*
- ▲ Refer the client for telemonitoring with a pulmonologist as appropriate, with use of an electronic spirometer, or an electronic peak flowmeter. **EB:** *A systematic review of home telemonitoring for conditions such as COPD, asthma, and lung transplantation found that use of telemonitoring resulted in early detection of deterioration of clients' respiratory status, and positive client receptiveness to the approach (Jaana, Paré, & Sicotte, 2009).*
- Teach the client and family the importance of maintaining the therapeutic regimen and having PRN drugs easily accessible at all times. *Appropriate and timely use of medications can decrease the risk of exacerbating ineffective breathing.* **EBN:** *Parents/family have been found to have inadequate knowledge about recognition of asthma attacks, triggers, and management (Navaie-Waliser et al, 2004).*
- Provide the client with emotional support in dealing with symptoms of respiratory difficulty. Provide family with support for care of a client with chronic or terminal illness. Refer to care plan for **Anxiety.** *Witnessing breathing difficulties and facing concerns of dealing with chronic or terminal illness can create fear in caregiver. Fear inhibits effective coping.*
- When respiratory procedures (e.g., apneic monitoring for an infant) are being implemented, explain equipment and procedures to family members, and provide needed emotional support. *Family members assuming responsibility for respiratory monitoring often find this stressful. They may not have been able to assimilate fully any instructions provided by hospital staff.*
- When electrically based equipment for respiratory support is being implemented, evaluate home environment for electrical safety, proper grounding, etc. Ensure that notification is sent to the local utility company, the emergency medical team, police and fire departments. *Notification is important to provide for priority service.*
- Refer to GOLD and ACP-ASIM/ACCP guidelines for management of home care and indications of hospital admission criteria (Chojnowski, 2003).
- Support clients' efforts at self-care. Ensure they have all the information they need to participate in care.
- Identify an emergency plan including when to call the physician or 911. *Having a ready emergency plan reassures the client and promotes client safety.*
- ▲ Refer to occupational therapy for evaluation and teaching of energy conservation techniques.
- ▲ Refer to home health aide services as needed to support energy conservation. *Energy conservation decreases the risk of exacerbating ineffective breathing.*
- ▲ Institute case management of frail elderly to support continued independent living.

Client/Family Teaching and Discharge Planning

- Teach pursed-lip and controlled breathing techniques. **EB:** *Studies have demonstrated that pursed-lip breathing was effective in decreasing breathlessness and improving respiratory function (Nield, Hoo, & Roper, 2007; Faager, Stahle, & Larsen, 2008).*
- Teach about dosage, actions, and side effects of medications. *Inhaled steroids and bronchodilators can have undesirable side effects, especially when taken in inappropriate doses.*
- Using a prerecorded tape, teach client progressive muscle relaxation techniques. **EB:** *Relaxation therapy can help reduce dyspnea and anxiety (National Lung Health Education Program, 2007; Langer et al, 2009).*
- Teach the client to identify and avoid specific factors that exacerbate ineffective breathing patterns, such as exposure to other sources of air pollution, especially smoking. If client smokes, refer to the smoking cessation section in the **Impaired Gas exchange** care plan.

Ⓔvolve   See the EVOLVE website for Weblinks for client education resource.

REFERENCES

Baker CF, Scholz JA: Coping with symptoms of dyspnea in chronic obstructive pulmonary disease, *Rehabil Nurs* 27(2):67, 2002.

Bailey PH: The dyspnea-anxiety-dypsnea cycle—COPD patients stories of breathlessness: "It's scary when you can't breathe," *Qual Health Res* 14(6):760, 2004.

Bailey PH, Colella T, Mossey S: COPD-intuition or template: nurses' stories of acute exacerbations of chronic obstructive pulmonary disease, *J Clin Nurs* 13(6):756, 2004.

Bickley LS, Szilagyi P: *Guide to physical examination*, ed 10, Philadelphia, 2009, Lippincott.

Carrieri-Kohlman V, Donesky-Cuenco D: Dyspnea management. An EBP guideline. In Ackley B, Ladwig, G, Swann BA et al, editors: *Evidence-based nursing care guidelines: medical-surgical Interventions*, Philadelphia, 2008, Mosby.

Chojnowski D: "GOLD" standards for acute exacerbation in COPD, *Nurs Pract* 28(5):26, 2003.

Clark AP, Giuliano K, Chen HM: Pulse oximetry revised, *Clin Nurse Spec* 20(6):268–272, 2006.

Considine J: The role of nurses in preventing adverse events related to respiratory dysfunction: literature review, *J Adv Nurs* 49(6):624–633, 2005.

Dechman G, Wilson CR: Evidence underlying breathing retraining in people with stable chronic obstructive pulmonary disease, *Phys Ther* 84(12):1189, 2004.

Faager G, Stahle A, Larsen FF: Influence of spontaneous pursed lips breathing on walking endurance and oxygen saturation in patients with moderate to severe chronic obstructive pulmonary disease, *Clin Rehabil* 22(8):675–683, 2008.

Fauci et al: *Harrison's principles of internal medicine*, ed 17, New York, 2008, McGraw-Hill.

Fletcher K: Immobility: geriatric self-learning module, *Medsurg Nurs* 14(1):35, 2005.

Hagle, M: Vital signs monitoring. An EBP guideline in: Ackley B, Ladwig, G, Swann BA et al, editors: *Evidence-based nursing care guidelines: medical-surgical interventions*, Philadelphia, 2008, Mosby.

Han J, Zhu Y, Li S et al: The language of medically unexplained dyspnea, *Chest* 133(4):961–968, 2008.

Jack S, Rossiter HB, Pearson MG et al: Ventilatory responses to inhaled carbon dioxide, hypoxia, and exercise in idiopathic hyper-ventilation, *Am J Respir Crit Care Med* 170(2):118, 2004.

Jaana M, Paré G, Sicotte C: Home telemonitoring for respiratory conditions: a systematic review, *Am J Manage Care* (5):313–320, 2009.

Kaptein AA, Scharloo M, Fischer MJ et al: 50 years of psychological research on patients with COPD—road to ruin or highway to heaven? *Resp Med* 103:3–11, 2008.

Kendrick KR, Baxi SC, Smith RM: Usefulness of the modified 1–10 Borg scale in assessing the degree of dyspnea in patients with COPD and asthma, *J Emerg Nurs* 26(3):216, 2000.

Langer D, Hendriks E, Burtin C et al: A clinical practice guideline for physiotherapists treating patients with chronic obstructive pulmonary disease based on a systematic review of available evidence, *Clinc Rehabil* 23(5):445–462, 2009.

Meuret AE, Wilhelm FH, Roth WT: Respiratory feedback for treating panic disorder, *J Clin Psychol* 60(2):197, 2004.

National Lung Health Education Program: a breath of fresh air, *Consum Rep Hlth* 19(2):3–6, 2007.

Navaie-Waliser M, Misener M, Mersman C et al: Evaluating the needs of children with asthma in home care: the vital role of nurses as caregivers and educators, *Public Health Nurs* 21(4):306, 2004.

Nield MA, Hoo GWS, Roper JM: Efficacy of pursed-lips breathing: a breathing pattern retraining strategy for dyspnea reduction, *J Cardiopul Rehabil Prev* 27(4):237–244, 2007.

Odencrants S, Ehnfors M, Ehrenbert A: Nutritional status and patient characteristics for hospitalized older patients with chronic obstructive pulmonary disease, *J Clin Nurs* 17(13):1771–1778, 2008.

Puhan M, Scharplatz M, Troosters T et al: Pulmonary rehabilitation following exacerbations of chronic obstructive pulmonary disease, *Cochrane Database Syst Rev* (1):CD005305, 2009.

Thomas L: Effective dyspnea management strategies identified by elders with end-stage chronic obstructive pulmonary disease, *Appl Nurs Res* 22(2):79–85, 2009.

Wong M, Elliott M: The use of medical orders in acute care oxygen therapy, *Br J Nurs* 18(8):462–464, 2009.

Decreased Cardiac output

Maryanne Crowther, MSN, APN, CCRN, and Lorraine A. Duggan, MSN, RN, APNC

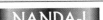

Definition

Inadequate volume of blood pumped by the heart per minute to meet metabolic demands of the body

Defining Characteristics

Altered Heart Rate/Rhythm

Arrhythmias; bradycardia; electrocardiographic changes; palpitations; tachycardia

Altered Preload

Edema; decreased central venous pressure (CVP); decreased pulmonary artery wedge pressure (PAWP); fatigue; increased central venous pressure (CVP); increased pulmonary artery wedge pressure (PAWP); jugular vein distention; murmurs; weight gain

Altered Afterload

Clammy skin; dyspnea; decreased peripheral pulses; decreased pulmonary vascular resistance (PVR); decreased systemic vascular resistance (SVR); increased pulmonary vascular resistance (PVR);

• = Independent   ▲ = Collaborative   **EBN** = Evidence-Based Nursing   **EB** = Evidence-Based

increased systemic vascular resistance (SVR); oliguria, prolonged capillary refill; skin color changes; variations in blood pressure readings

Altered Contractility

Crackles; cough; decreased ejection fraction; decreased left ventricular stroke work index (LVSWI); decreased stroke volume index (SVI); decreased cardiac index; decreased cardiac output; orthopnea; paroxysmal nocturnal dyspnea; S3 sounds; S4 sounds

Behavioral/Emotional

Anxiety; restlessness

Related Factors (r/t)

Altered heart rate; altered heart rhythm; altered stroke volume: altered preload, altered afterload, altered contractility

 (Nursing Outcomes Classification)

Suggested NOC Outcomes

Cardiac Pump Effectiveness, Circulation Status, Tissue Perfusion: Abdominal Organs, Peripheral, Vital Signs

Example NOC Outcome with Indicators
Cardiac Pump Effectiveness as evidenced by the following indicators: Blood pressure/Heart rate/Cardiac index/Ejection fraction/Activity tolerance/Peripheral pulses/NVD not present/Heart rhythm/Heart sounds/Angina not present/Peripheral edema not present/Pulmonary edema not present (Rate the outcome and indicators of **Cardiac Pump Effectiveness:** 1 = severe deviation from normal range, 2 = substantial deviation from normal range, 3 = moderate deviation from normal range, 4 = mild deviation from normal range, 5 = no deviation from normal range [see Section I].)

Client Outcomes

Client Will (Specify Time Frame):

- Demonstrate adequate cardiac output as evidenced by blood pressure and pulse rate and rhythm within normal parameters for client; strong peripheral pulses; and an ability to tolerate activity without symptoms of dyspnea, syncope, or chest pain
- Remain free of side effects from the medications used to achieve adequate cardiac output
- Explain actions and precautions to take for primary or secondary prevention of cardiac disease

NIC **(Nursing Interventions Classification)**

Suggested NIC Interventions

Cardiac Care, Cardiac Care: Acute

Example NIC Activities—Cardiac Care
Evaluate chest pain (e.g., intensity, location, radiation, duration, and precipitating and alleviating factors); Document cardiac dysrhythmias

Nursing Interventions and *Rationales*

- Monitor for symptoms of heart failure (HF) and decreased cardiac output; listen to heart sounds, lung sounds; note symptoms, including dyspnea, orthopnea, paroxysmal nocturnal dyspnea, Cheyne-Stokes respirations, fatigue, weakness, third and fourth heart sounds, crackles in lungs, increased venous pressure greater than 16 cm H2O, and positive hepatojugular reflex. *These are major criteria for diagnosis of HF—the Framingham Criteria (Kasper et al, 2005).*
- ▲ Administer oxygen as needed per physician's order. Supplemental oxygen increases oxygen availability to the myocardium. **EB:** *Clinical practice guidelines cite that oxygen should be administered to*

● = Independent   ▲ = Collaborative   **EBN** = Evidence-Based Nursing   **EB** = Evidence-Based

relieve symptoms related to hypoxemia (Jessup, et al, 2009). **EB:** *A study that assessed effectiveness of nasal cannula oxygen supplement for nocturnal obstructive sleep apnea found that 75% of HF clients had sleep apnea, and those who exhibited central sleep apnea had significantly reduced episodes when wearing nasal oxygen during sleep (Sakakibara et al, 2005).*

▲ If chest pain is present, have client lie down, monitor cardiac rhythm, give oxygen, check vital signs, run a monitor strip, medicate for pain, and notify the physician. *Prompt assessment of the client with acute coronary symptoms is critical because the incidence of ventricular fibrillation is 15 times greater during the first hour after symptoms of an acute myocardial infarction (Newberry, 2003).*

• Assess pulse oximetry regularly, using a forehead sensor if needed. **EBN:** *In a study that compared oxygen saturation values of arterial blood gases to various sensors, it was found that the forehead sensor was significantly better than the digit sensor for accuracy in clients with low cardiac output, while being easy to use and not interfering with client care (Fernandez et al, 2007).*

• Place client in semi-Fowler's or high Fowler's position with legs down or in a position of comfort. *Elevating the head of the bed and legs in down position may decrease the work of breathing and may also decrease venous return and preload.*

• During acute events, ensure client remains on short-term bed rest or maintains activity level that does not compromise cardiac output. *In severe HF, restriction of activity reduces the workload of the heart (Fauci et al, 2008).*

• Provide a restful environment by minimizing controllable stressors and unnecessary disturbances. Schedule rest periods after meals and activities. *Rest helps lower arterial pressure and reduce the workload of the myocardium by diminishing the requirements for cardiac output (Fauci et al, 2008).*

▲ Apply graduated compression stockings as ordered. Ensure proper fit by measuring accurately. Remove the stocking at least twice a day, then reapply. Assess the condition of the extremity frequently. **EBN:** *A study that assessed use of knee-length graduated compression stockings found they are as effective as thigh-length graduated compression stockings. They are more comfortable for clients, are easier for staff and clients to use, pose less risk of injury to clients, and are less expensive as recommended in this study (Hilleren-Listerud, 2009).* **EB:** *Graduated compression stockings, alone or used in conjunction with other prevention modalities, help promote venous return and prevent deep vein thrombosis in hospitalized clients (Amarigiri & Lees, 2005).*

▲ Check blood pressure, pulse, and condition before administering cardiac medications such as angiotensin-converting enzyme (ACE) inhibitors, digoxin, calcium channel blockers, and beta-blockers such as carvedilol. Notify physician if heart rate or blood pressure is low before holding medications. *It is important that the nurse evaluate how well the client is tolerating current medications before administering cardiac medications; do not hold medications without physician input. The physician may decide to have medications administered even though the blood pressure or pulse rate has lowered.*

• Observe for chest pain or discomfort; note location, radiation, severity, quality, duration, associated manifestations such as nausea, indigestion, and diaphoresis; also note precipitating and relieving factors. *Chest pain/discomfort is generally indicative of an inadequate blood supply to the heart, which can compromise cardiac output. Clients with HF can continue to have chest pain with angina or can reinfarct.*

• Recognize the effect of sleep disordered breathing in HF. **EB:** *A study that assessed effectiveness of nasal cannula oxygen supplement for nocturnal obstructive sleep apnea found that 75% of HF clients had sleep apnea, and those who exhibited central sleep apnea had significantly reduced episodes when wearing nasal oxygen during sleep (Sakakibara et al, 2005).* **EBN:** *Sleep-disordered breathing, including obstructive sleep apnea and Cheyne-Stokes with central sleep apnea, are common organic sleep disorders in clients with chronic HF and are a poor prognostic sign associated with higher mortality (Brostrom et al, 2004).*

▲ If intravenous fluid is ordered for circulatory failure, administer cautiously and observe for signs of fluid overload. Administering excessive volume is detrimental to cardiac output. **EB:** *The response to rapid fluid loading can be predicted noninvasively by changes in pulse pressure during passive leg raising in clients with acute circulatory failure who were receiving mechanical ventilation (Boulain et al, 2002).*

▲ Closely monitor fluid intake, including intravenous lines. *Maintain fluid restriction if ordered. In clients with decreased cardiac output, poorly functioning ventricles may not tolerate increased fluid volumes.*

• = Independent   ▲ = Collaborative   **EBN** = Evidence-Based Nursing   **EB** = Evidence-Based

- Monitor intake and output. If client is acutely ill, measure hourly urine output and note decreases in output **EB:** *Clinical practice guidelines cite that monitoring I&Os are useful for monitoring effects of diuretic therapy (Jessup et al, 2009). Decreased cardiac output results in decreased perfusion of the kidneys, with a resulting decrease in urine output.*
- ▲ Note results of electrocardiography and chest radiography. **EB:** *Clinical practice guidelines suggest that chest radiography and electrocardiogram are key tests in the assessment of HF (Jessup et al, 2009). HF is strongly suggested by the presence of cardiomegaly or pulmonary vascular congestion on the chest radiograph. The probability of HF is increased by anterior Q waves or left bundle branch block on the electrocardiogram (Dosh, 2004).*
- ▲ Note results of diagnostic imaging studies such as echocardiogram, radionuclide imaging, or dobutamine-stress echocardiography. **EB:** *Clinical practice guidelines state that the echocardiogram is a key test in the assessment of HF (Jessup et al, 2009). The ejection fraction (EF) is often quoted as a measure of left ventricular function, with an EF <40% indicating clinical HF (Williams & Kearney, 2002).*
- ▲ Watch laboratory data closely, especially arterial blood gases, electrolytes including potassium and magnesium, digoxin level, and B-type natriuretic peptide (BNP assay). **EB:** *A comparative study of aldosterone antagonists used for LVSD found that monitoring potassium and kidney function are essential to minimize the potential for life-threatening hyperkalemia that can occur from renal insufficiency, diabetes mellitus, advanced HF, advanced age, and concurrent drug therapy (Marcy & Ripley, 2006).* **EB:** *A systematic review that assessed addition of an ARB to ACE Inhibitors for control of HF from LVSD found that there was a significantly increased risk of hyperkalemia when agents from these two classes were combined (Lakhdar, Al-Mallah, & Lanfear, 2008).* **EB:** *Administering magnesium helps to control hypokalemia (Tang & Young, 2006).* **EB:** *In a study that assessed effects of serum digoxin concentrations on outcomes of HF clients at or over age 65, it was found that low serum digoxin concentrations (found with low-dose digoxin) reduced all-cause mortality and all-cause hospitalizations in older adults with HF and offered lower risk of digoxin toxicity (Ahmed, 2007). Client may be receiving cardiac glycosides and the potential for toxicity is greater with hypokalemia; hypokalemia is common in heart clients because of diuretic use (Fauci et al, 2008).* **EB:** *Clinical practice guidelines recommend that BNP or NTpro-BNP assay should be measured in clients when the contribution of HF is not known (Jessup et al, 2009).*
- ▲ Monitor laboratory work such as complete blood count (CBC), sodium level, and serum creatinine. Routine blood work can provide insight into the etiology of HF and extent of decompensation. **EB:** *In a randomized study to assess whether anemia is a risk factor for kidney dysfunction in HF clients, it was found that anemia was associated with a rapid decrease in kidney function in HF clients, especially in those with underlying chronic kidney disease. (Bansal et al, 2007).* **EB:** *A study assessed hyponatremia as a prognostic indicator in clients with preserved left ventricular function and found that hyponatremia at first hospitalization is a powerful predictor of long-term mortality in this group (Rusinaru et al, 2009). Serum creatinine levels will elevate in clients with severe HF because of decreased perfusion to the kidneys.*
- Gradually increase activity when client's condition is stabilized by encouraging slower paced activities or shorter periods of activity with frequent rest periods following exercise prescription; observe for symptoms of intolerance. Take blood pressure and pulse before and after activity and note changes. *Activity of the cardiac client should be closely monitored.* See **Activity intolerance.**
- ▲ Serve small, frequent, sodium-restricted, low-cholesterol meals. Sodium-restricted diets help decrease fluid volume excess. Low-cholesterol diets help decrease atherosclerosis, which causes coronary artery disease. *Clients with cardiac disease tolerate smaller meals better because they require less cardiac output to digest.* **EB:** *A study that assessed whether an association existed between breakfast cereal intake and HF found that over a 19–year period, higher intake of whole grain breakfast cereal was associated with lower risk of HF (Djousse & Graziano, 2007).* **EBN:** *A study that assessed gender differences in dietary sodium restriction found that women were more likely than men to recognize sodium buildup as fluid retention, and had a better understanding of what to take for a low sodium diet and were more adherent to the restriction (Chung et al, 2006).*
- Serve only small amounts of coffee or caffeine-containing beverages if requested (no more than four cups per 24 hours) if no resulting dysrhythmia. **EBN and EB:** *A review of studies on caffeine and cardiac arrhythmias concluded that moderate caffeine consumption does not increase the frequency or severity of cardiac arrhythmias (Schneider, 1987; Myers & Harris, 1990; Hogan, Hornick, & Bouchoux, 2002).*

● = Independent ▲ = Collaborative **EBN** = Evidence-Based Nursing **EB** = Evidence-Based

▲ Monitor bowel function. Provide stool softeners as ordered. Caution client not to strain when defecating. *Decreased activity can cause constipation, as well as pain medication. Straining when defecating that results in the Valsalva maneuver can lead to dysrhythmia, decreased cardiac function, and sometimes death.*

● Have clients use a commode or urinal for toileting and avoid use of a bedpan. *Getting out of bed to use a commode or urinal does not stress the heart any more than staying in bed to toilet. In addition, getting the client out of bed minimizes complications of immobility and is often preferred by the client (Winslow, 1992).*

● Weigh client at same time daily (after voiding). **EB:** *Clinical practice guidelines states that weighing at the same time daily is useful to assess effects of diuretic therapy (Jessup et al, 2009). Use the same scale if possible when weighing clients. Daily weight is also a good indicator of fluid balance. Increased weight and severity of symptoms can signal decreased cardiac function with retention of fluids.*

● Assess for presence of anxiety. See Nursing Interventions and Rationales for **Anxiety** to facilitate reduction of anxiety in clients and family. **EBN and EB:** *Descriptive studies have found higher complication rates following infarction in clients with increased anxiety (Moser & Dracup, 1996; Watkins, Blumenthal & Carney, 2002, Carpeggiani et al, 2005).*

▲ Refer for treatment if anxiety is present. **EB:** *In a study that assessed the association between client-reported difficulty taking medication, health status, and depression, it was found that difficulty taking medication is associated with worse health status which was explained in part by co-existing depression (Morgan et al, 2006). Depression is very common in HF clients and can result in increased mortality (Thomas et al, 2003).*

▲ Refer for treatment when depression is present. **EBN:** *A study that assessed health-related quality of life found that baseline depression, along with perceived control were strongest predictors of physical symptom status (Heo et al, 2008). **EB:** In a systematic review of HF clients it was found that 21% had clinically significant depression, which resulted in consistently higher rates of death, emergency department visits, hospitalizations, and health care use (Rutledge et al, 2006).*

▲ Refer to a cardiac rehabilitation program for education and monitored exercise. **EB:** *A study that analyzed baseline characteristics in HF clients for predicting cardiac events during exercise therapy found that a left ventricular end diastolic dimension at or over 65 mm at baseline was a significant predictor of cardiac events during the 12–week monitored exercise program (Nishi et al, 2007). **EB:** Exercise can help many clients with HF. Inactivity can worsen the skeletal muscle myopathy in these clients. A carefully monitored exercise program can improve both exercise capacity and quality of life in mild to moderate HF clients (Rees et al, 2004). Exercise-based cardiac rehabilitation is effective in reducing the number of cardiac deaths, decreasing cholesterol levels and systolic blood pressure, and reduced self-reported smoking (Jolliffe et al, 2001; Taylor et al, 2004).*

▲ Refer to HF program for education, evaluation, and guided support to increase activity and rebuild life. **EB:** *An assessment of a multidisciplinary HF center demonstrated that at 6 months, there were significant improvements in quality of life and significant reductions in HF hospitalizations (Omar et al, 2007). **EBN:** A study that assessed 3–year outcomes of a nurse practitioner–coordinated outpatient HF program found significantly reduced hospital readmissions, length of stay, and cost per case, as well as significantly improved quality of life, and functional status (Crowther & McCourt, 2004). **EBN:** A study assessing the 6–month outcomes of a nurse practitioner–coordinated HF Center found that readmissions, length of stay, and cost per case were all significantly reduced, while quality of life was significantly improved. (Crowther et al, 2002).*

▲ Be aware that cardiac resynchronization therapy improves cardiac output and may be ordered for appropriate clients. **EB:** *A meta-analyses found that both CRT-P and CRT-D devices significantly reduced mortality, HF hospitalizations and improved health-related quality of life in people with New York Heart Association (NYHA) class III and IV HF and evidence of dyssynchrony on optimal HF medications (Fox et al, 2007). **EB:** A study that quantified the effects of CRT on exercise pathophysiology of HF clients found that peak exercise cardiac output, stroke volume, maximal sustainable exercise capacity, and ventilation-perfusion mismatching all significantly improved with the device (Wasserman, Sun, & Hansen, 2007). **EB:** A systematic review of CRT of HF clients found that the device reduced all-cause mortality, HF hospitalizations and improved quality of life (Freemantle et al, 2006). **EB:** A study of both ischemic and nonischemic clients had increases in cardiac output after cardiac resynchronization therapy (Woo et al, 2005).*

▲ Be aware that chronic HF clients with LVSD may benefit from internal cardioverter defibrillators (ICDs). EB: A study comparing amiodarone to ICDs in NYHA class II and III HF clients found that ICDs were superior in their ability to decrease mortality by 23% (Bardy et al, 2005).

▲ Be aware that clients who have ICDs implanted are at risk for ventricular arrhythmias and internal defibrillation. **EBN:** *A study that assessed predictors of ICD shocks found that a history of ventricular tachycardia, HF, or COPD at implant were significant predictors of a defibrillation during the first year after implant (Dougherty & Hunziker, 2009).*

• Place electrode leads, defibrillator paddles, and transcutaneous medication away from the pacer or ICD implantation site. *This will help prevent damage to the devices that can affect their function.*

▲ Be aware that clients with refractory HF may have ultrafiltration ordered as a mechanical method to remove excess fluid volume **EB:** *Clinical practice guidelines cite that ultrafiltration is reasonable for clients with refractory HF not responsive to medical therapy (Jessup et al, 2009).* **EB:** *A study that assessed initial results of a small group of clients demonstrated that ultrafiltration variably removed fluid from clients with refractory advanced HF, although worsening renal function did occur in 45% of the sample (Liang et al, 2006).* **EB:** *A study that assessed ultrafiltraton to remove excess fluid volume in HF clients refractory to diuretics found that the procedure can safely and effectively be used to reduce length of hospitalization and readmissions (Costanzo et al, 2005).*

Critically III

▲ Observe for symptoms of cardiogenic shock, including impaired mentation, hypotension with blood pressure lower than 90 mm Hg, decreased peripheral pulses, cold clammy skin, signs of pulmonary congestion, and decreased organ function. If present, notify physician immediately. *Cardiogenic shock is a state of circulatory failure from loss from cardiac function associated with inadequate organ perfusion with a high mortality rate (Fuster et al, 2005).* **EBN:** *In a study the defining characteristics of decreased cardiac output were best indicated by decreased peripheral pulses and decreased peripheral perfusion (Oliva & Monteiro da Cruz, 2003).*

▲ If shock is present, monitor hemodynamic parameters for an increase in pulmonary wedge pressure, an increase in systemic vascular resistance, or a decrease in cardiac output and index. *Hemodynamic parameters give a good indication of cardiac function (Fauci et al, 2008).*

▲ Titrate inotropic and vasoactive medications within defined parameters to maintain contractility, preload, and afterload per physician's order. **EB:** *Clinical practice guidelines recommend that Intravenous inotropic drugs might be reasonable for HF clients presenting with low BP and low cardiac output to maintain systemic perfusion and preserve end-organ performance (Jessup et al, 2009). By following parameters, the nurse ensures maintenance of a delicate balance of medications that stimulate the heart to increase contractility, while maintaining adequate perfusion of the body.*

▲ Be aware that intraaortic balloon counterpulsation is implemented to treat cardiogenic shock by decreasing the workload of the left ventricle and improving myocardial perfusion (Reid & Cottrell, 2005).

▲ When using pulmonary arterial catheter technology, be sure to appropriately level and zero the equipment, use minimal tubing, maintain system patency, perform square wave testing, position the client appropriately, and consider correlation to respiratory and cardiac cycles when assessing waveforms and integrating data into client assessment. **EB:** *A clinical practice guideline recommends that invasive hemodynamic monitoring can be useful in acute HF with persistent symptoms when therapy is refractory, fluid status is unclear, systolic pressures are low, renal function is worsening, vasoactive agents are required, or when considering advanced device therapy or transplantation (Jessup et al, 2009).* **EB:** *Hemodynamic parameters are analyzed to assess cellular oxygen delivery, and cardiac output is a major determinant of oxygen delivery. Proper technique is imperative to accurate data collection (Adams, 2004).* **EBN:** *A study that assessed three different bed rest positions when measuring cardiac output by continuous method (using a heated filament in the PA catheter) at 0, 5, and 10 minutes after position changes demonstrated no differences in cardiac index across measurement conditions (Giuliano et al, 2003).*

▲ Recognize the importance of cardiac index estimated by thermodilution in the intensive care unit (ICU) client. **EBN:** *The cardiac index reflects with good precision the cardiac output of ICU clients and provides immediate results; in addition, the measurements are easy to repeat (Oliva & Monteiro da Cruz Dde, 2003).* **EB:** *Cardiac index is preferred to cardiac output to attenuate the effects of body mass index (BMI) (Stelfox et al, 2006).*

• = Independent   ▲ = Collaborative   **EBN** = Evidence-Based Nursing   **EB** = Evidence-Based

▲ Be aware of the utilization of other cardiac output techniques including the Fick Method and esophageal Doppler imaging. **EBN:** *A study assessing various methods for measuring cardiac output including bioimpedance, Fick, and thermodilution methods seem not to be interchangeable, although each can be trended separately, with the least accurate being the bioimpedance cardiography (Engoren & Barbee, 2005).* **EBN:** *There is good correlation between thermodilution and esophageal Doppler imaging methods (Iregui et al, 2003) and between thermodilution and bioimpedance methods for obtaining cardiac output (Albert, Hail, & Li, 2004).*

▲ Recognize that hemodynamic pressure and parameters can be obtained either before or after cardiac output measurement. **EBN:** *A study assessing hemodynamic parameter differences between precardiac and postcardiac output measurement found minimal differences between groups and concluded that hemodynamic parameters may be accurately obtained at either time (Urquhart & Jensen, 2003).* **EBN:** *A study assessing normal variations in hemodynamic parameters demonstrated normal fluctuations with values that vary under 8% for pulmonary artery systolic pressure, under 11% for pulmonary artery diastolic pressure, and under 12% for pulmonary artery wedge pressure in clients with left ventricular systolic dysfunction (Moser et al, 2002).*

▲ Be aware that clients with cardiogenic pulmonary edema may have noninvasive positive pressure ventilation (NPPV) ordered. **EB:** *A systematic review of NPPV for cardiogenic pulmonary edema found that use of NPPV significantly reduced mortality and intubation, while decreasing ICU stay by one day (Vital et al, 2009).*

▲ Be aware of the utilization of impedance cardiography in noninvasive hemodynamic monitoring of HF. **EB:** *A study that assessed ability of impedence cardiography to predict HF clinical deterioration found that the device was significantly accurate to identify clients at near-term risk of recurrent clinical decompensation (Packer et al, 2006).* **EB:** *Impedance cardiography has demonstrated diagnostic and prognostic value in emergent and chronic HF. It has been shown to aid in the diagnosis of cardiac versus noncardiac HF clients (Yancy & Abraham, 2003).* **EBN:** *Impedance cardiography has been well correlated with thermodilution in clients with decompensated complex HF (Albert, Hail, & Li, 2004).*

• Be aware that hypoperfusion from low cardiac output can lead to altered mental status. **EB:** *A study that assessed the relationship between hypoperfusion and neuropsychological performance found that among stable geriatric HF clients, executive functions of sequencing and planning were altered (Jefferson et al, 2007).*

Geriatric

• Observe for atypical pain; the elderly often have jaw pain instead of chest pain or may have silent myocardial infarctions (MIs) with symptoms of dyspnea or fatigue. *Symptoms, when present in older clients with an acute MI, may be extremely vague, and, as with myocardial ischemia, the diagnosis may be easily missed. Atypical symptoms of MI include dyspnea, neurologic symptoms, or gastrointestinal (GI) symptoms (Aronow & Silent, 2003).*

▲ If client has heart disease causing activity intolerance, refer for cardiac rehabilitation. **EB:** *The anxiety experienced after hospitalization is higher in elderly clients with heart disease compared to that of younger clients participating in exercise programs. (Twiss, Seaver, & McCaffrey, 2006).*

• Consider the use of graphic feedback with the elderly in exercise adherence. **EBN:** *The graphic format may be especially helpful because graphs provide a clear picture of the client's exercise goals and recent progress (Duncan & Pozehl, 2003).*

• Observe for syncope, dizziness, palpitations, or feelings of weakness associated with an irregular heart rhythm. *Dysrhythmias are common in the elderly.*

▲ Observe for side effects from cardiac medications. *The elderly have difficulty with metabolism and excretion of medications due to decreased function of the liver and kidneys; therefore toxic side effects are more common.*

Pediatrics

• Monitor heart rate continuously in the newborn and report abnormalities immediately. **EBN:** *Cardiac output in the newborn is dependent on heart rate, but has a decreased ability to maximize and vary heart rate (Sherman et al, 2002).*

Home Care

- Some of the above interventions may be adapted for home care use. Home care agencies may use specialized staff and methods to care for chronic HF clients. **EB:** *A study assessing HF outcomes over a 10–year period between a multidisciplinary home care intervention and usual care found significantly improved survival, and prolonged event-free survival and was both cost- and time-effective (Ingles et al, 2006).*

▲ Begin discharge planning as soon as possible upon admission to the emergency department (ED) with case manager or social worker to assess home support systems and the need for community or home health services. Consider referral for advanced practice nurse (APN) follow-up. Support services may be needed to assist with home care, meal preparations, housekeeping, personal care, transportation to doctor visits, or emotional support. *Case management begins in the ED and facilitates care throughout the client's stay (Conway, 2006).* **EB:** *A study to assess degree of social support as a predictor of HF readmission demonstrated that those without someone living with them had a greater readmission rate in a dose dependent response, but no correlation to death was found (Rodriguez-Artalejo et al, 2006). Clients often need help on discharge.* **EBN:** *In a randomized control trial, the assignment of an APN to assist with transition to the home for elders with HF resulted in greater length of time between hospitalizations, fewer total hospitalizations, and decreased health care costs. A study of transitional care using nonspecialist nurses found an improvement in the quality of life and a reduction in the number of emergency department visits with HF clients (Clark & Nadash, 2004).*

▲ Assess or refer to case manager or social worker to evaluate client ability to pay for prescriptions. *The cost of drugs may be a factor in filling prescriptions and adhering to a treatment plan.*

▲ Adopt a clinical pathway to address focused interventions with HF, coronary artery bypass graft (CABG). National Practice Guidelines for Cardiac Home Care are available to direct intervention for the client post-CABG who is recovering at home (Frantz & Walters, 2001). **EBN:** *Study of the outcome of a HF clinical pathway revealed a 45% reduction in rehospitalization (Hoskins et al, 2001; Young et al, 2004).*

▲ Continue to monitor client closely for exacerbation of HF when discharged home. *Transition to home can create increased stress and physiological instability related to diagnosis.* **EBN:** *Home visits and phone contacts that emphasize client education and recognition of early symptoms of exacerbation can decrease rehospitalization (Gorski & Johnson, 2003).*

▲ Monitor women for differential symptoms of MI and institute emergency treatment measures as indicated. **EBN:** *Continuing research is exploring differences in MI symptoms between men and women. A qualitative study of 40 women following MI noted prodromal symptoms. Most frequent were unusual fatigue, discomfort in the shoulder blade area, and chest sensations. Most common acute symptoms were chest sensations, shortness of breath, feeling hot and flushed, and unusual fatigue. Severe pain during the acute phase was experienced by only 11 women (McSweeney & Crane, 2000). African American and Caucasian women have different physical recovery trajectories from acute MI (prolonged) but similar psychosocial recovery trajectories (Rankin, 2002).*

- Instruct women in the differential symptoms of MI particular to women, and the need to take symptoms seriously and seek help as indicated. **EB:** *Women delay seeking help a median of 6.25 hours. Help-seeking behavior was influenced by beliefs about women's susceptibility to MI and differential symptom awareness. Symptoms presenting in this study were rarely consistent with those described in the health promotion literature (Holliday, Lowe, & Outram, 2000).*

- Assess client/family for understanding of and compliance with medical regimen, including medications, activity level, and diet. Client/family may need repetition of instructions received at hospital discharge, and may require reiteration as fear of a recent crisis decreases. *Fear interferes with the ability to assimilate new information.*

▲ Assess and monitor for signs of depression (particularly in adults age 65 years or older) or social isolation. Refer for mental health treatment as indicated. **EB:** *A study to assess changes in psychological, social, and spiritual needs of people with end-stage disease found that in advanced HF, social and psychological decline paralleled physical decline, while spiritual distress fluctuated (Murray et al, 2007).* **EB:** *A study that assessed depression in hospitalized HF clients found that depression is more common in elderly, especially women (Lesman-Leegte et al, 2006).* **EB:** *In a study that assessed the association between client-reported difficulty taking medication, health status, and depression, it was*

• = Independent ▲ = Collaborative **EBN** = Evidence-Based Nursing **EB** = Evidence-Based

found that difficulty taking medication is associated with worse health status which was explained in part by co-existing depression (Morgan et al, 2006). Depression is very common in HF clients and can result in increased mortality (Thomas et al, 2003). **EBN:** *Mood disturbance, social isolation, low socioeconomic status, and nonwhite ethnicity predicted lower functional status of clients with left ventricular dysfunction after 1 year (Clarke et al, 2000).* **EB:** *Depression has been noted as prevalent after acute MI in clients over age 65. Depression has been shown to be an independent risk factor for HF in elderly women but not in elderly men (Williams et al, 2002).*

- Assess for signs/symptoms of cognitive impairment. **EBN:** *Cognitive function may decline in late-stage HF (Quaglietti et al, 2004).*
- Assess for fatigue and weakness frequently. Assess home environment for safety, as well as resources/obstacles to energy conservation. Instruct client and family members on need for behavioral pacing and energy conservation. **EBN:** *Fatigue and weakness limit activity level and quality of life. Assistive devices and other techniques of work simplification can help the client participate in and respond to the health care regimen more effectively (Quaglietti et al, 2004).*
- Instruct family and client about the disease process, complications of disease process, information on medications, need for weighing daily, and when it is appropriate to call the doctor. *Early recognition of symptoms facilitates early problem solving and prompt treatment. Decreased cardiac output can be life threatening.* **EBN:** *Clients with HF need intensive education about these topics to help prevent readmission to the hospital (Moser, 2000).*
- Help family adapt daily living patterns to establish life changes that will maintain improved cardiac functioning in the client. Take the client's perspective into consideration, and use a holistic approach in assessing and responding to client planning for the future. *Transition to the home setting can cause risk factors such as inappropriate diet to reemerge.* **EBN:** *A study of women recovering from MI revealed that these women lived with a feeling of insecurity, based on a new inability to trust their bodies. Caring for women post-MI, researchers concluded, must approach health as being more than the absence of illness (Johansson, Dahlberg, & Ekebergh, 2003).*
- Assist client to recognize and exercise power in using self-care management to adjust to health change. **EBN:** *Women post-MI reported that not participating in their health process increased their suffering and left them feeling powerless (Johansson, Dahlberg, & Ekebergh, 2003).* Refer to care plan for **Powerlessness**.
- ▲ Explore barriers to medical regimen adherence. Review medications and treatment regularly for needed modifications. Take complaints of side effects seriously and serve as client advocate to address changes as indicated. *The presence of uncomfortable side effects frequently motivates clients to deviate from the medication regimen.*
- ▲ Refer for cardiac rehabilitation and strengthening exercises if client is not involved in outpatient cardiac rehabilitation. **EB:** *Exercise improves hemodynamic responsiveness in clients after uncomplicated acute myocardial infarction (Motohiro et al, 2005).*
- ▲ Refer to medical social services as necessary for counseling about the impact of severe or chronic cardiac disease. *Social workers can assist the client and family with acceptance of life changes.*
- ▲ Institute case management of frail elderly to support continued independent living.
- ▲ As client condition warrants, refer to hospice. *The multidisciplinary hospice team can reduce hospital readmission, increase functional capacity, and improve quality of life in end-stage HF (Coviello, Hricz, & Masulli, 2002).*
- Identify emergency plan, including use of cardiopulmonary resuscitation (CPR). Encourage family members to become certified in cardiopulmonary resuscitation. **EBN:** *CPR training significantly increased perceived control in spouses of recovering cardiac clients (Moser & Dracup, 2000).*

Client/Family Teaching and Discharge Planning

- Include significant others in client teaching opportunities. **EB:** *A study that assessed the influence of significant-other support in HF client care found that increased social support was moderately associated with medication and dietary adherence, among other aspects of self-care (Gwadry-Sridhar et al, 2008).*
- Teach symptoms of HF and appropriate actions to take if client becomes symptomatic.
- Teach importance of smoking cessation and avoidance of alcohol intake. Smoking is a well-established risk factor for coronary artery disease. Help clients who smoke stop by informing them

● = Independent ▲ = Collaborative   **EBN** = Evidence-Based Nursing   **EB** = Evidence-Based

of potential consequences and by helping them find an effective cessation method. **EB:** *Smoking cessation advice and counsel given by nurses can be effective, and should be available to clients to help stop smoking (Rice & Stead, 2000).* **EB:** *A study assessing right heart hemodynamic values and respiratory function among chronic smokers found that cardiac output and respiratory function worsened significantly in this sample (Gulbaran et al, 2004).*

- Teach stress reduction (e.g., imagery, controlled breathing, muscle relaxation techniques). **EBN:** *A study that assessed effects of relaxation or exercise In HF clients versus controls found that those who participated in regular relaxation therapy or exercise training reported greater improvements in psychological outcomes with the relaxation group significantly improving depression and the exercise training group more improving fatigue (Yu et al, 2007).*

- Explain necessary restrictions, including consumption of a sodium-restricted diet, guidelines on fluid intake, and the avoidance of Valsalva maneuver. Teach the importance of pacing activities, work simplification techniques, and the need to rest between activities to prevent becoming overly fatigued. *Sodium retention leading to fluid overload is a common cause of hospital readmission (Fauci et al, 2008).*

- ▲ Teach the client actions, side effects, and importance of consistently taking cardiovascular medications. **EB:** *Taking medication as directed can help prevent HF decompensation, rehospitalization. and morbidity (Jessup et al, 2009).* **EBN:** *A research study demonstrated that HF clients were not knowledgeable of the medications or for the need for weight monitoring and recognizing the definition for HF (Artinian et al, 2002).*

- Provide client/family with advance directive information to consider. Allow client to give advance directions about medical care or designate who should make medical decisions if he or she should lose decision-making capacity.

- ▲ Instruct the client on importance of getting a pneumonia shot (usually one per lifetime) and yearly influenza shots as prescribed by physician. *Clients with decreased cardiac output are considered higher risk for complications or death if they do not get immunization injections.*

- Instruct client/family on the need to weigh daily, take weights the same time daily and keep a weight log. Ask if client has a scale at home; if not, assist in getting one. Instruct on establishing baseline weight on own scale when gets home. **EB:** *Clinical practice guidelines suggests that daily weight monitoring leads to early recognition of excess fluid retention, which when reported, can be offset with additional medication to avoid hospitalization from HF decompensation (Jessup et al, 2009). Daily weighing is an essential aspect of self-management. A scale is necessary. Scales vary; the client needs to establish a baseline weight on his or her home scale.*

- Provide specific written materials and self-care plan for client/caregivers to use for reference.

- ▲ Consult dietitian or assist client in understanding the need for a sodium-restricted diet. Provide alternatives for salt such as spices, herbs, lemon juice, or vinegar. *Although the initial elimination of salt from the diet is very difficult, the taste of salt can be unlearned. The spices and seasonings above can enhance the taste appeal of food while the preference for salt is changing (Cataldo, DeBruyne, & Whitney, 2003). Taste sensation is often diminished as a function of age, producing a greater desire for salty foods (Forman & Rich, 2003).*

- Instruct family regarding cardiopulmonary resuscitation.

⊖volve   See the EVOLVE website for Weblinks for client education resources.

REFERENCES

Adams KL: Hemodynamic assessment: the physiologic basis for turning data into clinical information, *AACN Clinical Issues*, 15(4):534–546, 2004.

Ahmed A: Digoxin and reduction in mortality and hospitalization in geriatric heart failure: Importance of low doses and low serum concentrations, *J Gerontol* 62A(3): 323–329, 2007.

Albert NM, Hail MD, Li J: Equivalence of the bioimpedance and thermodilution methods in measuring cardiac output in hospitalized patients with advanced, decompensated chronic heart failure, *Am J Crit Care* 13(6):469, 2004.

Amarigiri SV, Lees TA: Elastic compression stockings for prevention of deep vein thrombosis, *Cochrane Database Syst Rev* (3):CD001484, 2005.

Aronow W, Silent MI: Prevalence and prognosis in older patients diagnosed by routine electrocardiograms, *Geriatrics* 58(1):24–26, 36–38, 40, 2003.

Artinian NT, Magnan M, Christian W et al: What do patients know about their heart failure? *Appl Nurs Res* 15(4):200, 2002.

Bansal N, Tighiourt H, Weiner D et al: Anemia as a risk factor for kidney function decline in individuals with heart failure, *Am J Cardiol* 99(8):1137–1142, 2007.

• = Independent   ▲ = Collaborative   **EBN** = Evidence-Based Nursing   **EB** = Evidence-Based

Bardy GH, Lee KL, Mark DB et al: Amiodarone or an implantable cardioverter-defibrillator for congestive heart failure, *N Engl J Med* 352(3):225–237, 2005.

Boulain T, Achard J, Teboul J et al: Changes in blood pressure induced by passive leg raising predict response to fluid loading in critically ill patients, *Chest* 121(4):1245–1253, 2002.

Brostrom A, Stromberg A, Dahlstrom U et al: Sleep difficulties, daytime sleepiness, and health-related quality of life in patients with chronic heart failure, *J Cardiovasc Nurs* 19(4):234, 2004.

Carpeggiani C, Emdin M, Bonaguidi F et al: Personality traits and heart rate variability predict long-term cardiac mortality after myocardial infarction. *Eur Heart J* 26(16):1612–1617, 2005.

Cataldo CB, DeBruyne LK, Whitney EN: *Nutrition and diet therapy*, ed 6, Belmont, CA, 2003, Thomson Wadsworth.

Chung ML, Moser DK, Lennie TA et al: Gender differences in adherence to the sodium-restricted diet in patients with heart failure, *J Card Fail* 12(8):628–634, 2006.

Clark A, Nadash P: The effectiveness of a nurse-led transitional care model for patients with congestive heart failure, *Home Healthc Nurs* 22(3):160, 2004.

Clarke SP, Frasure-Smith N, Lesperance F et al: Psychosocial factors as predictors of functional status at 1 year in patients with left ventricular dysfunction, *Res Nurs Health* 23:290–300, 2000.

Conway G: Case management for heart failure in the emergency department, *Crit Pathw Cardiol* 6(5):25–28, 2006.

Costanzo MR, Saltzberg M, O'Sullivan J et al: Early ultrafiltration in patients with decompensated heart failure and diuretic resistance, *J Am Coll Cardiol* 46(11):2047–2051, 2005.

Coviello JS, Hricz L, Masulli PS: Client challenge: accomplishing quality of life in end-stage heart failure: a hospice multidisciplinary approach, *Home Healthc Nurs* 20:195, 2002.

Crowther M, McCourt K: Three year outcomes: success of a hospital-based, nurse practitioner coordinated heart failure center. Poster Abstract, American Academy of Nurse Practitioners-19th National Conference for Nurse Practitioners, #26, 2004. http://66.219.50.180/NR/rdonlyres/epxs2t7owvhnlan5gpzvxvca2fe3hdlnfrhckb-cav6qjfk7nxmj2ktermbff5giicuav54lz4pd3op/NP%2BPoster%2B26.pdf. Accessed October 7, 2009.

Crowther M, Maroulis A, Shafer-Winter N et al: Evidence-based development of a hospital-based heart failure center, *Reflect Nurs Leadersh* 28(2):32–33, 2002.

Djousse L, Granziano M: Breakfast cereals and risk of heart failure in the physicians' health study I, *Arch Int Med* 167(19):2080–2085, 2007.

Dosh S: Diagnosis of heart failure in adults, *Am Fam Physician* 70(11):2145, 2004.

Dougherty CM, Hunziker J: Predictors of implantable cardioverter defibrillator shocks during the first year, *J Cardiovasc Nurs* 24(1):21–30, 2009.

Duncan K, Pozehl B: Effects of an exercise adherence intervention on outcomes in patients with heart failure, *Cardiac Rehab* 28(4):117, 2003.

Engoren M, Barbee D: Comparison of cardiac output determined by bioimpedance, thermodilution, and the Fick method, *Am J Crit Care* 14(1):40, 2005.

Fauci A, Braunwald E, Kasper DL et al: *Harrison's principles of internal medicine*, ed 17, New York, 2008, McGraw-Hill.

Fernandez M, Burns K, Calhoun B et al: Evaluation of a new pulse oximeter sensor, *Am J Crit Care* 16(2):146–152, 2007.

Forman D, Rich M: Heart failure in the elderly, *Congest Heart Fail* 9(6):311, 2003.

Fox M, Mealing S, Anderson R et al: The clinical effectiveness and cost-effectiveness of cardiac resynchronisation (biventricular pacing) for heart failure: systematic review and economic model, *Health Technol Assess* 11(47):iii-iv, ix-248, 2007.

Frantz AK, Walters JI: Recovery from coronary artery bypass grafting at home: is your practice current? *Home Healthc Nurs* 19:417, 2001.

Freemantle N, Tharmanathan P, Calvert MJ et al: Cardiac synchronization for patients with heart failure due to left ventricular systolic dysfunction—a systematic review and meta-analysis, *Eur J Heart Fail* 8(4):433–440, 2006.

Fuster V, Alexander RW, O'Rourke RA et al: *Hurst's the heart*, ed 11, vol 2, New York, 2005, McGraw Hill.

Giuliano KK, Scott SS, Brown V et al: Backrest angle and cardiac output measurement in critically ill patients, *Nurs Res* 52(4):242–248, 2003.

Gorski LA, Johnson K: A disease management program for heart failure: collaboration between a home care agency and a care management organization, *Home Healthc Nurs* 21(11):734, 2003.

Gulbaran M, Cagatay T, Gurman T et al: Right heart haemodynamic values and respiratory function test parameters in chronic smokers, *Eastern Mediterr Health J* 10(1/2):90–95, 2004.

Gwadry-Sridhar F, Guyatt G, O'Brien G et al: TEACH: Trial of Education And Compliance in heart dysfunction chronic disease and heart failure (HF) as an increasing problem, *Contemp Clin Trials* 29(6):905–918, 2008.

Heo S, Doering LV, Widener J et al: Predictors and effect of physical symptom status on health-related quality of life in patients with heart failure, *Am J Crit Care* 17:124–132, 2008.

Hilleren-Listerud AE: Graduated compression stocking and intermittent pneumatic compression device length selection, *Clin Nurse Spec* 23(1):21–24, 2009.

Hogan E, Hornick B, Bouchoux A: Communicating the message: clarifying the controversies about caffeine, *Nutr Today* 37(1):28, 2002.

Holliday JE, Lowe JM, Outram S: Women's experience of myocardial infarction, *Intl J Nurs Pract* 6:307, 2000.

Hoskins LM, Clark HM, Schroeder MA et al: A clinical pathway for congestive heart failure, *Home Healthc Nurs* 19:207, 2001.

Ingles SC, Pearson S, Treen S et al: Extending the horizon in chronic heart failure: effects of multidisciplinary, home-based intervention relative to usual care, *Circulation* 114(23):2466–73, 2006.

Iregui MG, Prentice D, Sherman G et al: Physicians' estimates of cardiac index and intravascular volume based on clinical assessment versus transesophageal Doppler measurements obtained by critical care nurses, *Am J Crit Care* 12(4):336–343, 2003.

Jefferson AL, Poppas A, Paul RH et al: Systemic hypoperfusion is associated with executive dysfunction In geriatric cardiac patients, *Neurobiol Aging* 28(3):477–483, 2007.

Jessup M, Abraham WT, Casey DE et al: 2009 focused update: ACCF/AHA guidelines for the diagnosis and management of heart failure in adults: a report of the American College of Cardiology Foundation/American Heart Association Task Force on Practice Guidelines: developed in collaboration with the International Society for Heart and Lung Transplantation, *Circulation* 119(14):1977–2016, 2009.

Johansson A, Dahlberg K, Ekebergh M: Living with experiences following a myocardial infarction, *Euro J Cardiovasc Nurs* 2:229, 2003.

Jolliffe JA, Rees K, Taylor RS et al: Exercise-based rehabilitation for coronary heart disease, *Cochrane Database Syst Rev* (1):CD001800, 2001.

Kasper DL, Braunwald E, Hauser S et al: *Harrison's principles of internal medicine*, ed 16, New York, 2005, McGraw-Hill.

Lakhdar R, Al-Mallah MH, Lanfear DE: Safety and tolerability of angiotensin-converting enzyme inhibitor versus the combination of angiotensin-converting enzyme inhibitor and angiotensin receptor blocker in patients with left ventricular dysfunction: a systematic review and meta-analysis of randomized control trials, *J Card Fail* 14(3):181–188, 2008.

Lesman-Leegte I, Jaarsma T, Sanderman R et al: Depressive symptoms are prominent among elderly hospitalised heart failure patients, *Eur J Heart Fail* 8(6):634–640, 2006.

Liang KV, Hiniker AR, Williams AW et al: Use of a novel ultrafiltration device as a treatment strategy for diuretic resistant, refractory heart failure: initial clinical experience in a single center, *J Card Fail* 12(9):707–714, 2006.

Marcy TR, Ripley TL: Aldosterone antagonists in the treatment of heart failure, Am J Health Syst Pharm 63(1): 49–58, 2006.

McSweeney JC, Crane PB: Challenging the rules: women's prodromal and acute symptoms of myocardial infarction, *Res Nurs Health* 23:135, 2000.

Morgan AL, Masoudi FA, Havranek EP et al: Difficulty taking medications, depression, and health status in heart failure patients, *J Card Fail* 12(1):54–60, 2006.

Moser DK: Heart failure management: optimal health care delivery programs, *Annu Rev Nurs Res* 18:91, 2000.

Moser DK, Dracup K: Is anxiety early after myocardial infarction associated with subsequent ischemic and arrhythmic events? *Psychosomat Med* 58(5):395–401, 1996.

Moser DK, Dracup K: Impact of cardiopulmonary resuscitation training on perceived control in spouses of recovering cardiac patients, *Res Nurs Health* 23:270, 2000.

Moser DK, Frazier SK, Woo MA et al: Normal fluctuations in pulmonary artery pressures and cardiac output in patients with severe left ventricular dysfunction, *Eur J Cardiovasc Nurs* 1(2):131–137, 2002.

Motohiro M, Yuasa F, Hattori T et al: Cardiovascular adaptations to exercise training after uncomplicated acute myocardial infarction, *Am J Phys Med Rehabil* 84(9):684–691, 2005.

Murray SA, Kendell M, Grant E et al: Patterns of social, psychological, and spiritual decline toward the end of life In lung cancer and heart failure, *J Pain Symptom Manage* 34(4):393–402, 2007.

Myers MG, Harris L: High dose caffeine and ventricular arrhythmias, *Can J Cardiol* 6(3):95, 1990.

Newberry L: *Sheehy's emergency nursing*, ed 5, St Louis, 2003, Mosby.

Nishi I, Noguchi T, Furuichi et al: Are cardiac events during exercise therapy for heart failure predictable from the baseline variables? *Circ J* 7(7):1035–1039, 2007.

Oliva AP, Monteiro da Cruz Dde A: Decreased cardiac output: validation with postoperative heart surgery patients, *Dimens Crit Care Nurs* 22(1):39–44, 2003.

Omar AR, Suppiah N, Chai P et al: Efficacy of community-based multi-disciplinary disease management of chronic heart failure, *Singapore Med J* 48(6):528–531, 2007.

Packer M, Abraham WT, Mehra MR et al: Utility of impedance cardiography for the identification of short-term risk of clinical decompensation in stable patients with chronic heart failure, *J Am Coll Cardiol* 47(11):2245–2252, 2006.

Quaglietti S, Lovett S, Hawthorne C et al: Management of the patient with congestive heart failure in the home care and palliative care setting, *Ann Long Term Care* 12(1):33, 2004.

Rankin SH: Women recovering from acute myocardial infarction: psychosocial and physical functioning outcomes for 12 months after acute myocardial infarction, *Heart Lung* 31(6):399, 2002.

Reid MB, Cottrell D: Nursing care of patients receiving intraaortic balloon counterpulsation, *Crit Care Nurse* 25(5):40–49, 2005.

Rees K, Taylor RS, Singh S et al: Exercise based rehabilitation for heart failure, *Cochrane Database Syst Rev* (3):CD003331, 2004.

Rice VH, Stead LF: Nursing interventions for smoking cessation, *Cochrane Database Syst Rev* (2):CD001188, 2000.

Rodriguez-Artalejo F, Guallar-Castillon P, Herrera MC et al: Social network as a predictor of hospital readmission and mortality among older patients with heart failure, *J Card Fail* 12(8):621–627, 2006.

Rusinaru D, Buiciuc O, Leborgne L et al: Relation of serum sodium level to long term outcome after a first hospitalization for heart failure with preserved ejection fraction, *Am J Cardiol* 103:405–410, 2009.

Rutledge T, Reis VA, Linke SE et al: Depression in heart failure a meta-analytic review of prevalence, intervention effects, and associations with clinical outcomes, *J Am Coll Cardiol* 48(8):1527–37, 2006.

Sakakibara M, Sakata Y, Usui K et al: Effectiveness of short-term treatment with nocturnal oxygen therapy for central sleep apnea in patients with congestive heart failure, *J Cardiol* 46(2):53–61, 2005.

Schneider JR: Effects of caffeine ingestion on heart rate, blood pressure, myocardial oxygen consumption, and cardiac rhythm in acute myocardial infarction patients, *Heart Lung* 16:167, 1987.

Sherman J, Young A, Sherman MP et al: Prenatal smoking and alterations in newborn heart rate during transition, *J Obstet Gynecol Neonatal Nurs* 31(6):680–687, 2002.

Stelfox H, Ahmed S, Ribeiro RA et al: Hemodynamic monitoring in obese patients: the impact of body mass index on cardiac output and stroke volume, *Crit Care Med* 34(4):1243–1246, 2006.

Tang WHW, Young JB: Chronic heart failure management. In Topol E, editor, *Textbook of cardiovascular medicine,* 3rd ed, Philadelphia, 2006, Lippincott, Williams and Wilkins.

Taylor RS, Brown A, Ebrahim S et al: Exercise-based rehabilitation for patients with coronary heart disease: systematic review and meta-analysis of randomized controlled trials, *Am J Med* 116(10):682, 2004.

Thomas SA, Friedmann E, Khatta M et al: Depression in patients with heart failure: physiologic effects, incidence, and relation to mortality, *AACN Clin Issues* 14(1):3, 2003.

Twiss E, Seaver J, McCaffrey R: The effects of music listening on older adults undergoing cardiovascular surgery, *Nurs Crit Care* 11(5):224–231, 2006.

Urquhart G, Jensen L: Timing of hemodynamic pressure measurements on derived hemodynamic parameters, *Dynamics* 14(3):13–20, 2003.

Vital FMR, Saconato M, Ladeira MT et al: Non-invasive positive pressure ventilation (CPAP or bilevel NPPV) for cardiogenic pulmonary edema, *Cochrane Database Syst Rev* (3): CD005351, 2009.

Wasserman K, Sun XG, Hansen JE: Effect of biventricular pacing on the exercise pathophysiology of heart failure, *Chest* 32(1):250–261, 2007.

Watkins L, Blumenthal JA, Carney R: Association of anxiety with reduced baroreflex cardiac control in patients after acute myocardial infarction, *Am Heart J* 143(3):460–466, 2002.

Williams H, Kearney M: Chronic heart failure, *Pharma J* 269:325, 2002.

Williams SA, Kasl SV, Heiat A et al: Depression and risk of heart failure among the elderly: a prospective community-based study, *Psychosom Med* 64(1):6, 2002.

Winslow EH: Panning bedpans, *Am J Nurs* 92:16G, 1992.

Woo GW, Petersen-Stejskal S, Johnson JW et al: Ventricular reverse remodeling and 6–month outcomes in patients receiving cardiac resynchronization therapy: analysis of the MIRACLE study, *J Interv Card Electrophysiol* 12(2):107–113, 2005.

Yancy C, Abraham W: Noninvasive hemodynamic monitoring in heart failure: utilization of impedance cardiography, *Congest Heart Fail* 9(5):241, 2003.

Young W, McShane J, O'Connor T et al: Registered nurses' experiences with an evidence-based home care pathway for myocardial infarction clients, *Can J Cardiovasc Nurs* 14(3):24, 2004.

Yu DS, Lee DT, Woo J et al: Non-pharmacological interventions in older people with heart failure: effects of exercise training and relaxation therapy, *Gerontology* 53(2):74–81, 2007.

Caregiver role strain   *Paula Reiss Sherwood, RN, CNRN, PhD, and Barbara Given, RN, PhD, FAAN*

NANDA-I

Definition

Difficulty in performing family caregiver role

Defining Characteristics

Caregiving Activities

Apprehension about care receiver's care if caregiver unable to provide care; apprehension about the future regarding care receiver's health; apprehension about the future regarding caregiver's ability to provide care; apprehension about possible institutionalization of care receiver; difficulty completing required tasks; difficulty performing required tasks; dysfunctional change in caregiving activities; preoccupation with care routine

Caregiver Health Status

Physical

Cardiovascular disease; diabetes; fatigue; GI upset; headaches; hypertension; rash; weight change

Emotional

Anger; disturbed sleep; feeling depressed; frustration; impaired individual coping; impatience; increased emotional lability; increased nervousness; lack of time to meet personal needs; somatization; stress

Socioeconomic

Changes in leisure activities; low work productivity; refuses career advancement; withdraws from social life

Caregiver–Care Receiver Relationship

Difficulty watching care receiver go through the illness; grief regarding changed relationship with care receiver; uncertainty regarding changed relationship with care receiver

Family Processes

Concerns about family members; family conflict

Related Factors (r/t)

Care Receiver Health Status

Addiction; codependence; cognitive problems; dependency; illness chronicity; illness severity; increasing care needs; instability of care receiver's health; problem behaviors; psychological problems; unpredictability of illness course

Caregiver Health Status

Addiction; codependency; cognitive problems; inability to fulfill one's own expectations; inability to fulfill other's expectations; marginal coping patterns; physical problems; psychological problems; unrealistic expectations of self

Caregiver–Care Receiver Relationship

History of poor relationship; mental status of elder inhibiting conversation, presence of abuse or violence; unrealistic expectations of caregiver by care receiver

Caregiving Activities

24–hour care responsibilities; amount of activities; complexity of activities; discharge of family members to home with significant care needs; ongoing changes in activities; unpredictability of care situation; years of caregiving

• = Independent   ▲ = Collaborative   **EBN** = Evidence-Based Nursing   **EB** = Evidence-Based

Family Processes

History of family dysfunction; history of marginal family coping

Resources

Caregiver is not developmentally ready for caregiver role; deficient knowledge about community resources; difficulty accessing community resources; emotional strength; formal assistance; formal support; inadequate community resources (e.g., respite services, recreational resources); inadequate equipment for providing care; inadequate physical environment for providing care (e.g., housing, temperature, safety); inadequate transportation; inexperience with caregiving; informal assistance; informal support; insufficient finances; insufficient time; lack of caregiver privacy; lack of support; physical energy

Socioeconomic

Alienation from others; competing role commitments; insufficient recreation; isolation from others

 (Nursing Outcomes Classification)

Suggested NOC Outcomes

Caregiver Adaptation to Patient Institutionalization, Caregiver Emotional Health, Caregiver Home Care Readiness, Caregiver Lifestyle Disruption, Caregiver-Patient Relationship, Caregiver Performance: Direct Care, Caregiver Performance: Indirect Care, Caregiver Physical Health, Caregiver Role Support, Caregiver Stressors, Caregiver Well-Being

Example NOC Outcome with Indicators
Caregiver Emotional Health with plans for a positive future as evidenced by the following indicators: Satisfaction with life/Sense of control/Self-esteem/Perceived social connectedness/Perceived spiritual well-being (Rate the outcome and indicators of **Caregiver Emotional Health:** 1 = severely compromised, 2 = substantially compromised, 3 = moderately compromised, 4 = mildly compromised, 5 = not compromised [see Section I].)

Client Outcomes

Caregiver Will (Specify Time Frame):

- Feel supported
- Report reduced or acceptable feelings of burden or distress
- Take part in self-care activities to maintain own physical and psychological/emotional health
- Identify resources available to help in giving care
- Verbalize mastery of the care situation; feel confident and competent to provide care

Care Receiver Will (Specify Time Frame):

- Obtain quality and safe care

 (Nursing Interventions Classification)

Suggested NIC Intervention

Caregiver Support

Example NIC Activities—Caregiver Support
Determine caregiver's acceptance of role; Accept expressions of negative emotion

Nursing Interventions and *Rationales*

- Watch for signs of depression and deteriorating physical health in the caregiver, especially if the marital relationship is poor, the care recipient has cognitive or neuropsychiatric symptoms, there is little social support available, the caregiver becomes enmeshed in the care situation, the caregiver is elderly, female, or has poor preexisting physical or emotional health. Refer to the care plan for

Hopelessness when appropriate. **EB:** *Caregiving may weaken the immune system and predispose the caregiver to illness, particularly cardiac illness and poor response to acquired infections in some situations (Gallagher et al, 2008; Gouin, Hantsoo, & Kiecolt-Glaser, 2008). The incidence of depression in family caregivers is estimated to be 40% to 50% (Schulz & Martire, 2004). Particular subgroups have been shown to be at high risk for becoming distressed as a result of providing care (Pinquart & Sorenson, 2007).*

- The impact of providing care on the caregiver's emotional health should be assessed at regular intervals using a reliable and valid instrument such as the Caregiver Strain Index, Caregiver Burden Inventory, Caregiver Reaction Assessment, Screen for Caregiver Burden, and the Subjective and Objective Burden Scale (Vitaliano et al, 1991; Given et al, 1992; Deeken et al, 2003). **EBN and EB:** *Research has validated the effectiveness of a number of evaluation tools for caregiver stress, including the Caregiver Reaction Assessment (Given et al, 1992), Burden Interview (Zarit et al, 1980), the Caregiver Strain Index (Robinson, 1983), and the Caregiver Burden Inventory (Novak & Guest, 1989). Caregiver assessment tools should be multidimensional and evaluate the impact of providing care on multiple aspects of the caregiver's life (Hudson & Hayman-White, 2006).*

- Identify potential caregiver resources such as mastery, social support, optimism, and positive aspects of care. **EB and EBN:** *Research has shown that caregivers can have simultaneous positive and negative responses to providing care. Positive responses may help to buffer the negative effects of providing care on caregivers' emotional health and may also increase the effectiveness of interventions to reduce strain (Hilgeman et al, 2007; Wilson, Filers, & Heermann, 2009).*

- Screen for caregiver role strain at the onset of the care situation, at regular intervals throughout the care situation, and with changes in care recipient status and care transitions. **EB and EBN:** *Care situations that last for several months or years can cause wear and tear that exhaust caregivers' coping mechanisms and available resources and that may continue after the care receiver has been institutionalized (te Boekhorst et al, 2008). In addition, changes in the care recipient's health status necessitate new skills and monitoring from the caregiver and affect the caregiver's ability to continue to provide care (Burton et al, 2003). Providing caregiver support throughout the care situation may decrease care recipient institutionalization (Mittelman et al, 2006).*

- Watch for caregivers who become enmeshed in the care situation (e.g., becoming overinvolved or unable to disentangle themselves from the caregiver role). **EB:** *Role training (assisting caregivers to understand and define their role) may prevent caregivers from becoming enmeshed, which can in turn prevent burden and depression (Hepburn et al, 2001).*

- Arrange for intervals of respite care for the caregiver; encourage use if available. **EB and EBN:** *Respite care provides time away from the care situation and can help alleviate distress (Beeber, Thorpe, & Clipp, 2008; Sussman & Regehr, 2009).*

- Help the caregiver to identify and utilize support systems. **EBN:** *Caregivers sometimes feel abandoned and need assistance to activate their support systems (Borg & Hallberg, 2006).*

- Encourage the caregiver to grieve over changes in the care receiver's condition and give the caregiver permission to share angry feelings in a safe environment. Refer to nursing interventions for **Grieving. EB:** *Caregivers grieve the loss of function of their loved one, especially when dementia is involved (Schulz et al, 2006; Holland, Currier, & Gallgher-Thompson, 2009).*

- Help the caregiver find personal time to meet his or her needs, learn stress management techniques, schedule regular health screenings, and schedule regular respite time. **EB and EBN:** *Self-care is important for the caregiver (Belle et al, 2006). Maintaining personal wellness can increase stamina, energy, and self-esteem and enhance the quality of care given, although caregivers with higher levels of burden may be less likely to engage in self-care activities (Lu & Wykle, 2007).*

- Encourage the caregiver to schedule and keep routine health care appointments (i.e., annual physicals and screening tests). **EBN:** *Caregivers who report being strained are at risk for lower perceptions of their own health status, increased risky behaviors such as smoking, and higher use of prescription drugs (Lu & Wykle, 2007).*

- Encourage the caregiver to talk about feelings, concerns, uncertainties, and fears. Acknowledge the frustration associated with caregiver responsibilities and recognize outlets (such as work) that may offset some of the negative effects of providing care. **EBN:** *Caregivers need a safe outlet for their feelings regarding the care situation (Stoltz, Andersson, & William, 2007).*

● = Independent   ▲ = Collaborative   **EBN** = Evidence-Based Nursing   **EB** = Evidence-Based

- Observe for any evidence of caregiver or care receiver violence or abuse, particularly verbal abuse; if evidence is present, speak with the caregiver and care receiver separately. **EB:** *Caregiver violence is possible, particularly when high levels of care demands or caregiver distress are present (Hansberry, Chen, & Gorbien, 2005; Cooper et al, 2009).*
- ▲ Involve the family in care transitions; use a multidisciplinary team to provide medical and social services for instruction and planning. **EBN:** *Caregivers who reported involvement in discharge planning, particularly when discharge planning was done by an interdisciplinary team, occurs well before discharge, and includes good communication between the family member and the health care team, report better acceptance of the caregiving role and better health (Bauer et al, 2009).*
- ▲ Encourage regular communication with the care recipient and with the health care team. **EB:** *Caregivers' preferential communication method and communication needs should be addressed at regular intervals to improve their sense of mastery over the care situation (Moore, 2008).*
- Help caregiver assess his/or her financial resources (services reimbursed by insurance, available support through community and religious organizations) and the impact of providing care on his or her financial status. **EB and EBN:** *Low incomes and limited financial resources can cause strain for the caregiver, particularly if there are substantial out-of-pocket costs involved in providing care (Siefert et al, 2008).*
- Help the caregiver identify competing occupational demands and potential ways to modify the work role in order to provide care (enact the Family Leave Act, change from full to part time, work from home, take a leave of absence or early retirement). **EB:** *Employed caregivers report missed days, interruptions at work, leaves of absence, and reduced productivity due to providing care (Ko, Aycock, & Clark, 2007).*
- When necessary, help the caregiver transition the care recipient to a long-term care facility. **EB:** *Placing a loved one in an extended-care facility can relieve the burden of care but does not relieve the stress resulting from financial concerns, guilt, loss of control, or lack of support (Schulz et al, 2004).*
- Help the caregiver problem solve to meet the care recipient's needs. **EBN:** *Using a problem solving intervention—helping the caregiver identify the problem, its sources, and generating potential solutions—has been shown to lower distress in caregivers of persons with cancer (Given et al, 2006).*

 Geriatric

- Monitor the caregiver for psychological distress and signs of depression, especially if caring for a mentally impaired elder or if there was an unsatisfactory marital relationship before caregiving. **EBN:** *A difficult marriage before caregiving predisposes the caregiver to depression (Hansberry, Chen, & Gorbien, 2005).* **EBN:** *Older adults in long-term marriages need to be considered as individuals as well as members of a couple in both assessment and planning interventions (Padula & Sullivan, 2006).*
- Assess the health of caregivers at intervals, especially if they have their own chronic illness in addition to caregiving role. **EB:** *Caregivers who report feeling burdened have an increased risk of mortality, risk that may be particularly high in elderly caregivers with comorbid conditions (Schulz & Beach, 1999; Beach et al, 2000).*
- Assess social support and encourage the use of secondary caregivers with elderly caregivers. **EBN:** *Older caregivers often become enmeshed in the care situation (often because they provide care by themselves) and isolate themselves from social and family support to become completely focused on providing care for their spouse (Borg & Hallberg, 2006).*
- Provide skills training related to direct care, performing complex monitoring tasks, supervision interpreting client symptoms, assisting with decision making, providing emotional support and comfort, and coordinating care. **EBN:** *Each task demands different skills and knowledge, organizational capacities, role demands, and social and psychological strengths from family members (Schumacher et al, 2000).*
- Teach symptom management techniques (assessment, potential causes, aggravating factors, potential alleviating factors, reassessment), particularly for fatigue, constipation, anorexia, and pain. **EB and EBN:** *Certain client symptoms such as fatigue, constipation, anorexia, pain, and depression have been associated with caregiver strain (Newton et al, 2002; Yurk et al, 2002; Kurtz et al, 2004).*

Multicultural

- Assess for the influence of cultural beliefs, norms, and values on the client's ability to modify health behavior. **EBN:** *What the client considers normal and abnormal health behavior may be based on cultural perceptions (Leininger & McFarland, 2002; Giger & Davidhizar, 2008).* **EBN:** *Each client should be assessed for ability to modify health behavior based on the phenomenon of communication, time, space, social organization, environmental control, and biological variations (Giger & Davidhizar, 2008).*
- Encourage spirituality as a source of support for coping. **EBN:** *Many African Americans and Latinos identify spirituality, religiousness, prayer, and church-based approaches as coping resources (Samuel-Hodge et al, 2000).* **EBN:** *Socioeconomic status, geographical location, and risks associated with health-seeking behavior all influence the likelihood that clients will seek health care and modify health behavior (Appel, Giger, & Davidhizar, 2005; Giger & Davidhizar, 2008).*
- Assess the role of fatalism on the client's ability to modify health behavior. **EB:** *Fatalistic perspectives, which involve the belief that you cannot control your own fate, influenced health behaviors in some African American, Asian, and Latino populations (Joiner et al, 2001; Powe & Finnie, 2003; Giger & Davidhizar, 2008). In addition, according to Gullatte and colleagues (2009), when fatalism is transferred to specific conditions such as cancer, the phenomenon is known as cancer fatalism. At its very essence, cancer fatalism occurs when the individual surrenders the human spirit to perception of hopelessness, powerlessness, worthlessness, and social despair.*
- Identify which family members the client can rely on for support. **EBN:** *A variety of different cultures rely on family members to cope with stress (White & Dorman, 2000; Aziz & Rowland, 2002; Donnelly, 2002; Gleeson-Kreig, Bernal, & Woolley, 2002). While families deliver most of health care and at one time being in a family was expected, today not being in a family is both common and accepted and has profound implications for health care delivery (Giorgianni, 2003).* **EBN:** *For clients from Afghanistan adjustment to the United States has been particularly difficult, and family members have needed to lean on the immediate family who are available for support (Giger & Davidhizar, 2002).*
- ▲ Assess for signs of depression and level of social support and make appropriate referrals. **EB:** *Increased depressed feelings and lower levels of available social support were reported by minorities following injury (Brown et al, 2004).*
- Assess for the presence of conflicting values within the culture. **EBN:** *Whereas sharing and caring is part of the Amish community, females with breast cancer were found to value privacy issues related to their body image and health status and to prefer this was shared in the closed community (Schwartz, 2008).*

Home Care

- Identify client and caregiver factors that necessitate the use of formal home care services, that may affect provision of care, or that need to be addressed before the client can be safely discharged from home care. **EBN:** *Although home care resources can be useful in decreasing caregiver distress, they are not used with regularity across client populations. Health care practitioners should assess for the need for support resources prior to discharge and at routine intervals throughout the care situation, particularly in the first 2 years following diagnosis and with changes in the care recipient's condition and should tailor caregiver education and services to particular caregiver needs (Davis, Weaver, & Habermann, 2006; King & Semik, 2006).*
- Collaborate with the caregiver and discuss the care needs of the client, disease processes, medications, and what to expect; use a variety of instructional techniques (e.g., explanations, demonstrations, visual aids) until the caregiver is able to express a degree of comfort with care delivery. **EB:** *Knowledge and confidence are separate concepts. Self-assurance in caregiving will decrease the amount of distress the caregiver perceives as a result of providing care (Gitlin et al, 2003).*
- Assist the caregiver and client in arranging care so that it is compatible with other household patterns. **EBN:** *Caregivers of elders have been identified as using home environmental modification strategies for specific purposes: organizing the home, supplementing the elder's function, structuring the elder's day, protecting the elder, working around limitations or deficits in the home environment, enriching the home environment, and transitioning to a new home setting (Messecar et al, 2002).*
- Assess family caregiving skill. The identification of caregiver difficulty with any of a core set of processes highlights areas for intervention. **EBN:** *The ability to engage effectively and smoothly in*

● = Independent   ▲ = Collaborative   **EBN** = Evidence-Based Nursing   **EB** = Evidence-Based

nine processes has been identified as constituting family caregiving skill: monitoring client behavior, interpreting changes accurately, making decisions, taking action, making adjustment to care, accessing resources, providing hands-on care, working together with the ill person, and negotiating the health care system (Schumacher et al, 2000). **EBN:** *Caregiver skills training has been shown to reduce caregivers' emotional distress, particularly when the care receiver has cognitive or neuropsychiatric symptoms (Farran et al, 2007).*

- Assess the client and caregiver at every visit for quality of relationship, and for the quality of caring that exists. **EB:** *Quality of the caregiver/care recipient relationship and the impact of the care situation on that relationship can be an important source of distress or support for the caregiver (Quinn, Clare, & Woods, 2009). Chronic illness, especially dementia, can represent a gradual and devastating loss of the marital relationship as it existed formerly. An understanding of the prior relationship is needed before the couple can be helped to anticipate continuing care needs or deterioration, as the dyadic relationship can be expected to change over the care situation (Langer et al, 2009).*

- Assess preexisting strengths and weaknesses the caregiver brings to the situation, as well as current responses, depression, and fatigue levels. **EB and EBN:** *Caregivers' personality type, mastery, self-efficacy, optimism, and social support have all been linked to the amount of distress the caregiver will perceive as a result of providing care (Campbell et al, 2008; Shirai et al, 2009).*

- Identify and support strengths and weaknesses of the caregiver and efforts to gain control of unpredictable situations. **EB:** *The use of external services may be helpful to gain control of the situation, and should be implemented when caregivers show signs of depressive symptomatology (Bookwala et al, 2004).*

- Form a trusting and supportive relationship with the caregiver. Allow the caregiver to verbalize frustrations. **EB:** *Building a supportive relationship between the health care provider and family caregiver is vital to meeting caregivers' needs (Kimberlin et al, 2004).*

- ▲ Refer the client to home health aide services for assistance with ADLs and light housekeeping. Allow the caregiver to gain confidence in the respite provider. *Home health aide services can provide physical relief and respite for the caregiver.* **EB:** *Caregiver burden increases as the care receiver's cognitive and functional ability decline (Ricci et al, 2009).*

- ▲ Refer to a caregivers' support group if available or recommend an online support group—see suggested websites listed on the Evolve website. **EBN:** *Sharing concerns with others can mitigate loneliness, particularly for caregivers who provide a high level of care (Wolff et al, 2009). Online support groups can alleviate caregiver distress by providing caregivers a sense of community and psychosocial support (Marziali & Donahue, 2006).*

- Be aware that physical and emotional demands on the caregiver tend to increase during the last 3 months of a care recipient's life, which may require more frequent or intense intervention. **EB:** *Families of terminally ill clients are especially vulnerable to caregiver role strain because the timing of the impending death is unpredictable, caregiver effort and resources are disproportionately spent early in the caregiving process, and increased physical care demands are associated with caregiver burden (Brazil et al, 2003).*

Client/Family Teaching and Discharge Planning

- Assess the caregiver's need for information such as information on symptom management, disease progression, specific skills, and available support. **EBN:** *Using problem solving to help the caregiver manage clients' symptoms has been shown to significantly lower caregiver distress (Given et al, 2006).*

- Teach the caregiver warning signs for burnout, depression, and anxiety. Help them identify a resource in case they begin to feel overwhelmed.

- Teach the caregiver methods for managing disruptive behavioral symptoms if present. Refer to the care plan for **Chronic Confusion.** *Multicomponent interventions can be particularly effective in caregivers of persons with neurologic sequelae (Pinquart & Sorenson, 2007).*

- Teach the caregiver how to provide the care needed and put a plan in place for monitoring the care provided.

- Provide ongoing support and evaluation of care skills as the care situation and care demands change.

• = Independent   ▲ = Collaborative   **EBN** = Evidence-Based Nursing   **EB** = Evidence-Based

- Provide information regarding the care recipient's diagnosis, treatment regimen, and expected course of illness. **EB:** *An Internet- and telephone-based education and support network for caregivers of individuals with progressive dementia has been developed (AlzOnline), and preliminary results demonstrate reductions in caregiver burden and improvements in caregiver mastery (Glueckauf et al, 2004).*
- ▲ Refer to counseling or support groups to assist in adjusting to the caregiver role and periodically evaluate not only the caregiver's emotional response to care but the safety of the care delivered to the care recipient.

ⓔvolve   See the EVOLVE website for Weblinks for caregiver education resources.

REFERENCES

Appel SJ, Giger JN, Davidhizar RE: Opportunity cost: the impact of contextual risk factors on the cardiovascular health of low-income rural southern African American women, *J Cardiovasc Nurs* 20:315–324, 2005.

Aziz NM, Rowland JH: Cancer survivorship research among ethnic minority and medically underserved groups, *Oncol Nurs Forum* 29(5):789–801, 2002.

Bauer M, Fitzgerald L, Haesler E et al: Hospital discharge planning for frail older people and their family, *J Clin Nurs* 18(18):2539–2546, 2009.

Beach S, Schulz R, Yee J et al: Negative and positive health effects of caring for a disabled spouse: longitudinal findings from the caregiver health effects study, *Psychol Aging* 15(2):259–271, 2000.

Beeber AS, Thorpe JM, Clipp EC: Community-based service use by elders with dementia and their caregivers: a latent class analysis, *Nurs Res* 57(5):312–21, 2008.

Belle SH, Burgio L, Burns R et al: Enhancing the quality of life of dementia caregivers from different ethnic or racial groups: a randomized, controlled trial, *Ann Intern Med* 145(10):727–738, 2006.

te Boekhorst S, Pot AM, Depla M et al: Group living homes for older people with dementia: the effects on psychological distress of informal caregivers, *Aging Ment Health* 12(6):761–768, 2008.

Bookwala J, Zdaniuk B, Burton L et al: Concurrent and long-term predictors of older adults' use of community-based long-term care services: the Caregiver Health Effects Study, *J Aging Health* 16(1):88–115, 2004.

Borg C, Hallberg I: Life satisfaction among informal caregivers in comparison with non-caregivers, *Scand J Caring Sci* 20(4):427–438, 2006.

Brazil K, Bedard M, Willison K et al: Caregiving and its impact on families of the terminally ill, *Aging Ment Health* 7(5):376–382, 2003.

Brown SA, McCauley SR, Levin HS et al: Perception of health and quality of life in minorities after mild-to-moderate traumatic brain injury, *Appl Neuropsychol* 11(1):54–64, 2004.

Burton LC, Zdaniuk B, Schulz R et al: Transitions in spousal caregiving, *Gerontologist* 43(2):230–241, 2003.

Campbell P, Wright J, Oyebode J et al: Determinants of burden in those who care for someone with dementia, *Int J Geriatr Psychiatry* 23(10):1078–1085, 2008.

Cooper C, Selwood A, Blanchard M et al: Abuse of people with dementia by family carers: representative cross sectional survey, *BMJ* 338:b155, 2009.

Davis LL, Weaver M, Habermann B: Differential attrition in a caregiver skill training trial, *Res Nurs Health* 29(5):498–506, 2006.

Deeken J, Taylor K, Mangan P et al: Care for the caregivers: a review of self-report instruments developed to measure the burden, needs, and quality of life of informal caregivers, *J Pain Symptom Manage* 26(4):922–953, 2003.

Donnelly TT: Contextual analysis of coping: implications for immigrants' mental health care, *Issues Ment Health Nurs* 23(7):715–732, 2002.

Farran CJ, Gilley DW, McCann JJ et al: Efficacy of behavioral interventions for dementia caregivers, *West J Nurs Res* 29(8):944–960, 2007.

Gallagher S, Phillips AC, Evans P et al: Caregiving is associated with low secretion rates of immunoglobulin A in saliva, *Brain Behav Immun* 22(4):565–572, 2008.

Giger J, Davidhizar R: Culturally competent care: emphasis on understanding the people of Afghanistan, Afghanistan Americans, and Islamic culture and religion, *Int Nurs Rev* 49(2):79–86, 2002.

Giger J, Davidhizar R: *Transcultural nursing: assessment and intervention,* St Louis, 2008, Mosby.

Giorgianni S: How families matter in health, *The Pfizer Journal* 7(1):1, 2003.

Gitlin LN, Winter L, Burke J et al: Tailored activities to manage neuropsychiatric behaviors in persons with dementia and reduce caregiver burden: a randomized pilot study, *Am J Geriatr Psychiatry* 16(3):229–239, 2008.

Given CW, Given B, Stommel M et al: The caregiver reaction assessment (CRA) for caregivers to persons with chronic physical and mental impairments, *Res Nurs Health* 15(4):271–383, 1992.

Given B, Given CW, Sikorskii A et al: The impact of providing symptom management assistance on caregiver reaction: results of a randomized trial, *J Pain Symptom Manage* 32(5):433–443, 2006.

Gleeson-Kreig J, Bernal H, Woolley S: The role of social support in the self-management of diabetes mellitus among a Hispanic population, *Public Health Nurs* 19(3):215–222, 2002.

Glueckauf R, Ketterson T, Loomis J et al: Online support and education for dementia caregivers: overview, utilization, and initial program evaluation, *Telemed J E Health* 10(2):223–232, 2004.

Gouin J, Hantsoo L, Kiecolt-Glaser JK: Immune dysregulation and chronic stress among older adults: a review, *Neuroimmunomodulation* 15(4–6):251–259, 2008.

Gullatte M, Brawley O, Kinney A et al: Religiosity, spirituality, and cancer fatalism beliefs on delay in breast cancer diagnosis in African American women, *J Relig Health* 2009, Epub ahead of print.

Hansberry MR, Chen E, Gorbien MJ: Dementia and elder abuse, *Clin Geriatr Med* 21(2):315–332, 2005.

Hepburn K, Tornatore J, Center B et al: Dementia family caregiver training: affecting beliefs about caregiving and caregiver outcomes, *J Am Geriatr Soc* 49(4):450–457, 2001.

Hilgeman MM, Allen RS, DeCoster J et al: Positive aspects of caregiving as a moderator of treatment outcome over 12 months, *Psychol Aging* 22(2):361–371, 2007.

Holland JM, Currier JM, Gallagher-Thompson D: Outcomes from the Resources for Enhancing Alzheimer's Caregiver Health (REACH) program for bereaved caregivers, *Psychol Aging* 24(1):190–202, 2009.

● = Independent   ▲ = Collaborative   **EBN** = Evidence-Based Nursing   **EB** = Evidence-Based

Hudson PL, Hayman-White K: Measuring the psychosocial characteristics of family caregivers of palliative care patients: psychometric properties of nine self-report instruments, *J Pain Symptom Manage* 31(3):215–228, 2006.

Joiner T, Perez M, Wagner K et al: On fatalism, pessimism, and depressive symptoms among Mexican-American and other adolescents attending an obstetrics-gynecology clinic, *Behav Res Ther* 39(8):887–896, 2001.

Kimberlin C, Brushwood D, Allen W et al: Cancer patient and caregiver experiences: communication and pain management issues, *J Pain Symptom Manage* 28(6):566–578, 2004.

King RB, Semik PE: Stroke caregiving: difficult times, resource use, and needs during the first 2 years, *J Gerontol Nurs* 32(4):37–44, 2006.

Ko JY, Aycock DM, Clark PC: A comparison of working versus nonworking family caregivers of stroke survivors, *J Neurosci Nurs* 39(4):217–225, 2007.

Kurtz M, Kurtz JC, Given CW et al: Depression and physical health among family caregivers of geriatric patients with cancer—a longitudinal view, *Med Sci Monit* 10(8):CR447–456, 2004.

Langer SL, Yi JC, Storer BE et al: Marital adjustment, satisfaction and dissolution among hematopoietic stem cell transplant patients and spouses: a prospective, five-year longitudinal investigation, *Psychooncology* 2009, Epub ahead of print.

Leininger MM, McFarland MR: *Transcultural nursing: concepts, theories, research and practices,* ed 3, New York, 2002, McGraw-Hill.

Lu YF, Wykle M: Relationships between caregiver stress and self-care behaviors in response to symptoms, *Clin Nurs Res* 16(1):29–43, 2007.

Marziali E, Donahue P: Caring for others: Internet video-conferencing group intervention for family caregivers of older adults with neurodegenerative disease, *Gerontologist,* 46(3):398–403, 2006.

Messecar DC, Archbold PG, Stewart BJ et al: Home environmental modification strategies used by caregivers of elders, *Res Nurs Health* 25(5):357–370, 2002.

Mittelman MS, Haley WE, Clay OJ et al: Improving caregiver well-being delays nursing home placement of patients with Alzheimer disease, *Neurology* 67(9):1592–1599, 2006.

Moore CD: Enhancing health care communication skills: preliminary evaluation of a curriculum for family caregivers, *Home Health Care Serv Q* 27(1):21–35, 2008.

Newton M, Bell D, Lambert S et al: Concerns of hospice patient caregivers, *ABNF J* 13(6):140–144, 2002.

Novak M, Guest C: Application of a multidimensional caregiver burden inventory, *Gerontologist* 29(6):798–803, 1989.

Padula C, Sullivan M: Long term married couples health promotion behaviors, *J Gerontol Nurs* 32(10):37–47, 2006.

Pinquart M, Sorensen S: Correlates of physical health of informal caregivers: a meta-analysis, *J Gerontol B Psychol Sci Soc Sci* 62(2):P126–37, 2007.

Powe BD, Finnie R: Cancer fatalism: the state of the science, *Cancer Nurs* 26(6):454–465, 2003.

Quinn C, Clare L, Woods B: The impact of the quality of relationship on the experiences and wellbeing of caregivers of people with dementia: a systematic review, *Aging Ment Health* 13(2):143–154, 2009.

Ricci M, Guidoni SV, Sepe-Monti M et al: Clinical findings, functional abilities and caregiver distress in the early stage of dementia with Lewy bodies (DLB) and Alzheimer's disease (AD), *Arch Gerontol Geriatr* 49(2):e101–104, 2009.

Robinson B: Validation of a Caregiver Strain Index, *J Gerontol* 38(3):344–348, 1983.

Samuel-Hodge CD, Headen SW, Skelly AH et al: Influences on day-to-day self-management of type 2 diabetes among African-American women: spirituality, the multi-caregiver role, and other social context factors, *Diabetes Care* 23(7):928–933, 2000.

Schulz R, Beach SR: Caregiving as a risk factor for mortality: the Caregiver Health Effects Study, *JAMA* 282(23):2215–2219, 1999.

Schulz R, Martire L: Family caregiving of persons with dementia: prevalence, health effects, and support strategies, *Am J Geriatr Psychiatry* 12(3):240–249, 2004.

Schulz R, Belle S, Czaja S et al: Long-term care placement of dementia patients and caregiver health and well-being, *JAMA* 292(8):961–967, 2004.

Schulz R, Boerner K, Shear K et al: Predictors of complicated grief among dementia caregivers: A prospective study of bereavement, *Am J Geriatr Psychiatr* 14(8):650–658, 2006.

Schumacher KL, Stewart BJ, Archbold PG et al: Family caregiving skill: development of the concept, *Res Nurs Health* 23(3):191–203, 2000.

Schwartz K: Breast cancer and health care beliefs, values, and practices of Amish women, *Diss Abstr* 29(1):587, 2008.

Shirai Y, Silverberg Koerner S et al: Reaping caregiver feelings of gain: the roles of socio-emotional support and mastery, *Aging Ment Health* 13(1):106–117, 2009.

Siefert ML, Williams AL, Dowd MF et al: The caregiving experience in a racially diverse sample of cancer family caregivers, *Cancer Nurs* 31(5):399–407, 2008.

Stoltz P, Andersson EP, William A: Support in nursing—an evolutionary concept analysis, *Int J Nurs Stud* 44(8):1478–89, 2007.

Sussman T, Regehr C: The influence of community-based services on the burden of spouses caring for their partners with dementia, *Health Soc Work* 34(1):29–39, 2009.

Vitaliano P, Russo J, Young H et al: The screen for caregiver burden, *Gerontologist* 31(1):76–83, 1991.

White MH, Dorman SM: Online support for caregivers: analysis of an internet Alzheimer mailgroup, *Comput Nurs* 18(4):168–176, 2000.

Wilson ME, Filers J, Heermann JA et al: The experience of spouses as informal caregivers for recipients of hematopoietic stem cell transplants, *Cancer Nurs* 32(3):E15–E23, 2009.

Wolff JL, Rand-Giovannetti E, Palmer S et al: Caregiving and chronic care: the guided care program for families and friends, *J Gerontol A Biol Sci Med Sci* 64(7):785–791, 2009.

Yurk R, Morgan D, Franey S et al: Understanding the continuum of palliative care for patients and their caregivers, *J Pain Symptom Manage* 24(5):459–470, 2002.

Zarit SH, Reever KE, Bach-Peterson J et al: Relatives of the impaired elderly: correlates of feelings of burden, *Gerontologist* 20(6):649–655, 1980.

Risk for Caregiver role strain   Betty J. Ackley, MSN, EdS, RN

NANDA-I

Definition

Caregiver is vulnerable for felt difficulty in performing the family caregiver role

● = Independent   ▲ = Collaborative   **EBN** = Evidence-Based Nursing   **EB** = Evidence-Based

Risk Factors

Addiction; amount of caregiving tasks; care receiver exhibits bizarre behavior; care receiver exhibits deviant behavior; caregiver's competing role commitments; caregiver health impairment; caregiver is female; caregiver is spouse; caregiver isolation; caregiver not developmentally ready for caregiver role; codependency; cognitive problems in care receiver; complexity of caregiving tasks; congenital defect; developmental delay of the care receiver; developmental delay of the caregiver; discharge of family member with significant home care needs; duration of caregiving required; family dysfunction prior to the caregiving situation; family isolation; illness severity of the care receiver; inadequate physical environment for providing care (e.g., housing, transportation, community services, equipment); inexperience with caregiving; instability in the care receiver's health; lack of recreation for caregiver; lack of respite for caregiver; marginal caregiver's coping patterns; marginal family adaptation; past history of poor relationship between caregiver and care receiver; premature birth; presence of abuse; presence of situational stressors that normally affect families (e.g., significant loss, disaster or crisis, economic vulnerability, major life events); presence of violence; psychological problems in care receiver; retardation of the care receiver; retardation of the caregiver; unpredictable illness course

NOC, NIC, Client Outcomes, Nursing Interventions, Client/Family Teaching and Discharge Planning, *Rationales,* and References

Refer to care plan for **Caregiver role strain.**

Readiness for enhanced Childbearing process *Gail B. Ladwig, MSN, RN, CHTP* ⊖volve

NANDA-I

Definition

A pattern of preparing for, maintaining, and strengthening a healthy pregnancy and childbirth process and care of newborn.

Defining Characteristics

During Pregnancy

Reports appropriate prenatal lifestyle (e.g., diet, elimination, sleep, bodily movement, exercise, personal hygiene); reports appropriate physical preparations; reports managing unpleasant symptoms in pregnancy; demonstrates respect for unborn baby; reports a realistic birth plan; prepares necessary newborn care items; seeks necessary knowledge (e.g., of labor and delivery, newborn care); reports availability of support systems; has regular prenatal health visits

During Labor and Delivery

Reports lifestyle (e.g., diet, elimination, sleep, bodily movement, personal hygiene) that is appropriate for the stage of labor; responds appropriately to onset of labor; is proactive in labor and delivery; uses relaxation techniques appropriate for the stage of labor; demonstrates attachment behavior to the newborn baby; utilizes support systems appropriately

After Birth

Demonstrates appropriate baby feeding techniques; demonstrates appropriate breast care; demonstrates attachment behavior to the baby; demonstrates basic baby care techniques; provides safe environment for the baby; reports appropriate postpartum lifestyle (e.g., diet, elimination, sleep, bodily movement, exercise, personal hygiene); utilizes support system appropriately

NOC   (Nursing Outcomes Classification)

Suggested NOC Outcomes

Knowledge: Pregnancy, Knowledge: Infant Care, Knowledge: Postpartum Maternal Health

 = Independent   ▲ = Collaborative   **EBN** = Evidence-Based Nursing   **EB** = Evidence-Based

> ### Example NOC Outcome with Indicators
>
> **Knowledge: Pregnancy** as evidenced by client conveying understanding of the following indicators: Importance of frequent prenatal care/Importance of prenatal education/Benefits of activity and exercise/Healthy nutritional practices/ Anatomic and physiological changes with pregnancy/Psychological changes associated with pregnancy/Birthing options/ Effective labor techniques/Signs and symptoms of labor (Rate the outcome and indicators of **Knowledge Pregnancy:** 1 = no knowledge, 2 = limited knowledge, 3 = moderate knowledge, 4 = substantial knowledge, 5 = extensive knowledge [See Section I].)

Client Outcomes

Client Will (Specify Time Frame):

During Pregnancy
- State importance of frequent prenatal care/education
- State knowledge of anatomic, physiological, psychological changes with pregnancy
- Report appropriate lifestyle choices prenatal: activity and exercise/healthy nutritional practices

During Labor and Delivery
- Report appropriate lifestyle choices during labor
- State knowledge of birthing options, signs and symptoms of labor, and effective labor techniques

After Birth
- Report appropriate lifestyle choices postpartum
- State normal physical sensations following delivery
- State knowledge of recommended nutrient intake, strategies to balance activity and rest, appropriate exercise, time frame for resumption of sexual activity, strategies to manage stress
- List strategies to bond with infant
- State knowledge of proper handling and positioning of infant/infant safety
- State knowledge of feeding technique and bathing of infant

NIC (Nursing Interventions Classification)

Suggested NIC Interventions

Prenatal Care, Intrapartal Care, Postpartal Care, Attachment Promotion, Newborn Care, Infant Care

> ### Example NIC Activities—Prenatal care
>
> Encourage parent(s) to attend prenatal classes; Instruct patient on nutrition needed during pregnancy; Instruct patient on appropriate exercises and rest during pregnancy; Assist patient to develop and use social support system; Refer patient to childbirth preparation class

Nursing Interventions and *Rationales*

Refer to care plans **Risk for impaired Attachment; Effective Breastfeeding; Readiness for enhanced family Coping; Readiness for enhanced Family processes; Risk for disproportionate Growth; Readiness for enhanced Nutrition; Readiness for enhanced Parenting; Ineffective Role performance.**

Prenatal Care

- Assess smoking status of pregnant client and offer effective smoking-cessation interventions **EB:** *The results of this study indicate that efforts to reduce smoking prevalence among female smokers before pregnancy have not been effective; however, efforts targeting pregnant women have met some success as rates have declined during pregnancy and after delivery. Smoking during pregnancy is associated with delivery of preterm infants, low infant birth weight, and increased infant mortality. After delivery, exposure to secondhand smoke can increase an infant's risk for respiratory tract infections and for dying of sudden infant death syndrome (Tong et al, 2009).*
- ▲ Assess for signs of depression and make appropriate referral: inadequate weight gain, underutilization of prenatal care, increased substance use, and premature birth. Past personal or family

---

• = Independent ▲ = Collaborative **EBN** = Evidence-Based Nursing **EB** = Evidence-Based

history of depression, single, poor health functioning, and alcohol use. **EB:** *These signs occurring during pregnancy may be associated with depression treatment. Engagement is important as untreated depression during pregnancy may have unfavorable outcomes for both women and children (Marcus, 2009).*

▲ Ensure that pregnant clients have an adequate diet and take multimicronutrient supplements during pregnancy. **EB:** *Nutrition plays an important role in the growth and development of the fetus. Overall, the diet of pregnant women has been reported to be deficient in calories and micronutrients. Both macronutrients and micronutrients are important for a woman to sustain pregnancy and for appropriate growth of the fetus. This systematic review demonstrated that prenatal supplementation with multimicronutrients was associated with a significantly reduced risk of low-birthweight infants and with improved birth weight (Shah, Ohlsson, & Knowledge Synthesis Group, 2009).*

• Consider a policy to fortify flour and pasta products with folate. **EB:** *In Quebec, Canada, public health measures to increase folic acid intake were followed by a decrease in the birth prevalence of severe congenital heart defects. These findings support the hypothesis that folic acid has a preventive effect on heart defects (Ionescu-Ittu et al, 2009).*

Intrapartal Care

• Encourage psychosocial support during labor. **EB:** *In a randomized control trial conducted at the University College Hospital Ibadan, Nigeria, women with anticipated vaginal delivery were recruited and randomized at the antenatal clinic. The experimental group had companionship in addition to routine care throughout labor until 2 hours after delivery, while the controls had only routine care. The primary outcome measure was caesarean section rate. Women with companionship had better labor outcomes compared to those without (Morhason-Bello et al, 2009).*

• Consider using aroma therapy during labor. **EB:** *Pain was reduced for nulliparae in this study (Burns et al, 2007).*

• Offer immersion bath during labor. **EBN:** *The present findings of this study suggest that use of an immersion bath is a suitable alternative form of pain relief for women during labor (da Silva, de Oliveira, & Nobre, 2009).*

• Provide massage and relaxation techniques during labor. **EB:** *The findings in this study suggest that regular massage with relaxation techniques from late pregnancy to birth is an acceptable coping strategy for pain relief (Kimber et al, 2008).*

• Offer the client in labor a light diet and water. **EB:** *In this study consumption of a light diet during labor did not influence obstetric or neonatal outcomes in participants, nor did it increase the incidence of vomiting. Women who are allowed to eat in labor have similar lengths of labor and operative delivery rates to those allowed water only (O'Sullivan et al, 2009).*

 ## Multicultural

Prenatal

• Provide prenatal care for black and white clients. **EB:** *Black-white disparities in infant mortality persist in the United States. In the years 2001 to 2004 Wisconsin had the highest black infant mortality rate (IMR) in the 40 states reporting. IMR have declined in Wisconsin from 2002 to 2007 despite national trends. Preliminary information suggests contributing factors may include improvement in adequate medical care and prenatal care for all (CDC, 2009).*

Intrapartal

• Consider the client's culture when assisting in labor and delivery. **EB:** *This study demonstrated the need for a culturally sensitive, reliable, and valid instrument to better understand the self-efficacy of childbirth as a basis for developing effective interventions to increase normal childbirth among Iranian pregnant women (Khorsandi et al, 2008).*

Postpartal

• Provide health and nutrition education for Chinese women after childbirth. Provide information and guidance on contemporary postpartum practices and take away common misconceptions about traditional dietary and health behaviors (e.g., fruit and vegetables should be restricted because of cold nature). Encourage a balanced diet and discourage unhealthy hygiene taboos.

• = Independent   ▲ = Collaborative   **EBN** = Evidence-Based Nursing   **EB** = Evidence-Based

EB: *"Sitting month" is the Chinese tradition for postpartum customs. Available studies indicate that some of the traditional postpartum practices are potentially harmful for women's health. Therefore, Chinese women are advised to follow a specific set of food choices and health care practices. For example, the puerperal women should stay inside and not go outdoors; all windows in the room should be sealed well to avoid wind. Bathing and hair washing should be restricted to prevent possible headache and body pain in later years. Foods such as fruits, vegetables, soybean products, and cold drinks that are considered "cold" should be avoided. In contrast, foods such as brown sugar, fish, chicken, and pig's trotter, which are considered "hot," should be encouraged. It is believed that if a woman does not observe these restrictions, she may suffer from poor health later in life. Several studies indicated that the incidences of postpartum health problems are high and these problems maybe have relation to traditional and unscientific dietary and behavior practices in the postpartum period. Available Chinese data also suggested that the incidences of constipation and hemorrhoids were associated with lack of exercise and a decreased intake of fruit and vegetables; the risk of oral problems were associated with no teethbrushing and excessive intake of sugar during the puerperium (Liu et al, 2009).*

- Health and nutrition education should include the Chinese family (particularly the relative who will be staying with the new mother) after the woman gives birth. **EB:** *The results of this study found that increased nutrition and health care knowledge did not lead to parallel dietary and health behavior changes. This lack of change is attributed to the fact that in China, the tradition to support a newly delivered woman and her baby for the first month after childbirth at home is still common. Most of the women had an elder female of the family such as her mother or mother-in-law as the support person. The elder female who takes care of the women may have hindered the changes due to traditional beliefs. The main problematic aspect of the study was the education intervention subjects aimed directly to the study of women, yet "sitting month" was usually recognized as an important event in the family and the postpartum woman has been taken care by her mother or mother-in-law (Liu et al, 2009).*

Home Care

Prenatal

▲ Involve pregnant drug users in drug treatment programs that include coordinated interventions in several areas: drug use, infectious diseases, mental health, personal and social welfare, and gynecological/obstetric care. **EB:** *This literature search revealed that involving pregnant drug users in drug treatment is likely to decrease the chances of prenatal and perinatal complications related to drug use and to increase access to prenatal care. Timely medical intervention can effectively prevent vertical transmission of human immunodeficiency virus and hepatitis B virus, as well as certain other sexually transmitted diseases, and would allow newborns infected with hepatitis C virus during birth to receive immediate treatment (Gyarmathy et al, 2009).*

Postpartal

- Provide video conferencing to support new parents. **EBN:** *The findings of this study indicate that VC equipment may be helpful for parents discharged from the hospital early after childbirth (Lindberg, Christensson, & Ohrling, 2009).*
- Consider reflexology for postpartum women to improve sleep quality. **EBN:** *In this RCT an intervention involving foot reflexology in the postnatal period significantly improved the quality of sleep in postpartum women (Li, Chen, & Li, 2009).*

Client/Family Teaching and Discharge Planning

Prenatal

- Provide dietary and lifestyle counseling as part of prenatal care to pregnant women. **EB:** *In this study an organized, consistent program of dietary and lifestyle counseling reduced weight gain in pregnancy (Asbee et al, 2009). Community-level interventions of improved perinatal care practices can bring about a reduction in maternal mortality (Kidney et al, 2009).*
- Provide the following information in parenting classes and via DVD: support mechanisms, information and antenatal education, breastfeeding, practical baby-care, and relationship changes. In-

---

• = Independent   ▲ = Collaborative   **EBN** = Evidence-Based Nursing   **EB** = Evidence-Based

clude fathers in the parenting classes. **EB:** *The men felt very involved with their partners' pregnancy but excluded from antenatal appointments and antenatal classes, and by the literature that was available. Parents had been unaware of, and surprised at, the changes in the relationship with their partners. They would have liked more information on elements of parenting and baby care, relationship changes and partners' perspectives prior to becoming parents. Parents suggested that information be provided on a DVD (Deave, Johnson, & Ingram, 2008).*

- Provide group prenatal care to families in the military. **EBN:** *Group PNC offers the potential for continuity of provider which the women were concerned was lacking. It also offers community with other women. In the process, women gain knowledge and power as a health care consumer (Kennedy et al, 2009).*

Postpartal

- Encourage physical activity in postpartum women; provide telephone counseling, pedometers, referral to community PA resources, social support, email advice on PA/pedometer goals, and newsletters. **EB:** *In this study these interventions were effective in increasing physical activity in postpartum women (Albright, Maddock, & Nigg, 2009).*
- Teach mothers of young children principles of a healthy lifestyle: substitute high fat foods with low fat foods such as fruits and vegetables, increase physical activity, consider a community-based self-management intervention to prevent weight gain. **EBN:** *Preventing weight gain rather than treating established obesity is an important economic and public health response to the rapidly increasing rates of obesity worldwide. In this study both a single health education session and interactive behavioral intervention resulted in a similar weight loss in the short term, although more participants in the interactive intervention lost or maintained weight. Self-monitoring appears to enhance weight loss when part of an intervention (Lombard et al, 2009).*

ⓔvolve   See the EVOLVE website for Weblinks for client education resources.

REFERENCES

Albright CL, Maddock JE, Nigg CR: Increasing physical activity in post-partum multiethnic women in Hawaii: results from a pilot study, *BMC Womens Health* 9:4, 2009.

Asbee SM, Jenkins TR, Butler JR et al: Preventing excessive weight gain during pregnancy through dietary and lifestyle counseling: a randomized controlled trial, *Obstet Gynecol* 113(2 Pt 1):305–312, 2009.

Burns E, Zobbi V, Panzeri D et al: Aromatherapy in childbirth: a pilot randomised controlled trial, *BJOG* 114(7):838–844, 2007.

Centers for Disease Control and Prevention (CDC): Apparent disappearance of the black-white infant mortality gap—Dane County, Wisconsin, 1990–2007, *MMWR Morb Mortal Wkly Rep* 58(20):561–565, 2009.

da Silva FM, de Oliveira SM, Nobre MR: A randomised controlled trial evaluating the effect of immersion bath on labour pain, *Midwifery* 25(3):286–294, 2009.

Deave T, Johnson D, Ingram J: Transition to parenthood: the needs of parents in pregnancy and early parenthood, *BMC Pregnancy Childbirth* 8:30, 2008.

Gyarmathy VA, Giraudon I, Hedrich D et al: Drug use and pregnancy—challenges for public health, *Euro Surveill* 4(9):33–36, 2009.

Ionescu-Ittu R, Marelli AJ, Mackie AS et al: Prevalence of severe congenital heart disease after folic acid fortification of grain products: time trend analysis in Quebec, Canada, *BMJ* 338:b1673, 2009.

Kennedy HP, Farrell T, Paden R et al: "I wasn't alone"—a study of group prenatal care in the military, *J Midwifery Womens Health* 54(3):176–183, 2009.

Khorsandi M, Ghofranipour F, Faghihzadeh S et al: Iranian version of childbirth self-efficacy inventory, *J Clin Nurs* 17(21):2846–2855, 2008.

Kidney E, Winter HR, Khan KS et al: Systematic review of effect of community-level interventions to reduce maternal mortality, *BMC Pregnancy Childbirth* 9:2, 2009.

Kimber L, McNabb M, McCourt C et al: Massage or music for pain relief in labour: a pilot randomised placebo controlled trial, *Eur J Pain* 12(8):961–969, 2008.

Li CY, Chen SC, Li CY: Randomised controlled trial of the effectiveness of using foot reflexology to improve quality of sleep amongst Taiwanese postpartum women, *Midwifery* 2009, Epub ahead of print.

Lindberg I, Christensson K, Ohrling K: Parents' experiences of using videoconferencing as a support in early discharge after childbirth, *Midwifery* 25(4):357–365, 2009.

Liu N, Mao L, Sun X et al: The effect of health and nutrition education intervention on women's postpartum beliefs and practices: a randomized controlled trial, *BMC Public Health* 9:45, 2009.

Lombard CB, Deeks AA, Ball K et al: Weight, physical activity and dietary behavior change in young mothers: short term results of the HeLP-her cluster randomized controlled trial, *Nutrition Journal* 8:17, 2009.

Marcus SM: Depression during pregnancy: rates, risks and consequences—Motherisk Update 2008, *J Clin Pharmacol* 16(1):e15–22, 2009.

Morhason-Bello IO, Adedokun BO, Ojengbede OA et al: Assessment of the effect of psychosocial support during childbirth in Ibadan, south-west Nigeria: a randomised controlled trial, *Aust N Z J Obstet Gynaecol* 49(2):145–150, 2009.

O'Sullivan G, Liu B, Hart D et al: Effect of food intake during labour on obstetric outcome: randomised controlled trial, *BMJ* 338:b784, 2009.

Shah PS, Ohlsson A: Knowledge Synthesis Group On Determinants Of Low Birth Weight And Preterm Births: Effects of prenatal multimicronutrient supplementation on pregnancy outcomes: a meta-analysis, *CMAJ* 180(12):E99–108, 2009.

Tong VT, Jones JR, Dietz PM et al: Trends in smoking before, during, and after pregnancy - Pregnancy Risk Assessment Monitoring System (PRAMS), United States, 31 sites, 2000–2005, *MMWR Surveill Summ* 58(4):1–29, 2009.

Impaired Comfort   *Katharine Kolcaba, PhD, RN*   evolve

NANDA-I

Definition

Perceived lack of ease, relief, and transcendence in physical, psychospiritual, environmental and social dimensions

Defining Characteristics

Anxiety; crying; disturbed sleep pattern; fear; illness-related symptoms; inability to relax; insufficient resources (e.g., financial, social support); irritability; lack of environmental control; lack of privacy; lack of situational control; moaning; noxious environmental stimuli; reports being uncomfortable; reports being cold; reports being hot; reports distressing symptoms; reports hunger; reports itching; reports lack of contentment in situation; reports lack of ease in situation; restlessness; treatment-related side effects (e.g., medication, radiation)

NOC   (Nursing Outcomes Classification)

Suggested NOC Outcomes

Client Satisfaction, Symptom Control, Comfort Status, Coping, Hope, Pain Control, Personal Well-Being, Spiritual Health

Example NOC Outcomes with Indicators
Comfort Status as evidenced by the following indicators: Physical and psychological well-being/Symptom control/Care consistent with needs (Rate the outcome and indicators of **Comfort Status:** 1 = severely compromised, 2 = substantially compromised, 3 = moderately compromised, 4 = mildly compromised, 5 = not compromised [see Section I].)

Client Outcomes

Client Will (Specify Time Frame):

- Provide evidence for improved comfort compared to baseline
- Identify strategies, with or without significant others, to improve and/or maintain acceptable comfort level
- Perform appropriate interventions, with or without significant others, as needed to improve and/or maintain acceptable comfort level
- Evaluate the effectiveness of strategies to maintain and/or acceptable comfort level
- Maintain an acceptable level of comfort when possible

NIC   (Nursing Interventions Classification)

Suggested NIC Interventions

Calming Techniques, Simple Massage, Hand Massage, Comfort Contract, Heat/Cold Application, Hope Inspiration, Humor, Meditation Facilitation, Music Therapy, Pain Management, Presence of Nurse and/or Significant Others, Relaxation Therapy, Spiritual Growth Facilitation, Distraction

Example NIC Activities—Hope Inspiration
Assist the client/significant others to identify areas of hope in life and/or to expand spiritual self; Involve the client/significant others in client care

● = Independent   ▲ = Collaborative   **EBN** = Evidence-Based Nursing   **EB** = Evidence-Based

Nursing Interventions and *Rationales*

- Assess client's current level of comfort. This is the first step in helping clients achieve improved comfort. *Sources of assessment data to determine level of comfort can be subjective, objective, primary, secondary, focused, or even special needs (Kolcaba, 2003; Wilkinson & VanLeuven, 2007).*
- Comfort is a holistic state under which pain management is included. Management of discomforts, however, can be better managed, and with less analgesics, by also addressing other comfort needs such as anxiety, insufficient information, social isolation, financial difficulties, etc. **EBN:** *One randomized study (N=53) found that female breast cancer clients undergoing radiation therapy rated their overall comfort as being greater than the sum of the hypothesized components of comfort, which lent support to the theory of the holistic nature of comfort (Kolcaba & Steiner, 2000).*
- Assist client to understand how to rate their current state of holistic comfort, utilizing institution's preferred method of documentation. *Documentation of comfort prenursing and postnursing interactions is essential to demonstrating the efficacy of nursing activities (Kolcaba, 2003; Kolcaba et al, 2004; Kolcaba, Tilton, & Drouin, 2006).*
- Enhance feelings of trust between the client and the health care provider. To attain the highest comfort level a client must be able to trust their nurse (Kolcaba, 2003; Kolcaba et al, 2004). **EBN:** *This randomized design (N=31) demonstrated the importance of promoting open relationships with clients which helps to acknowledge their individuality. Knowing the client/significant others is essential in the provision of to optimum palliative and terminal care (Kolcaba et al, 2004).*
- Manipulate the environment as necessary to improve comfort. **EBN:** *In two experimental studies, the protocol included that all clients be asked about preferences for light, furnishings, body position, television settings, etc. (Kolcaba, 2003; Kolcaba et al, 2004; Dowd et al, 2007).*
- Provide distraction techniques such as music, television, or games. These activities help to temporarily distract the client from discomforting sensations. **EBN:** *In an experiment, music therapy was found to reduce reported discomfort and anxiety compared to a control condition of no music in a study of individuals undergoing flexible sigmoidoscopy (Siedlecki & Good, 2006).*
- Encourage early mobilization and provide routine position changes to decrease physical discomforts associated with bed rest. **EBN:** *An experimental study of 420 individuals following nonemergency cardiac catheterization found consistently lower scores for back discomfort with no increase in bleeding in the intervention group, who were turned every hour (Chair et al, 2003). A review comparing the study by Chair et al found its results to be consistent with other studies which have found that backrest elevation, side lying, and early ambulation all improved comfort (Benson, 2004).*
- Provide simple massage. **EBN:** *Two experiments, one with 31 clients and one with 60, demonstrated that hand massage was helpful by reducing discomfort and anxiety, and promoting relaxation and sleep (Kolcaba, et al, 2004, Kolcaba, Schirm, & Steiner, 2006). In a descriptive study, reducing environmental stimuli in a critical care unit promoted client comfort (Honkus, 2003).*
- Provide healing touch, which may be well-suited for clients who cannot tolerate more stimulating interventions such as simple massage. **EBN:** *In an experiment (N=58), college students experienced enhanced comfort immediately after healing touch, compared to their baseline comfort level (Dowd et al, 2007).*
- Inform the client of options for control of discomfort such as self-hypnosis and guided imagery, and provide these interventions if appropriate. **EBN:** *A study found that female breast cancer clients (N=53) treated with guided imagery while undergoing radiation therapy had significant improvements in comfort compared with the control group (Kolcaba, 2003).*
- Utilize careful, safe technique when transferring clients in and out of beds or chairs. **EBN:** *A descriptive study of orthopedic nurses and their clients found that clients felt safer and more comfortable during transfers when the nurses used safe technique as measured by work technique score (Kjellberg, Lagerstrom, & Hagberg, 2004).*

 ### Geriatric

- Hand massage is helpful for elders because they respond well to touch and the provider's presence. **EBN:** *In an experiment (N=60), the effects of hand massage on comfort of nursing home residents was found to be significant immediately after the massage compared to residents who did not receive hand massage (Kolcaba, Schirm, & Steiner, 2006).*

• = Independent   ▲ = Collaborative   **EBN** = Evidence-Based Nursing   **EB** = Evidence-Based

- Frail elderly clients should be protected from cold discomfort and can be offered warmed blankets to decrease discomfort. **EBN:** *A pre-and post-design study of 49 clients found that clients receiving warmed blankets reported a significantly lower level of discomfort 1 hour after its application (Robinson & Benton, 2002). While not specifically focused on elderly clients, this study (N=126) found significantly increased comfort and decreased anxiety in clients who used self-controlled warming gowns (Wagner, Byrne, & Kolcaba 2006).*
- Increase fluid intake within cardiac or renal limits to a minimum of 1500 mL/day. *Dry skin is caused by loss of fluid through the skin; increasing fluid intake rehydrates the skin. Adequate hydration helps decrease itching.*
- Use a humidifier or place a container of water on a heat source to increase humidity in the environment, especially during winter. *Increasing moisture in the air helps to keep moisture in the skin.*

Multicultural

- Assess for the influence of cultural beliefs, norms, and values on the client's perceptions of skin and/or hair status and practices. *What the client considers normal and abnormal skin and hair condition may be based on cultural perceptions.*
- Identify and clarify cultural language used to describe skin and hair. *Clients may interchange words meaning discomfort and pain, may refer to minor discomforts as pain, or may not discuss nonpainful discomforts at all (Kolcaba, 2003).*
- Assess skin for ashy or yellow-brown appearance. *Black skin appears ashy and brown skin appears yellow-brown when clients have pallor sometimes associated with discomfort (Peters, 2007).*
- Encourage the use of lanolin-based lotions for clients with dry skin. Ask clients about their preferences. **EBN:** *In an experiment with 31 hospice clients, nonallergenic lotion soothed dry skin and promoted comfort (Kolcaba et al, 2004).*
- Offer hair oil and lanolin-based lotion for dry scalp and skin. *Black skin seems to produce less oil than lighter-colored skin; therefore African Americans may use more lubricants as a normal part of skin hygiene.*
- Use soap sparingly if the skin is dry. *Black skin tends to be dry and soap will exacerbate this condition.*

Home Care

- Assist the client and family in identifying and providing comfort measures that are effective and safe for the condition and situation.
- Encourage mobilization as frequently as is appropriate for the client.
- Keep the temperature of the home moderate to warm for frail clients.

Client/Family Teaching and Discharge Planning

- Teach techniques to use when the client is uncomfortable, including relaxation techniques, guided imagery, hypnosis, and music therapy. **EBN:** *Interventions such as progressive muscle relaxation training, guided imagery, and music therapy can effectively decrease the perception of uncomfortable sensations, including pain (Siedliecki & Good, 2006). Families want to learn how to provide comfort measures to their loved ones who are uncomfortable. (Kolcaba et al, 2004).*
- Instruct the client and family on prescribed medications and therapies that improve comfort.
- Teach the client to follow up with the physician or other practitioner if discomfort persists.

⊖volve   See the EVOLVE website for Weblinks for client education resources.

REFERENCES

Benson G: Changing patients' position in bed after non-emergency coronary angiography reduced back pain, *Evid Based Nurs* 7(1):19, 2004.

Chair SY, Taylor-Piliae RE, Lam G et al: Effect of positioning on back pain after coronary angiography, *J Adv Nurs* 42(5):470–478, 2003.

Dowd T, Kolcaba K, Steiner R et al: Comparison of healing touch and coaching on stress and comfort in young college students, *Holist Nurs Pract* 21(4):194–202, 2007.

Honkus V: Sleep deprivation in critical care units, *Crit Care Nurs Q* 26(3):179–189, 2003.

Kjellberg K, Lagerstrom M, Hagberg M: Patient safety and comfort during transfers in relation to nurses' work technique, *J Adv Nurs* 47(3):251–259, 2004.

Kolcaba K: *Comfort theory and practice: a holistic vision for health care,* New York, 2003, Springer.

● = Independent   ▲ = Collaborative   **EBN** = Evidence-Based Nursing   **EB** = Evidence-Based

Kolcaba K, Tilton C, Drouin C: Comfort theory: a unifying framework to enhance the practice environment, *J Nurs Admin* 36(11):538–544, 2006.

Kolcaba K, Steiner R: Empirical evidence for the nature of holistic comfort, *J Holist Nurs* 18(1):46–62, 2000.

Kolcaba K, Schirm V, Steiner R: Effects of hand massage on comfort of nursing home residents, *Geriatr Nurs* 27(2):85–91, 2006.

Kolcaba K, Dowd T, Steiner R et al: Efficacy of hand massage for enhancing comfort of hospice patients, *J Hospice Palliat Care* 6(2):91–101, 2004.

Peters J: Examining and describing skin conditions, *Practice Nurse* 34(8):39–40, 43, 45, 2007.

Robinson S, Benton G: Warmed blankets: an intervention to promote comfort for elderly hospitalized patients, *Geriatr Nurs* 23(6):320–323, 2002.

Siedliecki S, Good M: Effect of music on power, pain, depression and disability, *J Adv Nurs* 54(5):553–562, 2006.

Wagner D, Byrne M, Kolcaba K: Effect of comfort warming on preoperative patients, *AORN J* 84(3):1–13, 2006.

Wilkinson J, VanLeuven K: *Fundamentals of nursing*, Philadelphia, 2007, F.A. Davis.

Readiness for enhanced Comfort   *Natalie Fischetti, PhD, RN*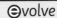

NANDA-I

Definition

A pattern of ease, relief and transcendence in physical, psychospiritual, environmental, and/or social dimensions that can be strengthened

Defining Characteristics

Expresses desire to enhance comfort; expresses desire to enhance feelings of contentment; expresses desire to enhance relaxation; expresses desire to enhance resolution of complaints

NOC   (Nursing Outcomes Classification)

Suggested NOC Outcomes

Client Satisfaction: Caring, Symptom Control, Comfort Level, Coping, Hope, Motivation, Pain Control, Participation in Healthcare Decisions, Spiritual Health

Example **NOC** Outcomes with Indicators
Comfort Level as evidenced by the following indicators: Physical well-being/Symptom control/Psychological well-being/Pain control (Rate the outcome and indicators of **Comfort Level:** 1 = not at all satisfied, 2 = somewhat satisfied, 3 = moderately satisfied, 4 = very satisfied, 5 = completely satisfied [See Section I].)

Client Outcomes

Client Will (Specify Time Frame):

- Assess current level of comfort as acceptable
- Express the need to achieve an enhanced level of comfort
- Identify strategies to enhance comfort
- Perform appropriate interventions as needed for increased comfort
- Evaluate the effectiveness of interventions at regular intervals
- Maintain an enhanced level of comfort when possible

NIC   (Nursing Interventions Classification)

Suggested NIC Interventions

Calming Technique, Cutaneous Stimulation, Environmental Management, Comfort, Heat/Cold Application, Hope Inspiration, Humor, Meditation Facilitation, Music Therapy, Pain Management, Presence, Simple Guided Imagery, Simple Massage, Simple Relaxation Therapy, Spiritual Growth Facilitation, Therapeutic Play, Therapeutic Touch, Touch, TENS, Distraction

---

Example NIC Activities—Spiritual Growth Facilitation
Assist the client with identifying barriers and attitudes that hinder growth or self-discovery; Assist the client to explore beliefs as related to healing of the body, mind, and spirit; Model healthy relating and reasoning skills

Nursing Interventions and *Rationales*

- Assess client's current level of comfort. *This is the first step in helping clients to achieve enhanced comfort. Sources of assessment data to determine level of comfort can be subjective, objective, primary, secondary, focused, or even special needs (Wilkinson & VanLeuven, 2007). While clinicians are assessing pain more frequently, this has not resulted in widespread pain reduction. A solution may be to establish comfort-function goals for clients, reminding clients to tell their nurse when pain interferes with function (Pasero & McCaffrey, 2004).*

- Help client understand that enhanced comfort is a desirable, positive, and achievable goal. *Human beings strive to have their basic comfort needs met, but comfort is more than just the absence of pain (Kolcaba, 2003). Comfort is best recognized when a person leaves the state of discomfort and nurses can enhance their client's comfort in everyday practice (Malinowski & Stamler, 2002).*

- ▲ Enhance feelings of trust between the client and the health care provider. **EBN:** *Clients had greater feelings of emotional comfort when they felt secure, informed, and valued (Williams, Dawson, & Kristjanson, 2009).* **EBN:** *Trust is an essential element in the nurse-client relationship (Bell & Duffy, 2009).*

- Use therapeutic massage for enhancement of comfort. **EBN:** *This study determined the effects of hand massage on clients near the end of life, with clients reporting feeling special and that the massage felt good. Also, meaningful connectedness was achieved (Kolcaba et al, 2004). Massage is helpful for low back pain and other orthopaedic problems (Dryden, Baskwill, & Preyde, 2004).* **EBN:** *Women who received massage in the latent labor period prior to delivery had less pain perception than women who did not (Yildirim & Sahin, 2004).*

- Teach and encourage use of guided imagery. *Guided imagery can be helpful on pain level, physical functional status, and self-efficacy in persons with fibromyalgia (Menzies, Taylor, & Bourguignon, 2006).*

- Foster and instill hope in clients whenever possible. **EBN:** *This study was the first to document the effectiveness of a brief hope intervention. The intervention produced a significant effect on pain tolerance. The increase in pain tolerance was stronger for females than males (Berg, Synder, & Hamilton, 2008).* See the care plan for **Hopelessness**.

- Provide opportunities for and enhance spiritual care activities. The need for comfort and reassurance may be perceived as spiritual needs. **EBN:** *To meet these needs, nurses engaged in interaction when they comforted assured clients. Participants also identified absolution as a spiritual need, and there is evidence that forgiveness may bring one feelings of joy, peace, elation, and a sense of renewed self-worth (Narayanasomy et al, 2004).* **EB:** *Individuals who practiced spiritual meditation were found to have a greater increase in pain tolerance (Wachholtz & Pargament, 2008).*

- Enhance social support and family involvement. **EBN:** *Methods to help terminally ill clients and their families transition from cure to comfort care included spending an increased amount of time with one's family, appointing one close friend to act as a contact person for other friends, and establishing an e-mail list serve for updates of a client's status and care (Duggleby & Berry, 2005).*

- Encourage mind-body therapies such as meditation as an enhanced comfort activity. **EB:** *The most common therapies used were meditation, imagery, and yoga. Research demonstrating the connection between the mind and body has therefore increased interest in the potential use of these therapies (Wolsko et al, 2004).* **EBN:** *Meditation has been shown to reduce anxiety, relieve pain, decrease depression, enhance mood and self-esteem, decrease stress, and generally improve clinical symptoms (Bonadonna, 2003).*

- Promote participation in creative arts and activity programs. **EBN:** *A creative arts program for caregivers of cancer clients was shown to lower anxiety and positive emotions were expressed (Walsh, Martin, & Schmidt, 2004).*

- ▲ Encourage clients to use Health Information Technology (HIT) as needed. Client services can now include management of medications, symptoms, emotional support, health education, and health information (Moody, 2005). **EBN:** *Injured car occupants experienced significantly lower dimensions of pain and discomfort with nursing intervention via telephone (Franzen et al, 2009).*

• = Independent   ▲ = Collaborative   **EBN** = Evidence-Based Nursing   **EB** = Evidence-Based

- Evaluate the effectiveness of all interventions at regular intervals and adjust therapies as necessary. **EBN:** *It is important for nurses to determine comfort and pain management goals because comfort goals will change with circumstances. Ask questions and ask them frequently, such as "How is your comfort?" Establish guidelines for frequency of assessment and document responses noting if goals are being met (Kolcaba, 2003).* **EB:** *A comprehensive palliative care project was conducted at 11 sites. The interdisciplinary review process built trust, endorsed creativity, and ultimately resulted in better meeting the needs of clients, families, and the community (London et al, 2005). Evaluation must be planned for, ongoing, and systematic. Evaluation demonstrates caring and responsibility on the part of the nurse (Wilkinson & VanLeuven, 2007).*
- Explain all procedures, including sensations likely to be experienced during the procedure. **EBN:** *Clients undergoing abdominal surgery in an experimental group received routine care and a preoperative nursing intervention which included: explaining the causes of pain that would occur due to the operation, explaining the influences of postoperative pain and the importance of early out-of-bed activities, teaching how to reduce pain using nonpharmacological methods, encouraging requesting pain medications after surgery, encouraging expression of feelings and concerns and setting a pain control goal. This group had a significant decrease in postoperative anxiety and a statistically significantly lower postoperative pain intensity 4 hours and 24 hours after the surgical procedure (Lin & Wang, 2004).*

Pediatric

- Assess and evaluate child's level of comfort at frequent intervals. *Comfort needs should be individually assessed and planned for. With assessment of pain in children, it is best to use input from the parents or a primary care provider. Use only accepted scales for standardized pain assessment (Remke & Chrastek, 2007).*
- Skin-to-skin contact (SSC) and selection of most effective method improves the comfort of newborns during routine blood draws. **EB:** *Premature infants who received skin-to-skin contact demonstrated a decrease in pain reaction during heel lancing (Castral et al, 2008).*
- Adjust the environment as needed to enhance comfort. *Environmental comfort measures include maintaining orderliness; quiet; minimizing furniture; special attention to temperature, light and sound, color, and landscape (Kolcaba & DeMarco, 2005).*
- Encourage parental presence whenever possible. The same basic principles for managing pain in adults and children apply to neonates. *In addition to other comfort measures, parental presence should be encouraged whenever possible (Pasero, 2004).* **EBN:** *This study reported the effects of co-residence and caregiving on the parents of children dying with AIDS. Although parents who did more caregiving did experience anxiety, insomnia, and fatigue, the caregiving experiences for many parents gave them an opportunity to fulfill their perceived duty as parents before their child died. This in turn resulted in better physical and emotional health outcomes (Kespichayawattana & VanLandingham, 2003).*
- Promote use of alternative comforting strategies such as positioning, presence, massage, spiritual care, music therapy, art therapy, and story-telling to enhance comfort when needed. In addition to oral sucrose, other comfort measures should be used to alleviate pain such as swaddling, skin-to-skin contact with mother, nursing, rocking, and holding (Pasero, 2004). **EBN:** *Building on the belief that parents are the primary care providers and health care resource for families, the blended infant massage parenting program is effective for both mother and infant (Porter & Porter, 2004).* **EB:** *In a study that examined the effects of music on pain in a pediatric burn unit during nursing procedures, the use of music during procedures reduced pain (Whitehead-Pleaux et al, 2007).*
- Support child's spirituality **EBN:** *Children are born with an intrinsic spiritual essence that can be enhanced. Spirituality promotes a sense of hope, comfort, and strength and creates a sense of being loved and nurtured by a higher power (Elkins & Cavendish, 2004).*

Geriatric

- Interventions described previously may be appropriate for geriatric client.
- Promote participation in creative arts and activity programs. **EBN:** *The use of an individualized music protocol program by elderly women was shown to promote and maintain sleep (Johnson, 2003).*

• = Independent   ▲ = Collaborative   **EBN** = Evidence-Based Nursing   **EB** = Evidence-Based

Multicultural

- Identify cultural beliefs, values, lifestyles, practices, and problem-solving strategies when assessing clients. **EBN:** *In a qualitative study that identified issues in pain management, cultural beliefs were cited as impediments or barriers to pain management, for example, some Moroccan physicians felt illness-related pain was inevitable, that suffering was normal, and that it had to be endured, especially by boys (McCarthy et al, 2004).* **EBN:** *In this study, focus groups were conducted with Moroccan pediatric oncology nurses and physicians to better understand how pain management was achieved in children with cancer. When no medication was available to relieve pain, other techniques were used to comfort clients. These included use of cold therapy, presence, holding a child's hand, utilizing distraction techniques, playing with them, story-telling, and encouraging parental engagement activities (McCarthy et al, 2004).*
- Enhance cultural knowledge by actively seeking out information regarding different cultural and ethnic groups. *Cultural knowledge is the process of actively seeking information about different cultural and ethnic groups such as their world views, health conditions, health practices, use of home remedies or self-medication, barriers to health care, and risk taking or health-seeking behaviors (Institute of Medicine, 2002).*
- Recognize the impact of culture on communication styles and techniques. *Communication and culture are closely intertwined and communication is the way culture is transmitted and preserved. It influences how feelings are expressed, decisions are made, and what verbal and nonverbal expressions are acceptable. By the age of 5, cultural patterns of communication can be identified in children (Giger & Davidhizar, 2004).*
- Provide culturally competent care to clients from different cultural groups. *Cultural competency requires health care providers to act appropriately in the context of daily interactions with people who are different from themselves. Providers need to honor and respect the beliefs, interpersonal styles, attitudes and behaviors of others. This level of cultural awareness requires providers to refrain from forming stereotypes and judgments based on one's own cultural framework (Institute of Medicine, 2002).* **EBN:** *The findings from a review of two studies of Japanese and American women suggest that although there were common ethical concerns between the two cultures, the cultural context of the underlying values may create very different meanings and result in different nursing practices (Wros, Doutrich, & Izumi, 2004). Visual imagery with mind body relaxation may be used for symptom control in Hispanic persons diagnosed with fibromyalgia (Menzies & Kim, 2008).*

Home Care

- The nursing interventions described previously in **Readiness for enhanced Comfort** may be used with clients in the home care setting. When needed, adaptations can be made to meet the needs of specific clients, families, and communities.
- ▲ Make appropriate referrals to other organizations or providers as needed to enhance comfort. *Referrals should have merit, be practical, timely, individualized, coordinated, and mutually agreed upon by all involved (Hunt, 2005).*
- ▲ Promote an interdisciplinary approach to home care. *Members of the interdisciplinary team who provide specialized care to enhance comfort can include the physician, physical therapist, occupational therapist, nutritionist, music therapist, social worker, etc. (Stanhope & Lancaster, 2006).*
- Evaluate regularly if enhanced comfort is attainable in the home care setting. *Home health agencies monitor client outcomes closely. Evaluation is an ongoing process and is essential for the provision of quality care (Stanhope & Lancaster, 2006).*

Client/Family Teaching and Discharge Planning

- Teach client how to regularly assess levels of comfort.
- Instruct client that a variety of interventions may be needed at any given time to enhance comfort.
- Help clients to understand that enhanced comfort is an achievable goal.
- Teach techniques to enhance comfort as needed.
- ▲ When needed, empower clients to seek out other health professionals as members of the interdisciplinary team to assist with comforting measures and techniques.

• = Independent   ▲ = Collaborative   **EBN** = Evidence-Based Nursing   **EB** = Evidence-Based

- Encourage self-care activities and continued self-evaluation of achieved comfort levels to ensure enhanced comfort will be maintained.

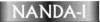 See the EVOLVE website for Weblinks for client education resources.

REFERENCES

Bell L, Duffy A: A concept analysis of nurse-patient trust, *BJN* 18(1):46–51, 2009.

Berg C, Snyder C, Hamilton N: The effectiveness of a hope intervention in coping with cold pressor pain, *J Health Psychol* 13:804–809, 2008.

Bonadonna R: Meditation's impact on chronic illness, *Holist Nurs Pract* 17(6):309–319, 2003.

Castral T, Warnock F, Leite A et al: The effects of skin-to-skin contact during acute pain in preterm newborns, *Eur J Pain* 12(4):464–471, 2008.

Dryden T, Baskwill A, Preyde M: Massage therapy for the orthopoedic patient: a review, *Orthop Nurs* 23:327–332, 2004.

Duggleby W, Berry P: Transitions and shifting goals of care for palliative patients and their families, *Clin J Oncol Nurs* 9(4):425–428, 2005.

Elkins M, Cavendish R: Developing a plan for pediatric spiritual care, *Holist Nurs Pract* 18(4):179–184, 2004.

Franzen C, Brulin C, Stenlund H et al: Injured road users' health-related quality of life after telephone intervention: a randomized controlled trial, *J Clin Nurs* 18(1):108–116, 2009.

Giger J, Davidhizar R: *Transcultural nursing: assessment and intervention,* ed 4, St Louis, 2004, Mosby.

Hunt R: *Introduction to community-based nursing,* ed 3, Philadelphia, 2005, Lippincott.

Institute of Medicine: *Speaking of health,* Washington, 2002, The National Academies Press.

Johnson J: The use of music to promote sleep in older women, *J Community Health Nurs* 20:27–35, 2003.

Kespichayawattana J, VanLandingham M: Effects of coresidence and caregiving on health of Thai parents of adult children with AIDS, *J Nurs Sch* 35(3):217–224, 2003.

Kolcaba K: *Comfort theory and practice,* New York, 2003, Springer.

Kolcaba K, DeMarco M: Comfort theory and application to pediatric nursing, *Pediatr Nurs* 31(3):187–194, 2005.

Kolcaba K, Dowd T, Steiner R et al: Efficacy of hand massage for enhancing the comfort of hospice patients, *Int J Palliat Nurs* 6(2):91–102, 2004.

Lin L, Wang R: Abdominal surgery, pain and anxiety, *J Adv Nurs* 51(3):252–260, 2004.

London M, McSkimming S, Drew N et al: Evaluation of a comprehensive, adaptable, life-affirming, longitudinal palliative care project, *J Palliat Med* 8(6):1214–1225, 2005.

Malinowski A, Stamler L: Comfort: exploration of the concept in nursing, *J Adv Nurs* 39(6):599–606, 2002.

McCarthy P, Chammas G, Wilimas J et al: Managing children's cancer pain in Morocco, *J Nurs Scholarsh* 36(1):11–15, 2004.

Menzies V, Kim S: Relaxation and guided imagery in Hispanic persons diagnosed with fibromyalgia: a pilot study, *Fam Community Health* 31(3):204–212, 2008.

Menzies V, Taylor A, Bourguignon C: Effects of guided imagery on outcomes of pain, functional status, and self-efficacy in persons diagnosed with fibromyalgia, *J Altern Complement Med* 12(1):23–30, 2006.

Moody L: E-health web portals: delivering holistic healthcare and making home the point of care, *Holist Nurs Pract* 19(4):156–160, 2005.

Narayanasomy A, Clissett P, Parumal L et al: Responses to the spiritual needs of older people, *J Adv Nurs* 48(1):6–16, 2004.

Pasero C: Pain relief for neonates, *Am J Nurs* 104(5):44–47, 2004.

Pasero C, McCaffrey M: Comfort—function goals, *Am J Nurs* 104(9):77–81, 2004.

Porter L, Porter B: A blended infant massage-parenting enhancement program for recovering substance abusing mothers, *Pediatr Nurs* 30(5):363–401, 2004.

Remke S, Chrastek J: Improving care in the home for children with palliative care needs, *Home Healthc Nurse* 25(1):45–51, 2007.

Stanhope M, Lancaster J: *Foundation of nursing in the community,* ed 2, St Louis, 2006, Mosby.

Wachholtz A, Pargament K: Migraines and meditation: does spirituality matter? *J Behav Med* 31(4):351–366, 2008.

Walsh S, Martin S, Schmidt L: Testing the efficacy of a creative-arts intervention with family caregivers of patients with cancer, *J Nurs Scholarsh* 36(3):214–219, 2004.

Whitehead-Pleaux AM, Zebrowski N, Baryza MJ et al: Exploring the effects of music therapy on pediatric pain: phase 1, *J Music Ther* 44(3):217–241, 2007.

Wilkinson J, VanLeuven K: *Fundamentals of nursing,* Philadelphia, 2007, F.A. Davis.

Williams A, Dawson S, Kristjanson L: Patients felt greater personal control and emotional comfort in hospital when they felt secure, informed, and valued, *Evid Based Nurs* 12(1):29, 2009.

Wolsko P, Eisenberg D, Davis R et al: Use of mind-body medical therapies, *J Gen Intern Med* 19:43–50, 2004.

Wros P, Doutrich D, Izumi S: Ethical concerns: comparison of values from two cultures, *Nurs Health Sci* 6(2):131–140, 2004.

Yildirim G, Sahin N: The effect of breathing and skin stimulation techniques on labour pain perception of Turkish women, *Pain Res Manag* 9(4):183–187, 2004.

Readiness for enhanced Communication   *Stacey M. Carroll, PhD, ANP-BC*

NANDA-I

Definition

A pattern of exchanging information and ideas with others that is sufficient for meeting one's needs and life's goals and can be strengthened

Defining Characteristics

Able to speak a language; able to write a language; expresses feelings; expresses satisfaction with ability to share ideas with others; expresses satisfaction with ability to share information with others;

• = Independent   ▲ = Collaborative   **EBN** = Evidence-Based Nursing   **EB** = Evidence-Based

expresses thoughts; expresses willingness to enhance communication; forms phrases; forms sentences; forms words; interprets nonverbal cues appropriately; uses nonverbal cues appropriately

 (Nursing Outcomes Classification)

Suggested NOC Outcomes

Communication, Communication: Expressive, Receptive

Example NOC Outcome with Indicators
Communication as evidenced by the following indicators: Use of spoken language/Use of written language/ Acknowledgment of messages received/Exchanges messages accurately with others (Rate the outcome and indicators of **Communication:** 1 = severely compromised, 2 = substantially compromised, 3 = moderately compromised, mildly compromised, 5 = not compromised [see Section I].)

Client Outcomes

Client Will (Specify Time Frame):

- Express willingness to enhance communication
- Demonstrate ability to speak or write a language
- Form words, phrases, and language
- Express thoughts and feelings
- Use and interpret nonverbal cues appropriately
- Express satisfaction with ability to share information and ideas with others

 (Nursing Interventions Classification)

Suggested NIC Interventions

Active Listening, Communication Enhancement: Hearing Deficit, Communication Enhancement: Speech Deficit

Example NIC Activity—Communication Enhancement: Hearing Deficit
Listen attentively; Validate understanding of messages by asking patient to repeat what was said

Nursing Interventions and *Rationales*

- Establish a therapeutic nurse-client relationship: provide appropriate education for the client, demonstrate caring by being present to the client. **EBN:** *Clients who were nonvocal and ventilated appreciated nursing care that was delivered in an individualized, caring manner (Carroll, 2004; Carroll, 2007).*
- Carefully assess the client's readiness to communicate, using an individualized approach. Avoid making assumptions regarding the client's preferred communication method. *A broad range of communication aids is available and should be considered on an individual basis (Higginbotham et al, 2007).*
- Assess the client's literacy level. *Low levels of health literacy negatively affect provider-client communication (Sparks & Nussbaum, 2008).*
- Listen attentively and provide a comfortable environment for communicating; use these practical guidelines to assist in communication: Slow down and listen to the client's story; use augmentative and alternative communication methods (such as lip-reading, communication boards, writing, body language, and computer/electronic communication devices) as appropriate; repeat instructions if necessary; limit the amount of information given; have the client "teach back" to confirm understanding; avoid asking, "Do you understand?"; be respectful, caring, and sensitive. **EBN:** *Alternative methods of communication are necessary when the client is unable to speak verbally (Happ, Roesch, & Kagan, 2005).* **EBN:** *Listening to the client, considering the client's feelings, and having a connected relationship with the client conveyed caring (Gregg, 2004).*
- ▲ Provide communication with specialty nurses such as clinical nurse specialists or nurse practitioners who have knowledge about the client's situation. **EBN:** *Clients report being well informed and having high satisfaction with nurse practitioner communication (Hayes, 2007).*

● = Independent ▲ = Collaborative **EBN** = Evidence-Based Nursing **EB** = Evidence-Based

▲ Refer couples in maladjusted relationships for psychosocial intervention and social support to strengthen communication; consider nurse specialists. **EB:** *Being part of a strong dyad may serve as a buffering factor; there is a need for psychosocial intervention for couples in maladjusted relationships (Banthia et al, 2003).*

• Consider using music to enhance communication between client who is dying and his/ her family. **EB:** *In clients with communication difficulties, music therapy may result in improvement in functional communication (Magee et al, 2006).*

• See care plan for **Impaired verbal Communication**.

Pediatric

▲ All individuals involved in the care and everyday life of children with learning difficulties need to have a collaborate approach to communication. **EBN:** *Collaboration has the potential to enable health professionals to adopt methods of communication that are familiar to the child, such as those used in the school setting (Kerzman & Smith, 2004).*

• See care plan for **Impaired verbal Communication**.

Geriatric

▲ Assess for hearing and vision impairments and make appropriate referrals for hearing aids. **EB:** *Each client's vision and conversational performance along with hearing thresholds should be assessed before considering directions for rehabilitation. During face-to-face interaction, many people with adequate vision can compensate for a high-frequency hearing loss through lip reading, which may preclude the need for hearing aids; many people with poor vision cannot compensate for a high-frequency hearing loss through lip reading and may require hearing aids (Erber, 2002).*

• Use touch if culturally acceptable when communicating with older clients and their families. **EBN:** *The use of touch by the nurse conveys caring to the client (Gregg, 2004).*

• Caregivers may sing when delivering care and instructions for clients with dementia. **EBN:** *During caregiver singing, the client with dementia communicated with an increased understanding of the situation, both verbally and behaviorally (Gotell, Brown, & Ekman, 2002).*

• See care plan for **Impaired verbal Communication**.

Multicultural

See care plan for **Impaired verbal Communication**.

Home Care, Client/Family Teaching and Discharge Planning

• The interventions described previously may be used in home care.
• See care plan for **Impaired verbal Communication**.

⊖volve   See the EVOLVE website for Weblinks for client education resources.

REFERENCES

Banthia R, Malcarne VL, Varni JW et al: The effects of dyadic strength and coping styles on psychological distress in couples faced with prostate cancer, *J Behav Med* 26(1):31–52, 2003.

Carroll SM: Nonvocal ventilated patients' perceptions of being understood, *West J Nurs Res* 26(1): 85–103, 2004.

Carroll SM: Silent, slow lifeworld: the communication experiences of nonvocal ventilated patients, *Qual Health Res* 17(9):1165–1177, 2007.

Erber NP: Hearing, vision, communication, and older people, *Semin Hear* 23(1):35–42, 2002.

Gotell E, Brown S, Ekman SL: Caregiver singing and background music in dementia care, *West J Nurs Res* 24(2):195–216, 2002.

Gregg MF: Values in clinical nursing practice and caring, *Japan J Nurs Sci* 1(1):11–18, 2004.

Happ MB, Roesch TK, Kagan SH: Patient communication following head and neck cancer surgery: a pilot study using electronic speech generating devices, *Oncol Nurs Forum* 32(6):1179–1187, 2005.

Hayes E: Nurse practitioners and managed care: Patient satisfaction and intention to adhere to nurse practitioner plan of care, *J Am Acad Nurse Pract* 19(8):418–426, 2007.

Higginbotham DJ, Shane H, Russell S et al: Access to AAC: present, past, and future, *Augment Alt Commun* 23(3):527–534, 2007.

• = Independent   ▲ = Collaborative   **EBN** = Evidence-Based Nursing   **EB** = Evidence-Based

Kerzman B, Smith P: Lessons from special education: enhancing communication between health professionals and children with learning difficulties, *Nurse Educ Pract* 4(4):230–235, 2004.

Magee WL, Brumfitt SM, Freeman M et al: The role of music therapy in an interdisciplinary approach to address functional communication in complex neuro-communication disorders: a case report, *Disabil Rehabil* 28(19):1221–1229, 2006.

Sparks L, Nussbaum JF: Health literacy and cancer communication with older adults, *Patient Educ Couns* 71(3):345–350, 2008.

Impaired verbal Communication   *Stacey M. Carroll, PhD, ANP-BC*   ⊖volve

NANDA-I

Definition

Decreased, delayed, or absent ability to receive, process, transmit, and/or use a system of symbols

Defining Characteristics

Absence of eye contact; cannot speak; difficulty in comprehending usual communication pattern; difficulty expressing thoughts verbally (e.g., aphasia, dysphasia, apraxia, dyslexia); difficulty forming sentences; difficulty forming words (e.g., aphonia, dyslalia, dysarthria); difficulty in maintaining usual communication pattern; difficulty in selective attending; difficulty in use of body expressions; difficulty in use of facial expressions; disorientation to person; disorientation to space; disorientation to time; does not speak; dyspnea; inability to speak language of caregiver; inability to use body expressions; inability to use facial expressions; inappropriate verbalization; partial visual deficit; slurring; speaks with difficulty; stuttering; total visual deficit; verbalizes with difficulty; willful refusal to speak

Related Factors (r/t)

Absence of significant others; altered perceptions; alteration in self-concept; alteration in self-esteem; alteration of central nervous system; anatomical defect (e.g., cleft palate, alteration of the neuromuscular visual system, auditory system, phonatory apparatus); brain tumor; cultural differences; decrease in circulation to brain; differences related to development age; emotional conditions; environmental barriers; lack of information; physical barrier (e.g., tracheostomy, intubation); physiological conditions; psychological barriers (e.g., psychosis, lack of stimuli); side effects of medication; stress; weakening of the musculoskeletal system

NOC   (Nursing Outcomes Classification)

Suggested NOC Outcomes

Communication, Communication: Expressive, Receptive

Example NOC Outcome with Indicators
Communication as evidenced by the following indicators: Use of spoken and written language/Acknowledgment of messages received/Exchanges messages accurately with others (Rate the outcome and indicators of **Communication:** 1 = severely compromised, 2 = substantially compromised, 3 = moderately compromised, 4 = mildly compromised, 5 = not compromised [see Section I].)

Client Outcomes

Client Will (Specify Time Frame):

- Use effective communication techniques
- Use alternative methods of communication effectively
- Demonstrate congruency of verbal and nonverbal behavior
- Demonstrate understanding even if not able to speak
- Express desire for social interactions

• = Independent   ▲ = Collaborative   **EBN** = Evidence-Based Nursing   **EB** = Evidence-Based

(Nursing Interventions Classification)

Suggested NIC Interventions

Active Listening, Communication Enhancement: Hearing Deficit, Communication Enhancement: Speech Deficit

Example NIC Activities—Communication Enhancement: Hearing Deficit
Listen attentively; Validate understanding of messages by asking client to repeat what was said

Nursing Interventions and *Rationales*

- Involve a familiar person when attempting to communicate with a client who has difficulty with communication, if accepted by the client. **EB:** *Conversation partners of individuals with aphasia, including health care professionals, families, and others, play a role that is important for communication for individuals with aphasia (Roth, 2004).*
- ▲ Identify the language spoken; obtain a language dictionary or interpreter if possible and accepted by the client. **EB:** *Professional interpreters are able to communicate medical terms while reducing the ever-present risk of breaching client privacy and confidentiality (Greenbaum & Flores, 2004). The CLAS Standards recommend asking individuals to rate their primary language and capacity in English, and to use qualified institutional interpreters (Pope, 2005).*
- Listen carefully. Validate verbal and nonverbal expressions particularly when dealing with pain. **EBN:** *Listening to a client was identified as a caring behavior of nurses (Gregg, 2004).* **EBN:** *Thirteen pain observation scales for use with older adults with communication difficulties, dementia, or both were reviewed and the Pain Assessment in Advanced Dementia Scale (PAINAD—Lane et al, 2003) was suggested as the most feasible for clinical practice in this population (van Herk et al, 2007).*
- Use therapeutic communication techniques: speak in a well-modulated voice, use simple communication, maintain eye contact at the client's level, get the client's attention before speaking, and show concern for the client. **EB:** *Effective communication between clients and health care professionals facilitates positive relations (Wain, Kneebone, & Billings, 2008).* **EB:** *Conditions that are tolerable for hearing adults in casual conversation can be intolerable for persons with deficits of hearing, language, attention, or processing. Sound-field amplification can improve the speech audibility index for all listeners in a noisy room (Boothroyd, 2004).*
- Use touch as appropriate. **EBN:** *The use of touch by the nurse conveys caring to the client (Gregg, 2004).*
- Use presence. Spend time with the client, allow time for responses, and make the call light readily available. *Relationship-centered care involves the art of nursing, presence, and caring (Finfgeld-Connett, 2008).*
- Explain all health care procedures. **EBN:** *Clients who were nonvocal and ventilated were attuned to everything occurring around them, and they appreciated explanations from the nurse (Carroll, 2004).*
- Be persistent in deciphering what the client is saying, and do not pretend to understand when the message is unclear. *When clients are truly understood, they experience greater satisfaction with nursing care (Shattell & Hogan, 2005).* **EBN:** *Persons who were nonvocal and ventilated appreciated persistence on the nurses' part with respect to being understood, and found it bothersome when others pretended to understand them (Carroll, 2004).*
- ▲ Obtain communication equipment such as electronic devices, letter boards, picture boards, magic slates, and intelligent keyboards. **EBN:** *Use of voice output communication aids may contribute to greater ease of communication, particularly with family members, during respiratory tract intubation (Happ, Roesch, & Garrett, 2004).* **EBN:** *Clients and nurses considered the "intelligent keyboard" to be significantly better than the traditional letter board (vanden Boogaard & van Grunsven, 2004).*
- ▲ Consider the use of a lipreader translator (LRT) for those who are intubated via a tracheostomy. *LRTs are proficient lipreaders who determine what a nonvocal client is mouthing and then verbalize the client's words verbatim to others, in order to facilitate communication (Carroll, 2003).*
- Using an individualized approach, establish an alternative method of communication such as writing or pointing to letters, word phrases, picture cards, or simple drawings of basic needs. **EBN:**

● = Independent   ▲ = Collaborative   **EBN** = Evidence-Based Nursing   **EB** = Evidence-Based

Alternative methods of communication are necessary when the client is unable to speak verbally (Happ, Roesch, & Kagan, 2005).

- Use consistent nursing staffing for those with communication impairments. **EBN:** *Consistent nursing care increased client-nurse communication and decreased client powerlessness (Carroll, 2007).*

▲ Consult a speech pathologist if appropriate. Supplement the work of the speech pathologist with appropriate exercises. *Speech pathologists consider interventions optimizing communication in people with hearing loss (Hickson, Worrall, & Donaldson-Scarinci, 2005).* **EB:** *Consultation and collaboration with a speech pathologist may provide the best approach to improving communication in clients with aphasia (Greener, Enderby, & Whurr, 2006).*

- Establish an understanding of the client's symbolic speech, especially with clients who have schizophrenia. Ask the client to clarify particular statements. **EB:** *Good communication with health care professionals was identified by people with schizophrenia as helping them learn to live with their illness (Schneider et al, 2004).*

▲ When the client is having difficulty communicating, assess and refer for consultation for hearing loss. Suspect hearing loss when:
  - Client frequently complains that people mumble, that others' speech is not clear, or client hears only parts of conversations.
  - Client often asks people to repeat what they said.
  - Client's friends or relatives state that client doesn't seem to hear very well, or plays the television or radio too loudly.
  - Client does not laugh at jokes due to missing too much of the story.
  - Client needs to ask others about the details of a meeting that the client attended.
  - Client cannot hear the doorbell or the telephone.
  - Client finds it easier to understand others when facing them, especially in a noisy environment.

  People with hearing loss do not hear sounds clearly. The loss may range from hearing speech sounds faintly or in a distorted way to profound deafness (American Speech-Language-Hearing Association, 2007b).

- When communicating with a client with a hearing loss:
  - Face toward his or her unaffected side or better ear while allowing client to see speaker's face at a reasonably close distance. *Correct positioning increases the client's awareness of the interaction and enhances the client's ability to communicate (Alexander Graham Bell Association for the Deaf and Hard of Hearing, 2007).*
  - Provide sufficient light and do not stand in front of window. *Light illuminates the speaker's face, making expressions and lip movements clearer. Standing in front of a window causes glare, which impedes the client's ability to clearly see the speaker (Alexander Graham Bell Association for the Deaf and Hard of Hearing, 2007).*
  - Remove masks if safe to do so, or use see-through masks and reduce background noise whenever possible. *Information on see-through masks: www.amphl.org.* **EB:** *Background noise had a negative effect on the ability to process speech and on perceived effort, especially for those with hearing loss (Larsby et al, 2005).*
  - Do not raise voice or overenunciate. *This practice distorts the voice and lips, inhibiting effective lip-reading. A loud voice can be frightening and inhibit communication (Lieu et al, 2007).*
  - Avoid making assumptions about the communication choice of those with hearing loss. **EB:** *Clients with hearing loss and their physicians had different perceptions about what constituted effective communication, and clients recommended that physicians ask them about their preferred communication approach (Iezonni et al, 2004).*

Pediatric

- Observe behavioral communication cues in infants. **EBN:** *Infant pain is encoded into observable manifestations through which an infant communicates behavioral and physiological changes such as altered vital signs, characteristic cries, and facial expressions (Byers & Thornley, 2004).*
- Identify and define variations of communication that may be used by children with significant disabilities. Teach at least two new forms of socially acceptable communication alternatives to teach as repairs when communication breaks down. Example: Teach use of one-word requests or teach

the child to point, reinforce appropriate responses. **EB:** *Young children with significant disability often have limited communicative repertoires. The means they have available to communicate with others might include natural gesturing, vocalizing, and occasionally challenging behavior (Halle, Brady, & Drasgow, 2004).*

- Teach children with severe disabilities functional communication skills. **EB:** *Children with severe disabilities can be taught new forms of communication to replace prelinguistic behaviors associated with escape or avoidance (Sigafoos et al, 2004).*
- ▲ Refer children with primary speech and language delay/disorder for speech and language therapy interventions. **EBN:** *Speech and language therapy interventions showed a positive effect on children with expressive phonological and expressive vocabulary difficulties (Law, Garrett, & Nye, 2003).*

Geriatric

- Carefully assess all clients for hearing difficulty using an audiometer. **EB:** *Healthy People 2010 encourages early identification of people with hearing loss. Despite a high prevalence of hearing loss in the elderly, there is a low incidence of audiological evaluation (Milstein & Weinstein, 2002).*
- Avoid use of "elderspeak." **EBN:** *Care providers unknowingly may communicate messages of dependence, incompetence, and control to older adults by using elderspeak, a speech style similar to baby talk that fails to communicate appropriate respect (Williams, Kemper, & Hummert, 2004).*
- Initiate communication with the client with dementia. *The responsibility to initiate communication with clients who have dementia lies with the clinician. Identifying the client's communication pattern and deficits is helpful in understanding the client (Frazier-Rios & Zembrzuski, 2005).*
- Encourage the client to wear hearing aids, if appropriate. **EB:** *Identifying individuals with hearing loss and supplying appropriate hearing aids or other listening devices and teaching coping strategies may have a positive effect on quality of life for older people (Dalton et al, 2003).* **EB:** *Disability from hearing impairment was reduced when clients with dementia were screened for hearing impairment and fitted with hearing aids (Allen et al, 2003).*
- Facilitate communication and reminiscing with remembering boxes that contain objects, photographs, and writings that have meaning for the client. **EB:** *These communication tools helped staff learn more about clients and enhanced interactions with staff and client's families (Hagens, Beaman, & Ryan, 2003). Reminiscence therapy is an appropriate intervention for communication and to relieve stress in elders (Stokes & Gordon, 2003).*

Multicultural

- Nurses should become more sensitive to the meaning of a culture's nonverbal communication modes, such as eye contact, facial expression, touching, and body language. *Nurses should realize that their good intentions and their usual nonverbal communication style may sometimes be interpreted as offensive and insulting by a specific cultural group.* **EBN:** *To give a client a positive signal during a therapy session, a nurse may display the American sign of thumbs up. In Iran, however, thumbs extended upward is considered a vulgar gesture (Campinha-Bacote, 1998).* **EBN:** *Years of watching animal behavior for survival needs have made the Eskimo people experts in the interpretation of nonverbal language. For the traditional Eskimo, a raised eyebrow may mean "yes" and a wrinkled nose "no." Disagreeing in public is seldom done. Nodding may not indicate agreement (Sanders & Davidhizar, 2004).*
- Assess for the influence of cultural beliefs, norms, and values on the client's communication process. **EBN:** *What the client considers normal and abnormal communication may be based on cultural perceptions (Leininger & McFarland, 2002; Giger & Davidhizar, 2008). The nurse must be aware of personal beliefs about communication and control personal reactions by a broadened understanding of the beliefs and behaviors of others (Giger & Davidhizar, 2008). An affirmative answer does not necessarily mean "yes"; a client may be showing respect to the caregiver or avoiding the embarrassment of saying "no" (Galanti, 1997).*
- Assess personal space needs, acceptable communication styles, acceptable body language, interpretation of eye contact, perception of touch, and use of paraverbal modes when communicating with the client. **EBN:** *Nurses need to consider multiple factors when interpreting verbal and nonverbal messages (Giger & Davidhizar, 2008). Native Americans may consider avoiding direct eye contact to be a*

• = Independent ▲ = Collaborative **EBN** = Evidence-Based Nursing **EB** = Evidence-Based

sign of respect and asking questions to be rude and intrusive (Seiderman et al, 1996). Empirical findings suggest that Chinese Americans and European Americans differ in the ways that they describe emotional experience, with Chinese Americans using more somatic and social words than Americans (Tsai, Simeonova, & Watanabe, 2004).

- Assess for how language barriers contribute to health disparities among ethnic and racial minorities. **EBN:** *Language barriers are associated with longer visit time per clinic visit, fewer frequent clinic visits, less understanding of physician's explanation, more laboratory tests, more emergency department visits, less follow-up, and less satisfaction with health services (Yeo, 2004).*

- Although touch is generally beneficial, there may be certain instances where it may not be advisable due to cultural considerations. **EBN:** *Touch is largely culturally defined (Leininger & McFarland, 2002). Touch is believed by some cultures to be a source of illness. Touching a baby's head requires parental permission in some Southeast Asian cultures. Many Latinos believe that excessive admiration of a child without touching will result in physical illness of the child* (mal de ojo—*"evil eye"*). *In some Islamic and Latino cultures, physical touch between a nurse and client is acceptable only if the individuals are of the same sex (Kelley, 1998). Some Asian cultures believe that touching the head is a sign of disrespect (Galanti, 1997).*

- Modify and tailor the communication approach in keeping with the client's particular culture. **EBN:** *Modification of communication will convey respect to the client and may increase client's satisfaction with care (Taylor & Lurie, 2004). Culturally tailored communication interventions were positively viewed by African American women (Kreuter et al, 2004).*

- Use reminiscence therapy as a language intervention. **EBN:** *Reminiscence therapy is well-suited as a language intervention for older adults from culturally and linguistically diverse backgrounds (Harris, 1997).*

- Use of the Office of Minority Health (OMH) of the U.S. Department of Health and Human Services (DHHS) standards on culturally and linguistically appropriate services (CLAS) in health care should be used as needed. **EB:** *The recommended standards cover three broad areas of competence requirements for health care for racial or ethnic minorities: (1) culturally competent care, (2) language access services, and (3) organizational support for cultural competence (CLAS, 2007).*

Home Care

The interventions described previously may be adapted for home care use.

Client/Family Teaching and Discharge Planning

- Teach the client and family techniques to increase communication, including the use of communication devices and tactile touch. *Clients and communication partners benefit from an individualized broad approach to communication access (Higginbotham et al, 2007).*

- ▲ Refer the client to a speech-language pathologist (SLP) or audiologist. *Audiological assessment quantifies and qualifies hearing in terms of the degree of hearing loss, the type of hearing loss, and the configuration of the hearing loss. Once a particular hearing loss has been identified, a treatment and management plan can be put into place by an SLP (American Speech-Language-Hearing Association, 2007a; Baumgartner, Bewyer & Bruner, 2008).*

- ▲ Refer to a specialist for possible surgical intervention when clients have surgical defects caused by cancer of the maxillary sinus and alveolar ridge. **EB:** *Obturators have been developed for surgical defects caused by cancer of the maxillary sinus and alveolar ridge. Clients' mean self-perceived communication effectiveness with the obturator in place was 75% of what it was before the diagnosis of cancer (Sullivan et al, 2002).*

ⓔvolve   See the EVOLVE website for Weblinks for client education resources.

REFERENCES

Alexander Graham Bell Association for the Deaf and Hard of Hearing: *Communicating with people who have a hearing loss.* Available at www.agbell.org/docs/CWPWHHL.pdf. Accessed on March 9, 2007.

Allen NH, Burns A, Newton V et al: The effects of improving hearing in dementia, *Age Ageing,* 32(2):189–193, 2003.

American Speech-Language-Hearing Association: *Hearing assessment.* Available atwww.asha.org/public/hearing/testing/assess.htm. Accessed on March 9, 2007a.

American Speech-Language-Hearing Association: *How do I know if I have a hearing loss?* Available at www.asha.org/public/hearing/disorders/how_know.htm. Accessed on March 9, 2007b.

Baumgartner CA, Bewyer E, Bruner D: Management of communication and swallowing in intensive care: the role of the speech pathologist, *AACN Adv Crit Care* 19(4):433–443, 2008.

Boothroyd A: Room acoustics and speech perception, *Semin Hear* 25(2):55–166, 2004.

Byers JF, Thornley K: Cueing into infant pain, *MCN Am J Matern Child Nurs* 29(2):84–91, 2004.

Campinha-Bacote J: *A model of practice to address cultural competence in rehabilitation nursing,* Continuing Education, Association of Rehabilitation Nurses, 1998. Available at www.rehabnurse.org/ce/010201/010201_a.htm. Accessed on March 9, 2007.

Carroll, SM: Lip-reading translating for non-vocal ventilated patients. *JAMPHL Online* 1(2): 2003. Available at www.amphl.org, accessed on November 26, 2006.

Carroll SM: Silent, slow lifeworld: the communication experiences of nonvocal ventilated patients, *Qual Health Res* 17(9):1165–1177, 2007.

CLAS (Culturally and appropriate Linguistic Services). Available at www.omhrc.gov/templates/browse.aspx?lvl52&lvlID515. Accessed on February 24, 2007.

Dalton DS, Cruickshanks KJ, Klein BE et al: The impact of hearing loss on quality of life in older adults, *Gerontologist* 43(5):661–668, 2003.

Finfgeld-Connett D: Qualitative convergence of three nursing concepts: art of nursing, presence and caring, *J Adv Nurs* 63(5):527–534, 2008.

Frazier-Rios D, Zembrzuski C: Try this: best practices in nursing care for hospitalized older adults with dementia. Communication difficulties: assessment and interventions, *Dermatol Nurs* 17(4):319–320, 2005.

Galanti G: *Caring for patients from different cultures: case studies from American hospitals,* ed 2, Philadelphia, 1997, University of Pennsylvania.

Giger J, Davidhizar R: Communication. In Giger J, Davidhizar R, editors: *Transcultural nursing: assessment and intervention,* St Louis, 2008, Mosby.

Greenbaum M, Flores G: Lost in translation. Professional interpreters needed to help hospitals treat immigrant patients, *Mod Healthc* 34(18):21, 2004.

Greener J, Enderby P, Whurr R: Speech and language therapy for aphasia following stroke, *Cochrane Database Syst Rev* (1):CD000425, 2006.

Gregg MF: Values in clinical nursing practice and caring, *Japan J Nurs Sci* 1(1):11–18, 2004.

Hagens C, Beaman A, Ryan EB: Reminiscing, poetry writing, and remembering boxes: personhood-centered communication with cognitively impaired older adults, *Activ Adapt Aging;* 27(3/4):97–112, 2003.

Halle J, Brady NC, Drasgow E: Enhancing socially adaptive communicative repairs of beginning communicators with disabilities, *Am J Speech Lang Pathol* 13(1):43–54, 2004.

Happ MB, Roesch TK, Garrett K: Electronic voice-output communication aids for temporarily nonspeaking patients in a medical intensive care unit: a feasibility study, *Heart Lung* 33(2):92–101, 2004.

Happ MB, Roesch TK, Kagan SH: Patient communication following head and neck cancer surgery: a pilot study using electronic speech generating devices, *Oncol Nurs Forum* 32(6):1179–1187, 2005.

Harris J: Silent voices: meeting the communication needs of older African Americans, *Top Lang Disorder* 19(4):23, 1997.

Hickson L, Worrall L, Donaldson-Scarinci N: Expanding speech-pathology services for older people with hearing impairment, *Adv Speech Lang Pathol* 7(4):203–210, 2005.

Higginbotham DJ, Shane H, Russell S et al: Access to AAC: present, past, and future, *Augment Altern Commun* 23(3):527–534, 2007.

Iezonni LI, O'Day BL, Killeen M et al: Communicating about health care: observations from persons who are deaf and hard of hearing, *Ann Int Med* 140(5):356–362, 2004.

Kelley J: Cultural and ethnic considerations. In Frisch NC, Frisch LE, editors: *Psychiatric mental health nursing,* Albany, NY, 1998, Delmar.

Kreuter MW, Skinner CS, Steger-May K et al: Responses to behaviorally vs. culturally tailored cancer communication among African American women, *Am J Health Behav* 28(3):195–207, 2004.

Lane P, Kuntupis M, MacDonald S et al: A pain assessment tool for people with advanced Alzheimer's and other progressive dementias, *Home Healthc Nurse* 21(1):32–37, 2003.

Larsby B, Hallgren M, Lyxell B et al: Cognitive performance and perceived effort in speech processing tasks: effects of different noise backgrounds in normal-hearing and hearing-impaired subjects, *Int J Audiol* 44(3):131–143, 2005.

Law J, Garrett Z, Nye C: Speech and language therapy interventions for children with primary speech and language delay or disorder, *Cochrane Database Syst Rev* (3):CD004110, 2003.

Leininger MM, McFarland MR: *Transcultural nursing: concepts, theories, research and practices,* ed 3, New York, McGraw-Hill, 2002.

Lieu CC, Sadler GR, Fullerton JT et al: Communication strategies for nurses interacting with patients who are deaf, *MedSurg Nurs* 16(4):239–244, 2007.

Milstein D, Weinstein BE: Effects of information sharing on follow-up after hearing screening for older adults, *J Acad Rehabil Audiol* 35:43–58, 2002.

Pope C: Addressing limited English proficiency and disparities for Hispanic postpartum women, *J Obstet Gynecol Neonatal Nurs* 34(4):512–520, 2005.

Roth EJ: Grand rounds. A set of observational measures for rating support and participation in conversation between adults with aphasia and their conversation partners, *Top Stroke Rehabil* 11(1):67–83, 2004.

Sanders N, Davidhizar R: American Eskimos: the Yup'ik and Inupiat. *Transcultural nursing: assessment and intervention,* St Louis, 2004, Mosby.

Schneider B, Scissons H, Arney L et al: Communication between people with schizophrenia and their medical professionals: a participatory research project, *Qual Health Res* 14(4):562–577, 2004.

Seiderman RY, Jacobson S, Primeaux M et al: Assessing American Indian families, *MCN Am J Matern Child Nurs* 21(6):274–279, 1996.

Shattell M, Hogan B: Facilitating communication: how to truly understand what patients mean, *J Psychosoc Nurs Ment Health Serv* 43(10):29–32, 2005.

Sigafoos J, Drasgow E, Reichle J et al: Tutorial: teaching communicative rejecting to children with severe disabilities, *Am J Speech Lang Pathol* 13(1):31–42, 2004.

Stokes SA, Gordon SE: Common stressors experienced by the well elderly. Clinical implications, *J Gerontol Nurs* 29(5):38–46, 2003.

Sullivan M, Gaebler C, Beukelman D et al: Impact of palatal prosthodontic intervention on communication performance of patients' maxillectomy defects: a multilevel outcome study, *Head Neck* 24(6):530–538, 2002.

Taylor SL, Lurie N: The role of culturally competent communication in reducing ethnic and racial healthcare disparities, *Am J Manag Care* 10:SP1–4, 2004.

Tsai JL, Simeonova DI, Watanabe JT: Somatic and social: Chinese Americans talk about emotion, *Pers Soc Psychol Bull* 30(9):1226–1238, 2004.

vanden Boogaard M, van Grunsven A: A new communication aid for mechanically ventilated patients, *Connect World Crit Care Nurs* 3(1):20–23, 2004.

● = Independent   ▲ = Collaborative   **EBN** = Evidence-Based Nursing   **EB** = Evidence-Based

van Herk R, van Dijk M, Baar FPM et al: Observation scales for pain assessment in older adults with cognitive impairments or communication difficulties, *Nurse Res* 56(1):34–43, 2007.

Wain HR, Kneebone II, Billings J: Patient experience of neurologic rehabilitation: a qualitative investigation, *Arch PhysMed Rehabil* 63(5):527–534, 2008.

Williams K, Kemper S, Hummert L: Enhancing communication with older adults: overcoming elderspeak, *J Gerontol Nurs* 30(10):17–25, 2004.

Yeo S: Language barriers and access to care, *Ann Rev Nurs Res* 22:59–73, 2004.

Decisional Conflict   *Dawn Fairlie, ANP, FNP, GNP, DNS(c)*

NANDA-I

Definition

Uncertainty about course of action to be taken when choice among competing actions involves risk, loss, or challenge to values and beliefs

Defining Characteristics

Delayed decision making; physical signs of distress or tension (e.g., increased heart rate, increased muscle tension, restlessness); questioning moral principles while attempting a decision; questioning moral rules while attempting a decision; questioning moral values while attempting a decision; questioning personal beliefs while attempting a decision; questioning personal values while attempting a decision; self-focusing; vacillation among alternative choices; verbalizes feeling of distress while attempting a decision; verbalizes uncertainty about choices; verbalizes undesired consequences of alternative actions being considered

Related Factors (r/t)

Divergent sources of information; interference with decision making; lack of experience with decision making; lack of relevant information; moral obligations require performing action; moral obligations require not performing action; moral principles support courses of action; moral rules support mutually inconsistent courses of action; moral values support mutually inconsistent courses of action; multiple sources of information; perceived threat to value system; support system deficit; unclear personal beliefs; unclear personal values

NOC   (Nursing Outcomes Classification)

Suggested NOC Outcomes

Decision Making, Information Processing, Participation in Healthcare Decisions

Example NOC Outcome with Indicators
Decision Making as evidenced by the following indicators: Identifies relevant information/Identifies alternatives/Identifies potential consequences of each alternative/Identifies needed resources to support each alternative (Rate the outcome and indicators of **Decision Making:** 1 = severely compromised, 2 = substantially compromised, 3 = moderately compromised, 4 = mildly compromised, 5 = not compromised [see Section I].)

Client Outcomes

Client Will (Specify Time Frame):

• State the advantages and disadvantages of choices
• Share fears and concerns regarding choices and responses of others
• Seek resources and information necessary for making an informed choice
• Make an informed choice

NIC   (Nursing Interventions Classification)

Suggested NIC Intervention

Decision-Making Support

• = Independent   ▲ = Collaborative   **EBN** = Evidence-Based Nursing   **EB** = Evidence-Based

Example NIC Activities—Decision-Making Support

Inform patient of alternative views or solutions in a clear and supportive manner; Provide information requested by patient.

Nursing Interventions and *Rationales*

- Observe for factors causing or contributing to conflict (e.g., value conflicts, fear of outcome, poor problem-solving skills). **EB:** *When studying client-provider dyads, it was found that the more unclear one member's expressed values, the greater their interpretation that the other member has made an ineffective choice, and this also correlated with both members experiencing personal uncertainty (Leblanc et al, 2009).*

- Work with and allow the client to make decisions in a way that is comfortable for the client, such as deferring (allowing others to decide), delaying (choosing an alternative that meets basic requirements), or deliberating (looking at all alternatives). **EB:** *Clients can be more involved in treatment decisions, and risks and benefits of treatment options can be explained in more detail, without adversely affecting client-based outcomes (Edwards et al, 2004).*

- Give the client time and permission to express feelings associated with decision making. **EB:** *The physician should take time to explore the client's values, concerns, and emotional and social needs (Whitney, McGuire, & McCullough, 2004).*

- Demonstrate reassurance with unconditional respect for and acceptance of the client's values, spiritual beliefs, and cultural norms. **EB:** *Trust in the client's physician is important in shared decision making. Supporting the client's autonomy is important (Kraetschmer et al, 2004).*

- ▲ Use decision aids or computer-based decision aid to assist clients in making decisions. **EB:** *An interactive computer program was more effective than standard genetic counseling for increasing knowledge of breast cancer and genetic testing among women at low risk of carrying a BRCA1 or BRCA2 mutation (Green et al, 2004a). In women at high risk for ovarian cancer, the group who received a decision aid package reported a significant decrease in decisional conflict compared to the group that received a pamphlet (Tiller et al, 2006). A study of pregnant women who received a decision-aid booklet had significantly improved decisional conflict scores (Shorten et al, 2005).*

- ▲ Initiate health teaching and referrals when needed. **EB:** *Male cancer clients who viewed a computerized education tool about sperm banking before their cancer treatment had significantly less decisional conflict about banking sperm than those who had not viewed it (Huyghe et al, 2008).* **EBN:** *Nurses' barriers to providing decision support was evaluated. It was found that helpline professionals have the potential to provide decision support which helps callers in understanding cancer information, as well as assisting in the clarification of their values which were associated with their options, and ultimately reduced decisional conflict (Stacey et al, 2008).*

- Facilitate communication between the client and family members regarding the final decision; offer support to the person actually making the decision. **EB:** *Family/HIV-positive adolescent-centered advance care planning demonstrated improved communication quality and congruence as well as decreased decisional conflict. Adolescents who received the intervention reported feeling significantly better informed about end-of-life decisions. Families were more willing to engage in end-of-life discussions (Lyon et al, 2009).*

- Provide detailed information on benefits and risks using functional terms and probabilities tailored to clinical risk, plus steps for considering the issues and means for making a decision, including values clarification and decision aids, when clients are faced with difficult treatment choices. **EB:** *Informed choices require information that is relevant, valid, and accessible (Oxman, 2004).*

- Encourage client to communicate values, beliefs, goals, and life plans and the ultimate decision with other health care providers, as appropriate. **EB:** *Clients who participated in an interactive workshop with feedback and point-of-care reminder had significantly similar decisional conflict scores than prior to attending the program (Légaré et al, 2006).*

Geriatric

- Carefully assess clients with dementia regarding ability to make decisions. *In evaluating reasoning it may be helpful to take the person through the reasoning process. Check if information is excluded*

• = Independent   ▲ = Collaborative   **EBN** = Evidence-Based Nursing   **EB** = Evidence-Based

because it was not remembered or because it was not important to the individual. **EB:** *Most adults with mild dementia can participate in medical decision making as defined by legal standards. In dementia, assessments of reasoning about treatment options should focus on whether a person can describe salient reasons for a specific choice (Moye et al, 2004).*

- If end-of-life discussions are being avoided, nurses can facilitate discussions of health care choices among older adults and their family members. **EB:** *Even though there has been an increase in the number of clients completing advance directives, multiple barriers to their intended implementation still exist largely due to inadequate communication. Client decision making and end-of-life care can improve if clinicians gain a better understanding of client's expectations. Better training in effective communication skills may help in eliciting client goals and in making appropriate recommendations (Saraiya et al, 2008).*
- Discuss the purpose of a living will and advance directives. **EBN:** *The literature indicates moderate to high stability of health care preferences into older adulthood. Renewing advance directives periodically may not be critical for certain groups of individuals (Martin & Roberto, 2006).*
- Discuss choices or changes to be made (e.g., moving in with children, into a nursing home, or into an adult foster care home). **EBN:** *A review of determinants of place of end-of-life cancer care identified that disease factors, the dying individual, and social environment influence place of end-of-life care for clients with cancer. Availability of social support, provider contact, social services and programs, and client preferences were the most important factors (Murray et al, 2009a).*

 ### Multicultural

- Assess for the influence of cultural beliefs, norms, and values on the client's decision-making conflict. **EB:** *Enhanced information regarding life-sustaining treatment decisions produced different patterns of desire for life-sustaining treatments in older, community-dwelling African Americans and Caucasians demonstrated different patterns for desire for treatment in the two groups. Decision aids may provide new information or knowledge and on decisional conflict in diverse cultural groups (Allen et al, 2008)* **EBN:** *African American women may use fatalistic and destiny beliefs to guide their health decisions (Green et al, 2004b).*
- Identify who will be involved in the decision-making process. **EB:** *Cultural and contextual factors can influence the experience of Latinos regarding participation in health care interactions and participation in decisions about mental health treatment (Cortes et al, 2009).*
- Use cross-cultural decision aids whenever possible to enhance an informed decision-making process. **EBN:** *African American women underwent immediate breast reconstruction at significantly lower rates compared with Caucasian, Hispanic, and Asian women. The decision pathways found that African American women were less likely to be offered referrals for reconstruction, were less likely to accept offered referrals, were less likely to be offered reconstruction, and were less likely to elect reconstruction if it was offered (Tseng et al, 2004).*
- Provide support for client's decision making. **EB:** *Intervention efforts designed to promote repeat human immunodeficiency (HIV) test acceptance among low-income African American women should focus on changing perceptions of barriers and enhancing supportive factors to enhance decision making (Bonney, Crosby, & Odenat, 2004).*

 ### Home Care

- The interventions described previously may be adapted for home care use.
- ▲ Before providing any home care, assess the client plan for advance directives (living will and power of attorney). If a plan exists, place a copy in the client file. If no plan exists, offer information on advance directives according to agency policy. Refer for assistance in completing advance directives as necessary. Do not witness a living will. *This is a legal requirement of the Consolidated Omnibus Budget Reconciliation Act (COBRA, 2009).*
- Assess the client and family for consensus (or lack thereof) regarding the issue in conflict. *When the conflict involves end-of-life decisions, work to shift the client's and family's expectations from curative to palliative.* **EBN:** *Clients, who have more choices about where to receive care as death approaches, often need help with decision making (Murray et al, 2009b).*

• = Independent   ▲ = Collaborative   **EBN** = Evidence-Based Nursing   **EB** = Evidence-Based

- Refer to the care plan for **Anxiety** as indicated.

 Client/Family Teaching and Discharge Planning

- Instruct the client and family members to provide advance directives in the following areas:
  - Person to contact in an emergency
  - Preference (if any) to die at home or in the hospital
  - Desire to sign a living will
  - Desire to donate an organ
  - Funeral arrangements (i.e., burial, cremation)

  EB: *Adolescents who received family-centered advance care planning reported feeling significantly better informed about end-of-life decisions. These adolescents and their surrogates were more likely to feel that their attitudes and wishes were known over time (Lyon et al, 2009).*
- Inform the family of treatment options; encourage and defend self-determination. **EB:** *A study of resuscitation preferences of older Irish inpatients revealed that most clients felt it was a good idea for doctors to discuss CPR routinely with clients (Cotter et al, 2009).*
- Identify reasons for family decisions regarding care. Explore ways in which family decisions can be respected. **EB:** *A significant percentage of cancer clients decline one or more conventional cancer treatments and use complementary and alternative medicine instead. This is a reflection of many personal factors. Accepting and respecting such decisions is vital for open communication (Verhoef et al, 2008).*
- Recognize and allow the client to discuss the selection of complementary therapies available, such as spiritual support, relaxation, imagery, exercise, lifestyle changes, diet (e.g., macrobiotic, vegetarian), and nutritional supplementation. **EB:** *Cognitive-behavioral strategies, such as relaxation and imagery, are recommended for cancer pain management. The clients who reported greater imaging ability, higher positive outcome expectancy, and fewer concurrent symptoms achieved greater improvement in pain (Kwekkeboom, Wanta, & Bumpus, 2008).*
- ▲ Provide the Physician Orders for Life-Sustaining Treatment (POLST) form for clients and families faced with end-of-life choices across the health care continuum. **EBN:** *The POLST form ensures end-of-life choices can be implemented in all settings, from the home through the health care continuum. The POLST form was congruent with residents' existing advance directives for health care (Meyers et al, 2004).*

⊖volve   See the EVOLVE website for Weblinks for client education resources.

REFERENCES

Allen RS, Allen JY, Hilgeman MM et al: End-of-life decision-making, decisional conflict, and enhanced information: race effects, *J Am Geriatr Soc* 56(10):1904–1909, 2008.

Bonney EA, Crosby R, Odenat L: Repeat HIV testing among low-income minority women: a descriptive analysis of factors influencing decisional balance, *Ethn Dis* 14(3):330–335, 2004.

COBRA The Consolidated Omnibus Budget Reconciliation Act, available at www.dol.gov/dol/topic/health-plans/cobra.htm. Accessed on April 15, 2009.

Cortes DE, Mulvaney-Day N, Fortuna L et al: Patient-provider communication: understanding the role of patient activation for Latinos in mental health treatment, *Health Educ Behav* 36(1):138–154, 2009.

Cotter PE, Simon M, Quinn C et al: Changing attitudes to cardiopulmonary resuscitation in older people: a 15–year follow-up study, *Age Ageing* 38(2):200–205, 2009.

Edwards A, Elwyn G, Hood K et al: Patient-based outcome results from a cluster randomized trial of shared decision making skill development and use of risk communication aids in general practice, *Fam Pract* 21(4):347–354, 2004.

Green BL, Lewis RK, Wang MQ et al: Powerlessness, destiny, and control: the influence on health behaviors of African Americans, *J Community Health* 29(1):15–27, 2004b.

Green MJ, Peterson SK, Baker MW et al: Effect of a computer-based decision aid on knowledge, perceptions, and intentions about genetic testing for breast cancer susceptibility: a randomized controlled trial, *JAMA* 292(4):442–452, 2004a.

Huyghe E, Martinetti P, Sui D et al: Banking on Fatherhood: pilot studies of a computerized educational tool on sperm banking before cancer treatment, *Psychooncology* 18(9):1011–1014 , 2008.

Kraetschmer N, Sharpe N, Urowitz S et al: How does trust affect patient preferences for participation in decision-making? *Health Expect* 7(4):317–326, 2004.

Kwekkeboom KL, Wanta B, Bumpus M: Individual difference variables and the effects of progressive muscle relaxation and analgesic imagery interventions on cancer pain, *J Pain Symptom Manage* 36(6):604–615, 2008.

Leblanc A, Kenny DA, O'Connor AM et al: Decisional conflict in patients and their physicians: a dyadic approach to shared decision making, *Med Decis Making* 29(1):61–68, 2009.

● = Independent   ▲ = Collaborative   **EBN** = Evidence-Based Nursing   **EB** = Evidence-Based

Légaré F, O'Connor AM, Graham ID et al: Impact of the Ottawa decision support framework on the agreement and the difference between patients' and physicians' decisional conflict, *Med Decis Making* 26(4):373–390, 2006.

Lyon ME, Garvie PA, McCarter R et al: Who will speak for me? Improving end-of-life decision-making for adolescents with HIV and their families, *Pediatrics* 123(2):e199–206, 2009.

Martin V, Roberto K: Assessing the stability of values and health care preferences of older adults: a long term comparison, *J Gerontol Nurs* 32(11):23–30, 2006.

Meyers JL, Moore C, McGrory A et al: Physician orders for life-sustaining treatment form: honoring end-of-life directives for nursing home residents, *J Gerontol Nurs* 30(9):37–46, 2004.

Moye J, Karel MJ, Azar AR et al: Capacity to consent to treatment: empirical comparison of three instruments in older adults with and without dementia, *Gerontologist* 44(2):166–175, 2004.

Murray MA, Wilson K, Kryworuchko J et al: Nurses' perceptions of factors influencing patient decision support for place of care at the end of life, *Am J Hosp Palliat Care* 26(4):254–263, 2009a.

Murray MA, Fiset V, Young S et al: Where the dying live: a systematic review of determinants of place of end-of-life cancer care, *Oncol Nurs Forum* 36(1):69–77, 2009b.

Oxman AD: You cannot make informed choices without information, *J Rehab Med* (43 Suppl):5–7, 2004.

Saraiya B, Bodnar-Deren S, Leventhal E et al: End-of-life planning and its relevance for patients' and oncologists' decisions in choosing cancer therapy, *Cancer* 113(12 Suppl):3540–3547, 2008.

Shorten A, Shorten B, Keogh J et al: Making choices for childbirth: a randomized controlled trial of a decision-aid for informed birth after cesarean, *Birth* 32(4):252–261, 2005.

Stacey D, Chambers SK, Jacobsen MJ et al: Overcoming barriers to cancer-helpline professionals providing decision support for callers: an implementation study, *Oncol Nurs Forum* 35(6): 961–969, 2008.

Tiller K, Meiser B, Gaff C et al: A randomized controlled trial of a decision aid for women at increased risk of ovarian cancer, *Med Decis Making* 26(4):360–372, 2006.

Tseng JF, Kronowitz SJ, Sun CC et al: The effect of ethnicity on immediate reconstruction rates after mastectomy for breast cancer, *Cancer* 101(7):1514–1523, 2004.

Verhoef MJ, Rose MS, White M et al: Declining conventional cancer treatment and using complementary and alternative medicine: a problem or a challenge? *Curr Oncol* 15(2 Suppl):S101–106, 2008.

Whitney SN, McGuire AL, McCullough LB: A typology of shared decision making, informed consent, and simple consent, *Ann Intern Med* 140(1):54–59, 2004.

Parental role Conflict   ⊖volve

Gail B. Ladwig, MSN, RN, CHTP; revised by Vanessa Sammons, MSN, APRN, BC, CNE

 NANDA-I

Definition

Parent's experience of role confusion and conflict in response to crisis

Defining Characteristics

Anxiety; demonstrated disruption in caretaking routines; expresses concern about perceived loss of control over decisions relating to his or her child; fear; parent(s) express(es) concern(s) about changes in parental role; parent(s) express(es) concern(s) about family (e.g., functioning, communication, health); parent(s) express(es) feeling(s) of inadequacy to provide for child's needs (e.g., physical, emotional); reluctant to participate in usual caretaking activities, verbalizes feelings of frustration, verbalizes feelings of guilt

Related Factors (r/t)

Change in marital status; home care of a child with special needs; interruptions of family life due to home care regimen (e.g., treatments, caregivers, lack of respite); intimidation with invasive modalities (e.g., intubation); intimidation with restrictive modalities (e.g., isolation); separation from child because of chronic illness; specialized care center

 NOC   (Nursing Outcomes Classification)

Suggested NOC Outcomes

Caregiver Lifestyle Disruption, Coping, Parenting Performance, Family Coping

Example NOC Outcome with Indicators

Family Coping as evidenced by the following indicators: Establishes role flexibility/Manages family problems/Uses family-centered stress reduction activities (Rate the outcome and indicators of **Family Coping:** 1 = never demonstrated, 2 = rarely demonstrated, 3 = sometimes demonstrated, 4 = often demonstrated, 5 = consistently demonstrated [see Section I].)

● = Independent   ▲ = Collaborative   **EBN** = Evidence-Based Nursing   **EB** = Evidence-Based

Client Outcomes

Client Will (Specify Time Frame):

- Express feelings and perceptions regarding impacts of illness, disability, and/or hospitalization on parental role
- Participate in hospital and home care as much as able given the availability of resources and support systems
- Exhibit assertiveness and responsibility in active family decision making regarding care of the child
- Describe and select available resources to support parental management of the child's and family's needs

NIC   (Nursing Interventions Classification)

Suggested NIC Interventions

Caregiver Support, Counseling, Decision-Making Support, Family Process Maintenance, Family Therapy, Role Enhancement

Example NIC Activities—Role Enhancement
Teach new behaviors needed by patient/parent to fulfill a role; Serve as role model for learning new behaviors as appropriate

Nursing Interventions and *Rationales*

- Assess and support parents' previous coping behaviors. **EBN:** *Support and caring can go a long way to ease the burden of parents caring for children with chronic illness (Coffey, 2006).*
- Determine parent/family sources of stress, usual methods of coping, and perceptions of illness/condition. Maximize on the strengths identified. **EBN:** *Parents of children with chronic illnesses/diseases find significant improvement to diminish stress and anxiety by utilizing support groups (Bragadottir, 2008).* **EB:** *Clinical assessment of parental stress, acknowledging a difference in parenting experiences for mothers and fathers is needed (Davis & Carter, 2008).*
- Evaluate the family's perceived strength of its social support system, including religious beliefs. Encourage the family to use social support. **EBN:** *A strong relationship has been identified between religiosity and positive coping behaviors (Elkin et al, 2007).*
- Determine the older childbearing woman's support systems and expectations for motherhood. **EBN:** *Nurses caring for the older childbearing woman must not forget that they need support and additional education during the peripartum period (Suplee, Dawley, & Bloch, 2007).*
- Consider the use of family-centered theory as the conceptual foundation to help guide interventions. **EB:** *The concept of family-centered care stresses the importance of the family in children's well-being (Bamm & Rosenbaum, 2008).*
- Be available to accept and support parents, listening and discussing concerns. **EBN:** *When parents feel accepted, supported, and not blamed by the health care professionals, their ability to reflect and make sense of their own thoughts, feelings, and behaviors seems to have a positive influence on the process of change (Levac et al, 2008).*
- ▲ Maintain parental involvement in shared decision making with regard to care by using the following steps: Incorporate parents' information concerning the child's typical routines, behaviors, fears, likes, and dislikes; provide clear and direct firsthand information concerning the child's condition and progress; normalize the home/hospital environment as much as possible; collaborate in care by providing choices when possible. **EBN:** *Developing an understanding of decision making within families prior to the informed consent process will increase health care knowledge of how to improve the health care experience for all families (Snethen et al, 2006).*
- Seek and support parental participation in care. **EBN:** *Environments that facilitate continual parental presence may reduce parental stress related to child's hospitalization (Smith, Hefley, & Anand, 2007).* **EBN:** *Promoting family-centered care enhances the overall quality of NICU resulting in less stress; parents become more informed and confident with the care of the infant (Cooper et al, 2007).*
- Provide support for each parent's primary coping strategies and needs. **EB:** *In this study of parents of ADHD children, mothers reported greater psychological distress and perceived less support from their*

● = Independent   ▲ = Collaborative   **EBN** = Evidence-Based Nursing   **EB** = Evidence-Based

families (Gau, 2007). **EBN:** *Parent support in a neonatal unit found nurses used more concrete guidance when dealing with fathers, while focusing on the emotional side with mothers (Inberg, Axelin, & Salantera, 2008).*

▲ Inform parents of financial resources, respite care, and home support to assist them in maintaining sufficient energy and personal resources to continue caregiving responsibilities. **EBN:** *If health professionals can make parents aware of the financial resources, respite care, and home support that are available to them early on in diagnosis, it may help to alleviate some of the emotional anxieties (Narramore, 2008).*

● Encourage the parent to meet his or her own needs for rest, nutrition, and hygiene. Provide parent bed spaces so that the parent may stay with the sick child. **EBN:** *Due to the potential for parental fatigue, it is essential for staff to promote parent self-care (Smith, Hefley, & Anand, 2007).*

● Provide family-centered care: allowing parents to touch and talk to the child, assisting in the handling of medical equipment, and offering a comfortable chair, preferably a rocking chair. Provide opportunities and offer praise for successful caregiving. **EBN:** *Establishing an emotionally safe and supportive neonatal unit where a trusting bond exits between parents and nurses may help decrease parents' stress level and their need to remain vigilant for the safety of their infant (Cleveland, 2008).*

● Refer parents to available telephone and/or Internet support groups. **EB:** *Parents reported that telephone support had improved their parenting (Ritchie, 2006).* **EBN:** *Participation in support groups can be an important source of emotional and informational support (Ahlberg & Nordner, 2006).*

● Involve new mother's partners or parents in clinical encounters and invite family members to discuss their expectations and parenting experiences. **EBN:** *Clinicians can validate their critical role in supporting the mother and child while having shared and contradictory meanings and habits that shape the mother's possibilities and her likelihood of following child-rearing advice disclosed (Smith-Battle, 2006).*

Multicultural

● Acknowledge racial/ethnic differences at the onset of care. **EBN:** *Acknowledgment of race/ethnicity issues will enhance communication, establish rapport, and promote treatment outcomes (Giger & Davidhizar, 2008).*

● Assess for the influence of cultural beliefs, norms, and values on the client's perceptions of the parental role. **EBN:** *What the client considers a normal or abnormal parental role may be based on cultural perceptions (Leininger & McFarland, 2002).* **EBN:** *What the client considers normal or abnormal when caring for other members of the family is also culturally related. Villarruel and Denyes (1997) reported that the importance and obligation of Mexican Americans in meeting the needs of others indicate that there may be a higher priority placed on promoting and supporting the development of abilities to care for others than on abilities to care for self. Two other patterns, the "accepted obligation to perform roles within the family" and the "willingness to bear the burden so as not to cause pain for others" further indicate that caring for others is both expected and rewarded (Villarruel & Denyes, 1997; Villarruel & Leininger, 2004). Some Mexican American families may engage in an intergenerational family ritual called* La Cuarentena, *which lasts for 40 days after birth and involves prescriptions for maternal food, clothing, and paternal role (Niska, Snyder, & Lia-Hoagberg, 1998).*

● Acknowledge that value conflicts arising from acculturation stresses may contribute to increased anxiety and significant conflict with the parental role. **EBN:** *This study indicates that helping family members retain traditional values may be protective for family functioning. Family conflict is particularly deleterious for youth, regardless of acculturation level. Thus, clinical intervention efforts geared toward preventing and reducing conflict relations among family members appears key to promoting adolescents' well-being (Pasch et al, 2006).*

● Promote the female parenting role by providing a treatment environment that is culturally based and woman-centered. **EBN:** *Pregnant and postpartum Asian and Pacific Islander women in substance abuse treatment identified provisions for the newborn, infant health care, parent education, and infant-mother bonding as conducive to their treatment (Morelli, Fong, & Oliveria, 2001). African American mothers of medically fragile infants reported the sights and sounds of the hospital environment as an additional stress (Miles et al, 2002).*

- Support the client's parenting role in their usual setting via social exchange. **EBN:** *Social exchange is a useful theory in support of the nurse-client relationship and is useful in accomplishing client outcomes (Byrd, 2006).*

Home Care

- The interventions described previously may be adapted for home care use.
- Assess family adjustment prenatally and postpartum; assist new parents to renegotiate parenting roles and responsibilities with co-parenting. Encourage the father to take an active role in infant care with the mother's support. **EB:** *Fathers' but not mothers' withdrawal during co-parenting negotiations was associated with greater disengagement and less warmth during triadic play and with fathers' feeling that mothers did not respect their parenting (Elliston et al, 2008).*

Client/Family Teaching and Discharge Planning

- Offer family-led education interventions to improve participants' knowledge about their condition and its treatment and decreasing their information needs. **EB:** *Family-led education interventions may provide families with the information they need to better cope with their relative's mental illness (Pickett-Schenk et al, 2008).*
- For children and their parents involved in bereavement support groups, identify the family's positive way of coping. **EBN:** *When assessing their group experiences, children and parents most appreciated the support and understanding they received, the freedom to express themselves, a diminished sense of isolation, and the normalization of their emotions (Davies et al, 2007).*
- ▲ Refer parents of children with behavioral problems to parenting programs. **EB:** *Parenting programs reduced disruptive behaviors in children with these improvements being maintained well over time, and further improvements in long-term follow-up (de Graaf et al, 2008).*
- Involve parents in formal and/or informal social support situations, such as Internet support groups. EBN: In this study, clients viewed Internet cancer support groups (ICSG) positively as an excellent source of social support. Participants wanted to use ICSG for emotional support, information, and interactions; they were able to reach out to other clients with cancer without traveling and without interrupting their busy schedules (Im et al, 2007).
- Teach the client about available community resources (e.g., therapists, ministers, counselors, self-help groups). **EB:** *Supporting caregivers over time and following up to ensure that they access needed services are critical ways to help them cope with care of a loved one (Dobrof et al, 2006).*
- Encourage parents with human immunodeficiency virus/acquired immune deficiency syndrome (HIV/AIDS) to implement custody plans for their children. **EBN:** *In this study, more than half of the children were not in custody of their HIV-infected parent at some time during the study period. Pediatricians and others taking care of children with HIV-infected parents may be able to offer counseling or referrals to assist parents with child custody issues (Cowgill et al, 2007).*

ⓔvolve   See the EVOLVE website for Weblinks for client education resources.

REFERENCES

Ahlberg K, Nordner A: The importance of participation in support groups for women with ovarian cancer, *Oncol Nurs Forum* 33(4): E53–E61, 2006.

Bamm EL, Rosenbaum P: Family-centered theory: origins, development, barriers, and supports to implementation in rehabilitation medicine, *Arch Phys Med Rehabil* 89(8):1618–1624, 2008.

Bragadottir H: Computer-mediated support group intervention for parents, *J Nurs Scholarsh* 40(1):32–38, 2008.

Byrd ME: Social exchange as a framework for client-nurse interaction during public health nursing maternal-child home visits, *Public Health Nurs* 23(3):271–276, 2006.

Cleveland LM: Parenting in the neonatal intensive care unit, *J Obstet Gynecol Neonatal Nurs* 37(6): 666–691, 2008.

Coffey JS: Parenting a child with chronic illness: a metasynthesis, *Pediatr Nurs* 32(1):51–59, 2006.

Cooper LG, Gooding JS, Gallagher J et al: Impact of family-centered care initiative on NICU care, staff and families, *J Perinatol*, 27(2 Suppl): S32–37, 2007.

Cowgill BO, Beckett MK, Corona R et al: Children of HIV-infected parents: custody status in a nationally representative sample, *Pediatrics* 120(3):e494–503, 2007.

Davies B, Collins J, Steele R et al: Parents' and children's perspectives of a children's hospice bereavement program, *J Palliat Care* 23(1):14–23, 2007.

Davis N, Carter A: Parenting stress in mothers and fathers of toddlers with autism spectrum disorders: associations with child characteristics, *J Autism Dev Disord* 38(7):1278–1291, 2008.

de Graaf I, Speetjens P, Smit F et al: Effectiveness of the Triple P Positive Parenting Program on behavioral problems in children: a meta-analysis, *Behav Modif* 32(5):714–735, 2008.

● = Independent   ▲ = Collaborative   **EBN** = Evidence-Based Nursing   **EB** = Evidence-Based

Dobrof J, Ebenstein H, Dodd S et al: Social work series. Caregivers and professionals partnership caregiver resource center: assessing a hospital support program for family caregivers, *J Palliat Med* 9(1):196–205, 2006.

Elkin TD, Jensen SA, McNeil L et al: Religiosity and coping in mothers of children diagnosed with cancer: an exploratory analysis, *J Pediatr Oncol Nurs* 24(5):274–278, 2007.

Elliston D, McHale J, Talbot J et al: Withdrawal from co-parenting interactions during early infancy, *Fam Process* 47(4):481–499, 2008.

Gau SS: Parental and family factors for attention-deficit hyperactivity disorder in Taiwanese children, *Aust Nz J Psychiatry* 41(8):688–696, 2007.

Giger J, Davidhizar R: Social organization. In Giger and Davidhizar's *Transcultural nursing: assessment and intervention,* St Louis, 2008, Mosby.

Im E, Chee W, Lim H et al: Patient's attitudes toward internet cancer support groups, *Oncol Nurs Forum* 34(3):705–712, 2007.

Inberg E, Axelin A, Salantera S: Supporting the early interaction between a premature baby and its parents with the help of nursing methods, *Hoitotiede* 20(4):192–202, 2008.

Leininger MM, McFarland MR: *Transcultural nursing: concepts, theories, research and practices,* ed 3, New York, McGraw-Hill, 2002.

Levac AM, McCay E, Merka P et al: Exploring parent participation in a parent training program for children's aggression: understanding and illuminating mechanisms of change, *J Child Adolesc Psychiatr Nurs* 21(2):78–88, 2008.

Miles MS, Burchinal P, Holditch-Davis D et al: Perceptions of stress, worry, and support in black and white mothers of hospitalized, medically fragile infants, *J Pediatr Nurs* 17(2):82–88, 2002.

Morelli PT, Fong R, Oliveria J: Culturally competent substance abuse treatment for Asian/Pacific Islander women, *J Hum Behav Soc Environ* 3(3/4):263, 2001.

Narramore N: Meeting the emotional needs of parents who have a child with complex needs, *J Child Young Peoples Nurs* 2(3):103–107, 2008.

Niska K, Snyder M, Lia-Hoagberg B: Family ritual facilitates adaptation to parenthood, *Public Health Nurs* 15(5):329–337, 1998.

Pasch LA, Deardorff J, Tschann JM et al: Acculturation, parent-adolescent conflict, and adolescent adjustment in Mexican American families, *Fam Process* 45(1):75–86, 2006.

Pickett-Schenk SA, Lippincott RC, Bennett C et al: Improving knowledge about mental illness through family-led education: the journey of hope, *Psychiatr Serv* 59(1):49–56, 2008.

Ritchie C: Can telephone support improve parent and child well-being? *J Soc Work* 6(3):361–374, 2006.

Smith AB, Hefley GC, Anand KJS: Parent bed spaces in the PICU: effect on parental stress, *Pediatr Nurs* 33(3):215–221, 2007.

Smith-Battle L: Family legacies in shaping teen mothers' caregiving practices over 12 years, *Qual Health Res* 16(8):1129–1144, 2006.

Snethen JA, Broome ME, Knafl K et al: Family patterns of decision-making in pediatric clinical trials, *Res Nurs Health* 29(3):223–232, 2006.

Suplee PD, Dawley K, Bloch JR: Tailoring peripartum nursing care for women of advanced maternal age, *J Obstet Gynecol Neonatal Nurs* 36(6):616–623, 2007.

Villarruel A, Denyes M: Testing Orem's theory with Mexican Americans, *J Nurs Scholarsh* 29(3):283–288, 1997.

Villarruel A, Leininger M: Culture care of Mexican Americans. In Leininger M (editor): *Transcultural nursing,* ed 3, New York, 2004, McGraw-Hill.

Acute Confusion   *Betty J. Ackley, MSN, EdS, RN*   ⊝volve

NANDA-I

Definition

Abrupt onset of reversible disturbances of consciousness attention, cognition, and perception that develop over a short period of time

Defining Characteristics

Fluctuation in cognition, level of consciousness, psychomotor activity; hallucinations; increased agitation; increased restlessness; lack of motivation to follow through with goal-directed behavior or purposeful behavior; lack of motivation to initiate goal-directed behavior or purposeful behavior; misperceptions

Related Factors (r/t)

Alcohol abuse; delirium; dementia; drug abuse, fluctuation in sleep-wake cycle, over 60 years of age, polypharmacy

NOC   (Nursing Outcomes Classification)

Suggested NOC Outcomes

Cognition, Distorted Thought Self-Control, Information Processing, Memory

Example **NOC** Outcome with Indicators
Cognition as evidenced by the following indicators: Communication clear for age/Comprehension of the meaning of situations/Attentiveness/Concentration/Cognitive orientation (Rate the outcome and indicators of **Cognition.** 1 = severely compromised, 2 = substantially compromised, 3 = moderately compromised, 4 = mildly compromised, 5 = not compromised [see Section I].)

Client Outcomes

Client Will (Specify Time Frame):

- Demonstrate restoration of cognitive status to baseline
- Be oriented to time, place, and person
- Demonstrate appropriate motor behavior
- Maintain functional capacity

NIC   (Nursing Interventions Classification)

Suggested NIC Interventions

Delirium Management, Delusion Management

Example NIC Activities—Delirium Management
Orient to time, place, and person; Present information in small, concrete portions

Nursing Interventions and *Rationales*

- Assess the client's behavior and cognition systematically and continually throughout the day and night, as appropriate. Utilize a validated tool to assess presence of delirium such as the Confusion Assessment Method (CAM) or the Mini-Mental State Examination (MMSE). **EB:** *Rapid onset and fluctuating course are hallmarks of delirium (Inouye, 2006). The CAM is sensitive, specific, reliable, and easy to use. Another tool to consider is the MMSE (Inouye, 2006).*
- Recognize that there are three distinct types of delirium (Bourne, 2008; Arend & Christensen, 2009):
  - Hyperalert: hyperactive delirium with symptoms of agitation; combative
  - Hypervigilant: uncooperative, paranoia, disorientation, hallucinations, and delusions
  - Hypoalert-Hypoactive: delirium with symptoms of withdrawn apathetic behavior, reduced alertness, confusion, slowed psychomotor function
  - Mixture of both hyper- and hypodelirium: the client fluctuates between both types of behaviors
  Clients who have delirium have higher mortality rates, and higher ICU and hospital costs (Sona, 2009).
- Perform an accurate mental status examination that includes the following:
  - Overall appearance, manner, and attitude
  - Behavior characteristics and level of psychomotor behavior
  - Mood and affect (presence of suicidal or homicidal ideation as observed by others and reported by the client)
  - Insight and judgment
  - Cognition as evidenced by level of consciousness, orientation (to time, place, and person), thought process, and content (perceptual disturbances such as illusions and hallucinations, paranoia, delusions, abstract thinking)
  - Level of attention
  New onset of delirium in adults warrants a thorough examination to determine cause and treatment (Cole et al, 2006). **EB:** *Early intervention in the case of delirium may decrease the severity and length of the delirious episode (Milisen et al, 2001). Clients discharged in delirium from the hospital with delirium had a high rate of institutionalization, and mortality over a 1–year follow-up (McAvay et al, 2006).*
- ▲ Assess for and report possible physiological alterations (e.g., sepsis, hypoglycemia, hypoxia, hypotension, infection, changes in temperature, fluid and electrolyte imbalance, and use of medications with known cognitive and psychotropic side effects). *Early attention to these risk factors may prevent delirium or shorten the length of the delirium episode (Inouye, 2006).*
- ▲ Treat the underlying causes of delirium in collaboration with the health care team:
  - Establish/maintain normal fluid and electrolyte balance; establish/maintain normal nutrition, normal body temperature, normal oxygenation (if the client experiences low oxygen saturation, deliver supplemental oxygen), normal blood glucose levels, normal blood pressure
  - Communicate client status, cognition, and behavioral manifestations to all necessary providers

● = Independent   ▲ = Collaborative   **EBN** = Evidence-Based Nursing   **EB** = Evidence-Based

- Monitor for any trends occurring in these manifestations
  EB: *Careful monitoring is needed to identify the potential etiologic factors for delirium (Foreman, Milisen, & Marcantonio, 2004)*
- ▲ Note results of all laboratory tests reporting abnormalities and follow-up with primary care physician. *Laboratory results should be closely monitored and physiological support given as appropriate.*
- Plan care that allows for an appropriate sleep-wake cycle. Please refer to the care plan for **Sleep deprivation**. *Both delirium and sleep deprivation are associated with disrupted neurotransmitters. It is sometimes difficult to tell which came first. It is known that benzodiazepines deplete melatonin in the body which is needed for normal sleep (Figueroa-Ramos et al, 2009).*
- ▲ Conduct a medication review. *Medication use is one of the most important modifiable factors that can cause or worsen delirium, especially the use of anticholinergics, benzodiazepines, and hypnotics (Inouye, 2006).*
- Modulate sensory exposure and establish a calm environment. *Lights and noise can give rise to agitation, especially if misunderstood. Sensory overload or sensory deprivation can result in increased confusion Clients with a hyperactive form of delirium often have increased irritability and startle responses and may be acutely sensitive to light and sound.*
- Provide reality orientation, including identifying self by name at each contact with the client, calling the client by their preferred name; using orientation techniques; providing familiar objects from home such as an afghan, providing clocks, calendars, and gently correcting misperceptions. **EBN:** *Use of reality orientation can help improve cognition in dementia clients (Forbes, 2008). A study found that use of reality orientation was deemed helpful by psychiatric nurses working with confused mentally ill elderly clients (Patton, 2006).*
- Avoid use of validation therapy with the confused client, other than to validate the feelings the client may be expressing. **EB:** *A Cochrane review demonstrated that there is no evidence that validation therapy is helpful for clients with cognitive impairment (Neal & Briggs, 2003).*
- Use gentle, caring communication with clients, provide reassurance of safety; give simple explanations of procedures as needed (Bourne, 2008). *Clients with delirium often respond to caring even though they may not understand the verbal message.*
- Provide supportive nursing care including meeting of basic needs such as feeding, toileting, and hydration. *Delirious clients are unable to care for themselves due to their confusion. Their care and safety needs must be anticipated by the nurse.*
- ▲ Identify, evaluate, and treat pain quickly (see care plans for **Acute Pain** or **Chronic Pain**). *Untreated pain is a potential cause of delirium, as is also excessive opioid administration (Bourne, 2008).*
- Facilitate appropriate sensory input by having clients use aids (e.g., glasses, hearing aids) as needed. *Sensory impairment contributes to misinterpretation of the environment and significantly contributes to delirium (Inouye, 2006).*
- ▲ Recognize that delirium is frequently treated with an antipsychotic medication. Administer cautiously as ordered, if there is no other way to keep the client safe. Watch for side effects of the medications. *Be aware of paradoxical effects and side effects such as extrapyramidal symptoms, agitation, sedation, and arrhythmias, because these may exacerbate the delirium (Bourne, 2008).* **EB:** *A Cochrane study found that there is insufficient evidence to guide use of medication for delirium in the terminally ill client (Jackson & Lipman, 2009).*

Critical Care

- Monitor for delirium in each client in critical care daily. Utilize the Confusion Assessment Method for the ICU (CAM-ICU) or the Intensive Care Delirium Screening Checklist (ICDSC). *Delirium is extremely common in critically ill clients (Sona, 2009). Both the CAM-ICU and the ICDSC are easy-to-use, reliable, and validated tools (Bergeron et al, 2001; Ely et al, 2001). Defined evaluation tools were needed for ICU clients because often clients were nonverbal or receiving mechanical ventilation (Sona, 2009). In years past, the term "ICU psychosis" was used and is now considered a misnomer. The behavior is not of psychiatric origin (Arend & Christensen, 2009).*
- ▲ Sedate critical care clients carefully. Ensure client receives a "sedation vacation" daily if possible. *Use of sedation is common in ventilated clients. Allowing the client to wake up daily has been associated with decreased incidence of ventilator-associated pneumonia.* NOTE: *A sedation vacation may not be appropriate for all clients, such as those receiving neuromuscular blockade (Bourne, 2008).*

• = Independent   ▲ = Collaborative   **EBN** = Evidence-Based Nursing   **EB** = Evidence-Based

Geriatric

▲ Evaluate all medications for potential to cause or exacerbate delirium. Review the Beers Criteria for Potentially Inappropriate Medication Use in Elderly. *Elderly are very prone to medication side effects that can include confusion. Polypharmacy is a frequent cause of delirium in the elderly (Fick & Mion, 2005).*

● Establish or maintain elimination patterns of urination and defecation. **EB and EBN:** *Urinary retention or a urinary tract infection resulting in urosepsis, as well as constipation, may lead to delirium in the elderly (Inouye, 2006; Faezah et al, 2008; Waardenburg, 2008).*

▲ Determine if the client is nourished, watch for possible protein-calorie malnutrition. Consult with physician, or dietitian as needed if malnutrition is present to ensure good nutrition. **EBN:** *A study found increased delirium in a group of extended care clients who had decreased body weight, possibly because of protein-binding from polypharmacy of medications (Culp & Cacchione, 2008).*

● Explain hospital routines and procedures slowly and in simple terms; repeat information as necessary.

● Provide continuity of care when possible (e.g., provide the same caregivers, avoid room changes) (Foreman, 2004).

● If clients know that they are not thinking clearly, acknowledge the concern. *Fear is frequently experienced by people with delirium.* **EBN:** *Confusion is very frightening, and the memory of the delirium can be equally frightening (Breitbart, Gibson, & Tremblay, 2002).*

● Keep the client's sleep-wake cycle as normal as possible (e.g., avoid letting the client take daytime naps, avoid waking the client at night, give sedatives but not diuretics at bedtime, provide pain relief and back rubs). **EB and EBN:** *Acute confusion is accompanied by disruption of the sleep-wake cycle (Inouye, 2006).*

Home Care

● Some of the interventions described previously may be adapted for home care use.

● Assess and monitor for acute changes in cognition and behavior. *An acute change in cognition and behavior is the classic presentation of delirium. It should be considered a medical emergency.*

● Delirium is reversible but can become chronic if untreated. The client may be discharged from the hospital to home care in a state of undiagnosed delirium. **EB:** *In a study of delirium among clients in a convalescent hospital following an acute care hospital stay for a variety of precipitating factors, 22% presented with delirium, and 93% of these had developed the delirium prior to convalescent home admission. Multiple precipitating factors were frequently present (Pi-Figueras et al, 2004).*

● Avoid preconceptions about the source of acute confusion; assess each occurrence on the basis of available evidence.

▲ Institute case management of frail elderly clients to support continued independent living if possible once delirium has resolved.

Client/Family Teaching and Discharge Planning

▲ Teach the family to recognize signs of early confusion and seek medical help.

● Counsel the client and family regarding the management of delirium and its sequelae. *Families experience a high degree of distress when observing a loved one in delirium (Arend & Christensen, 2009). Families should be told that symptoms of delirium may persist for months following a delirious episode so that appropriate plans can be made for continuing care (Marcantonio et al, 2003).*

ⓔvolve   See the EVOLVE website for Weblinks for client education resources.

REFERENCES

Arend E, Christensen M. Delirium in the intensive care unit: a review, *Br Assoc Crit Care Nurses* 14(3):145–154, 2009.

Bergeron N, Dubois MF, Dumont M et al: Intensive care delirium screening checklist: evaluation of a new screening tool, *Intensive Care Med* 27(5):859–864, 2001.

Bourne RS: Delirium and use of sedation agents in intensive care, *Crit Care Nurs* 13(4):195–202, 2008.

Breitbart W, Gibson C, Tremblay A: The delirium experience: delirium recall and delirium related distress in hospitalized patients with cancer, their spouses/caregivers, and their nurses, *Psychosomatics* 43(3): 183–194, 2002.

Cole CS, Williams ER, Williams RD: Assessment and discharge planning for hospitalized older adults with delirium, *Medsurg Nurs* 15(2):71–77, 2006.

● = Independent   ▲ = Collaborative   **EBN** = Evidence-Based Nursing   **EB** = Evidence-Based

Culp KR, Cacchione PZ: Nutritional status and delirium in long-term care elderly individuals, *Appl Nurs Res* 21(2):66–74, 2008.

Ely EW, Margolin R, Francis J et al: Evaluation of delirium in critically ill patients: validation of the confusion assessment method for the intensive care unit (CAM-ICU), *Crit Care Med* 29:1370–1379, 2001.

Faezah S, Zhang D, Yin LF: The prevalence and risk factors of delirium amongst the elderly in acute hospital, *Singapore Nurs J* 35(1):11–14, 2008.

Fick D, Mion L: Assessing and managing delirium in persons with dementia. Try this: best practices in nursing care for hospitalized older adults. *The John A. Hartford Institute for Geriatric Nursing and the Alzheimer's Association* 1(8):1–2, 2005.

Figueroa-Ramos, Arroyo-Novoa C, Lee D et al: Sleep and delirium in ICU patients: a review of mechanism and manifestations, *Intensive Care Med* 35(5):781–795, 2009.

Forbes D: Reality orientation. In Ackley, B, Ladwig, G, Swan B et al: *Evidence-based nursing guidelines: medical surgical interventions*, Philadelphia, 2008, Mosby.

Foreman MD, Milisen K, Marcantonio E: Prevention and treatment strategies for delirium, *Prim Psychiatry* 11(11):52–58, 2004.

Inouye SK: Current concepts: delirium in older persons, *N Engl J Med* 354(11):1157–65, 1217–20, 2006.

Jackson KC, Lipman AG: Drug therapy for delirium in terminally ill adult patients, *Cochrane Database System Rev* (2):CD004770, 2009.

Marcantonio ER, Simon SE, Bergmann MA et al: Delirium symptoms in post-acute care: prevalent, persistent, and associated with poor recovery, *J Am Geriatr Soc* 51(1):4–9, 2003.

McAvay GJ, Van Ness PH, Bogardus ST Jr et al: Older adults discharged from the hospital with delirium: 1–year outcomes, *J Am Geriatr Soc* 54(8):1245–1250, 2006.

Milisen K, Foreman MD, Abraham IL et al: A nurse-led interdisciplinary intervention program for delirium in elderly hip fracture patients, *J Am Geriatr Soc* 49(5):523–532, 2001.

Neal M, Briggs M: Validation therapy for dementia, *Cochrane Database Syst Rev* (3):CD001394, 2003.

Patton D: Reality orientation: its use and effectiveness within older person mental health care, *J Clin Nurs* 15(11):1440–1449, 2006.

Pi-Figueras M, Aguilera A, Arellano M et al: Prevalence of delirium in a geriatric convalescent hospital unit: patient's clinical characteristics and risk precipitating factor analysis, *Arch Gerontol Geriatr Suppl* (9):333–337, 2004.

Sona C: Assessing delirium in the intensive care unit, *Crit Care Nurs* 29(2):103–104, 2009.

Waardenburg IE: Delirium caused by urinary retention in elderly people: a case report and literature review on the "Cystocerebral syndrome," *J Am Geriatr Soc* 56(12):2371–2372, 2008.

Risk for acute Confusion   Betty J. Ackley, MSN, EdS, RN

NANDA-I

Definition

At risk for reversible disturbances of consciousness, attention, cognition, and perception that develop over a short period of time

Risk Factors

Alcohol use; decreased mobility; decreased restraints; dementia; fluctuation in sleep-wake cycle; history of stroke; impaired cognition; infection; male gender; medication/drugs: anesthesia, anticholinergics, diphenhydramine, multiple medications, opoids, psychoactive drugs; metabolic abnormalities: azotemia, decreased hemoglobin, dehydration, electrolyte imbalances, increased BUN/creatine, malnutrition; over 60 years of age; pain; sensory deprivation; substance abuse; urinary retention

NOC, NIC, Client Outcomes, Nursing Interventions, Client/Family Teaching and Discharge Planning, *Rationales*, and References

Refer to care plan for **Acute Confusion**.

⊖volve   See the EVOLVE website for Weblinks for client education resources.

Chronic Confusion   Rebecca Davis, RN, PhD   ⊖volve

NANDA-I

Definition

Irreversible, long-standing, and/or progressive deterioration of intellect and personality characterized by decreased ability to interpret environmental stimuli; decreased capacity for intellectual thought processes; and manifested by disturbances of memory, orientation, and behavior

• = Independent   ▲ = Collaborative   **EBN** = Evidence-Based Nursing   **EB** = Evidence-Based

Defining Characteristics

Altered interpretation; altered personality; altered response to stimuli; clinical evidence of organic impairment; impaired long-term memory; impaired short-term memory; impaired socialization; long-standing cognitive impairment; no change in level of consciousness; progressive cognitive impairment

Related Factors (r/t)

Alzheimer's disease; cerebral vascular attack; head injury; Korsakoff's psychosis; multiinfarct dementia

 (Nursing Outcomes Classification)

Suggested NOC Outcomes

Cognition, Cognitive Orientation, Distorted Thought Self-Control

Example NOC Outcome with Indicators
Cognition as evidenced by the following indicators: Cognitive orientation/Communicates clearly for age/Comprehends the meaning of situations/Attentiveness/Concentration (Rate the outcome and indicators of **Cognition**: 1 = severely compromised, 2 = substantially compromised, 3 = moderately compromised, 4 = mildly compromised, 5 = not compromised [see Section I].)

Client Outcomes

Client Will (Specify Time Frame):

- Remain content and free from harm
- Function at maximal cognitive level
- Participate in activities of daily living at the maximum of functional ability
- Have minimal episodes of agitation (as agitation occurs in up to 70% of clients with dementia)

NIC **(Nursing Interventions Classification)**

Suggested NIC Interventions

Dementia Management, Environmental Management, Surveillance: Safety

Example NIC Activities—Dementia Management
Use distraction rather than confrontation to manage behavior; Give one simple direction at a time

Nursing Interventions and *Rationales*

- Determine the client's cognitive level using a screening tool such as the Mini-Mental State Exam (MMSE) or Mini-Cog. **EB:** *Use of a standard evaluation tool such as the MMSE can help determine the client's abilities and assist in planning appropriate nursing interventions (Borson et al, 2005; Wilber et al, 2005; Borson et al, 2006).*
- If hospitalized, gather information about the client's pre-admission cognitive functioning. **EBN and EB:** *Individuals with a history of cognitive dysfunction are at higher risk for acute confusion (i.e., sundowner's syndrome) during acute illness (Fick et al, 2005; Voyer et al, 2006).*
- Assess the client for signs of depression: insomnia, poor appetite, flat affect, and withdrawn behavior. **EB:** *Up to 95% of individuals with dementia have some neuropsychiatric problems, with the most common being depression (Aalten et al, 2005; Steinberg et al, 2006).*
- Determine client's normal routines and attempt to maintain them. **EB:** *Activities that are designed to be consistent with past routines were effective at providing engagement and interest and enhancing quality of life (Cohen-Mansfield & Jensen, 2006).*
- Begin each interaction with the client by identifying yourself and calling the client by name. Approach the client with a caring, loving, and accepting attitude, and speak calmly and slowly. **EB:** *Dementia causes a loss of the ability to learn new things and remember people and places (episodic memory—thus clients will need reassurance and frequent reminding of the identity of caregivers). Reorienting people with dementia can be effective and help them with orientation (not during times of agitation) (Golby et al, 2005; Yu et al, 2009).*

● = Independent   ▲ = Collaborative   **EBN** = Evidence-Based Nursing   **EB** = Evidence-Based

- Use a calm approach, and attempt to address the emotional needs and reactions of the client. **EB:** *Emotion-centered care, including reminiscence and emotional support can help reduce anxiety and improve client satisfaction (Finnema et al, 2005).*
- Provide scheduled activities that are matched to the client's abilities and personality. **EB and EBN:** *Activities that are individualized to the client's abilities and personality can reduce agitation and improve quality of life (Kolanowski, Litaker, & Buettner, 2005; Richards et al, 2005; Phinney, Chaudhury, & O'Connor, 2007).*
- Give one simple direction at a time and repeat it as necessary. Use verbal and physical prompts, and model the desired action if needed and possible. **EB:** *There are a variety of communication problems in dementia, but with time and prompting people with dementia can make their needs known and improve well being (Perry et al, 2005; Bayles et al, 2006; Acton et al, 2007).*
- Break down self-care tasks into simple steps (e.g., instead of saying, "Take a shower," say to the client, "Please follow me. Sit down on the bed. Take off your shoes. Now take off your socks."). **EB:** *Verbal prompts, assistance with steps of a process, and cueing activities in sequential order can help those with dementia be more independent in activities of daily living (ADLs) (Giovannetti et al, 2007).*
- Engage the client in communication by individualizing the nurse's interactions to maximize client interaction and response. **EBN and EB:** *Individualized communication strategies that involve the client's interest have been shown to improve communication abilities in those with dementia to above the level that would be expected from their cognitive abilities (Perry et al, 2005; van Weert et al, 2005).*
- For anxious clients who are having problems relaxing enough to eat, try having them listen to music during meals. **EB:** *Clients who listen to music have been shown to have less agitation and consumed more foods (Hicks-Moore, 2005).*
- Assist clients in wayfinding, monitoring them so that they do not get lost in unfamiliar settings. **EB:** *Dementia and some related disorders cause impaired spatial learning, which results in wayfinding problems and incidences of getting lost, especially when environments are unfamiliar (Guariglia & Nitrini, 2006; deIpolyi et al, 2007).*
- Promote sleep by creating a restful environment, decreasing waking, and promoting quiet. **EB:** *Sleep disorders are very common in those with dementia, and a lack of sleep has been shown to be related to poorer memory. One study showed that naps in older people can improve sleep amounts without decreasing nighttime sleep and improve cognitive and psychomotor performance (Hatfield, Herbert, & Someren, 2004; Eeles, Stephens, & Benedict, 2006).*
- Provide structured social and physical activities that are individualized for the client. **EB:** *Social activities and exercise have been shown to improve sleep quality (Eggermont & Scherder, 2006) and structured activities can reduce agitated behaviors and promote well being (Volicer et al, 2006).*
- Provide quiet activities such as listening to music of the client's preference or introduce other cues that promote relaxation **EB and EBN:** *Many studies have shown a positive benefit of music therapy on promoting relaxation and well being in people with dementia (Sung, 2005; Svansdottir & Snaedal, 2006; Garland et al, 2007).*
- Provide simple activities for the client, such as folding washcloths and sorting or stacking activities or other hobbies the individual enjoyed prior to the onset of dementia. **EBN and EB:** *Activities such as folding washcloths, cooking, and gardening involve implicit memory and are thus something that the older adult can become engaged in, which can provide distraction and a sense of accomplishment (Golby et al, 2005; Harrison et al, 2007).*
- Use cues, such as picture boards denoting day, time, and location, to help client with orientation. **EBN and EB:** *Reality orientation, used not when clients are agitated, but as overall reminders of orientation, can help some clients remain more oriented (Leach, 2004; Farina et al, 2006; Yu et al, 2009).*
- Use reminiscence and life review therapeutic interventions; ask questions about the client's work, children, or time spent in military service. Ask questions such as, "What was really important to you as you look back?" to engage the client in storytelling. **EB:** *Reminiscence and life review can help an older person reframe and accept life events and provide social engagement (Herrmann, 2005; Kim & Whall, 2006; Woods et al, 2006).*
- ▲ If the client becomes increasingly confused and agitated, perform the following steps:
  - Assess the client for physiological causes, including acute hypoxia, pain, medication effects, malnutrition, infections such as urinary tract infection, fatigue, electrolyte disturbances, and constipation. *Clients with chronic confusion are at high risk for delirium (acute confusion) which*

• = Independent   ▲ = Collaborative   **EBN** = Evidence-Based Nursing   **EB** = Evidence-Based

may be caused by other physiologic problems such as infection or medication interactions. Nurses must assess the client and recognize any change in cognitive status and address underlying causes (Fick et al, 2005; Voyer et al, 2006; Voyer et al, 2007).

- Assess for psychological causes, including changes in the environment, caregiver, and routine; demands to perform beyond capacity; or multiple competing stimuli, including discomfort. **EBN:** *Agitated behaviors can be an expression of a need that is not being met (Kolanowski, Litaker, & Buetner, 2005; Kovach et al, 2005).*
- In clients with agitated behaviors, rather than confronting the client, provide divisional behaviors such as singing, games, and the provision of textured items to handle. **EB:** *Psychomotor and behavioral activities can reduce agitated episodes (Herrmann, 2005; Volicer et al, 2006; Phinney, Chaudhury, & O'Connor, 2007).*

• Decrease stimuli in the environment (e.g., turn off the television, take the client to a quiet place). Institute activities associated with pleasant emotions, such as playing soft music the client likes, looking through a photo album, providing favorite food, or using simulated presence therapy. **EB and EBN:** *Decreasing stimuli can decrease agitation (Tilly & Reed, 2005).*

• If clients with dementia become more agitated, assess for pain. **EB and EBN:** *A change in behavior may indicate pain, and pain is often undertreated in those with dementia. Treating pain can improve social interaction, engagement, and decrease agitation (Chibnall et al, 2005; Shega et al, 2006).*

• Avoid using restraints if at all possible. **EB:** *Restraints have been shown to cause decline in cognition, socialization, and depression in nursing home residents (Castle, 2006).*

▲ Use PRN or low-dose regular dosing of psychotropic or antianxiety drugs only as a last resort. They can be effective in managing symptoms of psychosis and aggressive behavior, but have undesirable side effects. Start with the lowest possible dose. **EB and EBN:** *Psychotropic medication use is variable in those with dementia and has many side effects, including sleep disturbances and medication interactions. Effective nursing interventions can reduce psychotropic medication usage (Coker, 2006; Kim & Whall, 2006; Simpson et al, 2006).*

▲ Avoid the use of anticholinergic medications such as Benadryl. *Anticholinergic medications have a high side-effect profile that includes disorientation, urinary retention, and excessive drowsiness, especially in those with decreased cognition. The anticholinergic side effects outweigh the antihistaminic effects (Artero et al, 2008; Uusvaara et al, 2009).*

• For predictable difficult times, such as during bathing and grooming, try the following:
  - Massage the client's hands lovingly or use therapeutic touch to relax the client. **EBN:** *Hand massage and therapeutic touch have been shown to induce relaxation that may allow care activities to take place without difficulty (Viggo Hansen, Jørgensen, & Ørtenblad, 2006).*
  - Approach the client in a client-centered framework as this offers a sense of control and promotes self-esteem (Hoeffer et al, 2006).
  - Involve family in care of the client. **EBN:** *Involving family in care of clients with dementia improved cognitive abilities (Jablonski, Reed, & Maas, 2005).*

• For care of early dementia clients with primarily symptoms of memory loss, see the care plan for **Impaired Memory.**

• For care of clients with self-care deficits, see the appropriate care plan (**Feeding Self-Care deficit; Dressing Self-Care deficit;** and **Toileting Self-Care deficit**).

Geriatric

NOTE: All interventions are appropriate with geriatric clients.

Multicultural

• Assess for the influence of cultural beliefs, norms, and values on the family's or caregiver's understanding of chronic confusion or dementia. **EBN:** *What the family considers normal and abnormal health behavior may be based on cultural perceptions (Leininger & McFarland 2002; Giger & Davidhizar, 2008). Research indicates that Caucasian older adults are significantly more knowledgeable about Alzheimer's disease (AD) than African American, Asian, and Latino older adults (Ayalon & Arean, 2004). Another study showed African Americans showed less awareness of facts about AD, reported fewer sources of information, and indicated less perceived threat of the disorder (Roberts et al, 2003).*

• = Independent   ▲ = Collaborative   **EBN** = Evidence-Based Nursing   **EB** = Evidence-Based

- Inform the client's family or caregiver of the meaning of and reasons for common behavior observed in clients with dementia. **EBN:** *An understanding of dementia behavior will enable the client's family or caregiver to provide the client with a safe environment. Black and Latino community-dwelling clients with moderate to severe dementia have a higher prevalence of dementia-related behaviors than whites (Sink et al, 2004).*
- Assist the family or caregiver in identifying barriers that would prevent the use of social services or other supportive services that could help reduce the impact of caregiving. **EBN:** *Expectations of discrimination, lack of knowledge about services, expectations embedded in familism, lack of sense of prevention, lack of health insurance, preference for traditional remedies, and neglect or abuse were barriers identified by researchers studying the low utilization of skilled home care nursing services by elderly Hispanic clients (Crist, 2002). Language may present another barrier to the access of supportive services (McGrath, Vun, & McLeod, 2001). The lack of health insurance and financial resources for a substantial proportion of Mexican American people means many do not receive medical care, so their Alzheimer's disease remains undiagnosed and untreated (Briones et al, 2002).*
- Assess the client for the presence of an instrumental activity of daily living (IADL) disability and chronic health conditions. **EBN:** *African American clients with cognitive impairments had higher IADL disability, poorer self-rated health, higher cognitive errors, and more chronic health conditions (Chumbler et al, 2001).*
- ▲ Refer the family to social services or other supportive services to assist in meeting the demands of caregiving for the client with dementia. **EBN:** *African American caregivers of dementia clients may evidence less desire than others to institutionalize their family members and are more likely to report unmet service needs (Hinrichsen & Ramirez, 1992). Families of dementia clients may report restricted social activity (Haley et al, 1995). Korean families reported waiting 3 to 4 years before seeking help for their family member with dementia. Help was sought when memory decline was accompanied by other problems (Watari & Gatz, 2004).*
- ▲ Encourage the family to make use of support groups or other service programs. **EBN:** *Studies indicate that some minority families of clients with dementia may use few support programs even though these programs could have a positive impact on caregiver well-being (Cox, 1999).*
- Validate the family members' feelings with regard to the impact of the client's behavior on family lifestyle. **EBN:** *Validation lets family members know that the nurse has heard and understood what was said, and it promotes the relationship between the nurse and family members (Heineken, 1998).*

NOTE: Black and Latino community-dwelling clients with moderate to severe dementia have a higher prevalence of dementia-related behaviors than Caucasian clients. Therefore, as the aging minority population grows, it will be especially important to target caregiver education, in-home support, and resources to minority communities (Sink et al, 2004).

Home Care

NOTE: Keeping the client as independent as possible is important. Because community-based care is usually less structured than institutional care, in the home setting the goal of maintaining safety for the client takes on primary importance.

- The interventions described previously may be adapted for home care use.
- ▲ Provide information to the family and home care client regarding advanced directives. *This is a legal requirement of the Consolidated Omnibus Budget Reconciliation Act (COBRA). Decision-making capacity depends on many factors such as stage of dementia. However, the client's autonomy should be valued (Menne & Whitlatch, 2007; Moye et al, 2006).*
- Assess the client's memory and executive function deficits before assuming the inability to make any medical decisions. **EB:** *A review of existing research on the decision-making competence of cognitively impaired older adults concluded that many persons with dementia are capable of decision making (Moye et al, 2006; Menne & Whitlatch, 2007).*
- Assess the home for safety features and client needs for assistive devices. Refer to the interventions for **Feeding Self-Care deficit, Dressing Self-Care deficit, Bathing Self-Care deficit** as needed.
- Elements of reality orientation therapy may be applied in the home, incorporating person-centered respect, reminiscence, validation, and sensory-motor stimulation. **EB:** *Reality orientation and cognitive stimulation can improve client outcomes (Leach, 2004; Woods et al, 2006).*

• = Independent ▲ = Collaborative **EBN** = Evidence-Based Nursing **EB** = Evidence-Based

- Provide education and support to the family of the client with a chronic and disabling condition; be prepared to offer support and information to family members who live at a distance as well. **EB:** *Increased self-efficacy for caregiving has been related to decreased caregiver stress and burden (Gonyea et al, 2005; Hepburn, Lewis, & Narayan, 2005).*
- Use familiar aspects of the environment (smells, music, foods, pictures) to cue the client, capitalizing on habit to remind the client of activities in which the client can participate (e.g., cooperating with medication administration). **EB and EBN:** *While clients with dementia are probably unable to learn new activities because of deteriorated explicit memory, preserved implicit memory or habit may be useful in maximizing functional ability (Harrison et al, 2007; Hong & Song, 2009).*
- Instruct the caregiver to provide a balanced activity schedule that does not stress the client nor deprive him or her of stimulation; avoid sustained low- or high-stimulation activity. **EB:** *Planned activities can decrease agitation and improve quality of life (Volicer et al, 2006; Phinney et al, 2007).*
- ▲ If the client will require extensive supervision on an ongoing basis, evaluate the client for day care programs. Refer the family to medical social services to assist with this process if necessary. *Day care programs provide safe, structured care for the client and respite for the family.* **EB:** *Adult Day programs have been shown to reduce stress associated with work, leisure, and family needs (Schacke & Zank, 2006).*
- Encourage the family to include the client in family activities when possible. Reinforce the use of therapeutic communication guidelines (see Client/Family Teaching and Discharge Planning) and sensitivity to the number of people present. *These steps help the client maintain dignity and lead to familial socialization of the client.*
- Assess family caregivers for caregiver stress, loneliness, and depression. **EBN:** *Caregiving is associated with poorer mental health. Increased burden (behavioral and health problems) is associated with more mental health problems in the caregiver (Willette-Murphy, Todero, & Yeaworth, 2006).*
- Refer to the care plan for **Caregiver role strain.**
- ▲ Refer the client to medical social services as necessary to evaluate financial resources and initiate benefits or access to providers. **EBN:** *Limited resources serve as barriers to effective use of community services (Scharlach et al, 2006; Beeber, Thorpe, & Clipp, 2008).*
- ▲ Institute case management for frail elderly clients to support continued independent living.

Client/Family Teaching and Discharge Planning

- In the early stages of confusion (e.g., initial period following stroke), provide the caregiver with information on illness processes, needed care, and likely trajectory of progress. **EBN:** *Caregiver education can help the caregiver feel supported (Hepburn et al, 2005).*
- Teach the family how to converse with a memory-impaired person. Individuals with dementia have a variety of communication difficulties. *Good assessment and individualized interventions are necessary to improve communication (Frazier-Rios & Zembrzuski, 2005).*
- Teach the family how to provide physical care for the client (bathing, feeding, and ADLs). **EB:** *Improved self-efficacy regarding how to care for loved ones has been shown to decrease caregiver burden (Gonyea et al, 2005).*
- Discuss with the family what to expect as the dementia progresses.
- ▲ Counsel the family about resources available regarding end-of-life decisions and legal concerns. **EB:** *Involving the caregivers in end-of-life decision making is important for satisfaction with the end-of-life process and in providing individualized care (Caron, Griffith, & Arcand, 2005; Engel, Kiely, & Mitchell, 2006).*
- ▲ Inform the family that as dementia progresses, hospice care may be available in the home in the terminal stages to help the caregiver. **EB:** *Clients who have hospice are more likely to die in the location of their choice and have improved caregiver satisfaction (Shega et al, 2008).*

NOTE: The nursing diagnoses **Impaired Environmental interpretation syndrome** and **Chronic Confusion** are very similar in definition and interventions. **Impaired Environmental interpretation syndrome** must be interpreted as a syndrome when other nursing diagnoses would also apply. **Chronic Confusion** may be interpreted as the human response to a situation or situations that require a level of cognition of which the individual is no longer capable. Further research is underway to make this distinction clear to the practicing nurse.

ⓔvolve   See the EVOLVE website for Weblinks for client education resources.

• = Independent   ▲ = Collaborative   **EBN** = Evidence-Based Nursing   **EB** = Evidence-Based

REFERENCES

Aalten P, de Vugt M, Jaspers N et al: The course of neuropsychiatric symptoms in dementia. Part I: findings from the two-year longitudinal Maasbed study, *Int J Geriatr Psychiatry* 20(6):523–530, 2005.

Acton GJ, Yauk S, Hopkins BA et al: Increasing social communication in persons with dementia, *Res Theory Nurs Pract* 21(1):32, 2007.

Artero S, Ancelin ML, Portet F et al: Risk profiles for mild cognitive impairment and progression to dementia are gender specific, *J Neurol Neurosurg Psychiatry* 79(9):979–984, 2008.

Ayalon L, Arean PA: Knowledge of Alzheimer's disease in four ethnic groups of older adults, *Int J Geriatr Psychiatry* 19(1):51–57, 2004.

Bayles K, Kim E, Chapman S et al: Evidence-based practice recommendations for working with individuals with dementia: simulated presence therapy, *J Med Speech Lang Pathol* 14(3):xiii-xxi, 2006.

Beeber AS, Thorpe JM, Clipp EC: Community-based service use by elders with dementia and their caregivers: a latent class analysis, *Nurs Res* 57(5):312, 2008.

Borson S, Scanlan J, Watanabe J et al: Simplifying detection of cognitive impairment: comparison of the Mini-Cog and Mini-Mental State Examination in a multiethnic sample, J Am Geriatr Soc 53(5):871–874, 2005.

Borson S, Scanlan J, Watanabe J et al: Improving identification of cognitive impairment in primary care, *Int J Geriatr Psychiatry* 21(4):349–355, 2006.

Briones DF, Ramirez AL, Guerrero M et al: Determining cultural psychosocial factors in Alzheimer disease among Hispanic populations, *Alzheimer Dis Assoc Disord* 16(Suppl 2):S86–88, 2002.

Caron CD, Griffith J, Arcand M: End-of-life decision making in dementia: the perspective of family caregivers, *Dementia* 4(1):113–136, 2005.

Castle N: Mental health outcomes and physical restraint among nursing homes, *Adm Policy Ment Health* 33:696–704, 2006.

Chibnall JT, Tait RC, Harman B et al: Effect of acetaminophen on behavior, well-being, and psychotropic medication use in nursing home residents with moderate-to-severe dementia, *J Am Geriatr* Soc 53(11):1921–1929, 2005.

Chumbler NR, Hartmann DJ, Cody M et al: Differences by race in the health status of rural cognitively impaired Arkansans, *Clin Gerontol* 24(1/2):103–121, 2001.

Cohen-Mansfield J, Jensen B: Do interventions bringing current self-care practices into greater correspondence with those performed premorbidly benefit the person with dementia? A pilot study, *Am J Alzheimers Dis Other Demen* 21(5):312–317, 2006.

Coker E: Training and support for nursing home staff reduced neuroleptic drug use and did not increase aggression in residents with dementia, *Evid Based Nurs* 9(4):122, 2006.

Cox C: Race and caregiving: patterns of service use by African-American and white caregivers of persons with Alzheimer's, *J Gerontol Soc Work* 32(2):5, 1999.

Crist JD: Mexican American elders' use of skilled home care nursing services, *Public Health Nurs* 19(5):366–376, 2002.

deIpolyi AR, Rankin KP, Mucke L et al: Spatial cognition and the human navigation network in AD and MCI, *Neurology* 69(10):986–997, 2007.

Eeles EM, Stephens M, Benedict C: Sleep in dementia assessment may require a multidisciplinary approach, *Am J Geriatr Psychiatry* 14(11):986, 2006.

Eggermont L, Scherder E: Physical activity and behavior in dementia: a review of the literature and implications for psychosocial intervention in primary care, *Dementia* 5:411–428, 2006.

Engel SE, Kiely DK, Mitchell SL: Satisfaction with end-of-life care for nursing home residents with advanced dementia, *J Am Geriatr Soc* 54(10):1567, 2006.

Farina E, Mantovani F, Fioravanti R et al: Evaluating two group programmes of cognitive training in mild-to-moderate AD: is there any difference between a 'global' stimulation and a 'cognitive-specific' one? *Aging Ment Health* 10(3):211–218, 2006.

Fick D, Kolanowski A, Waller et al: Delirium superimposed on dementia in a community-dwelling managed care population: a 3–year retrospective study of occurrence, costs, and utilization, *J Gerontol A Biol Sci Med Sci* 60A(6):748–753, 2005.

Finnema E, Dröes RM, Ettema T et al: The effect of integrated emotion-oriented care versus usual care on elderly persons with dementia in the nursing home and on nursing assistants: a randomized clinical trial, *Int J Geriatr Psychiatry* 20(4):330–343, 2005.

Frazier-Rios D, Zembrzuski C: Try this: best practices in nursing care for hospitalized older adults with dementia. Communication difficulties: assessment and interventions, *Dermatol Nurs* 17:319–320, 2005.

Garland K, Beer E, Eppingstall B et al: A comparison of two treatments of agitated behavior in nursing home residents with dementia: simulated family presence and preferred music, *Am J Geriatr Psychiatry* 15(6):514, 2007.

Giger J, Davidhizar R: *Transcultural nursing: assessment and intervention*, St Louis, 2008, Mosby.

Giovannetti T, Bettcher BM, Libon DJ et al: Environmental adaptations improve everyday action performance in Alzheimer's disease: empirical support from performance-based assessment, *Neuropsychology* 21(4):448–457, 2007.

Gonyea J, O'Connor M, Carruth A et al: Subjective appraisal of Alzheimer's disease caregiving: the role of self-efficacy and depressive symptoms in the experience of burden, *Am J Alzheimers Dis Other Demen* 20:273–280, 2005.

Golby A, Silverberg G, Race E et al: Memory encoding in Alzheimer's disease: an fMRI study of explicit and implicit memory, *Brain J Neurol* 128(Part 4):773–787, 2005.

Guariglia CC, Nitrini R: P2–109 Topographical disorientation in Alzheimer's disease, *Alzheimers Dement* (3S):265, 2006.

Haley WE, West CA, Wadley VG et al: Psychological, social, and health impact of caregiving: a comparison of black and white dementia family caregivers and noncaregivers, *Psychol Aging* 10(4):540, 1995.

Hatfield CF, Herbert J, Someren EJ: Disrupted daily activity/rest cycles in relation to daily cortisol rhythms of home-dwelling patients with early Alzheimer's dementia, *Brain* 127(PT 5):1061–1074, 2004.

Harrison BE, Son G, Kim J et al: Preserved implicit memory in dementia: a potential model for care, *Am J Alzheimers Dis Other Demen* 22(4):286–293, 2007.

Heineken J: Patient's silence is not necessarily client satisfaction: communication in home care nursing, *Home Healthc Nurs* 16(2):115, 1998.

Hepburn K, Lewis M, Narayan S et al: Partners in caregiving: a psychoeducation program affecting dementia family caregivers' distress and caregiving outlook, *Clin Gerontol* 29(1):53–69, 2005.

Herrmann N: Some psychosocial therapies may reduce depression, aggression, or apathy in people with dementia, *Evid Based Ment Health* 8(4):104, 2005.

Hicks-Moore S: Relaxing music at mealtime in nursing homes: effect on agitated patients with dementia, *J Gerontol Nurs* 31(12):26–32, 2005.

Hinrichsen GA, Ramirez M: Black and white dementia caregivers: a comparison of their adaptation, *Gerontologist* 32(3):375, 1992.

Hoeffer B, Talerico KA, Rasin J et al: Assisting cognitively impaired nursing home residents with bathing: effects of two bathing interventions on caregiving, *Gerontologist* 46(4):524–532, 2006.

Hong GR, Song JA: Relationship between familiar environment and wandering behaviour among Korean elders with dementia, *J Clin Nurs* 18(9):1365–1373, 2009.

● = Independent   ▲ = Collaborative   **EBN** = Evidence-Based Nursing   **EB** = Evidence-Based

Jablonski RA, Reed D, Maas ML: Care intervention for older adults with Alzheimer's disease and related dementias: effect of family involvement on cognitive and functional outcomes in nursing homes, *J Gerontol Nurs* 31(6):38–48, 2005.

Kim H, Whall A: Factors associated with psychotropic drug usage among nursing home residents with dementia, *Nurs Res* 55(4):252–258, 2006.

Kolanowski AM, Litaker M, Buettner L: Efficacy of theory-based activities for behavioral symptoms of dementia, *Nurs Res* 54(4):219–228, 2005.

Kovach C, Noonan PE, Schlidt AM et al: A model of consequences of need-driven, dementia-compromised behavior, *J Nurs Scholarsh* 37(2):134–140, 2005.

Leach L: Cognitive stimulation therapy improves cognition and quality of life in older people with dementia, *Evid Based Ment Health* 7(1):19, 2004.

Leininger MM, McFarland MR: *Transcultural nursing: concepts, theories, research and practices,* ed 3, New York, 2002, McGraw-Hill.

McGrath P, Vun M, McLeod L: Needs and experiences of non-English-speaking hospice patients and families in English-speaking country, *Am J Hosp Palliat Care* 18(5):305, 2001.

Menne HL, Whitlatch CJ: Decision-making involvement of individuals with dementia, *Gerontologist* 47(6):810–819, 2007.

Moye J, Karel MJ, Gurrera RJ et al: Neuropsychological predictors of decision-making capacity over 9 months in mild-to-moderate dementia, *J Gen Intern Med* 21(1):78–83, 2006.

Perry J, Galloway S, Bottorff J et al: Nurse-patient communication in dementia: improving the odds, *J Gerontol Nurs* 31(4):43–52, 2005.

Phinney A, Chaudhury H, O'Connor DL: Doing as much as I can do: the meaning of activity for people with dementia, *Aging Ment Health* 11(4):384–393, 2007.

Richards K, Beck C, O'Sullivan P et al: Effect of individualized social activity on sleep in nursing home residents with dementia, *J Am Geriatr Soc* 53(9):1510–1517, 2005.

Roberts JS, Connell CM, Cisewski D et al: Differences between African-Americans and whites in their perceptions of Alzheimer disease, *Alzheimer Dis Assoc Disord* 17(1):19–26, 2003.

Schacke C, Zank S: Measuring the effectiveness of adult day care as a facility to support family caregivers of dementia patients, *J Appl Gerontol* 25:65–81, 2006.

Scharlach AE, Kellam R, Ong N et al: Cultural attitudes and caregiver service use, *J Gerontol Social Work* 47(1):133–156, 2006.

Shega JW, Hougham GW, Stocking CB et al: Management of noncancer pain in community-dwelling persons with dementia, *J Am Geriatr Soc* 54(12):1892–1897, 2006.

Shega JW, Hougham GW, Stocking CB et al: Patients dying with dementia: Experience at the end of life and impact of hospice care, *J Pain Symptom Manag* 35(5):499–507, 2008.

Simpson K, Richards K, Enderlin C et al: Medications and sleep in nursing home residents with dementia, *J Am Psychiatric Nurses Assoc* 12(5):279–285, 2006.

Sink KM, Covinsky KE, Newcomer R et al: Ethnic differences in the prevalence and pattern of dementia-related behaviors, *J Am Geriatr Soc* 5(8):1277–1283, 2004.

Steinberg M, Corcoran C, Tschanz J et al: Risk factors for neuropsychiatric symptoms in dementia: the Cache County Study, *Int J Geriatr Psychiatry* 21(9):824–830, 2006.

Sung HC: Use of preferred music to decrease agitated behaviours in older people with dementia: a review of the literature, *J Clin Nurs* 14(9):1133–1140, 2005.

Svansdottir HB, Snaedal J: Music therapy in moderate and severe dementia of Alzheimer's type: a case–control study, *Int Psychogeriatr* 18(04):613–621, 2006.

Tilly J, Reed P: Interventions that optimize quality dementia care: a comprehensive literature search selects the best evidence-based interventions to improve quality dementia care in LTC facilities, *Can Nurs Home* 16:13–21, 2005.

Uusvaara J, Pitkala KH, Tienari PJ et al: Association between anticholinergic drugs and apolipoprotein E epsilon4 allele and poorer cognitive function in older cardiovascular patients: a cross-sectional study, *J Am Geriatr Soc* 57(3):427–431, 2009.

Viggo Hansen N, Jørgensen T, Ørtenblad L: Massage and touch for dementia, *Cochrane Database Syst Rev* (4):CD004989, 2006.

van Weert J, van Dulmen A, Spreeuwenberg P et al: Effects of snoezelen, integrated in 24h dementia care, on nurse-patient communication during morning care, *Patient Educ Couns* 58(3):312–326, 2005.

Volicer L, Simard J, Pupa JH et al: Effects of continuous activity programming on behavioral symptoms of dementia, *J Am Med Dir Assoc* 7(7):426–431, 2006.

Voyer P, McCusker J, Cole M et al: Influence of prior cognitive impairment on the severity of delirium symptoms among older patients, *J Neurosci Nurs* 38(2):90–101, 2006.

Voyer P, McCusker J, Cole MG et al: Factors associated with delirium severity among older patients, *J Clin Nurs* 16(5):819, 2007.

Watari KF, Gatz M: Pathways to care for Alzheimer's disease among Korean Americans, *Cultur Divers Ethnic Minor Psychol* 1(1):23–28, 2004.

Wilber S, Lofgren S, Mager T et al: An evaluation of two screening tools for cognitive impairment in older emergency department patients, *Acad Emerg Med* 12(7):612–616, 2005.

Willette-Murphy K, Todero C, Yeaworth R: Mental health and sleep of older wife caregivers for spouses with Alzheimer's disease and related disorders, *Issues Ment Health Nurs* 27(8):837–852, 2006.

Woods B, Thorgrimsen L, Spector A et al: Improved quality of life and cognitive stimulation therapy in dementia, *Aging Ment Health* 10(3):219–226, 2006.

Yu F, Rose KM, Burgener SC et al: Cognitive training for early-stage Alzheimer's disease and dementia, *J Gerontol Nurs* 35(3):23–29, 2009.

Constipation   *Marilee Schmelzer, PhD, RN*   ⊖volve

NANDA-I

Definition

Decrease in normal frequency of defecation, accompanied by difficult or incomplete passage of stool and/or passage of excessively hard, dry stool

• = Independent   ▲ = Collaborative   **EBN** = Evidence-Based Nursing   **EB** = Evidence-Based

Defining Characteristics

Feeling of rectal fullness; feeling of rectal pressure; straining with defecation; unable to pass stool; abdominal pain; abdominal tenderness; anorexia; atypical presentations in older adults (e.g., change in mental status, urinary incontinence, unexplained falls, elevated body temperature); borborygmi; change in bowel pattern; decreased frequency; decreased volume of stool; distended abdomen; generalized fatigue; hard, formed stool; headache; hyperactive bowel sounds; hypoactive bowel sounds; increased abdominal pressure; indigestion; nausea; oozing liquid stool; palpable abdominal or rectal mass; percussed abdominal dullness; pain with defecation; severe flatus; vomiting

Related Factors (r/t)

Functional

Abdominal muscle weakness; habitual denial; habitual ignoring of urge to defecate; inadequate toileting (e.g., timeliness, positioning for defecation, privacy); irregular defecation habits; insufficient physical activity; recent environmental changes

Psychological

Depression; emotional stress; mental confusion

Pharmacological

Aluminum-containing antacids; anticholinergics, anticonvulsants; antidiarrheal agents, antidepressants, antilipemic agents, bismuth salts, calcium carbonate, calcium channel blockers, diuretics, iron salts, laxative overdose, nonsteroidal antiinflammatory drugs (NSAIDs), opioids, phenothiazines, sedatives, and sympathomimetics

Mechanical

Neurological impairment; electrolyte imbalance; hemorrhoids; Hirschsprung's disease; obesity; post-surgical obstruction; pregnancy; prostate enlargement; rectal abscess; rectal anal fissures; rectal anal stricture; rectal prolapse; rectal ulcer; rectocele; tumors

Physiological

Change in eating patterns; change in usual foods; decreased motility of gastrointestinal tract; dehydration; inadequate dentition; inadequate oral hygiene; insufficient fiber intake; insufficient fluid intake; poor eating habits

NOC (Nursing Outcomes Classification)

Suggested NOC Outcomes

Bowel Elimination, Hydration

> **Example NOC Outcome with Indicators**
>
> **Bowel Elimination** as evidenced by the following indicators: Elimination pattern/Stool soft and formed/Passage of stool without aids/Ease of stool passage (Rate each indicator of **Bowel Elimination:** 1 = severely compromised, 2 = substantially compromised, 3 = moderately compromised, 4 = mildly compromised, 5 = not compromised [see Section I].)

Client Outcomes

Client Will (Specify Time Frame):

- Maintain passage of soft, formed stool every 1 to 3 days without straining
- State relief from discomfort of constipation
- Identify measures that prevent or treat constipation

NIC (Nursing Interventions Classification)

Suggested NIC Intervention

Constipation/Impaction Management

● = Independent ▲ = Collaborative **EBN** = Evidence-Based Nursing **EB** = Evidence-Based

Example NIC Activities—Constipation/Impaction Management
Identify factors (e.g., medications, bed rest, and diet) that may cause or contribute to constipation/impaction

Nursing Interventions and *Rationales*

- Assess usual pattern of defecation, including time of day, amount and frequency of stool, consistency of stool; history of bowel habits or laxative use; diet, including fiber and fluid intake; exercise patterns; personal remedies for constipation; obstetrical/gynecological history; surgeries; diseases that affect bowel motility; alterations in perianal sensation; present bowel regimen. *There often are multiple reasons for constipation; the first step is assessment of the usual patterns of bowel elimination (Bleser et al, 2005).*

- Have the client or family keep a 7–day diary of bowel habits, including information such as time of day; usual stimulus; consistency, amount, and frequency of stool; difficulty defecating; fluid consumption; and use of any aids to defecation. *Health care providers define constipation mainly in terms of frequency, but those affected are more concerned about hard stool and discomfort and straining when attempting to defecate (Wald et al, 2008).* **EBN:** *A diary of bowel habits is valuable in treatment of constipation; the use of a diary has proven to be more accurate than client recall in determining the presence of constipation (Andersen et al, 2006).*

- Use the Bristol Stool Scale to assess stool consistency. *The Bristol Stool scale is widely used as a more objective measure to describe stool consistency (Bleser et al, 2005; Kyle, 2007).*

- ▲ Review the client's current medications. **EB:** *Many medications are associated with chronic constipation including opioids, anticholinergics, antidepressants, antihypertensives (e.g. clonidine, calcium channel blockers), antispasmodics, diuretics, anticonvulsants, and psychotropics (Eoff & Lembo, 2008).*

- ▲ If clients are suffering from constipation and are taking constipating medications, consult with the health care provider (with prescriptive powers) about the possibilities of decreasing the medication dosages or finding an alternative medication that is less constipating.

- ▲ Recognize that opioids are especially problematic. If the client is receiving temporary opioids (e.g., for acute postoperative pain), request an order for routine stool softeners from the primary care practitioner, monitor bowel movements, and request a laxative if the client develops constipation. If the client is receiving round the clock opiates (e.g., for palliative care), request an order for Senokot-S and institute a bowel regimen. *Opioids lead to constipation because they decrease propulsive movement in the colon and enhance sphincter tone making it difficult to defecate. Senokot-S is recommended to prevent constipation when opioids are given round the clock (Kyle, 2007).* **EB:** *In a study of hip fracture clients who received opioids following surgery, clients who received prophylactic laxatives developed less constipation than those who did not receive prophylactic laxatives (Davies et al, 2008).*

- ▲ If the client is terminally ill and is receiving round the clock opioids for palliative care, speak with the health care provider (with prescriptive power) about prescribing methylnaltrexone or alvimopan, drugs that block the opioid effects on the gastrointestinal tract, without interfering with analgesia. *Both were approved by the FDA in 2008 (Eoff & Lembo, 2008).* **EB:** *In a RCT with subjects with opioid induced constipation, a significantly greater percentage of those who received methylnaltrexone had a bowel movement within 4 hours (without other laxatives) than those who received placebo (Thomas et al, 2008).*

- If new onset of constipation, determine if the client has recently stopped smoking. **EB:** *Constipation occurs in one in six people who stop smoking and in some people can be very severe (Hajek, Gillison, & McRobbie, 2003). Smoking was inversely related to constipation in a survey of women with constipation (Dukas, Willett, & Giovannucci, 2003). In a survey about perceived effects of various foods and beverages on constipation, cigarettes were the items that were most often perceived to have a laxative effect among smokers in all three groups (Müller-Lissner et al, 2005b).*

- Palpate for abdominal distention, percuss for dullness, and auscultate bowel sounds. *In clients with constipation the abdomen is often distended and tender, and stool in the colon produces a dull percussion sound. Bowel sounds will be present.*

- ▲ Check for impaction; if present, perform digital removal per physician's order. *An impaction is hard stool that is too large to move through the sphincter. Manual removal is necessary before a bowel routine can be instituted (Hinrichs et al, 2001). Some palliative care clients (e.g. those with spinal cord*

● = Independent   ▲ = Collaborative   **EBN** = Evidence-Based Nursing   **EB** = Evidence-Based

compression and advanced multiple sclerosis) may require regular digital removal of stool (Kyle, 2007).

▲ If the client is uncomfortable or in pain due to constipation or has acute or chronic constipation that does not respond to increased fiber, fluid, activity, and appropriate toileting, refer the client to the primary care practitioner for an evaluation of bowel function and health status. *There can be multiple causes of constipation, such as endocrine disorders (e.g. hypothyroidism), depression, neurological conditions (e.g. multiple sclerosis and Parkinson's disease), ano-rectal disorders, and Hirschsprung's disease (Eoff & Lembo, 2008).*

- Encourage fiber intake of 20 g/day (for adults) ensuring that the fiber is palatable to the individual and that fluid intake is adequate. Add fiber gradually to decrease bloating and flatus. *Larger stools move through the colon faster than smaller stools and dietary fiber makes stools bigger because it is undigested in the upper intestinal tract. Fiber fermentation by bacteria in the colon produces gas. The effectiveness of water-insoluble fibers (e.g. wheat bran) on bowel function is well supported by research, and there is growing evidence that water-soluble fibers (e.g., glucomannan and psyllium) also promote laxation (Vuksan et al, 2008). Psyllium is very hydrophilic and forms a moist, soft stool that promotes peristalsis; it may even be more effective than bran (Singh, 2007). EB: Analysis data from a women in the Nurses' Health Study Women found that those with a median fiber intake of 20 g/day were less likely to experience constipation than those with a median intake of 7 g/day (Dukas, Willett & Giovannucci, 2003). In a study of subjects receiving each of 5 treatments in a randomized design, the 5 treatments included: (1) bran cereal, (2) bran with corn cereal, (3) bran with psyllium cereal, (4) a cereal blend of 70% glucomannan and 30% xanthan, and (5) the low-fiber control diet. All four cereals produced significantly greater bowel movement than the low-fiber control diet and all were well tolerated (Vuksan et al, 2008). Researchers found that rye bread shortened intestinal transit time, softened the feces, and eased defecation of women with constipation, and that yogurt lessened the bloating and flatulence resulting from rye bread (Hongisto et al, 2006).*

▲ Use a mixture of bran cereal, applesauce, and prune juice; begin administration in small amounts and gradually increase amount. Keep refrigerated. Always check with the primary care practitioner before initiating this intervention. It is important that the client also ingest sufficient fluids. **EBN:** *This bran mixture has been shown to be effective even with short-term use in elderly clients recovering from acute conditions; however, it has not been tested with a RCT (Joanna Briggs Institute, 2008).* NOTE: *Giving fiber without sufficient fluid has resulted in worsening of constipation (Müller-Lissner et al, 2005). Additional dietary fiber and bulk-forming laxatives are inappropriate for those who have difficulty ingesting adequate fluids such as clients in palliative care (Kyle, 2007).*

- Provide prune or prune juice daily. *Each 100 g of prunes contain about 6 g of fiber and 15 g of sorbitol, and both are natural laxative (Müller-Lissner et al, 2005a). EB: In a study about the perceived effects of various foods and beverages on stool consistency, over half subjects surveyed reported that prunes had a softening effect on their stools (Müller-Lissner et al, 2005b).*

- Encourage a fluid intake of 1.5 to 2 L/day (6 to 8 glasses of liquids per day), unless contraindicated because of renal insufficiency. *Cereal fibers such as wheat bran add additional bulk by attracting water to the fiber, so adequate fluid intake is essential. EB: When dehydrated, the body absorbs additional water from stools resulting in dry, hard stools that are difficult to pass (Sykes, 2006). Increasing fluid intake is not helpful if the person is already well hydrated.*

- Encourage clients to resume walking and activities of daily living as soon as possible if their mobility has been restricted. Encourage turning and changing positions in bed, lifting the hips off the bed, performing range-of-motion exercises, alternately lifting each knee to the chest, doing wheelchair lifts, doing waist twists, stretching the arms away from the body, and pulling in the abdomen while taking deep breaths. *Bed rest and decreased mobility lead to constipation, but additional exercise does not help the constipated person who is already mobile. When the client has diminished mobility, even minimal activity increases peristalsis, which is necessary to prevent constipation (Joanna Briggs Institute, 2008; Kyle, 2007; Sykes, 2006). EB: Strenuous activity leads to gastrointestinal problems, but low to moderate levels of exercise seem to have beneficial effects on gastrointestinal function (Strid, 2005). Twelve weeks of physical activity significantly decreased symptoms of constipation and difficulty defecating in sedentary clients with chronic constipation, but transit time decreased only in subjects who had abnormally long transit time before starting the exercise program (DeSchryver et al, 2005).*

- Ask clients when they normally have a bowel movement and assist them to the bathroom at that same time every day to establish regular elimination. *An optimal time for many individuals is 30*

● = Independent ▲ = Collaborative **EBN** = Evidence-Based Nursing **EB** = Evidence-Based

minutes after breakfast because of the gastrocolic reflex (Godfrey & Rose, 2007). **EBN:** *When clients followed a bowel program that included adequate hydration, dietary fiber and regular toileting, most resumed normal bowel elimination patterns without laxatives (Benton et al, 1997). When subjects who had suffered a stroke were randomly scheduled for morning or evening defecation, those defecating in the morning after breakfast returned to regular elimination patterns significantly faster. Subjects whose defecation was scheduled for the same time of day as their normal, pre-stroke patterns, also resumed normal elimination patterns significantly faster (Venn, 1992).*

- Provide privacy for defecation. If not contraindicated, help the client to the bathroom and close the door. *Bowel elimination is a private act in Western cultures, and a lack of privacy can hinder the defecation urge thus contributing to constipation.*

- Help clients onto a bedside commode or toilet so they can either squat or lean forward while sitting. *Sitting upright allows gravity to aid defecation.* **EB:** *An experimental study of men found that flexing the hip to 90 degrees or more straightens the angle between the anus and the rectum and pulls the anal canal open, to decrease the resistance to the movement of feces from the rectum and the amount of pressure needed to empty the rectum. Hip flexion is greatest when squatting or when leaning forward while sitting (Tagart, 1966). In a repeated measures study involving volunteers, defecation required significantly less time and was significantly easier when squatting than when sitting (Sikirov, 2003). Researchers found significant differences in the ability of 25 subjects to defecate a water filled balloon in the lying position versus the sitting position and in the ability to defecate a silicone-filled device simulating normal stool while in the lying and the sitting positions. Fifteen subjects (60%) could not expel the water-filled balloon in the lying position, and four (16%) could not expel it in the sitting position. Eleven (44%) could not expel the simulated stool while lying down and only one could not expel it while sitting (Rao, Kavolic, & Rao, 2006).*

- Teach clients to respond promptly to the defecation urge. **EB:** *A study of male volunteers determined that the defecation urge can be delayed and that delaying defecation decreased bowel movement frequency, stool weight and transit time (Klauser et al, 1990).*

- ▲ Provide laxatives, suppositories, and enemas only as needed if other more natural interventions are not effective, and as ordered only; establish a client goal of eliminating their use. **EB:** *Moderate evidence exists for the efficacy of lactulose, laxatives containing polyethylene glycol, and bulking agents (e.g., psyllium and bran) for the treatment of constipation in the elderly (Joanna Briggs Institute, 2008). Use of stimulant laxatives should be avoided because they result in laxative dependence and loss of normal bowel function (Merli & Graham, 2003). Laxatives (e.g., bisacodyl) and enemas also damage the surface epithelium of the colon (Schmelzer et al, 2004).*

- ▲ When giving large-volume enema solutions (e.g., soapsuds or tapwater enemas), measure the amount of fluid given and the amount expelled, especially when giving repeated enemas. Use a low concentration of castile soap in the soapsuds enema. *Enema fluid can be retained, and this retained fluid can be harmful for the client prone to fluid overload.* **EBN:** *In studies comparing the effectiveness of soapsuds enemas in preoperative liver transplant clients (Schmelzer et al, 2000), and in healthy subjects (Schmelzer et al, 2004), the amount of enema solution given was often larger than the amount of returns, and some subjects retained large amounts of solution. Biopsies taken immediately after soapsuds and tap water enemas demonstrated damage to the surface epithelium of the colon (Schmelzer et al, 2004).*

 Geriatric

- Assess older adults for the presence of factors that contribute to constipation including: dietary fiber and fluid intake (less than 1.5 L/day), physical activity, use of constipating medications, and diseases that are associated with constipation.

- Explain the importance of adequate fiber intake, fluid intake, activity, and established toileting routines to ensure soft, formed stool. **EB:** *Strong evidence exists for the efficacy of adequate hydration and dietary fiber in the prevention of constipation in older adults; moderate evidence exists for the effectiveness of increased activity for those restricted to bedrest (Joanna Briggs Institute, 2008). In a RCT of elderly nursing home residents who were chronically ill and regularly used laxatives, those who received an additional 5.1 g of oat bran with their usual diets had significant reductions in laxative use when compared to those who did not (Sturtzel & Elmadfa, 2008).* **EBN:** *A study involving institutionalized elderly men with chronic constipation demonstrated that, with use of a bran mixture, clients were able to discontinue use of oral laxatives (Howard, West, & Ossip-Klein, 2000).*

• = Independent ▲ = Collaborative **EBN** = Evidence-Based Nursing **EB** = Evidence-Based

- Determine the client's perception of normal bowel elimination and laxative use; promote adherence to a regular schedule. **EB:** *In a survey of in the United States, United Kingdom, Germany, France, Italy, Brazil, and South Korea, elderly subjects reported more constipation and used laxatives more often than younger subjects (Wald et al, 2008).*
- Explain Valsalva maneuver and the reason it should be avoided. *Valsalva maneuver can cause bradycardia and even death in cardiac clients.*
- Respond quickly to the client's call for help with toileting.
- Avoid regular use of enemas in the elderly. *Enemas can cause fluid and electrolyte imbalances and damage to the colonic mucosa (Schmelzer et al, 2004).*
- ▲ Use opioids cautiously. If they are ordered, use stool softeners and bran mixtures to prevent constipation. *Use of opioids can cause constipation (Kurz & Sessler, 2003; Davies et al, 2008).*
- Position the client on the toilet or commode and place a small footstool under the feet. *Placing a small footstool under the feet increases intraabdominal pressure and makes defecation easier for clients with weak abdominal muscles (Kyle, 2007).*

 Home Care

- The interventions described previously may be adapted for home care use.
- Take complaints seriously and evaluate claims of constipation in a matter-of-fact manner. *Continued constipation can lead to bowel obstruction, a medical emergency. Use of a matter-of-fact manner will limit positive reinforcement of the behavior if actual constipation does not exist.* Refer to the care plan for **Perceived Constipation.**
- Assess the self-care management activities the client is already using. **EBN:** *Many older adults seek solutions to constipation, with laxative use a frequent remedy that creates its own problems (Annells & Koch, 2002).*
- The following treatment recommendations have been offered (Annells & Koch, 2002):
  - Acknowledge the client's lifelong experience of bowel function; respect beliefs, attitudes, and preferences, and avoid patronizing responses.
  - Make available comprehensive, useful written information about constipation and possible solutions.
  - Make available empathetic and accessible professional care to provide treatment and advice; a multidisciplinary approach (including physician, nurse, and pharmacist) should be used.
  - Institute a bowel management program.
  - Consider affordability when suggesting solutions to constipation; discuss cost-saving strategies.
  - Discuss a range of solutions to constipation and allow the client to choose the preferred options.
  - Have orders in place for a suppository and enema as the need may occur. *As part of a bowel management program, suppositories or enemas may become necessary (Annels & Koch, 2002).*
- Although the use of a bedside commode may be necessitated by the client's condition, allow the client to use the toilet in the bathroom when possible and provide assistance. *Bowel elimination is a very private act, and a lack of privacy can contribute to constipation.*
- In older clients, routinely advise consumption of fluids, fruits, and vegetables as part of the diet, and ambulation if the client is able. Introduce a bowel management program at the first sign of constipation. *Constipation is a major problem for terminally ill or hospice clients, who may need very high doses of opioids for pain management (Sykes, 2006).*
- ▲ Refer for consideration of the use of polyethylene glycol 3350 (PEG-3350) for constipation. **EBN:** *In a study of PEG-3350 use for idiopathic constipation, researchers concluded that it appeared to be safe and efficacious when dietary and lifestyle changes were ineffective. Clients reported increased perceived bowel control, with reduced complaints of straining, stool hardness, bloating, and gas (Stoltz et al, 2001).* **EB:** *There is good evidence to support the use of PEG for chronic constipation (Ramkumar & Rao, 2005).*
- Advise the client against attempting to remove impacted feces on his or her own. *Older or confused clients in particular may attempt to remove feces and cause rectal damage.*
- When using a bowel program, establish a pattern that is very regular and allows the client to be part of the family unit. *Regularity of the program promotes psychological and/or physiological readiness to*

• = Independent   ▲ = Collaborative   **EBN** = Evidence-Based Nursing   **EB** = Evidence-Based

evacuate stool. Families of home care clients often cannot proceed with normal daily activities until bowel programs are complete.

Client/Family Teaching and Discharge Planning

- Instruct the client on normal bowel function and the need for adequate fluid and fiber intake, activity, and a defined toileting pattern in a bowel program.
- Encourage the client to heed defecation warning signs and develop a regular schedule of defecation by using a stimulus such as a warm drink or prune juice. *Most cases of constipation are mechanical and result from habitual neglect of impulses that signal the appropriate time for defecation. The reflex that causes the urge to defecate diminishes after a few minutes and may remain quiet for several hours; as a result, the stool becomes hardened and more difficult to expel (American Academy of Family Physicians, 2005).*
- Encourage the client to avoid long-term use of laxatives and enemas and to gradually withdraw from their use if they are used regularly. *Use of stimulant laxatives should be avoided, and long-term use can result in dependence on laxative for defecation (American Academy of Family Physicians, 2005).*
- If not contraindicated, teach the client how to do bent-leg sit-ups to increase abdominal tone; also encourage the client to contract the abdominal muscles frequently throughout the day. Help the client develop a daily exercise program to increase peristalsis.

⊖volve   See the EVOLVE website for Weblinks for client education resources.

REFERENCES

American Academy of Family Physicians: Information from your family doctor: constipation, *Am Fam Physician* 71(3):539–540, 2005.

Andersen C, Adamsen L, Moeller T et al: The effect of a multidimensional exercise programme on symptoms and side-effects in cancer patient undergoing chemotherapy: the use of semi-structured diaries, *Eur J Oncol Nurs* 10:247–262, 2006.

Annells M, Koch T: Older people seeking solutions to constipation: the laxative mire, *J Clin Nurs* 11:603, 2002.

Benton JM, O'Hara PA, Chen H et al: Changing bowel hygiene practice successfully: a program to reduce laxative use in a chronic care hospital, *Geriatr Nurs* 18(1):12–17, 1997.

Bleser S, Brunton S, Carmichael B et al: Management of chronic constipation: recommendations from a consensus panel, *J Fam Pract* 54(8):692–698, 2005.

Davies EC, Green CF, Mottram DR et al: The use of opiods and laxatives, and incidence of constipation, in patients requiring neck-of-femur (NOF) surgery: a pilot study, *J Clin Pharm Ther* 33:561–566, 2008.

DeSchryver AM, Keulemans YC, Peters HP et al: Effects of regular physical activity on defecation pattern in middle-aged patients complaining of chronic constipation, *Scand J Gastroenterol* 40:422–429, 2005.

Dukas L, Willett WC, Giovannucci EL: Association between physical activity, fiber intake, and other lifestyle variables and constipation in a study of women, *Am J Gastroenterol* 98(8):1790–1796, 2003.

Eoff JC, Lembo AJ: Optimal treatment of chronic constipation in managed care: review and roundtable discussion, *J Manag Care Pharm* 14(9–a):S1–S17, 2008.

Godfrey JR, Rose S: Conversations with the experts: toward hoptimal health: Suzanne Rose, MD, M.S.E., discusses management of constipation in women, *J Womens Health* 16(9):1252–1257, 2007.

Hajek P, Gillison F, McRobbie H: Stopping smoking can cause constipation, *Addiction* 98(11):1563, 2003.

Hinrichs M, Huseboe J, Tang JH et al: Research-based protocol. Management of constipation, *J Gerontol Nurs* 27(2):17, 2001.

Hongisto S-M, Paajanen L, Saxelin et al: A combination of fibre-rich rye bread and yoghurt containing *Lactobacillus GG* improves bowel function in women with self-reported constipation, *Eur J Clin Nutr* 60:319–324, 2006.

Howard LV, West D, Ossip-Klein DJ: Chronic constipation management for institutionalized older adults, *Geriatr Nurs* 21(2):78, 2000.

Joanna Briggs Institute: Management of constipation in older adults, *Au Nurs J* 16(5):32–35, 2008.

Klauser AG, Voderholzer WA, Heinrich C et al: Behavioral modification of colonic function. Can constipation be learned? *Digest Dis Sci* 35(10):1271–1275, 1990.

Kurz A, Sessler DI: Opioid-induced bowel dysfunction: pathophysiology and potential new therapies, *Drugs* 63:7, 2003.

Kyle G: Constipation and palliative care—where are we now? *Int J Palliat Nurs* 13(1):6–16, 2007.

Merli GJ, Graham MG: Three steps to better management of constipation, *Patient Care*, 37:6, 2003.

Müller-Lissner SA, Kamm MA, Scarpignato C et al: Myths and misconceptions about constipation, *AM J Gastroenterol* 100(1): 232–242, 2005a.

Müller-Lissner SA, Kaatz V, Brandt W et al: The perceived effect of various foods and beverages on stool consistency, *Eur J Gastroentero Hepatol* 17:109–112, 2005b.

Ramkumar D, Rao SS: Efficacy and safety of traditional medical therapies for chronic constipation: systematic review, *Am J Gastro-enterol* 100(4):936–971, 2005.

Rao SSC, Kavolic R, Rao S: Influence of body position and stool characteristics on defecation in humans, *Am J Gastroenterol* 206(101):2790–2796, 2006.

Schmelzer M, Case P, Chappell SM et al: Colonic cleansing, fluid absorption, and discomfort following tap water and soapsuds enemas, *Appl Nurs Res* 13(2):83, 2000.

Schmelzer M, Schiller LR, Meyer R et al: Safety and effectiveness of large-volume enema solutions, *Appl Nurs Res* 17(4):265–274, 2004.

Sikirov D: Comparison of straining during defecation in three positions: results and implications for human health, *Digest Dis Sci* 48(7):1201–1205, 2003.

● = Independent   ▲ = Collaborative   **EBN** = Evidence-Based Nursing   **EB** = Evidence-Based

Singh B: Psyllium as therapeutic and drug delivery agent, *Int J Pharmaceut* 334(2007):1–14, 2007.

Strid H: The effects of physical activity on the gastrointestinal tract, *Int Sports Med J* 6(3):151–161, 2005.

Stolz R, Weiss LM, Merkin DH et al: An efficacy and consumer preference study of polyethylene glycol 3350 for the treatment of constipation in regular laxative users, *Home Healthc Consult* 8(2):21, 2001.

Sturtzel B, Elmadfa I: Intervention with dietary fiber to treat constipation and reduce laxative use in residents of nursing homes, *Ann Nutr Metabol* 52(suppl 1):54–56, 2008.

Sykes NP: The pathogenesis of constipation, *J Support Oncol* 4(5):213–218, 2006.

Tagart REB: The anal canal and rectum: their varying relationship and its effect on anal continence, *Dis Colon Rectum* 9(6):449–452, 1966.

Thomas J, Karver S, Coorney GA et al: Methylnaltrexone for opioid-induced constipation in advanced illness, *NEJM* 358(22):2332–2343, 2008.

Venn MR: The influence of timing and suppository use on efficiency and effectiveness of bowel training after a stroke, *Rehab Nurs* 17(3):116–121, 1992.

Vuksan V, Jenkins AL, Jenkins DJA et al: Using cereal to increase dietary fiber intake to the recommended level and the effect of fiber on bowel function in healthy persons consuming North American diets, *Am J Clin Nutr* 88:1256–1262, 2008.

Wald A, Scarpignato C, Mueller-Lissner S et al: A multinational survey of prevalence and patterns of laxative use among adults with self-defined constipation, *Aliment Pharmacol Ther* 28(7):917–930, 2008.

Perceived Constipation   *Marilee Schmelzer, PhD, RN*

 NANDA-I

Definition

Self-diagnosis of constipation and abuse of laxatives, enemas, and suppositories to ensure a daily bowel movement

Defining Characteristics

Expectation of a daily bowel movement that results in overuse of laxatives, enemas, and suppositories; expectation of a passage of stool at same time every day

Related Factors (r/t)

Cultural or family health beliefs, faulty appraisals, impaired thought processes

 NOC   **(Nursing Outcomes Classification)**

Suggested NOC Outcomes

Bowel Elimination, Health Beliefs, Health Beliefs: Perceived Threat

Example NOC Outcome with Indicators

Bowel Elimination as evidenced by the following indicators: Elimination pattern/Stool soft and formed/Passage of stool without aids/Ease of stool passage (Rate each indicator of **Bowel Elimination:** 1 = severely compromised, 2 = substantially compromised, 3 = moderately compromised, 4 = mildly compromised, 5 = not compromised [see Section I].)

Client Outcomes

Client Will (Specify Time Frame):

- Regularly defecate soft, formed stool without use of aids
- Explain the need to decrease or eliminate the use of stimulant laxatives, suppositories, and enemas
- Identify alternatives to stimulant laxatives, enemas, and suppositories for ensuring defecation
- Explain that defecation does not have to occur every day

 NIC   **(Nursing Interventions Classification)**

Suggested NIC Interventions

Bowel Management, Medication Management

Example NIC Activities—Bowel Management

Note preexistent bowel problems, bowel routine, and use of laxatives

• = Independent   ▲ = Collaborative   **EBN** = Evidence-Based Nursing   **EB** = Evidence-Based

Nursing Interventions and *Rationales*

- Have the client keep a 7-day diary of bowel habits, including information such as time of day; usual stimulus; consistency, amount, and frequency of stool; difficulty defecating; fluid consumption; and use of any aids to defecation. *Health care providers define constipation mainly in terms of frequency, but those affected are more concerned about hard stool and discomfort and straining when attempting to defecate (Wald et al, 2008).* **EBN:** *A diary of bowel habits is valuable in treatment of constipation; the use of a diary has proven to be more accurate than client recall in determining the presence of constipation (Andersen et al, 2006).*

- Determine the client's perception of an appropriate defecation pattern. *The client may need to be taught that one bowel movement every 1 to 3 days is normal (American Academy of Family Physicians, 2005).*

- Monitor the use of laxatives, suppositories, or enemas and suggest replacing them with increased fiber intake along with increased fluids to 2 L/day. *Use of stimulant laxatives should be avoided; long-term use can result in dependence on laxative for defecation (American Academy of Family Physicians, 2005). An increase in fiber intake to 20 to 30 g/day along with an increase in fluid intake can help clients with chronic constipation (Sturtzel & Elmadfa, 2008).*

- Encourage fiber intake of 20 g/day (for adults) ensuring that the fiber is palatable to the individual and that fluid intake is adequate. Add fiber gradually to decrease bloating and flatus. *Some people with eating disorders do not eat enough fiber to produce stools. Larger stools move through the colon faster than smaller stools and dietary fiber make stools bigger because it is undigested in the upper intestinal tract. Fiber fermentation by bacteria in the colon produces gas. The effectiveness of water insoluble fibers (e.g., wheat bran) on bowel function is well supported by research and there is growing evidence that water soluble fibers (e.g., glucomannan and psyllium) also promote laxation (Vuksan et al, 2008). Psyllium is very hydrophilic and forms a moist soft stool that promotes peristalsis; it may even be more effective than bran (Singh, 2007).* **EB:** *Analysis of data from the Nurses' Health Study found that those with a median fiber intake of 20 g/day were less likely to experience constipation than those with a median intake of 7 g/day (Dukas, Willett, & Giovannucci, 2003). In a study subjects received each of 5 treatments that included: (1) bran cereal, (2) bran with corn cereal, (3) bran with psyllium cereal, (4) a cereal blend of 70% glucomannan and 30% xanthan, and (5) the low-fiber control diet. All four cereals produced significantly greater bowel movement frequency than the low fiber control diet and all were well tolerated (Vuksan et al, 2008). Researchers found that rye bread shortened intestinal transit time, softened the feces, and eased defecation of women with constipation, and that yogurt lessened the bloating and flatulence resulting from rye bread (Hongisto et al, 2006).*

- ▲ Use a mixture of bran cereal, applesauce, and prune juice; begin administration in small amounts and gradually increase amount. Keep refrigerated. Always check with the primary care practitioner before initiating this intervention. It is important that the client also ingest sufficient fluids. **EBN:** *This bran mixture has been shown to be effective even with short-term use in elderly clients recovering from acute conditions; however, it has not been tested with a RCT (Joanna Briggs Institute, 2008). NOTE: Giving fiber without sufficient fluid has resulted in worsening of constipation (Müller-Lissner et al, 2005).*

- Teach clients to respond promptly to the defecation urge. **EB:** *A study of male volunteers determined that the defecation urge can be delayed and that delaying defecation decreased bowel movement frequency, stool weight and transit time (Klauser et al, 1990). The reflex that causes the urge to defecate diminishes after a few minutes and may remain quiet for several hours; as a result, the stool becomes hardened and more difficult to expel (American Academy of Family Physicians, 2005).*

- ▲ If the client is uncomfortable or in pain due to constipation or has chronic constipation that does not respond to increased fiber and fluid intake, activity, and appropriate toileting, refer the client to a gastroenterologist for an evaluation of bowel function and health status. *There can be multiple causes of constipation, such as endocrine disorders (e.g., hypothyroidism), depression, neurological conditions (e.g., multiple sclerosis and Parkinson's disease), ano-rectal disorders, and Hirschsprung's disease (Eoff & Lembo, 2008).*

- ▲ Obtain a referral to a dietician for analysis of the client's diet and input on how to improve the diet to ensure adequate fiber intake and nutrition.

- ▲ Assess for signs of depression, other psychological disorders, and a history of physical or sexual abuse. *These factors are prevalent in people with chronic constipation, but the pathophysiology is unclear (Canelli et al, 2001). Often, people with functional constipation have experienced physical or*

● = Independent   ▲ = Collaborative   **EBN** = Evidence-Based Nursing   **EB** = Evidence-Based

sexual abuse, and symptoms of constipation may arise from psychological problems (Mason, Serrano-Ikkos, & Kamm, 2000). **EB:** *In a survey of 47 women with idiopathic constipation, 28 healthy women, and 26 women with Crohn's disease, the women with idiopathic constipation had significantly more somatization and psychological problems (e.g., anxiety, depression, and social dysfunction than the other two groups of women (Mason, Serrano-Ikkos, & Kamm, 2000).*

- Encourage the client to increase activity, walking for at least 30 minutes at least 5 days a week as tolerated. *Decreased mobility leads to constipation, but additional exercise does not help the constipated person who is already mobile. When the client has diminished mobility, even minimal activity increases peristalsis, which is necessary to prevent constipation (Sykes, 2006; Kyle, 2007; Joanna Briggs Institute, 2008).* **EB:** *Strenuous activity leads to gastrointestinal problems, but low to moderate levels of exercise seem to have beneficial effects on gastrointestinal function (Strid, 2005). Twelve weeks of physical activity significantly decreased symptoms of constipation and difficulty defecating in sedentary clients with chronic constipation, but transit time decreased only in subjects who had abnormally long transit time before starting the exercise program (DeSchryver et al, 2005).*

▲ Observe for the presence of an eating disorder, and the use of laxatives to control or decrease weight; refer for counseling if needed. *People with eating disorders suffer from constipation and other gastrointestinal symptoms.* **EB:** *Laxative abuse is found in clients with both anorexia and bulimia nervosa, and may be associated with worsening of the eating disorder as a form of self-harm (Tozzi et al, 2006). In a study of 101 women with eating disorders, 21 abused laxatives (Boyd, Abraham, & Kellow, 2005).*

 Home Care

- The interventions described previously may be adapted for home care use.
- Take complaints seriously and evaluate claims of constipation in a matter-of-fact manner. *Continued constipation can lead to bowel obstruction, a medical emergency. Presence of a pattern of perceived constipation does not mean actual constipation cannot occur. However, use of a matter-of-fact manner will limit positive reinforcement of the behavior.*
- Obtain family and client histories of bowel or other patterned behavior problems. *History may reveal a psychological cause for the constipation (e.g., withholding).*
- Observe family cultural patterns related to eating and bowel habits. *Cultural patterns may control bowel habits.*
- Encourage a mindset and program of self-care management. Elicit from the client the self-talk he or she uses to describe body perceptions; correct fatalistic interpretations.
- Instruct the client in a healthy lifestyle that supports normal bowel function (e.g., activity, fluid intake, diet) and encourage progressive inclusion of these elements into daily activities. *A study of cognitive patterns in individuals with somatization syndrome showed that body perceptions were assumed to be a sign of catastrophic occurrence (e.g., "physical complaints are always signs of disease") and concepts of health were very restrictive. Somatizing individuals were acutely aware of bodily sensations that would normally be considered automatic and would seek help immediately to obtain medications or other solutions. They did not participate in other types of health-seeking behavior (Rief, Hiller, & Margraf, 1998).*
- Discuss the client's self-image. Help the client to reframe the self-concept as capable. *Somatizing individuals tend to see themselves as weak and therefore avoid exercise (Rief, Hiller, & Margraf, 1998). Developing the ability to see themselves as capable of self-care management may take time, as will making lifestyle changes.*
- Instruct the client and family in appropriate expectations for having bowel movements.
- Offer instruction and reassurance regarding explanations for variation from the previous pattern of bowel movements. *The client may have unrealistic expectations regarding the frequency or type of bowel movements and may assume that constipation exists when there is a reasonable explanation for deviation from the past pattern. The client may resort to the use of laxatives inappropriately.*
- Contract with the client and/or a responsible family member regarding the use of laxatives. Have the client maintain a bowel pattern diary. Observe for diarrhea or frequent evacuation. *Intermittent care does not allow for 24–hour supervision. Contracting allows guided control of care by the client in partnership with the nurse, and the diary promotes more accurate reporting.*

● = Independent ▲ = Collaborative **EBN** = Evidence-Based Nursing **EB** = Evidence-Based

▲ Teach the family to carry out the bowel program per the physician's orders.

▲ Refer for home health aide services to assist with personal care, including the bowel program, if appropriate.

• Identify a contingency plan for bowel care if the client is dependent on outside persons for such care.

Client/Family Teaching and Discharge Planning

• Explain normal bowel function and the necessary ingredients for a regular bowel regimen (e.g., fluid, fiber, activity, and regular schedule for defecation).

• Work with the client and family to develop a diet that fits the client's lifestyle and includes increased fiber.

• Teach the client that it is not necessary to have daily bowel movements and that the passage of anywhere from three stools each day to three stools each week is considered normal.

• Explain to the client the harmful effects of the continual use of defecation aids such laxatives and enemas.

• Encourage the client to gradually decrease the use of the usual laxatives and or enemas, and recognize it may take months for the process to do it gradually (American Academy of Family Physicians, 2005).

• Determine a method of increasing the client's fluid intake and fit this practice into client's lifestyle.

• Explain what Valsalva maneuver is and why it should be avoided.

• Work with the client and family to design a bowel training routine that is based on previous patterns (before laxative or enema abuse) and incorporates the consumption of warm fluids, increased fiber, and increased fluids; privacy; and a predictable routine.

Additional Nursing Interventions and *Rationales*, Client/Family Teaching and Discharge Planning

See care plan for **Constipation**.

   See the EVOLVE website for Weblinks for client education resources.

REFERENCES

American Academy of Family Physicians: Information from your family doctor: constipation, *Am Fam Physician* 71(3):539–540, 2005.

Andersen C, Adamsen L, Moeller T et al: The effect of a multidimensional exercise programme on symptoms and side-effects in cancer patient undergoing chemotherapy: the use of semi-structured diaries, *Eur J Oncol Nurs* 10:247–262, 2006.

Boyd C, Abraham S, Kellow J: Psychological features are important predictors of functional gastrointestinal disorders in patients with eating disorders, *Scand J Gastroenterol* 40:929–935, 2005.

Canelli M, Nista EC, Zocco MA et al: Idiopathic chronic constipation: pathophysiology, diagnosis and treatment, *Hepato Gastroenterol* 48:1050–1057, 2001.

DeSchryver AM, Keulemans YC, Peters HP et al: Effects of regular physical activity on defecation pattern in middle-aged patients complaining of chronic constipation, *Scand J Gastroenterol* 40:422–429, 2005.

Dukas L, Willett WC, Giovannucci EL: Association between physical activity, fiber intake, and other lifestyle variables and constipation in a study of women, *Am J Gastroenterol* 98(8):1790–1796, 2003.

Eoff JC, Lembo AJ: Optimal treatment of chronic constipation in managed care: review and roundtable discussion, *J Manag Care Pharm* 14(9–a):S1–S17, 2008.

Hongisto S-M, Paajanen L, Saxelin et al: A combination of fibre-rich rye bread and yoghurt containing *Lactobacillus GG* improves bowel function in women with self-reported constipation, *Eur J Clin Nutr* 60:319–324, 2006.

Joanna Briggs Institute: Management of constipation in older adults, *Au Nurs J* 16(5):32–35, 2008.

Klauser AG, Voderholzer WA, Heinrich C et al: Behavioral modification of colonic function. Can constipation be learned? *Digest Dis Sci* 35(10):1271–1275, 1990.

Kyle G: Constipation and palliative care—where are we now? *Int J Palliat Nurs* 13(1):6–16, 2007.

Mason HJ, Serrano-Ikkos E, Kamm MA: Psychological morbidity in women with idiopathic constipation, *Am J Gastroenterol* 95(1):2852–2857, 2000.

Müller-Lissner SA, Kamm MA, Scarpignato C et al: Myths and misconceptions about constipation, *Am J Gastroenterol* 100(1):232–242, 2005.

Rief W, Hiller W, Margraf J: Cognitive aspects of hypochondriasis and somatization syndrome, *J Abnorm Psychol* 107:587, 1998.

Singh B: Psyllium as therapeutic and drug delivery agent, *Int J Pharmaceut* 334(1–2):1–14, 2007.

Strid H: The effects of physical activity on the gastrointestinal tract, *Int Sports Med J* 6(3):151–161, 2005.

Sturtzel B, Elmadfa I: Intervention with dietary fiber to treat constipation and reduce laxative use in residents of nursing homes, *Ann Nutr Metabol* 52(suppl 1):54–56, 2008.

Sykes NP: The pathogenesis of constipation, *J Support Oncol* 4(5):213–218, 2006.

• = Independent   ▲ = Collaborative   **EBN** = Evidence-Based Nursing   **EB** = Evidence-Based

Tozzi F, Thornton LM, Mitchell J et al: Features associated with laxative abuse in individuals with eating disorders, *Psychosom Med* 68(3):470–477, 2006.

Vuksan V, Jenkins AL, Jenkins DJA et al: Using cereal to increase dietary fiber intake to the recommended level and the effect of fiber on bowel function in healthy persons consuming North American diets, *Am J Clin Nutr* 88:1256–1262, 2008.

Wald A, Scarpignato C, Müller-Lissner S et al: A multinational survey of prevalence and patterns of laxative use among adults with self-defined constipation, *Aliment Pharmacol Ther* 28:917–930, 2008.

Risk for Constipation   *Betty J. Ackley, MSN, EdS, RN*

NANDA-I

Definition

At risk for a decrease in normal frequency of defecation accompanied by difficult or incomplete passage of stool and/or passage of excessively hard, dry stool

Risk Factors

Functional

Habitual denial/ignoring of urge to defecate; recent environmental changes; inadequate toileting (e.g., timeliness, positioning for defecation, privacy); irregular defecation habits; insufficient physical activity; abdominal muscle weakness

Psychological

Depression; emotional stress; mental confusion

Physiological

Change in usual eating patterns; change in usual foods; decreased motility of gastrointestinal tract; dehydration; inadequate dentition; inadequate oral hygiene; insufficient fiber intake; insufficient fluid intake; poor eating habits

Pharmacological

Aluminum containing antiacids; anticholinergics; anticonvulsants; antidepressants; antilipemic agents; bismuth salts; calcium carbonate; calcium channel blockers; diuretics; iron salts; laxative overuse; nonsteroidal antiinflammatory drugs; opiads; phenothiazines; sedatives; and sympathomimetics

Mechanical

Electrolyte imbalance; hermorrhoids; Hirschsprung's disease; neurological impairment; obesity; post-surgical obstruction; pregnancy; prostate enlargement; rectal abscess; rectal anal fissures; rectal anal stricture; rectal prolapse; rectal ulcer; rectocele; tumors

NOC, NIC, Client Outcomes, Nursing Interventions, Client/Family Teaching and Discharge Planning, *Rationales*, and References

Refer to care plans for **Constipation** or **Perceived Constipation**

⊖volve   See the EVOLVE website for Weblinks for client education resources.

Contamination   *Laura V. Polk, PhD, RN, and Pauline M. Green, PhD, RN, CNE*

NANDA-I

Definition

Exposure to environmental contaminants in doses sufficient to cause adverse health effects

Defining Characteristics

Pesticides

Dermatological effects of pesticide exposure; gastrointestinal effects of pesticide exposure; neurological effects of pesticide exposure; pulmonary effects of pesticide exposure; renal effects of pesticide

• = Independent   ▲ = Collaborative   **EBN** = Evidence-Based Nursing   **EB** = Evidence-Based

exposure; major categories of pesticides: insecticides, herbicides, fungicides, antimicrobials, rodenticides; major pesticides: organophosphates, carbamates, oranochlorines, pyrethrum, arsenic, glycophosphates, bipyridyls, chlorophenoxy

Chemicals

Dermatological effects of chemical exposure; gastrointestinal effects of chemical exposure; immunologic effects of chemical exposure; neurological effects of chemical exposure; pulmonary effects of chemical exposure; renal effects of chemical exposure; major chemical agents: petroleum-based agents, anticholinesterases type I agents act on proximal trachebronchial portion of the respiratory tract, type II agents act on alveoli; type III agents produce systemic effects

Biologicals

Dermatological effects of exposure to biologics; gastrointestinal effects of exposure to biologics; pulmonary effects of exposure to biologics; neurological effects of exposure to biologics; renal effects of exposure to biologics (toxins from organisms [bacteria, viruses, fungi])

Pollution

Neurological effects of pollution exposure; pulmonary effects of pollution exposure (major locations: air, water, soil; major agents: asbestos, radon, tobacco, heavy metal, lead, noise, exhaust)

Waste

Dermatological effects of waste exposure; gastrointestinal effects of waste exposure; hepatic effects of waste exposure; pulmonary effects of waste exposure (categories of waste: trash, raw sewage, industrial waste)

Radiation

External exposure through direct contact with radioactive material; genetic effects of radiation exposure; immunologic effects of radiation exposure; neurological effects of radiation exposure; oncological effects of radiation exposure

Related Factors (r/t)

External

Chemical contamination of food; chemical contamination of water; exposure to bioterrorism; exposure to disasters (natural or man-made); exposure to radiation (occupation in radiology; employment in nuclear industries and electrical generating plants; living near nuclear industries and/or electrical generating plants); exposure through ingestion of radioactive material (e.g., food/water contamination); flaking; peeling paint in presence of young children; flaking; peeling plaster in presence of young children; floor surface (carpeted surfaces hold contaminant residue more than hard floor surfaces); geographic area (living in area where high level of contaminants exist); household hygiene practices; inadequate municipal services (trash removal, sewage treatment facilities); inappropriate use of protective clothing; lack of breakdown of contaminants once indoors (breakdown is inhibited without sun and rain exposure); lack of protective clothing; lacquer in poorly ventilated areas; lacquer without effective protection; living in poverty (increases potential for multiple exposure, lack of access to health care, poor diet); paint in poorly ventilated areas; paint without effective protection; personal hygiene practices; playing in outdoor areas where environmental contaminants are used; presence of atmospheric pollutants; use of environmental contaminants in the home (e.g., pesticides, chemicals, environmental tobacco smoke); unprotected contact with chemicals (e.g., arsenic); unprotected contact with heavy metals (e.g., chromium, lead)

Internal

Age (children <5 years, older adults); concomitant exposures; developmental characteristics of children; female gender; gestational age during exposure; nutritional factors (e.g., obesity, vitamin and mineral deficiencies); preexisting disease states; pregnancy; previous exposures; smoking

(Nursing Outcomes Classification)

Suggested NOC Outcomes

Community Health Status, Family Physical Environment, Anxiety Level, Fear Level

Example NOC Outcome with Indicators
Community Health Status as evidenced by the following indicators: Evidence of health protection measures/ Compliance with environmental health standards/Health Status of population (Rate the outcome and indicators of **Community Health Status:** 1 = poor, 2 = fair, 3 = good, 4 = very good, 5 = excellent [See Section I].)

Client Outcomes

Client Will (Specify Time Frame):

- Have minimal health effects associated with contamination
- Cooperate with appropriate decontamination protocol
- Participate in appropriate isolation precautions

Community Will (Specify Time Frame):

- Utilize health surveillance data system to monitor for contamination incidents
- Utilize disaster plan to evacuate and triage affected members
- Have minimal health effects associated with contamination

NIC **(Nursing Interventions Classification)**

Suggested NIC Interventions

Triage: Disaster, Infection Control, Anxiety Reduction, Crisis Intervention, Health Education

Example NIC Activities—Triage: Disaster
Initiate appropriate emergency measures, as indicated; Monitor for and treat life-threatening injuries or acute needs

Nursing Interventions and *Rationales*

▲ Help individuals cope with contamination incident by doing the following:
  - Use groups that have survived terrorist attacks as useful resource for victims
  - Provide accurate information on risks involved, preventive measures, use of antibiotics, and vaccines
  - Assist to deal with feelings of fear, vulnerability, and grief
  - Encourage individuals to talk to others about their fears
  - Assist victims to think positively and to move toward the future

  EB: *Interventions aimed at supporting an individual's coping help the person deal with feelings of fear, helplessness, and loss of control that are normal reactions in a crisis situation (Boscarino et al, 2006).*

- Triage, stabilize, transport, and treat affected community members. **EB:** *Accurate triage and early treatment provides the best chance of survival to affected persons (Murdoch & Cymet, 2006; Veenema, 2007).*

- Utilize approved procedures for decontamination of persons, clothing, and equipment. *Victims may first require decontamination prior to entering health facility to receive care in order to prevent the spread of contamination (U.S. Army Medical Research Institute of Infectious Diseases, 2005).*

- Utilize appropriate isolation precautions: universal, airborne, droplet, and contact isolation. *Proper use of isolation precautions prevents cross-contamination by contaminating agents (U.S. Army Medical Research Institute of Infectious Diseases, 2005).*

- Monitor individual for therapeutic effects, side effects, and compliance with postexposure drug therapy. *Drug therapy may extend over a long period of time and will require monitoring for compliance as well as therapeutic and side effects (Veenema, 2007).*

• = Independent   ▲ = Collaborative   **EBN** = Evidence-Based Nursing   **EB** = Evidence-Based

▲ Collaborate with other agencies (local health department, emergency medical service [EMS], state and federal agencies). *Communication among agencies increases ability to handle crisis efficiently and correctly (Veenema, 2007; CDC, 2009).*

Geriatric

- Help the client identify age-related factors that may affect response to contamination incidents.
- Encourage family members to acknowledge and validate the client's concerns. *Validation alleviates anxiety and increases client's ability to cope (Boscarino et al, 2006).*

Pediatric

- Provide environmental health hazard information. *Developing children are more vulnerable to environmental toxicants due to greater and longer exposure and particular susceptibility windows (Children's Environmental Health Network, 2006).*

Home Care

- Assess current environmental stressors and identify community resources. *Accessing resources decreases stress and increases ability to cope (Boscarino et al, 2006).*

Client/Family Teaching and Discharge Planning

- Provide truthful information to the person or family affected
- Discuss signs and symptoms of contamination
- Explain decontamination protocols
- Explain need for isolation procedures
  Well-managed efforts at communication of contamination information ensures that messages are correctly formulated, transmitted, and received and that they result in meaningful actions (ATSDR, 2006).

ⓔvolve   See the EVOLVE website for Weblinks for client education resources.

REFERENCES

Agency for Toxic Substances and Disease Registry (ATSDR): *A primer on health risk communication: principles and practices. Overview of issues and guiding principles*, 2006, available at www.atsdr.cdc.gov/risk/riskprimer/vision.html. Accessed April 1, 2009.

Boscarino J, Adams R, Figley C et al: Fear of terrorism and preparedness in New York City 2 years after the attacks: implications for disaster planning and research, *J Public Health Manag Pract* 12(6):505–513, 2006.

Centers for Disease Control and Prevention: *Emergency preparedness & response*, available at www.bt.cdc.gov. Accessed March 19, 2009.

Children's Environmental Health Network: *Resource guide on children's environmental health*, 2006, available at www.cehn.org/cehn/resourceguide/rgtoc.html. Accessed March 19, 2009.

Murdoch S, Cymet TC: Treating victims after disaster: physical and psychological effects, *Compr Ther* 32(1):39–42, 2006.

U.S. Army Medical Research Institute of Infectious Diseases: *USAMRIID's medical management of biological casualties handbook*, ed 6, Fort Detrick, MD, 2005, Author.

Veenema TG: *Disaster nursing and emergency preparedness for chemical, biological and radiological terrorism and other hazards*, ed 2, New York, 2007, Springer.

Risk for Contamination   *Laura V. Polk, PhD, RN, and Pauline M. Green, PhD, RN, CNE*

NANDA-I

Definition

Accentuated risk of exposure to environmental contaminants in doses sufficient to cause adverse health effects

Risk Factors

See Related Factors in **Contamination** care plan.

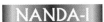

• = Independent   ▲ = Collaborative   **EBN** = Evidence-Based Nursing   **EB** = Evidence-Based

NOC (Nursing Outcomes Classification)

Suggested NOC Outcomes

Risk Control, Health Beliefs: Perceived Threat, Knowledge: Health Resources, Knowledge: Health Behavior, Community Disaster Readiness, Community Health Status

See **Contamination** for other possible NOC outcomes.

Example NOC Outcome with Indicators
Risk Control as evidenced by the following indicators: Monitors environmental risk factors/Avoids exposure to health threats/Follows selected risk control strategies (Rate the outcome and indicators of **Risk Control:** 1 = never demonstrated, 2 = rarely demonstrated, 3 = sometimes demonstrated, 4 = often demonstrated, 5 = consistently demonstrated [See Section I].)

Client Outcomes

Client Will (Specify Time Frame):

- Remain free of adverse effects of contamination

Community Will (Specify Time Frame):

- Utilize health surveillance data system to monitor for contamination incidents
- Participate in mass casualty and disaster readiness drills
- Remain free of contamination-related health effects
- Minimize exposure to contaminants

NIC (Nursing Interventions Classification)

Suggested NIC Interventions

Environmental Risk Protection, Bioterrorism Preparedness, Environmental Management: Safety, Health Education, Health Screening, Immunization/Vaccination Management, Risk Identification, Surveillance: Safety, Community, Communicable Disease Management, Community Disaster Preparedness, Health Policy Monitoring

Example NIC Activities—Environmental Risk Protection
Assess environment for potential and actual risk; Monitor incidents of illness and injury related to environmental hazards; Collaborate with other agencies to improve environmental safety

Nursing Interventions and *Rationales*

- ▲ Conduct surveillance for environmental contamination. Notify agencies authorized to protect the environment of contaminants in the area. *Early surveillance and detection are critical components of preparation (Murdoch & Cymet, 2006; Veenema, 2007)*
- Assist individuals to modify the environment to minimize risk or assist in relocating to safer environment. *Modification of the environment will decrease the risk of actual contamination occurring (Veenema & Tōke, 2006).*
- Schedule mass casualty and disaster readiness drills. *Practice in handling contamination occurrences will decrease the risk of exposure during actual contamination events (Chung & Shannon, 2005).*
- Provide accurate information on risks involved, preventive measures, use of antibiotics, and vaccines. *Well-managed efforts at communication of contamination information ensure that messages are correctly formulated, transmitted, and received, and that they result in meaningful actions (ATSDR, 2006).*
- Assist to deal with feelings of fear and vulnerability. **EB:** *Interventions aimed at supporting an individual's coping help the person deal with feelings of fear, helplessness, and loss of control that are normal reactions in a crisis situation (Boscarino et al, 2006).*
- Assist with decontamination of persons, clothing, and equipment using approved procedure. *Victims may first require decontamination prior to entering health facility to receive care in order to*

• = Independent   ▲ = Collaborative   **EBN** = Evidence-Based Nursing   **EB** = Evidence-Based

prevent the spread of contamination (U.S. Army Medical Research Institute of Infectious Diseases, 2005).

- Utilize appropriate isolation precautions: universal, airborne, droplet, and contact isolation. *Proper use of isolation precautions prevents cross-contamination by contaminating agent (U.S. Army Medical Research Institute of Infectious Diseases, 2005).*
- Monitor individual for therapeutic effects, side effects, and compliance with postexposure drug therapy. *Drug therapy may extend over a long period of time and will require monitoring for compliance as well as therapeutic and side effects (Veenema, 2007).*
- ▲ Collaborate with other agencies (local health department, emergency medical service [EMS], state and federal agencies). *Communication among agencies increases ability to handle crisis efficiently and correctly (Veenema, 2007; CDC, 2009).*

Geriatric

- Help the client identify age-related factors that may affect response to contamination incidents.
- Encourage family members to acknowledge and validate the client's concerns. *Validation alleviates anxiety and increases client's ability to cope (Boscarino et al, 2006).*

Pediatric

- Provide environmental health hazard information relevant to children. *Developing children are more vulnerable to environmental toxicants due to greater and longer exposure and particular susceptibility windows (Children's Environmental Health Network, 2006).*

Home Care

- Assess current environmental stressors and identify community resources. *Accessing resources decreases stress and increases ability to cope (Boscarino et al, 2006).*

Client/Family Teaching and Discharge Planning

- Provide truthful information to the person or family.
- Discuss signs and symptoms of contamination.
- Explain decontamination protocols.
- Explain need for isolation procedures.
  Well-managed efforts at communication of contamination information ensure that messages are correctly formulated, transmitted, and received, and that they result in meaningful actions (ATSDR, 2006).

⊖volve   See the EVOLVE website for Weblinks for client education resources.

REFERENCES

Agency for Toxic Substances and Disease Registry (ATSDR): *A primer on health risk communication: principles and practices. Overview of issues and guiding principles*, 2006, available at www.atsdr.cdc.gov/risk/riskprimer/vision.html. Accessed April 1, 2009.

Boscarino J, Adams R, Figley C et al: Fear of terrorism and preparedness in New York City 2 years after the attacks: implications for disaster planning and research, *J Public Health Manag Pract* 12(6):505–513, 2006.

Centers for Disease Control and Prevention: *Emergency preparedness & response*, available at www.bt.cdc.gov. Accessed March 19, 2009.

Children's Environmental Health Network: *Resource guide on children's environmental health*, 2006, available at www.cehn.org/cehn/resourceguide/rgtoc.html. Accessed March 19, 2009.

Chung S, Shannon M: Hospital planning for acts of terrorism and other public health emergencies involving children, *Arch Dis Child* 90(12):1300–1307, 2005.

Murdoch S, Cymet TC: Treating victims after disaster: physical and psychological effects, *Compr Ther* 32(1):39–42, 2006.

U.S. Army Medical Research Institute of Infectious Diseases: *USAMRIID's medical management of biological casualties handbook*, ed 6, Fort Detrick, MD, 2005, Author.

Veenema TG: *Disaster nursing and emergency preparedness for chemical, biological and radiological terrorism and other hazards*, ed 2, New York, 2007, Springer.

Veenema T, Tóke J: Early detection and surveillance for biopreparedness and emerging infectious diseases, *Online J Issues Nurs* 11(1):3, 2006.

Ineffective community Coping　*Dawn Fairlie, ANP, FNP, GNP, DNS(c)*　ⓔvolve

NANDA-I

Definition

Pattern of community activities for adaptation and problem-solving that is unsatisfactory for meeting the demands or needs of the community

Defining Characteristics

Community does not meet its own expectations; deficits in community participation; excessive community conflicts; expressed community powerlessness; expressed vulnerability; high illness rates; increased social problems (e.g., homicides, vandalism, arson, terrorism, robbery, infanticide, abuse, divorce, unemployment, poverty, militancy, mental illness); stressors perceived as excessive

Related Factors (r/t)

Deficits in community social support services; deficits in community social support resources; natural disasters; man-made disasters; inadequate resources for problem solving; ineffective community systems (e.g., lack of emergency medical system, transportation system, or disaster planning systems); nonexistent community systems

NOC　(Nursing Outcomes Classification)

Suggested NOC Outcomes

Community Competence, Community Health Status, Community Violence Level

> ### Example NOC Outcome with Indicators
>
> **Community Competence** as evidenced by the following indicators: Participation rates in community activities/Consideration of common and competing interests among groups when solving community problems/Representation of all segments of the community in problem solving/Effective use of conflict management strategies (Rate the outcome and indicators of **Community Competence:** 1 = poor, 2 = fair, 3 = good, 4 = very good, 5 = excellent [see Section I].)

Community Outcomes

A Broad Range of Community Members Will (Specify Time Frame):

- Participate in community actions to improve power resources
- Develop improved communication among community members
- Participate in problem solving
- Demonstrate cohesiveness in problem solving
- Develop new strategies for problem solving
- Express power to deal with change and manage problems

NIC　(Nursing Interventions Classification)

Suggested NIC Interventions

Community Health Development, Program Development

> ### Example NIC Activities—Community Health Development
>
> Enhance community support networks; Identify and mentor potential community leaders; Unify community members behind a common mission; Ensure that community members maintain control over decision making

Nursing Interventions and *Rationales*

NOTE: The diagnosis of **Ineffective Coping** does not apply and should not be used when stress is being imposed by external sources or circumstance. If the community is a victim of circumstances, using the

---

• = Independent　▲ = Collaborative　**EBN** = Evidence-Based Nursing　**EB** = Evidence-Based

nursing diagnosis **Ineffective Coping** is equivalent to blaming the victim. See the care plan for and **Readiness for enhanced community Coping**.

▲ Establish a collaborative partnership with the community (see the care plan for **Readiness for enhanced community Coping** for additional references). **EB:** *In a study conducted by Mt. Sinai researchers and clinicians with community leaders of east and central Harlem, the collaborative partnerships of researchers, clinicians, and community leaders were key assets to accomplishing community health goals (Horowitz et al, 2004). Community participation with health providers is an essential aspect of health and development (Sule, 2004).*

• Assist the community with team building. **EBN:** *Local nurses in Cape Winelands, South Africa established a collaborative partnership between farm workers and their families, employers, the public health sector, and various nongovernmental organizations to develop an intervention to train peer-selected lay health workers (LHWs) (Dick et al, 2007).*

• Participate with community members in the identification of stressors and assessment of distress; for example, observe and participate in faith-based organizations that want to improve community stress management. **EBN:** *Health programs in faith-based organizations made a significant difference in health outcomes (DeHaven et al, 2004).*

• Assist community members to articulate the local perspective based on years of experience with the issue or concern. **EB:** *Scientific information may be used to resolve intractable conflicts, but the local experience is also very important but needs to be adequately described (Ozawa, 2006).*

▲ Identify the health services and information resources that are currently available in the community. **EBN:** *Gynecological cancer survivors in Queensland were studied to identify awareness of, utilization of, and factors associated with use of community support services. Seventy-two percent were aware of the primary cancer support organization, Cancer Council Queensland, 74% were aware of booklets, 66% were aware of helplines, 56% were aware of support groups, and 50% were aware of Internet resources. Less than half were aware of other services (Beesley et al, 2009).*

▲ Consult with community mediation services, for example, the National Association of Community Mediation. **EB:** *In a review of community mediation research, it was shown that using community mediation services effectively resolves conflicts, and many of the resolutions are durable and cost-efficient (Hedeen, 2004).*

• Work with community members to increase awareness of ineffective coping behaviors (e.g., conflicts that prevent community members from working together, anger and hate that paralyze the community, health risk behaviors of adolescents). **EBN:** *Problem solving is essential for effective coping. Community members in partnership with providers can modify behaviors that interfere with problem solving (Chinn, 2004; Anderson & McFarlane, 2006).* **EB:** *In a study of 319 college-age students, health risk behaviors were significantly higher for students who were exposed to community violence (Brady, 2006).*

• Provide support to the community and help community members to identify and mobilize additional supports. **EBN:** *Often people need help in mobilizing supports that are available (Pender, Murdaugh, & Parsons, 2006).*

• Advocate for the community in multiple arenas (e.g., television, newspapers, and governmental agencies). **EBN:** *Advocacy is a specific form of caring that enhances power resources for community coping (Anderson & McFarlane, 2006).*

• Work with community groups to improve the economic status and reduce unemployment. **EB:** *Analysis of population and labor force data from 1992 to 2002 indicated a strong significant correlation of penetrating trauma/crime indices and economic conditions, including unemployment (Cinat et al, 2004).*

• Write grant proposals to help community members obtain funds for programs that reduce stress or improve coping. (See Coley & Scheinberg, 2007, for program proposal-writing methods.) **EBN:** *The programs that are necessary may be expensive, and often funds may not be available without the assistance of public or privately funded grants (Anderson & McFarlane, 2006).*

• Work with members of the community to identify and develop coping strategies that promote a sense of power (e.g., obtaining sources for funding, collaborating with other communities). **EBN:** *A first step in power enhancement is for the community to identify and develop its own coping strategies (Anderson & McFarlane, 2006).*

• Engage emotions during conflict mediation. **EB:** *An experienced mediator recommended that specific strategies can be used to engage the emotions that are present in conflict. Suggested strategies in the*

• = Independent   ▲ = Collaborative   **EBN** = Evidence-Based Nursing   **EB** = Evidence-Based

realm of art, rituals, and joking help to create a space in which new understandings can develop (Maiese, 2006).

- Protect children from exposure to community conflicts. **EB:** *Children exposed to community conflict have permanent negative effects from exposure to community conflicts, including increased health risk behaviors (Brady, 2006) and increased physical symptoms (Wilson, Rosenthal, & Austin, 2005).*

 Multicultural

- Acknowledge the stressors unique to racial/ethnic communities. **EBN:** *Socioeconomic status, geographical location, and risks associated with health-seeking behavior all influence the likelihood that clients will seek health care and be compliant with a regimen they are given (Appel, Giger, & Davidhizar, 2005).*
- Identify community strengths with community members. **EB:** *Latino men from three urban housing communities in the southeastern USA identified Latino community strengths and general community strengths as factors that promote health and prevent risk (Rhodes et al, 2009).*
- Work with members of the community to prioritize and target health goals specific to the community. **EB:** *Such prioritization and targeting will increase feelings of control over and sense of ownership of programs (Chinn, 2004; Anderson & McFarlane, 2006).*
- Establish and sustain partnerships with key individuals within communities when developing and implementing programs. **EB:** *Public health officials in Georgia and members of the Business Executives for National Security collaborated to develop a model for collaboration in emergency mass dispensing of pharmaceuticals (Buehler, Whitney, & Berkelman, 2006).*
- Use mentoring strategies for community members. **EB:** *In a study of child vaccination in Haiti, it was found that mother's use of traditional healer services was negatively associated with vaccination of their children, underscoring the potential of enlisting the support of traditional healers in promoting child health by mentoring and educating traditional healers in supporting vaccination efforts (Muula et al, 2009).*
- Use community church settings as a forum for advocacy, teaching, and program implementation. **EBN:** *Participant and pastor feedback supported the feasibility of ongoing faith-based screening and education programs as one way to reduce risk factors for diabetes, cardiovascular disease, and stroke in Southern, rural African Americans (Frank & Grubbs, 2008).*

Community Teaching

- Teach strategies for stress management.
- Explain the relationship between enhancing power resources and coping.

⊖volve   See the EVOLVE website for Weblinks for client education resources.

REFERENCES

Anderson ET, McFarlane J: *Community as partner: theory and practice in nursing,* ed 5, Philadelphia, 2006, Lippincott Williams & Wilkins.

Appel SJ, Giger JN, Davidhizar RE: Opportunity cost: the impact of contextual risk factors on the cardiovascular health of low-income rural southern African-American women, *J Cardiovasc Nurs* 20:315–324, 2005.

Beesley VL, Janda M, Eakin EG et al: Gynecological cancer survivors and community support services: referral, awareness, utilization and satisfaction, *Psychooncology,* Feb 10, 2009, Epub ahead of print.

Brady SS: Lifetime community violence exposure and health risk behavior among young adults in college, *J Adolesc Health* 39:610–613, 2006.

Buehler JW, Whitney EA, Berkelman RL: Business and public health collaboration for emergency preparedness in Georgia: a case study, *BMC Public Health* 20(6):285, 2006.

Chinn PL: *Peace and power: creative leadership for building community,* ed 6, Boston, 2004, Jones and Bartlett.

Cinat ME, Wilson SE, Lush S et al: Significant correlation of trauma epidemiology with economic conditions of a community, *Arch Surg* 139(12):1350–1355, 2004.

Coley SM, Scheinberg CA: *Proposal writing,* ed 3, Thousand Oaks, CA, 2007, Sage.

DeHaven MJ, Hunter IB, Wilder L et al: Health programs in faith-based organizations: are they effective? *Am J Pubic Health* 94:1030–1036, 2004.

Dick J, Clarke M, van Zyl H et al: Primary health care nurses implement and evaluate a community outreach approach to health care in the South African agricultural sector, *Int Nurs* 54 (4):383–90, 2007.

Frank D, Grubbs L: A faith-based screening/education program for diabetes, CVD, and stroke in rural African Americans, *ABNF J* 19(3):96–101, 2008.

Hedeen T: The evolution and evaluation of community mediation: limited research suggests unlimited progress, *Conflict Resolut Q* 22(1/2):101–113, 2004.

• = Independent   ▲ = Collaborative   **EBN** = Evidence-Based Nursing   **EB** = Evidence-Based

Horowitz CR, Arniella A, James S et al: Using community-based participatory research to reduce health disparities in East and Central Harlem, *Mt Sinai J Med* 71(6):368–374, 2004.

Maiese M: Engaging the emotions in conflict intervention, *Conflict Resolut Q* 24(2):187–195, 2006.

Muula AS, Polycarpe MY, Job J et al: Association between maternal use of traditional healer services and child vaccination coverage in Pont-Sonde, Haiti, *Int J Equity Health* 8:1, 2009.

Ozawa CP: Science and intractable conflict, *Conflict Resolut Q* 24:197–205, 2006.

Pender NJ, Murdaugh CL, Parsons MA: *Health promotion in nursing practice,* ed 5, Upper Saddle River, NJ, 2006, Prentice Hall.

Rhodes SD, Hergenrather KC, Griffith DM et al: Sexual and alcohol risk behaviours of immigrant Latino men in the southeastern USA, *Cult Health Sex* 11(1):17–34, 2009.

Sule SS: Community participation in health and development, *Niger J Med* 13:276–281, 2004.

Wilson WC, Rosenthal BS, Austin S: Exposure to community violence and upper respiratory illness in older adolescents, *J Adolesc Health* 36:313–319, 2005.

Readiness for enhanced community Coping   *Dawn Fairlie, ANP, FNP, GNP, DNS(c)*

NANDA-I

Definition

Pattern of community activities for adaptation and problem solving that is satisfactory for meeting the demands or needs of the community but that can be improved for management of current and future problems/stressors

Defining Characteristics

One or more characteristics that indicate effective coping:

Active planning by community for predicted stressors; active problem solving by community when faced with issues; agreement that community is responsible for stress management; positive communication among community members; positive communication between community/aggregates and larger community; programs available for recreation; programs available for relaxation; resources sufficient for managing stressors

NOC   (Nursing Outcomes Classification)

Suggested NOC Outcomes

Community Competence, Community Health Status

Example NOC Outcome with Indicators

Community Health Status as evidenced by the following indicators: Prevalence of health promotion programs/Health status of infants, children, adolescents, adults, elders/Participation rates in community health programs (Rate the outcome and indicators of **Community Health Status:** 1 = poor, 2 = fair, 3 = good, 4 = very good, 5 = excellent [see Section I].)

Community Outcomes

Community Will (Specify Time Frame):

- Develop enhanced coping strategies
- Maintain effective coping strategies for management of stress

NIC   (Nursing Interventions Classification)

Suggested NIC Interventions

Environmental Management: Community, Health Policy Monitoring: Program Development

Example NIC Activities—Program Development

Assist the group or community in identifying significant health needs or problems; Identify alternative approaches to address the need(s) or problem(s)

 = Independent   ▲ = Collaborative   **EBN** = Evidence-Based Nursing   **EB** = Evidence-Based

Nursing Interventions and *Rationales*

NOTE: Interventions depend on the specific aspects of community coping that can be enhanced (e.g., planning for stress management, communication, development of community power, community perceptions of stress, community coping strategies). Nursing interventions are conducted in collaboration with key members of the community, community/public health nurses, and members of other disciplines (Anderson & McFarlane, 2006).

- Describe the roles of community/public health nurses in working with healthy communities. **EBN:** *Nurses at general and specialists' levels (bachelor's and master's degrees) have significant roles in helping communities to achieve optimum health, including coping with stress (Chinn, 2004; Logan, 2005; Stanhope & Lancaster, 2006).*
- Help the community to obtain funds for additional programs. (See Coley & Scheinberg, 2007, for proposal-writing methods.) **EBN:** *Healthy communities may need additional funding sources to strengthen community resources (Chinn, 2004; Anderson & McFarlane, 2006).*
- Encourage positive attitudes toward the community through the media and other sources. **EB:** *Negative attitudes or stigmas create additional stress and deficits in social support (Chinn, 2004; Anderson & McFarlane, 2006; Stanhope & Lancaster, 2006).*
- Help community members to collaborate with one another for power enhancement and coping skills. **EBN:** *Community members may not have sufficient skills to collaborate for enhanced coping. Health care providers can promote effective collaboration skills (Chinn, 2004; Anderson & McFarlane, 2006).*
- Assist community members with cognitive skills and habits of mind for problem solving. **EBN:** *The cognitive skills and habits of mind of critical thinking support problem-solving ability (Rubenfeld & Scheffer, 2006).*
- Demonstrate optimum use of the power resources. **EBN:** *Optimum use of power resources and working for community empowerment supports coping (Chinn, 2004).*
- Reduce poverty whenever possible. **EB:** *Public health studies in most countries of the world show that poverty is an important predictor of health status in all categories (Wagstaff et al, 2004). Socioeconomic inequalities are most likely relevant to the health of people in all age groups.*
- ▲ Collaborate with community members to improve educational levels within the community. **EBN:** *In many population level studies, educational levels were associated with stress, health disparities, and increased illness (Park et al, 2007). For example, in an analysis of mortality data in Wisconsin from 1990 to 2000, there was a graded associated between education and premature mortality (Reither et al, 2006).*

 ## Multicultural

- Refer to care plan **Ineffective community Coping**.

Community Teaching

- Review coping skills, power for coping, and the use of power resources.

⊖volve See the EVOLVE website for Weblinks for client education resources.

REFERENCES

Refer to **Ineffective community Coping** for additional references.

Anderson ET, McFarlane J: *Community as partner: theory and practice in nursing*, ed 4, Philadelphia, 2006, Lippincott Williams & Wilkins.

Chinn PL: *Peace and power: creative leadership for building community*, ed 6, Boston, 2004, Jones and Bartlett.

Coley SM, Scheinberg CA: *Proposal writing*, ed 3, Thousand Oaks, CA, 2007, Sage.

Logan L: The practice of certified community health CNSs, *Clin Nurse Spec* 19(1):43–48, 2005.

Park MJ, Yun KE, Lee GE et al: A cross-sectional study of socioeconomic status and the metabolic syndrome in Korean adults, *Ann Epidemiol* 17(4):320–326, 2007.

Reither EN, Peppard PE, Remington PL et al: Increasing educational disparities in premature adult mortality, Wisconsin, 1990–2000, *WMJ* 105(7):38–41, 2006.

Rubenfeld MG, Scheffer BK: *Critical thinking TACTICS for nurses*, Boston, 2006, Jones and Bartlett.

Stanhope M, Lancaster J: *Foundations of nursing in the community: community-oriented approach*, ed 2, St Louis, 2006, Mosby.

Wagstaff A, Bustreo F, Bryce J et al: Child health: reaching the poor, *Am J Public Health* 94(5):726–736, 2004.

● = Independent   ▲ = Collaborative   **EBN** = Evidence-Based Nursing   **EB** = Evidence-Based

Defensive Coping

Patricia Ferreira, RN, MSN, Michelangelo Juvenale, BSc, MSc, PhD, and Gail B. Ladwig, MSN, RN, CHTP

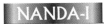

Definition

Repeated projection of falsely positive self-evaluation based on a self-protective pattern that defends against underlying perceived threats to positive self-regard

Defining Characteristics

Denial of obvious problems; denial of obvious weaknesses; difficulty establishing relationships; difficulty maintaining relationships; difficulty in perception of reality testing; grandiosity; hostile laughter; hypersensitivity to criticism; hypersensitivity to slight; lack of follow-through in therapy; lack of follow-through in treatment; lack of participation in therapy; lack of participation in treatment; projection of blame; projection of responsibility; rationalization of failures; reality distortion; ridicule of others; superior attitude toward others

Related Factors (r/t)

Conflict between self-perception and value system; deficient support system; fear of failure; fear of humiliation; fear of repercussions; lack of resilience; low level of confidence in others; low level of self-confidence; uncertainty; unrealistic expectations of self

NOC (Nursing Outcomes Classification)

Suggested NOC Outcomes

Coping, Decision Making, Impulse Self-Control, Information Processing

Example NOC Outcome with Indicators
Coping as evidenced by the following indicators: Identifies effective and ineffective coping patterns/Modifies lifestyle to reduce stress (Rate the outcome and indicators of **Coping:** 1 = never demonstrated, 2 = rarely demonstrated, 3 = sometimes demonstrated, 4 = often demonstrated, 5 = consistently demonstrated [see Section I].)

Client Outcomes

Client Will (Specify Time Frame):

- Acknowledge need for change in coping style
- Accept responsibility for own behavior
- Establish realistic goals with validation from caregivers
- Solicit caregiver validation in decision making

NIC (Nursing Interventions Classification)

Suggested Nursing Interventions:

Body Image Enhancement, Complex Relationship Building, Coping Enhancement, Patient Contracting, Self-Awareness Enhancement, Self-Esteem Enhancement, Socialization Enhancement, Surveillance: Safety

Example NIC Activities—Self-Awareness Enhancement
Encourage patient to recognize and discuss thoughts and feelings; Assist patient in identifying behaviors that are self-destructive

Nursing Interventions and *Rationales*

- Assess for the presence of denial as a coping mechanism. **EB:** *A thorough assessment for behaviors indicating the presence of denial is necessary in order to address issues of nonadherence in persons with human immunodeficiency virus (HIV) (Power et al, 2003).*

• = Independent   ▲ = Collaborative   **EBN** = Evidence-Based Nursing   **EB** = Evidence-Based

- Assess for possible symptoms associated with defensive coping: Depressive symptoms, excessive self-focused attention, negativism and anxiety, hypertension, posttraumatic stress disorder (PTSD) (e.g., exposure to terrorism), unjust world beliefs. *Depression is often associated with use of defensive coping (Hobfoll, Canetti-Nisim, & Johnson, 2006).* **EB:** *The heightened self-focused attention might result from automatically instigated states of self-focused attention and paradoxical effects of defensive efforts to avoid self-focus (Höping, de Jong-Meyer, & Abrams, 2006). This study demonstrated, in group comparisons, that negative affect group obtained higher scores on the "Self-reflectiveness scale" than the control group (p<0.03) (Höping, de Jong-Meyer, and Abrams, 2006). Repressive (or defensive) coping has been associated with elevated blood pressure levels, essential hypertension, and paroxysmal hypertension. Cardiovascular clients who use a repressive style have shown mixed results during recuperation. Repressive coping describes the capacity to render events and feelings inaccessible to consciousness. Intrapsychic conflicts involving unacceptable wishes, fantasies, and impulses can be hidden from conscious awareness (Gleiberman, 2007). In this study, authors related that exposure to terrorism was significantly related to greater loss and gain of psychosocial resources and to greater posttraumatic stress disorder (PTSD) and depressive symptoms (Hobfoll, Canetti-Nisim, & Johnson, 2006). In two studies, the Unjust World Views scale (UJVS) was developed. Belief in an unjust world was related to defensive coping, anger, and perceived future risk. These findings contribute to theory development and suggest that a belief in an unjust world may serve a self-protective function. Clinical implications are discussed as unjust world views also were found to be potentially maladaptive (Lench and Chang, 2007).*
- Stimulate cognitive behavioral stress management (CBSM). **EB:** *Although denial may be an effective means of distress reduction in the short term, reliance on this coping strategy may result in a decreased capacity to effectively manage a variety of disease-related stressors in the long term. CBSM addresses this potentially detrimental pattern by teaching stress reduction skills that may decrease depressed mood via reduced reliance on denial coping (Carrico et al, 2006).*
- Ask appropriate questions to assess whether denial (defensive coping) is being used in association with alcoholism. **EB:** *Alcohol abuse is a major problem in the United States, but individuals are not getting treatment. In this survey, denial or refusal to admit severity and fear of social embarrassment were the top two reasons for not seeking help (To & Vega, 2006).*
- Promote the client's positive feelings by using multisensory therapy on clients with developmental disability. **EB:** *Multisensory therapy could be used to provide leisure and promote psychological well-being, rather than for reducing problem behavior (Chan et al, 2005).*
- Empower the client/caregiver's self-knowledge. **EB:** *Theory of therapist resilience: the theory that was constructed included a central category (Integration of Self with Practice), a paradigm (Trust in Self), and two main categories (Career Development and Practice of Therapy). The process involved an initial calling, a positive agency experience, career corrections, the influence of relationships, and a move to a more flexible environment (Clark, 2009).*
- Assess an individual's sociocultural backgrounds in teaching self-management and self-regulation as a means of supporting hope and coping with a diagnosis of type 2 diabetes. **EBN:** *Findings obtained from the themes of this study illustrated that self-management of clients with diabetes is highly related to their own sociocultural environment and experiences (Lin et al, 2008).*
- Develop professional's self-protective mechanisms (related to coping enhancement). **EB:** *Situations that compromise empathy can be particularly worrisome in health delivery practices like pain medicine that are highly relational and that seek to use relationships therapeutically (Banja, 2008).*

 Geriatric

- Assess the client for anger and identify previous outlets for anger. *Nurses can help individuals to cope effectively with a change in health status by teaching them alternative methods of coping (Reynaud & Meeker, 2002).*
- Assess the client for dementia or depression. *A thorough assessment must be conducted to determine if the aberrant behavior has an organic origin (Green, 2002). Clients may not readily admit to psychological or substance abuse symptoms (Boyd & Stanley, 2002).*
- ▲ Identify problems with alcohol in the elderly with the appropriate tools and make suitable referrals. *Tools such as the Alcohol Use Disorders Identification Test (AUDIT), Michigan Alcohol Screening Test-Geriatric Version (MAST-G), and the Alcohol-Related Problems Survey (ARPS) may have additional use in this population. Brief interventions have been shown to be effective in producing sustained ab-*

• = Independent   ▲ = Collaborative   **EBN** = Evidence-Based Nursing   **EB** = Evidence-Based

stinence or reducing levels of consumption, thereby decreasing hazardous and harmful drinking (Culberson, 2006).

- Encourage exercise for positive coping. **EBN:** *After a 10–week period, the elderly participants in this exercise group reported significant improvements in stress, mood, and several quality-of-life indices (Starkweather, 2007).*
- Stimulate individual reminiscence therapy. **EB:** *After eight sessions, elderly woman had a happier expression on her face, was willing to express herself more verbally, had more interaction with others, and required medication less frequently to help her sleep (Chou, Lan & Chao, 2008).*
- Stimulate group reminiscence therapy. **EB:** *Participation in reminiscence activities can be a positive and valuable experience for demented older persons. Consequently, the development of a structured care program for elderly persons with cognitive impairment and the need for long-term care is essential. Thus, health providers in long-term care facilities should be trained in reminiscence group therapy, and to be able to deliver such a program to the targeted group (Wang, 2007).*

 ### Multicultural

- Encourage the client to use spiritual coping mechanisms such as faith and prayer. **EBN:** *Prayer is a powerful way of coping and is practiced by all Western religions and several Eastern traditions (Mohr, 2006). Spirituality inspired hope among caregivers of stroke clients (Pierce et al, 2008).*
- Encourage spirituality as a source of support for coping. **EB:** *The association among spirituality/religiosity, positive appraisals, and internal adaptive coping strategies indicate that the utilization of spirituality/religiosity goes far beyond fatalistic acceptance, but can be regarded as an active coping process (Büssing et al, 2009).*
- Acknowledge racial/ethnic differences at the onset of care. **EBN:** *Acknowledgment of race/ethnicity issues will enhance communication, establish rapport, and promote treatment outcomes (D'Avanzo et al, 2001). African American parents who denied experiences of racism reported higher rates of behavior problems in their children, in contrast to African American parents who actively coped with racism and reported lower levels of behavior problems in their children (Caughy, O'Campo, & Muntaner, 2004).*

 ### Home Care

- ▲ Refer the client for a behavioral program that teaches coping skills via "Lifeskills" workshop and/or video. **EB:** *Commercially available, facilitator- or self-administered behavioral training products can have significant beneficial effects on psychosocial well-being in a healthy community sample (Kirby et al, 2006).*

 ### Client/Family Teaching and Discharge Planning

- Teach coping skills to family caregivers of cancer clients. **EBN:** *A coping skills intervention was effective in improving caregiver quality of life, reducing burden related to client's symptoms, and caregiving tasks compared with hospice care alone or hospice plus emotional support (McMillan et al, 2006).*
- Teach caregivers the COPE intervention (creativity, optimism, planning, expert information) to assist with symptom management. **EBN:** *Symptom distress, a measure that encompasses client suffering along with intensity, was significantly decreased in the group in which caregivers were trained to better manage client symptoms (McMillan & Small, 2007).*

Ⓔvolve   See the EVOLVE website for Weblinks for client education resources.

REFERENCES

Refer to **Ineffective Coping** for additional references.
Banja JD: Toward a more empathic relationship in pain medicine, *Pain Med* 9(8):1125–1129, 2008.
Boyd MA, Stanley M: Mental health assessment of the elderly. In Boyd MA, editor: *Psychiatric nursing in contemporary practice*, ed 2, Philadelphia, 2002, Lippincott.

Büssing A, Michalsen A, Balzat HJ et al: Are spirituality and religiosity resources for patients with chronic pain conditions? *Pain Med* 10(2):327–339, 2009.
Carrico AW, Antoni MH, Duran RE et al: Reductions in depressed mood and denial coping during cognitive behavioral stress management

● = Independent   ▲ = Collaborative   **EBN** = Evidence-Based Nursing   **EB** = Evidence-Based

with HIV-positive gay men treated with HAART, *Ann Behav Med* 31(2):155–164, 2006.

Caughy MO, O'Campo PJ, Muntaner C: Experiences of racism among African American parents and the mental health of their preschool-aged children, *Am J Public Health* 94(12):2118–2124, 2004.

Chan S, Fung MY, Tong CW et al: The clinical effectiveness of a multi-sensory therapy on clients with developmental disability, *Res Dev Disabil* 26(2):131–142, 2005.

Chou YC, Lan YH, Chao SY: Application of individual reminiscence therapy to decrease anxiety in an elderly woman with dementia, *Hu Li Za Zhi* 55(4):105–110, 2008.

Clark P: Resiliency in the practicing marriage and family therapist, *J Marital Fam Ther* 35(2):231–247, 2009.

Culberson JW: Alcohol use in the elderly: beyond the CAGE. Part 2: Screening instruments and treatment strategies, *Geriatrics*, 61(11):20–26, 2006.

D'Avanzo CE et al: Developing culturally informed strategies for substance-related interventions. In Naegle MA, D'Avanzo CE, editors: *Addictions and substance abuse: strategies for advanced practice nursing*, St Louis, 2001, Mosby.

Gleiberman L: Repressive/defensive coping, blood pressure, and cardiovascular rehabilitation, *Curr Hypertens Rep* 9(1):7–12, 2007.

Green GC: Guidelines for assessing and diagnosing acute psychosis: a primer, *J Emerg Nurs* 28(6):S1–6, 2002.

Hobfoll SE, Canetti-Nisim D, Johnson RJ: Exposure to terrorism, stress-related mental health symptoms, and defensive coping among Jews and Arabs in Israel, *J Consult Clin Psychol* 74(2):207–218, 2006.

Höping W, de Jong-Meyer R, Abrams D: Excessive self-focused attention and defensiveness among psychiatric patients: a vicious cycle? *Psychol Rep* 98(2):307–317, 2006.

Kirby ED, Williams VP, Hocking MC et al: Psychosocial benefits of three formats of a standardized behavioral stress management program, *Psychosom Med* 68(6):816–823, 2006.

Lench HC, Chang ES: Belief in an unjust world: when beliefs in a just world fail, *J Pers Assess* 89(2):126–135, 2007.

Lin CC, Anderson RM, Hagerty BM et al: Diabetes self-management experience: a focus group study of Taiwanese patients with type 2 diabetes, *J Clin Nurs* 17(5a):34–42, 2008.

McMillan SC, Small BJ, Weitzner M et al: Impact of coping skills intervention with family caregivers of hospice patients with cancer: a randomized clinical trial, *Cancer* 106(1):214–222, 2006.

McMillan SC, Small BJ: Using the COPE intervention for family caregivers to improve symptoms of hospice homecare patients: a clinical trial, *Oncol Nurs Forum* 34(2):313–321, 2007.

Mohr WK: Spiritual issues in psychiatric care, *Perspect Psychiatr Care* 42(3):174–183, 2006.

Pierce LL, Steiner V, Havens H et al: Spirituality expressed by caregivers of stroke survivors, *West J Nurs Res* 30(5):606–619, 2008.

Power R, Koopman C, Volk J et al: Social support, substance use, and denial in relationship to antiretroviral treatment adherence among HIV-infected persons, *Aids Patient Care* 17(5):245, 2003.

Reynaud SN, Meeker BJ: Coping styles of older adults with ostomies, *J Gerontol Nurs* 28(5):30, 2002.

Starkweather AR: The effects of exercise on perceived stress and IL-6 levels among older adults, *Biol Res Nurs* 8(3):186–194, 2007.

To SE, Vega CP: Alcoholism and pathways to recovery: new survey results on views and treatment options, *MedGenMed* 8(1):2, 2006.

Wang JJ: Group reminiscence therapy for cognitive and affective function of demented elderly in Taiwan, *Int J Geriatr Psychiatry* 22(12):1235–1240, 2007.

Compromised family Coping   *Katherina A. Nikzad Terhune, MSW*   ⊝volve

NANDA-I

Definition

Usually supportive primary person (family member or close friend) provides insufficient, ineffective, or compromised support, comfort, assistance, or encouragement that may be needed by client to manage or master adaptive tasks related to his or her health challenge

Defining Characteristics

Objective

Significant person attempts assistive behaviors with unsatisfactory results; significant person attempts supportive behaviors with unsatisfactory results; significant person displays protective behavior disproportionate to client's abilities; significant person displays protective behavior disproportion to client's need for autonomy; significant person enters into limited personal communication with client; significant person withdraws from client

Subjective

Client expresses a complaint about significant person's response to health problem; client expresses a concern about significant person's response to health problem; significant person expresses an inadequate knowledge base, which interferes with effective supportive behaviors; significant person expresses an inadequate understanding, which interferes with supportive behaviors; significant person describes preoccupation with personal reaction (e.g., fear, anticipatory grief, guilt, anxiety) to client's needs

Related Factors (r/t)

Coexisting situations affecting the significant person; developmental crises that the significant person may be facing; exhaustion of supportive capacity of significant people; inadequate information by a

• = Independent   ▲ = Collaborative   **EBN** = Evidence-Based Nursing   **EB** = Evidence-Based

primary person; inadequate understanding of information by a primary person; incorrect information by a primary person; incorrect understanding of information by a primary person; lack of reciprocal support; little support provided by client, in turn, for primary person; prolonged disease that exhausts supportive capacity of significant people; situational crises that the significant person may be facing; temporary family disorganization; temporary family role changes; temporary preoccupation by a significant person

NOC   (Nursing Outcomes Classification)

Suggested NOC Outcomes

Caregiver Emotional Health, Caregiver-Patient Relationship, Family Coping, Family Participation in Professional Care, Family Support During Treatment

Example NOC Outcome with Indicators

Family Coping as evidenced by the following indicators: Confronts family problems/Manages family problems/Seeks family assistance when appropriate (Rate each indicator of **Family Coping:** 1 = never demonstrated, 2 = rarely demonstrated, 3 = sometimes demonstrated, 4 = often demonstrated, 5 = consistently demonstrated [see Section I].)

Client Outcomes

Family/Significant Person Will (Specify Time Frame):

- Verbalize internal resources to help deal with the situation
- Verbalize knowledge and understanding of illness, disability, or disease
- Provide support and assistance as needed
- Identify need for and seek outside support

NIC   (Nursing Interventions Classification)

Suggested NIC Interventions

Caregiver Support, Coping Enhancement, Family Involvement Promotion, Family Mobilization, Family Support, Mutual Goal Setting, Normalization Promotion, Sibling Support

Example NIC Activities—Family Support

Appraise family's emotional reaction to client's condition; Promote trusting relationship with family

Nursing Interventions and *Rationales*

- Assess the strengths and deficiencies of the family system. **EBN:** *Thorough and comprehensive assessments offer valuable information regarding how problems evolve within the family context over time. Assessments also allow for anticipatory care and guidance to help family members acquire and maintain support and coping strategies, which are associated with fewer distress indices (McGoldrick, Gerson, & Petry, 2008).*
- Assess how family members interact with each other; observe verbal and nonverbal communication; individual and group responses to stress; and discern how individuals cope with stress when health concerns are present. **EBN:** *Understanding how families cope with stress is important and relevant for subsequent interventions (Lewandowska et al, 2009).*
- Establish rapport with families by providing accurate communication. **EBN:** *Families in psychiatric settings indicated that family care can be improved by focusing on building rapport and communicating problems and concerns between families and health professionals (Watson, Kieckhefer, & Olshansky, 2006).*
- Consider the use of family theory as a framework to help guide interventions (e.g., family stress theory, role theory, social exchange theory, family systems theory). **EBN:** *Involving concepts from theoretical frameworks, such as family systems theory, can be helpful and effective when dealing with critical medical situations within the family (Leon & Knapp, 2008).*
- Help family members recognize the need for help and teach them how to ask for it.

● = Independent   ▲ = Collaborative   **EBN** = Evidence-Based Nursing   **EB** = Evidence-Based

- Encourage expression of positive thoughts and emotions. **EB:** *Cognitive behavioral therapeutic approaches can be utilized to help positively impact emotions, thoughts, and behaviors. A great deal of research supports the efficacy of this therapeutic approach, which has been found to improve self-efficacy, self-esteem, symptoms of depression, symptoms of anxiety, and various mental health symptomology (Bramham et al, 2009; Hyer et al, 2009; Schmidt, 2009).*
- Encourage family members to verbalize feelings. Spend time with them, sit down and make eye contact, and offer coffee and other nourishment.
- Provide opportunities for families to discuss spirituality. **EB:** *Results from a recent study revealed that African American young adult males connected and identified with spirituality as a strong form of coping (Page, 2009).*
- Mothers may require additional support in their role of caring for chronically ill children. **EB:** *A recent literature review examining gender differences in the experiences of parents of children with cancer found a tendency toward traditional gender roles regarding parental tasks. Findings also revealed mixed results regarding parent psychological distress and preferences in coping strategies, with mothers tending to experience increased distress, more emotion-focused coping, and more social support-seeking behaviors (Clarke et al, 2009).*
- Provide privacy during family visits. If possible, maintain flexible visiting hours to accommodate more frequent family visits. If possible, arrange staff assignments so the same staff members have contact with the family. Familiarize other staff members with the situation in the absence of the usual staff member. *Providing privacy, maintaining flexible hours, and arranging consistent staff assignments will reduce stress, enhance communication, and facilitate the building of trust.*
- Determine whether the family is suffering from additional stressors (e.g., child care issues, financial problems, parental mental health issues). **EB:** *Children of mothers with depression demonstrated significantly poorer adaptive skills compared to children of mothers without depression (Riley et al, 2009).*
- Examine antecedent factors within the family system (e.g., existing mental health issues, substance abuse, past traumas) that may be exacerbating the current situation. **EBN:** *Brook, Zhang & Brook (2009) found a strong relationship between internalizing behaviors in later adolescence and adverse health outcomes later in adulthood.*
- ▲ Refer the family with ill family members to appropriate resources for assistance as indicated (e.g., counseling, psychotherapy, financial assistance, or spiritual support).

 Pediatric

- Assess the adolescent's perception of support from family and friends during crisis and illness. Also thoroughly assess adolescent's needs and concerns. **EB:** *A qualitative study focusing on the self-identified needs of adolescents living with chronic pain found that the adolescents were experiencing common stressors and concerns, including the struggle to be "normal," and coping with the pain (Forgeron & McGrath, 2009).*
- Provide educational and psychosocial interventions such as coping skills training in treatment for families and their adolescents who have Type 1 diabetes. **EB:** *Understanding parent/child dynamics and the influence of anxiety on behalf of the parents may help predict autonomy development and self-management behaviors of adolescents with diabetes (Dashiff et al, 2009).*
- Focus on the communication dynamics of families coping with chronic illness. Identify communication barriers, and ways in which to enhance the communication process among parents, siblings, and other family members involved. **EBN:** *A recent qualitative study identified four communication themes present among siblings, parents, and others within families of children with chronic illnesses: Communication as a reflection of family roles and relationships; giving voice; staying connected; and struggling for normalcy (Branstetter et al, 2008).*
- Encourage the use of family rituals such as connection, spirituality, love, recreation, and celebration, especially in single parent families. **EBN:** *Family routines and meaningful rituals provide predictability that can positively impact behaviors and emotions within the family unit. Family routines can also influence early development (Spagnola & Fiese, 2007).*
- Staff should involve the family in decision making processes, especially during hospital discharge planning. **EBN:** *Increasing parental involvement in caregiving procedures and including them in hos-*

---

pital discharge processes has been identified as an effective way to increase feelings of competence and confidence in family caregivers (Griffin & Abraham, 2006).

- Transitioning into parenthood is a major life event for individuals. Providing effective strategies and education to first-time parents can help them feel more prepared, confident, and supported during this transition. **EBN:** *Research indicates that positive experiences during the transitional period into parenthood contribute to parents feeling more confident and educated prior to the postnatal period. Programs such as "Coming ready or not!" provide innovative educational and supportive strategies to those preparing for the parenthood role (McKellar, Pincombe, & Henderson, 2009).*
- Teenage mothers may experience a variety of psychosocial complications during and after their pregnancy, including conflicts due to poor relational boundaries with their own mothers. This type of conflict may exacerbate maternal stress and negatively impact mother-infant interactions (Stiles, 2008). **EBN:** *Interventions, including cognitive behavioral therapy interventions, may help improve relational boundaries between teenage mothers and their mothers. This may subsequently improve mother-infant relationships (Stiles, 2008).*

Geriatric

- Perform a holistic assessment of all needs of informal spousal caregivers. **EBN:** *The role of informal spousal caregivers has increased as the population ages. Community based services can positively impact the stress process for family caregivers (Sussman & Regehr, 2009).*
- Help caregivers believe in themselves and their ability to handle the situation, taking life one day at a time, looking for positive aspects in each situation, and relying on their own individual expertise and experience. Encourage caregivers to establish their priorities and concentrate on caring for their own physical and emotional well-being. **EBN:** *Utilizing respite care services is an effective coping mechanism for family caregivers (Salin, Kaunonen, & Astedt-Kurki, 2009).*
- ▲ Refer caregivers of clients with Alzheimer's disease to a monthly psychoeducational support group (i.e., the Alzheimer's Association). **EB:** *Nonpharmacologic interventions, including manual based interventions, and weekly sessions with clinicians, have been shown to reduce symptoms of depression and anxiety in family caregivers compared to caregivers in control groups (Lopez, Crespo, & Zarit, 2007).*
- ▲ Consider the use of telephone support for caregivers of family members with illnesses such as cancer and dementia. **EBN:** *Family caregivers can be helped through a variety of social support mechanisms including telephone support (Radziewicz et al, 2009).*
- Assist in finding transportation to enable family members to visit. **EB:** *If a family member is homebound and unable to visit, encourage alternative contact (e.g., telephone, cards and letters, e-mail) to provide ongoing scheduled progress reports. Reducing loneliness and isolation has many positive psychosocial and physical health benefits (Drentea et al, 2006).*

Multicultural

- Acknowledge racial/ethnic differences at the onset of care. **EBN:** *Acknowledgment of race/ethnicity issues will enhance communication, establish rapport, and promote treatment outcomes (Mokuau et al, 2008).*
- Assess for the influence of cultural beliefs, norms, and values on the family's/community's perceptions of coping. **EB:** *What the family/community considers normal and abnormal coping behavior may be based on cultural perceptions (von Peter, 2009).*
- Use culturally competent assessment procedures when working with families with different racial/ethnic backgrounds in order to avoid discrepancies and diagnostic errors (Zayas, Torres, & Cabassa, 2009). **EBN:** *A study by Mandell et al (2009) revealed that significant racial/ethnic disparities were present in regard to recognizing autism spectrum disorders in children. Professionals and clinicians must continue to culturally educate themselves in order to avoid such disparities, and to provide the most effective assessments and interventions needed within the given cultural context.*
- Provide culturally relevant interventions by understanding and utilizing treatment strategies that are acceptable and effective for a particular culture. **EBN:** *Terminology and therapeutic strategies must reflect and adhere to the values of one's culture (Hodge & Nadir, 2008).* **EB:** *Clinicians have a responsibility to take into consideration the many factors present in culturally diverse situations,*

• = Independent   ▲ = Collaborative   **EBN** = Evidence-Based Nursing   **EB** = Evidence-Based

including epidemiological knowledge in relation to specific cultures; awareness of how culture influences thoughts and behaviors; taking into consideration one's cultural and social context; relaying information in an appropriate manner; and recognizing one's own biases and prejudices toward a specific culture (Seeleman, Suurmond, & Stronks, 2009).

- Determine how the family's cultural context impacts their decisions in regard to managing and coping with a child's illness. Recognize and validate the cultural context. **EBN:** *Nurses and other clinicians working with families must include cultural variables when assisting family members with ill children. Research indicates that when working with Asian cultures, health beliefs, communication beliefs, religious practice, and family structure are strong cultural influences on families (Thibodeaux & Deatrick, 2007).*

Home Care

- The interventions described previously may be adapted for home care use.
- Assess the reason behind the breakdown of family coping. *Knowledge of the reasons behind compromised coping will assist in identification of appropriate interventions.* Refer to the care plan for **Caregiver role strain**.
- During the time of compromised coping, increase visits to ensure the safety of the client, support of the family, and assistance with coping strategies. Provide reassurance regarding expectations for prognosis as appropriate. **EBN:** *Caregivers of heart failure clients require adequate support to help them cope effectively with burden, stress, and poor health outcomes (Pressler et al, 2009).*
- ▲ Assess the needs of the caregiver in the home. Intervene to meet needs as appropriate, and explore all available resources that may be used to provide adequate home care (e.g., parish nursing as an effective adjunct, home health aide services to relieve the caregiver's fatigue). Encourage caregivers to attend to their own physical, mental, and spiritual health and give more specific information about the client's needs and ways to meet them. *Meeting the needs of caregivers supports their ability to meet the needs of the client. Assess the client and caregiver separately and in interaction.* **EBN:** *Caregivers of individuals with heart failure report poor physical and emotional health. Physical health conditions of the caregivers and the perceived difficulty of caregiving procedures predicted physical health-related quality of life. Depressive symptoms reported by the caregiver were predictors of emotional health-related quality of life. Caregivers of individuals with heart failure may be a vulnerable population of caregivers requiring appropriate interventions and support for enhancing caregiver outcomes (Pressler et al, 2009).*
- ▲ Refer the family to medical social services for evaluation and supportive counseling. *Dedicating time for nurturing the caregivers and reassuring the client allows them to express feelings and feel hope.*
- ▲ Serve as an advocate, mentor, and role model for caregiving. Write down or contract for the care needed by the client. *Therapeutic use of self by the nurse and concrete task definition and assignment reinforce positive coping strategies and allow caregivers to feel less guilty when tasks are delegated to multiple caregivers.*
- ▲ When a terminal illness is the precipitating factor for ineffective coping, offer hospice services and support groups as possible resources. *Nonjudgmental support from helpers with no agenda allows verbalization of feelings. The hospice paradigm addresses the physical, emotional, and spiritual needs of the dying and their loved ones.* **EB:** *Research has indicated that hospice care has the potential to mediate the effects of burden caused by caregiving, and positively impact quality of life for caregivers (McMillan et al, 2006).*
- With a cancer client, encourage family discussion of stressors (including the meaning of the illness, fear of recurrence, the client's employment status) and resources (family social support). **EBN:** *Stressors and resources have been shown to play an important role in determining family quality of life among cancer survivors (Woodgate, 2006).*
- Encourage the client and family to discuss changes in daily functioning and routines created by the client's illness. Validate discomfort resulting from changes. *Individuals who live together for a long period tend to become familiar with each others' patterns: meals are expected at certain times, a spouse becomes accustomed to the client's sleep habits.*
- Support positive individual and family coping efforts. *Positive feedback reinforces desired behaviors and supports the family unit.*

● = Independent   ▲ = Collaborative   **EBN** = Evidence-Based Nursing   **EB** = Evidence-Based

▲ If compromised family coping interferes with the ability to support the client's treatment plan, refer for psychiatric home health care services for family counseling and implementation of a therapeutic regimen. **EBN:** *Psychiatric home care nurses can address issues related to family members' ability to adjust to changes in the client's health status. Behavioral interventions in the home can help the family to participate more effectively in the treatment plan (Oneal et al, 2006).*

Client/Family Teaching and Discharge Planning

- Provide truthful information and support for the family and significant people regarding the client's specific illness or condition. Address grief issues that arise in the process, including anticipatory grief. **EB:** *Family caregivers, especially spouses and adult children, of individuals with Alzheimer's disease and other forms of dementia often experience anticipatory grief during the caregiving process. Assessing for this type of grief, and providing appropriate support and interventions may help improve various aspects of caregiving (Frank, 2008).*

▲ Refer women with breast cancer and their family caregivers to support groups and other services which provide assistance with daily coping. **EBN:** *Many women require emotional, social, cognitive, and physical support following cancer, especially in instances of partial and total mastectomies (Skrzypulec et al, 2009).*

- Promote individual and family relaxation and stress-reduction strategies. *The immune system weakens in response to stress; relaxation elicits the opposite, healthful response (Cass, 2006).*

▲ Provide a parent support and education group to provide opportunities for parents to access support, learn new parenting skills, and, ultimately, optimize their relationships with their children in families of children in residential care. **EB:** *Parent support groups are increasingly utilized to help prevent various forms of child maltreatment. Positive results have been shown in regard to the parental functioning of those who participated in these support groups (Falconer et al, 2008).*

ⓔvolve   See the EVOLVE website for Weblinks for client education resources.

REFERENCES

Bramham J, Young S, Bickerdike A et al: Evaluation of group cognitive behavioral therapy for adults with ADHD, *J Atten Disord* 12(5):434–441, 2009.

Branstetter JE, Domian EW, Williams PD et al: Communication themes in families of children with chronic conditions, *Issues Compr Pediatr Nurs* 31(4):171–184, 2008.

Brook JS, Zhang C, Brook DW: Psychosocial antecedents and adverse health consequences related to substance use, *Am J Public Health* 99(3):563–568, 2009.

Cass H: Stress and the immune system, *Total Health* 27(6):24–25, 2006.

Clarke NE, McCarthy MC, Downie P et al: Gender differences in the psychosocial experience of parents of children with cancer: a review of the literature, *Psychooncology* 18(9):907–915, 2009.

Dashiff C, Vance D, Abdullatif H et al: Parenting, autonomy and self-care of adolescents with Type 1 diabetes, *Child Care Health Dev* 35(1):79–88, 2009.

Drentea P, Clay O, Roth D et al: Predictors of improvement in social support: five-year effects of a structured intervention for caregivers of spouses with Alzheimer's disease, *Soc Sci Med* 63(4):957–67, 2006.

Falconer MK, Haskett ME, McDaniels L et al: Evaluation of support groups for child abuse prevention: outcomes of four state evaluations, *Soc Work Groups* 31(2):165–182, 2008.

Forgeron P, McGrath PJ: Self-identified needs of youth with chronic pain, *J Pain Manag* 1(2):163–172, 2009.

Frank J: Evidence for grief as the major barrier faced by Alzheimer caregivers: a qualitative analysis, *Am J Alzheimers Dis Other Demen* 22(6):516–527, 2008.

Griffin T, Abraham M: Transition to home from the newborn intensive care unit: applying the principles of family-centered care to the discharge process, *J Perinat Neonatal Nurs* 20(3):243–249, 2006.

Hodge D, Nadir A: Moving toward culturally competent practice with Muslims: modifying cognitive therapy with Islamic tenets, *Social Work* 53(1):31–39, 2008.

Hyer L, Yeager C, Hilton N et al: Group, individual, and staff therapy: an efficient and effective cognitive behavioral therapy in long-term care, *Am J Alzheimers Dis Other Demen* 23(6):528–539, 2009.

Leon AM, Knapp S: Involving family systems in critical care nursing: challenges and opportunities, *Dimen Crit Care Nurs* 27(6):255–262, 2008.

Lewandowska K, Specjalski K, Jassem E et al: [Style of coping with stress and emotional functioning in patients with asthma] [Article in Polish], *Pneumonal Alergol Pol* 77(1):31–36, 2009.

Lopez J, Crespo M, Zarit SH: Assessment of the efficacy of a stress management program for informal caregivers of dependent older adults, *Gerontologist*, 47(2):205–214, 2007.

Mandell DS, Wiggins LD, Carpenter LA et al: Racial/ethnic disparities in the identification of children with autism spectrum disorders, *Am J Public Health* 99(3):493–498, 2009.

McGoldrick M, Gerson R, Petry S: *Genograms: assessment and intervention*, ed 3, New York, 2008, WW Norton.

McKellar L, Pincombe J, Henderson A: Coming ready or not! Preparing parents for parenthood, *Br J Midwif* 17(3):160–167, 2009.

McMillan SC, Small BJ, Weitzner J et al: Impact of coping skills intervention with family caregivers of hospice patients with cancer: a randomized trial, *Cancer* 106(1):214–222, 2006.

Mokuau N, Braun K, Wong L et al: Development of a family intervention for native Hawaiian women with cancer: a pilot study, *Soc Work* 53(1):9–19, 2008.

Oneal B, Reeb R, Korte J et al: Assessment of home-based behavior modification programs for autistic children: reliability and validity of the behavioral summarized evaluation, *Prev Interv Community* 32(1–2):25–39, 2006.

Page T: Spirituality and coping of the African American young adult male: a phenomenological study, *Diss Abstr Int B Sci Engin* 69 (7–B):4405, 2009.

Pressler S, Gradus-Pizlo I, Chubinski S et al: Family caregiver outcomes in heart failure, *Am J Crit Care* 18(2):149–159, 2009.

Radziewicz RM, Rose JH, Bowman KF et al: Establishing treatment fidelity in a coping and communication support telephone intervention for aging patients with advanced cancer and their family caregivers, *Cancer Nurs* 32(3):193–220, 2009.

Riley AW, Coiro MJ, Broitman M et al: Mental health of children of low-income depressed mothers: influences of parenting, family environment, and raters, *Psychiatr Serv* 60(3):329–336, 2009.

Salin S, Kaunonen M, Astedt-Kurki P: Informal carers of older family members: how they manage and what support they receive from respite care, *J Clin Nurs* 18(4):492–501, 2009.

Schmidt U: Cognitive behavioral approaches in adolescent anorexia and bulimia nervosa, *Child Adolesc Psychiatr Clin North Am* 18(1):147–158. 2009.

Seeleman C, Suurmond J, Stronks K: Cultural competence: a conceptual framework for teaching and learning, *Med Educ* 43(3):229–237, 2009.

Skrzypulec V, Tobor E, Drosdzol A et al: Biopsychosocial functioning of women after mastectomy, *J Clin Nurs* 18(4):613–619, 2009.

Spagnola M, Fiese BH: Family routines and rituals: a context for development in the lives of young children, *Infants Young Child* 20(4):284–299, 2007.

Stiles AS: A pilot study to test the feasibility and effectiveness of an intervention to help teen mothers and their mothers clarify relational boundaries, *J Pediatr Nurs* 23(6):415–428, 2008.

Sussman T, Regehr C: The influence of community-based services on the burden of spouses caring for their partners with dementia, *Health Social Work* 34(1):29–39, 2009.

Thibodeaux AG, Deatrick JA: Cultural influence on family management of children with cancer, *J Pediatr Oncol Nurs* 24(4):227–233, 2007.

von Peter S: The concept of "mental trauma" and its transcultural application, *Anthropol Med* 16(1):13–25, 2009.

Watson K, Kieckhefer G, Olshansky, E: Striving for therapeutic relationships: parent-provider communication in the developmental treatment setting, *Qual Health Res* 16(5):647–663, 2006.

Woodgate R: The importance of being there: perspectives of social support by adolescents with cancer, *J Pediatr Oncol Nurs* 23(3):122–134, 2006.

Zayas LH, Torres LR, Cabassa LJ: *Community Ment Health J* 45(2):97–105, 2009.

Disabled family Coping   *Dena L. Jarog, DNP, RN, CCNS*

Definition

Behavior of significant person (family member or other primary person) that disables his or her capacities and the client's capacities to effectively address tasks essential to either person's adaptation to the health challenge.

Defining Characteristics

Abandonment; aggression; agitation; carrying on usual routines without regard for client's needs; client's development of dependence; depression; desertion; disregarding client's needs; distortion of reality regarding client's health problem; family behaviors that are detrimental to well-being; hostility; impaired individualization; impaired restructuring of a meaningful life for self; intolerance; neglectful care of client in regard to basic human needs; neglectful care of client in regard to illness treatment; neglectful relationships with other family members; prolonged over-concern for client; psychosomaticism; rejection; taking on illness signs of client

Related Factors (r/t)

Arbitrary handling of family's resistance to treatment; dissonant coping styles for dealing with adaptive tasks by the significant person and client; dissonant coping styles among significant people; highly ambivalent family relationships; significant person with chronically unexpressed feelings (e.g., guilt, anxiety, hostility, despair)

NOC   (Nursing Outcomes Classification)

Suggested NOC Outcomes

Caregiver Well-Being, Family Coping, Family Normalization, Neglect Recovery

---

Example NOC Outcome with Indicators

Family Normalization as evidenced by the following indicators: Adapts family routines to accommodate needs of affected member/Meets physical and psychosocial needs of family members/Provides activities appropriate to age and ability for affected family member/Uses community support groups. (Rate the outcome and indicators of **Family Normalization:** 1 = never demonstrated, 2 = rarely demonstrated, 3 = sometimes demonstrated, 4 = often demonstrated, 5 = consistently demonstrated [See Section I].)

Client Outcomes

Family/Significant Person Will (Specify Time Frame):

- Identify normal family routines that will need to be adapted
- Participate positively in the client's care within the limits of his or her abilities
- Identify responses that are harmful
- Acknowledge and accept the need for assistance with circumstances
- Identify appropriate activities for affected family member

NIC   (Nursing Interventions Classification)

Suggested NIC Interventions

Family Process Maintenance, Caregiver Support, Family Support, Family Therapy, Respite Care

---

Example NIC Activities—Family Process Maintenance

Determine typical family processes; Minimize family routine disruption by facilitating family routines and rituals such as private meals together or family discussions for communication and decision making; Design schedules of home care activities that minimize disruption of family routine.

Nursing Interventions and *Rationales*

- Identify current roles of family members. **EB:** *The most important predictors of caregivers' well-being were child behavior, caregiving demands, and family role function (Raina et al, 2005).*
- Assist families to identify physical and mental health effects of caregiving. **EBN:** *Evidence over the last two decades shows that caregiving is a major public health issue. Caregiving has features of a chronic stress experience with high levels of unpredictability and uncontrollability leading to secondary stress in multiple life domains (Schulz & Sherwood, 2008).*
- Evaluate the family's perceived strength of its social support system. Encourage the family to use social support to increase its resiliency and to moderate stress. **EBN:** *Nurses use professional communications to encourage families to engage in social activities, build up their social network, and master the chronic condition (Mu, 2005).*
- Encourage family members to participate in appropriate support programs (e.g., chronic obstructive pulmonary disease [COPD] support groups, Arthritis I Can Cope groups, Alzheimer's support groups, asthma support groups, cancer survivor support groups). **EBN:** *The stress of caregivers of clients with cancer was reduced when they attended an art-making class (Walsh et al, 2007).* **EB:** *Older caregivers in telesupport groups reported lower depression than control group caregivers (Winter & Gitlin, 2007).*
- Assist family members to find professional assistance for primary stressors such as financial issues and insurance coverage, or communicating with professionals. **EBN:** *In a focus group interview respondents identified a spectrum of needs including information about navigating financial and communication barriers (Yedidia & Tiedemann, 2008).*

 Pediatric

▲ Report any actual, potential, or suspected child abuse or neglect to the appropriate agency. **EBN:** *Physical child abuse is a significant social and medical problem (Bull, 2006). The United Nations (UN) and the World Health Organization (WHO) cast the problem of child abuse and neglect as a major public health issue (Giardino, 2009).*

• = Independent   ▲ = Collaborative   **EBN** = Evidence-Based Nursing   **EB** = Evidence-Based

• Work with fathers of children with chronic conditions to help them develop sufficient coping capacities and understanding of the medical condition. **EBN:** *Nurses can assist fathers in their development of sufficient coping capacities while caring for a child with a chronic condition (Mu, 2005).*

Geriatric

▲ Observe for and report any symptoms of elder abuse or neglect. Prompt reporting of abuse according to local and state law is necessary. **EB:** *Elders need to be assessed for signs of abuse and neglect. Types of elder abuse existing in our society include physical, sexual, emotional, psychological, and exploitation (Roman, 2004). All who provide care to an elder must be aware of the potential signs of abuse and the remedies available (Birke, 2004).*

• Work with the family to manage common challenges related to normal aging. **EB:** *Maltreatment of elders is less likely when caregivers are trained to cope with the stress of caregiving of elders and potentially abusive elders (Nadien, 2006).*

▲ Refer the family to appropriate senior community resources (e.g., senior centers, Medicare assistance, meal programs, parish nursing services, charitable organizations). *This study demonstrates the importance of social support among visually impaired elders (Lee & Brennan, 2006).*

• Provide support for family caregivers of persons with dementia and related disorders: Encourage pleasant event therapies (i.e., interventions that teach caregivers to identify and pursue experiences that give them pleasure on a regular basis). Provide dietary and physical activity interventions. Screen for signs of depression. *Collaborative care models are essential for treating physical and psychiatric conditions in caregivers. Such models should be adapted to caregivers' needs (Vitaliano & Katon, 2006).*

Multicultural

• Work to provide caregivers who understand the importance of cultural beliefs and values the family may hold. **EBN:** *Cultures can differ with regard to health beliefs, practices, and values (Vitaliano & Katon, 2006). There is a stigma to having a family member with mental illness in China (Chang & Horrocks, 2006).*

• Develop programs to prevent injury from abuse and suffocation for the African American community. **EB:** *This study demonstrated that African American infants have 3.5 times increased risk of death from preventable injuries compared to white infants (Falcone, Brown, & Garcia, 2007).*

Home Care

• The interventions described previously may be adapted for home care use.

• Assess for strain in family caregivers. **EBN:** *Utilizing a tool such as the Modified Caregiver Strain Index gives the nurse information about a caregiver's abilities. It also could identify a need to evaluate the care recipient's living situation (Onega, 2008).*

▲ If disabled family coping interferes with the family member's ability to support the client's treatment plan, refer for psychiatric home health care services for family and client counseling and implementation of a therapeutic regimen. **EBN:** *Psychiatric home care nurses can address issues related to family members' ability to adjust to changes in the client's health status. Behavioral interventions in the home can help the family to participate more effectively in the treatment plan (Logsdon, McCurry, & Teri, 2005; Oneal et al, 2006).*

Client/Family Teaching and Discharge Planning

• Involve the client and family in the planning of care as often as possible; mutual goal setting is considered part of "client safety." *Major changes in the fifth annual issuance of National Patient Safety Goals include home care, assisted living, and disease-specific care programs in 2009. An expectation is to "encourage patients' active involvement in their own care as a patient safety strategy" (Joint Commission, 2009).*

• Discuss with the family appropriate ways to demonstrate feelings such as reminiscence. *This study demonstrated the positive effects of reminiscence therapy among student nurses and older adults (Shellman, 2006).*

• = Independent ▲ = Collaborative **EBN** = Evidence-Based Nursing **EB** = Evidence-Based

- Educate family members regarding stress management techniques including massage and alternative therapies. **EBN:** *Education, support, psychotherapy, and respite interventions have demonstrated the greatest effect in reducing caregiver strain and burden. A significant decline was observed in the depression and anxiety scores of caregivers in the treatment group receiving massage therapy (Honea et al, 2008).*

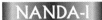 See the EVOLVE website for Weblinks for client education resources.

REFERENCES

Birke MG: Elder law, Medicare, and legal issues in older patients, *Semin Oncol* 31(2):282–292, 2004.

Bull L: Children's non-accidental injuries at an accident and emergency department: does the age of the child and the type of injury matter? *Accid Emerg Nurs* 14(3):155–159, 2006.

Chang KH, Horrocks S: Lived experiences of family caregivers of mentally ill relatives, *J Adv Nurs* 53(4):435–443, 2006.

Falcone RA, Brown RL, Garcia VF, The epidemiology of infant injuries and alarming health disparities, *J Pediatr Surg* 42(1):172–176, 2007.

Giardino AP: Child maltreatment: is the glass half full yet? *J Forensic Nurs* 5(1):1–4, 2009.

Honea NJ, Brintanall R, Given B et al: Putting evidence into practice: nursing assessment and interventions to reduce family caregiver strain and burden, *Clin J Oncol Nurs* 12(3):507–516, 2008.

Joint Commission (2009): *National Patient Safety Goals*, available at www.jointcommission.org/NR/rdonlyres/DB3D6A66–DA79–412B–97E5–6FC400663127/0/OME_NPSG_Outline.pdf. Accessed on March 31, 2009.

Lee EK, Brennan M: Stress constellations and coping styles of older adults with age-related visual impairment, *Health Soc Work* 31(4):289–298, 2006.

Logsdon RG, McCurry SM, Teri L: A home health care approach to exercise for persons with Alzheimer's disease, *Care Manag J* 6(2):90–97, 2005.

Mu PF: Paternal reactions to a child with epilepsy: uncertainty, coping strategies, and depression, *J Adv Nurs* 49(4):367–376, 2005.

Nadien MB: Factors that influence abusive interactions between aging women and their caregivers, *Ann N Y Acad Sce* 1087:158–169, 2006.

Oneal BJ, Reeb RN, Korte JR et al: Assessment of home-based behavior modification programs for autistic children: reliability and validity of the behavioral summarized evaluation, *J Prev Interv Community* 32(1–2):25–39, 2006.

Onega L: Helping those who help others: the modified caregiver strain index, *Am J Nurs* 108(9):62–69, 2008.

Raina P, O'Donnell M, Rosenbaum P et al: The health and well-being of caregivers of children with cerebral palsy, *Pediatrics* 115(6):e626–e636, 2005.

Roman M: Elder abuse, *Medsurg Matters* 13(3):10–12, 2004.

Schulz R, Sherwood PR: Physical and mental health effects of family caregiving, *Am J Nurs* 108(9 Suppl):23–27, 2008.

Shellman J: "Making a connection": BSN students' perceptions of their reminiscence experiences with older adults, *J Nurs Educ* 45(12):497–503, 2006.

Vitaliano PP, Katon WJ: Effects of stress on family caregivers: recognition and management, *Psychiatr Times* 23(7):24, 2006.

Walsh S, Radcliffe RS, Castillo L et al: A pilot study to test the effects of art-making classes for family caregivers of patients with cancer, *Oncol Nurs Forum* 34(1):E9–E16, 2007.

Winter L, Gitlin LN: Evaluation of a telephone-based support group intervention for female caregivers of community-dwelling individuals with dementia, *Am J Alzheimers Dis Other Demen* 21(6):391–397, 2007.

Yedidia MJ, Tiedemann A: How do family caregivers describe their needs for professional help? *Am J Nurs* 108(9):35–37, 2008.

Readiness for enhanced family Coping   *Keith A. Anderson, PhD*

NANDA-I

Definition

Effective management of adaptive tasks by family member involved with client's health challenge, who now exhibits desire and readiness for enhanced health and growth in regard to self and in relation to the client

Defining Characteristics

Chooses experiences that optimize wellness; family member attempts to describe growth impact of crisis; family member moves in directions of enriching lifestyle; family member moves in direction of health promotion; individual expresses interest in making contact with others who have experienced a similar situation

NOC   (Nursing Outcomes Classification)

Suggested NOC Outcomes

Family Coping, Health-Seeking Behavior, Participation in Healthcare Decisions

• = Independent   ▲ = Collaborative   **EBN** = Evidence-Based Nursing   **EB** = Evidence-Based

> ### Example NOC Outcome with Indicators
>
> **Family Coping** as evidenced by the following indicator: Confronts and manages family problems/Cares for needs of all family members (Rate the outcome and indicators of **Family Coping**: 1 = never demonstrated, 2 = rarely demonstrated, 3 = sometimes demonstrated, 4 = often demonstrated, 5 = consistently demonstrated [See Section I].)

Client Outcomes

Client Will (Specify Time Frame):

- State a plan indicating strengths and areas for growth
- Perform tasks needed for change
- Evaluate changes and continually re-evaluate plan for continued growth

NIC (Nursing Interventions Classification)

Suggested NIC Interventions

Family Integration Promotion, Family Involvement Promotion, Family Support, Mutual Goal Setting

> ### Example NIC Activities—Family Support
>
> Facilitate communication of concerns and feelings between clients and family or among family members; Respect and support adaptive coping mechanisms used by family

Nursing Interventions and *Rationales*

- Assess the structure, resources, and coping abilities of families. **EBN:** *It is critical to understand the resiliency and coping capabilities of families; the utilization of established assessment instruments (e.g., Calgary Family Assessment Model) can provide insight into family dynamics and the coping styles and resources of family systems (Black & Lobo, 2008; Wright & Leahey, 2009).*
- Acknowledge, assess and support the spiritual needs and resources of families and clients. **EBN:** *Spirituality has been found to be an important, yet often overlooked, coping resource for families and clients during illness and recovery (Tanyi, 2006).*
- Establish rapport with families and empower their decision making through effective and accurate communication. **EBN:** *Effective engagement and communication between health care providers and clients' families can help to establish rapport, provide timely and desired information to families, and empower families in their caregiving activities and decision-making capacities (Lowey, 2008; Bowman et al, 2009).*
- Provide family members with educational and skill-building interventions to alleviate caregiving stress and to facilitate adherence to prescribed plans of care. **EBN:** *The provision of educational interventions can help family members gain a sense of control in the caregiving role and to become more comfortable in making informed decisions (McMillan et al, 2006; White et al, 2008).* **EB:** *Comprehensive educational interventions that include family, friends, and clients can benefit caregivers and improve the well-being of clients (Sutherland et al, 2008).*
- ▲ Develop, provide, and encourage family members to use counseling services and interventions. **EBN:** *Family-level counseling interventions have been shown to be effective, particularly in psychiatric nursing settings (Goodman & Happell, 2006).* **EB:** *Behavioral management interventions of modest length have also been found to be effective in addressing burden in family caregivers (Selwood et al, 2007).*
- ▲ Identify and refer to support groups that discuss experiences and challenges similar to those faced by the family (e.g., Alzheimer's Association; Leukemia & Lymphoma Society). **EB:** *While there is wide diversity in the format of support groups and methodological concerns exist, a systematic review found that group-based supportive interventions may be effective in reducing psychological morbidity in family caregivers (Thompson et al, 2007).*
- Incorporate the use of emerging technologies to increase the reach of interventions to support family coping. **EB and EBN:** *Emerging computer and Internet-based supportive and educational interventions may hold promise in enhancing family members satisfaction with care (Salonen et al,*

• = Independent   ▲ = Collaborative   **EBN** = Evidence-Based Nursing   **EB** = Evidence-Based

2008), and addressing family caregiver stress (Marziali & Donahue, 2006) and informational needs (Feil et al, 2008).
- Refer to **Compromised family Coping** for additional interventions.

Pediatric

- Implement developmentally supportive family-centered services for infants and their caregivers. **EBN:** *Developmentally supportive family care interventions that individualized to the specific needs of families have been found to be associated with higher levels of well-being and lower levels of medication use in infants (Byers et al, 2006; Turan, Basbakkal, & Ozbek, 2008).*
- Identify the management styles of families and facilitate the use more effective ways of coping with childhood illness. **EBN:** *Understanding the dominant characteristics of each family's coping styles and resources and helping them to use more effective management styles can result in better family functioning and treatment outcomes (Conlon et al, 2008).*
- Provide educational and supportive interventions for families caring for children with illness and disability. **EB and EBN:** *Providing information, training parents in care management, and offering supportive programs can reduce stress levels in parents and lead to better outcomes for children (Barlow et al, 2008; Burns, Gray, & Henry, 2008; Cummins, 2008).*

Geriatric

- Encourage family caregivers to participate in counseling and support groups. **EBN:** *While a wide variety of programs exist, certain counseling and support group programs have been found to be effective in lowering caregiver burden and depression and decreasing family conflict (Gaugler et al, 2008; Logsdon, McCurry & Teri, 2006).*
- Provide educational interventions to family caregivers that focus on knowledge- and skill-building. **EBN:** *Educational interventions that are accessible and tailored to individual needs can be highly valued and useful to family caregivers (Curry, Walker & Hogstel, 2006).*
- Older adults should be provided with opportunities to engage their families and their communities. **EB:** *Programs that support and facilitate family interaction and intergenerational exchange can be important to the maintenance of family relationships (Heyman & Guthreil, 2008).*

Multicultural

- Acknowledge the importance of cultural influences in families and ensure that assessments and assessment tools account for such cultural differences. **EBN:** *Families react to illness and crisis in diverse ways that are often influenced by culture. Culture may impact the fit, reliability, and validity of family functioning assessment tools (Aarons et al, 2008).*

ⓔvolve   See the EVOLVE website for Weblinks for client education resources.

REFERENCES

Aarons GA, McDonald EJ, Connelly CD et al: Assessment of family functioning in Caucasian and Hispanic Americans: reliability, validity, and factor structure of the Family Assessment Device, *Fam Proc* 46(4):557–569, 2008.

Barlow JH, Powell LA, Gilchrist M et al: The effectiveness of the Training and Support Program for parents of children with disabilities: a randomized controlled trial, *J Psychosom Res* 64(1):55–62, 2008.

Black K, Lobo M: A conceptual review of family resilience factors, *J Fam Nurs* 14(1)S33–55, 2008.

Bowman KF, Rose JH, Radziewicz RM et al: Family caregiver engagement in a coping and communication support intervention tailored to advanced cancer patients and families, *Cancer Nurs* 32(1):73–81, 2009.

Burns C, Gray M, Henry R: The development, dissemination and evaluation of written information as a component of asthma management for parents of children with asthma, *Neonatal Paediatr Child Health Nurs* 11(3):9–12, 2008.

Byers JF, Lowman LB, Francis J et al: A quasi-experimental trial on individualized developmentally supportive family-centered care, *J Obstec Gynecol Neonatal Nurs* 35(1):105–115, 2006.

Conlon KE, Strassle CG, Vinh D et al: Family management styles and ADHD, *J Fam Nurs* 14(2):181–200, 2008.

Cummins A: Parents' need for information and support following their child's diagnosis of epilepsy, *J Child Young Peoples Nurs* 2(1), 37–41, 2008.

Curry LC, Walker C, Hogstel MO: Educational needs of employed caregivers of older adults: evaluation of a workplace project, *Geriatr Nurs* 27(3):166–173, 2006.

Feil EG, Bagget KM, Davis B et al: Expanding the reach of preventative interventions: Development of an Internet-based training for parents of infants, *Child Maltreat* 13(4):334–346, 2008.

Gaugler JE, Roth DL, Haley WE et al: Can counseling and support reduce burden and depressive symptoms in caregivers of people with

Alzheimer's disease during the transition to institutionalization? Results from the New York University Caregiver Intervention Study. *J Am Geriatr Soc* 56(3):421–428, 2008.

Goodman D, Happell B: The efficacy of family intervention in adolescent mental health, *Int J Psychiatr Nurs Res* 12(1):1–9, 2006.

Heyman JC, Guthreil IA: "They touch our hearts": the experiences of shared site intergenerational program participants, *J Intergen Relat* 6(40):397–412, 2008.

Logsdon RG, McCurry SM, Teri L: Time-limited support groups for individuals with early stage dementia and their care partners: preliminary outcomes from a controlled clinical trial, *Clin Gerontol* 30(2):5–19, 2006.

Lowey SE: Communication between the nurse and family caregiver in end-of-life care: a review of the literature, *J Hospice Palliat Care* 10(1):35–48, 2008.

Marziali E, Donahue P: Caring for others: Internet video-conferencing group intervention for family caregivers of older adults with neurodegenerative disease, *Gerontologist* 46(3):398–403, 2006.

McMillan SC, Small BJ, Weitzner M et al: Impact of coping skills intervention with family caregivers of hospice patients with cancer: a randomized clinical trial, *Cancer* 106(1):214–222, 2006.

Salonen AH, Kaunonen M, Astedt-Kurki P et al: Development of an internet-based intervention for parents of infants, *J Adv Nurs* 64(1):60–72, 2008.

Selwood A, Johnston K, Katona C et al: Systematic review of the effect of psychological interventions on family caregivers of people with dementia, *J Affect Disord* 101:75–89, 2007.

Sutherland G, Hoey L, White V et al: How does a cancer education program impact on people with cancer and their family and friends? *J Cancer Educ* 23(2):126–132, 2008.

Tanyi RA: Spirituality and family nursing: Spiritual assessment and interventions for families, *J Adv Nurs* 53(3):287–294, 2006.

Thompson CA, Spilsbury K, Hall J et al: Systematic review of information and support interventions for caregivers of people with dementia, *BMC Geriatrics* 7:18, 2007.

Turan T, Basbakkal Z, Ozbek S: Effect of nursing interventions on stressors of parents of premature infants in neonatal intensive care unit, *J Clin Nurs* 17(21):2856–2866, 2008.

White K, D'Abrew N, Auret K et al: Learn now; live well: an educational programme for caregivers, *Int J Palliat Nurs* 14(10):497–501, 2008.

Wright LM, Leahey M: *Nurses and families: a guide to family assessment and intervention,* ed 5, Philadelphia, 2009, F.A. Davis.

Ineffective Coping   *Arlene T. Farren, RN, PhD, AOCN®, CTN-A*   ⊝volve

NANDA-I

Definition

Inability to form a valid appraisal of the stressors, inadequate choices of practiced responses, and/or inability to use available resources

Defining Characteristics

Abuse of chemical agents; change in usual communication patterns; decreased use of social support; destructive behavior toward others; destructive behavior toward self; difficulty organizing information; fatigue; high illness rate; inability to attend to information; inability to meet basic needs; inability to meet role expectations; inadequate problem solving; lack of goal-directed behavior; lack of resolution of problem; poor concentration; risk taking; sleep disturbance; use of forms of coping that impede adaptive behavior; verbalization of inability to ask for help; verbalization of inability to cope

Related Factors (r/t)

Disturbance in pattern of appraisal of threat; disturbance in pattern of tension release; gender differences in coping strategies; high degree of threat; inability to conserve adaptive energies; inadequate level of confidence in ability to cope; inadequate level of perception of control; inadequate opportunity to prepare for stressor; inadequate resources available; inadequate social support created by characteristics of relationships; maturational crisis; situational crisis; uncertainty

NOC   (Nursing Outcomes Classification)

Suggested NOC Outcomes

Coping, Decision Making, Impulse Self-Control, Information Processing

Example NOC Outcome with Indicators
Coping as evidenced by the following indicator: Identifies effective and ineffective coping patterns/Modifies lifestyle to reduce stress (Rate the outcome and indicators of **Coping:** 1 = never demonstrated, 2 = rarely demonstrated, 3 = sometimes demonstrated, 4 = often demonstrated, 5 = consistently demonstrated [see Section I].)

• = Independent   ▲ = Collaborative   **EBN** = Evidence-Based Nursing   **EB** = Evidence-Based

Client Outcomes

Client Will (Specify Time Frame):

- Use effective coping strategies
- Use behaviors to decrease stress
- Remain free of destructive behavior toward self or others
- Report decrease in physical symptoms of stress
- Report increase in psychological comfort
- Seek help from a health care professional as appropriate

NIC (Nursing Interventions Classification)

Suggested NIC Interventions

Coping Enhancement, Decision-Making Support

Example NIC Activities—Coping Enhancement
Assist the patient in developing an objective appraisal of the event; Explore with the client previous methods of dealing with life problems

Nursing Interventions and *Rationales*

- Observe for contributing factors of ineffective coping such as poor self-concept, grief, lack of problem-solving skills, lack of support, recent change in life situation, or gender differences in coping strategies. **EBN:** *Ineffective coping strategies such as disengagement with others have been found to be predictors of greater distress in a sample of palliative care nurses (Desbiens & Fillion, 2007).* **EB:** *Males and females differ in appraisal of health and lifestyle choices and use of coping behavior (Goodwin, 2006; Dawson et al, 2007).*
- Use verbal and nonverbal therapeutic communication approaches including empathy, active listening, and confrontation to encourage the client and family to express emotions such as sadness, guilt, and anger (within appropriate limits); verbalize fears and concerns; and set goals. **EBN:** *Clinicians' communication skills contribute to the well-being of clients and minimizes psychosocial problems (Duff et al, 2009).*
- Collaborate with the client to identify strengths such as the ability to relate the facts and to recognize the source of stressors. **EBN:** *In a group of family caregivers of elderly living at home, an intervention that included collaboration between caregivers and case managers was found to be effective in managing stress and increasing caregiver empowerment (Ducharme et al, 2006).*
- Encourage the client to describe previous stressors and the coping mechanisms used. **EBN:** *A psychoeducation intervention that included clients' identification of symptoms, types of coping strategies used before and after the event, and ways to select alternative strategies was accompanied by medication intervention for participants with posttraumatic stress disorder (PTSD) statistically significantly improved PTSD and depression (Oflaz, Haitpoglu, & Ayan, 2008).*
- Be supportive of coping behaviors; allow the client time to relax. **EBN:** *The supportive relationship the nurse has with the client/couple has a positive effect on coping during the cancer experience (Morgan, 2009). Supporting hope may be essential to individuals coping with a threatening process (Giske & Gjengedal, 2007).*
- Provide opportunities for the client to discuss the meaning the situation might have for the client. **EBN:** *Participants in this study shared the importance of framing the illness experience in ways that enabled a sense of normalcy. Clinicians should offer support as clients search for meanings (Houldin & Lewis, 2006). When facing uncertainty, a meaning-making intervention significantly improved self-esteem and sense of security (Lee et al, 2006).*
- Assist the client to set realistic goals and identify personal skills and knowledge. **EBN:** *Researchers found that participants who were four months after myocardial infarction experiencing fatigue described fumbling coping strategies. The researchers concluded that nursing interventions to assist clients to identify and reduce stressors and increase clients' ability to cope with stressors would be useful (Alsen, Brink, & Persson, 2008).* **EB:** *In one correlational study, adjusting goals was found to be an effective coping strategy in childless people (Kraaij, Garnefski, & Schroevers, 2009).*

- Provide information regarding care before care is given. **EBN:** *Providing information regarding what to expect during hospitalization and about symptoms being experienced was important to participants in a qualitative study of individuals awaiting a gastric diagnosis (Giske & Gjengedal, 2007).* **EB:** *In a clinical trial of families responsible for taking care of a relative with mental illness, a family-led education intervention resulted in significant differences in coping and decreased information needs between the intervention and control group (Pickett-Schenk et al, 2008).*
- Discuss changes with the client before making them. **EBN:** *Nurses guided older persons with heart failure during the transition from hospital to home and self-management and coordinated community care, which resulted in positive client outcomes and cost savings (McCauley, Bixby, & Naylor, 2006).*
- Provide mental and physical activities within the client's ability (e.g., reading, television, radio, crafts, outings, movies, dinners out, social gatherings, exercise, sports, games). **EBN:** *In a pilot study of a nurse-based, in-home transitional care intervention for seriously mentally ill persons, researchers found that one of the factors of importance to community transition was involvement in daily activities (Rose, Gerson, & Carbo, 2007).*
- Discuss the client's and family's power to change a situation or the need to accept a situation. **EBN:** *A basic process of coping for significant others of persons living with HIV includes facing the change and dealing with it (Kylmä, 2005/2006).*
- Offer instruction regarding alternative coping strategies. **EBN:** *Mindfulness meditation intervention assisted coping with unpleasant symptoms for hospitalized clients receiving hematopoietic stem cell transplantation (Bauer-Wu, Sullivan, & Rosenbaum, 2008).* **EB:** *Meditative approaches (mindfulness meditation, relaxation response, yoga, etc.) have multifaceted effects on psychologic and biologic functions via the psychoneuroendrocrine/immune and autonomic nervous system pathway and are efficacious and safe (Arias et al, 2006).*
- Encourage use of spiritual resources as desired. **EBN:** *Spiritual activities such as prayer, meditation, and doing good deeds played a major role in coping with living with HIV in a sample of Thai women practicing Buddhism (Ross, Sawatphanit, & Suwansujarid, 2007). The strength to cope was identified as a major theme reflecting what spirituality provided African American breast cancer survivors (Gibson & Hendricks, 2006). HeartTouch technique (HRTT) is an internal method for changing thoughts and feelings through centered awareness, loving connections with others, and connecting to a higher power; the experimental group of nurses using HRTT statistically significantly increased spiritual well-being (Walker, 2006).*
- Encourage use of social support resources. **EBN:** *In a study of family caregivers in hospice care, participants who perceived support from the hospice team also used other types of coping strategies (Raleigh et al, 2006).* **EB:** *Better adjustment in children of a parent with multiple sclerosis was related to higher levels of social support and approach coping strategies (Pakenham & Bursnall, 2006).*
- ▲ Refer for additional or more intensive therapies as needed. **EBN:** *More complex interventions are available to assist with coping, for example, a nurse-delivered intervention for depression in clients with cancer (Forchuk, 2009).*

 Pediatric

- Monitor the client's risk of harming self or others and intervene appropriately. See care plan for **Risk for Suicide. EBN:** *Adolescents may use self-harming behaviors as a means of communication or way of coping (Murray & Wright, 2006).*
- Support adolescent and children's individual coping styles. **EB:** *In this study of youth with type I diabetes the following coping skills were observed: Younger children used more coping that involved choosing an alternate activity, helping others, and an emotional response (taking personal responsibility), whereas adolescents used more coping that involved persistence, alternate thinking, and talking things over (taking personal responsibility) (Hema et al, 2009).*
- Encourage moderate aerobic exercise (as appropriate). **EB:** *Exercise was found to decrease the likelihood of depressive feelings when used as a positive coping strategy for school-age children with angry feelings (Goodwin, 2006).*

 Geriatric

- ▲ Assess and report possible physiological alterations (e.g., sepsis, hypoglycemia, hypotension, infection, changes in temperature, fluid and electrolyte imbalances, and use of medications with known

---

• = Independent   ▲ = Collaborative   **EBN** = Evidence-Based Nursing   **EB** = Evidence-Based

cognitive and psychotropic side effects). **EB:** *A reversible pathophysiological process may be causing symptoms (Rocchiccioli & Sanford, 2009).*

- Screen for elder neglect or other forms of elder mistreatment. **EB:** *Abuse of older people is a serious and growing social problem (Wang, Tseng, & Chen, 2007).*
- Encourage the client to make choices (as appropriate) and participate in planning care and scheduled activities. **EBN:** *Older persons with heart failure transitioning to home from the hospital made choices about participation in the therapeutic regimen based on their individual goals for community living during a nursing intervention study, which resulted in positive client outcomes and cost savings (McCauley, Bixby, & Naylor, 2006).* **EBN:** *In a pilot study examining depression care preferences of older home care clients, researchers concluded client preferences during care planning may improve participation in geriatric depression care management (Fyffe et al, 2008).*
- Target selected coping mechanisms for older persons based on client features, use, and preferences. **EBN:** *Health, routine tasks, family issues, financial management, and living conditions are thought to improve support measures (Ark et al, 2006). Elders with arthritis reported cognitive efforts, diversional activities, and assertive actions were useful in dealing with daily stress (Tak, 2006). Additional relevant research: Nokes, Chew, & Altman, 2003; Tryssenaar, Chui, & Finch, 2003; Boerner, Reinhardt, & Horowitz, 2006.*
- Increase and mobilize support available to older persons by encouraging a variety of mechanisms involving family, friends, peers, and health care providers. **EBN:** *Relationships are pivotal in supporting coping in older adults. Social support was thought to be one of the dynamics in a peer-counseling program that was successful in terms of improving perceived health status, level of depression, and personal growth (Ho, 2007). Mobilizing religious coping styles has been found to be one way to measure health service use and length of stay for older persons (Ark et al, 2006). While limitations to telephone support groups for older HIV-positive persons may be difficult, it was found to facilitate connections with others and decrease geographical and logistical isolation (Nokes et al, 2003).*
- Actively listen to complaints and concerns. **EBN:** *The quality of care provided to elderly chronic pain clients living at home could be improved by active listening (Blomquist & Edberg, 2002).*
- Engage the client in reminiscence. **EBN:** *Life review as an intervention had a significant effect of lowering depression in individuals with cerebral vascular accident (Davis, 2004).* **EB:** *Reminiscence activates positive memories and evokes well-being (Puentes, 2002).*

Multicultural

- Assess for the influence of cultural beliefs, norms, and values on the client's perceptions of effective coping. *"Healthcare providers must recognize, respect, and integrate clients' cultural beliefs and practices into health prescriptions" (Purnell & Paulanka, 2005).* **EBN:** *The client's coping behavior may be based on cultural perceptions of normal and abnormal coping behavior (Sterling & Peterson, 2003).* **EBN:** *Chinese women may be less likely to seek mental health services for postnatal depression (Chan et al, 2002). Gender and age mediate a woman's response to signs and symptoms of cardiac disease (Lefler & Bondy, 2004). For Mexican American adolescents, positive reinterpretation, focusing and venting emotions, instrumental social support, active coping, religious, restraint, emotional support, acceptance, and planning were all forms of coping and were all associated with positive psychological and physical health (Vaughn & Roesch, 2003).*
- Assess the influence of fatalism on the client's coping behavior. **EBN:** *Fatalistic perspectives, which involve the belief that one cannot control one's own fate, may influence health behaviors in some Asian American, African American, and Latino populations (Chen, 2001).* **EBN:** *Clients with non–small cell lung cancer in Taiwan yielded that one response was to accept the outcome as fate (Kuo & Ma, 2002).*
- Assess the influence of cultural conflicts that may affect coping abilities. **EBN:** *It may be necessary to help the client to identify and find coping strategies that do not conflict with cultural expectations (Shibusawa & Mui, 2001).*
- Assess for intergenerational family problems that can overwhelm coping abilities. **EBN:** *Family assessment is integral to nursing care of clients (Northouse et al, 2002).*
- Encourage spirituality as a source of support for coping. **EBN:** *Many African Americans and Latinos identify spirituality, religiousness, prayer, and church-based approaches as coping resources (Abrums, 2004; Coon et al, 2004; Weaver & Flannelly, 2004). A sense of faith is an important component of*

• = Independent   ▲ = Collaborative   **EBN** = Evidence-Based Nursing   **EB** = Evidence-Based

psychosocial well-being in individuals with advanced cancer (Lin & Bauer-Wu, 2003). Spirituality has a positive effect on coping (Kelly, 2004).

- Negotiate with the client with regard to the aspects of coping behavior that will need to be modified. **EBN:** *As a part of the assessment of coping behaviors, alternate methods may be introduced and offered to the client as a possible choice in new coping strategies (Wassem, Beckham, & Dudley, 2001).*
- Encourage moderate aerobic exercise (as appropriate). **EBN:** *In a group of African American elders with chronic health conditions, exercise was used as a coping strategy for effectively managing chronic health conditions (Loeb, 2006).*
- Identify which family members the client can count on for support. **EBN:** *In a variety of different cultures family members are relied on to cope with stress (Donnelly, 2002; Gleeson-Kreig, Bernal, & Woolley, 2002; White et al, 2002).*
- Support the inner resources that clients use for coping. **EBN:** *African American women in one study used inner resources to develop self-help strategies to cope with reactions following involuntary pregnancy loss (Van & Meleis, 2003).*
- Use an empowerment framework to redefine coping strategies. **EB:** *Empowerment strategies are important for people with severe mental illness (Linhorst et al, 2002).*

 Home Care

- The interventions described previously may be adapted for home care use.
- ▲ Assess for suicidal tendencies. Refer for mental health care immediately if indicated.
- Identify an emergency plan should the client become suicidal. *Ineffective coping can occur in a crisis situation and can lead to suicidal ideation if the client sees no hope for a solution. A suicidal client is not safe in the home environment unless supported by professional help. Refer to the care plan for* **Risk for Suicide**.
- Observe the family for coping behavior patterns. Obtain family and client history as possible. **EB:** *Family assessment is necessary to guide interventions and activate appropriate resources (Ellenwood & Jenkins, 2007).*
- ▲ Assess for effective symptoms after cerebrovascular accident (CVA) in the elderly, particularly emotional lability and depression. Refer for evaluation and treatment as indicated. **EBN:** *In a study of older persons poststroke, researchers found a range of physical and psychological concerns; with some clients expressing fears of getting worse while others expressed hope for recovery. In either case, nurses can assist with the needs and promote the use of effective coping (Popovich, Fox, & Bandagi, 2007).*
- Encourage the client to use self-care management to increase the experience of personal control. Identify with the client all available supports and sense of attachment to others. Refer to the care plan for **Powerlessness. EBN:** *In a study of coping strategies of Latino women spouses of stroke survivors, women maintained a sense of spousal obligation to care and used emotion focused coping to preserve their own physical and psychological health (Arabit, 2008).*
- ▲ Refer the client and family to support groups. **EBN:** *Predictors of participation in support groups by cancer clients include trusted others' views of support groups, support received from special others, and the person's own beliefs about support groups (Grande, Myers, & Sutton, 2006).*
- ▲ If monitoring medication use, contract with the client or solicit assistance from a responsible caregiver. *Elders with arthritis identified taking medications as an assertive action coping strategy (Tak, 2006).*
- ▲ Institute case management for frail elderly clients to support continued independent living. **EBN:** *Case management provides home-based care of frail elderly using a process of assessment and medication review leading to new diagnoses, coordination of care, and tailoring of services that match individual needs (Elwyn et al, 2008).*
- ▲ If the client is homebound, refer for psychiatric home health care services for client reassurance and implementation of a therapeutic regimen. **EBN:** *Researchers found a therapeutic life review intervention delivered by home care workers enhanced mood in women participants (Symes et al, 2007).* **EB:** *An intervention study of a peer-based and regular case management for community-dwelling adults with severe mental illness demonstrated that improved positive regard at 6 months predicted and sustained treatment motivation for psychiatric, alcohol, and drug use problems and attendance at Alcoholics and Narcotics Anonymous meetings (Sells et al, 2006).*

Client/Family Teaching and Discharge Planning

- Teach the client to problem solve. Have the client define the problem and cause, and list the advantages and disadvantages of the options. **EB:** *A systematic review regarding healthy coping in diabetes management suggested there is evidence from well-controlled intervention studies about coping/problem solving interventions, which support their use (Fisher et al, 2007).*

- Provide the seriously ill client and his or her family with needed information regarding the condition and treatment. **EB:** *Researchers concluded that seriously ill hospitalized clients have poor knowledge of CPR and would benefit from improved understanding of CPR and their role (clients and family) in the decision-making process (Heyland et al, 2006).*

- Teach relaxation techniques. **EBN:** *Mindfulness meditation (MBSR) was taught to community-dwelling adults who found the intervention promoted health awareness, personal self-care, and overall well-being (Matchim, Armer, & Stewart, 2008).*

- Work closely with the client to develop appropriate educational tools that address individualized needs. **EB:** *Researchers developed a purpose-based information assessment (PIA) tool to evaluate how effective the information met the clients' individual needs; findings included estimates supporting the validity, reliability, and sensitivity of the PIA. Researchers concluded that the PIA can be used to identify strengths and limitations in meeting an individual's information needs (Feldman-Stewart, Brennestuhl, & Brundage, 2007).*

- ▲ Teach the client about available community resources (e.g., therapists, ministers, counselors, self-help groups). **EB and EBN:** *While research suggests that persons needing community services are interested in using them, not all who need services use them, due in part to the need for more information about resources, how to use them more effectively, or availability of services (Cohen-Mansfield & Frank, 2008; Janda et al, 2008).*

⊖volve   See the EVOLVE website for Weblinks for client education resources.

REFERENCES

Abrums M: Faith and feminism: how African American women from a storefront church resist oppression in healthcare, *ANS Adv Nurs Sci* 27(3):187–201, 2004.

Alsen P, Brink E, Persson L: Living with incomprehensible fatigue after recent myocardial infarction, *J Adv Nurs* 64(5): 459–468, 2008.

Arabit LD: Coping strategies of Latino women caring for a spouse recovering from stroke: A grounded theory, *J Theory Construct* 12(2):42–49, 2008.

Arias AJ, Steinberg K, Banga A et al: Systematic review of the efficacy of meditation techniques as treatments for medical illness, *J Alt Comp Med* 12(8):817–832, 2006.

Ark PD, Hull PC, Husaini BA et al: Religiosity, religious coping styles, and health service use, *J Geront Nurs* 32(8):20–29, 2006.

Bauer-Wu S, Sullivan AM, Rosenbaum E: Facing the challenges of hematopoietic stem cell transplantation with mindfulness meditation: a pilot study, *Integr Cancer Ther* 7(2):62–69, 2008.

Blomquist K, Edberg AK: Living with persistent pain: experiences of older people receiving home care, *J Adv Nurs* 40(3):297–306, 2002.

Boerner K, Reinhardt JP, Horowitz A: The effect of rehabilitation service use on coping patterns over time among older adults with age-related vision loss, *Clin Rehab* 20(6):478–487, 2006.

Chan SW, Levy V, Chung TK et al: A qualitative study of a group of Hong Kong Chinese women diagnosed with postnatal depression, *J Adv Nurs* 39(6):571–579, 2002.

Chen YC: Chinese values, health, and nursing, *J Adv Nurs* 36(2):270–273, 2001.

Cohen-Mansfield J, Frank J: Relationship between perceived needs and assessed needs for services in community-dwelling older persons, *Gerontologist* 48(4):505–516, 2008.

Coon DW, Rubert M, Solano N et al: Well-being, appraisal, and coping in Latina and Caucasian female dementia caregivers: findings from the REACH study, *Aging Ment Health* 8(4):330–345, 2004.

Davis MC: Life review therapy as an intervention to manage depression and enhance life satisfaction in individuals with right hemisphere cerebral vascular accidents, *Issues Ment Health Nurs* 25(5):503–515, 2004.

Dawson KA, Schneider MA, Fletcher PC et al: Examining gender differences in the health behaviors of Canadian university students, *J R Soc Health* 127(1):38–44, 2007.

Desbiens J, Fillion L: Coping strategies, emotional outcomes, and spiritual care nurses, *Intl J Pal Nurs* 13(6):291–300, 2007.

Donnelly TT: Contextual analysis of coping: implications for immigrants' mental health care, *Issues Ment Health Nurs* 23:715–732, 2002.

Duff E, Firth M, Barr K et al: A follow-up study of oncology nurses after communication skills training, *Ca Nurs Pract* 8(1):27–31, 2009.

Ducharme F, Lebel P, Lachance L et al: Implementation and effects of an individual stress management intervention for family caregivers of an elderly relative living at home: a mixed research design, *Res Nurs Health* 29(5):427–441, 2006.

Ellenwood AE, Jenkins JE: Unbalancing the effects of chronic illness: non-traditional family therapy assessment and intervention approach, *Am J Fam Ther* 35(3):265–277, 2007.

Elwyn G, Williams M, Roberts C et al: Case management by nurses in primary care: analysis of 73 "success stories," *Qual Prim Care* 16(2):75–82, 2008.

Feldman-Stewart D, Brennestuhl S, Brundage MD: A purpose-based evaluation of information for patients: An approach to measuring effectiveness, *Patient Educ Couns* 65(3):311–319, 2007.

Fisher EB, Thorpe CT, Devellis BM et al: Healthy coping, negative emotions, and diabetes management: a systematic review, *Diabetes Educ* 33(6):1080–1103, 2007.

Forchuk C: A nurse-delivered intervention was effective for depression in patients with cancer, *Evid Based Nurs* 12(1):17, 2009.

● = Independent   ▲ = Collaborative   **EBN** = Evidence-Based Nursing   **EB** = Evidence-Based

Fyffe DC, Brown EL, Sirey JA et al: Older home care patients preferred approaches to depression care: a pilot study, *J Gerontol Nurs* 34(8):17–22, 2008.

Gibson LM, Hendricks CS: Integrative review of spirituality in African American breast cancer survivors, *ABNF J* 17(2):67–72, 2006.

Giske T, Gjengedal E: "Preparative waiting" and coping theory with patients going through gastric diagnosis, *J Adv Nurs* 57(1): 87–94, 2007.

Gleeson-Kreig J, Bernal H, Woolley S: The role of social support in the self-management of diabetes mellitus among a Hispanic population, *Public Health Nurs* 19(3):215–222, 2002.

Goodwin RD: Association between coping with anger and feelings of depression among youths, *AM J Publ Health* 96(4): 664–669, 2006.

Grande GE, Myers LB, Sutton SR: How do patients who participate in cancer support groups differ from those who do not? *Psychooncology* 15(4):321–334, 2006.

Hema DA, Roper SO, Nehring JW et al: Daily stressors and coping responses of children and adolescents with type 1 diabetes, *Child Care Health Dev* 35(3):330–339, 2009.

Heyland DK, Frank C, Groll D et al: Understanding cardiopulmonary resuscitation decision making: perspectives of seriously ill hospitalized patients and family members, *Chest* 130(2):419–428, 2006.

Ho APY: A peer counseling program for the elderly with depression living in the community, *Aging Ment Health* 11(1):69–74, 2007.

Houldin AD, Lewis FM: Salvaging their normal lives: a qualitative study of patients with recently diagnosed advanced colorectal cancer, *Oncol Nurs Forum* 33(4):719–725, 2006.

Janda M, Steginga S, Dunn J et al: Unmet supportive care needs and interest in services among patients with a brain tumor and their carers, *Patient Educ Couns* 71(2):251–258, 2008.

Kelly J: Spirituality as a coping mechanism, *Dimen Crit Care Nurs* 23(4):162–168, 2004.

Kraaij V, Garnefski N, Schroevers MJ: Coping, goal adjustment, and positive and negative effect in definitive infertility, *J Health Psychol* 14(1):18–26, 2009.

Kuo TT, Ma FC: Symptoms distresses and coping strategies in patients with non-small cell lung cancer, *Cancer Nurs* 25(4):309–317, 2002.

Kylmä J: Hope, despair and hopelessness in significant others of adult persons living with HIV, *J Theory Construct Test* 9(2):49–54, 2005/2006.

Lee V, Cohen SR, Edgar L et al: Meaning-making and psychological adjustment to cancer: development of an intervention and pilot results, *Oncol Nurs Forum* 33(2):291–302, 2006.

Lefler L, Bondy KN: Women's delay in seeking treatment with myocardial infarction: a meta-synthesis, *J Cardiovasc Nurs* 19(4):251–268, 2004.

Lin HR, Bauer-Wu SM: Psycho-spiritual well-being in patients with advanced cancer: an integrative review of the literature, *J Adv Nurs* 44(1):69–80, 2003.

Linhorst DM, Hamilton G, Young E et al: Opportunities and barriers to empowering people with severe mental illness through participation in treatment planning, *Soc Work* 47(4):425–434, 2002.

Loeb SJ: African American older adults coping with chronic health conditions, *J Transcult Nurs* 17(2): 139–147, 2006.

Matchim Y, Armer JM, Stewart BR: IOS new scholar paper: a qualitative study of participants perceptions of the effect of mindfulness meditation practice on self care and overall well-being, *Self Care Depend Care Nurs* 16(2):46–53, 2008.

McCauley KM, Bixby MB, Naylor MD: Advanced practice nurses strategies to improve outcomes and reduce costs in elders with heart failure, *Dis Manag* 9(5): 302–310, 2006.

Morgan MA: Considering the patient-partner relationship in cancer care: coping strategies for couples, *Clin J Oncol Nurs* 13(1):65–72, 2009.

Murray BL, Wright K: Integration of a suicide risk assessment and intervention approach: the perspective of youth, *J Psychiatr Ment Health Nurs* 13(2):157–164, 2006.

Nokes KM, Chew L, Altman C: Using telephone support group for HIV-positive persons aged 50+ to increase social support and health-related knowledge, *AIDS Patient Care STDS* 17(7):345–351, 2003.

Northouse L, Walker J, Schafenacker A et al: A family-based program of care for women with recurrent breast cancer and their family members, *Oncol Nurs Forum* 29(10):1411–1419, 2002.

Oflaz F, Haitpoglu S, Ayan H: Effectiveness of psychoeducation intervention on post-traumatic stress disorder and coping styles of earthquake survivors, *J Clin Nurs* 17(5):677–687, 2008.

Pakenham KI, Bursnall S: Relations between social support, appraisal, and coping and both positive and negative outcomes for children of a parent with multiple sclerosis and comparisons with children of healthy parents, *Clin Rehab* 20(8):709–723, 2006.

Pickett-Schenk SA, Lippincott RC, Bennett C et al: Improving knowledge about mental illness through family-led education: the journey of hope, *Psychiatr Serv* 59(1):49–56, 2008.

Popovich JM, Fox PG, Bandagi R: Coping with stroke: psychological and social dimensions in U.S. patients, *Int J Psychiatr Nurs Res* 12(3): 1474–1487, 2007.

Puentes WJ: Simple reminiscence: a stress-adaptation model of the phenomenon, *Issues Ment Health Nurs* 23(5):497–511, 2002.

Purnell LD, Paulanka BJ: *Guide to culturally competent health care,* Philadelphia, 2005, F.A. Davis.

Raleigh EDH, Robinson JH, Marold K et al: Family caregiver perception of hospice support, *J Hospice Palliat Nurs* 8(1):25–33, 2006.

Rocchiccioli JT, Sanford JT: Revisiting geriatric failure to thrive: a complex and compelling clinical condition, *J Gerontol Nurs* 35(1):18–24, 2009.

Rose LE, Gerson L, Carbo C: Transitional care for seriously mentally ill persons: a pilot study *Arch Psychiatr Nurs* 21(6):297–308, 2007.

Ross R, Sawatphanit W, Suwansujarid T: Finding peace (Kwam Sa-ngob): a Buddhist way to live with HIV, *J Holistic Nurs* 25(4):228–235, 2007.

Sells D, Davidson L, Jewell C et al: The treatment relationship in peer-based and regular case management for clients with severe mental illness, *Psychiatr Serv* 57(8):1179–1184, 2006.

Shibusawa T, Mui AC: Stress, coping and depression among Japanese American elders, *J Gerontol Soc Work* 36(1/2):63, 2001.

Sterling YM, Peterson JW: Characteristics of African American women caregivers of children with asthma, *MCN Am J Matern Child Nurs* 28(1):32–38, 2003.

Symes L, Mastel-Smith B, Hersch C et al: The feasibility of home care workers delivering an intervention to decrease depression among home-dwelling older women, *Issues Ment Health Nurs* 28(7):799–810, 2007.

Tak SH: An insider perspective of daily stress and coping in elders with arthritis, *Orthop Nurs* 25(2): 27–32, 2006.

Tryssenaar J, Chui A, Finch L: Growing older: the lived experience of older persons with serious mental illness, *Can J Community Ment Health* 22(1):21–36, 2003.

Van P, Meleis AI: Coping with grief after involuntary pregnancy loss: perspectives of African American women, *J Obstet Gynecol Neonatal Nurs* 32(1):28–39, 2003.

Vaughn AA, Roesch SC: Psychological and physical health correlates of coping in minority adolescents, *J Health Psychol* 8(6): 671–683, 2003.

Walker MJ: The effects of nurses' practicing of the HealthTouch Technique on perceived stress, spiritual well-being, and hardiness, *J Holistic Nurs* 24(3):164–175, 2006.

Wang J, Tseng H, Chen K: Development and testing of screening indicators for psychological abuse of older people, *Arch Psychiatr Nurs* 21(1):40–47, 2007.

• = Independent   ▲ = Collaborative   **EBN** = Evidence-Based Nursing   **EB** = Evidence-Based

Wassem R, Beckham N, Dudley W: Test of a nursing intervention to promote adjustment to fibromyalgia, *Orthop Nurs* 20(3):33–45, 2001.

Weaver AJ, Flannelly KJ: The role of religion/spirituality for cancer patients and their caregivers, *South Med J* 97(12):1210–1214, 2004.

White N, Bichter J, Koeckeritz J et al: A cross-cultural comparison of family resiliency in hemodialysis clients, *J Transcult Nurs* 13(3):218–227, 2002.

Readiness for enhanced Coping   *Gail B. Ladwig, MSN, RN, CHTP*

NANDA-I

Definition

A pattern of cognitive and behavioral efforts to manage demands that is sufficient for well-being and can be strengthened

Defining Characteristics

Acknowledges power; aware of possible environmental changes; defines stressors as manageable; seeks knowledge of new strategies; seeks social support; uses a broad range of emotion-oriented strategies; uses a broad range of problem-oriented strategies; uses spiritual resources

NOC (Nursing Outcomes Classification)

Suggested NOC Outcomes

Coping, Personal Well-Being, Social Interaction Skills, Quality of life

Example NOC Outcome with Indicators
Coping as evidenced by the following indicator: Identifies effective coping patterns/Uses effective coping strategies (Rate the outcome and indicators of **Coping:** 1 = never demonstrated, 2 = rarely demonstrated, 3 = sometimes demonstrated, 4 = often demonstrated, 5 = consistently demonstrated [see Section I].)

Client Outcomes

Client Will (Specify Time Frame):

- Acknowledge personal power
- State awareness of possible environmental changes that may contribute to decreased coping
- State that stressors are manageable
- Seek new effective coping strategies
- Seek social support for problems associated with coping
- Demonstrate ability to cope, using a broad range of coping strategies
- Use spiritual support of personal choice

NIC (Nursing Interventions Classification)

Suggested NIC Interventions

Coping Enhancement, Decision-Making Support

Example NIC Activities—Coping Enhancement
Assist client in developing an objective appraisal of the event; Explore with client previous methods of dealing with life problems

Nursing Interventions and *Rationales*

- Assess and support family strengths of commitment, appreciation and affection towards each other, positive communication, time together, a sense of spiritual well-being, and the ability to cope with stress and crisis. **EBN:** *With the family strengths approach, nurses help families cope by defining their visions and hopes for the future instead of looking at what factors contribute to family problems (Sittner, Hudson, & Defrain, 2007).*

● = Independent   ▲ = Collaborative   **EBN** = Evidence-Based Nursing   **EB** = Evidence-Based

- Use empathetic communication and encourage the client and family to verbalize fears, express emotions, and set goals. Be present for clients physically or by telephone. **EBN:** *This study of social support by telephone demonstrated that therapeutic presence facilitated Outcomes that include problem solving, adaptive behavior change, and diminished distress (Finfgeld-Connett, 2005). Presence involves knowing the uniqueness of the person, listening intently, and mutually defining changes in the provision of confident caring (Caldwell et al, 2005).*
- Empower the client to set realistic goals and to engage in problem solving. **EBN:** *This case study assesses how individuals who have had a stroke use continued problem-solving and goal-setting. It demonstrates that health care workers need to empower individuals to make decisions about their care so they can achieve life satisfaction (Western, 2007).*
- Encourage expression of positive thoughts and emotions. **EB:** *A technique that may help clients with bi-polar diagnosis to cope with their illness (Straughan, 2007).* **EBN:** *Clients believe that coping is important to their well-being (Edgar & Watt, 2004).*
- Encourage the client to use spiritual coping mechanisms such as faith and prayer. **EBN:** *Prayer is a powerful way of coping and is practiced by all Western religions and several Eastern traditions (Mohr, 2006). Spirituality inspired hope among caregivers of stroke clients (Pierce et al, 2008).*
- Encourage the client to visit favorite natural settings. **EB:** *Change toward positive feelings was associated in particular with natural favorite places and relaxing in them (Korpela & Ylén, 2007).*
- Help the clients with serious and chronic conditions such as depression, cancer diagnosis, and chemotherapy treatment to maintain social support networks or assist in building new ones. **EBN:** *Health care providers can encourage social support networks to help clients cope with the negative aspects of cancer and chemotherapy (Mattioli, Repinski, & Chappy, 2008).* **EB:** *Decades of research has shown that individuals with more social ties have better health outcomes and lower mortality rates across many illnesses and diseases (Voils et al, 2007).*
- ▲ Refer women facing diagnostic and curative breast cancer surgery for psychosocial support. **EB:** *Psychological distress is a central experience for women facing diagnostic and curative breast cancer surgery. Psychosocial interventions are recommended for both groups (Schnur et al, 2008).*
- ▲ Refer for cognitive behavioral therapy (CBT). **EBN:** *CBT approaches in adult acute inpatient settings can help clients to cope by facilitating client-caregiver engagement and improving hope-inspiring interventions to reduce distress (Forsyth et al, 2008).*
- Refer to the care plans for **Readiness for enhanced Communication** and **Readiness for enhanced Spiritual well-being**.

Pediatric

- Encourage exercise for children and adolescents to promote positive self-esteem, to enhance coping, and to prevent behavioral and psychological problems. **EBN:** *Exercise has positive short-term effects on self-esteem in children and young people (Ekeland et al, 2004). Physical activity helped to decrease depression and anxiety and to increase coping skills in adolescents (Beauchemin & Manns, 2008).*
- Suggest that parents with children diagnosed with cancer use computer mediated support groups to exchange messages with other parents. **EBN:** *Using computer technology for support was particularly useful for this dispersed group with limited time, helping to decrease depression and anxiety in fathers and mothers (Bragadóttir, 2008).*

Geriatric

- Consider the use of telephone support for caregivers of family members with dementia. **EB and EBN:** *Family caregivers of clients with dementia experience caregiver burden and need holistic nursing interventions, such as telephone support (Belle et al, 2006; Mason & Harrison, 2008).* **EBN:** *This study shows that families provide a considerable amount of informal care and support for older adults. Best practice is to involve families in setting goals and recommendations for plan of care (Bradway & Hirschman, 2008).*
- Support a positive sense of humor and social support. **EB:** *Social support and a sense of humor may play an important role in reinforcing self-efficacious approaches to the management of health issues in older adults (Marziali, McDonald, & Donahue, 2008).*

- Refer the older client to self-help support groups, (e.g., suggest the "Red Hat Society" for older women). **EB:** *A leisure-focused group (Red Hat Society) helped the members to cope with stressors associated with the challenges and losses of old age (Hutchinson et al, 2008).*
- ▲ Refer the client with Alzheimer's disease who is terminally ill to hospice. **EB:** *The National Institute of Clinical Excellence (NICE) and the National Council for Palliative Care (NCPC) have highlighted the importance of palliative care for people with dementia (Chatterjee, 2008).*

Multicultural

- Assess an individual's sociocultural backgrounds in teaching self-management and self-regulation as a means of supporting hope and coping with a diagnosis of type 2 diabetes. **EBN:** *Findings obtained from the themes of this study illustrated that self-management of clients with diabetes is highly related to their own sociocultural environment and experiences (Lin et al, 2008).*
- Encourage spirituality as a source of support for coping. **EBN:** *Many African Americans and Latinos may identify spirituality, religiousness, prayer, and church-based approaches as coping resources (Abrums, 2004; Coon et al, 2004; Weaver & Flannelly, 2004).*
- Refer to care plans for **Ineffective Coping**.

Home Care

- The interventions described previously may be adapted for home care use.
- Provide an Internet-based health coach to encourage self-management for clients with chronic conditions such as depression, impaired mobility and chronic pain. **EBN:** *Clients who have higher self-efficacy and participate actively in their care have better disease management. Client-provider Internet portals offer a new venue for empowering and engaging clients in better management of chronic conditions (Allen et al, 2008).*
- ▲ Refer the client to mutual health support groups. *Participating in mutual health support groups led to enhanced coping by improving psychological and social functioning (Pistrang, Barker, & Humphreys, 2008).*
- ▲ Refer the client for a behavioral program that teaches coping skills via "Lifeskills" workshop and/or video. **EB:** *Commercially available, facilitator- or self-administered behavioral training product can have significant beneficial effects on psychosocial well-being in a healthy community sample (Kirby et al, 2006).*
- ▲ Refer prostate cancer clients and their spouses to family programs that include family-based interventions of communication, hope, coping, uncertainty, and symptom management. **EBN:** *Men with prostate cancer and their spouses reported positive outcomes from a family intervention that offered them information and support (Northouse et al, 2007).*
- ▲ Refer combat veterans and service members directly involved in combat as well as those providing support to combatants, including nurses for mental health services. **EBN:** *Early identification and treatment of mental health problems may decrease the psychosocial impact of combat and thus prevent progression to more chronic and severe psychopathology such as depression and posttraumatic stress disorder (PTSD) (Gaylord, 2006; Jones et al, 2008).* **EB:** *Combat duty in Iraq was associated with high utilization of mental health services and attrition from military service after deployment (Hoge, Auchterlonie, & Milliken, 2006).*

Client/Family Teaching and Discharge Planning

- Teach the client about available community resources (e.g., therapists, ministers, counselors, self-help groups, family-education groups). **EB:** *Families need assistance in coping with health changes (Pickett-Schenk et al, 2008).*
- Teach coping skills to family caregivers of cancer clients. **EBN:** *A coping skills intervention was effective in improving caregiver quality of life, reducing burden related to client's symptoms, and caregiving tasks compared with hospice care alone or hospice plus emotional support (McMillan et al, 2006).*
- Teach caregivers the COPE intervention (creativity, optimism, planning, expert information) to assist with symptom management. **EBN:** *Symptom distress, a measure that encompasses client*

suffering along with intensity, was significantly decreased in the group in which caregivers were trained to better manage client symptoms (McMillan & Small, 2007).

ⓔvolve   See the EVOLVE website for Weblinks for client education resources.

REFERENCES

Refer to **Ineffective Coping** for additional references.

Abrums M: Faith and feminism: how African American women from a storefront church resist oppression in healthcare, *Adv Nurs Science* 27(3):187–201, 2004.

Allen M, Iezzoni LI, Huang A et al: Improving patient-clinician communication about chronic conditions: description of an internet-based nurse e-coach intervention, *Nurs Res* 57(2):107–112, 2008.

Beauchemin J, Joleen Manns J: Walking talking therapy, *Ment Health Today,* Apr:34–35, 2008.

Belle S, Burgio L, Burns R et al: Enhancing the quality of life of dementia caregivers from different ethnic or racial groups: a randomized, controlled trial, *Ann Intern Med* 145(10):727–738, 2006.

Bradway C, Hirschman KB: Working with families of hospitalized older adults with dementia: caregivers are useful resources and should be part of the care team, *Am J Nurs* 108(10):52–60, 2008.

Bragadóttir H: Computer-mediated support group intervention for parents, *J Nurs Scholarsh* 40(1):32–38, 2008.

Caldwell B, Dolye M, Morris M et al: Presencing: channeling therapeutic effectiveness with the mentally ill in a state psychiatric hospital, *Issues Ment Health Nurs* 26:853–871, 2005.

Chatterjee J: End-of-life care for patients with dementia, *Nurs Older People* 20(2):29–34, 2008.

Coon DW, Rubert M, Solano N et al: Well-being, appraisal, and coping in Latina and Caucasian female dementia caregivers: findings from the REACH study, *Aging Ment Health* 8(4):330–345, 2004.

Edgar L, Watt S: Nucare, a coping skills training intervention for oncology patients and families: participants' motivations and expectations, *Can Oncol Nurs J* 14(2):84–95, 2004.

Ekeland E, Heian F, Hagen KB et al: Exercise to improve self-esteem in children and young people, *Cochrane Database Syst Rev* (1): CD003683, 2004.

Finfgeld-Connett D: Telephone social support or nursing presence? Analysis of a nursing intervention, *Qual Health Res* 15(1):19–29, 2005.

Forsyth A, Weddle R, Drummond A et al: Implementing cognitive behaviour therapy skills in adult acute inpatient settings, *Mental Health Pract* 11(5):24–27, 2008.

Gaylord KM: The psychosocial effects of combat: the frequently unseen injury, *Crit Care Nurs Clin North Am* 18(3):349–357, 2006.

Hoge CW, Auchterlonie JL, Milliken CS: Mental health problems, use of mental health services, and attrition from military service after returning from deployment to Iraq or Afghanistan, *JAMA* 295(9):1023–1032, 2006.

Hutchinson SL, Yarnal CM, Staffordson J et al: Beyond fun and friendship: the Red Hat Society as a coping resource for older women, *Ageing Soc* 28(7):979–999, 2008.

Jones DE, Perkins K, Cook JH et al: Intensive coping skills training to reduce anxiety and depression for forward deployed troops, *Milit Med* 173(3):241–246, 2008.

Kirby ED, Williams VP, Hocking MC et al: Psychosocial benefits of three formats of a standardized behavioral stress management program, *Psychosom Med* 68(6):816–823, 2006.

Korpela KM, Ylén M: Perceived health is associated with visiting natural favorite places in the vicinity, *Health & Place* 13(1):138–151, 2007.

Lin C, Anderson R, Hagerty B et al: Diabetes self-management experience: a focus group study of Taiwanese patients with type 2 diabetes, *J Clin Nurs* 17(5a):34–52, 2008.

Marziali E, McDonald L, Donahue P: The role of coping humor in the physical and mental health of older adults, *Aging Ment Health* 12(6):713–718, 2008.

Mason BJ, Harrison BE: Telephone interventions for family caregivers of patients with dementia: what are best nursing practices? *Holist Nurs Pract* 22(6):348–354, 2008.

Mattioli JL, Repinski R, Chappy SL: The meaning of hope and social support in patients receiving chemotherapy, *Oncol Nurs Forum* 35(5):822–829, 2008.

McMillan SC, Small BJ: Using the COPE intervention for family caregivers to improve symptoms of hospice homecare patients: a clinical trial, *Oncol Nurs Forum* 34(2):313–321, 2007.

McMillan SC, Small BJ, Weitzner M et al: Impact of coping skills intervention with family caregivers of hospice patients with cancer: a randomized clinical trial, *Cancer* 106(1):214–222, 2006.

Mohr WK: Spiritual issues in psychiatric care, *Perspect Psychiatr Care* 42(3)174–183, 2006.

Northouse LL, Mood DW, Schafenacker A et al: Randomized clinical trial of a family intervention for prostate cancer patients and their spouses, *Cancer* 110(12):2809–2818, 2007.

Pickett-Schenk SA, Lippincott RC, Bennett C et al: Improving knowledge about mental illness through family-led education: the journey of hope, *Psychiatr Serv* 59(1):49–56, 2008.

Pierce L, Steiner V, Havens H et al: Spirituality expressed by caregivers of stroke survivors *West J Nurs Res* 30(5):606–619, 2008.

Pistrang N, Barker C, Humphreys K: Mutual help groups for mental health problems: a review of effectiveness studies, *Am J Community Psychol* 42(1–2):110–121, 2008.

Schnur JB, Montgomery GH, Hallquist MN et al: Anticipatory psychological distress in women scheduled for diagnostic and curative breast cancer surgery, *Int J Behav Med* 15(1):21–28, 2008.

Sittner B, Hudson D, Defrain John J: Using the concept of family strengths to enhance nursing care, *MCN Am J Matern Child Nurs* 32(6):353–357, 2007.

Straughan H: Learning to cope together, *Ment Health Today,* Oct:34–36, 2007.

Voils CI, Allaire JC, Olsen MK et al: Five-year trajectories of social networks and social support in older adults with major depression, *Int Psychogeriatr* 19(6):1110–11124, 2007.

Weaver AJ, Flannelly KJ: The role of religion/spirituality for cancer patients and their caregivers, *South Med J* 97(12):1210–1214, 2004.

Western H: Altered living: coping, hope and quality of life after stroke, *Br J Nurs* 16(20):1266–1270, 2007.

• = Independent   ▲ = Collaborative   **EBN** = Evidence-Based Nursing   **EB** = Evidence-Based

Risk for sudden infant Death syndrome

Mary E. B. Stahl, RN, MSN, CEN, and Betty J. Ackley, MSN, EdS, RN

NANDA-I

Definition

Presence of risk factors for sudden death of an infant under 1 year of age

Risk Factors

Modifiable

Delayed prenatal care; infant overheating; infant overwrapping; infants placed to sleep in the prone position; infants placed to sleep in the side-lying position; bed sharing; lack of prenatal care; postnatal infant smoke exposure; prenatal infant smoke exposure; soft underlayment (loose articles in the sleep environment)

Potentially Modifiable

Low birth weight, prematurity, young maternal age

Nonmodifiable

Ethnicity (e.g., African American or Native American), male gender, seasonality of SIDS deaths (e.g., winter and fall months), infant age of 2–4 months, possible gene mutation resulting in Brugada (QT) syndrome.

NOC   (Nursing Outcomes Classification)

Suggested NOC Outcomes

Knowledge: Child Physical Safety, Parenting Performance, Safe Home Environment, Safe Sleep Environment

Example **NOC Outcome with Indicators**
Knowledge: Child Physical Safety as evidenced by the following indicators: Description of methods to prevent SIDS/Description of first aid techniques (Rate the outcome and indicators of **Knowledge: Child Physical Safety:** 1 = none, 2 = limited, 3 = moderate, 4 = substantial, 5 = extensive [see Section I].)

Client Outcomes

Client Will (Specify Time Frame):

- Explain appropriate measures to prevent SIDS
- Demonstrate correct techniques for positioning and blanketing the infant, protecting the infant from harm

NIC   (Nursing Interventions Classification)

Suggested NIC Interventions

Infant Care, Teaching: Infant Safety 0–3 months

Example **NIC Activities—Teaching: Infant Safety**
Instruct parent/caregiver to place infant on back to sleep and keep loose bedding, pillows, and toys out of crib; Avoid holding infant while smoking

Nursing Interventions and *Rationales*

- Position infant on back to sleep, do not position in the prone position. **EB:** *The prone position for sleeping infants is a risk factor for SIDS (Malloy & Freeman, 2004). There is a striking trend in decreased incidence of SIDS since parents have been taught not to place infants in the prone position. Side*

● = Independent   ▲ = Collaborative   **EBN** = Evidence-Based Nursing   **EB** = Evidence-Based

sleeping is not as safe as supine sleeping and is not advised (American Academy of Pediatrics, 2005; Dwyer & Ponsonby, 2009).

- Avoid use of loose bedding, such as blankets and sheets for sleeping. If blankets are used, they should be tucked in around the crib mattress so the infant's face is less likely to become covered by bedding. *One strategy is to make up the bedding so that the infant's feet are able to reach the foot of the crib with the blankets tucked in around the crib mattress and reaching only the level of the infant's chest.* **EB:** *A strong interaction was found between prone sleep position and soft bedding surface, indicating that these two factors together are very hazardous. Soft surfaces have also been implicated in infant deaths occurring on adult beds (American Academy of Pediatrics, 2005).*
- To avoid overbundling and overheating the infant, lightly clothe the child for sleep. The infant should not feel hot to touch. **EB:** *Overheating the infant has been associated with increased risk of SIDS. "Head covering precedes the death and is not an agonal event and is causally related to SIDS. This supports the recommendation to avoid head covering as part of the SIDS prevention strategies" (Mitchell et al, 2008).*
- Provide the infant a certain amount of time in prone position, or "tummy time," while the infant is awake and observed. "Provide 'tummy time' when your baby is awake and someone is watching; change the direction that your baby lies in the crib from one week to the next; and avoid too much time in car seats, carriers, and bouncers" (National Institute of Childhood Health and Human Development, 2006).
- Consider offering the infant a pacifier during sleep times. **EB:** *A pacifier given at bedtime enhances the infant's ability to maintain a more adequate oral airflow. The reduced risk of SIDS associated with pacifier use during sleep is compelling, and the evidence that pacifier use inhibits breastfeeding or causes later dental complications is not (American Academy of Pediatrics, 2005). Use of a pacifier was associated with decreased incidence of SIDS (Vennemann et al, 2009).*
- ▲ Use electronic respiratory or cardiac monitors to detect cardiorespiratory arrest only if ordered. **EB:** *There is no evidence that infants prone to SIDS can be identified by monitoring of respiratory or cardiac function in the hospital. There is no evidence that use of such home monitors decreases the incidence of SIDS (American Academy of Pediatrics, 2005).*

 ### Home Care

- Most of the interventions above are relevant to home care.
- Evaluate home for potential safety hazards, such as inappropriate cribs, cradles, or strollers.
- Determine where and how the child sleeps, and provide instructions on safe sleeping positions and environments as needed.

 ### Multicultural

- Discuss cultural norms with families to provide care that is appropriate for promoting safety for the infant in sleeping arrangements and care. *Misinterpretation of parenting behaviors can occur when the nurse and parent are from different cultures.*
- Encourage American Indian mothers to avoid drinking alcoholic beverages and to avoid wrapping infants in excessive blankets or clothing. **EB:** *In the American Indian population, an association has been shown between binge drinking during pregnancy and having two or more layers of clothing on the infant (Iyasu et al, 2002).*
- Encourage African American mothers to find alternatives to bed sharing and to avoid placing pillows, soft toys, and soft bedding in the sleep environment. **EB:** *A higher incidence of SIDS occurs in African American infants. There appears to be a relationship between SIDS, race, genetics, and deaths noted in African American infants. In African Americans, there appears to be a non-synonymous single nucleotide polymorphism within exon 2 of PACAP which appears to be significantly associated with SIDS (Cummings et al, 2009). Nonetheless, among the infants that died of SIDS, most are commonly found in the supine position, but are more likely to be sharing a bed with another person (Unger et al, 2003). The greatest impact for SIDS reduction in the African American population is the need to change behaviors regarding sleep locations by reducing the instances of placing infants for sleep on adult beds, sofas, or cots (Hauck et al, 2003; Rasinski et al, 2003).*

● = Independent   ▲ = Collaborative   **EBN** = Evidence-Based Nursing   **EB** = Evidence-Based

Client/Family Teaching and Discharge Planning

- Teach families to position infants to sleep on their back rather than in the prone position. **EB:** *The prone position for sleeping infants is a risk factor for SIDS (Malloy & Freeman, 2004).*
- Teach the parents to place the infant supine to sleep with the head rotated to one side for a week, and then to the other side for the next week. Parents should also change the orientation of the crib at intervals, so the infant turns the head in alternate directions. *This is necessary to prevent the infant from developing a flat area on the back of the head.*
- Recommend the following infant care practices to parents:
  - Infants should not be put to sleep on soft surfaces such as waterbeds, sofas, or soft mattresses.
  - Avoid placing soft materials in the infant's sleeping environment such as pillows, quilts, and comforters. Do not use sheepskins under a sleeping infant.
  - Avoid the use of loose bedding, such as blankets and sheets.

  EB: *Placing an infant to sleep on a soft surface is a strong independent risk factor for SIDS (National Institute of Childhood Health and Human Development, 2006). A study of infants who were found dead in bassinets found that soft bedding was found in 74% of the cases (Pike & Moon, 2008)*
- Teach parents the need to obtain a crib that conforms to the safety standards of the Consumer Product Safety Commission. *Although many cradles and bassinets may also provide safe sleeping enclosures, safety standards have not been established for these items.*
- Teach parents not to place the infant in an adult bed to sleep, or a sofa or chair. Infants should sleep in a crib. *Sleep surfaces designed for adults have the risk of trapping the baby between the mattress and the structure of the bed (e.g., the headboard, footboard, side rails, and frame), the wall, or adjacent furniture, as well as between railings in the headboard or footboard.* **EB:** *A European study found that bed sharing with mothers who did not smoke was a significant risk factor among infants up to 8 weeks of age. Similarly, a study conducted in Scotland (Tappin, Ecob, & Brooke, 2005) found that the risk of bed sharing was greatest for infants younger than 11 weeks, and this association remained among infants with nonsmoking mothers. The risk of SIDS seems to be particularly high when there are multiple bed sharers and also may be increased when the bed sharer has consumed alcohol or is overtired (American Academy of Pediatrics Task Force, 2005).*
- Teach parents not to sleep with an infant, especially if alcohol or medications/illicit drugs are used by the parents. *"Bed sharing may increase the risk in certain circumstances from overheating, rebreathing, and exposure to tobacco smoke, all of which are known risk factors for SIDS" (Fu et al, 2008).* **EB:** *Parents under the influence of alcohol or illicit drugs or who smoke are more likely to have a SIDS result. Mothers who consume three or more alcoholic drinks in the previous 24 hours increase the risk of SIDS when bed sharing with an infant (Carpenter et al, 2004).* **EBN:** *In a study of mothers of 3–month-old infants, 39 of almost 300 mothers reported incidences when they had rolled partially or fully over the infant in the bed (Ateah & Hamelin, 2008).*
- Recommend an alternative to sleeping with an infant; parents might consider placing the infant's crib near their bed to allow for more convenient breastfeeding and parent contact. *There is growing evidence that room sharing (infant sleeping in the parent's room) without bed sharing is associated with a reduced risk of SIDS (American Academy of Pediatrics, 2005).*
- Recommend the mother breastfeed the infant. **EB:** *In a study, breastfeeding was associated with a 50% reduction in incidence of SIDS (Vennemann et al, 2009).*
- Teach parents to avoid overbundling and overheating the infant by lightly clothing the child for sleep. The infant should not feel hot to touch. The bedroom temperature should be comfortable for an adult wearing light bedclothing.
- Question parents regarding following recommendations for the prevention of SIDS at each well-baby visit or visit with a health care practitioner for illness. Strongly encourage compliance with precautions to prevent SIDS. **EB:** *Although a majority of British mothers knew the precautions, 25% of mothers were not following the recommended practice (Roberts & Upton, 2000).*
- Teach the need to stop smoking during pregnancy and to not smoke around the infant, because smoking is a risk factor for SIDS. **EBN:** *Newborns whose mothers smoke have a limited ability to maximize and vary their heart rate, which can result in the infant being unable to maximize cardiac output during stress. This increases the infant's risk for morbidity and possibly mortality (Sherman et al, 2002).* **EB:** *Smoke in the environment after birth is considered a risk factor for SIDS. Mothers should be informed of the twofold increased rate of SIDS associated with maternal cigarette consumption (Anderson, Johnson, & Batal, 2005).*

● = Independent   ▲ = Collaborative   **EBN** = Evidence-Based Nursing   **EB** = Evidence-Based

- Recommend that parents with infants in child care make it very clear to the employees that the infant must always be placed in the supine position to sleep, not prone or in a side-lying position. **EB:** *Only 14.3% of licensed child care facilities are in compliance with the recommendation that infants be placed in the supine position to sleep. Temporary caretakers who change an infant's usual sleeping position increase the risk of SIDS, because infant sleep physiology differs when they are sleeping in the prone position rather than the supine position (Li et al, 2003).*

▲ Suggest speaking with a physician about genetic counseling. *In light of recent genetic research, it is reasonable to suggest that families that have lost an infant to SIDS or who have a family history of other unexplained deaths, fainting episodes, or seizures seek consultation (Mayo Clinic, 2006).*

- Teach child care employees how best to position infants for sleeping and the dangers of a too soft environment. **EB:** *A 60–minute educational experience designed for child care providers may be effective in increasing the compliance with guidelines and increasing the number of written sleep position policies at the child care centers (Moon & Oden, 2003).*

▲ Involve family members in learning and practicing rescue techniques, including treatment of choking, breathing, and cardiopulmonary resuscitation (CPR). Initiate referral to formal training classes. *Family members need adequate preparation to deal with emergency situations and should take part in the AHA Basic Lifesaving Course or the American Red Cross Infant/Child CPR Course. "Ventricular fibrillation has been newly considered as an important cause of cardiac arrest in children and adolescents in several recent studies, which underscores the importance of basic life support training for the public, because cardiopulmonary resuscitation (CPR) is needed before attempted defibrillation"* (Pyles et al, 2004). **EBN:** *Concerns about CPR training resulting in increased anxiety for parents are unsupported by scientific data (Pyles et al, 2004).*

ⓔvolve   See the EVOLVE website for Weblinks for client education resources.

REFERENCES

American Academy of Pediatrics Task Force on Sudden Infant Death Syndrome: The changing concept of sudden infant death syndrome: diagnostic coding shifts, controversies regarding the sleeping environment, and new variables to consider in reducing risk, *Pediatrics* 116(5):1245–1255, 2005.

Anderson M, Johnson D, Batal HL: Sudden infant death syndrome and prenatal maternal smoking: rising attributed risk in back to sleep era, *BMC Med* 3:4, 2005.

Ateah CA, Hamelin KJ: Maternal bedsharing practices, experiences, and awareness of risks, *J Obstet Gynecol Neonatal Nurs* 37(3):274–281, 2008.

Carpenter RG, Irgens LM, Blair PS et al: Sudden unexplained infant death in 20 regions in Europe: case control study, *Lancet* 363(9404):185–191, 2004.

Cummings KJ, Klotz C, Liu WQ et al: Sudden infant death syndrome (SIDS) in African Americans: polymorphisms in the gene encoding the stress peptide pituitary adenylate cyclase-activating polypeptide (PACAP), *Acta Paediatr* 98(3):482–489, 2009.

Dwyer T, Ponsonby AL: Sudden infant death syndrome and prone sleeping position, *Ann Epidemiol* 19(4):245–249, 2009.

Fu L, Colson E, Corwin M et al: Infant sleep location: associated maternal and infant characteristics with sudden infant death syndrome prevention recommendations, *J Pediatr* 153(4):503–508, 2008.

Hauck FR, Herman SM, Donovan M et al: Sleep environment and the risk of sudden infant death syndrome in an urban population: the Chicago infant mortality study, *Pediatrics* 111(5 part 2):1207–1214, 2003.

Iyasu S, Randall LL, Welty TK et al: Risk factors for sudden infant death syndrome among northern plains Indians, *JAMA* 288(21):2717–2723, 2002.

Li DK, Petitti DB, Willinger M et al: Infant sleeping position and the risk of sudden infant death syndrome in California, *Am J Epidemiol* 157(5):446–455, 2003.

Malloy MH, Freeman DH: Age at death, season, and day of death as indicators of the effect of the back to sleep program on sudden infant death syndrome in the United States, 1992–1999, *Arch Pediatr Adolesc Med* 158(4):359–365, 2004.

Mayo Clinic in Rochester: *Researchers link two more genes to sudden infant death syndrome,* Rochester, MN, 2006, Mayo Clinic. Accessed June 8, 2009 from www.mayoclinic.org/news2006–rst/3408.html.

Mitchell EA, Thompson JMD, Becroft DMO et al: Head covering and the risk for SIDS: findings from the New Zealand and German SIDS case-controlled studies, *Pediatrics* 121(6):e1478–1483, 2008.

Moon RY, Oden RP: Back to sleep: can we influence child care providers? *Pediatrics* 112(4):878–882, 2003.

National Institute for Childhood Health and Human Development (Updated 9/15/06): *Safe sleep for your baby: ten ways to reduce the risk of sudden infant death syndrome,* www.nichd.nih.gov/publications/pubs/safe_sleep_gen.cfm. Accessed March 27, 2009.

Pike J, Moon RY: Bassinet use and sudden unexpected death in infancy, *J Pediatr* 153(4):509–512, 2008.

Pyles L, Knaff J, American Academy of Pediatrics Committee on Pediatric Emergency Medicine: Role of pediatricians in advocating life support training courses for parents and the public, *Pediatrics* 114(6):e761–765, 2004.

Rasinski KA, Kuby A, Bzdusek SA et al: Effect of a sudden infant death syndrome risk reduction education program on risk factor compliance and information sources in primarily black urban communities, *Pediatrics* 111(4 Pt 1):E347–E354, 2003.

Roberts H, Upton D: New mother's knowledge of sudden infant death syndrome risk reduction education program on risk factor compliance and information sources in primarily back urban communities, *Pediatrics* 111(4Pt1): E347–E354, 2000.

Sherman J, Young A, Sherman MP et al: Prenatal smoking and alterations in newborn heart rate during transition, *J Obstet Gynecol Neonatal Nurs* 31(6):680–687, 2002.

Tappin D, Ecob R, Brooke H: Bedsharing, roomsharing, and sudden infant death syndrome in Scotland: a case-control study, *J Pediatr* 147(1):32–32, 2005.

Unger B, Kemp JS, Wilkins D et al: Racial disparity and modifiable risk factors among infants dying suddenly and unexpectedly, *Pediatrics* 111(2):E127–E131, 2003.

● = Independent   ▲ = Collaborative   **EBN** = Evidence-Based Nursing   **EB** = Evidence-Based

Vennemann MM, Bajanowski T, Brinkmann B et al: The GeSID Study Group. Sleep environment risk factors for sudden infant death syndrome: the German Sudden Infant Death Syndrome Study, *Pediatrics* 123(4):1162–1170, 2009.

Readiness for enhanced Decision-Making

Dawn Fairlie, ANP, FNP, GNP, DSN(c), and Marie Giordano, RN, MS

Definition

A pattern of choosing courses of action that is sufficient for meeting short- and long-term health-related goals and can be strengthened

Defining Characteristics

Expresses desire to enhance decision making; expresses desire to enhance congruency of decisions with goals; expresses desire to enhance congruency of decisions with personal values; expresses desire to enhance congruency of decisions with sociocultural goals; expresses desire to enhance congruency of decisions with sociocultural values; expresses desire to enhance risk benefit analysis of decisions; expresses desire to enhance understanding of choices for decision making, expresses desire to enhance understanding of the meaning of choices expresses desire to enhance use of reliable evidence for decisions.

 (Nursing Outcomes Classification)

Suggested NOC Outcomes

Decision Making, Participation in Health Care Decisions, Personal Autonomy

Example NOC Outcome with Indicators
Participation in Health Care Decisions as evidenced by the following indicators: Claims decision making responsibility/Exhibits self-direction in decision making/Seeks reputable information/Specifies health outcome preferences (Rate the Outcome and Indicators of **Participation in Health Care Decisions** as 1 = never demonstrated, 2 = rarely demonstrated; 3 = sometimes demonstrated, 4 = often demonstrated, 5 = consistently demonstrated [see Section I].)

Client Outcomes

Client Will (Specify Time Frame):

- Review treatment options with providers
- Ask questions about the benefits and risks of treatment options
- Communicate decisions about treatment options to providers in relation to personal preferences, values and goals

 (Nursing Interventions Classification)

Suggested NIC Interventions

Decision-Making Support, Mutual Goal Setting, Support System Enhancement, Values Clarification

Example NIC Activities—Decision-Making Support
Help patient to identify the advantages and disadvantages of each alternative; Facilitate collaborative decision making; Help patient to explain decisions to others, as needed

Nursing Interventions and *Rationales*

- Support and encourage clients and their representatives to engage in health care decisions. **EB:** *"A number of research studies have concluded that there is a positive link between the practice of patient-centered healthcare in clinical settings and positive outcomes."* The positive health outcomes

• = Independent   ▲ = Collaborative   **EBN** = Evidence-Based Nursing   **EB** = Evidence-Based

of client-centered care include "patient satisfaction, emotional health, symptom resolution, function, physiological measures, quality of life . . ." (Harkness, 2005).

- Respect personal preferences, values, needs, and rights. **EB:** *Only the client and family for whom treatment is intended can know how the treatment will affect them (Harkness, 2005).*
- Determine the degree of participation desired by the client. **EBN:** *In a study of 80 nurse-client dyads, it was found that nurses were not always aware of their clients' perspectives and tended to overestimate the clients' willingness to participate (Florin, Ehrenberg, & Ehnfors, 2006).*
- Provide access to health care services as needed. One type of access to consider is interactive, Internet-based decision supports. **EB:** *Decision making related to health care services is directly affected by access to such services (Harkness, 2005).* **EB:** *Traditional formats such as verbal instructions and reading materials with intense amounts of information often do not work (Evans, Elwyn, & Edwards, 2004). The Internet can offer clients a range of opportunities to ask complex questions related to health and illness (Evans, Elwyn, & Edwards, 2004).*
- Provide information that is appropriate, relevant, and timely. **EB:** *This "enables patients [and their representatives] to make informed decisions and to take effective action to improve their health" (Harkness, 2005).*
- Determine the health literacy of clients and their representatives prior to helping with decision making. **EB:** *Communication skills are crucial in shared decision making, especially for clients with low literacy. Tailoring information and communication to clients' individual needs is beneficial (Shaw et al, 2009).*
- Tailor information to the specific needs of individual clients, according to principles of health literacy. **EB:** *The format of relevant information should be adapted in consideration of the individual's condition, language, age, understanding, abilities, and culture (Harkness, 2005).*
- Motivate clients to be as independent as possible in decision making. **EB:** *Clients should be the leaders in their own health care decisions (Harkness, 2005).*
- Identify the client's level of choice in decision making. **EB:** *Some clients want to be completely involved in all decisions; other clients prefer to have less involvement (Harkness, 2005).*
- Focus on the positive aspects of decision making, rather than decisional conflicts. **EBN:** *Numerous studies conducted during development of the health promotion model show that promotion differs from prevention and requires a positive rather than negative approach (Pender, Murdaugh, & Parsons, 2006).*
- Design educational interventions for decision support. **EBN:** *Helpline nurses' barriers to providing decision support were decreased by specific educational and institutional interventions (Stacey et al, 2008).*
- Provide clients with the benefits of decisions at the same time as helping them to identify strategies to reduce the barriers for healthful decisions. **EB:** *The attrition in programs for the prevention of mother-to-child-transmission of HIV is partially due the attitude of the male partner toward involvement and a low participation rate, suggesting that external barriers play a large role in this decision-making process and that partner's needs should be addressed more specifically when providing services (Theuring et al, 2009).*
- Acknowledge the complexity of everyday self-care decisions related to self-management of chronic illnesses. **EB:** *Individual's participation in day-to-day life is influenced by personal characteristics as well as the environment, and these influence a person's decision to return to walking in their community after stroke (Corrigan & McBurney, 2008).*

Geriatric

- The above interventions may be adapted for geriatric clients.
- See care plan for **Decisional Conflict**.

Multicultural

- Use existing decision aids for particular types of decisions, or develop decision aids as indicated. **EBN:** *A decision-making tree predicted 13 criteria that Taiwanese women use to make decisions about hysterectomy (Wu et al, 2005).*

● = Independent   ▲ = Collaborative   **EBN** = Evidence-Based Nursing   **EB** = Evidence-Based

Home Care

- The above interventions may be adapted for home care use.
- Develop clinical practice guidelines that include shared decision making. **EBN:** *An intervention study using a pretest/posttest design with both an intervention and control group demonstrated that clinical practice guidelines, which focused on client autonomy and shared decision making, were effective in helping older adults to improve their use of assistive devices (Roelands et al, 2004).*

Client/Family Teaching and Discharge Planning

- Before teaching, identify client preferences in involvement with decision making. **EB:** *This study compared clients' desire regarding their level of involvement in decision making about their care with the perceptions of their doctors regarding the clients' desire to be involved. Results showed an underestimation by the physician in the clients' desire to be involved in decision making (Cox et al, 2007).*

See the EVOLVE website for Weblinks for client education resources.

REFERENCES

Corrigan R, McBurney H: Community ambulation: influences on therapists and clients reasoning and decision making, *Disabil Rehabil* 30(15):1079–1087, 2008.

Cox K, Britten N, Hooper R et al: Patients' involvement in decisions about medicines: GPs' perceptions of their preferences, *Br J Gen Pract* 57(543):777–84, 2007.

Evans R, Elwyn G, Edwards A: Making interactive decision support for patients a reality, *Inform Prim Care* 12:109–113, 2004.

Florin J, Ehrenberg A, Ehnfors M: Patient participation in clinical decision-making in nursing: a comparative study of nurses' and patients' perceptions, *J Clin Nurs* 15(12):1498–1508, 2006.

Harkness J: Patient involvement: a vital principle for patient-centered health care, *World Hosp Health Serv* 41(2):12–16, 2005.

Pender NJ, Murdaugh CL, Parsons MA: *Health promotion in nursing practice*, ed 5, Upper Saddle River, NJ, 2006, Pearson Prentice Hall.

Roelands M, Van Oost P, Stevens V et al: Clinical practice guidelines to improve shared decision-making about assistive device use in home care: a pilot interventions study, *Patient Educ Couns* 55:252–264, 2004.

Shaw A, Ibrahim, S, Reid F et al: Patients' perspectives of the doctor-patient relationship and information giving across a range of literacy levels, *Patient Educ Couns* 75:114–120, 2009.

Stacey D, Chambers SK, Jacobsen MJ et al: Overcoming barriers to cancer-helpline professionals providing decision support for callers: an implementation study, *Oncol Nurs Forum* 35:961–969, 2008.

Theuring S, Mbezi P, Luvanda H et al: Male involvement in PMTCT Services in Mbeya Region, Tanzania, *AIDS Behav* 13(Suppl 1):92–102, 2009.

Wu S-M, Yu Y-MC, Yang C-F et al: Decision-making tree for women considering hysterectomy, *J Adv Nurs* 51(4):361–368, 2005.

Ineffective Denial   *Mary T. Shoemaker, RN, MSN, SANE*

NANDA-I

Definition

Conscious or unconscious attempt to disavow the knowledge or meaning of an event to reduce anxiety/fear, but leading to the detriment of health

Defining Characteristics

Delays seeking health care attention to the detriment of health; displaces fear of impact of the condition; displaces source of symptoms to other organs; displays inappropriate affect; does not admit fear of death; does not admit fear of invalidism; does not perceive personal relevance of danger; does not perceive personal relevance of symptoms; makes dismissive comments when speaking of distressing events; makes dismissive gestures when speaking of distressing events; minimizes symptoms; refuses health care attention to the detriment of health; unable to admit impact of disease on life pattern; uses self-treatment

Related Factors (r/t)

Anxiety; fear of death; fear of loss of autonomy; fear of separation; lack of competency in using effective coping mechanisms; lack of control of life situation; lack of emotional support from others; overwhelming stress; threat of inadequacy in dealing with strong emotions; threat of unpleasant reality

• = Independent   ▲ = Collaborative   **EBN** = Evidence-Based Nursing   **EB** = Evidence-Based

(Nursing Outcomes Classification)

Suggested NOC Outcomes

Acceptance: Health Status, Anxiety Self-Control, Health Beliefs: Perceived Threat, Symptom Control

Example NOC Outcome with Indicators
Anxiety Self-Control as evidenced by the following indicators: Eliminates precursors of anxiety/Monitors physical manifestations of anxiety/Controls anxiety response (Rate the outcome and indicators of **Anxiety Self-Control:** 1 = never demonstrated, 2 = rarely demonstrated, 3 = sometimes demonstrated, 4 = often demonstrated, 5 = consistently demonstrated [see Section I].)

Client Outcomes

Client Will (Specify Time Frame):

- Seek out appropriate health care attention when needed
- Use home remedies only when appropriate
- Display appropriate affect and verbalize fears
- Actively engage in treatment program related to identified "substance" of abuse
- Remain substance-free
- Demonstrate alternate adaptive coping mechanism

NIC **(Nursing Interventions Classification)**

Suggested NIC Intervention

Anxiety Reduction

Example NIC Activities—Anxiety Reduction
Use a calm, reassuring approach; Stay with the patient to promote safety and reduce fear

Nursing Interventions and *Rationales*

- Determine the client's understanding of symptoms of illness, treatments, and expected outcomes. **EBN:** *The themes of shame and social stigma related to personal beliefs about self, personal relationships, and social relationships intersected with the theme of denial and difficulty in accepting the HIV diagnosis (Konkle-Parker, Erlen, & Dubbert, 2008).*
- Spend time with the client and allow time for responses. *Nursing presence and one-on-one interaction support the nurse-client relationship. Nurses must understand that presence provides meaning; engenders feelings of comfort and peacefulness; diminishes anxiety, loneliness, and vulnerability; and reassures when no words exist (Stanley, 2006).*
- Assess whether the use of denial is helping or hindering the client's care. Provide support for clients who are using denial as a way of coping. **EBN:** *Denial may be used as an adaptive mechanism during times of illness and stress. Patience, understanding, and self-awareness are crucial for providing a safe, trusting environment for clients who are experiencing denial (Stephenson, 2004).*
- Allow the client to express and use denial as a coping mechanism. **EBN:** *To meet health requirements, assess the coping mechanism of denial of illness and support the client in examining/developing appropriate strategies in order to assist in their implementation of self-management (McGann, Sexton, & Chyun, 2008).*
- Avoid confrontation and consider the client as an equal partner in health care. **EBN:** *The crucial attitude is a respectful listening to the person with a desire to understand his or her perspectives on care decisions (Cook, 2008).*
- Support the client's spiritual coping measures. **EBN:** *Most religious coping is considered positive (Meisenhelder, 2002). Physical and mental health is interrelated with spiritual health (Taylor, 2002).*
- Develop a trusting, therapeutic relationship with the client/family. **EBN:** *Nurses who develop trusting relationships demonstrate a holistic approach to caring; show their understanding of clients' suffer-*

● = Independent   ▲ = Collaborative   **EBN** = Evidence-Based Nursing   **EB** = Evidence-Based

ing; are aware of their unvoiced needs; provide comfort without actually being asked; and are reliable, proficient, competent, and dedicated in their care (Mok & Chui, 2004).

- Encourage individual family members to share their concerns and worries. **EBN:** *This communication may help reframe the experience in a way that is acceptable, and allows the nurse to identify possible misperceptions and/or questions (Goossens, Knoppert-van der Klein, & van Achterberg, 2008).*
▲ Explain signs and symptoms of illness; as necessary, reinforce use of the prescribed treatment plan. **EBN:** *A straightforward education on the effects of mental illness is integral to the client's motivation (Goossens, Knoppert-van der Klein, & van Achterberg 2008).*
- Have the client make choices regarding treatment and actively involve him or her in the decision-making process. **EB:** *"Forced retention" is not linked to positive results for drug-addicted offenders (Brochu et al, 2006).*
- Help the client recognize existing and additional sources of support; allow time for adjustment. **EBN:** *The use of caring behaviors supports active participation in one's treatment regiment (Owens, 2006).*
- Refer to care plans **Defensive Coping** and **Dysfunctional Family processes**.

Geriatric

- Identify recent losses of the client, because grieving may prolong denial. Encourage the client to take one day at a time. *Older adult clients often have experienced significant, multiple losses in a variety of domains. This may complicate adaptation to an individual change in health status, because the resources formerly used for successful adaptation are no longer available (Boyd & Stanley, 2002).*
- Encourage the client to verbalize feelings. **EBN:** *Bereaved individuals benefit from individual, family and group therapy to discuss losses (Douglas, 2004).*
- Encourage communication among family members. *Communication problems within families are pivotal in the development of family adjustment to a change in health status and/or adaptation to a life change (Hanson et al, 2002).*
- Recognize denial. **EB:** *Older adults selected more avoidance-denial strategies than young adults when solving interpersonal problems (Blanchard-Fields, Mienaltowski, & Seay, 2007).*
- Use reality-focusing techniques. Wherever possible, provide realistic feedback, allowing the client to validate his or her perceptions. *Providing validation of actual stressors and available resources aids in a positive adaptation (Pakenham, 2001).*

Multicultural

- Assess for the influence of cultural beliefs, norms, and values on the client's understanding of and ability to acknowledge health status. **EBN:** *Willingness to acknowledge health status may be based on cultural perceptions (Giger & Davidhizar, 2008).*
- Discuss with the client those aspects of his or her health behavior/lifestyle that will remain unchanged by health status. **EBN:** *Aspects of the client's life that are meaningful and valuable to him or her should be understood and preserved without change (Leininger & McFarland, 2002).*
- Negotiate with the client regarding the aspects of health behavior that will need to be modified as a result of health status. **EBN:** *Give and take with the client will lead to culturally congruent care (Leininger & McFarland, 2002).*
- Assess the role of fatalism in the client's ability to acknowledge health status. **EBN:** *Fatalistic perspectives, which involve the belief that you cannot control your own fate, may influence health behaviors in some Asian, African American, and Latino populations (Chen, 2001). A culturally appropriate way to deal with fatalistic views is to communicate to the family that it is also fate that the best care is available (Munet-Vilaro, 2004; Gullatte et al, 2009).*
- Validate the client's feelings of anxiety and fear related to health status. **EBN:** *Validation lets family members know that the nurse has heard and understood what was said, and it promotes the relationship between nurse and family members (Spiers, 2002).*

Home Care

- Previously mentioned interventions may be adapted for home care use.

- Observe family interaction and roles. Assess whether denial is being used to meet the needs of another family member. *Communication problems within families are pivotal in the development of family adjustment to a change in health status and/or adaptation to a life change (Hanson et al, 2002).*
- ▲ Refer the client/family for follow-up if prolonged denial is a risk. *Family therapy has been demonstrated to enhance treatment adherence and facilitate implementation and monitoring of contingency contracts with opioid-dependent clients (Work Group on Substance Use Disorders, 2006).*
- Encourage communication between family members, particularly when dealing with the loss of a significant person. **EBN:** *An understanding of the family structure, patterns of communication, health care history, and cultural influences will facilitate effective nursing interventions. In the context of some family patterns of communication, defensive coping may be a learned behavior (Hellemann, Lee & Kary, 2002).*

Client/Family Teaching and Discharge Planning

- Teach signs and symptoms of illness and appropriate responses (e.g., taking medication, going to the emergency department, calling the physician). Provide a list of names and numbers. *Family members should be involved at all points of care to ensure that the necessary care will be provided in a safe, accurate manner (Harmon, 2001).*
- Teach family members that denial may continue throughout the adjustment to treatment and they should not be confrontational. *These individuals often are in denial of their substance abuse problem—a normal part of their disease—and require behavioral modification therapy for effective treatment (Spolarich, 2006).*
- ▲ If the problem is substance abuse, refer to an appropriate community agency (e.g., Alcoholics Anonymous). **EBN:** *Families need assistance in coping with health changes. The nurse is often perceived as the individual who can help them obtain necessary social support (Northouse et al, 2002; Tak & McCubbin, 2002).*
- Teach families of clients with brain injuries that denial has been associated with damage to the right hemisphere. *The client may exhibit inappropriate affect and anxiety.*
- Inform family of available community support resources. *Mutual support groups can have a positive effect not only in Western cultures but also in Eastern cultures (Fung & Chien, 2002).*

ⓔvolve   See the EVOLVE website for Weblinks for client education resources.

REFERENCES

See **Defensive Coping** for additional references.

Blanchard-Fields F, Mienaltowski A, Seay RB: Age differences in everyday problem-solving effectiveness: older adults select more effective strategies for interpersonal problems, *J Gerontol B Psychol Sci Soc Sci* 62(1):P61–P64, 2007.

Boyd MA, Stanley M: Mental health assessment of the elderly. In Boyd MA, editor: *Psychiatric nursing in contemporary practice*, ed 2, Philadelphia, 2002, Lippincott.

Brochu S, Cournoyer LG, Tremblay J et al: Understanding treatment impact on drug-addicted offenders, *Subst Use Misuse* 41(14):1937–1949, 2006.

Chen YC: Chinese values, health and nursing, *J Adv Nurs* 36(2):270, 2001.

Cook P: Patients' and health care practitioners' attributions about adherence problems as predictors of medication adherence, *Res Nurs Health* 31(3):261–173, 2008.

Douglas DH: The lived experience of loss: a phenomenological study, *J Am Psychiatr Nurses Assoc* 10(1):24–32, 2004.

Fung WY, Chien WT: The effectiveness of a mutual support group for family caregivers of a relative with dementia, *Arch Psychiatr Nurs* 16(3):134, 2002.

Giger J, Davidhizar R: *Transcultural nursing: assessment and intervention*, ed 5, St Louis, 2008, Mosby.

Goossens P, Knoppert-van der Klein E, van Achterberg T: Coping styles of outpatients with a bipolar disorder, *Arch Psychiatric Nurs* 22(5):245–53, 2008.

Gullatte M, Brawley O, Kinney A et al: Religiosity, spirituality, and cancer fatalism beliefs on delay in breast cancer diagnosis in African American women, *J Relig Health* Jan 30, 2009 [Epub ahead of print].

Hanson E, Andersson BA, Magnusson L et al: Information center: responding to needs of older people and carers, *Br J Nurs* 11(14):935–940, 2002.

Harmon SMH: *Family health care nursing*, Philadelphia, 2001, FA Davis.

Hellemann MS V, Lee KA, Kary FS: Strengths and vulnerabilities of women of Mexican descent in relation to depressive symptoms, *Nurs Res* 51(3):175, 2002.

Konkle-Parker D, Erlen J, Dubbert P: Barriers and facilitators to medication adherence in a southern minority population with HIV disease, *J Assoc Nurses AIDS Care* 19(2):98–104, 2008.

Leininger MM, McFarland MR: *Transcultural nursing: concepts, theories, research and practices*, ed 3, New York, 2002, McGraw-Hill.

Meisenhelder JB: Terrorism, posttraumatic stress, and religious coping, *Issues Ment Health Nurs* 23:771, 2002.

McGann E, Sexton D, Chyun D: Denial and compliance in adults with asthma, *Clin Nurs Res*, 17(3):151–170, 2008.

● = Independent   ▲ = Collaborative   **EBN** = Evidence-Based Nursing   **EB** = Evidence-Based

Mok E, Chui PC: Nurse-patient relationships in palliative care, *J Adv Nurs* 48(5):475–483, 2004.

Munet-Vilaro F: Delivery of culturally competent care to children with cancer and their families—the Latino experience, *J Pediatr Oncol Nurs* 21(3):155–159, 2004.

Northouse LL, Walker J, Schafenacker A et al: A family-based program of care for women with recurrent breast cancer and their family members, *Oncol Nurs Forum* 29(10):1411–1419, 2002.

Owens R: The caring behaviors of the home health nurse and influence on medication adherence, *Home Healthc Nurse* 24(8):517–26, 2006.

Pakenham KI: Application of a stress and coping model to caregiving in multiple sclerosis, *Psychol Health Med* 6(1):13, 2001.

Spiers J: The interpersonal contexts of negotiating care in home care nurse-patient interactions, *Qual Health Res* 12(8):1033–1057, 2002.

Spolarich A: Addressing addiction, *Mod Hyg* 2(9):22–25, 2006.

Stanley K: The healing power of presence: respite from the fear of abandonment, *Oncol Nurs Forum* 33(4):J935–J942, 2006.

Stephenson PS: Understanding denial, *Oncol Nurs Forum* 31(5):985–988, 2004.

Tak YR, McCubbin M: Family stress, perceived social support and coping following the diagnosis of a child's congenital heart disease, *J Adv Nurs* 39(2):190–198, 2002.

Taylor EJ: *Spiritual care: nursing theory, research and practice*, Upper Saddle River, NJ, 2002, Prentice-Hall.

Work Group on Substance Use Disorders: Treatment of patients with substance use disorders, second edition. American Psychiatric Association, *Am J Psychiatry* 163(suppl 8):5–82, 2006.

Impaired Dentition   *Betty J. Ackley, MSN, EdS, RN*

NANDA-I

Definition

Disruption in tooth development/eruption patterns or structural integrity of individual teeth

Defining Characteristics

Abraded teeth, absence of teeth; asymmetrical facial expression; crown caries; erosion of enamel; excessive calculus; excessive plaque; halitosis; incomplete eruption for age (may be primary or permanent teeth); loose teeth; malocclusion; missing teeth; premature loss of primary teeth; root caries; tooth enamel discoloration; tooth fracture(s); tooth misalignment; toothache; worn-down teeth

Related Factors (r/t)

Barriers to self-care; bruxism; chronic use of coffee; chronic use of tea; chronic use of red wine; chronic use of tobacco; chronic vomiting; deficient knowledge regarding dental health; dietary habits; economic barriers to professional care; excessive use of abrasive cleaning agents; excessive intake of fluorides; genetic predisposition; ineffective oral hygiene; lack of access to professional care; nutritional deficits; selected prescription medications; sensitivity to cold; sensitivity to heat

NOC   (Nursing Outcomes Classification)

Suggested NOC Outcomes

Oral Hygiene, Self-Care: Oral Hygiene

Example NOC Outcome with Indicators
Oral Hygiene as evidenced by the following indicators: Cleanliness of teeth/Cleanliness of gums/Cleanliness of dentures/Tongue integrity/Gum integrity (Rate the outcome and indicators of **Oral Hygiene:** 1 = severely compromised, 2 = substantially compromised, 3 = moderately compromised, 4 = mildly compromised, 5 = not compromised [see Section I].)

Client Outcomes

Client Will (Specify Time Frame):

- Have clean teeth, healthy pink gums
- Be free of halitosis
- Explain how to perform oral care
- Demonstrate ability to masticate foods without difficulty
- State free of pain in mouth

• = Independent   ▲ = Collaborative   **EBN** = Evidence-Based Nursing   **EB** = Evidence-Based

NIC   (Nursing Interventions Classification)

Suggested NIC Interventions

Oral Health Maintenance, Oral Health Promotion, Oral Health Restoration

Example NIC Activities—Oral Health Maintenance
Establish a mouth care routine; Arrange for dental check-ups as needed

Nursing Interventions and *Rationales*

▲ Inspect oral cavity/teeth at least once daily and note any discoloration, presence of debris, amount of plaque buildup, presence of lesions, edema, or bleeding, intactness of teeth. Refer to a dentist or periodontist as appropriate. *Systematic inspection can identify impending problems.*

• If the client is free of bleeding disorders and is able to swallow, encourage the client to brush teeth with a soft toothbrush using fluoride-containing toothpaste at least two times per day and to floss teeth daily. **EB:** *A Cochrane review demonstrated that the benefits of fluoride toothpaste in preventing caries in children and adolescents has been firmly established (Marinho et al, 2003). A study demonstrated that use of flossing daily resulted in decreased plaque and gingivitis, as compared to brushing teeth alone (Schiff et al, 2006).* **EBN:** *The toothbrush is the most important tool for oral care; toothbrushing is the most effective method of reducing plaque and controlling periodontal disease; foam swabs are not effective in removing plaque (Pearson & Hutton, 2002).*

• Use a rotation-oscillation power toothbrush for removal of dental plaque. **EB:** *Multiple studies have found a rotation-oscillation power toothbrush more effective than an ultrasonic toothbrush (Biesbrock, Walters, & Bartizek, 2008; He et al, 2008; Williams et al, 2008). A Cochrane systematic review found that use of powered toothbrushes with a rotation oscillation action reduced plaque and incidence of gingivitis versus a manual toothbrush (Robinson et al, 2005).*

• Determine the client's mental status and manual dexterity; if the client is unable to care for self, nursing personnel must provide dental hygiene.

• If the client is unable to brush own teeth, follow this procedure:
  ▪ Position the client sitting upright or on side.
  ▪ Use a soft-bristle baby toothbrush.
  ▪ Use fluoride toothpaste and tap water or saline as a solution.
  ▪ Brush teeth in an up-and-down manner.
  ▪ Suction as needed.
  Each client must receive oral care including toothbrushing two times every day to maintain healthy teeth and mouth, and to prevent complications associated with periodontitis (the advanced form of gum disease that can cause tooth loss), which is associated with health problems such as cardiovascular disease, stroke, and bacterial pneumonia (ADA, 2009).

• Monitor the client's nutritional and fluid status to determine if adequate. Recommend the client eat a balanced diet and limit between meal snacks. *Poor nutrition predisposes clients to dental disease (ADA, 2009).*

• Recommend the client decrease or preferably stop intake of soft drinks. *Sugar containing soft drinks can cause cavities and the low pH of the drink can cause erosion in teeth (ADA, 2009).* **EB:** *A study demonstrated a much higher incidence of caries in children who drank soft drinks, as well as increased processed foods (Llena & Forner, 2008).*

• If client has halitosis, review good oral care with the client including brushing teeth, using floss, and brushing the tongue. *Halitosis can be a beginning sign of gingivitis, and can be eradicated by a good program of dental hygiene (Obesity, Fitness & Wellness Week, 2006; ADA, 2009).*

• Instruct the client with halitosis to clean the tongue when performing oral hygiene. Brush tongue with tongue scraper and follow with a mouth rinse. *Tongue brushing and mouth rinsing are basic treatment measures for halitosis (Krepsi, Shrime, & Kacker, 2006).* **EB:** *A Cochrane review found that tongue cleaning was effective for short-term control of halitosis (Outhouse et al, 2006).*

• Assess the client for underlying medical condition that may be causing halitosis. *Causes of halitosis can be subdivided into three categories: oral origin where good mouth care can help prevent halitosis from the upper respiratory tract including the sinuses and nose, and halitosis from systemic diseases*

• = Independent   ▲ = Collaborative   **EBN** = Evidence-Based Nursing   **EB** = Evidence-Based

that are blood-borne, volatilized in the lungs, and expelled from the lower respiratory tract. Potential sources of blood-borne halitosis are some systemic diseases, metabolic disorders, medication, and certain foods (Tangerman, 2005; ADA, 2009).

- Determine the client's usual method of oral care. Whenever possible, build on the client's existing knowledge base and current practices to develop an individualized plan of care.
- Tell the client to direct the toothbrush vertically toward the tooth surfaces, not horizontally (ADA, 2009).
- ▲ Use an antimicrobial mouthwash as ordered or tap water or saline only for a mouth rinse. Avoid the use of hydrogen peroxide, lemon-glycerin swabs, or alcohol-based mouthwashes. *Some antimicrobial mouthwashes have demonstrated effective action in decreasing bacterial counts in plaque and decreasing gingivitis (ADA, 2009).* **EBN:** *Hydrogen peroxide can cause mucosal damage and is extremely foul tasting to clients (Tombes & Gallucci, 1993). Lemon-glycerin swabs can result in decreased salivary amylase and oral moisture, as well as erosion of tooth enamel (Poland, 1987; Foss-Durant & McAffee, 1997).*
- If the client does not have a bleeding disorder, encourage the client to floss daily with approximately 18 inches of floss, using a gentle rubbing up and down motion. *Floss is useful to remove plaque buildup between the teeth and should be done daily (ADA, 2009).*
- ▲ Recommend client see a dentist at prescribed intervals, generally two times per year if teeth are in satisfactory condition. *It is important to see a dentist at regular intervals for preventative dental care (ADA, 2009).*
- ▲ If there are any signs of bleeding when the teeth are brushed, refer the client to a dentist or if obvious signs of inflamed gums, a periodontist. Bleeding, along with halitosis, is associated with gingivitis. *Beginning gingivitis can often be reversed with good oral hygiene; with more advanced cases a peridontist may be needed to correct the condition (Obesity, Fitness & Wellness Week, 2006).*
- If platelet numbers are decreased, or if the client is edentulous, use moistened toothettes or a specially made very soft toothbrush for oral care. *A toothbrush can cause soft tissue injury and bleeding in clients with low numbers of platelets.*
- Recognize that good dental care/oral care can be effective in preventing hospital-acquired (or extended care–acquired) pneumonia (Garcia, 2005; Wetzel, 2006; Ishikawa et al, 2008; Sarin et al, 2008; Arpin, 2009).
- Provide scrupulous dental care to critically ill clients, including ventilated clients to prevent ventilator-associated pneumonia. **EBN:** *Numerous studies have demonstrated decreased incidence of ventilator-associated pneumonia with good oral care (Fields, 2008; Panchabhai et al, 2009).*
- If teeth are nonfunctional for chewing, modification of oral intake (e.g., edentulous diet, soft diet) may be necessary. The nursing diagnosis **Imbalanced Nutrition: less than body requirements** may apply.
- If the client is unable to swallow, keep suction nearby when providing oral care. See care plan for **Impaired Swallowing**.
- See care plan for **Impaired Oral mucous membrane**.

Pregnant Client

- Encourage the expectant mother to eat a healthy, balanced diet that is rich in calcium. *The teeth usually start to form in the gums during the second trimester of pregnancy. To encourage the development of good, strong teeth, expectant mothers should eat a healthy, balanced diet that is rich in calcium (ADA, 2009).*
- Advise the pregnant mother not to smoke. **EB:** *Maternal smoking during pregnancy has been associated with increased caries in the teeth of the child (Iida et al, 2007).*
- Advise the expentant mother to practice good care of her teeth, to protect her child's teeth once born. *Dental caries in children are associated with high levels of mutans streptococci; this bacterium is commonly spread from the mother with infected teeth to the infant by tasting of food and sharing of utensils once the child is born (Kagihara, Niederhauser, & Stark, 2009).*

Infant Oral Hygiene

- Gently wipe the baby's gums with a washcloth or sterile gauze at least once a day. *Wiping gums prevents bacterial buildup in the mouth.*
- Never allow the child to fall asleep with a bottle containing milk, formula, fruit juice, or sweetened liquids. If the child needs a comforter between regular feedings, at night, or during naps, fill a bottle

• = Independent ▲ = Collaborative **EBN** = Evidence-Based Nursing **EB** = Evidence-Based

with cool water or give the child a clean pacifier recommended by the dentist or physician. Never give child a pacifier dipped in any sweet liquid. Avoid filling child's bottle with liquids such as sugar water and soft drinks. *Decay occurs when sweetened liquids such as milk, formula, and fruit juice are given and are left clinging to an infant's teeth for long periods. Bacteria in the mouth use these sugars as food to produce acids that attack the teeth (ADA, 2007; Kagihara, Niederhauser, & Stark, 2009).*

▲ When multiple teeth appear, brush with a small toothbrush with a small (pea-size) amount of fluoride toothpaste. Recommend that child either use a fluoride gel or fluoride varnish. Use of topical fluoride (mouth rinses, gels, or varnishes) in addition to toothpaste containing fluoride resulted in a modest reduction of cavity formation versus use of fluoride toothpaste only (Marinho et al, 2003).

▲ Advise parents to begin dental visits at 1 year of age. The goal is to prevent caries and find any problems *with teeth early. Caries and infection of the first set of teeth have been associated with problems of alignment of permanent teeth, difficulty chewing, problems speaking, sleeping, concentrating, and learning, as well as problems with self-esteem (Kagihara, Niederhauser, & Stark, 2009).*

Older Children

▲ Encourage the family to talk with the dentist about dental sealants, which can help prevent cavities in permanent teeth. **EB:** *A Cochrane review found that use of dental sealants on the molars of children was effective in preventing caries (Ahovuo-Saloranta et al, 2008).*

• Recommend the child use dental floss to help prevent gum disease. The dentist will give guidelines on when to start using floss.

• Recommend to parents that they not permit the child to smoke or chew tobacco, and stress the importance of setting a good example by not using tobacco products themselves.

• Recommend the child drink fluoridated water when possible. *The American Dental Association strongly endorses use of fluoridated water, based on scientific research that validates the effectiveness in preventing cavities (ADA, 2009).*

Geriatric

▲ Provide dentists with accurate medication history to avoid drug interactions and client harm. *If the client is taking anticoagulants, the INR should be reviewed before providing dental care (Little et al, 2002).*

• Carefully observe oral cavity and lips for abnormal lesions when providing oral care.

• Ensure that dentures are removed and cleaned regularly, preferably after every meal and before bedtime. *Dentures left in the mouth at night impede circulation to the palate and predispose the client to oral lesions.*

• Support other caregivers providing oral hygiene. *Physical and cognitive impairment in older adults can interfere with the client's ability to perform oral hygiene. In many cases caregivers take over these procedures. If no caregiver is available, the client is prone to dental problems such as dental caries, tooth abscess, tooth fracture, gingival, and periodontal disease.*

Multicultural

• Assess for the influence of cultural beliefs, norms, and values on the client's understanding of dental care. **EBN:** *What the client considers normal and abnormal dental care may be based on cultural perceptions (Leininger & McFarland, 2002; Giger & Davidhizar, 2008).*

• Assess for barriers to access to dental care, such as lack of insurance. *Children from racial minority groups may have significantly more difficulty in accessing dental care (Savage et al, 2004).* **EBN:** *Poverty and lack of dental care insurance may prevent the obtainment of dental care (Woolfolk et al, 1999). African Americans and persons of lower socioeconomic status reported more new dental symptoms, were less likely to obtain dental care, and reported more tooth loss (Gilbert, Duncan, & Shelton, 2003).*

Home Care

• Assess client patterns for daily and professional dental care and related patterns (e.g., smoking, nail biting). Assess for environmental influences on dental status (e.g., fluoride).

• = Independent   ▲ = Collaborative   **EBN** = Evidence-Based Nursing   **EB** = Evidence-Based

- Assess client facilities and financial resources for providing dental care. *Lack of appropriate facilities or financial resources is a barrier to positive dental care patterns. Provision for dental care may be missing from health care plans or unavailable to the uninsured.*
- Request dietary log from the client, adding column for type of food (i.e., soft, pureed, regular).
- Observe a typical meal to assess firsthand the impact of impaired dentition on nutrition. *Clients, especially the elderly, are often hesitant to admit nutritional changes that may be embarrassing because of poor dentition.*
- Identify mechanical needs for food preparation and ease of ingestion/digestion to meet the client's dental/nutritional needs.
- Assist the client with accessing financial or other resources to support optimum dental and nutritional status.

Client/Family Teaching and Discharge Planning

- Teach how to inspect the oral cavity and monitor for problems with the teeth and gums.
- Teach how to implement a personal plan of dental hygiene, including appropriate brushing of teeth and tongue and use of dental floss.
- Advise the client to change their toothbrush every 3 to 4 months, because after that toothbrushes are less effective in removing plaque (ADA, 2009).
- Teach the client the value of having an optimal fluoride concentration in drinking water, and to brush teeth twice daily with fluoride toothpaste.
- Teach clients of all ages the need to decrease intake of sugary foods and to brush teeth regularly.
- Inform individuals who are considering tongue piercing of the potential complications, such as chipping and cracking of teeth and possible trauma to the gingiva. If piercing is done, teach the client how to care for the wound and prevent complications. **EB:** *Complications identified in the literature from tongue piercing include postoperative swelling, infection, and bleeding; damage to the teeth; and trauma to the soft tissues (Knox, 2002).* **EB:** *A study demonstrated that 74% of adolescents with tongue piercing had complications or alterations (Firoozmand, Paschotto, & Almeida, 2009). Another study demonstrated that gingival recession was associated with oral piercing (Slutzkey & Levin, 2008).*

ⓔvolve   See the EVOLVE website for Weblinks for client education resources.

REFERENCES

American Dental Association (ADA): *Oral health topics A-Z,* www.ada .org/public/index.asp. Accessed on July 3, 2009.

Ahovuo-Saloranta A, Hiiri A, Nordblad A et al: Pit and fissure sealants for preventing dental decay in the permanent teeth of children and adolescents, *Cochrane Database Syst Rev* (4):CD001830, 2008.

Arpin S: Oral hygiene in elderly people in hospitals and nursing homes, *Evid Based Dent* 10(2):46, 2009.

Biesbrock AR, Walters PA, Bartizek RD: Plaque removal efficacy of an advanced rotation-oscillation power toothbrush versus a new sonic toothbrush, *Am J Dent* 21(3):185–188, 2008.

Fields LB: Oral care intervention to reduce incidence of ventilator-associated pneumonia in the neurologic intensive care unit, *J Neurosci Nurs* 40(5):291–298, 2008.

Firoozmand LM, Paschotto DR, Almeida JD: Oral piercing complications among teenage students, *Oral Health Prev Dent* 7(1):77–81, 2009.

Foss-Durant AM, McAffee A: A comparison of three oral care products commonly used in practice, *Clin Nurs Res* 6:1, 1997.

Garcia R: A review of the possible role of oral and dental colonization on the occurrence of health care-associated pneumonia: underappreciated risk and a call for interventions, *Am J Infect Control* 33(9):527–541, 2005.

Giger J, Davidhizar, R: *Transcultural nursing: assessment and intervention,* ed 5, St Louis, 2008, Mosby.

Gilbert GH, Duncan RP, Shelton BJ: Social determinants of tooth loss, *Health Serv Res* 38(6 Pt 2), 2003.

He T, Biesbrock AR, Walters PA et al: A comparative clinical study of the plaque removal efficacy of an oscillating/rotating power toothbrush and an ultrasonic toothbrush, *J Clin Dent* 19(4):138–142, 2008.

Iida H, Auinger P, Billings RJ et al: Association between infant breast-feeding and early childhood caries in the United States, *Pediatrics* 120(4):e944–952, 2007.

Ishikawa, Yoneyama T, Hirota K et al: Professional oral health care reduces the number of oropharyngeal bacteria, *J Dent Res* 87(6):594–598, 2008.

Kagihara LE, Niederhauser VP, Stark M: Assessment, management, and prevention of early childhood caries, *J Am Acad Nurse Pract* 21(1):1–10, 2009.

Knox KT: The potential complications of intra-oral and peri-oral piercing, *Dent Health* 41:3, 2002.

Krespi YP, Shrime MG, Kacker A: The relationship between oral malodor and volatile sulfur compound-producing bacteria, *Otolaryngol Head Neck Surg* 135(5):671–676, 2006.

Leininger MM, McFarland MR: *Transcultural nursing: concepts, theories, research and practices,* ed 3, New York, 2002, McGraw-Hill.

Little J, Falace D, Miller C et al: *Dental management of the medically compromised patient,* ed 6, St Louis, 2002, Mosby.

Llena C, Forner L: Dietary habits in a child population in relation to caries experience, *Caries Res* 42(5):387–393, 2008.

• = Independent   ▲ = Collaborative   **EBN** = Evidence-Based Nursing   **EB** = Evidence-Based

Marinho VC, Higgins JP, Sheiham A, et al: Fluoride toothpastes for preventing dental caries in children and adolescents, *Cochrane Database Syst Rev* (1):CD002278, 2003.

[No author]: Dental research: gingival bleeding and halitosis are greatly reduced after a two-week oral hygiene program, *Obesity, Fitness & Wellness Week* Aug 26:843, 2006.

Outhouse TL, Fedorowicz Z, Keenan JV et al: A Cochrane systematic review finds tongue scrapers have short-term efficacy in controlling halitosis, *Gen Dent* 54(5):352–359; 360, 367–368, 2006.

Panchabhai TS, Dangayach NS, Krishnan A et al: Oropharyngeal cleansing with 0.2% chlorhexidine for prevention of nosocomial pneumonia in critically ill patients: an open-label randomized trial with 0.01% potassium permanganate as control, *Chest* 135(5):1150–1156, 2009.

Pearson LS, Hutton JL: A controlled trial to compare the ability of foam swabs and toothbrushes to remove dental plaque, *J Adv Nurs* 39(5):480, 2002.

Poland JM: Comparing Moi-Stir to lemon-glycerin swabs, *Am J Nurs* 87(4):422, 1987.

Robinson PG, Deacon SA, Deery C et al: Manual versus powered toothbrushing for oral health, *Cochrane Database Syst Rev* (2):CD002281, 2005.

Sarin J, Balasubramaniam R, Corcoran A et al: Reducing the risk of aspiration pneumonia among elderly patients in long-term care facilities through oral health interventions. *J Am Med Dir Assoc* 9(2):128–135, 2008.

Savage MF, Lee JY, Kotch JB et al: Early preventive dental visits: effects on subsequent utilization and costs, *Pediatrics* 114(4): e418–423, 2004.

Schiff, T, Proskin, HM, Zhang, YP et al: A clinical investigation for the efficacy of three different treatment regimens for the control of plaque and gingivitis. *J Clin Dent* 17(5):138–144, 2006.

Slutzkey S, Levin L: Gingival recession in young adults: occurrence, severity, and relationship to past orthodontic treatment and oral piercing, *Am J Orthod Dentofacial Orthop* 134(5):652–656, 2008.

Tangerman A: Halitosis in medicine: a review, *Int Dent J* 52(Suppl 3):201–206, 2005.

Tombes MB, Gallucci B: The effects of hydrogen peroxide rinses on the normal oral mucosa, *Nurs Res* 42:332, 1993.

Wetzel T: Preventing nosocomial pneumonia: routine oral care reduced the risk of infection at one facility, *Am J Nurs* 106(9):72A-B, 72 E-G, 2006.

Williams K, Rapley K, Huan J et al: A study comparing the plaque removal efficacy of an advanced rotation-oscillation power toothbrush to a new sonic toothbrush, *J Clin Dent* 19(4):154–158, 2008.

Woolfolk MW, Lang WP, Borgnakke WS et al: Determining dental checkup frequency, *J Am Dent Assoc* 130(5):715–723, 1999.

Risk for delayed Development   *Dena L. Jarog, DNP, RN, CCNS*

NANDA-I

Definition

At risk for delay of 25% or more in one or more of the areas of social or self-regulatory behavior, or in cognitive, language, gross, or fine motor skills

Risk Factors

Prenatal

Endocrine disorders; genetic disorders; illiteracy; inadequate nutrition; infections; lack of prenatal care; late prenatal care; maternal age <15 years; maternal age >35 years; inadequate prenatal care; poverty; substance abuse; unplanned pregnancy; unwanted pregnancy

Individual

Adopted child; behavior disorders; brain damage (e.g., hemorrhage in postnatal period, shaken baby, abuse, accident); chemotherapy; chronic illness; congenital disorders; failure to thrive; foster child; frequent otitis media; genetic disorders; hearing impairment; inadequate nutrition; lead poisoning; natural disasters; positive drug screen(s); prematurity; radiation therapy; seizures; substance abuse; technology-dependent; vision impairment

Environmental

Poverty; violence

Caregiver

Abuse; learning disabilities; mental illness; severe learning disability

NOC   (Nursing Outcomes Classification)

Suggested NOC Outcomes

Abuse Recovery, Child Development: 1 Month, 2 Months, 4 Months, 6 Months, 12 Months, 2 Years, 3 Years, 4 Years, 5 Years, Middle Childhood, Adolescence, Development: Late Adulthood, Middle Adulthood, Young Adulthood, Neglect Recovery, Knowledge: Parenting.

• = Independent   ▲ = Collaborative   **EBN** = Evidence-Based Nursing   **EB** = Evidence-Based

---

Example NOC Outcome with Indicators

Child Development as evidenced by the following indicators: Appropriate milestones of physical, cognitive, and psychosocial age–appropriate progression (Rate the outcome and indicators of **Child Development:** 1 = never demonstrated, 2 = rarely demonstrated, 3 = sometimes demonstrated, 4 = often demonstrated, 5 = consistently demonstrated [see Section I].)

Client Outcomes

Client/Parents/Primary Caregiver Will (Specify Time Frame):

- Describe realistic, age-appropriate patterns of development
- Promote activities and interactions that support age-related developmental tasks

NIC   (Nursing Interventions Classification)

Suggested NIC Interventions

Developmental Enhancement: Child, Adolescent, Emotional Support, Kangaroo Care, Teaching: Stimulation-Infant, Teaching: Infant Nutrition 0–3 months, 4–6 months, 7–9 months, 10–12 months, Teaching: Safety-Infant, Toddler, Parent Education: Child rearing family, Parenting promotion

---

Example NIC Activities—Developmental Enhancement: Child

Teach caregivers about normal developmental milestones and associated behaviors; Establish one-on-one interaction with child; Demonstrate activities that promote development to caregivers; Offer age-appropriate toys or materials; Redirect attention when needed

---

Nursing Interventions and *Rationales*

- Refer to care plan for **Delayed Growth and development.**

Preconception/Pregnancy

- Males and females should avoid exposure to organic solvents before and during pregnancy. **EB:** *Exposure in utero to organic solvents is associated with poorer performance on some specific subtle measures of neurocognitive function, language, and behavior (Laslo-Baker et al, 2004). There is some indication of an increased risk of functional developmental disorders in offspring among painters with intermediate and high model-predicted exposures (Hooiveld et al, 2006).*
- Avoid exposure to heavy metals, pesticides, herbicides, sterilants, anesthetic gases, and anticancer drugs used in health care. **EB:** *Many toxicants with unambiguous reproductive and developmental effects are still in regular commercial or therapeutic use and thus present exposure potential to workers. Caregivers must be aware of their clients' potential environmental and workplace exposures (McDiarmid & Gehle, 2006). Increased maternal lead concentration at third trimester of pregnancy, especially around week 28, was associated with decreased intellectual child development (Schnaas et al, 2006).*
- ▲ Encourage mothers to abstain from alcohol and cocaine use during pregnancy; refer them to treatment programs for substance abuse. **EBN:** *Prenatal exposure to cocaine had an outcome of poorer gross and fine neuromotor performance among infants exposed to cocaine prenatally at 4 and 7 months using the Alberta Infant Motor Scale (AIMS) and Movement Assessment of Infants (MAI) (Schiller & Allen, 2005).*
- Encourage adequate antepartum and postpartum care for both mother and child. A*ccess to prenatal and postnatal health care promotes optimal growth and development (Bland et al, 2000).*

 Multicultural

Parents

- Assess for the influence of cultural beliefs, norms, and values on the client's perceptions of child development. **EBN:** *Latino mothers of children with developmental disabilities viewed their child as not being responsible for the behavior problem (Chavira et al, 2000). Latino mothers of developmentally disabled adults reported their relationship with the educational and service delivery systems to be*

• = Independent   ▲ = Collaborative   **EBN** = Evidence-Based Nursing   **EB** = Evidence-Based

characterized by poor communication, low effort in providing services, negative attitudes of professionals toward the client/children, and negative treatment of parents by professionals (Shapiro et al, 2004). Where disabilities are concerned, it is essential to remember that parents with children with disabilities should be told that it is reported that there is a two to three times greater likelihood that individuals with disabilities could suffer from each of 16 secondary condition including falls or other injuries, respiratory infections, asthma, sleep problems, chronic pain, and periods of depression, and children would not be an exception to these data (Kinne, Patrick & Doyle, 2004).

Infants

- Carefully assess Pakistani and Bangladeshi infants for developmental milestones, and supply appropriate preventive interventions, such as adequate nutrition. *Deprivation among these groups must be addressed to reduce the likelihood of developmental delay and possible longer term behavioral and cognitive problems and consequent opportunities throughout life (Kelly et al, 2006).*

Pediatric/Parenting

- ▲ Encourage mothers with postpartum depression to seek assistance and support as appropriate. *The overall incidence of developmental delay at 18 months in children of women displaying depression following pregnancy was 9% (Deave et al, 2008).*
- Teach new mothers the importance of breastfeeding. **EB:** *Prolonged and exclusive breastfeeding improves children's cognitive development (Kramer et al, 2008).*
- Teach the parents to provide toys and books and read aloud to young children in the home. *Reading aloud and providing toys are associated with better child cognitive and language development (Tomopoulos et al, 2006).*
- Counsel parents, and caregivers about the importance of smoking cessation and the necessity of eliminating all secondhand smoke exposure. *Smoking affects development not only during intrauterine life but also during the early stage of extrauterine life (Bottini et al, 2004).*
- Teach caregivers of children appropriate developmental interactions; use anticipatory guidance to facilitate preparation for developmental milestones. **EBN:** *Maternal interaction variables were the more potent predictors of cognitive, linguistic, and problem-solving outcomes (McGrath, Sullivan, & Seifer, 1998).*
- Provide developmental care interventions to preterm infants to improve neurodevelopmental outcomes. **EB:** *Developmental care is effective to improve outcomes (Symington & Pinelli, 2002).*
- Provide information on support groups and education on human immunodeficiency virus (HIV) and caring for infants with this diagnosis. *Developmental delay has been well documented in infants with HIV (Potterton & Eales, 2001).*
- Teach parents to identify safety hazards in the home and environment. **EB:** *Injuries are often preventable yet remain the most common cause of death in children age 1 to 19, and many children require the need for rehabilitation services following a significant injury (Joffe & Lalani, 2006).*

⊖volve   See the EVOLVE website for Weblinks for client education resources.

REFERENCES

Bland M, Vermillion ST, Soper DE et al: Late third trimester treatment of rectovaginal group B streptococci with benzathine penicillin G, *Am J Obstet Gynecol* 183(2):372, 2000.

Bottini N, Gloria-Bottini F, Magrini A et al: Maternal cigarette smoking, metabolic enzyme polymorphism, and developmental events in the early stages of extrauterine life, *Hum Biol* 76(2):289–297, 2004.

Chavira V, Lopez SR, Blacher J et al: Latina mothers' attributions, emotions, and reactions to the problem behaviors of their children with developmental disabilities, *J Child Psychol Psychiatry* 41(2):245–252, 2000.

Deave T, Heron J, Evans J et al: The impact of maternal depression in pregnancy on early child development, *Obstet Gynecol Surv* 63(10):626–628, 2008.

Hooiveld M, Haveman W, Roskes K et al: Adverse reproductive outcomes among male painters with occupational exposure to organic solvents, *Occup Environ Med* 63(8):538–544, 2006.

Joffe AR, Lalani A: Injury admissions to pediatric intensive care are predictable and preventable: a call to action, *J Intens Care Med* 21(4):227–234, 2006.

Kelly Y, Sacker A, Schoon I et al: Ethnic differences in achievement of developmental milestones by 9 months of age: the Millennium Cohort Study, *Dev Med Child Neurol* 48(10):825–830, 2006.

Kinne S, Patrick DL, Doyle DL: Prevalence of secondary conditions among people with disabilities, *Am J Pub Health* 94(3):443–445, 2004.

Kramer MS, Aboud F, Mironova E et al: Breastfeeding and child cognitive development: new evidence from a large randomized trial, *Arch Gen Psychiatry* 65(5):578–584, 2008.

Laslo-Baker D, Barrera M, Knittel-Keren D et al: Child neurodevelopmental outcome and maternal occupational exposure to solvents, *Arch Pediatr Adolesc Med* 158(10):956–961, 2004.

● = Independent   ▲ = Collaborative   **EBN** = Evidence-Based Nursing   **EB** = Evidence-Based

McDiarmid MA, Gehle K: Preconception brief: occupational/environmental exposures, *Matern Child Health J* 10(suppl 5):123–128, 2006.

McGrath MM, Sullivan MC, Seifer R: Maternal interaction patterns and preschool competence in high-risk children, *Nurs Res* 47(6):309–317, 1998.

Potterton J, Eales C: Prevalence of developmental delay in infants who are HIV positive, *S Afr J Physiother* 57(3):11, 2001.

Schiller C, Allen PJ: Follow-up of infants prenatally exposed to cocaine, *Pediatr Nurs* 31(5):427–436, 2005.

Schnaas L, Rothenberg S, Flores M et al: Reduced intellectual development in children with prenatal lead exposure, *Environ Health Perspect* 114(5):791–797, 2006.

Shapiro J, Monzo LD, Rueda R et al: Alienated advocacy: perspectives of Latina mothers of young adults with developmental disabilities on service systems, *Ment Retard* 42(1):37–54, 2004.

Symington A, Pinelli J: Developmental care for promoting development and preventing morbidity in preterm infants, *Cochrane Database Syst Rev* (3):CD001814, 2002.

Tomopoulos S, Dreyer BP, Tamis-LeMonda C et al: Books, toys, parent-child interaction, and development in young Latino children, *Ambul Pediatr* 6(2):72–78, 2006.

Diarrhea   *Nancy Albright Beyer, RN, CEN, MS, and Betty J. Ackley, MSN, EdS, RN*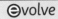

NANDA-I

Definition

Passage of loose, unformed stools

Defining Characteristics

Abdominal pain; at least three loose liquid stools per day; cramping; hyperactive bowel sounds; urgency

Related Factors (r/t)

Psychological

Anxiety; high stress levels

Situational

Adverse effects of medications; alcohol abuse; contaminants; travel; laxative abuse; radiation; toxins; tube feedings

Physiological

Infectious processes; inflammation; irritation; malabsorption; protozoal, gastrointestinal disorders

NOC   (Nursing Outcomes Classification)

Suggested NOC Outcomes

Bowel Elimination, Electrolyte and Acid-Base Balance, Fluid Balance, Hydration, Treatment Behavior: Illness or Injury

Example **NOC** Outcome with Indicators
Bowel Elimination as evidenced by the following indicators: Elimination pattern/Stool soft and formed/Diarrhea not present/Control of bowel movements/Comfort of stool passage/Pain with passage of stool not present (Rate the outcome and indicators of **Bowel Elimination:** 1 = severely compromised, 2 = substantially compromised, 3 = moderately compromised, 4 = mildly compromised, 5 = not compromised [see Section I].)

Client Outcomes

Client Will (Specify Time Frame):

- Defecate formed, soft stool every day to every third day
- Maintain a rectal area free of irritation
- State relief from cramping and less or no diarrhea
- Explain cause of diarrhea and rationale for treatment
- Maintain good skin turgor and weight at usual level
- Contain stool appropriately (if previously incontinent)

● = Independent   ▲ = Collaborative   **EBN** = Evidence-Based Nursing   **EB** = Evidence-Based

NIC (Nursing Interventions Classification)

Suggested NIC Intervention

Diarrhea Management

Example NIC Activities—Diarrhea Management
Evaluate medication profile for gastrointestinal side effects; Suggest trial elimination of foods containing lactose

Nursing Interventions and *Rationales*

- Assess pattern of defecation, or have the client keep a diary that includes the following: time of day defecation occurs; usual stimulus for defecation; consistency, amount, and frequency of stool; type of, amount of, and time food consumed; fluid intake; history of bowel habits and laxative use; diet; exercise patterns; obstetrical/gynecological, medical, and surgical histories; medications; alterations in perianal sensations; and present bowel regimen. *Assessment of defecation pattern will help direct treatment.*
- ▲ Use an evidence-based bowel management protocol and consistently monitor and report bowel activity. **EB:** *After the protocol was implemented, diarrhea was decreased in an Australian ICU setting with fewer ICU days occurrences of diarrhea (Ferrie & East, 2007).*
- Assess stool consistency and its influence on risk for stool loss. *Several classification systems for stool have been developed including the Hart and Dobb Diarrhea Scale, the Guenther and Sweed Stool Output Assessment Tool, and the Bristol Stool scale (Kyle, 2007; Sabol & Carlson, 2007).* **EBN:** *A study of stool consistency found good reliability when evaluated by professional nurses, student nurses, and clients. Word-only descriptors yielded equivocal consistency when assessed by subjects as did tools that combined words with illustrations of various stool consistencies (Bliss et al, 2001).*
- Inspect, auscultate, palpate, and percuss the abdomen in that order. *Expect increased frequency of bowel sounds with diarrhea (Bickley & Szilagyi, 2009).*
- ▲ Identify cause of diarrhea if possible based on history (e.g., rotavirus or norovirus exposure; HIV infection; food poisoning; medication effect; radiation therapy; protein malnutrition; laxative abuse; stress). See Related Factors (r/t). *Identification of the underlying cause is important, because the treatment often depends on it (Thielman & Guerrant, 2004).*
- ▲ Obtain stool specimens as ordered, to either rule out or diagnose an infectious process (e.g., ova and parasites, *C. difficile* infection, bacterial cultures for food poisoning).
- ▲ If the client has watery diarrhea, a low-grade fever, abdominal cramps, and a history of antibiotic therapy, consider possibility of *C. difficile* infection. C. difficile *infections have become common because of the frequent use of broad-spectrum antibiotics, and now there is a hypervirulent form of* C. difficile *causing increased morbidity and mortality (Gravel et al, 2009). The workup is based on clinical history and presentation, a stool specimen, but may also include blood cultures and a complete blood cell count with differential if the client is febrile (Sabol & Carlson, 2007).*
- Use standard precautions when caring for clients with diarrhea to prevent spread of infectious diarrhea; use gloves and handwashing. C. difficile *and viruses causing diarrhea have been shown to be highly contagious.* C. difficile *is difficult to eradicate because of spore formation (Poutanen & Simor, 2004).* **EBN and EB:** *A nursing review of the most recent development in client care related to* C. difficile *summarizes care to include: contact isolation, soap and water handwashing (alcohol rubs are not effective), use of disposable equipment, and intensive housekeeping using hypochlorite-based products for disinfection (Todd, 2006). A medical review of prevention of spread of* C. difficile *recommended additional guidelines of avoiding rectal temperatures, placing clients in private rooms, and using full barrier precautions (Dubberke et al, 2008). Bacterial spores, such as* C. difficile, *are not destroyed by alcohol, chlorhexidine, or triclosan products. Even vigorous hand-washing is minimally effective. Vegetative cells of* C. difficile *can survive for at least 24 hours on inanimate surfaces, and spores can survive up to 5 months (Kampf & Kramer, 2004).*
- ▲ If the client has diarrhea associated with antibiotic therapy, consult with the primary care practitioner regarding the use of probiotics, such as yogurt, with active cultures to treat diarrhea, or preferably use probiotics to prevent diarrhea when first beginning antibiotic therapy. **EB:** *Probiotics*

• = Independent   ▲ = Collaborative   **EBN** = Evidence-Based Nursing   **EB** = Evidence-Based

have been shown to be helpful to prevent antibiotic-associated diarrhea in some clients (Rohde, Barto-lini & Jones, 2009; Guarino, Lo Vecchio & Canani, 2009).

▲ If the diarrhea is related to inflammatory bowel disease (IBD) (Crohns or ulcerative colitis), interventions may include the use of complementary or alternative treatment, such as probiotics. **EB:** *Probiotics enhance the normal intestinal microflora and decrease the symptom of diarrhea (Savard & Sawatzky, 2007).*

• Ask the client to examine intake of high fructose corn syrup and fructose sweeteners in relation to onset of diarrhea symptoms. If diarrhea is associated with fructose ingestion, intake should be limited or eliminated. **EB:** *High fructose corn syrup or fructose sweeteners from fruit juices can cause gastrointestinal (GI) symptoms of bloating, rumbling, flatulence, and diarrhea at amounts of 25 to 50 g. Malabsorption is demonstrated in clients after 25 g fructose, and most clients develop symptoms with 50 g fructose (Beyer, Caviar, & McCallum, 2005).*

▲ If the client has infectious diarrhea, avoid using medications that slow peristalsis. *If an infectious process is occurring, such as C.* difficile *infection or food poisoning, medication to slow peristalsis should generally not be given. The increase in gut motility helps eliminate the causative factor, and use of antidiarrheal medication could result in a toxic megacolon (Sunenshine & McDonald, 2006).*

• Assess for dehydration by observing skin turgor over sternum and inspecting for longitudinal furrows of the tongue. Watch for excessive thirst, fever, dizziness, lightheadedness, palpitations, excessive cramping, bloody stools, hypotension, and symptoms of shock. *Severe diarrhea can cause deficient fluid volume with extreme weakness (Mentes, 2006). Acutely ill clients are at risk for hemodynamic and metabolic instability because of fluid and electrolyte imbalances caused by diarrhea (Thorson, Bliss, & Savik, 2008).*

• Observe for symptoms of sodium and potassium loss (e.g., weakness, abdominal or leg cramping, dysrhythmia). Note results of electrolyte laboratory studies. *Stool contains electrolytes; excessive diarrhea causes electrolyte abnormalities that can be especially harmful to clients with existing medical conditions. Laboratory test results assist in the monitoring of a person's physiologic response and hydration status. The results can also provide useful information in determining the cause of the diarrhea (Sabol & Carlson, 2007).*

• Monitor and record intake and output; note oliguria and dark, concentrated urine.

• Measure specific gravity of urine if possible. *Dark, concentrated urine, along with a high specific gravity of urine, is an indication of deficient fluid volume.*

• Weigh the client daily and note decreased weight. *An accurate daily weight is an important indicator of fluid balance in the body.*

• Give dilute clear fluids as tolerated; serve at lukewarm temperature. *Most episodes of acute diarrhea typically warrant supportive therapies such as fluids (oral or intravenous) (Sabol & Carlson, 2007).*

▲ If the client has chronic diarrhea causing fecal incontinence at intervals, consider suggesting use of dietary fiber from psyllium or gum arabic after consultation with primary practitioner. **EBN and EB:** *Use of a fiber supplement decreases the number of incontinent stools and improves stool consistency (Bliss et al, 2001). The use of soluble dietary fiber is useful for controlling diarrhea and normalizing the intestinal flora (Nakao et al, 2002).*

▲ If diarrhea is chronic and there is evidence of malnutrition, consult with primary care practitioner for a dietary consult and possible use of a hydrolyzed formula (a clear liquid supplement containing increased protein and calories) such as Ensure Alive, Resource Breeze Fruit Beverage, or citrotein (Lutz & Przytulski, 2010) to maintain nutrition while the gastrointestinal system heals.

• Encourage the client to eat small, frequent meals, to consume foods that are easy to digest (e.g., bananas, crackers, pretzels, rice, potatoes, clear soups, applesauce), and to avoid milk products, foods high in fiber, and caffeine (dark sodas, tea, coffee, chocolate). *The BRAT diet has been traditionally recommended but if used, should be used for only short periods of time as it is nutritionally incomplete (Centers for Disease Control and Prevention, 2003).*

• Provide a readily available bathroom, commode, or bedpan.

• If the client has diarrhea and incontinence, consider use of a Perineal Assessment Tool to measure the risk for perineal skin injury. **EBN:** *The Perineal Assessment Tool has been developed to determine the risk of perineal skin injury. The initial results of the study are encouraging, and further studies are needed (Nix, 2002).*

• = Independent   ▲ = Collaborative   **EBN** = Evidence-Based Nursing   **EB** = Evidence-Based

- Thoroughly cleanse and dry the perianal and perineal skin daily and as needed (PRN) using a cleanser capable of stool removal. Select a product with a slightly acidic pH designed to preserve the skin's acid mantle, and designed to remove irritants from the skin with minimal physical force. Avoid vigorous scrubbing with water, soap, and a washcloth. Consider selection of a product with a built-in moisturizer and also skin protectant. *Traditional soaps tend to be alkaline, interfering with the natural acid mantle of the integument and increasing its susceptibility to irritant dermatitis and secondary infection. Brisk scrubbing may exacerbate skin erosion and further increase the risk of irritation and infection (Gray, 2004).*
- ▲ If the client has enteral tube feedings and diarrhea, consider infusion rate, position of feeding tube, tonicity of formula, and formula contamination. Consider changing the formula to a lower osmolarity, lactose-free, peptide-based, or high-fiber feeding. *Slowing the infusion rate and using formula at room temperature helps avoid the abdominal cramping and diarrhea sometimes seen with rapid delivery methods and chilled formula (Sabol & Carlson, 2007).*
- Do not administer bolus feedings into the small bowel. *The stomach has a larger capacity for large fluid volumes while the small bowel can usually only tolerate up to 150 mL/hr (Sabol & Carslon, 2007).*
- ▲ Dilute liquid medications before administration through the enteral tube and flush enteral feeding tube with sufficient water before and after medication administration. *Since many liquid medications contain sorbitol or are hyperosmotic, diluting the medication may help decrease occurrence of diarrhea (Sabol & Carlson, 2007).*
- Assess whether the cause of the diarrhea may be the combination factor of concurrent administration of tube feeding and sorbitol medications. **EBN:** *Both of these given concurrently can increase the incidence of diarrhea in the tube-fed client (Thorson, Bliss, & Savik, 2008).*

 Pediatric

- ▲ Recommend the parents give the child oral rehydration fluids to drink in the amounts specified by the physician, especially during the first 4 to 6 hours to replace lost fluid. Once the child is rehydrated, an orally administered maintenance solution should be used along with food. **EB:** *A Cochrane review found that children admitted to the hospital with diarrhea receiving reduced osmolarity–oral rehydration solutions had fewer stools, less stool volume, less vomiting, and less use of intravenous fluids (Hahn, Kim, & Garner, 2002). Treatment with oral rehydration fluids for children is generally as effective as intravenous (IV) fluids; IV fluids do not shorten the duration of gastroenteritis and are more likely to cause adverse effects than oral rehydration therapy (Banks & Meadows, 2005).*
- Recommend the mother resume breastfeeding as soon as possible.
- Recommend parents not give the child flat soda, fruit juices, gelatin dessert, or instant fruit drink. *These fluids have a high osmolality from carbohydrate contents and can exacerbate diarrhea. In addition they have low sodium concentrations that can aggravate existing hyponatremia (Behrman, Kliegman, & Jensen, 2004).*
- Recommend parents give children foods with complex carbohydrates, such as potatoes, rice, bread, cereal, yogurt, fruits, and vegetables. Avoid fatty foods, foods high in simple sugars, and milk products (Behrman, Kliegman, & Jensen, 2004). *The BRAT diet has been traditionally recommended but if used, should be used for only short periods of time as it is nutritionally incomplete (Centers for Disease Control and Prevention, 2003). When a child has diarrhea, dietary modification includes avoiding dairy products, because viral or bacterial infections can cause a transient lactase deficiency (Amerine & Keirsy, 2004).*

 Geriatric

- ▲ Evaluate medications the client is taking. Recognize that many medications can result in diarrhea, including digitalis, propranolol, angiotensin-converting enzyme (ACE) inhibitors, histamine-receptor antagonists, nonsteroidal antiinflammatory drugs (NSAIDs), anticholinergic agents, oral hypoglycemia agents, antibiotics, and others. **EB:** *A study found that multiple medications can cause diarrhea in the elderly client including: antibiotics, proton pump inhibitors, allopurinol, psycholeptics, selective serotonin reuptake inhibitors, and angiotensin II receptor blockers (Pilotto et al, 2008).*

• = Independent   ▲ = Collaborative   **EBN** = Evidence-Based Nursing   **EB** = Evidence-Based

▲ Monitor the client closely to detect whether an impaction is causing diarrhea; remove impaction as ordered. *Clients with fecal impaction commonly experience leakage of mucus or liquid stool from rectum, rectal irritation, distention, and impaired anal sensation (Butcher, 2004).*

▲ Seek medical attention if diarrhea is severe or persists for more than 24 hours, or if the client has history of dehydration or electrolyte disturbances, such as lassitude, weakness, or prostration. *Older adult clients can dehydrate rapidly; especially serious is development of hypokalemia with dysrhythmias. C. difficile is a common cause of diarrhea in older adult clients when they have been subjected to long-term antibiotic therapy. Proper infection control practices should be maintained within the home to avoid cross contamination.*

• Provide emotional support for clients who are having trouble controlling unpredictable episodes of diarrhea. *Diarrhea can be a great source of embarrassment to older clients and can lead to social isolation and a feeling of powerlessness.*

Home Care

• Previously mentioned interventions may be adapted for home care use.

• Assess the home for general sanitation and methods of food preparation. Reinforce principles of sanitation for food handling. *Poor sanitation or mishandling of food may cause bacterial infection or transmission of dangerous organisms from utensils to food.*

• Assess for methods of handling soiled laundry if the client is bed bound or has been incontinent. Instruct or reinforce Universal Precautions with family and blood-borne pathogen precautions with agency caregivers. *The Bloodborne Pathogen Regulations of the Occupational Safety and Health Administration (OSHA) identify legal guidelines for caregivers.*

• When assessing medication history, include over-the-counter (OTC) drugs, both general and those currently being used to treat the diarrhea. Instruct clients not to mix OTC medications when self-treating. *Mixing OTC medications can further irritate the gastrointestinal system, intensifying the diarrhea or causing nausea and vomiting.*

• Evaluate current medications for indication that specific interventions are warranted. *Blood levels of medications may increase during prolonged episodes of diarrhea, indicating the need for close monitoring of the client or direct intervention.*

▲ Consult with physician regarding need for blood work or stool specimens. *Laboratory tests may be needed to identify presence of a bacterial pathogen or assess for electrolyte imbalance.*

▲ Evaluate the need for a home health aide or homemaker service referral. *Caregiver may need support for maintaining client cleanliness to prevent skin breakdown.*

• Evaluate the need for durable medical equipment in the home. *The client may need bedside commode, call bell, or raised toilet seat to facilitate prompt toileting.*

Client/Family Teaching and Discharge Planning

• Encourage avoidance of coffee, spices, milk products, and foods that irritate or stimulate the gastrointestinal tract.

• Teach appropriate method of taking ordered antidiarrheal medications; explain side effects.

• Explain how to prevent the spread of infectious diarrhea (e.g., careful handwashing, appropriate handling and storage of food, and thoroughly cleaning the bathroom and kitchen. **EB:** *A Cochrane review found that careful hand-washing with infectious disease can reduce diarrhea episodes by about one third (Ejemot et al, 2008).*

• Help the client to determine stressors and set up an appropriate stress reduction plan, if stress is the cause of diarrhea.

• Teach signs and symptoms of dehydration and electrolyte imbalance.

• Teach perirectal skin care.

▲ Consider teaching clients about complementary therapies such as probiotics, after consultation with primary care practitioner.

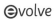 See the EVOLVE website for Weblinks for client education resources.

• = Independent   ▲ = Collaborative   **EBN** = Evidence-Based Nursing   **EB** = Evidence-Based

REFERENCES

Amerine E, Keirsy M: Managing acute diarrhea, *Nursing* 3(9):64, 2004.

Banks JB, Meadows S: Intravenous fluids for children with gastroenteritis, *Am Fam Physician* 71(1):121, 2005.

Behrman RE, Kliegman RM, Jenson HB: *Nelson textbook of pediatrics*, ed 17, Philadelphia, 2004, Saunders.

Beyer PL, Caviar EM, McCallum RW: Fructose intake at current levels in the United States may cause gastrointestinal distress in normal adults, *J Am Diet Assoc* 105(10):1559–1566, 2005.

Bickley LS, Szilagyi P: *Guide to physical examination*, ed 10, Philadelphia, 2009, Lippincott.

Bliss DZ, Jung HJ, Savik K et al: Supplementation with dietary fiber improves fecal incontinence, *Nurs Res* 50(4):203, 2001.

Butcher L: Clinical skills: nursing considerations in patients with faecal incontinence, *Br J Nurs* 13(13):760, 2004.

Centers for Disease Control and Prevention: *Managing acute gastroenteritis among children,* Vol. 52/No. RR-16, 2003.

Dubberke E, Gerding D, Classen D et al: Strategies to prevent *clostridium difficile* infections in acute care hospitals, *Infect Control Hosp Epidemiol* 29(Suppl 1):S81–S92, 2008.

Ejemot RI, Ehiri JE, Meremikwu MM et al: Hand washing for preventing diarrhea, *Cochrane Database Syst Rev* (1):CD004265, 2008.

Ferrie S, East V: Managing diarrhoea in intensive care, *Aust Crit Care* 20(1):7–13, 2007.

Gravel D, Gardam M, Taylor G et al: Infection control practices related to *Clostridium difficile* infection in acute care hospitals in Canada, *Am Infect Control* 37(1):9–14, 2009.

Gray M: Preventing and managing perineal dermatitis: a shared goal for wound and continence care, *J Wound Ostomy Continence Nurs* 31(suppl 1):S2–S9, 2004.

Guarino A, Lo Vecchio A, Canani RB: Probiotics as prevention and treatment for diarrhea, *Curr Opin Gastroenterol* 25(1):18–23, 2009.

Hahn S, Kim S, Garner P: Reduced osmolarity oral rehydration solution for treating dehydration caused by acute diarrhea in children, *Cochrane Database Syst Rev* (1):CD002847, 2002.

Kampf G, Kramer A: Epidemiologic background of hand hygiene and evaluation of the most important agents for scrubs and rubs, *Clin Microbiol Rev* 17(4):863–893, 2004.

Kyle G: Constipation and palliative care—where are we now? *Int J Palliat Nurs* 13(1):6–16, 2007.

Lutz C, Przytulski K: *Nutrition and diet therapy,* ed 5, Philadelphia, 2010, FA Davis.

Mentes J: Oral hydration in older adults: greater awareness is needed in preventing, recognizing, and treating dehydration, *Am J Nurs* 106(6):40–49, 2006.

Nakao M, Ogura Y, Satake S et al: Usefulness of soluble dietary fiber for the treatment of diarrhea during general nutrition in elderly patients, *Nutrition* 18(1):35, 2002.

Nix DH: Validity and reliability of the Perineal Assessment Tool, *Ostomy Wound Manage* 48:2, 2002.

Pilotto A, Franceschi M, Vitale D et al: The prevalence of diarrhea and its association with drug use in elderly outpatients: a multicenter study, *Am J Gastroenterol* 103(11):2816–2823, 2008.

Poutanen SM, Simor AE: *Clostridium difficile*-associated diarrhea in adults, *CMAJ* 171(1):51, 2004.

Rohde CL, Bartolini V, Jones N: The use of probiotics in the prevention and treatment of antibiotic-associated diarrhea with special interest in *Clostridium difficile*-associated diarrhea, *Nutr Clin Pract* 24(1):33–40, 2009.

Sabol VK, Carlson KK: Diarrhea: applying research to bedside practice, *AACN Adv Crit Care* 18(1):32–44, 2007.

Savard J, Sawatzky JA: The use of a nursing model to understand diarrhea and the role of probiotics in patients with inflammatory bowel disease, *Gastroenterol Nurs* 30(6):418–23, 2007.

Sunenshine RH, McDonald LC: Clostridium difficile-associated disease: new challenges from an established pathogen, *Cleve Clin J Med* 73(2):187–197, 2006.

Thielman NM, Guerrant RL: Clinical practice. Acute infectious diarrhea, *N Engl J Med* 350(1):38, 2004.

Thorson MA, Bliss DZ, Savik K: Re-examination of risk factors for non-*Clostridium difficile*-associated diarrhea in hospitalized patients, *J Adv Nurs* 62(3):354–64, 2008.

Todd B: *Clostridium difficile:* familiar pathogen, changing epidemiology: a virulent strain has been appearing more often, even in patients not taking antibiotics, *Am J Nurs* 106(5):33–36, 2006.

Risk for compromised human Dignity   ⊝volve

Shari Froelich, MSN, MSBA, APRN, BC, ACHPN, and Betty J. Ackley, MSN, EdS, RN

NANDA-I

Definition

At risk for perceived loss of respect and honor

NOTE: Honoring an individual's dignity is imperative and consists of the following elements:

- Physical comfort (bathing, positioning, pain and symptom relief, touch, and a peaceful environment). Encompasses aspects of privacy, respect, and autonomy. Also includes staff expertise, effectiveness, and safety of care
- Psychosocial comfort (listening, sharing fears, giving permission, presence, not dying alone, family support and presence). Includes elements of client participation and choice. Clients feel at ease, safe, and protected; neither intimidated nor threatened
- Spiritual comfort (sharing love and caring words, being remembered, validating their lives, praying with and for, reading scripture and Bible, clergy and referral to other providers [i.e. hospice]) (Touhy, Brown & Smith, 2005; Groenewoud et al, 2008)

Risk Factors

Cultural incongruity; disclosure of confidential information; exposure of the body; inadequate participation in decision making; loss of control of body functions; perceived dehumanizing treatment;

• = Independent   ▲ = Collaborative   **EBN** = Evidence-Based Nursing   **EB** = Evidence-Based

perceived humiliation; perceived intrusion by clinicians; perceived invasion of privacy; stigmatizing label; use of undefined medical terms

 (Nursing Outcomes Classification)

Suggested NOC Outcomes

Health Beliefs: Perceived Control, Decision-Making, Spiritual Control, Perceived Social Support

Example **NOC Outcome with Indicators**
Health Beliefs: Perceived Control as evidenced by the following indicators: Perceived responsibility for health decisions/Requested involvement in health decisions/Efforts at gathering information/Belief that own decisions control health outcomes/Willingness to designate surrogate decision maker (Rate the outcome and indicators of **Health Beliefs: Perceived Control:** 1 = very weak, 2 = weak, 3 = moderate, 4 = strong, 5 = very strong [see Section I].)

Client-Based Outcome

Client/Caregiver Will (Specify Time Frame):

- Perceive that dignity is maintained throughout hospitalization
- Consistently call client by name of choice
- Maintain client's privacy

 (Nursing Interventions Classification)

Suggested NIC Interventions

Presence, Decision-Making Support, Spiritual Support, Hope Instillation

Example **NIC Activities—Presence**
Demonstrate accepting attitude; Listen to client's concerns

Nursing Interventions and *Rationales*

- Be authentically present when with the client, try to limit extraneous thoughts of self or others, and concentrate on the well-being of the client. *Helping the client feel important is a core value in the nursing profession. Respect for human dignity includes self-worth, autonomy, self-determination, individuality, and client rights (Coventry, 2006; DiBartolo, 2006). The nurse attempts to enter into and stay within the other's frame of reference to connect with the inner life world of meaning and spirit of the other; together they join in a mutual search for meaning and wholeness of being and becoming to potentiate comfort measures, pain control, a sense of well-being, wholeness, or even spiritual transcendence of suffering (Cara, 2003).* **EBN:** *The mutual act of intentionally focusing on the client through attentiveness to their needs by offering of one's whole self to be with the client for the purpose of healing (Tavernier, 2009).*
- Accept the client as is, with unconditional positive regard. *The person is viewed as whole and complete, regardless of illness or social situation. Dignity is an inherent characteristic of being human (DiBartolo, 2006). Being treated with unconditional love is a healing experience in itself. Essential to the client-centered relationship are unconditional regard, empathy, and genuineness (Dossey & Keegan, 2009).*
- Use loving, appropriate touch based on the client's culture. When first meeting the client, shake hands with younger clients; touch the arm or shoulder of older clients. *Ideally the caring relationship with client and family begins on hospital admission and is carried through to discharge and into the home if possible.* **EBN:** *Touch can lower anxiety (Maville, Bowen, & Benham, 2008). Touch can help build interpersonal relationships (Salzmann-Erikson & Eriksson, 2005).*
- Determine the client's perspective about their health. Example questions include: "Tell me about your health." "What is it like to be in your situation?" "Tell me how you perceive yourself in this situation." "What meaning are you giving to this situation?" "Tell me about your health priorities." "Tell me about the harmony you wish to reach." *Such questions usually contribute to helping people find meaning to the crisis in their life (Watson, 2008).*

● = Independent   ▲ = Collaborative   **EBN** = Evidence-Based Nursing   **EB** = Evidence-Based

- Create a loving, healing environment for the client to help meet physical, psychological, and spiritual needs as possible. *The goal is to develop a healing environment where wholeness, beauty, comfort, dignity, and peace are potentiated (Watson & Foster, 2003; Dossey & Keegan, 2009).*
- Determine the client's preferences for when and how nursing care is needed and follow the client's guidelines if at all possible. *The client's autonomy must be recognized as part of dignified nursing care (Coventry, 2006).* **EBN:** *Summary of older adults' perceptions of the most important nurse caring behaviors are (Marini, 1999):*
  - *Knowing what they are doing*
  - *Know when it's necessary to call the medical provider*
  - *Treat me as an individual*
  - *Give my treatments and medications on time*
  - *Check my condition very closely*
  - *Give my pain medication on time*
  - *Know how to handle equipment*
  - *Keep my family informed of my progress*
  - *Don't give up on me when I am difficult to get along with*
- Include the client in all decision making; if the client does not choose to be part of the decision, or is no longer capable of making a decision, use the named surrogate decision maker. *The Patient Self-Determination Act, effective in 1991, requires that all individuals receiving medical care also receive written information about their right to accept or refuse medical or surgical treatment and their right to initiate advance directives. Advance Directives are instructions that indicate health care interventions to initiate or withhold or that designate someone who will act as a surrogate in making such decisions in the event that decision-making capacity is lost (Dossey & Keegan, 2009).*
- Encourage the client to share his or her feelings, both positive and negative as appropriate and as the client is willing. *Being present to, and supportive of the expression of positive and negative feelings is a connection with deeper spirit of self and the one-being-cared-for (Watson, 2008).*
- Ask the client what they would like to be called and use that name consistently.
- Maintain privacy at all times.
- Avoid authoritative care where the nurse knows what should be done, and the client is powerless. *Authoritative practice does not acknowledge the rights and dignity of others, those who have power must constrain themselves and use caution in applying care based on own judgments (Matiti & Cotrel-Gibbons, 2006).*
- Sit down when talking to clients in the bed; establish appropriate eye contact. *Towering over a client makes communication difficult; the nurse is displaying power behaviors that make the client uncomfortable and decrease communication.* **EBN:** *Fewer visits, less eye contact, and increasingly meaningless conversations reflect emotional abandonment; community is denied. Suffering is devaluing and causes people to retreat from dehumanizing experiences (Stanley, 2002).* **EB:** *Body language often indicates a lack of openness to questions—as demonstrated by lack of eye contact, moving towards the door before concluding the assessment and a hesitance to touch the client are nonverbal actions that give clients a "rushed" and uneasy feeling, which causes anxiety, tension, and forgetfulness (Vieder, Krafchick, & Kovach, 2002).*
- Actively listen to what the client is saying both verbally and nonverbally. **EBN:** *We must quiet our "inner dialog" so that we may hear more clearly, allow others to tell the whole story, listen without judgment or advice, and bear witness to the experience. Attentive silence is a communicative act in its own right, an act of compassion. It signifies respect, legitimizes what is said, and creates an atmosphere in which self-discovery can occur (Stanley, 2002).*
- Encourage the client to share thoughts about spirituality as desires. *The care of the soul remains the most powerful aspect of the art of caring in nursing. The caring occasion becomes "transpersonal" when "it allows for the presence of the spirit of both—then the event of the moment expands the limits of openness and has the ability to expand human capabilities" (Watson, 2008).*
- Utilize interventions to instill increased hope; see the care plan **Readiness for enhanced Hope. EB:** *When hope for a cure is no longer possible, help clients to recognize that the relationships change between clients, families, and caregivers but do not end. Hope continues, but now has a different focus (Erlen, 2003). Caring does not end but is rather transformed when intensive treatment ends.*
- For further interventions on spirituality, see the care plan for **Readiness for enhanced Spiritual well-being.**

● = Independent   ▲ = Collaborative   **EBN** = Evidence-Based Nursing   **EB** = Evidence-Based

Geriatrics

- Always ask the client how he or she would like to be addressed. Avoid calling elderly clients "sweetie," "honey," "Gramps" or other terms that can be demeaning unless this is acceptable in the client's culture, or requested by the client. *Appropriate forms of address must be used with the elderly to maintain dignity (Woolhead et al, 2006).*
- Treat the elderly client with the utmost respect, even if delirium or dementia is present with confusion. *Confused clients respond positively to caregivers who approach gently, with positive regard, and treat the confused client with respect and dignity.*
- Avoid use of restraints. Consider all aspects of restraint use including IVs, foleys, and chemicals. *The paternalistic use of physical restraints is morally unjustified and a violation of the client's autonomy. Dignity is not maintained (Cheung & Yam, 2005).*

Multicultural

- Assess for the influence of cultural beliefs, norms, and values on the client's way of communicating, and follow the client's lead in communicating in matters of eye contact, amount of personal space, voice tones, and amount of touching. If in doubt, ask the client. *What the client considers normal and appropriate communication that maintains and facilitates dignity is based on cultural perceptions (Leininger & McFarland, 2002; Giger & Davidhizar, 2004).*

Home Care

- Most of the interventions described previously may be adapted for home care use.
- Recognize that the client with the caregiver has complete autonomy in the home. *The nurse's role is to provide the care needed and desired. The client and caregiver determine if the care offered is acceptable.*

Client/Family Teaching and Discharge Planning

- Teach family and caregivers the need for the dignity of the client to be maintained at all times. *How an individual cognitively perceives and emotionally deals with the illness can depend on the person's family and social relationships and ultimately can affect the ability to heal.*

NOTE: Caring is integral to maintaining dignity. According to Jean Watson (2008), a caring occasion is the moment (focal point in space and time) when the nurse and another person come together in such a way that an occasion for human caring is created. Both the one cared-for and the one caring can be influenced by the caring moment through the choices and actions decided within the relationship, thereby, influencing and becoming part of their own life history (Watson, 2008).

⊖volve   See the EVOLVE website for Weblinks for client education resources.

REFERENCES

Cara CJ: A pragmatic view of Jean Watson's caring theory, *Int J Hum Caring* 7(3):51–61, 2003.

Cheung PP, Yam BM: Patient autonomy in physical restraint, *J Clin Nurs* 14(Suppl 1):34–40, 2005.

Coventry ML: Care with dignity: a concept analysis, *J Gerontol Nurs* 32(5):42–49, 2006.

DiBartolo MC: Respect and dignity: enduring concepts, enduring challenges, *J Gerontol Nurs* 32(5):12, 2006.

Dossey B, Keegan L: *Holistic nursing: a handbook for practice,* ed 5, Sudbury, MA, 2009, Jones and Bartlett.

Erlen J: Caring doesn't end, *Orthop Nurs* 22(5):446–449, 2003.

Giger J, Davidhizar R: *Transcultural nursing: assessment and intervention.* St Louis, 2004, Mosby.

Groenewoud A, Job N, van Exel A et al: Building quality report card for geriatric care in the Netherlands: Using concept mapping to identify the appropriate "building blocks" from the consumer's perspective, *Gerontologist* 48(1):79–92, 2008.

Leininger MM, McFarland MR: *Transcultural nursing: concepts, theories, research and practices,* ed 3, New York, 2002, McGraw-Hill.

Marini B: Institutionalized older adults' perception of nursing caring behaviors: a pilot study, *J Gerontol Nurs* 25(5):10–16, 1999.

Matiti M, Cotrel-Gibbons L: Patient dignity—promoting good practice, *Dev Pract Improv Care* 3(5):1–4, 2006.

Maville J, Bowen J, Benham G: Effect of healing touch on stress perception and biological correlates, *Holistic Nurs Pract* 22(2):103–110, 2008.

Salzmann-Erikson M, Eriksson H: Encouraging touch: a path to affinity in psychiatric care, *Issues Ment Health Nurs* 26(8):843–852, 2005.

Stanley K: The healing power of presence: respite from the fear of abandonment, *Oncol Nurs Forum* 39(6):935–940, 2002.

Tavernier S: An evidence-based conceptual analysis of presence. In Dossey B et al: *Holistic nursing: a handbook for practice,* ed 5, Sudbury, MA, 2009, Jones and Bartlett.

Touhy T, Brown C, Smith C: Spiritual caring: end of life in a nursing home, *J Gerontol Nurs* 31(9):27–35, 2005.

Vieder JN, Krafchick MA, Kovach AC: Physician-patient interaction: what do elders want? *J Am Osteopath Assoc* 102(2):73–8, 2002.

Watson J: *Nursing: the philosophy and science of caring,* Boulder, CO, 2008, University Press of Colorado.

Watson J, Foster R: The Attending Nurse Caring Model: integrating theory, evidence and advanced caring-healing therapeutics for transforming professional practice, *J Clin Nurs* 12(3):360–365, 2003.

Woolhead G, Tadd W, Boix-Ferrer JA et al: "Tu" or "vous?" A European qualitative study of dignity and communication with older people in health and social care settings, *Patient Educ Couns* 61(3):363–371, 2006.

Moral Distress   *Beverly Kopala, PhD, RN, and Lisa Burkhart, PhD, RN*

NANDA-I

Definition

Response to the inability to carry out one's chosen ethical/moral decision/action

Defining Characteristics

Expresses anguish (e.g., powerlessness, guilt, frustration, anxiety, self-doubt, fear) over difficulty acting on one's moral choice

Related Factors (r/t)

Conflict among decision makers; conflicting information guiding ethical decision making; conflicting information guiding moral decision making; cultural conflicts; end-of-life decisions; loss of autonomy; physical distance of decision maker; time constraints for decision making; treatment decisions

NOC   (Nursing Outcomes Classification)

Suggested NOC Outcomes

Personal Autonomy, Client Satisfaction: Protection of Rights

Example NOC Outcomes with Indicators
Client Satisfaction: Protection of Rights as evidenced by the following indicators: Requests respected/ Included in decisions about care/Care consistent with religious and spiritual needs (rate the outcome and indicators of **Client Satisfaction: Protection of Rights**: 1 = not at all satisfied, 2 = somewhat satisfied, 3 = moderately satisfied, 4 = very satisfied, 5 = completely satisfied [see Section I].)

Client Outcomes

Client Will (Specify Time Frame):

- Be able to act in accordance with values, goals, and beliefs
- Regain confidence in the ability to make decisions and/or act in accord with values, goals, and beliefs
- Expresses satisfaction with the ability to make decisions consistent with values, goals, and beliefs
- Have choices respected

NIC   (Nursing Interventions Classification)

Suggested NIC Intervention

Patient Rights Protection, Emotional Support

Example NIC Activities—Patient Rights Protection
Provide environment conductive for private conversations between patient, family, and health care professionals

Nursing Interventions and *Rationales*

- Examine the source of moral distress. *Rushton's model of 4 A's to Rise Above Moral Distress (2006) identifies the first step as determining the exact nature of the problem (Rushton, 2006).*

● = Independent   ▲ = Collaborative   **EBN** = Evidence-Based Nursing   **EB** = Evidence-Based

- Affirm and validate the client's feelings and perceptions of others (Rushton, 2006). *The second phase of Rushton's model (2006) is to affirm distress, commitment, feelings, perceptions of others, and obligations (Rushton, 2006). A qualitative study of eight pediatric nurses working with children in a persistent vegetative state found the pediatric nurses tried to respect the client's family's values even when inconsistent with their own (Montagnino & Ethier, 2007).*
- ▲ Provide adequate information and emotional and psychological support to assist in coping and making collaborative decisions with the health care team. *Expert opinion recommends providing accurate information and discussing decisions throughout hospitalization (Gutierrez, 2005). Recognize that families seek more involvement (McClendon & Buckner, 2007).*
- Assess personal source of distress to contemplate ability to act. *The third phase of Rushton's model (2006) is to identify source and severity of distress and readiness to act on the distress (Rushton, 2006).*
- Implement strategies to initiate changes to resolve moral distress. *The fourth phase of Rushton's model (2006) is to take action on the moral distress (Rushton, 2006). Negativity may be lessened by focusing on the positive aspects of the situation (Montagnino & Ethier, 2007).*
- Confront the barrier. *A review of the literature on moral distress and the pediatric intensive care unit suggests sharing of stories to eliminate a culture of silence (Austin et al, 2009). A qualitative data analysis produced a substantive grounded theory of a three-stage process of moral reckoning in nursing that challenges nurses to examine conflicts and be partners in moral decision making (Nathaniel, 2006).*
- ▲ Improve communication and collaboration between client, family, and health care team. *Expert opinion recommends ethics rounds to discuss moral issues and related client treatment goals to resolve or prevent conflicts (Gutierrez, 2005). The findings of ethnographic research focused on a multidisciplinary, home health agency team caring for clients with mental illness note the benefits resulting from team members sharing perspectives with one another (Sturm, 2007).*
- Advocate for the client (Ferrell, 2006). *Develop a forum for ethical discussions. Expert opinion encourages the nurse to voice moral distress issues regularly in an established forum (Gutierrez, 2005).*
- Develop a support system. *A descriptive study of nine nurses working in an intensive care unit suggests that individuals can receive support from others including chaplains (McClendon & Buckner, 2007); individual and group support was found to be a useful coping strategy (Mobley et al, 2007).*
- ▲ Consult with other health care providers that may include the family. *Implications and recommendations from a study of moral distress in 260 medical and surgical nurses working in an adult acute tertiary care hospital include using client care conferences to increase communication among health care providers and families (Rice et al, 2008).*
- ▲ Contact an ethicist or the ethics committee to ensure the client's rights are protected. *A retrospective review of 255 ethics consultations conducted at the Mayo Clinic revealed that nurses are among those requesting consults and that events capable of causing moral distress were listed among reasons for the requests (Swetz et al, 2007).*

Pediatric

- Consider the developmental age of children when evaluating decisions and conflict. *This study of children's emotional consequences of desire fulfillment versus desire inhibition demonstrated differences in psychological, deontic, and future-oriented reasoning about emotions as well as the development of self-control (Lagattuta, 2005).*

Multicultural

- Acknowledge and understand that cultural differences may influence a client's moral choices. *In this study it was demonstrated that African Americans and Caucasians differ in beliefs about genetic testing and the basis for moral decision making (Zimmerman et al, 2006). Our beliefs about morality are culturally embedded in social, religious, and political ideologies that influence individuals and communities. Attention to the meaning of concepts and their cultural contexts is crucial in fostering mutual respect and understanding for different cultural frames of reference (Andersson, Mendes, & Trevizan, 2002).*

• = Independent   ▲ = Collaborative   **EBN** = Evidence-Based Nursing   **EB** = Evidence-Based

Geriatric and Home Care

- Previous interventions may be adapted for geriatric or home care use.

⊖volve   See the EVOLVE website for Weblinks for client education resources.

REFERENCES

Andersson M, Mendes IA, Trevizan MA: Universal and culturally dependent issues in health care ethics, *Med Law* 21(1):77–85, 2002.

Austin W, Kelecevic J, Goble E et al: An overview of moral distress and the paediatric intensive care team, *Nurs Ethics* 16:57–68, 2009.

Ferrell BR: Understanding the moral distress of nurses witnessing medically futile care, *Oncol Nurs Forum* 33(5):922–930, 2006.

Gutierrez KM: Critical care nurses' perception of responses to moral distress, *Dimen Crit Care Nurs* 24(5):229–241, 2005.

Lagattuta KH: When you shouldn't do what you want to do: young children's understanding of desires, rules, and emotions, *Child Dev* 76(3):713–733, 2005.

McClendon H, Buckner EB: Distressing situations in the intensive care unit: a descriptive study of nurses' responses, *Dimens Crit Care Nurs* 26:199–206, 2007.

Mobley MJ, Rady MY, Verheijde JL et al: The relationship between moral distress and perception of futile care in the critical care unit, *Intens Crit Care Nurs* 23:256–263, 2007.

Montagnino BA, Ethier AM: The experiences of pediatric nurses caring for children in a persistent vegetative state, *Pediatr Crit Care Med* 8:440–446, 2007.

Nathaniel AK: Moral reckoning in nursing, *West J Nurs Res* 28:419–441, 2006.

Rice EM, Rady MY, Hamrick A et al: Determinants of moral distress in medical and surgical nurses at an adult acute tertiary care hospital. *J Nurs Manag* 16:360–373, 2008.

Rushton CH: Defining and addressing moral distress: tools for critical care nursing leaders, *AACN Adv Crit Care* 17(2):161–168, 2006.

Sturm BA: Issues of ethics and care in psychiatric home care: multidisciplinary perspectives revealed through ethnographic research, *Home Healthc Manag Pract* 19:94–103, 2007.

Swetz KM, Crowley ME, Hook CC et al: Report of 255 clinical ethics consultations and review of the literature, *Mayo Clin Proc* 82(6):686–691, 2007.

Zimmerman RK, Tabbarah M, Nowalk MP et al: Racial differences in beliefs about genetic screening among patients at inner-city neighborhood health centers, *J Natl Med Assoc* 98(3):370–377, 2006.

Risk for Disuse syndrome   *Betty J. Ackley, MSN, EdS, RN*

NANDA-I

Definition

At risk for a deterioration of body systems as the result of prescribed or unavoidable musculoskeletal inactivity

Risk Factors

Altered level of consciousness; mechanical immobilization; paralysis; prescribed immobilization; severe pain

NOTE: Complications from immobility can include pressure ulcer, constipation, stasis of pulmonary secretions, thrombosis, urinary tract infection and/or retention, decreased strength or endurance, orthostatic hypotension, decreased range of joint motion, disorientation, disturbed body image, and powerlessness.

NOC   (Nursing Outcomes Classification)

Suggested NOC Outcomes

Endurance, Immobility Consequences: Physiological, Mobility, Neurological Status: Consciousness; Pain Level

Example NOC Outcome with Indicators
Immobility Consequences: Physiological as evidenced by the following indicators: Pressure sores/ Constipation/Compromised nutrition status/Urinary calculi/Compromised muscle strength (Rate the outcome and indicators of **Immobility Consequences: Physiological:** 1 = severe, 2 = substantial, 3 = moderate, 4 = mild, 5 = none [see Section I].)

Client Outcomes

Client Will (Specify Time Frame):
- Maintain full range of motion in joints
- Maintain intact skin, good peripheral blood flow, and normal pulmonary function
- Maintain normal bowel and bladder function
- Express feelings about imposed immobility
- Explain methods to prevent complications of immobility

 (Nursing Interventions Classification)

Suggested NIC Interventions

Energy Management, Exercise Therapy: Joint Mobility, Muscle Control

Example NIC Activities—Energy Management
Determine the client's physical limitations; Determine the client's significant other's perception of causes of fatigue

Nursing Interventions and *Rationales*

- Once client's condition is stable, screen for mobility skills in the following order: (1) bed mobility; (2) supported and unsupported sitting; (3) transition movements such as sit to stand, sitting down, and transfers; and (4) standing and walking activities. Use a tool such as the Assessment Criteria and Care Plan for Safe Patient Handling and Movement (Sedlak et al, 2009).
- Assess for quality of movement, ability to walk and move, gait pattern, ADL function, presence of spasticity, activity tolerance, and activity order (Kneafsey, 2007). Additional measures of physical function to assess strength of muscle groups include: unassisted leg stand, use of a balance platform, elbow flexion and knee extension strength, grip strength, timed chair stands, and the 6–minute walk. **EBN:** *The nursing assessment should include factors related to mobility problems (e.g., ability to walk and move), with nursing goals and interventions developed to promote maximum mobility (Kneafsey, 2007). The abilities of the client should be assessed to determine how best to facilitate movement and protect the nurse from harm (Nelson et al, 2003; Curb et al, 2006).*
- ▲ Have the client do exercises in bed if possible and not contraindicated (e.g., flexing and extending feet and quadriceps, performing gluteal and abdominal sitting exercises, lifting small weights to maintain muscle strength). *In-bed exercises help maintain muscle strength and tone (Kasper & Talbor, 2002).*
- Position clients as close to the upright position as possible several times per day. *Almost all clients can get out of bed now with use of the stretcher-chair, which converts from a stretcher to a chair (Nelson et al, 2003). Deconditioning of the cardiovascular system occurs within days and involves fluid shifts, fluid loss, decreased cardiac output, decreased peak oxygen uptake, and increased resting heart rate (Fletcher, 2005; Fauci et al, 2008). Bed rest is almost always harmful to clients; early mobilization is better than bed rest for most health conditions (Perme & Chandrashekar, 2009).*
- ▲ If not contraindicated by the client's condition, obtain referral to physical therapy for use of tilt table to provide weight bearing on long bones. *The upright position helps maintain bone strength, increase circulation, and prevent postural hypotension (Fauci et al, 2008).*
- Perform range of motion exercises for all possible joints at least twice daily; perform passive or active range of motion exercises as appropriate. *If not used, muscles weaken and shorten from fibrosis of the muscle (Wagner et al, 2008).* **EBN:** *Range of motion exercises are effective in maintaining joint mobility and muscle integrity (Gillis & MacDonald, 2008; Summers et al, 2009).*
- Use high-top sneakers or specialized boots to prevent pressure ulcers on the heels and footdrop; remove shoes twice daily to provide foot care. *Sneakers or boots help keep the foot in normal anatomical alignment; footdrop can make it difficult or impossible to walk after bed rest.* **EBN:** *A study found that when using a protocol, the incidence of heel ulcers was reduced 95% (Burda, 2007). Another study found that use of a wedge shaped viscoelastic bed-sized support surface was more effective than use of a pillow to prevent heel ulcers (Heyneman et al, 2009).*
- Position the client so that joints are in normal anatomical alignment at all times. *Improper positioning can damage peripheral nerves and blood vessels, as well as cause joint deformities (Fried & Fried, 2001).*

• = Independent   ▲ = Collaborative   **EBN** = Evidence-Based Nursing   **EB** = Evidence-Based

- When positioning a client on the side, tilt client 30 degrees or less while lying on side. *Full (versus tilt) side-lying position places higher pressure on trochanter, predisposing to skin breakdown though there is not a good evidence base (van Rijswijk, 2009).*
- Assess skin condition at least daily and more frequently if needed. Utilize a risk assessment tool such the Braden Scale or the Norton Scale to predict the risk of developing pressure ulcers. **EBN:** *Use of a risk assessment tool is possibly effective to predict the risk of developing a pressure ulcer (Gillis & MacDonald, 2008). Refer to care plan for* **Risk for impaired Skin integrity.**
- Initiate a "No Lift" policy in which appropriate assistive devices are utilized for manual lifting. **EBN:** *A "No Lift" policy along with other measures such as the Back Injury Resource Nurses and an algorithm on safe client handling resulted in decreased workers' compensation expenses with reduced lost and modified work days, along with nurse and client satisfaction (Nelson et al, 2006).*
- Turn clients at high risk for pressure/shear/friction frequently. Turn clients **at least** every 2 to 4 hours on a pressure-reducing mattress/every 2 hours on standard foam mattress. *These are general guidelines given for turning, but they do not have a good evidence base. Preferably base the turning schedule on close assessment of the client's condition and predisposing conditions (van Rijswijk, 2009; Krapfl & Gray, 2008).* Provide the client with a pressure-relieving horizontal support surface. For further interventions on skin care, refer to the care plan for **Impaired Skin integrity.**
- Help the client out of bed as soon as able. *Early mobilization reduces risk of atelectasis, pneumonia, DVT, and pulmonary embolism, and decreases orthostatic hypotension (Summers et al, 2009).*
- When getting the client up after bed rest, do so slowly and watch for signs of postural (orthostatic) hypotension, tachycardia, nausea, diaphoresis, or syncope. Take the blood pressure lying, sitting, and standing, waiting 2 minutes between each reading. *Sitting or standing after 3 or 4 days of bed rest results in postural hypotension because of cardiovascular reflex dysfunction (Fletcher, 2005).*
- Obtain assistive devices such as braces, crutches, or canes to help the client reach and maintain as much mobility as possible. *Assistive devices can help increase mobility (Nelson et al, 2004; Yoem, Keller, & Fleury, 2009).*
- ▲ Apply graduated compression stockings as ordered. Ensure proper fit by measuring accurately. Remove the stocking at least twice a day, in the morning with the bath and in the evening to assess the condition of the extremity, then reapply. Knee-length is preferred rather than thigh length. **EBN and EB:** *The use of graduated compression stockings reduced the incidence of deep vein thrombosis in a high-risk orthopedic surgical population. Implementation of additional antithrombotic measures along with stocking use decreased the incidence even further (Joanna Briggs Institute, 2001). Graduated compression stockings, alone or used in conjunction with other prevention modalities, help prevent deep vein thrombosis in hospitalized clients (Amarigiri & Lees, 2005).* **EBN:** *A study that assessed use of knee-length graduated compression stockings found they are as effective as thigh-length graduated compression stockings. They are more comfortable for clients, are easier for staff and clients to use, pose less risk of injury to clients, and are less expensive as recommended in this study (Hilleren-Listerud, 2009).*
- Observe for signs of deep vein thrombosis, including pain, tenderness, swelling in the calf and thigh, and redness in the involved extremity. Take serial leg measurements of the thigh and calf circumferences. In some clients a tender venous cord can be felt in the popliteal fossa. Do not rely on Homans' sign. *Thrombosis with clot formation is usually first detected as swelling of the involved leg and then as pain. Homans' sign is not reliable. Symptoms of existing deep vein thrombosis are nonspecific and cannot be used alone to determine the presence of DVT (Fauci et al, 2008).*
- Have the client cough and deep breathe or use incentive spirometry every 2 hours while awake. *Bed rest compromises breathing because of decreased chest expansion, decreased cilia activity, and pooling of mucus (Fletcher, 2005).*
- Monitor respiratory functions, noting breath sounds and respiratory rate. Percuss for new onset of dullness in lungs. *Immobility results in hypoventilation, which predisposes the client to atelectasis, the pooling of respiratory secretions, and thus pneumonia (Fletcher, 2005).*
- Note bowel function daily. Provide increased fluids, fiber, and natural laxatives such as prune juice as needed. *Constipation is common in immobilized clients because of decreased activity and fluid and food intake.*
- Increase fluid intake to 2000 mL/day within the client's cardiac and renal reserve. *Adequate fluids helps prevent kidney stones and constipation both of which are associated with bed rest.*
- Encourage intake of a balanced diet with adequate amounts of fiber and protein. *Reduced muscular activity and lowered metabolism generally reduce the appetite of a client on bed rest (Fletcher, 2005).*

● = Independent   ▲ = Collaborative   **EBN** = Evidence-Based Nursing   **EB** = Evidence-Based

Critical Care

▲ Recognize that the client who has been in an intensive care environment may develop a neuromuscular disorder resulting in extreme weakness. The client may need a workup to determine the cause before satisfactory ambulation can begin. *Critical care clients can develop disorders such as critical illness myopathy, or a polyneuropathy due to ischemia, pressure, prolonged recumbency, compartment syndrome, or hematomas (Maramattom & Wijdicks, 2006).*

▲ Consider use of a continuous lateral rotation therapy bed. **EBN:** *Implementing kinetic therapy in the ICU resulted in improved oxygenation and decreased length of stay for clients with pulmonary disorders (Powers & Daniels, 2004; Swadener-Culpepper, Skaggs, & Vangilder, 2008).*

▲ For the stable client in the intensive care unit, consider mobilizing the client in a four-phase method from dangling at the side of the bed to walking if there is sufficient knowledgeable staff available to protect the client from harm. *Even intensive care unit clients receiving mechanical ventilation can be mobilized safely if a multidisciplinary team is present to support, protect, and monitor the client for intolerance to activity (Perme & Chandrashekar, 2009).* **EB:** *A study found that whole-body rehabilitation consisting of interruption of sedation and physical and occupational therapy in the early days of critical illness was safe and well tolerated, and resulted in better functional outcomes at discharge (Schweickert et al, 2009).* **EBN:** *Critical-care clients are at high risk for complications related to immobility such as ventilator-associated pneumonia (VAP), atelectasis, and long-lasting functional limitations, therefore once hemodynamically stable, use progressive mobilization to dangle legs, sit in a chair, stand and bear weight, and walk. Use rotation therapy (kinetic and continuous lateral) to reduce risk of VAP for clients on mechanical ventilation (Rauen et al, 2008).*

Geriatric

• Help the mostly immobile client achieve mobility as soon as possible, depending on physical condition. *In the elderly, mobility impairment can predict increased mortality and dependence; however, this can be prevented by physical exercise (Fletcher, 2005). Functional decline from hospital-associated deconditioning is common in the elderly, and acute inpatient rehabilitation can be effective in preventing this condition (Kortebein, 2009).*

• Use the Outcome Expectation for Exercise Scale to determine client's self-efficacy expectations and outcomes expectations toward exercise. **EBN:** *Use of self-efficacy–based interventions resulted in increased exercise (Resnick et al, 2007).*

▲ Refer the client to physical therapy for resistance strength exercise training. **EB:** *Clients in an extended care facility were put on a strength, balance, and endurance training program; the clients' balance and mobility improved significantly (Rydwik, Kerstin & Akner, 2005). A Cochrane review found that progressive resistance training is effective in increasing strength in older people (Liu & Latham, 2009).*

• Monitor for signs of depression: flat affect, poor appetite, insomnia, many somatic complaints. *Depression can commonly accompany decreased mobility and function in the elderly (Fletcher, 2005).*

• Keep careful track of bowel function in the elderly; do not allow the client to become constipated. *The elderly can easily develop impactions as a result of immobility.*

Home Care

• Some of the previous interventions may be adapted for home care use.

▲ Begin discharge planning as soon as possible with case manager or social worker to assess need for home support systems and community or home health services.

▲ Become oriented to all programs of care for the client before discharge from institutional care.

▲ Confirm the immediate availability of all necessary assistive devices for home.

• Perform complete physical assessment and recent history at initial visit.

▲ Refer to physical and occupational therapies for immediate evaluations of the client's potential for independence and functioning in the home setting and for follow-up care.

• Allow the client to have as much input and control of the plan of care as possible. *Client perception of control increases self-esteem and motivation to follow medical plan of care.*

• Assess knowledge of all care with caregivers. Review as necessary. *Having the necessary knowledge and skills to perform care decreases caregiver role strain and supports safety of the client.*

• = Independent   ▲ = Collaborative   **EBN** = Evidence-Based Nursing   **EB** = Evidence-Based

▲ Support the family of the client in assumption of caregiver activities. Refer for home health aide services for assistance and respite as appropriate. Refer to medical social services as appropriate.

▲ Institute case management of frail elderly to support continued independent living, if possible in the home environment.

Client/Family Teaching and Discharge Planning

• Teach client/family how to perform range-of-motion exercises in bed if not contraindicated.

• Teach the family how to turn and position the client and provide all care necessary.

NOTE: Nursing diagnoses that are commonly relevant when the client is on bed rest include **Constipation, Risk for impaired Skin integrity, Disturbed Sensory perception, Disturbed Sleep pattern, Adult Failure to thrive,** and **Powerlessness.**

⊖volve   See the EVOLVE website for Weblinks for client education resources.

REFERENCES

Amarigiri SV, Lees TA: Elastic compression stockings for prevention of deep vein thrombosis, *Cochrane Database Syst Rev* (3):CD001484, 2005.

Burda V: *A successful heel ulcer prevention program resulting in 95% reduction of heel ulcer incidence.* Poster presented at the Symposium on Advanced Wound Care, Tampa, FL, April, 2007.

Curb JD et al: Performance-based measures of physical function for high-function populations, *J Am Geriatr Soc* 54(5):737–742, 2006.

Fauci A, Braunwald E, Kasper DL et al: *Harrison's principles of internal medicine,* ed 17, New York, 2008, McGraw-Hill.

Fletcher K: Immobility: geriatric self-learning module, *Medsurg Nurs* 14(1):35, 2005.

Fried KM, Fried GW: Immobility. In Derstine JB, Hargrove SD, editors: *Comprehensive rehabilitation nursing,* Philadelphia, 2001, WB Saunders.

Gillis AJ, MacDonald BC: Bedrest care guideline. In Ackley B Ladwig G, Swan BA et al: *Evidence-based nursing care guidelines: medical-surgical interventions,* Philadelphia, 2008, Mosby.

Heyneman A, Vanderwee K, Grypdonck M et al: Effectiveness of two cushions in the prevention of heel pressure ulcers, *Worldviews Evid Based Nurs* 6(2):114–120, 2009.

Hilleren-Listerud AE: Graduated compression stocking and intermittent pneumatic compression device length selection, *Clin Nurse Spec* 23(1):21–24, 2009.

Joanna Briggs Institute: Best practice: graduated compression stockings for the prevention of post-operative venous thromboembolism, *Evidenced Based Practice Information Sheets for Health Professions* 5:2, 2001.

Kasper CE, Talbor LA: Skeletal muscle damage and recovery, *AACN Clin Issues* 13(2):237, 2002.

Kneafsey R: A systematic review of nursing contributions to mobility rehabilitation: examining the quality and content of the evidence, *J Clin Nurs* 16(11C):325–340, 2007.

Kortebein P: Rehabilitation for hospital-associated deconditioning, *Am J Phys Med Rehabil* 88(1):66–77, 2009.

Krapfl LA, Gray M: Does regular repositioning prevent pressure ulcers? *J Wound Ostomy Continence Nurs* 35(6):571–577, 2008.

Liu CJ, Latham NK: Progressive resistance strength training for improving physical function in older adults, *Cochrane Database Syst Rev* (3): CD002759, 2009.

Maramattom BV, Wijdicks EF: Acute neuromuscular weakness in the intensive care unit, *Crit Care Med* 34(11):2835–2841, 2006.

Nelson A, Owen B, Lloyd JD et al: Safe patient handling and movement, *Am J Nurs* 103(3):32–43, 2003.

Nelson A, Matz M, Chen F et al: Development and evaluation of a multifaceted ergonomics program to prevent injuries associated with patient handling tasks, *Int J Nurs Stud* 43(6):717–733, 2006.

Nelson A, Powell-Cope G, Gavin-Dreschnack D et al: Technology to promote safe mobility in the elderly, *Nurs Clin North Am* 39:649, 2004.

Perme C, Chandrashekar R: Early mobility and walking program for patients in intensive care units: creating a standard of care, *Am J Crit Care* 18(3):212–221, 2009.

Powers J, Daniels D: Turning points: implementing kinetic therapy in the ICU, *Nurs Manage* 35(5):1, 2004.

Rauen CA, Chulay M, Bridges E et al: Seven evidence-based practice habits: putting some sacred cows out to pasture, *Crit Care Nurse* 28(2):98–113, 2008.

Resnick B, Orwig D, D'Adamo C et al: Factors that influence exercise activity among women post hip fracture participating in the Exercise Plus Program, *Clin Interv Aging* 2(3):413–27, 2007.

Rydwik E, Kerstin F, Akner G: Physical training in institutionalized elderly people with multiple diagnoses—a controlled pilot study, *Arch Gerontol Geriatr* 40(1):29, 2005.

Schweickert WD, Pohlman MC, Pohlman AS et al: Early physical and occupational therapy in mechanically ventilated, critically ill patients: a randomised controlled trial, *Lancet* 373(9678):1874–1882, 2009.

Sedlak CA, Doheny MO, Nelson A et al: Development of the National Association of Orthopaedic Nurses guidance statement on safe patient handling and movement in the orthopaedic setting, *Orthop Nurs* 28(2 Suppl):S2–8, 2009.

Summers D, Leonard A, Wentworth D et al: Comprehensive overview of nursing and interdisciplinary care of the acute ischemic stroke patient, *Stroke* 40:2911, 2009.

Swadener-Culpepper L, Skaggs RL, Vangilder CA: The impact of continuous lateral rotation therapy in overall clinical and financial outcomes of critically ill patients, *Crit Care Nurs Q* 31(3):270–279, 2008.

Van Rijswijk L: Pressure ulcer prevention updates, *Am J Nurs* 109(8):56, 2009.

Wagner L, Capezuti E, Brush B et al: Contractures in frail nursing home residents, *Geriatr Nurs* 29(4):259–265, 2008.

Yoem HA, Keller C, Fleury J: Interventions for promoting mobility in community-dwelling older adults, *J Am Acad Nurse Pract* 21:95–100, 2009.

Deficient Diversional activity   *Betty J. Ackley, MSN, EdS, RN*

NANDA-I

Definition

Decreased stimulation from (or interest or engagement in) recreational or leisure activities

Defining Characteristics

Client's statements regarding boredom (e.g., wish there was something to do, to read, etc.); usual hobbies cannot be undertaken in hospital

Related Factors (r/t)

Environmental lack of diversional activity

NOC   (Nursing Outcomes Classification)

Suggested NOC Outcomes

Leisure Participation, Play Participation, Social Involvement

Example **NOC Outcome with Indicators**
Leisure Participation as evidenced by the following indicators: Expresses satisfaction with leisure activities/Feels relaxed from leisure activities/Enjoys leisure activities (Rate the outcome and indicators of **Leisure Participation:** 1 = never demonstrated, 2 = rarely demonstrated, 3 = sometimes demonstrated, 4 = often demonstrated, 5 = consistently demonstrated [see Section I].)

Client Outcomes

Client Will (Specify Time Frame):

- Engage in personally satisfying diversional activities

NIC   (Nursing Interventions Classification)

Suggested NIC Interventions

Recreation Therapy, Self-Responsibility Facilitation

Example **NIC Activities—Recreation Therapy**
Assist the client to identify meaningful recreational activities; Provide safe recreational equipment

Nursing Interventions and *Rationales*

- Observe for signs of deficient diversional activity: restlessness, unhappy facial expression, and statements of boredom and discontent.
- Observe ability to engage in activities that require good vision and use of hands. *Diversional activities must be tailored to the client's capabilities.*
- Discuss activities with clients that are interesting and feasible in the present environment.
- Encourage the client to share feelings about situation of inactivity away from usual life activities. *Work and hobbies provide structure and continuity to life; the client can feel a sense of loss when unable to engage in usual activities.*
- Encourage the client to participate in any available social or recreational opportunities in the health care environment. **EB:** *Spinal cord injury clients who experienced increased frequency of recreational experiences had increased levels of well-being (Lee & McCormick, 2004). A creative art-making experience helped women with chronic disease develop increased satisfaction in daily life, a positive self-image, increased hope, and contact with the outside world (Reynolds, Vivat, & Prior, 2008).*
- Encourage a mix of physical and mental activities if possible (e.g., crafts, crossword puzzles).
- Provide videos and or DVDs of movies for recreation and distraction.

● = Independent   ▲ = Collaborative   **EBN** = Evidence-Based Nursing   **EB** = Evidence-Based

- Provide magazines of interest, books of interest.
- Provide books on CD and CD player.
- Set up a puzzle in a community space, or provide individual puzzles as desired.
- Provide access to a portable computer so that the client can access e-mail and the Internet. Give client a list of interesting websites, including games and directions on how to perform Web searches if needed.
- Help client find a support group for the appropriate condition on the Internet if interested, and if support group is available.
- Use "bread therapy" in long-term or mental health units—clients/staff bake bread with an automatic bread maker as desired. *Assembling the ingredients is a group activity and can be therapeutic. The smell of bread baking gives a homelike, loving atmosphere to a health care environment.*
- ▲ Arrange animal-assisted therapy if desired, with a dog, cat, or bird for the client to interact with and care for, if possible. **EBN:** *A study demonstrated decreased passivity and improved mood in extended care clients (Kawamura, Niiyama, & Niiyama, 2009). Another study in hospitalized clients with heart failure found decreased cardiopulmonary pressures, decreased stress hormones, and decreased anxiety with use of animal-assisted therapy (Cole et al, 2007). In a study on animal-assisted therapy for clients with cancer, clients reported decreased anxiety but no measurable difference in mood, sense of coherence, or self-perceived health (Johnson et al, 2008). Clients receiving a canary had fewer depressed symptoms and increased perception of quality of life (Colombo et al, 2006).*
- Encourage the client to schedule visitors so that they are not all present at once or at inconvenient times. *A schedule prevents the client from becoming exhausted from frequent company.*
- If clients are able to write, help them keep journals; if clients are unable to write, have them record thoughts on tape, or on videotape. *Writing is personal freedom. It frees people as an individual apart from the masses. Writing helps people survive as individuals (Quindlen, 2007).*
- ▲ Request recreational or art therapist to assist with providing diversional activities. *Recreational therapists specialize in helping people have fun.*
- Provide a change in scenery; get the client out of the room as possible. *A lack of sensory stimulation has significant adverse effects on clients.*
- Help the client to experience nature through looking at a nature scene from a window, or walking through a garden if possible. **EBN:** *Exposure to a natural environment can be helpful to promote relaxation, stress recovery, and mental restoration (Jones & Haight, 2002). Listening to birds and feeling the sun on their faces can be a wonderful experience for long-term clients (Fioravanti, 2004).*
- Structure the environment as needed to promote optimal comfort and sensory diversity (e.g., have family bring in posters, banners, or a sound system; change lighting; change direction bed faces). *Modification of the environment is sometimes necessary for the well-being of the client.*
- Work with family to provide music that is enjoyable to the client. **EBN:** *Music can help decrease anxiety in clients before surgery (Cooke et al, 2005) after surgery (Sendelbach et al, 2006), and in clients with an acute myocardial infarction (Winters, 2005, 2008).*
- Structure the client's schedule around personal wishes for time of care, relaxation, and participation in fun activities. *Increased client control fosters increased client self-esteem.*
- Spend time with the client when possible, giving the client full attention and being present in the moment or arrange for a friendly visitor. *Presence involves knowing the uniqueness of the person, listening intently, involving the person, mobilizing resources, and mutually defining changes in the provision of confident caring (Caldwell et al, 2005).*

 Pediatric

- ▲ Request an order for a child life specialist or, if not available, a play therapist for children.
- Provide activities such as video projects and use of computer-based support groups for children, such as Starbright World, a computer network where children interact virtually, sharing their experiences and escaping hospital routines. www.starbrightworld.org. **EB:** *Starbright World was shown to significantly reduce loneliness and withdrawn behavior in chronically ill children (Battles & Wiener, 2002).*
- Provide computer games and virtual reality experiences for children, which can be used as distraction techniques during venipuncture or other procedures. *Augmented reality programs (where vir-*

tual reality programs are overlayed on existing reality) were shown to be effective in decreasing the amount of pain during burn dressing changes (Mott et al, 2008).

Geriatric

- If the client is able, arrange for him or her to attend a group senior citizen activities. **EBN:** *Participation in social behavior improved performance of older adults in activities of daily living. Social behaviors included communicating, concentration skills, and fulfilling occupational tasks (Patton, 2006).*
- Encourage involvement in senior citizen activities (e.g., AARP, YMCA, church groups). Arrange transportation to activities as needed.
- Encourage clients to use their ability to help others by volunteering. *Assisting others can help the client grow as a generative human being.*
- Provide an environment that promotes activity (e.g., one that has adequate lighting for crafts, large-print books).
- Allow periods of solitude and privacy. *Periods of solitude are important for emotional well-being in the elderly.*
- ▲ Use reminiscence therapy in conjunction with the expression of emotions. Refer to a reminiscence group if available. **EBN:** *Participation in a reminiscence group reduced symptoms of depression (Zauszniewski et al, 2004). A systematic review of studies found that reminiscence therapy research demonstrated possibly effective results (Puentes, 2008).*
- Use the Eden Alternative with the elderly; bring in appropriate plants for the elderly client to care for, animals such as birds, fish, dogs, and cats as appropriate for the client and children to visit. **EB:** *A study in clients with Alzheimer's found that animal-assisted therapy was more effective in reducing physiological stress than watching a humorous video or listening to music and viewing fish in a digital tank (Petterson & Loy, 2008). See further rationales for animal-assisted therapy above. The Eden Alternative offers a more natural human habitat where the quality of life is improved (Baumann, 2008).*
- For clients who love gardening, bring in seeds, soil, and pots for indoor gardening experiences. Use seeds such as sunflower, pumpkin, and zinnia seeds that grow rapidly. *Nursing home residents who participated in a weekly gardening experience demonstrated increased socialization and increased physical functioning (Brown et al, 2004).*
- For clients in assisted-living facilities, provide leisure educational programs. **EB:** *Participation in leisure education programs resulted in increased perception of quality of life (Janssen, 2004).*
- Prescribe activities to engage passive dementia clients based on their extraversion and openness. *With onset of dementia, the underlying personality does not completely disintegrate, and knowing this allows the professional to more effectively prescribe activities to engage the client (Kolanowski & Buettner, 2008).*
- ▲ Provide recreational therapy exercises in the morning for clients with dementia in the extended care facility, and in geropsychiatric programs. **EB:** *Morning recreational exercises resulted in decreased agitation and passivity and also increased strength and flexibility (Buetttner & Fitzsimmons, 2004). A therapeutic recreation service in a geropsychiatric program resulted in decreased depress scores, increased mini-mental exam scores, and decreased dependency (McHugh & Smith, 2008).*

Home Care

- Many of the previously listed interventions may be administered in the home setting.
- Explore with the client previous interests; consider related activities that are within the client's capabilities.
- ▲ Assess the client for depression. Refer for mental health services as indicated. *Lack of interest in previously enjoyed activities, is part of the syndrome of depression.*
- Assess the family's ability to respond to the client's psychosocial needs for stimulation. Assist as able.
- ▲ Refer to occupational therapy to assist the client and family with identifying diversional activities within the capability of the client and family.

- Introduce (or continue) friendly volunteer visitors if the client is willing and able to have the company. If transportation is an issue or if the client does not want visitors in the home, consider alternatives (e.g., telephone contacts, computer messaging).
- For clients who are interested and capable, suggest involvement in a community gardening experience through the senior center. *A community elder gardening experience in ambulatory people resulted in decreased depression, and increased level of functioning (Austin et al, 2006).*
- If the client is dying, and is interested, assist in making a videotape, audiotape, or memory book for family members with treasured stories, memoirs, pictures, and video clips. *"Wouldn't all of us love to have a journal, a memoir, a letter, from those we have loved and lost? Shouldn't all of us leave a bit of that behind (Quindlen, 2007)?"*

Client/Family Teaching and Discharge Planning

- Work with the client and family on learning diversional activities that the client is interested in (e.g., knitting, hooking rugs, writing memoirs).
- If the client is in isolation, give the client complete information on why isolation is needed and how it should be accomplished, especially guidelines for visitors. **EBN:** *Clients who were in isolation identified their greatest needs, which were for more information about the isolation regulations and the need for guidelines for visitors so that visitors would be comfortable and continue to visit (Ward, 2000).*

⊝volve   See the EVOLVE website for Weblinks for client education resources.

REFERENCES

Austin et al: Community gardening in a senior center: a therapeutic intervention to improve the health of older adults, *Ther Recreation J* 40(1):48–58, 2006.

Battles HB, Weiner LS: Effects of an electronic network on the social environment of children with life-threatening illness, *Childrens Healthc* 31(1):47–68, 2002.

Baumann SL: How do you keep the music playing? *Nurs Sci Q* 21(4):363–364, 2008.

Brown VM, Allen AC, Dwozan M et al: Indoor gardening and older adults : effects on socialization, activities of daily living, and loneliness, *J Gerontol Nurs* 30(10):34–42, 2004.

Buettner LL, Fitzsimmons S: Recreational therapy exercise on the special care unit: impact on behaviors, *Am J Recreation Ther* 3(4):8–24, 2004.

Caldwell B, Dolye M, Morris M et al: Presencing: channeling therapeutic effectiveness with the mentally ill in a state psychiatric hospital, *Issues Mental Health Nurs* 26:853–871, 2005.

Cole KM, Gawlinski A, Steers N et al: Animal-assisted therapy in patients hospitalized with heart failure, *Am J Crit Care* 16(6):575–585, 2007.

Colombo G, Buono MD, Smania K et al: Pet therapy and institutionalized elderly: a study on 144 cognitively unimpaired subjects, *Arch Gerontol Geriatr* 42(2):207–16, 2006.

Cooke M, Chaboyer W, Schluter P et al: The effect of music on preoperative anxiety in day surgery, *J Adv Nurs* 52(1):47–55, 2005.

Fioravanti MA: Helping patients break the boredom, *RN* 67(1):46–49, 2004.

Janssen MA: The use of leisure education in assisted living facilities, *Am J Recreation Ther* 3(4):25–30, 2004.

Johnson, RA, Meadows RL, Haubner JS et al: Animal-assisted activity among patients with cancer: effects on mood, fatigue, self-perceived health, and sense of coherence, *Oncol Nurs Forum* 35(2):225–232, 2008.

Jones MM, Haight BK: Environmental transformations: an integrative review, *J Gerontol Nurs* 28(3):23, 2002.

Kawamura N, Niiyama M, Niiyama H: Animal-assisted activity: experiences of institutionalized Japanese older adults, *J Psychosoc Nurs Ment Health Serv* 47(1):41–47, 2009.

Kolanowski A, Buettner L: Prescribing activities that engage passive residents, *J Gerontol Nurs* 34(1):13–18, 2008.

Lee Y, McCormick B: Subjective well-being of people with spinal cord injury: does leisure contribute? *J Rehabil* 70(3), 2004.

McHugh M, Smith RW: Comparison of treatment outcomes in geropsychiatric programs with and without therapeutic recreation services, *Ann Ther Recreation* 16:81–90, 2008.

Mott J, Bucolo S, Cuttle L et al: The efficacy of an augmented virtual reality system to alleviate pain in children undergoing burns dressing changes: a randomised controlled trial, *Burns* 34(6):803–808, 2008.

Patton D: The value of reality orientation with older adults, *J Gerontol Nurs* 32(12):6–13, 2006.

Petterson M, Loy DP: Comparing the effectiveness of animal interaction, digital music relaxation, and humor on the galvanic skin response of individuals with Alzheimer's disease: implications for creational therapy, *Annu Ther Recreation* 16:129–145, 2008.

Puentes WJ: Reminiscence therapy. In Ackley BJ, Ladwig GB, Swan BA et al: *Evidence-based nursing care guidelines: medical-surgical interventions,* Philadelphia, 2008, Mosby.

Quindlen A: The last word, *Newsweek,* 149(3):74, 2007.

Reynolds F, Vivat B, Prior S: Women's experiences of increasing subjective well-being in CFS/ME through leisure-based arts and crafts activities: a qualitative study, *Disabil Rehabil* 30(17)1279–1288, 2008.

Sendelbach SE, Halm MA, Doran KA et al: Effects of music therapy on physiological and psychological outcomes for patients undergoing cardiac surgery, *J Cardiovasc Nurs* 21(3):194–200, 2006.

Ward D: Infection control: reducing the psychological effects of isolation, *Br J Nurs* 9(3):162, 2000.

Winters J: Effects of timing and frequency of relaxing music interventions during acute recovery from acute myocardial infarction, *Am J Crit Care* 14(3):254–255, 2005.

Winters J: Music therapy guideline. In Ackley B, Ladwig G, Swann BA, et al: *Evidence-based nursing care guidelines: medical-surgical interventions,* Philadelphia, 2008, Mosby.

Zauszniewski JA, Eggenschwiler K, Preechawong S et al: Focused reflection reminiscence group for elders: implementation and evaluation, *Appl Gerontol* 23(4):429–442, 2004.

• = Independent   ▲ = Collaborative   **EBN** = Evidence-Based Nursing   **EB** = Evidence-Based

Risk for Electrolyte imbalance

Jennifer Hafner, RN, BSN, TNCC, and Joan Klehr, RNC, BS, MPH

 ⊖volve

NANDA-I

Definition

At risk for change in serum electrolyte levels that may compromise health

Risk Factors

Diarrhea; endocrine dysfunction; fluid imbalance (e.g., dehydration, water intoxication); impaired regulatory mechanisms (e.g., diabetes insipidus, syndrome of inappropriate secretion of antidiuretic hormone); renal dysfunction; treatment-related side effects (e.g., medications, drains); vomiting

NOC　(Nursing Outcomes Classification)

Suggested NOC Outcomes

Electrolyte & Acid Base Balance, Fluid Balance, Hydration, Nutritional Status: Biochemical Measures, Nutritional Status: Food & Fluid Intake, Nutritional Status: Nutrient Intake, Kidney Function

Example NOC Outcome with Indicators
Electrolyte & Acid/Base Balance as evidenced by: Apical heart rate/Apical heart rhythm/Serum potassium/ Serum sodium/Serum calcium (Rate the outcome and indicators of **Electrolyte & Acid/Base Balance:** 1 = Severe deviation from normal range, 2 = substantial deviation from normal range, 3 = Moderate deviation from normal range, 4 = mild deviation from normal range, 5 = No deviation from normal range [See Section I].)

Client Outcomes

Client Will (Specify Time Frame):

- Maintain a normal sinus heart rhythm with a regular rate
- Have a decrease in edema
- Maintain an absence of muscle cramping
- Maintain normal serum potassium, sodium, and calcium
- Maintain normal serum pH

NIC　(Nursing Interventions Classification)

Suggested NIC Interventions

Electrolyte Monitoring, Electrolyte Management: Hypokalemia, Electrolyte Management: Hyponatremia, Fluid/Electrolyte Management, Laboratory Data Interpretation

Example NIC Activities—Electrolyte Monitoring
Identify possible causes of electrolyte imbalances; Monitor the serum level of electrolytes

Nursing Interventions and *Rationales*

▲ Monitor vital signs at least three times a day. Notify provider of significant deviation from baseline. *Electrolyte imbalance can lead to changes in vital signs including orthostatic hypotension, bradycardia, tachycardia, respiratory depression, and EKG changes (Elgart, 2004).*

▲ Monitor cardiac rate and rhythm. Report changes to provider. *Hyperkalemia can result in EKG changes that include tall peaked T waves, prolonged PR interval, and widened QRS interval, and can lead to cardiac arrest from complete heart block, or ventricular dysrhythmias (Elgart, 2004; Muller & Bell, 2008). Hypokalemia can result in EKG changes that include flat or inverted T waves, U waves, depressed ST segments, or premature ventricular or atrial complexes, and may lead to ventricular tachycardia (Muller & Bell, 2008). Magnesium has been shown to affect the QT interval and has been used to treat ventricular tachycardia (Weglicki et al, 2005).*

• = Independent　　▲ = Collaborative　　**EBN** = Evidence-Based Nursing　　**EB** = Evidence-Based

- Monitor intake and output and daily weights. *Weight gain is a sensitive and consistent sign of fluid volume excess (Elgart, 2004).*
- Monitor for abdominal distension and discomfort. *Fluid and electrolyte imbalance can cause an adverse effect on GI function due to changes in GI mucosal perfusion and GI tract edema (Macafee, Allison, & Lobo, 2005).*
- Assess neurological status including level of consciousness and mental status. *Electrolyte imbalances can cause changes in neurologic status including confusion, seizures, agitation, delirium, and coma (Trimarchi, 2006; Muller & Bell, 2008; Wedro, 2008).*
- ▲ Review laboratory data as ordered and report deviations to provider. *Laboratory studies may include serum electrolytes: potassium, chloride, sodium, bicarbonate, magnesium, phosphate, calcium; serum pH; comprehensive metabolic panel; and atrial natiuretic peptide (Trimarchi, 2006; Muller & Bell, 2008).*
- Review the client's medical and surgical history. *Certain conditions place the client at increased risk of electrolyte imbalance. Periods of excess fluid loss can lead to dehydration and resulting loss of electrolytes; and fluid can be lost through gastrointestinal illness, hyperthermia, blood loss, and perspiration due to strenuous exercise. Other risk factors for fluid and electrolyte imbalance include endocrine disorders such as diabetes insipidus, diabetes mellitus, or aldosterone insufficiency (Trimarchi, 2006), medications including diuretics, trauma, renal disease, diabetic ketoacidosis, extensive surgeries, and changes in acid-base balance (O'Neill, 2007; Muller & Bell, 2008).*
- ▲ Complete pain assessment. Assess and document the onset, intensity, character, location, duration, aggravating factors, and relieving factors. Notify the provider for any increase in pain or discomfort or if comfort measures are not effective. *Symptoms of electrolyte imbalance and dehydration can include muscle cramps, paresthesias, abdominal cramps, and tetany (O'Neill, 2007; Muller & Bell, 2008; Wedro, 2008).*
- ▲ Monitor the effects of ordered medications such as diuretics and heart medications. *Medications can have adverse effects on electrolyte balance; for example, diuretics can deplete potassium levels (Muller & Bell, 2008) Other medications can increase potassium levels such as potassium-sparing diuretics and ACE inhibitors (Elgart, 2004).*
- ▲ Administer parenteral fluids as ordered and monitor their effects. *Fluid requirements for fluid resuscitation must be adequate to restore intravascular volume, and aggressive replacement with crystalloids is necessary to restore hemodynamic stability and tissue perfusion. During the recovery period, excess fluid administration can lead to water and electrolyte imbalance with adverse effects to the client (Macafee, Allison, & Lobo, 2005).*

Geriatric

- Monitor electrolyte levels carefully, including sodium levels and potassium levels, with both increased and decreased levels possible. *Elderly are prone to electrolyte abnormalities because of failure of regulatory mechanisms associated with heart and kidney disease, plus the large number of medications that are taken that can affect electrolyte levels (Zarowitz & Lefkovitz, 2008). Many elderly clients are receiving selective serotonin reuptake inhibitors for treatment of depression, which can result in hyponatremia (Bowen, 2009).*

Client/Family Teaching and Discharge Planning

- Teach client/family the signs of low potassium and the risk factors. *Signs and symptoms of low potassium include muscle weakness, leg cramps, decreased or absent deep tendon reflexes, orthostatic hypotension, and decreased gastrointestinal motility (O'Neill, 2007).*
- Teach client/family signs of high potassium and the risk factors. *Signs and symptoms of high potassium include restlessness; GI symptoms such as nausea, vomiting, diarrhea and cramping; and skeletal muscle weakness (O'Neill, 2007).*
- Teach client/family the signs of low sodium and the risk factors. *Early signs of low sodium include nausea, muscle cramps, disorientation and may mimic those of dehydration. More severe signs of low sodium include lethargy (fatigue, listlessness), agitation, confusion, and seizures (Stöppler, 2007).*
- Teach client/family the signs of high sodium and the risk factors. *Signs of high sodium include thirst, dry mucous membranes, rapid heartbeat, low blood pressure, and cool extremities. Symptoms can progress to confusion, delirium, and seizures (Elgart, 2004).*

• = Independent   ▲ = Collaborative   **EBN** = Evidence-Based Nursing   **EB** = Evidence-Based

- Teach client/family the importance of hydration during exercise. *Dehydration occurs when the amount of water leaving the body is greater than the amount consumed. The body can lose large amounts of fluid when it tries to cool itself by sweating (Wedro, 2008).*
- Teach client/family the warning signs of dehydration. *Early signs of dehydration include thirst and decreased urine output. As dehydration increases, symptoms may include dry mouth, eyes stop tearing, cessation of perspiration, muscle cramps, nausea and vomiting, lightheadedness, and orthostatic hypotension. Severe dehydration can cause confusion, weakness, coma, and organ failure (Wedro, 2008).*
- Teach client about any medications prescribed. Medication teaching includes the drug name, its purpose, administration instructions such as taking it with or without food, and any side effects to be aware of. *Diuretic use remains a primary cause of low serum potassium levels (Muller & Bell, 2008).*
- ▲ Instruct the client to report any adverse medication side effects to his/her provider. *Assessing and instructing clients about medications and focusing on important details can help prevent client medication errors (Polzien, 2007).*

⊝volve   See the EVOLVE website for Weblinks for client education resources.

REFERENCES

Bowen P: Use of selective serotonin reuptake inhibitors in the treatment of depression in older adults: identifying and managing potential risk for hyponatremia, *Geriatr Nurs* 30(2):85–89, 2009.

Elgart HN: Assessment of fluids and electrolytes, *AACN Clin Issues* 15(4):607–621, 2004.

Macafee D, Allison S, Lobo D: Some interactions between gastrointestinal function and fluid and electrolyte homeostasis, *Curr Opin Clin Nutr Metab Care* 8(2):197–203, 2005.

Muller AC, Bell AE: Electrolyte update: potassium, chloride, and magnesium, *Nurs Crit Care* 3(1):5–7, 2008.

O'Neill P: Helping your patient to restrict potassium, *Nursing 2007* 37(4):6–8, 2007.

Polzien G: Prevent medication errors: a new year's resolution teaching patients about their medications, *Home Healthc Nurse* 25(1):59–62, 2007.

Stöppler M: *Exercise-associated hyponatremia: who's at risk?,* www.medicinenet.com/script/main/art.asp?articlekey=47388, 2007. Accessed March 24, 2009.

Trimarchi T: Endocrine problems in critically ill children: an overview, *AACN Clin Issues* 17(1):66–78, 2006.

Wedro B: *Dehydration,* www.medicinenet.com/dehydration/article.htm, 2008. Accessed March 24, 2009.

Weglicki W, Quamme G, Tucker K et al: Potassium, magnesium, and electrolyte imbalance and complications in disease management, *Clin Exp Hypertens* 1:95–112, 2005.

Zarowitz B, Lefkovitz A: Recognition and treatment of hyperkalemia, *Geriatr Nurs* 29(5):333–339, 2008.

Disturbed Energy field   *Gail B. Ladwig, MSN, RN, CHTP, and Diane Wardell, PhD, RN, WHNP-BC*    ⊝volve

NANDA-I

Definition

Disruption of the flow of energy surrounding a person's being results in disharmony of the body, mind, and/or spirit

Defining Characteristics

Perceptions of changes in patterns of energy flow, such as movement (wave, spike, tingling, density, flowing); sounds (tone, words); temperature change (warmth, coolness); visual changes (image, color); disruption of the field (deficit, hole, spike, bulge, obstruction, congestion, diminished flow in energy field)

Related Factors (r/t)

Slowing or blocking of energy flows secondary to:

Maturational Factors

Age-related developmental crisis, age-related developmental difficulties

Pathophysiologic Factors

Illness, injury, pregnancy

● = Independent   ▲ = Collaborative   **EBN** = Evidence-Based Nursing   **EB** = Evidence-Based

Situational Factors

Anxiety, fear, grieving, pain

Treatment-Related Factors

Chemotherapy, immobility, labor and delivery, perioperative experience

 (Nursing Outcomes Classification)

Suggested NOC Outcomes

Personal Well-Being, Personal Health Status

Example NOC Outcome with Indicators
Personal Well-Being as evidenced by the following indicators: Psychological health/Spiritual life/Ability to relax/Level of happiness (Rate the outcome and indicators of **Personal Well-Being:** 1 = not all satisfied, 2 = somewhat satisfied, 3 = moderately satisfied, 4 = very satisfied, 5 = completely satisfied [see Section I].)

Client Outcomes

Client Will (Specify Time Frame):

- State sense of well-being
- State feeling of relaxation
- State decreased pain
- State decreased tension
- Demonstrate evidence of physical relaxation (e.g., decreased blood pressure, pulse, respiration rate, muscle tension)

 (Nursing Interventions Classification)

Suggested NIC Intervention

Therapeutic Touch (TT), Hope Inspiration

Example NIC Activities—Therapeutic Touch (TT)
Focus awareness on the inner self; Focus on the intention to facilitate wholeness and healing at all levels of consciousness

Nursing Interventions and *Rationales*

- Consider using Therapeutic Touch (TT) and/or Healing Touch (HT) for clients with anxiety, tension, pain, or other conditions that indicate a disruption in the flow of energy. **EBN:** *TT and HT, when provided in the clinical setting, promote comfort, calmness, and well-being among hospitalized clients (Danhauer et al, 2008; MacIntyre et al, 2008; Wardell, Rintala, & Tan, 2008).* **EBN:** *TT and HT may be effective treatments for relieving pain and improving quality of life in this specific population of persons with fibromyalgia syndrome (Denison, 2004). HT may also decrease length of stay in those undergoing coronary artery bypass surgery (MacIntyre et al, 2008). Gentle touch used with clients with cancer showed significant improvements in psychological and physical functioning, quality of life, stress and relaxation, severe pain/discomfort, and depression/anxiety (Weze, Leathard, & Grange, 2004). HT has been used in a variety of cancer studies showing improved quality of life, decreased pain and anxiety, better symptom management (Cook, Guerrerio, & Slater, 2004; Wardell & Weymouth, 2004) and decreased fatigue and nausea (Danhauer et al, 2008).*
- Consider HT treatments for clients with psychological depression. **EBN:** *HT can be a complementary approach to help in the reconnection process to self and others (Van Aken, 2004).*
- Administer TT and/or HT as described in the following discussion (may also include Reiki practice). **EB:** *The research relating to therapeutic touch's effect on pain and anxiety in clients with cancer indicates that the therapy does help reduce pain and anxiety (Jackson et al, 2008).* **EBN:** *HT may reduce stress, anxiety, and pain; facilitate healing; have some improvement in biochemical and physiological markers; and give a greater sense of well-being. Nurses may provide safe, noninvasive care to*

• = Independent   ▲ = Collaborative   **EBN** = Evidence-Based Nursing   **EB** = Evidence-Based

promote healing with HT (Wardell & Weymouth, 2004). HT reduced anxiety in clients undergoing first-time elective coronary artery bypass surgery (MacIntyre et al, 2008).

- Refer to care plans for **Anxiety**, **Acute Pain**, and **Chronic Pain**.

Guidelines for Therapeutic Touch and Healing Touch

- TT and HT may be practiced by anyone with the requisite preparation, desire, and commitment. *TT requires completion of a minimum 12–contact hour basic workshop by a TT practitioner who meets Nurse Healer–Professional Associates International, Inc. criteria. HT requires completion of a minimum 16–contact hour level 1 workshop (out of five levels needed for program completion) by a Certified HT Instructor.*
- Those who are not licensed health care professionals may practice TT and HT within their families, religious or spiritual community, and with friends.
- NOTE: Nurses who are not trained in TT or HT should consider spending quiet time with clients listening to their concerns. **EBN:** *Nurses who are not trained in the administration of TT may use quiet time and dialogue to enhance feelings of calmness and relaxation in clients with breast cancer (Kelly et al, 2004).*
- TT is conducted according to the standards for its practice developed by Dolores Krieger (1997) and Dora Kuntz (2004). *It is used in accordance with guidelines provided by the Nurse Healers Professional Associates (NH-PAI, 2006).*
- HT is conducted according to the code of ethics and standards of practice developed by Healing Touch International, Inc. *(Healing Touch International, 2009).*
- Administer TT and HT according to the guidelines established by the prospective therapies and programs. *A description of HT is found at Healing Touch International at www.HealingTouchInternational .org and for TT at Therapeutic Touch at www.therapeutic-touch.org.*

Pediatric

- Consider using TT or HT for pediatric clients with adjunct therapies to decrease stress, anxiety, and pain. **EBN:** *HT and TT are unique touch techniques. They are widely available in pediatric hospitals. Practitioners, as well as clients, may notice improved sense of well-being during and after treatments. These therapies are safe and readily available (Kemper & Kelly, 2004).*
- Teach that when working with the very young, old, or ill, or in the head area, TT should be gentle and used only for short periods. *Exercise caution when using TT with clients who may exhibit an extreme sensitivity to the process (e.g., premature infants, frail elderly, psychotic clients) (Sayer-Adams, 1994).* **EBN:** *This study revealed no adverse effects of TT administered for 5 minutes in preterm infants daily for 3 days (Whitley & Rich, 2008).*

Geriatric

- Consider TT and HT for agitated clients with Alzheimer's disease. **EBN:** *TT and HT may be an effective technique to alleviate agitation in people with Alzheimer's disease (Hawranik, Deatrich, & Johnston, 2004; Wang & Hermann, 2006).*
- Consider TT for elderly with postsurgical pain. **EB:** *The elderly clients in this study who received TT demonstrated a statistically significant decrease in pain intensity scores, pretreatment and posttreatment (McCormack, 2009). Use of therapeutic touch for older adults with diabetic neuropathy can improve quality of life.* **EBN:** *Several clinical trials and double blind studies have indicated that further research is needed to determine the use of therapeutic touch to reduce pain in clients with diabetic neuropathy. The study indicates that using therapeutic touch can improve quality of life as well as improve ability to perform ADLs and the ability to walk (Gillespie, 2007).*

Multicultural

- Assess for the influence of cultural beliefs, norms, and values on the client's sense of disharmony of mind and spirit. **EBN:** *The client's sense of disharmony may have cultural roots (Leininger & McFarland, 2002; Giger & Davidhizar, 2004). Nurses can increase their knowledge about other health* *systems through assessment and incorporate these into the plan of care for clients as needed (Snyder & Niska, 2003).*

- Assess for the presence of specific culture-bound syndromes that may manifest as disturbances in energy or spirit. **EBN:** *Voodoo death, evil eye, and trance dissociation are some of the culture-bound syndromes that have symptoms of disharmony of mind and spirit (Arnault, 1998).*
- Validate the client's feelings and concerns related to sense of disharmony or energy disturbance. **EBN:** *Validation lets family members know that the nurse has heard and understood what was said, and it promotes the relationship between nurse and family members (Spiers, 2002).*

 ## Home Care

- See Guidelines for TT and HT.
- Help the client and family accept TT and HT as healing interventions. *Consultation and collaboration with a specialist may be the best approach to nursing care. Numerous studies have reported positive outcomes of HT as a noninvasive complementary therapy (Umbreit, 2000). HT has been used in the home care setting for chronic pain clients and for hospice care (Ziembroski et al, 2004; Wardell et al, 2006).*
- Assist the family with providing an appropriate space in which TT and or HT can be administered.
- ▲ Assess clients with bipolar disorder for the occurrence of social rhythm disruption, particularly during periods of stressful life events. Refer for mental health treatment. *Stressful life events, particularly those involving social rhythm disruption, appear to play a role in initiating manic episodes (Malkoff-Schwartz et al, 2000).*
- ▲ In the presence of a psychiatric disorder, refer for psychiatric home health care services for client reassurance and implementation of therapeutic regimen. **EBN:** *Psychiatric home visit nursing provides an important role in community care for people with mental disorders. Several reports indicated that home visits were associated with rate reduction of readmission to psychiatric wards and reduced hospital stays (Setoya et al, 2008).*

 ## Client/Family Teaching and Discharge Planning

- Teach the TT and/or specific HT technique to clients and family members. **EBN:** *Helping clients while using touch therapy related to Ki (a Korean type of energy therapy) was found to be a dynamic process with each participant actively engaged in increasing the activating, potential power of the human being (Chang, 2003). HT was taught to caregivers of veterans experiencing chronic pain from spinal cord injury (Wardell et al, 2006).*
- Teach that when working with the very young, old, or ill, or in the head area, TT should be gentle and used only for short periods. *Exercise caution when using TT with clients who may exhibit an extreme sensitivity to the process (e.g., premature infants, frail elderly, psychotic clients) (Sayer-Adams, 1994).*
- Teach the client how to use guided imagery. **EBN:** *Imagery is harmless, is time- and cost-effective, and creates a healing partnership between the nurse and client (Reed, 2007).*
- Teach the client to use deep breathing to relax. Ask the client to create an image of the disease, affected organ, or symptom. After the image has been identified, ask the client to speak with the image to address an unresolved issue. *By describing a previously unacknowledged part of the self, liberated energy can transform resistance, defenses, and disease into self-acceptance, peace, and wholeness (Remen, 1994).*

Ⓔvolve   See the EVOLVE website for Weblinks for client education resources.

REFERENCES

Arnault DS: Framework for culturally relevant psychiatric nursing. In Varcarolis EM, editor: *Foundations of psychiatric mental health nursing,* ed 3, Philadelphia, 1998, WB Saunders.

Chang SO: The nature of touch therapy related to K: practitioners' perspective, *Nurs Health Sci* 5(2):103–114, 2003.

Cook CAL, Guerrerio JF, Slater VE: Healing touch and quality of life in women receiving radiation treatment for cancer: a randomized controlled trial, *Alt Ther Health Med* 10(3):24–41, 2004.

Danhauer SC, Tooze JA, Holder P et al: Healing touch as a supportive intervention for adult acute leukemia patients: a pilot investigation of effects on distress and symptoms, *J Soc Integrat Oncol* (6)3:89–97, 2008.

Denison B: Touch the pain away: new research on therapeutic touch and persons with fibromyalgia syndrome, *Holist Nurs Pract* 18(3):142–151, 2004.

Giger JN, Davidhizar RE: *Transcultural nursing: assessment and intervention,* ed 4, St Louis, 2004, Mosby.

● = Independent   ▲ = Collaborative   **EBN** = Evidence-Based Nursing   **EB** = Evidence-Based

Gillespie: Painful diabetic neuropathy: impact of an alternative approach, *Diabetes Care* 30(4):999–101, 2007.

Hawranik P, Deatrich J, Johnston P: Therapeutic touch: another approach for the management of agitation, *Can Nurs Home* 15(1):46–48, 2004.

Healing Touch International, Inc. www.healingtouchinternational.org. Accessed Nov. 3, 2009.

Jackson E, Kelley M, McNeil P et al: Does therapeutic touch help reduce pain and anxiety in patients with cancer? *Clin J Oncol Nurs* 12(1):113–20, 2008.

Kelly AE, Sullivan P, Fawcett J et al: Therapeutic touch, quiet time, and dialogue: perceptions of women with breast cancer, *Oncol Nurs Forum* 31(3):625–631, 2004.

Kemper KJ, Kelly EA: Treating children with therapeutic and healing touch, *Pediatr Ann* 33(4):248–252, 2004.

Krieger D: *Therapeutic touch inner workbook*, Santa Fe, NM, 1997, Bear and Company.

Kuntz D, Kreiger D: *The spiritual dimension of therapeutic work*, 2004, Inner Traditions International, Limited.

Leininger MM, McFarland MR: *Transcultural nursing: concepts, theories, research and practices*, ed 3, New York, 2002, McGraw-Hill.

MacIntyre B, Hamilton J, Fricke T et al: The efficacy of healing touch in coronary artery bypass surgery recovery: a randomized clinical trial, *Altern Ther Healing Med* 14(4):24–32, 2008.

Malkoff-Schwartz S, Frank E, Anderson BP et al: Social rhythm disruption and stressful life events in the onset of bipolar and unipolar episodes, *Psychol Med* 30:1005, 2000.

McCormack GL: Using non-contact therapeutic touch to manage post-surgical pain in the elderly, *Occup Ther Int* 16(1):44–56, 2009.

Nurse Healers-Professional Associates International: *Guidelines of recommended standards and scope of practice for therapeutic touch*, www.therapeutic-touch.org/content/guidelines.asp. Accessed March 15, 2006.

Reed T: Imagery in the clinical setting: a tool for healing, *Nurs Clin North Am* 42(2):261–277, 2007.

Remen N: Psychosynthesis and healing, *J Holist Nurs* 12:150, 1994.

Sayer-Adams J: Complementary therapies: therapeutic touch nursing function, *Nurs Stand* 8:25, 1994.

Setoya N, Kayama M, Miyamoto Y et al: Nursing interventions provided by psychiatric home visit nurses in Japan, *J Japan Acad Nurs Sci* 28(1):41–51, 2008.

Snyder M, Niska K: Cultural related complementary therapies: their use in critical care units, *Crit Care Nurs Clin North Am* 15(3):341–346, 2003.

Spiers J: The interpersonal contexts of negotiating care in home care nurse-patient interactions, *Qual Health Res* 12(8):1033–1057, 2002.

Umbreit AW: Healing touch: applications in the acute care setting, *AACN Clin Issues* 11(1):105, 2000.

Van Aken R: *The experiential process of healing touch for people with moderate depression*, Lismore, NSW, Australia, 2004, Southern Cross University.

Wang K, Hermann C: Pilot study to test the effectiveness of healing touch on agitation levels in people with dementia, *Geriatr Nurs* 27(1):34–40, 2006.

Wardell D, Rintala D, Tan G et al: Pilot study of healing touch and progressive relaxation for chronic neuropathic pain in persons with spinal cord injury, *J Holist Nurs* 24(4):231–240, 2006.

Wardell D, Rintala D, Tan G: Study description of Healing Touch with veterans experiencing chronic neuropathic pain from spinal cord injury, *J Explore* 4(3):187–95, 2008.

Wardell DW, Weymouth KF: Review of studies of healing touch, *J Nurs Scholarship* 36(2):147–154, 2004.

Weze C, Leathard HL, Grange J: Evaluation of healing by gentle touch in 35 clients with cancer, *Eur J Oncol Nurs* 8(1):40–49, 2004.

Whitley JA, Rich BL: A double-blind randomized controlled pilot trial examining the safety and efficacy of therapeutic touch in premature infants, *Adv Neonatal Care* 8(6):315–333, 2008.

Ziembroski J, Gilbert N, Bossarte R et al: Healing touch and hospice care: examining outcomes at the end of life, *Altern Complement Ther* 9(3):146–151, 2004.

Impaired Environmental interpretation syndrome   *Betty J. Ackley, MSN, EdS, RN*

NANDA-I

Definition

Consistent lack of orientation to person, place, time, or circumstances for more than 3 to 6 months, necessitating a protective environment

Defining Characteristics

Chronic confusional states; consistent disorientation; inability to concentrate; inability to follow simple directions; inability to reason; loss of occupation; loss of social functioning; slow in responding to questions

Related Factors (r/t)

Dementia; depression; Huntington's disease

NOC, NIC, Client Outcomes, Nursing Interventions, Client/Family Teaching and Discharge Planning, *Rationales*, and References

Refer to care plan for **Chronic Confusion.**

⊖volve   See the EVOLVE website for Weblinks for client education resources.

• = Independent   ▲ = Collaborative   **EBN** = Evidence-Based Nursing   **EB** = Evidence-Based

Adult Failure to thrive   *Gail B. Ladwig, MSN, RN, CHTP*

 ⓔvolve

NANDA-I

Definition

Progressive functional deterioration of a physical and cognitive nature. The individual's ability to live with multisystem diseases, cope with ensuing problems, and manage his or her care is remarkably diminished.

Defining Characteristics

Altered mood state; anorexia; apathy; cognitive decline: demonstrated difficulty responding to environmental stimuli; demonstrated difficulty in concentration; demonstrated difficulty in decision making; demonstrated difficulty in judgment; demonstrated difficulty in memory; demonstrated difficulty in reasoning; decreased perception; consumption of minimal-to-no food at most meals (i.e., consumes <75% of normal requirements); decreased participation in activities of daily living; decreased social skills; expresses loss of interest in pleasurable outlets; frequent exacerbations of chronic health problems; inadequate nutritional intake; neglect of home environment; neglect of financial responsibilities; physical decline (e.g., fatigue, dehydration, incontinence of bowel and bladder); self-care deficit; social withdrawal; unintentional weight loss (e.g., 5% in 1 month, 10% in 6 months); verbalizes desire for death

Related Factor (r/t)

Depression

NOC   (Nursing Outcomes Classification)

Suggested NOC Outcomes

Physical Aging, Psychosocial Adjustment: Life Change, Will to Live

Example NOC Outcome with Indicators
Will to Live as evidenced by the following indicators: Expression of determination to live/Expression of hope/Use of strategies to compensate for problems associated with disease (Rate the outcome and indicators of **Will to Live:** 1 = severely compromised, 2 = substantially compromised, 3 = moderately compromised, 4 = mildly compromised, 5 = not compromised [see Section I].)

Client Outcomes

Client Will (Specify Time Frame):

- Resume highest level of functioning possible
- Express feelings
- Participate in ADLs
- Participate in social interactions
- Consume adequate dietary intake for weight and height
- Maintain usual weight
- Have adequate fluid intake with no signs of dehydration
- Maintain clean personal and home environment

NIC   (Nursing Interventions Classification)

Suggested NIC Interventions

Hope Inspiration, Mood Management, Self-Care Assistance

Example NIC Activities—Hope Inspiration
Assist patient/family to identify areas of hope in life; Involve the patient actively in own care

● = Independent   ▲ = Collaborative   **EBN** = Evidence-Based Nursing   **EB** = Evidence-Based

Nursing Interventions and *Rationales*

Psychosocial

- Elderly clients who have failure to thrive (FTT) should be evaluated by review of their ADLs, cognitive function, and mood; a targeted history and physical examination; selected laboratory studies and screening for alcohol and substance abuse. **EB:** *A mental status examination is crucial in the diagnosis of delirium. It is precipitated by medial illness, substance intoxication/withdrawal, or medication effect and is a leading presenting symptom of illness in the elderly (Nassisi et al, 2006).* **Adult Failure to thrive** *is characterized by lower-than-expected physical function and needs to be identified and treated early to enhance a positive outcome (Higgins & Daly, 2005).* **EBN:** *Alcoholism is frequently missed in older adults because they drink in private (Rocchiccioli & Sanford, 2009). Early identification of geriatric* **Adult Failure to thrive** *may lead to appropriate supportive treatment before an advanced level of deterioration occurs (Rocchiccioli & Sanford, 2009).*

- Assess for depression with a geriatric depression scale. Be alert for depression in clients newly admitted to nursing homes. **EBN:** *Depression was identified in 52% of the homebound elderly adults according to the Geriatric Depression Scale (Loughlin, 2004).* **EBN:** *Clients admitted to nursing homes may have lack of perceived social support and signs of depression. (Rocchiccioli & Sanford, 2009).* **EB:** *Depression is the most common silent killer in geriatrics (Chakraborty, 2009).*

- Screen for depression in persons with adult macular degeneration and low vision or vision loss. **EB:** *Rates of depression in AMD are substantially greater than those found in the general population of older people (Casten & Rovner, 2008).*

- ▲ Carefully assess for elder abuse and refer for treatment. **EB:** *Abuse of older people is a serious and growing social problem (Wang, Tseng, & Chen, 2007).*

- Provide reality orientation for clients with mild dementia. **EBN:** *Reality orientation is effective in improving cognitive ability (Bates, Boote, & Beverly, 2004).*

- Instill hope and encourage the expression of positive thoughts. **EBN:** *Hope is central to life and is essential in dealing with illness and preparing for death (Miller, 2007).*

- Provide music for clients with dementia, pain, acute confusion, and functional defcits. **EBN:** *In this study music therapy improved cognition, behavior problems, and depression in adults with dementia (Tung & Chen, 2007). Music is a safe, inexpensive, and easy-to-use intervention that nurses can implement independently to help older adults cope (McCaffrey, 2008).*

- ▲ Consider the use of light therapy. **EBN:** *Bright light therapy is effective for the treatment of seasonal affective disorder (Holland, 2009).*

- ▲ Provide opportunities for visitation from animals. **EBN:** *Animal visitation programs have been used in a wide variety of clinical settings, with predominantly positive outcomes reported anecdotally (Smith & Buckwalter, 2006). In cognitively intact residents of a nursing home, the group that received a canary had fewer depressed symptoms and an increased perception of quality of life (Colombo et al, 2005).*

- Encourage clients to reminiscence and share and compile life histories. **EBN:** *Reflecting on the past and sharing memories with others is an excellent way of facilitating communication. Be sensitive that some people do not like to look back but prefer to enjoy the present and look forward (Swann, 2008).*

- Support client's spirituality, encourage clients to pray if they wish. **EB:** *Prayer can be used as a coping strategy (Ai et al, 2004). Clients with dementia have spiritual needs (Dakin, 2009).*

- Encourage elderly clients to take part in activities and social relationships according to their capacity and wishes. **EBN:** *The specific behaviors that were found to ameliorate loneliness included utilizing friends and family as an emotional resource, engaging in eating and drinking rituals as a means of maintaining social contacts, and spending time constructively by reading and gardening (Pettigrew & Roberts, 2008).*

- Help clients identify and practice activities that promote usefulness. **EB:** *Older adults with persistently low perceived usefulness or feelings of usefulness may be a vulnerable group with increased risk for poor health outcomes in later life (Gruenewald et al, 2009).*

- Provide physical touch for clients. Touch the client's hand or arm when speaking with him or her; offer hugs with permission. **EBN:** *Appropriate use of touch by nurses has the potential to significantly improve the health status of older adults (Bush, 2001; Edvardsson, Sandman, & Rasmussen, 2003).*

- Administer TT. **EBN:** *TT can improve overall well-being, provide pain relief, reduce stress and anxiety, and decrease and prevent disruptive behavior for aged residents in an aged care environment (Gregory & Verdouw, 2005). TT may be an effective technique to alleviate agitation in people with Alzheimer's disease (Hawranik, Deatrich, & Johnston, 2004).*

• = Independent ▲ = Collaborative **EBN** = Evidence-Based Nursing **EB** = Evidence-Based

Physiological

- Assess possible causes for adult FTT and treat any underlying problems such as malnutrition, diarrhea, renal failure, and illnesses caused by physical and cognitive changes. **EBN:** *Weight loss is one of the most important indicators of malnutrition. Both low body weight and weight loss are highly predictive of morbidity and death in elderly persons (Levinson et al, 2005; Hickson, 2006).* **EB:** *Physicians who care for elderly clients should be alert to the possible presence of diarrhea and malabsorption if there is unexplained weight loss and FTT. Older clients may not admit to having chronic diarrhea, particularly if they also are incontinent (Holt, 2001).* **EB:** *The elderly client with renal failure is more often admitted for failure to thrive (Van den Noortgate et al, 2001). A reversible pathophysiologic process may be causing symptoms (Rocchiccioli & Sanford, 2009).*

- Assess for signs of fatigue and sensory changes that may indicate an infection is present that may be related to undetected diabetes mellitus, human immunodeficiency virus (HIV), or *Staphylococcus aureus* bacteremia. **EB:** *A substantial proportion of group care home residents not known to have diabetes and able to undergo testing had undetected diabetes based on a 2–hour postglucose load (Sinclair et al 2001).* **EB:** *Many older adults are sexually active and often demonstrate risky sexual behavior, such as dispensing with the use of condoms, and the isolation that frequently accompanies old age can lead to alcoholism and injectable drug use (Lieberman, 2000). S. aureus bacteremia should be suspected in elderly adults with previous hospitalization (3 months), residence in a long-term care facility, and altered mental status (Bader, 2006).*

- Monitor weight loss, leaving 25% or more of food uneaten at most meals, psychiatric/mood diagnoses, and deteriorated ability to participate in activities of daily living. **EBN:** *The above criteria are significant predictors of protein calorie malnutrition (Higgins & Daly, 2005). Diagnosis and intervention of malnutrition can prevent loss of function and independence and decrease morbidity and mortality in the elderly (Ennis, Saffel-Shrier, & Verson, 2001).*

- Assess for signs of dehydration. **EBN:** *Dehydration is the most common fluid and electrolyte imbalance in older adults (Hodgkinson, Evans, & Wood, 2003; Mentes, 2006).*

- Play soothing music during mealtimes to increase the amount of food eaten and promote decreased agitation. **EBN:** *Soothing music selections have beneficial effects on relaxation in community-residing elderly people (Lai, 2004). Relaxing music played during the evening meal may reduce the overall level of agitation among nursing home residents with severe cognitive impairment (Hicks-Moore, 2005).*

- Decrease noise and increase lighting in the dining area. **EB:** *Lighting enhancement and noise reduction may further improve dietary intake, which in turn may promote improved nutritional status (McDaniel et al, 2001; Dorner, 2005).*

- Serve "family-style" meals. **EBN:** *Family-style meals may result in modest increases in mealtime participation and communication of residents with dementia (Altus, Engelman, & Mathews, 2002).*

- ▲ Refer to a dietician for individualized nutrition therapy. **EB:** *For the obese older person, modest weight reduction can possibly result in health benefits. For the undernourished older person, early recognition of inadequate nutrition and declining weight with timely intervention is critical (Callahan & Jensen, 2004).*

- Refer to care plan **Readiness for enhanced Nutrition** for additional interventions.

- Assess how often the frail elder living at home goes outdoors. (Ask, "How often do you go outside the house?" Examples include shopping, taking a walk, working in the garden.) Encourage outside activities. **EB:** *Frail elders living at home in Japan who went outdoors less than once a week were part of a high-risk group for functional decline, intellectual activity, and self-efficacy. This question may be a useful and simple indicator to predict these changes (Kono et al, 2004).*

- Provide opportunities for interaction with the natural environment. **EB:** *Interaction with the natural world is a vital part of biopsychosocial-spiritual well-being (Irvine & Warber, 2002). Garden walks were helpful in older clients with mild to moderate depression (McCaffrey, 2007).*

- Assess grip strength. **EB:** *Grip strength may prove a more useful single marker of frailty for older people of similar age than chronological age alone (Syddall, Cooper, & Martin, 2003).*

- Frail elderly clients should also participate in carefully supervised group exercise as well as balance and gait programs accompanied by music. **EB:** *Exercise preserves lean body mass and energy intake and helps improve or maintain physical fitness and functioning vital for independent living (De Jong & Franklin, 2004).* **EB:** *In long-term care residents with dementia using wheelchair bicycle riding, depression levels were significantly reduced. Improvements were also found in sleep and levels of activ-*

ity engagement (Buettner & Fitzsimmons, 2002). **EBN:** *Residents reported significantly enhanced mood while exercising to music (Van de Winckel et al, 2004).* **EB:** *Balance exercises led to improvements in static balance function and gait exercises resulted in improvements to dynamic balance and gait functions in the very frail elderly (Shimada, Uchiyama, & Kakurai, 2003).*

- Implement dance therapy. *Exercise slows the progression of cognitive symptoms. Dance as an exercise also increases self-esteem and social involvement (Purshouse & Mukaetova-Ladinska, 2009).*
- ▲ Refer for possible pharmacological intervention. **EB:** *A client with multiple myeloma with FTT was successfully treated with modafinil and mirtazapine. By using combination pharmacotherapy, immediate results were achieved in a gravely ill client (Schillerstrom & Seaman, 2002).*
- Refer to care plans for **Imbalanced Nutrition: less than body requirements, Hopelessness,** and **Disturbed Energy field.**

Multicultural

- Assess for the influence of cultural beliefs, norms, and values on the family's or caregiver's understanding of FTT. **EBN:** *What the family considers normal and abnormal health behavior may be based on cultural perceptions (Leininger & McFarland, 2002).*
- Actively listen and be sensitive to how communication is shared culturally. Some cultures combine communication with eye contact, and some avoid eye contact. **EBN:** *The nurse who actively listens encourages sharing of thoughts and feelings, communicates respect, and provides clients with feedback about things they might not be aware of. Finally, active listening involves attention to cultural bias (Davidhizar, 2004).*
- ▲ Refer culturally diverse clients to appropriate social, medical, mental health, and long-term care services. **EB:** *In a system providing access to and coordination of comprehensive medical and long-term care services for frail older people, black clients showed a lower mortality rate than white clients (Tan, Lui, & Eng, 2003). Being black was associated with moderately high and very high levels of nutritional risk (Sharkey & Schoenberg, 2002).*

Home Care

- The above interventions may be adapted for home care use.
- If FTT is attributable to a dementing illness, refer to care plan for **Chronic Confusion.**
- ▲ Institute case management and refer for care housing of frail elderly to support continued independent living. *With the number of people needing long-term care services, the care housing model is needed for people until they are restored and discharged to a less costly level of care and a more productive quality of life. The case management systems automatically trigger standard interventions for their standard needs, and customize interventions for their special needs, using templates for personalizing them into a problem-driven action plan (Newcomer et al, 2004; Rhoades, 2007).*
- ▲ Refer for individualized care management for home health care services, such as homemaker or psychiatric home health care services for respite, client reassurance, and implementation of therapeutic regimen. **EB:** *There is a need for individualized care management assessment and service planning (Alkema, Reyes, & Wilber, 2006).*

Client/Family Teaching and Discharge Planning

- ▲ Consider use of a nurse-managed telehealth system with clients who have been discharged early from the hospital to monitor symptoms, provide education, and make referrals if necessary. *This system helps the client/family manage their own care, reinforces change, and moves clients toward optimum functioning (Martin & Coyle, 2006).* **EBN:** *Videophones were useful in educating clients with Parkinson's disease about complicated medication regimens (Fincher et al, 2009).*
- ▲ Refer for medical evaluation when cognitive changes are noticed. **EB:** *The combination of functional imaging and neuropsychological tests can diagnose with high sensitivity and specificity if a client is suffering cognitive impairment in its early stages and may aid in predicting the risk of developing dementia (Cabranes et al, 2004).*
- Encourage family to provide social interaction with the client. **EBN:** *The importance of family involvement may be effective in enhancing the lives of frail elders (Gosline, 2003). Positive social*

● = Independent   ▲ = Collaborative   **EBN** = Evidence-Based Nursing   **EB** = Evidence-Based

relationships contribute to the well-being of older adults with osetoarthritis (Ferreira & Sherman, 2007).

- Instruct the family to monitor the elder person's weight. **EBN:** *Monitoring the elder's weight regularly is a surveillance measure of nutritional status (Cowan, Roberts, & Fitzpatrick, 2004).*
- ▲ Provide referral for evaluation of hearing and appropriate hearing aids. **EB:** *Residents older than 65 years (mean age, 79 years) living in nursing homes demonstrated that hearing loss affects the communication, sociability, and psychological aspects of quality of life (Tsuruoka et al, 2001).*
- ▲ Refer for psychotherapy and possible medication if the etiology is depression. *Geriatric depression is a common but frequently unrecognized or inadequately treated condition in the elderly population. Nonpharmacological and pharmacological treatment options for managing depression are available (Lapid & Rummans, 2003).*
- ▲ Refer for possible medication therapy when the diagnosis is dementia. **EB:** *Residents with dementia in nursing homes showed that Tacrine was associated with lower mortality (Ott & Lapane, 2002).*

ⓔvolve   See the EVOLVE website for Weblinks for client education resources.

REFERENCES

Ai AL, Peterson C, Tice TN et al: Faith-based and secular pathways to hope and optimism subconstructs in middle-aged and older cardiac patients, *J Health Psychol* 9(3):435–450, 2004.

Alkema G, Reyes J, Wilber K: Characteristics associated with home- and community-based service utilization for Medicare managed care consumers, *Gerontologist* 46(2):173–183, 2006.

Altus DE, Engelman KK, Mathews RM: Using family-style meals to increase participation and communication in persons with dementia, *J Gerontol Nurs* 28(9):47–53, 2002.

Bader MS: *Staphylococcus aureus* bacteremia in older adults: predictors of 7–day mortality and infection with a methicillin-resistant strain, *Infect Control Hosp Epidemiol* 27(11):219–225, 2006.

Bates J, Boote J, Beverley C: Psychosocial interventions for people with a milder dementing illness: a systematic review, *J Adv Nurs* 45(6):644–658, 2004.

Buettner LL, Fitzsimmons S: AD-venture program: therapeutic biking for the treatment of depression in long-term care residents with dementia, *Am J Alzheimers Dis Other Demen* 17(2):121–127, 2002.

Bush E: The use of human touch to improve the well-being of older adults: a holistic nursing intervention, *J Holist Nurs* 19(3):256–270, 2001.

Cabranes JA, De Juan R, Encinas M et al: Relevance of functional neuroimaging in the progression of mild cognitive impairment, *Neurol Res* 26(5):496–501, 2004.

Callahan E, Jensen G: Weight issues in later years, *Generations* 28(3):39–45, 2004.

Casten RJ, Rovner BW: Depression in age-related macular degeneration, *J Visual Impair Blind* 102(10):591–599, 2008.

Chakraborty M: Depression: a silent killer of the old age: an overview, *Homoeopath Herit* 34(1):29–32, 2009.

Colombo G, Buono MD, Smania K et al: Pet therapy and institutionalized elderly: a study on 144 cognitively unimpaired subjects, *Arch Gerontol Geriatr* 42:207–216, 2005.

Cowan DT, Roberts JD, Fitzpatrick JM: Nutritional status of older people in long term care settings: current status and future directions, *Int J Nurs Stud* (3):225–237, 2004.

Dakin C: Spiritual care and dementia: pilgrims on a journey, J Dement Care 17(1):24–27, 2009.

Davidhizar R: Listening: a nursing strategy to transcend culture, *J Pract Nurs* 54(2):22, 2004.

De Jong AA, Franklin BA: Prescribing exercise for the elderly: current research and recommendations, *Curr Sports Med Rep* 3(6):337–343, 2004.

Dorner B: Nutrition for the dementia resident, *Nurs Homes* 54(5):29–31, 2005.

Edvardsson JD, Sandman P, Rasmussen RH: Meanings of giving touch in the care of older patients: becoming a valuable person and professional, *J Clin Nurs* 12(4):601–609, 2003.

Ennis BW, Saffel-Shrier S, Verson H: Diagnosing malnutrition in the elderly, *Nurse Pract* 26(3):52, 2001.

Ferreira VM, Sherman AM: The relationship of optimism, pain and social support to well-being in older adults with osteoarthritis, *Aging Ment Health* 11(1):89–98, 2007.

Fincher L, Ward C, Dawkins V et al: Using telehealth to educate Parkinson's disease patients about complicated medication regimens, *J Gerontol Nurs* 35(2):16–24, 2009.

Gosline MB: Client participation to enhance socialization for frail elders, *Geriatr Nurs* 24(5):286–289, 2003.

Gregory S, Verdouw J: Therapeutic touch: its application for residents in aged care, *Aus Nurs J* 12(7):23–26, 2005.

Gruenewald TL, Karlamangla AS, Greendale GA et al: Increased mortality risk in older adults with persistently low or declining feelings of usefulness to others, *J Aging Health* 21(2):398–425, 2009.

Hawranik P, Deatrich J, Johnston P: Therapeutic touch: another approach for the management of agitation, *Can Nurs Home* 15(1):46–48, 2004.

Hicks-Moore SL: Relaxing music at mealtime in nursing homes, *J Gerontol Nurs* 31(12):26–33, 2005.

Hickson M: Malnutrition and aging, *Postgrad Med J* 82(963):2–8, 2006.

Higgins P, Daly B: Adult failure to thrive in the older rehabilitation patient, *Rehab Nurs* 30(4):152–160, 2005.

Hodgkinson B, Evans D, Wood J: Maintaining oral hydration in older adults: a systematic review, *Int J Nurs Pract* 9(3):S19–S28, 2003.

Holland R: Somatic therapies for seasonal affective disorder, *J Psychosoc Nurs Men Health Serv* 47(1):17–20, 2009.

Holt PR: Diarrhea and malabsorption in the elderly, *Gastroenterol Clin North Am* 30(2):427, 2001.

Irvine KN, Warber SL: Greening healthcare: practicing as if the natural environment really mattered, *Altern Ther Health Med* 8(5):76, 2002.

Kono A, Kai I, Sakato C et al: Frequency of going outdoors: a predictor of functional and psychosocial change among ambulatory frail elders living at home, *J Gerontol A Biol Sci Med Sci* 59(3):275–280, 2004.

Lai H: Music preference and relaxation in Taiwanese elderly people, *Geriatr Nurs* 25(5):286–291, 2004.

Lapid MI, Rummans TA: Evaluation and management of geriatric depression in primary care, *Mayo Clin Proc* 78(11):1423–1429, 2003.

Leininger MM, McFarland MR: *Transcultural nursing: concepts, theories, research and practices,* ed 3, New York, 2002, McGraw-Hill.

● = Independent   ▲ = Collaborative   **EBN** = Evidence-Based Nursing   **EB** = Evidence-Based

Levinson Y, Dwolatzky T, Epstein A et al: Is it possible to increase weight and maintain the protein status of debilitated elderly residents of nursing homes? *J Gerontol A Biol Sci Med Sci* 60(7):878–881, 2005.

Lieberman R: HIV in older Americans: an epidemiologic perspective, *J Midwifery Womens Health* 45(2):176, 2000.

Loughlin A: Depression and social support: effective treatments for homebound elderly adults, *J Gerontol Nurs* 30(5):11–15, 2004.

Martin E, Coyle M: Nursing protocol for telephonic supervision of clients, *Rehab Nurs* 31(2):54–59, 2006.

McCaffrey R: Music listening: its effects in creating a healing environment, *J Psychosoc Nurs Ment Health Serv* 46(10):39–44, 2008.

McCaffrey R: The effect of healing gardens and art therapy on older adults with mild to moderate depression, *Holist Nurs Pract* 21(2):79–84, 2007.

McDaniel JH, Hunt A, Hackes B et al: Impact of dining room environment on nutritional intake of Alzheimer's residents: a case study, *Am J Alzheimers Dis Other Demen* 16(5):297, 2001.

Mentes J: Oral hydration in older adults: greater awareness is needed in preventing, recognizing, and treating dehydration, *Am J Nurs* 106(6):40–49, 2006.

Miller JF: Hope: a construct central to nursing, *Nurs Forum* 42(1):12–19, 2007.

Nassisi D, Korc B, Hahn S et al: The evaluation and management of the acutely agitated elderly patient, *Mt Sinai J Med* 73(7):976–984, 2006.

Newcomer R, Maravilla V, Faculijak P et al: Outcomes of preventive case management among high-risk elderly in three medical groups: a randomized clinical trial, *Eva Health Prof* 27(4):323, 2004.

Ott BR, Lapane KL: Tacrine therapy is associated with reduced mortality in nursing home residents with dementia, *J Am Geriatr Soc* 50(1):35, 2002.

Pettigrew S, Roberts M: Addressing loneliness in later life, *Aging Ment Health* 12(3):302–309, 2008.

Purshouse K, Mukaetova-Ladinska E: Dance therapy for Alzheimer's disease, *Stud BMJ* 17:b595, 2009.

Rhoades J: Cultural dysfunction, *Nurs Homes* 56(1):10–11, 2007.

Rocchiccioli JT, Sanford JT: Revisiting geriatric failure to thrive: a complex and compelling clinical condition, *J Gerontol Nurs* 35(1):18–24, 2009.

Schillerstrom JE, Seaman JS: Modafinil augmentation of mirtazapine in a failure-to-thrive geriatric inpatient, *Int J Psychiatry Med* 32(4):405–410, 2002.

Sharkey JR, Schoenberg NE: Variations in nutritional risk among black and white women who receive home-delivered meals, *J Women Aging* 14(3–4):99–119, 2002.

Shimada H, Uchiyama Y, Kakurai S: Specific effects of balance and gait exercises on physical function among the frail elderly, *Clin Rehabil* 17(5):472–479, 2003.

Sinclair AJ, Gadsby R, Penfold S et al: Prevalence of diabetes in care home residents, *Diabetes Care* 24(6):1066–1068, 2001.

Smith M, Buckwalter K: Behaviors associated with dementia, *Clin J Oncol Nurs* 10(2):183–192, 2006.

Swann J: Preserving memories: using reminiscence techniques, *Nurs Resident Care* 10(12):611–613, 2008.

Syddall H, Cooper C, Martin F: Is grip strength a useful single marker of frailty? *Age Ageing* 32(6):650–656, 2003.

Tan EJ, Lui LY, Eng C: Differences in mortality of black and white patients enrolled in the program of all-inclusive care for the elderly, *J Am Geriatr Soc* 51(2):246–251, 2003.

Tsuruoka H, Masuda S, Ukai K et al: Hearing impairment and quality of life for the elderly in nursing homes, *Auris Nasus Larynx* 28(1):45–54, 2001.

Tung H, Chen K: Effects of music therapy on cognition, behavior problems, and depression among demented older adults in long-term care facilities [Chinese]. *J Evid Based Nurs* 3(4):309–318, 2007.

Van de Winckel A, Feys H, De Weerdt W et al: Cognitive and behavioural effects of music-based exercises in patients with dementia, *Clin Rehabil* 18(3):253–260, 2004.

Van den Noortgate NJ, Janssens WH, Afschrift MB et al: Renal function in the oldest-old on an acute geriatric ward, *Int Urol Nephrol* 32(4):531–537, 2001.

Wang J, Tseng H, Chen K: Development and testing of screening indicators for psychological abuse of older people, *Arch Psychiatr Nurs* 21(1):40–47, 2007.

Risk for Falls   Sherry A. Greenberg, MSN, GNP-BC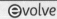

NANDA-I

Definition

Increased susceptibility to falling that may cause physical harm

Risk Factors (Intrinsic and Extrinsic)

Adults

Age 65 or older; history of falls; lives alone; lower limb prosthesis; use of assistive devices (e.g., walker, cane); wheelchair use

Children

Less than 2 years of age; bed located near window; lack of automobile-restraints; lack of gate on stairs; lack of window guard; lack of parental supervision; male gender when less than 1 year of age; unattended infant on elevated surface (e.g., bed/changing table)

Cognitive

Diminished mental status

• = Independent   ▲ = Collaborative   **EBN** = Evidence-Based Nursing   **EB** = Evidence-Based

Environment

Cluttered environment; dimly lit room; no antislip material in bath; no antislip material in shower; restraints; throw rugs; unfamiliar room; weather conditions (e.g., wet floors, ice)

Medications

Angiotensin-converting enzyme (ACE) inhibitors; alcohol use; antianxiety agents; antihypertensive agents; diuretics; hypnotics; narcotics/opiates; tranquilizers; tricyclic antidepressants

Physiological

Anemias; arthritis; diarrhea; decreased lower extremity strength; difficulty with gait; faintness when extending neck; foot problems; hearing difficulties; impaired balance; impaired physical mobility; incontinence; neoplasms (i.e., fatigue; limited mobility); neuropathy; orthostatic hypotension; post-operative conditions; postprandial blood sugar changes; presence of acute illness; proprioceptive deficits; sleeplessness; urgency; vascular disease; visual difficulties

NOC   (Nursing Outcomes Classification)

Suggested NOC Outcomes

Fall Prevention Behavior, Knowledge: Child Physical Safety

> #### Example NOC Outcome with Indicators
>
> **Fall Prevention Behavior** as evidenced by the following indicators: Uses assistive devices correctly/Eliminates clutter, spills, glare from floors/Uses safe transfer procedures (Rate each indicator of **Fall Prevention Behavior:** 1 = never demonstrated, 2 = rarely demonstrated, 3 = sometimes demonstrated, 4 = often demonstrated, 5 = consistently demonstrated [see Section I].)

Client Outcomes

Client Will (Specify Time Frame):

- Remain free of falls
- Change environment to minimize the incidence of falls
- Explain methods to prevent injury

NIC   (Nursing Interventions Classification)

Suggested NIC Interventions

Dementia Management, Fall Prevention, Post-Fall Assessment, Surveillance: Safety

> #### Example NIC Activities—Fall Prevention
>
> Assist unsteady individual with ambulation; Monitor gait, balance, and fatigue level with ambulation

Nursing Interventions and *Rationales*

- Safety Guidelines. Complete a fall-risk assessment for older adults in acute care using a valid and reliable tool such as the Hendrich II Model. Recognize that risk factors for falling include recent history of falls, confusion, depression, altered elimination patterns, cardiovascular/respiratory disease impairing perfusion or oxygenation, postural hypotension, dizziness or vertigo, primary cancer diagnosis, and altered mobility (Gray-Miceli, 2008). *The Hendrich II Fall Risk Model is quick to administer and provides a determination of risk for falling based on gender, mental and emotional status, symptoms of dizziness, and known categories of medications increasing risk (Hendrich, 2006). This tool screens for primary prevention of falls and is integral in a post-fall assessment for the secondary prevention of falls (Gray-Miceli, 2007).*
- Screen all clients for balance and mobility skills (supine to sit, sitting supported and unsupported, sit to stand, standing, walking and turning around, transferring, stooping to floor and recovering, and sitting down). Use tools such as the Balance Scale by Tinetti or the Get Up and Go Scale. *It is*

• = Independent   ▲ = Collaborative   **EBN** = Evidence-Based Nursing   **EB** = Evidence-Based

helpful to determine the client's functional abilities and then plan for ways to improve problem areas or determine methods to ensure safety (Gray-Miceli, 2008).

- Recognize that when people attend to another task while walking, such as carrying a cup of water, clothing, or supplies, they are more likely to fall. **EB:** *Those who slow down when given a carrying task are at a higher risk for subsequent falls (Lundin-Olsson, Nysberg, & Gustafson, 1998).*
- Be careful when getting a mostly immobile client up. Be sure to lock the bed and wheelchair and have sufficient personnel to protect the client from falls. When rising from a lying position, have the client change positions slowly, dangle legs, and stand next to the bed prior to walking to prevent orthostatic hypotension.
- Use a "high-risk fall" armband/bracelet and Fall Risk room sign to alert staff for increased vigilance and mobility assistance. *These steps alert the nursing staff of the increased risk of falls (McCarter-Bayer, Bayer, & Hall, 2005).*
- ▲ Evaluate the client's medications to determine whether medications increase the risk of falling; consult with physician regarding the client's need for medication if appropriate. *Polypharmacy, or taking more than four medications, has been associated with increased falls. Medications such as benzodiazepines and antipsychotic and antidepressant medications given to promote sleep actually increase the rate of falls (Capezuti et al, 1999).* **EB:** *Short-to-intermediate-acting benzodiazepine and tricyclic antidepressants may produce ataxia, impaired psychomotor function, syncope, and additional falls (Fick et al, 2003).* NOTE: See Molony (2008).
- Thoroughly orient the client to environment. Place the call light within reach and show how to call for assistance; answer call light promptly.
- Use one quarter– to one half–length side rails only, and maintain bed in a low position. Ensure that wheels are locked on bed and commode. Keep dim light in room at night. *Use of full side rails can result in the client climbing over the rails, leading with the head, and sustaining a head injury. Side rails with widely spaced vertical bars and side rails not situated flush with the mattress have been associated with asphyxiation deaths because of rail and in bed entrapment and should not be used (Capezuti, 2004).*
- Routinely assist the client with toileting on his or her own schedule. Always take the client to bathroom on awakening and before bedtime (McCarter-Bayer, Bayer & Hall, 2005). Keep the path to the bathroom clear, label the bathroom, and leave the door open.
- ▲ Avoid use of restraints if at all possible. Obtain a physician's order if restraints are deemed necessary, and use the least restrictive device. *The use of restraints has been associated with serious injuries including rhabdomyolysis, brachial plexus injury, neuropathy, and dysrhythmias, as well as strangulation, asphyxiation, traumatic brain injuries, and all the consequences of immobility (Capezuti, 2004; Evans & Cotter, 2008).* **EBN and EB:** *A study demonstrated that there was no increase in falls or injuries in a group of clients that were not restrained, versus a similar group that was restrained in a nursing home (Capezuti et al, 1999).* **EB:** *A study in two acute care hospitals demonstrated that when restraints were not used, there was no increase in client falls, injuries, or therapy disruptions (Mion et al, 2001).*
- In place of restraints, use the following:
  - Well-staffed and educated nursing personnel with frequent client contact with careful consideration during shift changes
  - Nursing units designed to care for clients with cognitive or functional impairments
  - Non-skid footwear, sneakers preferable
  - Adequate lighting, night-light in bathroom
  - Toilet frequently
  - Frequently assess need for invasive devices, tubes, IVs
  - Hide tubes with bandages to prevent pulling of tubes
  - Consider alternative IV placement site to prevent pulling out IV
  - Alarm systems with ankle, above-the-knee, or wrist sensors
  - Bed or wheelchair alarms
  - Wedge cushions on chairs to prevent slipping
  - Increased observation of the client
  - Locked doors to unit
  - Low or very low height beds

• = Independent ▲ = Collaborative **EBN** = Evidence-Based Nursing **EB** = Evidence-Based

■ Border-defining pillow/mattress to remind the client to stay in bed
These alternatives to restraints can be helpful to prevent falls (McCarter-Bayer, Bayer, & Hall, 2005; Cotter & Evans, 2007).

- If the client has an acute change in mental status (delirium), recognize that the cause is usually physiological and is a medical emergency. Consider possible causes for delirium. Consult with the physician or health care provider immediately. Note: See Fick & Mion (2007). See interventions for **Acute Confusion**.

- If the client has chronic confusion due to dementia, implement individualized strategies to enhance communication. *Assessment of specific receptive and expressive language abilities is needed in order to understand the client's communication difficulties and facilitate communication.* Note: See interventions for **Chronic Confusion.** See Frazier-Rios D & Zembrzuski (2007).

- Ask family to stay with the client to assist with ADLs and prevent the client from accidentally falling or pulling out tubes.

▲ If the client is unsteady on feet, have two nursing staff members alongside when walking the client. Consider referral to physical therapy for gait training and strengthening. *The client can walk independently, but the nurse can rapidly ensure safety if the knees buckle. Interdisciplinary care is most comprehensive and beneficial to the client.*

- Place a fall-prone client in a room that is near the nurses' station. *Such placement allows more frequent observation of the client.*

- Help clients sit in a stable chair with arm rests. Avoid use of wheelchairs except for transportation as needed. *Clients are likely to fall when left in a wheelchair because they may stand up without locking the wheels or removing the footrests. Wheelchairs do not increase mobility; people just sit in them the majority of the time (Simmons et al, 1995).*

- Avoid use of wheelchairs as much as possible because they can serve as a restraint device. Most people in wheelchairs do not move. *Wheelchairs unfortunately serve as a restraint device.* **EB:** *A study has shown that only 4% of residents in wheelchairs were observed to propel them independently and only 45% could propel them, even with cues and prompts. Another study showed that no residents could unlock wheelchairs without help, the wheelchairs were not fitted to residents, and residents were not trained in propulsion (Simmons et al, 1995).*

▲ Refer to physical therapy or other programs for exercise programs that target strength, balance, flexibility, or endurance. **EB:** *Programs with at least two of these components have been shown to decrease the rate of falling and number of people falling, (Gillespie et al, 2009).*

 Geriatric

- Assess ability to move using the Hendrich II Fall Risk Model, which includes the Get Up and Go test. Ask the client to rise from a sitting position, walk 10 feet, turn, and return to the chair to sit. *Performance on this screening exam demonstrates the client's mobility and ability to leave the house safely. If the client completes the test in less than 20 seconds, they usually can live independently. If completing the test takes longer than 30 seconds, the client is more likely to be dependent on others, and more likely to sustain a fall (Gray-Miceli, 2007).*

- Complete a fall-risk assessment for older adults in acute care using a valid and reliable tool such as the Hendrich II Fall Risk Model. *It is quick to administer and provides a determination of risk for falling based on gender, mental and emotional status, symptoms of dizziness, and known categories of medications increasing risk (Hendrich, et al, 2003). This tool screens for primary prevention of falls and is integral in a post-fall assessment for the secondary prevention of falls (Gray-Miceli, 2007).*

▲ If new onset of falling, assess for lab abnormalities, and signs and symptoms of infection and dehydration, and check blood pressure and pulse rate supine, sitting, and standing for hypotension and orthostatic hypotension. If the client has a borderline high blood pressure, the risk of falling due to administration of antihypertensives may outweigh the benefits of the antihypertensive medication. Discuss with the health care provider on a client-to-client basis. *If orthostatic hypotension is present and there is minimal change in the heart rate, most likely the baroreceptors are not working to maintain blood pressure on arising. This is common in the elderly and may be caused by hypovolemia resulting from the excessive use of diuretics, vasodilators, or other types of drugs; dehydration; or prolonged bed rest as well as cardiovascular disease, neurological disease, or another medication's adverse effect (NINDS, 2007). Insertion of a pacemaker can reduce falls in people with frequent falls associated with carotid sinus hypersensitivity, a condition that may cause changes in heart rate and blood pressure (Gillespie, 2009).*

- Encourage the client to wear glasses and use walking aids when ambulating.
- If the client experiences dizziness because of orthostatic hypotension when getting up, teach methods to decrease dizziness, such as rising slowly, remaining seated several minutes before standing, flexing feet upward several times while sitting, sitting down immediately if feeling dizzy, and trying to have someone present when standing. *Always have the client dangle at the bedside before trying standing to evaluate for postural hypotension. Watch the client closely for dizziness during increased activity. Postural hypotension can be detected in up to 30% of elderly clients. These methods can help prevent falls as well as maintain adequate fluid intake (Tinetti, 2003).*
- ▲ If the client is experiencing syncope, determine symptoms that occur before syncope, and note medications that the client is taking. Refer for medical care. *The circumstances surrounding syncope often suggest the cause. Use of many medications, including diuretics, antihypertensives, digoxin, beta-blockers, and calcium channel blockers can cause syncope. Use of the tilt table can be diagnostic in incidences of syncope (Fick et al, 2007).*
- ▲ Observe client for signs of anemia, and refer to primary care practitioner for testing if appropriate. **EB:** *One study demonstrated that elderly clients with mild anemia had a three times increased incidence of falls (Dharmarajan & Norkus, 2004).*
- Evaluate client for chronic alcohol intake, as well as mental health and neurologic function. **EBN:** *A study of falls in a community of older adults found that age, gender, neurological disease, mental health, and regular use of alcohol significantly influenced the rate of falls (Resnick & Junlapeeya, 2004).*
- ▲ Refer to physical therapy for strength training, using free weights or machines and suggest participation in exercise programs. *Exercise can prevent falls in older people. Greater relative effects are seen in programs that include exercises that challenge balance, use a higher dose of exercise, and do not include a walking program. Service providers can use these findings to design and implement exercise programs for falls prevention (Sherrington et al, 2008).*
- ▲ If an elderly woman has symptoms of urge incontinence, refer to a urologist or nurse specialist in incontinence for evaluation and ensure the path to the bathroom is well lit and free of obstructions. *Urge urinary incontinence was associated with an increased incidence of falls and non-supine, non-traumatic fractures in older women (Brown et al, 2000).*

Home Care

- Some of the above interventions may be adapted for home care use.
- Implement evidence-based fall prevention practices to older adults in community settings and home health care programs (Fortinsky et al, 2008).
- If the client was identified as a fall risk in the hospital, recognize that there is a high incidence of falls after discharge, and use all measures possible to reduce the incidence of falls. **EBN:** *The rate of falls is substantially increased in the geriatric client who has been recently hospitalized, especially during the first month after discharge (Mahoney et al, 2000).*
- ▲ If delirium is present, assess for cause of delirium and/or falls with the use of an interdisciplinary team. Consult with the physician immediately. Assess and monitor for acute changes in cognition and behavior. *An acute and fluctuating change in cognition and behavior is the classic presentation of delirium. Delirium is reversible and should be considered a medical emergency. Delirium can become chronic if untreated, and clients may be discharged from hospitals to home care in states of undiagnosed delirium.* **EBN:** *Falls may be a precipitating event or an indication of frailty consistent with acute confusion (Mentes et al, 1999).* NOTE: *See Waszynski (2007).*
- Assess for additional factors leading to risk for falls. **EB:** *A study of individuals receiving home care services found that risk factors included medical history (neurological and cardiovascular impairments); medication usage (antipsychotic and tricyclic antidepressant medications); and fall history (fall recurrence during the preceding 3 months) (Lewis et al, 2004).*
- Assess home environment for threats to safety including clutter, slippery floors, scatter rugs, and other potential hazards. Additionally, assess external environment (e.g., uneven pavement, un-leveled stairs/steps). *Clients suffering from impaired mobility, impaired visual acuity, and neurological dysfunction, including dementia and other cognitive functional deficits, are all at risk for injury from common hazards. These recommendations were shown to be effective to reduce falls (Tinetti, 2003).*

• = Independent   ▲ = Collaborative   **EBN** = Evidence-Based Nursing   **EB** = Evidence-Based

▲ Institute a home-based, nurse-delivered exercise program to reduce falls or refer to physical therapy services for client and family education of safe transfers and ambulation and for strengthening exercises (for the client). **EBN:** *A metaanalysis of studies demonstrated a 4% reduction in the rate of falls in individuals who received fall prevention programs (Hill-Westmoreland, Soeken & Spellbring, 2002).*

▲ Instruct the client and family or caregivers on how to correct identified hazards for those with visual impairment. Refer to physical and occupational therapy services for assistance if needed. **EB:** *Interventions to improve home safety were shown to be effective in people at high risk, such as those with severe visual impairment (Gillespie et al, 2009).*

▲ Use a multifactorial assessment along with interventions targeted to the identified risk factors. Key components of the interventions include evaluating need for all medications, balance, gait and strength training, use of strategies to deal with postural hypotension if present, home safety evaluation with needed modifications, and any needed cardiovascular treatment. **EB:** *As people age, they may fall more often for a multiple of reasons including problems with balance, poor vision, and dementia. Fear of falling can result in self-restricted activity levels (Gillespie et al, 2009).*

• Encourage the client to eat a balanced diet, with particular inclusion of vitamin D and calcium. *Vitamin D deficiency and hypocalcemia are common in older adults, contributing to falls, musculoskeletal complaints, and functional and mobility deficits. Results show that Vitamin D and calcium were superior to calcium supplementation alone in regard to fall prevention, musculoskeletal function, and bone metabolism, especially in recurrent falls and frail, older women with Vitamin D deficiency (Bischoff et al, 2003). Older adults with unexplained falls, pain, and gait imbalance may have osteomalacia due to vitamin D deficiency (Dharmarajan, 2005).*

• If the client lives alone or spends a lot of time alone, teach the client what to do if he or she falls and cannot get up, and make sure he or she has a personal emergency response system or a mobile phone that is available from the floor (Tinetti, 2003). If the client is at risk for falls, use gait belt and additional persons when ambulating. *Gait belts decrease the risk of falls during ambulation.* **EBN:** *Be aware that clients may react ambivalently to a personal emergency response system. A study showed that, while the system alleviated some anxiety about ability to receive help, concern was also expressed about being shocked by hearing strangers enter the home (Porter, 2003).*

• Ensure appropriate non-glare lighting in the home. Ask the client to install indoor strip or "runway" type of lighting to baseboards to help clients balance. Install motion-sensitive lighting that turns on automatically when the client gets out of bed to go to the bathroom.

• Have the client wear supportive, low-heeled shoes with good traction when ambulating. Avoid use of slip-on footwear. Wear appropriate footwear in inclement weather. *Supportive shoes provide the client with better balance and protect the client from instability on uneven surfaces. Antislip shoe devices worn in icy conditions have been shown to reduce falls (Gillespie et al, 2009).*

• Provide a signaling device for clients who wander or are at risk for falls. *Orienting a vulnerable client to a safety net relieves anxiety of the client and caregiver and allows for rapid response to a crisis situation.*

• Provide medical identification bracelet for clients at risk for injury from dementia, diabetes, seizures, or other medical disorders.

• Suggest a tai chi class designed for the elderly to selected clients who have sufficient balance to participate. **EB:** *Participation in once per week tai chi classes for 16 weeks can prevent falls in relatively healthy community-dwelling older people (Voukelatos et al, 2007).*

 Client/Family Teaching and Discharge Planning

• Safety Guidelines. Teach the client and the family about the fall reduction measures that are being used to prevent falls (Joint Commission, 2009).

• Teach the client how to safely ambulate at home, including using safety measures such as hand rails in bathroom, and need to avoid carrying things or performing other tasks while walking. *Walking more slowly in response to a visual-spatial decision task may identify individuals at risk for multiple falls (Faulkner et al, 2007).*

• Teach the client the importance of maintaining a regular exercise program. If the client is afraid of falling while walking outside, suggest they walk the length of a local mall. *Exercise can prevent falls*

• = Independent   ▲ = Collaborative   **EBN** = Evidence-Based Nursing   **EB** = Evidence-Based

in older people. Greater relative effects are seen in programs that include exercises that challenge balance and use a higher dose of exercise than just walking programs (Sherrington et al, 2008).

℮volve   See the EVOLVE website for Weblinks for client education resources.

REFERENCES

Bischoff HA, Stahelin HB, Dick W et al: Effects of Vitamin D and calcium supplementation on falls: a randomized controlled trial, *J B Mineral Res* 18:343–351, 2003.

Brown JS, Vittinghoff E & Wyman JF et al: Urinary incontinence: does it increase risk for falls and fractures? Study of Osteoporotic Fracture Research Group, *J Am Geriatr Soc* 48(7):721, 2000.

Capezuti E: Minimizing the use of restrictive devices in dementia patients at risk for falling, *Nurs Clin North Am* 39:625, 2004.

Capezuti E, Strumph N Evans I et al: Outcomes of nighttime physical restrain removal for severely impaired nursing home residents, *Am J Alzheimers Dis Other Deme* 14(3):157, 1999.

Cotter VT, Evans L: Try this: best practices in nursing care to older adults. In: The John A. Hartford Institute for Geriatric Nursing and the Alzheimer's Association: *Avoiding restraints in older adults with dementia*, 2007. www.consultgerirn.org/uploads/File/trythis/dementia.pdf. Accessed March 15, 2009.

Evans LK, Cotter VT: Avoiding restraints in patients with dementia: understanding, prevention, and management are the keys, *Am J Nurs* 108(3):40–49, 2008.

Dharmarajan TS: Vitamin D deficiency in community older adults with falls of gait imbalance: an under-recognized problem in the inner city, J Nutr Elderly 25(1):7–19, 2005.

Dharmarajan TS, Norkus EP: Mild anemia and the risk of falls in older adults from nursing homes and the community, *J Am Med Dir Assoc* 5(6):395–400, 2004.

Faulkner KA, Redfern MS, Cauley JA et al: Multitasking: association between poorer performance and a history of recurrent falls, *J Am Geriatr Soc* 55(4):570–576, 2007.

Fick D, Mion L: Try this: best practices in nursing care to older adults. In: The John A. Hartford Institute for Geriatric Nursing: *Assessing and managing delirium in older adults with dementia*, 2007. www.consultgerirn.org/uploads/File/trythis/AssesMange DeleriumWDementia.pdf. Accessed March 15, 2009.

Fick DM, Cooper JW, Wade WE et al: Updating the Beers Criteria for potentially inappropriate medication use in older adults: results of a US consensus panel of experts, *Arch Intern Med* 163(22): 2716–2724, 2003.

Fortinsky RH, Baker D, Gottschalk M et al: Extent of implementation of evidence-based fall prevention practices for older patients in home health care, *J Am Geriatr Soc* 56(4):737–743, 2008.

Frazier-Rios D, Zembrzuski C: Try this: best practices in nursing care to older adults. In: The John A. Hartford Institute for Geriatric Nursing: *Communication difficulties: assessment and interventions in hospitalized older adults with dementia*, 2007. www.consultgerirn.org/uploads/File/trythis/communication.pdf. Accessed March 15, 2009.

Gillespie LD, Robertson MC, Gillespie WJ et al: Interventions for preventing falls in older people living in the community, *Cochrane Database Syst Rev* (2):CD007146, 2009.

Gray-Miceli D: Try this: best practices in nursing care to older adults. In: The John A. Hartford Institute for Geriatric Nursing. Fall risk assessment in older adults: The Hendrich II Model, 2007. www.consultgerirn.org/uploads/File/trythis/issue08.pdf. Accessed March 15, 2009.

Gray-Miceli D: Delirium: preventing falls in acute care. In: Capezuti E, Zwicker D, Mezey M et al, editors: *Geriatric nursing protocols,* ed 3, New York, 2008, Springer.

Gray-Miceli D, Johnson J, Strumpf N: A step-wise approach to a comprehensive post-fall assessment, *Annals of Long-Term Care* 13(12):16–24, 2005.

Hendrich A: Inpatient falls: lessons from the field, *Patient Saf Qual Healthc* May/June:26–30, 2006.

Hendrich AL, Bender PS, Nyhuis A: Validation of the Hendrich II Fall Risk Model: a large concurrent CASE/control study of hospitalized patients, *Appl Nurs Res* 16(1):9–21, 2003.

Hill-Westmoreland EE, Soeken K, Spellbring AM: A meta-analysis of fall prevention programs for the elderly: how effective are they? *Nurs Res* 51(1):1, 2002.

The Joint Commission on Accreditation of Healthcare Organizations: Accreditation program: home care. 2010 national patient safety goals. Goal 9. Reduce the risk of patient harm resulting from falls, 2009. www.jointcommission.org/NR/rdonlyres/E07E8A63–5867–4090–A5AC-210D9565BCDB/0/RevisedChapter_OME_NPSG_20090924.pdf. Accessed on October 8, 2009.

Lewis CL, Moutoux M, Slaughter M et al: Characteristics of individuals who fell while receiving home health services, *Phys Ther* 84(1):23, 2004.

Lundin-Olsson L, Nyberg L, Gustafson Y: Attention, frailty, and falls: the effect of a manual task on basic mobility, *J Am Geriatr Soc* 46(6):758–761, 1998.

Mahoney JE, Palta M, Johnson J et al: Temporal association between hospitalization and rate of falls after discharge, *Arch Intern Med* 160(18):2788, 2000.

McCarter-Bayer A, Bayer F, Hall K: Preventing falls in acute care: an innovative approach, *J Gerontol Nurs* 31(3):25, 2005.

Mentes J, Culp K, Maas M et al: Acute confusion indicators: risk factors and prevalence using MDS data, *Res Nurs Health* 22(2):95–105, 1999.

Mion LC, Fogel J, Sandhu S et al: Outcomes following physical restraint reduction programs in two acute care hospitals, *Jt Comm J Qual Improv* 27(11):605–618, 2001.

Molony S: Try this: best practices in nursing care to older adults. In: The John A. Hartford Institute for Geriatric Nursing. *Beers Criteria for potentially inappropriate medication use in older adults: Part II: 2002 Criteria Considering Diagnoses or Conditions,* 2008. www.consultgerirn.org/uploads/File/trythis/issue16_2.pdf. Accessed March 15, 2009.

National Institute of Neurological Disorders and Stroke: NINDS orthostatic hypotension information page, 2007. www.ninds.nih.gov/disorders/orthostatic_hypotension/orthostatic_hypotension.htm. Accessed April 15, 2009.

Porter EJ: Moments of apprehension in the midst of a certainty: some frail older widows' lives with a personal emergency response system, *Qual Health Res* 13(9):1311, 2003.

Resnick B, Junlapeeya P: Falls in a community of older adults: findings and implications for practice, *Appl Nurs Res* 17(2):81–91, 2004.

Sherrington C, Whitney JC, Lord SR et al: Effective exercise for the prevention of falls: a systematic review and meta-analysis, *J Am Geriatr Soc* 56(12):2234–2243, 2008.

Simmons SF, Schnelle JF, MacRae PG et al: Wheelchairs as mobility restraints: predictors of wheelchair activity in non-ambulatory nursing home residents, *J Am Geriatr Soc* 43(4):384–388, 1995.

• = Independent   ▲ = Collaborative   **EBN** = Evidence-Based Nursing   **EB** = Evidence-Based

Tinetti ME: Preventing falls in elderly persons, *N Engl J Med* 348(1):42–49, 2003.

Voukelatos A, Cumming RG, Lord SR et al: A randomized controlled trial of tai chi for the prevention of falls: the Central Sydney tai chi trial, *J Am Geriatr Soc* 55(8):1185–1191, 2007.

Waszynski CM: Try this: best practices in nursing care to older adults. In: The John A. Hartford Institute for Geriatric Nursing: *Confusion Assessment Method* (CAM), 2007. www.consultgerirn.org/uploads/File/trythis/issue13_cam.pdf. Accessed March 15, 2009.

Dysfunctional Family processes*
Gail B. Ladwig, MSN, RN, CHTP, and Debora Y. Fields, RN, BSN, MA, LICDC, CARN

Definition

Psychosocial, spiritual, and physiological functions of the family unit are chronically disorganized, which leads to conflict, denial of problems, resistance to change, ineffective problem solving, and a series of self-perpetuating crises

Defining Characteristics

Behavioral

Alcohol abuse; agitation; blaming; broken promises; chaos; contradictory communication; controlling communication; criticizing; deficient knowledge about alcoholism; denial of problems; dependency; difficulty having fun; difficulty with intimate relationships; difficulty with life cycle transitions; diminished physical contact; disturbances in academic performance in children; disturbances in concentration; enabling maintenance of alcoholic drinking pattern; escalating conflict; failure to accomplish developmental tasks; family special occasions are alcohol-centered; harsh self-judgment; immaturity; impaired communication; inability to accept health; inability to accept help; inability to accept a wide range of feelings; inability to deal constructively with traumatic experiences; inability to express a wide range of feelings; inability to meet emotional needs of its members; inability to meet security needs of its members; inability to meet spiritual needs of its members; inability to receive help appropriately; inadequate understanding of alcoholism; inappropriate expression of anger; ineffective problem-solving skills; isolation; lack of dealing with conflict; lack of reliability; lying; manipulation; nicotine addiction; orientation toward tension relief rather than achievement of goals; paradoxical communication; power struggles; rationalization; refusal to get help; seeking affirmation; seeking approval; self-blaming; stress-related physical illnesses; substance abuse other than alcohol; unresolved grief; verbal abuse of children; verbal abuse of parent; verbal abuse of spouse

Feelings

Abandonment; anger; anxiety; being different from other people; being unloved; confused love and pity; confusion; decreased self-esteem; depression; dissatisfaction; distress; embarrassment; emotional control by others; emotional isolation; failure; fear; frustration; guilt; hopelessness; hostility; hurt; insecurity; lack of identity; lingering resentment; loneliness; loss; mistrust; misunderstand; moodiness; powerlessness; rejection; repressed emotions; responsibility for alcoholic's behavior; suppressed rage; shame; tension; unhappiness; vulnerability; worthlessness

Roles and Relationships

Altered role function; chronic family problems; closed communication systems; deterioration in family relationships/disrupted family rituals; disrupted family roles; disturbed family dynamics; economic problems; family denial; family does not demonstrate respect for autonomy of its members; family does not demonstrate respect for individuality of its members; inconsistent parenting; ineffective spouse communication; intimacy dysfunction; lack of cohesiveness; lack of skills necessary for relationships; low perception of parental support; marital problems; neglected obligations; pattern of rejection; reduced ability of family members to relate to each other for mutual growth and maturation; triangulating family relationships

*This diagnosis formerly held the label, Dysfunctional Family processes: alcoholism.

Related Factors (r/t)

Abuse of alcohol; addictive personality; biochemical influences; family history of alcoholism; family history of resistance to treatment; genetic predisposition; inadequate coping skills; lack of problem-solving skills

 (Nursing Outcomes Classification)

Suggested NOC Outcomes

Family Coping, Family Functioning, Family Health Status, Substance Addiction Consequences

Example NOC Outcome with Indicators
Family Coping as evidenced by the following indicators: Confronts/manages family problems/Obtains family assistance (Rate the outcome and indicators of **Family Coping:** 1 = never demonstrated, 2 = rarely demonstrated, 3 = sometimes demonstrated, 4 = often demonstrated, 5 = consistently demonstrated [see Section I].)

Client Outcomes

Family/Client Will (Specify Time Frame):

- State one way that alcoholism has affected the health of the family
- Identify three healthy coping behaviors that family members can employ to facilitate a shift toward improved family functioning
- Identify one Al-Anon meeting from Al-Anon meeting schedule that family members express a desire to attend

 (Nursing Interventions Classification)

Suggested NIC Interventions

Family Process Maintenance, Substance Use Treatment

Example Activities—Family Process Maintenance
Identify effects of role changes on family process; Assist family members to use existing support mechanisms

Nursing Interventions and *Rationales*

- Refer to care plans for **Ineffective Denial** and **Defensive Coping** for additional interventions.
- When completing a family assessment, assess behaviors of alcohol abuse, loss of control of drinking, denial, nicotine and other drug addiction, impaired communication, inappropriate expression of anger, and enabling behaviors. **EB:** *A set of standard measures is available for helping assess the needs of concerned and affected family members, derived from an explicit model of the family in relation to excessive drinking, drug taking, or gambling (Orford et al, 2005).*
- Screen clients for at-risk drinking during routine primary care visits. **EB:** *Researchers from the United States and the United Kingdom believe the Alcohol Use Disorders Identification Test (AUDIT) is now one of the most effective and cost-efficient means for identifying hazardous and harmful drinkers in the primary care setting. AUDIT is a 10–item questionnaire specifically developed for use as a short screening instrument for the identification of hazardous, harmful, or dependent alcohol users (Babor, Higgins-Biddle, & Saunders, 2001). In this study of Spanish adults, the high criterion-related validity of AUDIT was proven (de Torres et al, 2009).*
- Provide brief (5– to 10–minute) education and individual counsel as a routine part of primary care. *This practice, along with alcohol screening, can reduce alcohol consumption by high-risk drinkers (Reiff-Hekking et al, 2005). Give family materials from anonymous affiliations. Educate about ways family members may be affected by the alcoholic's drinking and explore effective coping strategies that improve families' ability to function.* **EB:** *Alcoholism is a family disease, and the entire family requires support while they learn about the disease of alcoholism and as they adjust to a new way of living (Center for Substance Abuse Treatment, 2004).*

- Instill hope and encourage the expression of positive thoughts. **EB:** *Hopefulness appears to be central to a family's coping with the impact of mental illness. Nurses should be mindful of their capacity to sustain or diminish the hopes of family members (Bland & Darlington, 2002).*
- Stress early treatment and brief intervention to resolve the problem. **EBN:** *This study demonstrated cost-effectiveness of the early treatment model (project TrEAT; Trial for Early Alcohol Treatment) (Mundt, 2006).*
- Assist with stabilization and maintenance of positive change in the family. Instruct the alcoholic's family members before the client's discharge to give verbal messages that convey concern about the alcoholic's problem drinking, their observations of the alcoholic's past episodes of drinking, and wishes and support for abstinence. **EB:** *This intervention method can help the alcoholic face the reality of his or her drinking problem and alcohol dependence and thus remain longer in long-term rehabilitation programs, which is a prerequisite for successful recovery from alcohol dependence (Ino & Hayasida, 2000).*
- Provide activities that are physical in nature, such as adventure therapy and therapeutic camping, as part of a substance abuse treatment program. **EBN:** *Mental health promotion is considered a strategy to promote health (Epstein, 2004).*
- ▲ Consider alternative therapies such as acupuncture. *Acupuncture may be helpful in detoxification and is valuable when used in combination with counseling (Serrano, 2003).*
- ▲ Refer for possible use of medications to control problem drinking. *Currently, four agents are approved by the Food and Drug Administration for this purpose: disulfiram, acamprosate, oral naltrexone, and the once-monthly injectable, extended-release naltrexone.* **EB:** *All four agents have demonstrated some ability to reduce drinking and/or increase time spent abstinent, but results have not always been consistent (Garbutt, 2009).* **EB:** *Pharmacotherapy, in conjunction with psychosocial interventions, is emerging as a valuable tool for alcohol dependence treatment (Buri et al, 2007).*

Pediatric

- Educate family members about available educational and support programs and encourage no/limited alcohol use in the home. **EBN:** *The family remains a strong factor in moderating adolescent substance use (Kingon & O'Sullivan, 2001). Both individual and multiperson interventions exert an influential role in family-based therapy for treatment of adolescent drug abuse (Hoque et al, 2006).*
- Use closed-ended questions when questioning adolescents about drinking behavior. *Student reports of specific beverage type use were higher when using closed-ended questions compared with open-ended questions. The adolescent drinking amount self-reports seem reasonably reliable and valid both on a population and individual level (Lintonen, Ahlstro, & Metso, 2004).*
- Provide a brief motivational interviewing and cognitive/behavioral-based alcohol intervention group program for young people at risk of developing a problem with alcohol. **EB:** *Participants showed an increase in readiness to reduce their alcohol consumption and a reduction in their frequency of drinking at posttreatment and the first follow-up assessment (Bailey et al, 2004).*
- Encourage parent involvement with adolescents for both supervision and emotional support. *The results of this study indicate that inadequate parent involvement may be a form of neglect, which leads to adolescent alcohol involvement. Neglected adolescents were more likely to develop alcohol use disorders (Duncan, Duncan, & Stryker, 2003).*
- Work at strengthening adolescents' relationships in and out of the home. *Prevention interventions focusing on increasing socially conforming attitudes and on strengthening relationships both in and out of the home during adolescence are likely to be effective in reducing aspects of alcohol involvement for women in the general community (Locke & Newcomb, 2004).*
- Provide school-based prevention programs using peer leaders at an early age. **EB:** *Targeting middle school–aged children and designing programs that can be delivered primarily by peer leaders will increase the effectiveness of school-based substance-use prevention programs (Gottfredson & Wilson, 2003).*
- Provide a school-based drug-prevention program to junior high students. **EB:** *Students who received the drug-prevention program during junior high school were less likely to have violations and points on their driving records (Griffin, Botvin, & Nichols, 2004; Warner, White, & Johnson, 2007).*

Geriatric

- Include assessment of possible alcohol abuse when assessing elderly family members. **EB:** *Alcohol abuse and alcoholism are common but underrecognized problems among older adults (Rigler, 2000).* **EB:** *Alcohol abuse and dependence in older people are important problems that frequently remain undetected by health services (Beullens & Aertgeerts, 2004). The majority of elderly alcoholics are married, have low education levels, and do not belong to high social classes (Shahpesandy et al, 2006).*
- ▲ Provide alcohol treatment programs for geriatric clients in primary care settings. **EB:** *Older primary care clients were more likely to accept collaborative mental health treatment within primary care than in mental health/substance abuse clinics. These results suggest that integrated service arrangements improve access to mental health and substance abuse services for older adults who underuse these services (Bartels et al, 2004).*

Multicultural

- Acknowledge racial/ethnic differences at the onset of care. **EBN:** *Acknowledgment of race/ethnicity issues will enhance communication, establish rapport, and promote treatment outcomes (D'Avanzo et al, 2001; Giger & Davidhizar, 2008).*
- Approach families of color with respect, warmth, and professional courtesy. **EBN:** *Instances of disrespect and lack of caring have special significance for families of color (Kritek et al, 2002; D'Avanzo et al, 2001).*
- Give rationale when assessing African American families about alcohol use and misuse. **EBN:** *Many blacks may expect white caregivers to hold negative and preconceived ideas. Giving a rationale for questions asked will help alleviate this perception (D'Avanzo et al, 2001).*
- Use a family-centered approach when working with Latino, Asian American, African American, and Native American clients. **EBN:** *Latinos may perceive family as a source of support, solver of problems, and source of pride. Asian Americans may regard the family as the primary decision maker and influence on individual family members (D'Avanzo et al, 2001). American Indian families may be extended structures that could exert powerful influences over functioning (Kopera-Frye, 2009). Family therapy is important in addressing the needs of Hispanic families with adolescent substance abusers (Santisteban et al, 2006; Kopera-Frye, 2009). When working with Asian American clients, provide opportunities for the family to adhere to what is considered a normal family structure when working through issues related to alcoholism, and allow the family to save face?* **EBN:** *This will allow the family to not have to own the shame of the alcohol problem. Asian American families may avoid situations that bring shame on the family unit (Chen, 2001; D'Avanzo et al, 2001). In addition, remember to involve the entire family structure in working through the problem. This is essential because some Asian-American families are perceived as patriarchal. For example, Sue (2004) described the family lifestyle of Chinese and Japanese Americans as patriarchal, with authority and communication exercised from the top down. Sue (2004) also noted that within these families there is a need for interdependent roles, strict adherence to traditional norms, and minimization of conflict by suppression of overt emotion.*
- Some less-acculturated Latino families may be unwilling to discuss family issues with health care providers until they perceive a close personal relationship with the provider. **EBN:** *Some Latino families may believe that personal problems should be kept private and may not respond to the health care provider until there is an established personal relationship (Galanti, 2003; Kopera-Frye, 2009).*
- Use family strengthening interventions such as behavioral parent training, family skills training, in-home family support, brief family therapy, and family education when working with culturally diverse families. **EB:** *Comprehensive prevention programs combining multiple approaches produced large positive effects when used with different cultural groups and with different ages of children (Kumpfer, Alvarado, & Whiteside, 2003). Increased alcohol use is strongly related to increased separation from family and increased family conflict in both Mexican American and African American adolescents (Bray et al, 2001).*
- Work with families in a way that incorporates cultural elements. **EB:** *Activities such as tundra walks and time with elders supported in treatment were used successfully for substance abuse treatment with Yup'ik and Cup'ik Eskimos (Mills, 2003).*

- • = Independent   ▲ = Collaborative   **EBN** = Evidence-Based Nursing   **EB** = Evidence-Based

Home Care

NOTE: In the community setting, alcoholism as cause of dysfunctional family processes must be considered in two categories: (1) when the client suffers personally from the illness, and (2) when a significant other suffers from the illness, that is, the client is not the active alcoholic but may depend on the alcoholic for caregiving. The following considerations apply to both situations with appropriate adaptation for the circumstances.

- The previous interventions may be adapted for home care use.
- Work with family members to support a sense of valued fit on their part; include them in treatment planning and identify the importance of their roles in the client's care. At the same time, encourage their pursuit of positive outside activities that enhance their sense of belonging. **EBN:** *Sense of belonging (valued fit) has been identified as a buffer to depression among both depressed and nondepressed individuals with a family history of alcoholism. A buffering effect was not found for individuals with a family history of drug abuse (Sargent et al, 2002).*
- Educate client and family regarding the interactions of alcohol use with medications and the therapeutic regimen. *Increased awareness of drug interactions decrease the chance of relapse due to over the counter and other medications (Weisberg & Hawes, 2005).*
- Alcoholism is a family disease. *If everyone participates in recovery everyone can be healed (Buddy, 2007).*
- ▲ Refer for psychiatric home health care services for client reassurance and implementation of therapeutic regimen. **EB:** *Twelve studies (five randomized controlled trials, one quasi-experimental study, and six uncontrolled cohort studies) found that home and community-based treatment of psychiatric symptoms of socially isolated older adults with mental illness, were associated with improved or maintained psychiatric status. All randomized controlled trials reported improved depressive symptoms, and one reported improved overall psychiatric symptoms (Van Citters & Bartells, 2004).*
- Provide telephone prompting for clients to start alcohol treatment. **EB:** *This study demonstrated that telephone prompting was a simple and effective way to improve attendance for the start of treatment and retention in alcohol treatment (Jackson et al, 2009).*

 Client/Family Teaching and Discharge Planning

- Suggest the client complete a confidential Internet self-screening test for identification of problems and suggestions for treatment if a problem with alcohol is suspected. Many tools are available. *The website www.AlcoholScreening.org helps individuals assess their own alcohol consumption patterns to determine if their drinking is likely harming their health or increasing their risk for future harm. Through education and referral, the site urges those whose drinking is harmful or hazardous to take positive action and informs all adults who consume alcohol about guidelines and caveats for lower risk drinking (Boston University School of Public Health, 2005).*
- Provide education for family. **EB:** *Family Education facilitates understanding of the disease and its causes, effects, and treatment (U.S. Department of Health and Human Services, 2005).*

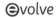 See the EVOLVE website for Weblinks for client education resources.

REFERENCES

Babor TF, Higgins-Biddle JC, Saunders JB et al: *AUDIT. The Alcohol Use Disorders Identification Test: guidelines for use in primary care*, ed 2, Geneva, Switzerland, 2001, World Health Organization.

Bailey KA, Baker AL, Webster RA et al: Pilot randomized controlled trial of a brief alcohol intervention group for adolescents, *Drug Alcohol Rev* 23(2):157–166, 2004.

Bartels SJ, Coakley EH, Zubritsky C et al: Improving access to geriatric mental health services: a randomized trial comparing treatment engagement with integrated versus enhanced referral care for depression, anxiety, and at-risk alcohol use, *Am J Psychiatry* 161(8):1455–1462, 2004.

Beullens J, Aertgeerts B: Screening for alcohol abuse and dependence in older people using DSM criteria: a review, *Aging Ment Health* 8(1):76–82, 2004.

Bland R, Darlington Y: The nature and sources of hope: perspectives of family caregivers of people with serious mental illness, *Perspect Psychiatr Care* 38(2):61, 2002.

Boston University School of Public Health: *How much is too much?* www.alcoholscreening.org. Accessed January 18, 2005.

Bray JH, Adams GJ, Getz JG et al: Developmental, family, and ethnic influences on adolescent alcohol usage: a growth curve approach, *J Fam Psychol* 15(2):301–314, 2001.

Buddy T: Alcoholism is a family disease why do I need help? He's the alcoholic! *About.com*, updated December 24, 2007. http://alcoholism.about.com/cs/info2/a/aa030597.htm. Accessed August 19, 2009.

Buri C, Moggi F, Giovanoli A et al: Prescription procedures in medication for relapse prevention after inpatient treatment for alcohol use disorders in Switzerland, *Alcohol Alcohol* 42(4):333–339, 2007.

Center for Substance Abuse Treatment: *What is substance abuse treatment? A booklet for families*, DHHS Publication No. (SMA) 04–3955. Rockville, MD, 2004, Substance Abuse and Mental Health Services Administration.

Chen YC: Chinese values, health and nursing, *J Adv Nurs* 36(2):270, 2001.

D'Avanzo CE et al: Developing culturally informed strategies for substance-related interventions. In: Naegle MA, D'Avanzo CE, editors: *Addictions and substance abuse: strategies for advanced practice nursing*, St Louis, 2001, Mosby.

de Torres LA, Rebollo EM, Ruiz-Moral R et al: Diagnostic usefulness of the Alcohol Use Disorders Identification Test (AUDIT) questionnaire for the detection of hazardous drinking and dependence on alcohol among Spanish patients, *Eur J Gen Pract* 15(1):15–21, 2009.

Duncan SC, Duncan TE, Stryker LA: Family influences on youth alcohol use: a multiple-sample analysis by ethnicity and gender, *J Ethn Subst Abuse* 2(2):17–33, 2003.

Epstein I: Adventure therapy: a mental health promotion strategy in pediatric oncology, *J Pediatr Oncol Nurs* 21(2):103–110, 2004.

Galanti GA: The Hispanic family and male-female relationships: an overview, *J Transcult Nurs* 14(3):180–185, 2003.

Garbutt JC: The state of pharmacotherapy for the treatment of alcohol dependence, *J Subst Abuse Treat* 36(1):S15–23, 2009.

Giger J, Davidhizar R: *Transcultural nursing: assessment and intervention*, ed 4, St Louis, 2008, Mosby.

Gottfredson DC, Wilson DB: Characteristics of effective school-based substance abuse prevention, *Prev Sci* 4(1):27, 2003.

Griffin KW, Botvin GJ, Nichols TR: Long-term follow-up effects of a school-based drug abuse prevention program on adolescent risky driving, *Prev Sci* 5(3):207–212, 2004.

Hoque A, Dauber S, Samuolis J et al: Treatment techniques and outcomes in multidimensional family therapy for adolescent behaviour problems, *J Fam Psychol* 20(4):535–543, 2006.

Ino A, Hayasida M: Before-discharge intervention method in the treatment of alcohol dependence, *Alcohol Clin Exp Res* 24(3):373, 2000.

Jackson KR, Booth PG, Salmon P et al: The effects of telephone prompting on attendance for starting treatment and retention in treatment at a specialist alcohol clinic, *Br J Clin Psychol* 2009, Epub ahead of print.

Kingon YS, O'Sullivan AL: The family as a protective asset in adolescent development, *J Holist Nurs* 19(2):102–121, 2001.

Kopera-Frye K: Strengths and challenges within a needs and issues of Latino and Native American nonparental relative caregivers: strengths and challenges within a cultural context, *Fam Consumer Sci Res J* 37:394, 2009.

Kritek P, Hargraves M, Cuellar K et al: Eliminating health disparities among minority women: a report on conference workshop process and outcomes, *Am J Public Health* 92(4):580–587, 2002.

Kumpfer KL, Alvarado R, Whiteside HO: Family-based interventions for substance use and misuse prevention, *Subst Use Misuse* 38(11–13):1759–1787, 2003.

Lintonen T, Ahlstro MS, Metso L: The reliability of self-reported drinking in adolescence, *Alcohol Alcohol* 39(4):362–368, 2004.

Locke TF, Newcomb MD: Adolescent predictors of young adult and adult alcohol involvement and dysphoria in a prospective community sample of women, *Prev Sci* 5(3):151–168, 2004.

Mills PA: Incorporating Yup'ik and Cup'ik Eskimo traditions into behavioral health treatment, *J Psychoactive Drugs* 35(1):85–88, 2003.

Mundt M: Analyzing the costs and benefits of brief intervention, *Alcohol Res Health* 29(1):34–36, 2006.

Orford J, Templeton L, Velleman R et al: Family members of relatives with alcohol, drug and gambling problems: a set of standardized questionnaires for assessing stress, coping and strain, *Addiction* 100(11):1611–1624, 2005.

Reiff-Hekking S, Ockene JK, Hurley TG et al: Brief physician and nurse practitioner-delivered counseling for high-risk drinking. Results at 12–month follow-up, *J Gen Intern Med* 20(1):96–97, 2005.

Rigler SK: Alcoholism in the elderly, *Am Fam Physician* 61(6):1710, 2000.

Santisteban DA, Suarez-Morales L, Robbins MS et al: Brief strategic family therapy: lessons learned in efficacy research and challenges to blending research and practice, *Fam Process* 45(2):259–271, 2006.

Sargent J, Williams RA, Hagerty B et al: Sense of belonging as a buffer against depressive symptoms, *J Am Psychiatr Nurs Assoc* 8(4):120–129, 2002.

Serrano R: *Solution focused addictions counseling, acupuncture treatment for substance abuse.* www.holisticwebs.com/solution/sfac4.html. Accessed January 18, 2003.

Shahpesandy H, Pristasova J, Janikova Z et al: Alcoholism in the elderly: a study of elderly alcoholics compared with healthy elderly and young alcoholics, *Neuro Endocrinol Lett* 27(5):651–657, 2006.

Sue DW: Ethnic identity: the impact of two cultures on the psychological development of Asians in America. In: Atkinson DR, Morton G, Sue DW, editors: *Counseling American minorities: a cross cultural perspective*, ed 6, Boston, 2004, McGraw-Hill.

U.S. Department of Health and Human Services. *What is substance abuse treatment? A booklet for families*, 2005. www.samhsa.gov. Accessed December 10, 2009.

Van Citters AD, Bartels SJ: A systematic review of the effectiveness of community-based mental health outreach services for older adults, *Psychiatr Serv* 55(11):1237–1249, 2004.

Warner LA, White HR, Johnson V: Alcohol initiation experiences and family history of alcoholism as predictors of problem-drinking trajectories, *J Stud Alcohol* 68(1):56–65, 2007.

Weisberg J, Hawes G: *Safe medicine for sober people: how to avoid relapsing on pain, sleep, cold, or any other medication*, New York, 2005, St. Martin's Griffin.

Interrupted Family processes   *Vanessa Sammons, MSN, APRN, BC, CNE*

NANDA-I

Definition

Change in family relationships and/or functioning

Defining Characteristics

Changes in assigned tasks; changes in availability for affective responsiveness; changes in availability for emotional support; changes in communication patterns; changes in effectiveness in completing assigned tasks; changes in expressions of conflict with community resources; changes in expressions of isolation from community resources; changes in expressions of conflict within family; changes in intimacy; changes in mutual support; changes in patterns; changes in participation in problem solving; changes in participation in decision making; changes in power alliances; changes in rituals; changes in satisfaction with family; changes in somatic complaints; changes in stress-reduction behaviors

Related Factors (r/t)

Developmental crises; developmental transition; family-roles shift; interaction with community; modification in family finances; modification in family social status; power shift of family members; shift in health status of a family member; situation transition; situational crises

 (Nursing Outcomes Classification)

Suggested NOC Outcomes

Family Coping, Family Functioning, Family Normalization, Psychosocial Adjustment: Life Change, Role Performance

Example NOC Outcome with Indicators
Family Coping as evidenced by the following indicators: Confronts/manages family problems/Involves family members in decision making (Rate the outcome and indicators of **Family Coping:** 1 = never demonstrated, 2 = rarely demonstrated, 3 = sometimes demonstrated, 4 = often demonstrated, 5 = consistently demonstrated [see Section I].)

Client Outcomes

Family/Client Will (Specify Time Frame):

- Express feelings (family)
- Identify ways to cope effectively and use appropriate support systems (family)
- Treat impaired family member as normally as possible to avoid overdependence (family)
- Meet physical, psychosocial, and spiritual needs of members or seek appropriate assistance (family)
- Demonstrate knowledge of illness or injury, treatment modalities, and prognosis (family)
- Participate in the development of the plan of care to the best of ability (significant person)

NIC **(Nursing Interventions Classification)**

Suggested NIC Interventions

Family Integrity Promotion, Family Process Maintenance, Normalization Promotion

Example NIC Activities—Family Integrity Promotion
Collaborate with family in problem solving and decision making; Counsel family members on additional effective coping skills for their own use

Nursing Interventions and *Rationales*

- Motivate family members to speak openly about illnesses. **EB:** *Open communications can improve the quality of life to allow family members to derive solutions and face challenges (Silva, Galera, & Morena, 2007).*
- Acknowledge the range of emotions and feelings that may be experienced when the health status of a family member changes; counsel family members that it is normal to be angry and afraid. **EBN:** *Nurses should provide care for the critically ill client while attending to the needs of the stressed family members (Maxwell, Stuenkel, & Saylor, 2007).*
- Encourage family members to list their personal strengths. *A list of strengths provides information that family members can refer to for positive feedback.*
- Establish relationships among clients, their families, and health care professionals. **EBN:** *Insights gained may inform nurses' of the possible provisions needed during end-of-life care (McWilliam et al, 2008).*

• = Independent   ▲ = Collaborative   **EBN** = Evidence-Based Nursing   **EB** = Evidence-Based

- Encourage family to visit the client; adjust visiting hours to accommodate family's schedule. **EBN:** *Unrestricted visitation in the intensive care unit was found to decrease anxiety of the client's family members (Garrouste-Orgeas et al, 2008).*
- Allow and encourage family members to assist in the client's treatment. **EBN:** *Families of critical care clients focus on their decision making, spiritual and emotional support, and continuity of care at the end of life (Kirchhoff & Faas, 2007).*
- Consider the use of different instruction methods in assisting inexperienced older adults through interactive training systems. **EB:** *Video-supported knowledge acquisition is better than text (Gram & Struve, 2009).*
- Refer to the care plan **Readiness for enhanced Family processes** for additional interventions.

Pediatric

- Carefully assess potential for reunifying children placed in foster care with their birth parents. **EB:** *Reunifying children placed in foster care with their birth parents is a primary goal of the child welfare system (Wulczyn, 2004).*
- Allow and encourage family to assist in the client's care. **EBN:** *Parents need to be able to negotiate with health staff what this participation will involve and negotiate new roles for themselves in sharing care of their sick child. Parents should be involved in the decision-making process (Corlett & Twycross, 2006).*
- ▲ Refer children and mothers exposed to violence in the home to theraplay: an attachment-based intervention that uses the four core elements of nurturing, engagement, structure, and challenge in interactions between mother and her child. **EBN:** *This family connections program improves the quality of life for mothers and children during a short shelter stay; it has the potential to improve the long-term quality of life (Bennett, Shiner, & Ryan, 2006).*

Geriatric

- Encourage family members to be involved in the care of relatives who are in residential care settings. **EB:** *Family involvement in residential long-term care is important (Gaugler et al, 2004). If family satisfaction is to be achieved, family presence in a nursing home needs to give caregivers a sense of positive involvement and influence over the care of their relative (Tornatore & Grant, 2004).*
- Support group problem solving among family members and include the older member. *Problem solving is an effective method to manage stressors for family members of all ages.*
- ▲ Refer family for counseling with a psychotherapist who is knowledgeable about gerontology.
- Refer to care plan for **Readiness for enhanced Family processes** for additional interventions.

Multicultural

- Refer to the care plan **Readiness for enhanced Family processes** for additional interventions.

Home Care

- The nursing interventions described in the care plan for **Compromised family Coping** should be used in the home environment with adaptations as necessary.
- Encourage family members to find meaning in a serious illness. **EBN:** *Letting go before the death of a loved one involves a shift in thinking in which there is acknowledgement of impending loss without impeding its natural progression (Lowey, 2008).*

Client/Family Teaching and Discharge Planning

- Refer to Client/Family Teaching and Discharge Planning in **Compromised family Coping** and **Readiness for enhanced family Coping** for suggestions that may be used with minor adaptations.

⊖volve   Go to the Evolve website for Weblinks for client education resources.

● = Independent   ▲ = Collaborative   **EBN** = Evidence-Based Nursing   **EB** = Evidence-Based

REFERENCES

Bennett L, Shiner S, Ryan S: Using Theraplay in shelter setting with mothers and children who have experienced violence in the home, *J Psychosoc Nurs Ment Health Serv* 44(10):38–48, 2006.

Corlett J, Twycross A: Negotiation of parental roles within family-centred care: a review of the research, *J Clin Nurs* 15(10):1308–1316, 2006.

Garrouste-Orgeas M, Philippart F, Timsit JF et al: Perceptions of a 24–hour visiting policy in the intensive care unit, *Crit Care Med* 36(1):30–35, 2008.

Gaugler JE, Anderson KA, Zarit SH et al: Family involvement in nursing homes: effects on stress and well-being, *Aging Ment Health* 8(1):65–75, 2004.

Gram D, Struve D: Instructional videos for supporting older adults who use interactive systems, *Educ Gerontol* 35(2):164–176, 2009.

Kirchhoff KT, Faas AI: Family support at end of life, *AACN Adv Crit Care* 18(4):426–435, 2007.

Lowey SE: Letting go before a death: a concept analysis, *J Adv Nurs* 63(2): 208–215, 2008.

Maxwell KE, Stuenkel D, Saylor C: Needs of family members of critically ill patients: a comparison of nurse and family perceptions, *Heart Lung* 36(5):367–376, 2007.

McWilliam CL, Ward-Griffin C, Oudshoorn A et al: Living while dying/dying while living: older clients' sociocultural experience of home-based palliative care, *J Hosp Palliat Nurs* 10(6):338–349, 2008.

Silva L, Galera SAF, Morena V: Meeting at home: a proposal of home attendance for families of dependent seniors, *Acta Paul Enfermagem* 20(4):397–403, 2007.

Tornatore JB, Grant LA: Family caregiver satisfaction with the nursing home after placement of a relative with dementia, *J Gerontol B Psychol Sci Soc Sci* 59(2):S80–S88, 2004.

Wulczyn F: Family reunification, *Future Child* 14(1):94–113, 2004.

Readiness for enhanced Family processes   *Vanessa Sammons, MSN, APRN, BC, CNE*

NANDA-I

Definition

A pattern of family functioning that is sufficient to support the well-being of family members and can be strengthened

Defining Characteristics

Activities support the growth of family members; activities support the safety of family members; balance exists between autonomy and cohesiveness; boundaries of family members are maintained; communication is adequate; energy level of family supports activities of daily living; expresses willingness to enhance family dynamics; family adapts to change; family functioning meets needs of family members; family resilience is evident; family roles are appropriate for developmental stages; family roles are flexible for developmental stages; family tasks are accomplished; interdependent with community; relationships are generally positive; respect for family members is evident

NOC   (Nursing Outcomes Classification)

Suggested NOC Outcomes

Family Coping, Health-Promoting Behavior, Health-Seeking Behavior, Parent-Infant Attachment, Parenting Performance

---

Example NOC Outcome with Indicators

Family Coping as evidenced by the following indicators: Confronts/manages family problems/Involves family members in decision making (Rate the outcome and indicators of **Family Coping:** 1 = never demonstrated, 2 = rarely demonstrated, 3 = sometimes demonstrated, 4 = often demonstrated, 5 = consistently demonstrated [see Section I].)

Client Outcomes

Family/Client Will (Specify Time Frame):

- Identify ways to cope effectively and use appropriate support systems (family)
- Meet physical, psychosocial, and spiritual needs of members or seek appropriate assistance (family)
- Demonstrate knowledge of potential environmental, lifestyle, and genetic risks to health and use appropriate measures to decrease possibility of risk (family)
- Focus on wellness, disease prevention, and maintenance (family and individual)
- Seek balance among exercise, work, leisure, rest, and nutrition (family and individual)

• = Independent   ▲ = Collaborative   **EBN** = Evidence-Based Nursing   **EB** = Evidence-Based

NIC   (Nursing Interventions Classification)

Suggested NIC Interventions

Coping Enhancement, Decision-Making Support, Family Integrity Promotion, Family Involvement Promotion, Family Mobilization, Family Process Maintenance, Parent Education: Adolescent, Child-rearing Family, Risk Identification, Role Enhancement

Example NIC Activities—Risk Identification
Determine community support systems; Determine presence and quality of family support

Nursing Interventions and *Rationales*

- Assess the family's stress level and coping abilities during the initial nursing assessment. **EBN:** *Comprehensive assessments of family members' psychosocial needs are important to plan appropriate interventions to alleviate their stress and strengthen their coping skills (Chui & Chan, 2007).*
- Consider the use of family-centered theory as the conceptual foundation to help guide interventions. **EB:** *The concept of family-centered care stresses the importance of the family in children's well-being (Bamm & Rosenbaum, 2008).*
- Use family-centered care and role modeling for holistic care of families. **EBN:** *In this study, data showed nurses helping burned children to heal holistically while simultaneously supporting families to heal holistically by role-modeling ways of being with and caring for the children (Zengerle-Levy, 2006).*
- Discuss with family members and identify the perceptions of the health care experience. **EBN:** *Nurses should explore perceptions of the needs of family members of critically ill clients and identify to the extent these needs can be met to improve quality of nursing care (Maxwell, Stuenkel, & Saylor, 2007).*
- Support family needs, strengths, and resourcefulness through family interviews. **EBN:** *Family interviews both affirm and give greater understanding of individual family member's issues and concerns (Eggenberger & Nelms, 2007).*
- Spend time with family members; allow them to verbalize their feelings. **EBN:** *In this study, families emphasized the importance of feeling that health professionals cared for them and their loved one and that this caring could be made visible in a number of simple, small gestures (Brysiewicz, 2008).*
- Encourage family members to find meaning in a serious illness. **EBN:** *Letting go before the death of a loved one involves a shift in thinking in which there is acknowledgment of impending loss without impeding its natural progression (Lowey, 2008).*
- Provide family-centered care to explore and use all available resources appropriate for the situation (e.g., counseling, social services, self-help groups, pastoral care). **EBN:** *Family-centered care has become a cornerstone of pediatric practice (Shields, Pratt, & Hunter, 2006).*
- Consider focus groups to provide insight to family perceptions of illness and/or disease prevention. **EBN:** *Focus groups provide insight into doctor-client communications and can inform efforts to improve primary prevention in the clinical setting (Sege et al, 2006).*

 Pediatric

- Provide a parenting class series based on individual and couple changes in meaning and identity, roles, and relationships and interaction during the transition to parenthood. Address mother and father roles, infant communication abilities, and patterns of the first 3 months of life in a mutually enjoyable, possibility focused manner. **EBN:** *Interventions that enhance mutual parent-child interaction through increased sensitivity to cues and responsiveness to infant needs or signals are important avenues for facilitating secure attachment, father and mother involvement, optimal development, and prevention of child abuse and neglect (Bryan, 2000).*
- Encourage families with adolescents to have family meals. *Eating family meals may enhance the health and well-being of adolescents. Public education on the benefits of family mealtime is recommended (Eisenberg et al, 2004).*
- ▲ Consider the use of adventure therapy for adolescents with cancer. **EBN:** *This mental health promotion is considered a strategy to promote health (Epstein, 2004).*

• = Independent   ▲ = Collaborative   **EBN** = Evidence-Based Nursing   **EB** = Evidence-Based

Geriatric

- Carefully listen to residents and family members in the long-term care facility. **EBN:** *Nurses can improve life and dignity for residents by listening to residents and family members (Iwasiw et al, 2003).*
- Support caregivers' awareness of the positive effects of their contribution to the well-being of parents. **EBN:** *Client-focused and family-focused care requires attention to design. One successful model is the Caring Model, which demonstrates the difference between direct caregivers and indirect caregivers within the family (Dossey, Keegan, & Guzzetta, 2005).*
- Teach family members about the impact of developmental events (e.g., retirement, death, change in health status, and household composition). *Knowledge regarding normative developmental challenges of aging can reduce the stress such challenges place on families.*
- Encourage social networks; social integration; and social engagement with friends, children, and relatives of the elderly. **EB:** *A longitudinal study indicated that few social ties, poor integration, and social disengagement are risk factors for cognitive decline among community-dwelling elderly persons (Zunzunegui et al, 2003).*

Multicultural

- Assess for the influence of cultural beliefs, norms, and values on the family's perceptions of normal functioning. **EBN:** *What the family considers normal and abnormal family functioning may be based on cultural perceptions (Giger & Davidhizar, 2004). Latino families who express a higher degree of familism are characterized by positive interpersonal familial relationships, high family unity, social support, interdependence in the completion of daily activities, and close proximity with extended family members (Romero et al, 2004).*
- Identify and acknowledge the stresses unique to racial/ethnic families. **EBN:** *Women in Turkey perceive themselves as wives sharing everything within the family; their decision-making rate was lower than that of men, except for selecting clothes (Erci, 2003). Access to care, financial means, and mistrust of the health care system are significant obstacles for low-income Southern, black American women (Appel, Giger, & Davidhizar, 2005).*
- Assess and support spiritual needs of families. **EBN:** *A study of African American mothers demonstrated that spirituality helped them cope during the time of their infants' hospitalization for a serious illness (Wilson & Miles 2001).*
- With the client's consent, facilitate a group meeting for family members to discuss how the family is functioning. **EBN:** *A family meeting opens communication and lets each family member know it is okay to talk about what is happening (Rivera-Andino & Lopez, 2000). Focus groups with African Americans found that families could benefit from help with placement of family members in nursing homes and hospitals and the process of family decision making (Turner et al, 2004).*
- Facilitate modeling and role playing for the client and family regarding healthy ways to start a discussion about the client's prognosis. **EBN:** *It is helpful for families and the client to practice communication skills in a safe environment before trying them in a real-life situation (Rivera-Andino & Lopez, 2000).*
- Encourage family mealtimes. **EB:** *Frequency of family meals was inversely associated with tobacco, alcohol, and marijuana use; low grade point average; depressive symptoms; and suicide involvement of diverse adolescents (Eisenberg et al, 2004).*

Home Care

- The previous nursing interventions should be used in the home environment with adaptations as necessary.
- ▲ Encourage virtual support groups to family caregivers. **EB:** *Positive participant responses were identified as learning to use computers, negotiating the website links, obtaining disease-specific information from the website, using technology to communicate, bonding with group members, providing mutual guidance and support, and benefiting in terms of coping with the stresses of caregiving (Marziali, Damianakis, & Donahue, 2006).*
- ▲ Encourage caregivers of elderly clients with chronic obstructive pulmonary disease (COPD) receiving long-term oxygen therapy (LTOT) to seek additional services such as social services, respite

• = Independent   ▲ = Collaborative   **EBN** = Evidence-Based Nursing   **EB** = Evidence-Based

care, and additional home health visits. **EB:** *More convenient family resources for severe COPD clients may improve the stress among caregivers (Takata et al, 2008).*

Client/Family Teaching and Discharge Planning

- Refer to Client/Family Teaching and Discharge Planning in **Readiness for enhanced family Coping** for suggestions that may be used with minor adaptations.

⊖volve   Go to the Evolve website for Weblinks for client education resources.

REFERENCES

Appel SJ, Giger JN, Davidhizar RE: Opportunity cost: the impact of contextual risk factors on the cardiovascular health of low-income rural southern African American women, *J Cardiovasc Nurs* 20:315–324, 2005.

Bamm EL, Rosenbaum P: Family-centered theory: origins, development, barriers, and supports to implementation in rehabilitation medicine, *Arch Phys Med Rehabil* 89(8):1618–1624, 2008.

Bryan AA: Enhancing parent-child interaction with a prenatal couple intervention, *MCN Am J Matern Child Nurs* 25(3):139, 2000.

Brysiewicz P: The lived experience of losing a loved one to a sudden death in KwaZulu-Natal, South Africa, *J Clin Nurs* 17(2): 224–231, 2008.

Chui WY, Chan SW: Stress and coping of Hong Kong Chinese family members during a critical illness, *J Clin Nurs* 16(2): 372–381, 2007.

Dossey B, Keegan L, Guzzetta C: *Holistic nursing*, ed 4, Boston, 2005, Jones & Bartlett.

Eggenberger SK, Nelms TP: Family interviews as a method for family research, *J Adv Nurs* 58(3):282–292, 2007.

Eisenberg ME, Olson RE, Neumark-Sztainer D et al: Correlations between family meals and psychosocial well-being among adolescents, *Arch Pediatr Adolesc Med* 158(8):792–796, 2004.

Epstein I: Adventure therapy: a mental health promotion strategy in pediatric oncology, *J Pediatr Oncol Nurs* 21(2):103–110, 2004.

Erci B: Women's efficiency in decision making and their perception of their status in the family, *Public Health Nurs* 20(1):65, 2003.

Giger JN, Davidhizar RE: *Transcultural nursing: assessment & intervention*, ed 4, St Louis, 2004, Mosby.

Iwasiw C, Goldenberg D, Bol N et al: Resident and family perspectives: the first year in a long-term care facility, *J Gerontol Nurs* 29(1):45, 2003.

Lowey SE: Letting go before death: a concept analysis, *J Adv Nurs* 63(2):208–215, 2008.

Marziali E, Damianakis T, Donahue P: Internet-based clinical services: virtual support groups for family caregivers, *J Technol Hum Serv*, 24(2/3): 39–54, 2006.

Maxwell KE, Stuenkel D, Saylor C: Needs of family members of critically ill patients: a comparison of nurse and family perceptions, *Heart Lung* 36(5): 367–376, 2007.

Rivera-Andino J, Lopez L: When culture complicates care, *RN* 63(7):47, 2000.

Romero AJ, Robinson TN, Haydel KF et al: Associations among familism, language preference, and education in Mexican-American mothers and their children, *J Dev Behav Pediatr* 25(1):34–40, 2004.

Sege RD, Hatmaker-Flanigan E, De Vos E et al: Anticipatory guidance and violence prevention: results from family and pediatrician focus groups, *Pediatrics* 117(2):455–463, 2006.

Shields L, Pratt J, Hunter J: Family centered care: a review of qualitative studies, *J Clin Nurs* 15(10):1317–1323, 2006.

Takata S, Washio M, Moriwaki A et al: Burden among caregivers of patients with chronic obstructive pulmonary disease with long-term oxygen therapy, *Int Med J* 15(1):53–57, 2008.

Turner WL, Wallace BR, Anderson JR et al: The last mile of the way: understanding caregiving in African American families at the end-of-life, *J Marital Fam Ther* 30(4):427–438, 2004.

Wilson SM, Miles MS: Spirituality in African-American mothers coping with a seriously ill infant, *J Soc Pediatr Nurs* 6(3):116–122, 2001.

Zengerle-Levy K: The inextricable link in caring for families of critically burned children, *Qual Health Res* 16(1):5–26, 2006.

Zunzunegui MV, Alvarado BE, Del Ser T et al: Social networks, social integration, and social engagement determine cognitive decline in community-dwelling Spanish older adults, *Gerontol B Psychol Sci Soc Sci* 58(2):S93, 2003.

Fatigue   *Paula Riess Sherwood, RN, CNRN, PhD, and Barbara Given, RN, PhD, FAAN*

NANDA-I

Definition

An overwhelming, sustained sense of exhaustion and decreased capacity for physical and mental work at usual level

Defining Characteristics

Compromised concentration; compromised libido; decreased performance; disinterest in surroundings; drowsy; feelings of guilt for not keeping up with responsibilities; inability to maintain usual level of physical activity; inability to maintain usual routines; inability to restore energy even after sleep; increase in physical complaints; increase in rest requirements; introspection; lack of energy; lethargic; listless; perceived need for additional energy to accomplish routine tasks; tired; verbalization of an unremitting lack of energy; verbalization of an overwhelming lack of energy

---

• = Independent   ▲ = Collaborative   **EBN** = Evidence-Based Nursing   **EB** = Evidence-Based

Related Factors (r/t)

Psychological

Anxiety; boring lifestyle; depression

Physiological

Anemia; disease states (e.g., cancer, multiple sclerosis, respiratory diseases, coronary diseases); increased physical exertion; malnutrition; poor physical condition; pregnancy; sleep deprivation

Environmental

Humidity; lights; noise; temperature

Situational

Negative life events; occupation

 (Nursing Outcomes Classification)

Suggested NOC Outcomes

Concentration, Endurance, Energy Conservation, Nutritional Status, Energy, Vitality

Example NOC Outcome with Indicators
Endurance as evidenced by the following indicators: Performance of usual routine/Activity/Rested appearance/Blood oxygen level/Muscle endurance (Rate the outcome and indicators of **Endurance:** 1 = severely compromised, 2 = substantially compromised, 3 = moderately compromised, 4 = mildly compromised, 5 = not compromised [see Section I].)

Client Outcomes

Client Will (Specify Time Frame):

- Identify potential factors that aggravate and relieve fatigue
- Describe ways to assess and track patterns of fatigue
- Describe ways in which fatigue affects the ability to accomplish goals
- Verbalize increased energy and improved well-being
- Explain energy conservation plan to offset fatigue
- Explain energy restoration plan to offset fatigue

NIC **(Nursing Interventions Classification)**

Suggested NIC Intervention

Energy Management (including conservation and restoration)

Example NIC Activities—Energy Management
Assess patient's physiologic status for deficits resulting in fatigue within the context of age and development; Determine patient/significant other's perception of causes of fatigue

Nursing Interventions and *Rationales*

- Assess severity of fatigue on a scale of 0 to 10 (average fatigue, worst and best levels); assess frequency of fatigue (number of days per week and time of day), activities and symptoms associated with increased fatigue (e.g., pain), ability to perform ADLs and instrumental ADLs, interference with social and role function, times of increased energy, ability to concentrate, mood, and usual pattern of activity. Consider use of an instrument such as the Profile of Mood State Short Form Fatigue Subscale, the Multidimensional Assessment of Fatigue, the Lee Fatigue Scale, the Multidimensional Fatigue Inventory, the HIV-Related Fatigue Scale, the Brief Fatigue Inventory, or the Dutch Fatigue Scale to assess fatigue accurately. **EBN:** *These assessments have all been shown to have good internal reliability. The Fatigue Severity Scale, Fatigue Impact Scale, and Brief Fatigue Inventory are relatively short with good psychometric properties, making them clinically useful. These measures, along with the Multidimensional Assessment of Fatigue, have shown the ability to detect changes in fatigue over time (Whitehead, 2009).*

● = Independent   ▲ = Collaborative   **EBN** = Evidence-Based Nursing   **EB** = Evidence-Based

The Revised Schwartz Cancer Fatigue Scale and the M.D. Anderson Symptom Inventory have demonstrated value in assessing fatigue in clients with cancer (Cleeland et al, 2000; Schwartz & Meek, 1999).

- Evaluate adequacy of nutrition and sleep hygiene (napping throughout the day, inability to fall asleep or stay asleep). Encourage the client to get adequate rest, limit naps (particularly in the late afternoon or evening), use a routine sleep/wake schedule, avoid caffeine in the late afternoon or evening, and eat a well-balanced diet with at least eight glasses of water a day. Refer to **Imbalanced Nutrition: less than body requirements** or **Insomnia** if appropriate. **EBN:** *A commonly suggested treatment for fatigue is rest, although excessive sleep can aggravate fatigue (Pigeon, Sateia, & Ferguson, 2003; Carpenter et al, 2004). Inadequate nutrition can also contribute to fatigue, particularly if anemia is present (Minton et al, 2008).*

▲ Collaborate with the primary care practitioner to identify physiological and/or psychological causes of fatigue that could be treated, such as anemia, pain, electrolyte imbalance (e.g., altered potassium levels), hypothyroidism, depression, or medication effect. **EB and EBN:** *The presence of fatigue can be associated with multiple biological, psychological, social, and personal factors (Craig & Kakumanu, 2002; Barsevick et al, 2004; Forlenza et al, 2005; Ranjith, 2005). If an etiology for fatigue can be determined, the condition should be treated according to the underlying cause. Depression and anxiety have been significantly correlated with fatigue (Phillips et al, 2004). Anemia is highly correlated with fatigue, particularly in clients with cancer (Minton et al, 2008).*

▲ Work with the primary care practitioner to determine if the client has chronic fatigue syndrome, paying attention to risk factors in particular populations. *Chronic fatigue syndrome is unexplained fatigue lasting 6 months or longer that is not associated with a diagnosed physical or psychological condition and has been shown to be more frequent and severe in African Americans and Native Americans (Dinos et al, 2009).*

- Encourage the client to express feelings about fatigue, including potential causes of fatigue, and possible interventions to alleviate fatigue such as setting small, easily achieved, short-term goals and developing energy management techniques; use active listening techniques and help identify sources of hope. **EBN and EB:** *Problem-solving interventions have been shown to lower the incidence of fatigue (Given et al, 2002; Vanage, Gilbertson, & Mathiowetz, 2003; Mathiowetz et al, 2005). In particular, cognitive behavioral therapy has been shown to be moderately effective when compared to usual care and to relaxation, counseling, and education/support, although these effects have not been maintained over time (Malouff et al, 2008; Price et al, 2008).*

- Encourage the client to keep a journal of activities, symptoms of fatigue, and feelings, including how fatigue affects the client's normal activities and roles. **EBN:** *The journal can increase the client's awareness of symptoms and sense of control and facilitate communication with health care practitioners (Given et al, 2002; Schumacher et al, 2002).*

- Help the client identify sources of support and essential and nonessential tasks to determine which tasks can be delegated to whom. Give the client permission to limit social and role demands if needed (e.g., switch to part-time employment, hire cleaning service). **EBN:** *Problem solving can improve the client's sense of mastery by helping the client problem solve to decrease the impact of fatigue on daily activities (Given et al, 2002). Psychoeducational interventions that include fatigue education, self-care, coping techniques, and activity management have been shown to be effective in reducing cancer-related fatigue (Goedendorp et al, 2009).*

▲ Collaborate with the primary care practitioner regarding the appropriateness of referrals to physical therapy for carefully monitored aerobic exercise program and possible physical aids, such as a walker or cane. **EB and EBN:** *Aerobic exercise and physical therapy may reduce fatigue in cancer clients, although not all metaanalyses have replicated this finding (Jacobsen et al, 2007) and the effect of exercise has not been shown to be better than psychological interventions (Conn et al, 2006; Kangas, Bovbjerg, & Montgomery, 2008). **EB and EBN:** An exercise program for clients receiving chemotherapy or radiation treatments for breast cancer helped improve levels of fatigue (Mock et al, 2005). An exercise program may also reduce fatigue and improve energy in clients with other medical conditions, such as cardiac disease (Gary et al, 2004; Puetz, Beasman, & O'Connor, 2006). **EB and EBN:** Supervised aerobic exercise training has beneficial effects on physical capacity and fibromyalgia symptoms as well as in clients with multiple sclerosis, rheumatoid arthritis, and systemic lupus erythematosus (Busch et al, 2002; Neill, Belan, & Ried, 2006; Motl & Gosney, 2008).*

- Clients may desire multiple strategies to relieve fatigue rather than one single intervention, particularly when there are multiple potential etiologies present. **EB:** *Participants often used multiple*

• = Independent ▲ = Collaborative **EBN** = Evidence-Based Nursing **EB** = Evidence-Based

strategies to alleviate their fatigue, possibly because of their tendency to attribute it to multiple causes (Seigel, Brown-Bradley, & Lekas, 2004).

▲ Refer the client to diagnosis-appropriate support groups such as National Chronic Fatigue Syndrome Association, Multiple Sclerosis Association, or cancer fatigue websites such as the Oncology Nurses Association *(www.ons.org)* or the *National Comprehensive Cancer Network.* **EB:** *Support groups can help clients legitimize their symptoms and cope with the frequent depression that accompanies fatigue (Friedberg, Leung & Quick, 2005).*

▲ For a cardiac client, recognize that fatigue is common after a myocardial infarction or chronic cardiac insufficiency. Refer to cardiac rehabilitation for carefully prescribed and monitored exercise program. **EBN:** *Carefully monitored exercise is thought to decrease symptoms of fatigue in cardiac clients (Gary et al, 2004).*

• For fatigue associated with multiple sclerosis, encourage energy conservation, "recharging efforts," and excellent self-care; consider use of a cooling suit because fatigue increases in a warm environment. **EBN:** *Use of a cooling suit by individuals with multiple sclerosis may decrease their sense of fatigue (Flensner & Lindencrona, 2002; Puetz, Beasman, & O'Connor, 2006).*

• If fatigue is associated with cancer or cancer-related treatment, assess for other symptoms that may enhance fatigue (e.g., pain or depression). **EBN:** *Clients with cancer who reported both pain and fatigue reported three times as many other symptoms as clients who reported neither pain nor fatigue; fatigue was linked to the presence of pain, multiple comorbid conditions, and site of cancer (Given et al, 2001; NCCN, 2009).*

▲ Collaborate with primary care practitioners to identify attentional fatigue, which may manifest itself as the inability to direct attention necessary to perform usual activities. **EBN:** *Reduced performance in cognitive function was observed before treatment and found to persist over time in older women newly diagnosed with breast cancer (Cimprich & Ronis, 2003; Simoneau, Begin, & Teasdale, 2006).*

▲ Collaborate with primary care practitioners to identify potential pharmacologic treatment for fatigue. **EB and EBN:** Pharmacologic therapy has been shown to be effective in reducing fatigue in clients with diseases such as multiple sclerosis, cancer, and depression (Papakostas et al, 2006; Pucci et al, 2007; Minton et al, 2008)

Geriatric

• Review comorbid conditions that may contribute to fatigue, such as congestive heart failure, arthritis, and cancer.

• Identify recent losses; monitor for depression as a possible contributing factor to fatigue. **EBN:** *There is a high correlation between depression and fatigue (Sugahara et al, 2004).*

▲ Review medications for side effects. *Certain medications (e.g., antihistamines, pain medications, anticonvulsants, chemotherapeutic agents) may cause fatigue, particularly in the elderly.*

Home Care

• The above interventions may be adapted for home care use.

• Assess the client's history and current patterns of fatigue as they relate to the home environment and environmental and behavioral triggers of increased fatigue. **EBN and EB:** *Fatigue may be more pronounced in specific settings for physical, environmental (e.g., stairs required to reach bathroom, patterns of movement around home, cleaning activities that require high energy), or psychological (e.g., rooms associated with loss of loved ones) reasons (Sugahara et al, 2004; Gitlin et al, 2006).*

▲ Refer to occupational and/or physical therapy if substantial intervention is needed to assist the client in adapting to home and daily patterns. **EB:** *Interventions in the elderly led by occupational and physical therapists have been associated with less difficulty in ADLs and instrumental ADLs, which may lead to lower levels of fatigue (Gitlin et al, 2006).*

• For clients receiving chemotherapy, intervene to:
  ▪ Relieve symptom distress (negative mood, nausea, difficulty sleeping)
  ▪ Encourage as much physical activity as possible
  ▪ Support a positive attitude for the future

• = Independent   ▲ = Collaborative   **EBN** = Evidence-Based Nursing   **EB** = Evidence-Based

- Support adequate recovery time between treatments

The above factors have been identified as associated with fatigue, particularly during early stages of chemotherapy (NCCN, 2009).

- Teach the client and family the importance of and methods for setting priorities for activities, especially those with high energy demand (e.g., home or family events). Instruct in realistic expectations and behavioral pacing. **EBN:** *The client and/or family may assume a more rapid rate of energy recovery than actually occurs. Assistance may be needed to ensure accuracy of expectations for the client. Unrealistic expectations provoke guilt feelings in the client, leading to efforts that can exceed the client's energy capacity (Patusky, 2002). Prioritization of activities can be effective in restoring energy (Goedendorp et al, 2009).*

- Assess effect of fatigue on the client's relatedness; recognize that the client's fatigue affects the whole family. Initiate the following interventions:

  - Avoid dismissing reports of fatigue; validate the client's experience and foster hope for eventual treatment, if not resolution, of the fatigue.
  - Identify with the client ways in which he or she continues to be a valued part of his or her social environment.
  - Identify with the client ways in which he or she continues to participate in equitable exchange with others.
  - Encourage the client to maintain regular family routines (e.g., meals, sleep patterns) as much as possible.
  - Initiate cognitive restructuring to refute the client's guilt-producing and negative thought patterns.
  - Assess and intervene with family's and friends' contributions to guilt-inducing self-talk.
  - Work with the client to inoculate against the negative thinking of others.
  - Explore family life and demands to identify accommodations.
  - Support the client's efforts at limit setting on the demands of others.
  - Assist the client to move toward a state of parallelism by working to identify and relieve sources of physical or emotional discomfort. Degree of involvement, limited by fatigue, need not be changed.

Based on reports of fatigued women, the above interventions have been suggested as addressing problem areas. Parallelism is a state of comfortable noninvolvement and was described by some fatigued women as achievable and relatively positive state, given their fatigue (Patusky, 2002). Clients with fatigue may perceive a sense of disconnect with health care practitioners who do not recognize the impact of the symptom on client and family functioning (Larun & Malterud, 2007).

- ▲ Refer for family therapy in the event the client's fatigue interferes with normal family functioning. **EBN:** *Family therapy may be necessary to address underlying problems that may be magnified by the influence of fatigue (Patusky, 2002).*

- ▲ If fatigue has affected the client's ability to participate in relationships effectively, refer for psychiatric home health care services for client reassurance and implementation of therapeutic regimen. **EBN:** *Psychiatric home care nurses can address issues relating to the client's ability to adjust to changes in health status. Behavioral interventions in the home can help the client participate more effectively in the treatment plan (Patusky, 2002).*

Client/Family Teaching and Discharge Planning

- Help client to reframe cognitively; share information about fatigue and how to live with it, including need for positive self-talk. **EBN:** *Cognitive behavioral approaches to managing fatigue enhance the client's sense of control over the symptom (Given et al, 2001; Malouff et al, 2008; Price et al, 2008).*

- Teach strategies for energy conservation (e.g., sitting instead of standing during showering, storing items at waist level). **EB:** *Energy conservation strategies can decrease the amount of energy used (Vanage, Gilbertson, & Mathiowetz, 2003; Goedendorp et al, 2009).*

- Teach the client to carry a pocket calendar, make lists of required activities, and post reminders around the house. **EBN:** *Fatigue is often associated with memory loss and sometimes difficulty thinking. Fatigue can also result in the inability to direct attention to a certain task, such as cooking or paying bills (i.e., attentional fatigue) (Cimprich & Ronis, 2003).*

• = Independent ▲ = Collaborative **EBN** = Evidence-Based Nursing **EB** = Evidence-Based

- Teach the importance of following a healthy lifestyle with adequate nutrition, fluids, and rest; pain relief; insomnia correction; and appropriate exercise to decrease fatigue (i.e., energy restoration).
- See **Hopelessness** care plan if appropriate. **EB:** *Depression is correlated with increased fatigue (Phillips et al, 2004).*

ⓔvolve   See the EVOLVE website for Weblinks for client education resources.

REFERENCES

Barsevick A, Dudley W, Beck S et al: A randomized clinical trial of energy conservation for patients with cancer-related fatigue, *Cancer* 100(6):1302, 2004.

Busch A, Schachter CL, Peloso PM et al: Exercise for treating fibromyalgia syndrome, *Cochrane Database Syst Rev* (3):CD003786, 2002.

Carpenter J, Elan J, Ridner S et al: Sleep, fatigue, and depressive symptoms in breast cancer survivors and matched healthy women experiencing hot flashes, *Oncol Nurs Forum* 31(3):591, 2004.

Cimprich B, Ronis D: An environmental intervention to restore attention in women with newly diagnosed breast cancer, *Cancer Nurs* 26(4):284, 2003.

Cleeland CS, Mendoza TR, Wang XS et al: Assessing symptom distress in cancer patients: the MD Anderson Symptom Inventory, *Cancer* 89(7):1634, 2000.

Conn V, Hafdahl A, Porock D et al: A meta-analysis of exercise interventions among people treated for cancer, *Support Care Cancer* 14(7):699–712, 2006.

Craig T, Kakumanu S: Chronic fatigue syndrome: evaluation and treatment, *Am Fam Physician* 65(5):1083, 2002.

Dinos S, Khoshaba B, Ashby D et al: A systematic review of chronic fatigue, its syndromes and ethnicity: prevalence, severity, co-morbidity and coping, *Int J Epidemiol* 2009, Epub ahead of print.

Flensner G, Lindencrona C: The cooling-suit: case studies of its influence on fatigue among eight individuals with multiple sclerosis, *J Adv Nurs* 37(6):541, 2002.

Forlenza MJ, Hall P, Lichtenstein P et al: Epidemiology of cancer-related fatigue in the Swedish twin registry, *Cancer* 104(9):2022–2031, 2005.

Friedberg F, Leung DW, Quick J: Do support groups help people with chronic fatigue syndrome and fibromyalgia? *J Rheumatol* 32(12):2416–2420, 2005.

Gary RA, Sueta CA, Dougherty M et al: Home-based exercise improves functional performance and quality of life in women with diastolic heart failure, *Heart Lung* 33(4):210–218, 2004.

Gitlin L, Winter L, Dennis M et al: A randomized trial of a multicomponent home intervention to reduce functional difficulties in older adults, *J Am Geriatr Soc* 54:809–816, 2006.

Given C, Given B, Azzouz F et al: Predictors of pain and fatigue in the year following diagnosis among elderly cancer patients, *J Pain Symptom Manage* 21(6):456, 2001.

Given B, Given CW, McCorkle R et al: Pain and fatigue management: Results of a nursing randomized clinical trial, *Oncol Nurs Forum* 29(6):949–956, 2002.

Goedendorp MM, Gielissen MF, Verhagen CA et al: Psychosocial interventions for reducing fatigue during cancer treatment in adults, *Cochrane Database Syst Rev,* (1): CD006953, 2009.

Jacobsen PB, Donovan KA, Vadaparampli ST et al: Systematic review and meta-analysis of psychological and activity-based interventions for cancer related fatigue, *Health Psychol* 26(6):660–667, 2007.

Kangas M, Bovbjerg DH, Montgomery GH: Cancer-related fatigue: a systematic and meta-analytic review of non-pharmacological therapies for cancer patients, *Psychol Bull* 134(5):700–741, 2008.

Larun L, Malterud K: Identity and coping experiences in Chronic Fatigue Syndrome: a synthesis of qualitative studies, *Patient Educ Couns* 69(1–3):20–28, 2007.

Malouff JM, Thorsteinsson EB, Rooke SE et al: Efficacy of cognitive behavioral therapy for chronic fatigue syndrome: a meta-analysis, *Clin Psychol Rev* 28(5):736–745, 2008.

Mathiowetz V, Finlayson M, Matuska K et al: Randomized controlled trial of an energy conservation course for persons with multiple sclerosis, *Mult Scler* 11(5):592–601, 2005.

Minton O, Richardson A, Sharpe M et al: A systematic review and meta-analysis of the pharmacological treatment of cancer-related fatigue, *J Natl Cancer Inst* 100(16): 1155–1166, 2008.

Mock V, Frangakis C, Davidson NE et al: Exercise manages fatigue during breast cancer treatment: a randomized controlled trial, *Psychooncology* 14(6):464–477, 2005.

Motl RW, Gosney JL: Effect of exercise training on quality of life in multiple sclerosis: a met-analysis, *Mult Scler* 14(1):129–135, 2008.

National Comprehensive Cancer Network. *Cancer related fatigue, v.1.* Author: 2009.

Neill J, Belan I, Ried K: Effectiveness of non-pharmacological interventions for fatigue in adults with multiple sclerosis, rheumatoid arthritis, or systemic lupus erythematosus: a systematic review, *J Adv Nurs,* 56(6): 617–635, 2006.

Papakostas GI, Nutt DJ, Hallett LA et al: Resolution of sleepiness and fatigue in major depressive disorder: A comparison of bupropion and the selective serotonin reuptake Inhibitors, *Biol Psychiatry* 60(12):1350–1355, 2006.

Patusky KL: Relatedness theory as a framework for the treatment of fatigued women, *Arch Psychiatr Nurs* 5:224, 2002.

Phillips K, Sowell R, Rojas M et al: Physiological and psychological correlates of fatigue in HIV disease, *Biol Res Nurs* 6(1):59, 2004.

Pigeon W, Sateia M, Ferguson R: Distinguishing between excessive daytime sleepiness and fatigue: toward improved detection and treatment, *J Psychosom Res* 54(1):61, 2003.

Price JR, Mitchell E, Tidy E et al: Cognitive behavior therapy for chronic fatigue syndrome in adults, *Cochrane Database Syst Rev* 16(3), 2008.

Pucci E, Branas P, D'Amico R et al: Amantadine for fatigue in multiple sclerosis, *Cochrane Database Syst Rev* (1), 2007.

Puetz TW, Beasman KM, O'Connor PJ: The effect of cardiac rehabilitation exercise programs on feelings of energy and fatigue: a meta-analysis of research from 1945 to 2005, *Eur J Cardiovasc Prev Rehabil* 13(6):886–893, 2006.

Ranjith G: Epidemiology of chronic fatigue syndrome, *Occup Med* 55(1):13–19, 2005.

Schumacher A, Wewers D, Heinecke A et al: Fatigue as an important aspect of quality of life in patients with acute myeloid leukemia, *Leuk Res* 26(4):355, 2002.

Schwartz A, Meek P: Additional construct validity of the Schwartz Cancer Fatigue Scale, *J Nurs Meas* 7(1):35, 1999.

Seigel K, Brown-Bradley C, Lekas H: Strategies for coping with fatigue among HIV-positive individuals fifty years and older, *AIDS Patient Care* 18(5):275, 2004.

Simoneau M, Begin F, Teasdale N: The effects of moderate fatigue on dynamic balance control and attentional demands, *J Neuroeng Rehabil* 3:22, 2006.

Sugahara H, Adamine M, Kondo T et al: Somatic symptoms most often associated with depression in an urban hospital medical setting in Japan, *Psychiatry Res* 128(3):305–311, 2004.

● = Independent   ▲ = Collaborative   **EBN** = Evidence-Based Nursing   **EB** = Evidence-Based

Vanage S, Gilbertson K, Mathiowetz V: Effects of an energy conservation course on fatigue impact for persons with progressive multiple sclerosis, *Am J Occup Ther* 57(3):315, 2003.

Whitehead L: The measurement of fatigue in chronic illness: a systematic review of unidimensional and multidimensional fatigue measures, *J Pain Symptom Manage* 37(1):107–28, 2009.

Fear   *Ruth McCaffrey, DNP, ARNP*   ⊖volve

NANDA-I

Definition

Response to perceived threat that is consciously recognized as a danger

Defining Characteristics

Report of alarm; apprehension; being scared; increased tension; decreased self-assurance; dread; excitement; jitteriness; panic; terror

Cognitive

Diminished productivity; learning ability; problem-solving ability; identifies object of fear; stimulus believed to be a threat

Behaviors

Attack or avoidance behaviors; impulsiveness; increased alertness; narrowed focus on the source of fear

Physiological

Anorexia; diarrhea; dry mouth; dyspnea; fatigue; increased perspiration, pulse, respiratory rate, systolic blood pressure; muscle tightness; nausea; pallor; pupil dilation; vomiting

Related Factors (r/t)

Innate origin (e.g., sudden noise, height, pain, loss of physical support); innate releasers (neurotransmitters); language barrier; learned response (e.g., conditioning, modeling from or identification with others); phobic stimulus; sensory impairment; separation from support system in potentially stressful situation (e.g., hospitalization, hospital procedures); unfamiliarity with environmental experience(s)

NOC   (Nursing Outcomes Classification)

Suggested NOC Outcome

Fear Self-Control

Example NOC Outcome with Indicators
Fear Self-Control as evidenced by the following indicators: Eliminates precursors of fear/Seeks information to reduce fear/Plans coping strategies for fearful situations (Rate the outcome and indicators of **Fear Self-Control:** 1 = never demonstrated, 2 = rarely demonstrated, 3 = sometimes demonstrated, 4 = often demonstrated, 5 = consistently demonstrated [see Section I].)

Client Outcomes

Client Will (Specify Time Frame):

- Verbalize known fears
- State accurate information about the situation
- Identify, verbalize, and demonstrate those coping behaviors that reduce own fear
- Report and demonstrate reduced fear

 • = Independent   ▲ = Collaborative   **EBN** = Evidence-Based Nursing   **EB** = Evidence-Based

NIC (Nursing Interventions Classification)

Suggested NIC Interventions

Anxiety Reduction, Coping Enhancement, Security Enhancement

Example NIC Activities—Anxiety Reduction
Use a calm, reassuring approach; Stay with the patient to promote safety and reduce fear

Nursing Interventions and *Rationales*

- Assess source of fear with the client. **EB:** *The capacity to experience fear is adaptive, enabling rapid and energetic response to imminent threat or danger (Stephanos & Edwards, 2009).*
- Assess for a history of anxiety. **EB:** *Participants in a study of older adults who had anxiety were found to have a higher level of fear of pain (Asmundson et al, 2009).*
- Have the client draw the object of his or her fear. **EBN:** *Drawing can be used as an assessment tool to better understand the experience of the client to facilitate better nursing and professional practice in valuing the experience of others (Osborn, 2007).*
- Discuss the situation with the client and help distinguish between real and imagined threats to well-being. **EB:** *Fear activation occurs before conscious cognitive analysis of the stimulus can occur (Stephanos & Edwards, 2009).*
- Encourage the client to explore underlying feelings that may be contributing to the fear. *Exploring underlying feelings may help the client confront unresolved conflicts and develop coping abilities (Bowman et al, 2009).*
- Stay with clients when they express fear; provide verbal and nonverbal (touch and hug with permission and if culturally acceptable) reassurances of safety if safety is within control. **EBN:** *Healing touch may reduce stress, anxiety, and pain and provide a greater sense of well-being (Marville, Bowen, & Benham, 2008).*
- Explore coping skills previously used by the client to deal with fear; reinforce these skills and explore other outlets. **EBN:** *Recounting previous experiences that were perceived by the client as having been dealt with successfully strengthens effective coping and helps eliminate ineffective coping mechanisms (Olsson et al, 2005).*
- Provide backrubs and massage for clients to decrease anxiety. **EB:** *Massage is effective in reducing distress and pain (Currin & Meister, 2008).*
- Use TT and HT techniques. **EBN:** *Nurses may offer TT, quiet time, or quiet, relaxing music or dialogue when feelings of calmness and relaxation are desired (Marville, Bowen, & Benham, 2008).*
- ▲ Refer for cognitive behavior therapy. **EB:** *The use of cognitive behavioral therapy reduced anxiety, worry, and fear among a group of older adults during and after acute care hospitalization (Stanley et al, 2009). Exposure-based cognitive behavioral therapy was successful at reducing fear and symptoms of PTSD in trauma clients (Bryant et al, 2008).*
- ▲ Animal-assisted therapy can be incorporated into the care of perioperative clients. **EB:** *Animal visitation reduced fear in hospitalized children (Sabo, Eng, & Kassity-Kritch, 2006). Pet therapy reduced fear and aggressive behaviors in 144 cognitively impaired older adults (Colombo et al, 2006).*
- Encourage clients to express their fears in narrative form. **EB:** *One of the main ways in which people adjust to threats associated with serious illness is through the use of narrative, which helps make sense of illness (Heliker, 2007).*
- Refer to care plans for **Anxiety** and **Death Anxiety**.

 Pediatric

- Use draw-and-tell conversations with children about fear. **EB:** *The draw-and-tell conversation as a child-centered and child-directed approach to data collection provides new insight into how children describe and experience fear (Driessnack, 2006).*
- Explore coping skills previously used by the client to deal with fear. *Children generally rate their coping behaviors as helpful. A variety of coping behaviors reported were seeking support from parents, avoidance, distraction, trying to sleep, and clinging to stuffed animals (Justus et al, 2006).*

● = Independent ▲ = Collaborative **EBN** = Evidence-Based Nursing **EB** = Evidence-Based

- Teach parents to use cognitive-behavioral strategies such as positive coping statements ("I am a brave girl [boy]. I can take care of myself in the dark.") and rewards of bravery tokens for appropriate behavior. *Cognitive behavioral therapy undertaking by parents decreased separation anxiety, social phobia, and fear in children at the time of the intervention and throughout a 1–year follow-up period (Kendall et al, 2008).*
- Screen for depression in clients who report social or school fears (Roy-Byrne et al, 2005).
- Teach relaxation techniques to children to induce calmness. **EB:** *Relaxation training may reduce somatic or psychological symptoms and support children's ability to cope with emotional reactions (Williams et al, 2006).*

Geriatric

- Establish a trusting relationship so that all fears can be identified. *An elderly client's response to a real fear may be immobilizing. In a study of community-dwelling elders, a group of nurses from a faith community were able to significantly reduce anxiety and fear (Rydholm et al, 2008).*
- Monitor for dementia and use appropriate interventions. *Fear may be an early indicator of disorientation or impaired reality testing in elderly clients (Colombo et al, 2006).*
- Provide a protective and safe environment, use consistent caregivers, and maintain the accustomed environmental structure. *Elderly clients tend to have more perceptual impairments and adapt to changes with more difficulty than younger clients, especially during an illness (Colombo et al, 2006).*
- Observe for untoward changes if antianxiety drugs are taken. *Advancing age renders clients more sensitive to both the clinical and toxic effects of many agents (Singh, 2009).*
- Assess for fear of falls in hospitalized clients with hip fractures to determine risk of poor health outcomes. **EBN:** *Fear of falls correlated with poor health outcomes and has a major impact on function, especially with regard to walking (Lee, MacKenzie, & James, 2008).*
- Encourage exercises to improve physical skills and levels of mobility to decrease fear of falling. *Improving physical skills and levels of mobility counteracts excessive fear during activity performance (Singh, 2009).*
- Assist the client in identifying and reducing risk factors of falls, including environmental hazards in and out of the home, the importance of good nutrition and activity, proper footwear, and how to stand up after a fall. **EB:** *Clients receiving education focused on identifying and reducing risk factors for falls were found to have a significant reduction in their fear of falling (Singh, 2009).*

Multicultural

- Assess for the presence of culture-bound anxiety and fear states. **EBN:** *The context in which anxiety and fear is experienced, its meaning, and responses to it are culturally mediated (Emery, 2006).*
- Assess for the influence of cultural beliefs, norms, and values on the client's perspective of a stressful situation. **EBN:** *What the client considers stressful may be based on cultural perceptions (Nadel & Muir, 2008).*
- Identify what triggers fear response. **EBN:** *Arab Muslim clients may express a high correlation between fear and pain (Hammoud, White, & Fetters, 2005).*
- Identify how the client expresses fear. **EBN:** *Research indicates that the expression of fear may be culturally mediated (Connor & Zhang, 2006).*
- Validate the client's feelings regarding fear. **EBN:** *Validation is a therapeutic communication technique that lets the client know that the nurse has heard and understands what was said, and it promotes the nurse-client relationship (de Hoog, Stroebe, & de Wit, 2007).*
- Assess for fears of racism in culturally diverse clients. **EB:** *Findings suggest that, independent of the effects of gender, age, and household social class, being worried about being a victim of racial harassment could have an important impact on an individual's health experience (Buchanan & Fitzgerald, 2008).*

Home Care

- The previous interventions may be adapted for home care use.
- Assess to differentiate the presence of fear versus anxiety.

● = Independent   ▲ = Collaborative   **EBN** = Evidence-Based Nursing   **EB** = Evidence-Based

- Refer to care plan for **Anxiety**.
- During initial assessment, determine whether current or previous episodes of fear relate to the home environment (e.g., perception of danger in the home or neighborhood or of relationships that have a history in the home). *Fear and anxiety are predictors of depression. When depression is assessed, a thorough discussion about fears and anxiety are warranted (Warner, Wickramaratne & Weissman, 2008).*
- Identify with the client what steps may be taken to make the home a "safe" place to be. *Identifying a given area as a safe place reduces fear and anxiety when the client is in that area.*
- ▲ Encourage the client to seek or continue appropriate counseling to reduce fear associated with stress or resolve alterations in irrational thought processes. *Correcting mistaken beliefs reduces anxiety.*
- ▲ Encourage the client to have a trusted companion, family member, or caregiver present in the home for periods when fear is most prominent. Pending other medical diagnoses, a referral to homemaker or home health aide services may meet this need. *Creating periods when fear and anxiety can be reduced allows the client periods of rest and supports positive coping.*
- ▲ Offer to sit quietly with a terminally ill client as needed by the client or family, or provide hospice volunteers to do the same. **EB:** *Terminally ill clients and their families often fear the dying process. The presence of a nurse or volunteer lets clients know they are not alone (McKee, Kelley & Guirguis-Younger, 2007).*

Client/Family Teaching and Discharge Planning

- Teach the client the difference between warranted and excessive fear. *Different interventions are indicated for rational and irrational fears.*
- Teach clients to use guided imagery when they are fearful; have them use all senses to visualize a place that is "comfortable and safe" for them. *Imagery makes use of subjective symbolism bypassing the rational mind and making the areas "safe" that the client may otherwise be reluctant to face (Bowman et al, 2009).*
- Teach use of appropriate community resources in emergency situations (e.g., hotlines, emergency departments, law enforcement, judicial systems). *Serious emergencies need immediate assistance to ensure the client's safety.*
- Encourage use of appropriate community resources in nonemergency situations (e.g., family, friends, neighbors, self-help and support groups, volunteer agencies, churches, recreation clubs and centers, seniors, youths, others with similar interests).
- If fear is associated with bioterrorism, provide accurate information and ensure that health care personnel have appropriate training and preparation. *Clear, consistent, accessible, reliable, and redundant information (received from trusted sources) will diminish public uncertainty about the cause of symptoms that might otherwise prompt persons to seek unnecessary treatment. Training for providers is essential.*

⊖volve   See the EVOLVE website for Weblinks for client education resources.

REFERENCES

Asmundson G, Hadjistavropoulos T, Bernstein A et al: Anxiety and illness behaviors. *Eur J Pain* 13(4):419–425, 2009.

Bowman K, Rose J, Radziewicz R et al: Family caregiver engagement in a coping and communication support intervention tailored to advanced cancer patients and families, *Cancer Nurs* 32(1):73–81, 2009.

Bryant R, Mastrodomenico M, Felmingham K et al: Treatment for acute stress disorder: a randomized controlled trial, *Arch Gen Psychiatr* 65(6):659–667, 2008.

Buchanan N, Fitzgerald L: Effects of racial and sexual harassment on work and the psychological well-being of African American women, *J Occup Health Psychol* 13(2):137–151, 2008.

Colombo G, Buono K, Raviola R et al: Pet therapy and institutionalized elderly: a study of 144 cognitively unimpaired subjects, *Arch Gerontol Geriatr* 42(2):207–216, 2006.

Connor K, Zhang W: Resilience: determinants, measurements, and treatment responsiveness, *Int J Neuropsychiatr Med* 11(10) Suppl 12:5–12, 2006.

Currin J, Meister E: A hospital-based intervention using massage to reduce distress among oncology patients, *Cancer Nurs* 31(3):214–221, 2008.

de Hoog N, Stroebe W, de Wit J: The impact of vulnerability to and severity of a health risk on processing and acceptance of fear-arousing communications: a meta analysis, *Rev Gen Psychol* 11(3):258–285, 2007.

Driessnack M: Draw and tell conversations with children about fear, *Qual Health Res* 16(10):1414–1435, 2006.

Emery P: Building a new culture of aging: revolutionizing long-term care, *J Christ Nurs* 23(1):16–24, 2006.

● = Independent   ▲ = Collaborative   **EBN** = Evidence-Based Nursing   **EB** = Evidence-Based

Hammoud M, White C, Fetters M: Opening cultural doors: providing culturally sensitive healthcare to Arab American and American Muslim patients, *Am J Obstet Gynecol* 193(4):1307–1311, 2005.

Heliker D: Story sharing: restoring the reciprocity of caring in long-term care, *J Psychosoc Nurs Ment Health Serv* 45(7):20–23, 2007.

Justus R, Wyles D, Wilson J et al: Preparing children and families for surgery: Mount Sinai's multidisciplinary perspective, *Pediatr Nurs* 32(1):35–43, 2006.

Kendall P, Hudson J, Gosch E et al: Cognitive-behavioral therapy for anxiety disordered youth: a randomized clinical trial evaluating child and family modalities, *J Consult Clin Psychol* 76(2):282–297, 2008.

Lee F, Mackenzie L, James C: Perceptions of older people living in the community about their fear of falling, *Disabil Rehabil* 30(23):1803–18011, 2008.

Marville J, Bowen J, Benham G: Effect of healing touch on stress perception and biological correlates, *Holist Nurs Pract* 22(2):103–110, 2008.

McKee M, Kelley ML, Guirguis-Younger M: So no one dies alone: a study of hospice volunteering with rural seniors, *J Palliat Care* 23(3):163–172, 2007.

Nadel J, Muir D: *Emotional development*, London, 2008, Oxford University.

Olsson A, Elbert J, Banaji M et al: The role of social groups in the persistence of learned fear, *Science* (5735):785–787, 2005.

Osborn K: Children deal with fear using art therapy. 2007. www.ptcweb.org/pdfs/ArtTherapy.pdf. Accessed May 12, 2009.

Roy-Byrne P, Craske M, Stein M et al: A randomized effectiveness trial for cognitive-behavioral therapy and medication for primary care panic disorder, *Arch Gen Psychiatr* 62(3):290–298, 2005.

Rydholm L, Moone R, Thornquis L et al: Care of community-dwelling older adults by faith community nurses, *J Gerontol Nurs* 34(4):18–29, 2008.

Sabo E, Eng B, Kassity-Kritch N: Canine visitation (pet) therapy, *J Holist Nurs* 24(1):51–57, 2006.

Singh J: Informing practice: polypharmacy in older adults is increasing, *Am J Nurs* 109(4):72–75, 2009.

Stanley M, Wilson M, Novy D et al: Cognitive behavior therapy for generalized anxiety disorder among older adults in primary care: a randomized clinical trial, *JAMA* 301(14):1460–1467, 2009.

Stephanos P, Edwards W: Adaptive and maladaptive self-focus: a pilot extension study with individuals high and low in fear of negative evaluation, *Behav Ther* 40(2):181–189, 2009.

Warner V, Wickramaratne P, Weissman M: The role of fear and anxiety in the familial risk for major depression: a three-generation study, *Psychol Med* 38(11):1543–1556, 2008.

Williams P, Schmideskamp J, Ridder L et al: Symptom monitoring and dependent care during cancer treatment in children: pilot study, *Cancer Nurs* 29(3):188–197, 2006.

Ineffective infant Feeding pattern   *Teresa Ferguson, MSN, RN*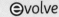

NANDA-I

Definition

Impaired ability of an infant to suck or coordinate the suck/swallow response resulting in inadequate oral nutrition for metabolic needs

Defining Characteristics

Inability to coordinate sucking, swallowing, and breathing; inability to initiate an effective suck; inability to sustain an effective suck

Related Factors (r/t)

Anatomic abnormality; neurological delay; neurological impairment; oral hypersensitivity; prematurity; prolonged NPO status

NOC   (Nursing Outcomes Classification)

Suggested NOC Outcomes

Breastfeeding Establishment: Infant, Maternal, Breastfeeding: Maintenance, Hydration, Nutritional Status: Food and Fluid Intake

Example **NOC Outcome with Indicators**
Breastfeeding Establishment: Infant as evidenced by the following indicators: Proper alignment and latch-on/Correct suck and tongue placement/Urinations per day appropriate for age/Weight gain appropriate for age (Rate the outcome and indicators of **Breastfeeding Establishment: Infant:** 1 = not adequate, 2 = slightly adequate, 3 = moderately adequate, 4 = substantially adequate, 5 = totally adequate [see Section I].)

Client Outcomes

Infant Will (Specify Time Frame):

● Consume adequate calories that will result in appropriate weight gain and optimal growth and development

● = Independent   ▲ = Collaborative   **EBN** = Evidence-Based Nursing   **EB** = Evidence-Based

- Have opportunities for skin-to-skin (kangaroo care) experiences
- Have opportunities for "trophic" (i.e., small volume of breastmilk/formula) enteral feedings prior to full oral feedings
- Progress to stable, neurobehavioral organization (i.e., motor, state, self-regulation, attention-interaction)
- Demonstrate presence of mature oral reflexes that are necessary for safe feeding
- Progress to safe, self-regulated oral feedings
- Coordinate the suck-swallow-breathe sequence while nippling
- Display clear behavioral cues related to hunger and satiety
- Display approach/engagement cues, with minimal avoidance/disengagement cues
- Have opportunities to pace own feeding, taking breaks as needed
- Display evidence of being in the "quiet-alert" state while nippling
- Progress to and engage in mutually positive parent/caregiver-infant/child interactions during feedings

Parent/Family Will (Specify Time Frame):

- Recognize necessity of adequate calories for appropriate weight gain and optimal growth and development
- Learn to read and respond contingently to infant's behavioral cues (e.g., hunger, satiety, approach/engagement, stress/avoidance/disengagement)
- Learn strategies that promote organized infant behavior
- Learn appropriate positioning and handling techniques
- Learn effective ways to relieve stress behaviors during nippling
- Learn ways to help infant coordinate suck-swallow-breathe sequence (i.e., external pacing techniques)
- Engage in mutually positive interactions with infant during feeding
- Recognize ways to facilitate effective feedings: feed in quiet-alert state; keep length of feeding appropriate; burp; prepare/structure environment; recognize signs of sensory overload; encourage self-regulation; respect need for breaks and breathing pauses; avoid pulling and twisting nipple during pauses; allow infant to resume sucking when ready; provide oral support (cheek and/or jaw) as needed; use appropriate nipple hole size and flow rate

 (Nursing Interventions Classification)

Suggested NIC Interventions

Bottle Feeding, Breastfeeding Assistance, Fluid Monitoring, Kangaroo Care, Lactation Counseling, Teaching: Infant Safety

Example NIC Activities—Lactation Counseling
Provide information about advantages and disadvantages of breastfeeding; Discuss alternative methods of feeding

Nursing Interventions and *Rationales*

- Refer to care plans for **Disorganized Infant behavior, Risk for disorganized Infant behavior,** and **Effective, Ineffective,** and **Interrupted Breastfeeding** and assess as needed.
- Interventions follow a sequential pattern of implementation that can be adapted as appropriate.
- Assess coordination of infant's suck, swallow, and gag reflex. *Infants are at increased risk for aspiration with a poor gag, suck, and/or swallow reflex (Ladewig, London, & Davidson, 2010).*
- ▲ Provide developmentally supportive neonatal intensive care for preterm infants. **EBN:** *Parents are more confident in providing care for their infant with assistance from the nursing staff (Cleveland, 2008).*
- Provide opportunities for kangaroo (i.e., skin-to-skin) care. *Very early skin-to-skin contact enhanced breastfeeding success during the early postpartum period. No significant differences were found at 1 month (Moore & Anderson, 2007).*
- ▲ Before the infant is ready for oral feedings, implement gavage feedings (or other alternative) as ordered, using breast milk whenever possible. *Gavage feeding is the method used to feed preterm*

• = Independent ▲ = Collaborative **EBN** = Evidence-Based Nursing **EB** = Evidence-Based

infants or infants with inadequate suck/swallow during feeding (Ladewig, London, & Davidson, 2010).

- Provide a naturalistic environment for tube feedings (naso-oro-gastric, gavage, or other) that approximates a pleasurable oral feeding experience: hold in semi-upright/flexed position; offer NNS; pace feedings; allow for semi-demand feedings contingent with infant cues; offer rest breaks; burp, as appropriate. *Nonnutritive sucking during gavage feeding is comforting for the infant and stimulates the suck reflex (Ladewig, London, & Davidson, 2010).*
- Consider trophic (i.e., small volume) feedings for high-risk hospitalized infants if appropriate. *Trophic feeding decrease the development of complications associated with parenteral feeding (Ladewig, London, & Davidson, 2010).*
- Allow parent(s) to feed the infant when possible. *Parent involvement in feeding promotes bonding and promotes positive coping behaviors (Ladewig, London, & Davidson, 2010).*
- Position preterm infant in semi-upright position, with head in neutral alignment, chin slightly tucked, back straight, shoulders/arms forward, hands in midline, hips flexed 90 degrees. **EBN:** *Inappropriate positioning during feeding can lead to apnea and bradycardia (Walker, 2008).*
- Feed infant in the quiet-alert state. **EBN:** *The infant feeding in a quiet alert state is more successful at latching and breastfeeding (Shannon, O'Donnell, & Skinner, 2007).*
- Determine the appropriate shape, size, and hole of nipple to provide flow rate for preterm infants. **EBN:** *Premature infants using single-hole nipples for feeding had an increased milk intake and less respiratory difficulties with feeding (Chang et al, 2007).*
- Implement pacing for infants having difficulty coordinating breathing with sucking and swallowing. *Paced feedings decreases risk of fatigue and oxygen desaturation of the infant (Walker, 2008).*
- Provide infants with jaw and/or cheek support, as needed. *Jaw or cheek support during breastfeeding may enhance the infant's ability to latch onto breast for feeding (Walker, 2008).*
- Allow appropriate time for nipple feeding to ensure infant's safety, limiting to 15 to 20 minutes for bottle feeding. *Limiting feeding time decreases the expenditure of energy used during the feeding (Ladewig, London, & Davidson, 2010).*
- Monitor length of breastfeeding so that it does not exceed 30 minutes. **EBN:** *Limiting breastfeeding time will decrease infant fatigue (Shannon, O'Donnell, & Skinner, 2007).*
- Encourage transitioning from scheduled to semi-demand feedings, contingent with infant behavior cues. *Flexible feeding schedules allow infants to feed during awake and alert periods (Ladewig, London, & Davidson, 2010).*
- ▲ Refer to a multidisciplinary team (e.g., neonatal/pediatric nutritionist, physical or occupational therapist, speech pathologist, lactation specialist) as needed. **EB:** *Parents will need referrals from the primary care provider to meet the multiple needs of their premature infants after discharge (Vanderbilt, Wang, & Parker, 2007).*

Home Care

- The above appropriate interventions may be adapted for home care use.
- ▲ Infants with risk factors and clinical indicators of feeding problems present prior to hospital discharge should be referred to appropriate community early-intervention service providers (e.g., community health nurses, Early-On, occupational therapy, speech pathologists, feeding specialists) to facilitate adequate weight gain for optimal growth and development. *Late preterm infants are at greater risk for readmission when being breastfed (Tomashek et al, 2006). Late preterm infants are susceptible to multiple complications including feeding and sucking problems (Walker, 2008).*

Client/Family Teaching and Discharge Planning

- Provide anticipatory guidance for infant's expected feeding course. *Health care providers need to educate mothers using evidence-based infant feeding practices in order for mothers to make informed decisions on how to feed their infants (Lawson, 2007).*
- Teach various effective feeding methods and strategies to parent(s). *Health care providers need to educate parents using evidence-based infant feeding practices in order for parents to make informed decisions on how to feed their infants (Lawson, 2007).*

● = Independent   ▲ = Collaborative   **EBN** = Evidence-Based Nursing   **EB** = Evidence-Based

- Teach parents how to read, interpret, and respond contingently to infant cues. *Parents ability to recognize and react quickly and consistently to their infant's state or cues leads to parental confidence in providing care (Tedder, 2008).*
- Help parents identify support systems prior to hospital discharge. *This should include immediate and extended family members and friends; if necessary, include these persons in family teaching sessions (Griffin & Abraham, 2006).*
- Provide anticipatory guidance for the infant's discharge. *Health care providers need to educate mothers using evidence-based infant feeding practices in order for mothers to make informed decisions on how to feed their infants (Lawson, 2007).*

 See the EVOLVE website for Weblinks for client education resources.

REFERENCES

Chang YJ, Lin CP, Lin YJ et al: Effects of single-hole and cross-cut nipple units on feeding efficiency and physiological parameters in premature infants, *J Nurs Res* 15(3):215–222, 2007.

Cleveland LM: Parenting in the neonatal intensive care unit, *J Obstet Gynecol Neonatal Nurs* 37(6):666–691, 2008.

Griffin T, Abraham M: Transition to home from the newborn intensive care unit: applying the principles of family-centered care in the discharge process, *J Perinatal Neonatal Nurs* 20(3):243–249, 2006.

Ladewig PW, London ML, Davidson MR: Contemporary maternal-newborn nursing care, ed 7, Upper Saddle River NJ, 2010, Pearson Education Inc.

Lawson M: Contemporary aspects of infant feeding, *Paediatr Nurs* 19(2):39–45, 2007.

Moore ER, Anderson GC: Randomized controlled trial of very early mother-infant skin-to-skin contact and breastfeeding status, *J Midwifery Womens Health* 52(2):116–125, 2007.

Shannon T, O'Donnell MJ, Skinner K: Breastfeeding in the 21st century: overcoming barriers to help women and infants, *Nurs Womens Health* 11(6):568–575, 2007.

Tedder JL: Give them the HUG: an innovative approach to helping parents understand the language of their newborn, *J Perinatal Educ* 17(2):14–20, 2008.

Tomashek KM, Shapiro-Mendoza CK, Weiss J et al: Early discharge among late preterm and term newborns and risk of neonatal morbidity, *Semin Perinatol* 30:61–68, 2006.

Vanderbilt D, Wang CJ, Parker S: The do's in preemie neurodevelopment, *Contemp Pediatr* 24(9):84–92, 2007.

Walker M: Breastfeeding the late preterm infant, *J Obstet Gynecol Neonatal Nurs* 37:692–701, 2008.

Readiness for enhanced Fluid balance   *Betty J. Ackley, MSN, EdS, RN*

NANDA-I

Definition

A pattern of equilibrium between fluid volume and chemical composition of body fluids that is sufficient for meeting physical needs and can be strengthened

Defining Characteristics

Dehydration; expresses willingness to enhance fluid balance; good tissue turgor; intake adequate for daily needs; moist mucous membranes; no evidence of edema; no excessive thirst; specific gravity within normal limits; stable weight; straw-colored urine; urine output appropriate for intake

NOC   (Nursing Outcomes Classification)

Suggested NOC Labels

Fluid Balance, Electrolyte and Acid-Base Balance, Hydration

Example NOC Outcome with Indicators
Maintains **Fluid Balance** as evidenced by the following indicators: BP/Peripheral pulses palpable/Skin turgor/Moist mucous membranes/Serum electrolytes/Hematocrit/Body weight stable/24–hour intake and output balanced/Urine specific gravity (Rate each indicator of **Fluid Balance:** 1 = severely compromised, 2 = substantially compromised, 3 = moderately compromised, 4 = mildly compromised, 5 = not compromised [see Section I].)

• = Independent   ▲ = Collaborative   **EBN** = Evidence-Based Nursing   **EB** = Evidence-Based

Client Outcomes

Client Will (Specify Time Frame):

- Maintain light-yellow urine output
- Maintain elastic skin turgor, moist tongue, and mucous membranes
- Explain measure that can be taken to improve fluid intake

NIC   (Nursing Interventions Classification)

Suggested NIC Interventions

Fluid Management, Fluid Monitoring

Example NIC Activities—Fluid Management
Monitor hydration status as appropriate; Monitor food/fluid ingested and calculate daily caloric intake, as appropriate

Nursing Interventions and *Rationales*

- Discuss normal fluid requirements. *A guideline is 1 to 1.5 mL of fluid per each calorie needed, so an average intake would be between 2000 and 3000 mL/day, or at least 8 cups of fluid. The adequate intake recommendation is 3 L for the 19– to 30–year-old male and 2.2 L for the 19– to 30–year-old female. Water balance studies suggest that adult men require 2.5 L per day (Institute of Medicine, 2004).* **EB:** *Increased daily fluid intake by 1.5 L has no negative effect in healthy men aged 55 to 75 years. On average, intervention subjects increased daily intake by 1 L, with no significant changes in blood pressure, sodium level, glomerular filtration rate, or quality of life (Spigt et al, 2006).*
- Recommend the client choose mainly water to meet fluid needs, although fruit juices and milk are also useful for hydration. The intake of beverages containing caffeine or alcohol is no longer thought to cause dehydration. *While caffeinated drinks and alcohol can cause mild diuresis, intake of these beverages is not associated with dehydration, and these fluids do contribute to the body fluid needs (Institute of Medicine, 2004).*
- Recommend the client choose and prepare foods with less salt, aiming for a maximum of 1500 mg per day, less than a teaspoon. The CDC (2009) recommends that all salt-sensitive Americans, including everyone 40 years or older, should decrease daily sodium intake. *The amount of sodium in the body helps determine fluid balance, in addition to other factors.* **EB:** *A study found that decreased sodium intake helped lower blood pressure, as well as increase flexibility in blood vessels, improving the health of the blood vessels (CDC, 2009).*
- Recommend the client avoid intake of soft drinks with sugar; instead, encourage the client to drink water. *Most carbonated beverages and also flavored waters contain excessive amounts of sugar that is a source of empty calories, as well as a cause of significant damage to the teeth (ADA, 2009).*
- Recommend the client note the color of urine at intervals when voiding. Normal urine is straw-colored or amber. *Dark-colored urine reflects increased urine concentration, and fluid deficit (Scales & Pilsworth, 2008).* **EBN:** *Because it is correlated to urine specific gravity and urine osmolality, observing urine color is an effective and low-cost method of monitoring for possible dehydration and need for more water (Wakefield et al, 2002).*
- Recommend client monitor weight at intervals for alterations. *Decreases in weight may be caused by inadequate fluid intake, whereas increases in weight are often due to increased salt intake.*

 Geriatric

- Encourage the elderly client to develop a pattern of drinking water regularly. *Thirst sensation diminishes with aging: dehydration is common in the elderly (Mentes, 2004). Some geriatric clients limit fluid intake due to fear of incontinence, inability to drink on their own, altered sensorium/cognition, or decreased thirst as a part of the aging process. Due to the aging process causing a decrease in thirst, once a geriatric client experiences thirst, they may have a severe water deficit (Ferry, 2005).*
- Ensure that when food intake is reduced or limited, it is compensated with an increase in water/fluid intake. **EB:** *Food contains water, thus any reduction in food intake also involves a reduction in*

water intake. Anorexia increases the risk of dehydration—the geriatric client is frequently anorexic (Ferry, 2005).

- Incorporate regular hydration into daily routines, such as providing an extra glass of fluid with medication or during social activities. Consider using a beverage cart and a hydration assistant to routinely offer beverages to clients in extended care facilities. (Wotton, Crannitch & Munt, 2008). **EBN:** *A study demonstrated that institution of a beverage cart with a trained hydration assistant resulted in increased number of bowel movements, less use of laxatives, decreased number of falls, fewer urinary tract infections and respiratory infections, and less skin breakdown (Robinson & Rosher, 2002).*

⊖volve   See the Evolve website for Weblinks for client education resources.

REFERENCES

American Dental Association (ADA): *Oral health topics A-Z.* Available at www.ada.org/public/index.asp. Accessed on July 3, 2009.

Centers for Disease Control and Prevention (CDC): Application of lower sodium intake recommendations to adults—United States, 1999–2006. *MMWR Morb Mortal Wkly Rep*; 58(11):281–283, 2009.

Ferry M: Strategies for ensuring good hydration in the elderly, *Nutr Rev* 63(6 Part 2):S22–S29, 2005.

Institute of Medicine: *Applications of dietary reference intakes for electrolytes and water*, National Academy of Sciences, 2004, National Academies.

Mentes JC: *Hydration management*, Iowa City IA, 2004, University of Iowa Gerontological Nursing Interventions Research Center.

Robinson SB, Rosher RB: Can a beverage cart help improve hydration? *Geriatr Nurs* 23:4, 2002.

Scales K, Pilsworth J: The importance of fluid balance in clinical practice, *Nurs Standard* 22(47):50–57, 2008.

Spigt MG, Knottnerus JA, Westerterp KR et al: The effects of 6 months of increased water intake on blood sodium, glomerular filtration rate, blood pressure, and quality of life in elderly (aged 55–75) men, *J Am Geriatr Soc* 54(3):438–443, 2006.

Wakefield B, Mentes J, Diggelmann L et al: Monitoring hydration status in elderly veterans, *West J Nurs Res*, 24(2):132–142, 2002.

Wotton K Crannitch K, Munt R: Prevalence, risk factors and strategies to prevent dehydration in older adults, *Contemp Nurse* 31(1):44–56, 2008.

Deficient Fluid volume   *Betty J. Ackley, MSN, EdS, RN*   ⊖volve

NANDA-I

Definition

Decreased intravascular, interstitial, and/or intracellular fluid. This refers to dehydration, water loss alone without change in sodium level

Defining Characteristics

Change in mental state; decreased blood pressure, pulse pressure and pulse volume; decreased skin and tongue turgor; decreased urine output; decreased venous filling; dry mucous membranes; dry skin; elevated hematocrit; increased body temperature; increased pulse rate; increased urine concentration; sudden weight loss (except in third spacing); thirst; weakness

Related Factors (r/t)

Active fluid volume loss; failure of regulatory mechanisms

NOC   (Nursing Outcomes Classification)

Suggested NOC Outcomes

Fluid Balance, Hydration, Nutritional Status: Food and Fluid Intake

Example **NOC** Outcome with Indicators
Fluid Balance as evidenced by the following indicators: Skin turgor/Moist mucous membranes/Orthostatic hypotension not present/24–hour intake and output balanced/Urine specific gravity (Rate each indicator of **Fluid Balance: 1** = severely compromised, 2 = substantially compromised, 3 = moderately compromised, 4 = mildly compromised, 5 = not compromised [see Section I].)

● = Independent   ▲ = Collaborative   **EBN** = Evidence-Based Nursing   **EB** = Evidence-Based

Client Outcomes

Client Will (Specify Time Frame):

- Maintain urine output more than 1300 mL/day (or at least 30 mL/hr)
- Maintain normal blood pressure, pulse, and body temperature
- Maintain elastic skin turgor; moist tongue and mucous membranes; and orientation to person, place, and time
- Explain measures that can be taken to treat or prevent fluid volume loss
- Describe symptoms that indicate the need to consult with health care provider

NIC   (Nursing Interventions Classification)

Suggested NIC Interventions

Fluid Management, Hypovolemia Management, Shock Management: Volume

Example NIC Activities—Fluid Management
Monitor hydration status (e.g., moist mucous membranes, adequacy of pulses, and orthostatic blood pressure) as appropriate; Administer intravenous fluids at room temperature

Nursing Interventions and *Rationales*

- Watch for early signs of hypovolemia, including thirst, restlessness, headaches, and inability to concentrate. Thirst is often the first sign of dehydration (Scales & Pilsworth 2008). **EB:** *A study of healthy volunteers who experienced a fluid restriction of up to 37 hours reported symptoms of headache, decreased alertness, and inability to concentrate (Shirreffs et al, 2004).*
- Recognize symptoms of cyanosis, cold clammy skin, weak thready pulse, confusion, and oliguria as late signs of hypovolemia. *These symptoms occur after the body has compensated for fluid loss by moving fluid from the interstitial space into the vascular compartment, several liters of fluid may be lost from the body (Scales & Pilsworth, 2008).*
- Monitor pulse, respiration, and blood pressure of clients with deficient fluid volume every 15 minutes to 1 hour for the unstable client, every 4 hours for the stable client. *Vital sign changes seen with fluid volume deficit include tachycardia, tachypnea, decreased pulse pressure first, then hypotension, decreased pulse volume, and increased or decreased body temperature (Scales & Pilsworth, 2008).* **EB:** *A systematic review demonstrated that hypotension and tachycardia, and occasionally fever, are clinical signs of dehydration (Ferry, 2005).*
- Check orthostatic blood pressures with the client lying, sitting, and standing. *A 20 mm Hg drop when upright or an increase of 15 beats/min in the pulse rate are seen with deficient fluid volume (Kasper et al, 2005). If the systolic blood pressure drops 20 mm Hg and the pulse rate does not change, the baroreceptors in the body are not working, and the cause can be cardiovascular, neurologic, or a medication effect (Sclater & Kannayiram, 2004).*
- Note skin turgor over bony prominences such as the hand or shin.
- Monitor for the existence of factors causing deficient fluid volume (e.g., vomiting, diarrhea, difficulty maintaining oral intake, fever, uncontrolled type 2 diabetes, diuretic therapy). *Early identification of risk factors and early intervention can decrease the occurrence and severity of complications from deficient fluid volume.*
- Observe for dry tongue and mucous membranes, and longitudinal tongue furrows. *These are symptoms of decreased body fluids.*
- Recognize that checking capillary refill may not be helpful in identifying fluid volume deficit. *Capillary refill can be normal in clients with sepsis, increased body temperature dilates peripheral blood vessels, and capillary return may be immediate (Scales & Pilsworth, 2008).* **EBN:** *A systematic review found capillary refill not helpful to determine hypovolemia (Dufault et al, 2008).*
- Weigh client daily and watch for sudden decreases, especially in the presence of decreasing urine output or active fluid loss. *Body weight changes reflect changes in body fluid volume (Kasper et al, 2005).* **EB:** *Systematic reviews demonstrated that measurement of body mass change is a safe technique to assess hydration status (Armstrong, 2005; Wakefield, 2008).*
- Monitor total fluid intake and output every 8 hours (or every hour for the unstable client). Recognize that urine output is not always an accurate indicator of fluid balance. *A urine output of less*

than 30 mL/hr is insufficient for normal renal function and indicates hypovolemia or onset of renal damage (Scales & Pilsworth, 2008).

- Note the color of urine and specific gravity. *Normal urine is straw-colored or amber. Dark-colored urine with increasing specific gravity reflects increased urine concentration, and fluid deficit. Increasing specific gravity of urine also reflects fluid deficit (Scales & Pilsworth, 2008).*
- Provide frequent oral hygiene, at least twice a day (if mouth is dry and painful, provide hourly while awake). *Oral hygiene decreases unpleasant tastes in the mouth and allows the client to respond to the sensation of thirst.*
- Provide fresh water and oral fluids preferred by the client (distribute over 24 hours [e.g., 1200 mL on days, 800 mL on evenings, and 200 mL on nights]); provide prescribed diet; offer snacks (e.g., frequent drinks, fresh fruits, fruit juice); instruct significant other to assist the client with feedings as appropriate. *The oral route is preferred for maintaining fluid balance). Distributing the intake over the entire 24–hour period and providing snacks and preferred beverages increases the likelihood that the client will maintain the prescribed oral intake.*
- ▲ Provide oral replacement therapy as ordered and tolerated with a hypotonic glucose-electrolyte solution when the client has acute diarrhea or nausea/vomiting. Provide small, frequent quantities of slightly chilled solutions. *Maintenance of oral intake stabilizes the ability of the intestines to digest and absorb nutrients; glucose-electrolyte solutions increase net fluid absorption while correcting deficient fluid volume. Use diluted carbohydrate-electrolyte solutions such as sports replacement drinks, and ginger ale, which are often tolerated better than other solutions, sometimes even with vomiting and diarrhea (Suhayda & Walton, 2002).* **EB:** *A study demonstrated that decreasing the osmolality of standard glucose-electrolyte oral replacement solutions improves the absorption of water, and results in decreased stool volume (Farthing, 2002).*
- ▲ Administer antidiarrheals and antiemetics as ordered and appropriate. *The goal is to stop the loss that results from vomiting or diarrhea.* Refer to care plan for **Diarrhea** or **Nausea.**
- ▲ Hydrate the client with ordered isotonic intravenous (IV) solutions if prescribed. *Isotonic intravenous fluids such as 0.9% normal saline or lactated Ringer's allow replacement of in-travascular volume (Fauci et al, 2008).*
- Assist with ambulation if the client has postural hypotension. *Hypovolemia causes postural hypotension, which can result in syncope, and increased risk for injury (Fauci et al, 2008).*

Critically Ill

- Monitor central venous pressure, right atrial pressure, and pulmonary wedge pressure for decreases. *Hemodynamic parameters are sensitive indicators of intravascular fluid volume, and hemodynamic measurements are especially needed in the client with cardiac or renal problems (Fauci et al, 2008).*
- Monitor serum and urine osmolality, serum sodium, BUN/creatinine ratio, and hematocrit for elevations. *These are all measures of concentration and will be elevated with decreased intravascular volume (Fauci et al, 2008).*
- Utilize a sublingual capnometry device if available to determine level of tissue hypoxia caused by lack of fluid volume. *Recognizing decreased perfusion during resuscitation from blood loss can help avoid onset of multiple organ failure (Boswell & Scalea, 2003).*
- ▲ Insert a foley catheter if ordered and measure urine output hourly. Notify physician if less than 30 mL/hr. *A decrease in urine output is seen with increasing severity of shock in the client with normal kidney function, and if action is taken early, can prevent further deterioration of the client (Scales & Pilsworth, 2008).*
- ▲ When ordered, initiate a fluid challenge of crystalloids (0.9% normal saline or lactated Ringer's) for replacement of intravascular volume; monitor the client's response to prescribed fluid therapy and fluid challenge, especially noting central venous pressure and pulmonary capillary wedge pressure readings, vital signs, urine output, blood lactate concentrations, and lung sounds. *A fluid challenge can help the client with deficient fluid volume regain intravascular volume quickly, but the client must be carefully observed to ensure that he or she does not go into fluid volume overload (Fauci et al, 2008).*
- Position the client flat with legs elevated when hypotensive, if not contraindicated. *This position enhances venous return, thus contributing to the maintenance of cardiac output (Fauci et al, 2008).*

• = Independent   ▲ = Collaborative   **EBN** = Evidence-Based Nursing   **EB** = Evidence-Based

▲ Monitor trends in serum lactic acid levels and base deficit obtained from blood gasses as ordered. *A trend of increasing lactic acid levels and increasing base deficit can help identify hypoperfusion, which results in decreased survival and increased incidence of organ failure (Fauci et al, 2008).*

▲ Consult physician if signs and symptoms of deficient fluid volume persist or worsen. *Prolonged deficient fluid volume increases the risk for development of complications, including shock, multiple organ failure, and death.*

Pediatric

- Monitor the child for signs of deficient fluid volume, including capillary refill time, skin turgor, and respiratory pattern along with other symptoms. **EB:** *A metaanalysis of the literature identified these factors as more significant in identifying dehydration, but these are still imprecise and it is difficult to determine the exact degree of dehydration (Steiner et al, 2004).*

▲ Re-enforce the physician's recommendation for the parents to give the child oral rehydration fluids to drink in the amounts specified, especially during the first 4 to 6 hours to replace fluid losses. Once the child is rehydrated, an orally administered maintenance solution should be used along with food. **EB:** *A study demonstrated that treatment with oral rehydration fluids for children were generally as effective as intravenous fluids, and IV fluids did not shorten the duration of gastroenteritis and are more likely to cause adverse effects than oral rehydration therapy (Banks & Meadows, 2005). A Cochrane review found that children admitted to the hospital with diarrhea receiving reduced osmolarity oral rehydration solutions had less stool volume, less vomiting, and less use of intravenous fluids (Hahn, Kim, & Garner, 2002).*

- Recommend the mother resume breastfeeding as soon as possible.

- Recommend parents not give the child decarbonated soda, fruit juices, gelatin dessert, or instant fruit drink mix. *These fluids have a high osmolality due to carbohydrate contents and can exacerbate diarrhea. In addition they have low sodium concentrations, which can aggravate existing hyponatremia (Behrman, Kliegman, & Jenson, 2004).*

- Recommend parents give children foods with complex carbohydrates, such as potatoes, rice, bread, cereal, yogurt, fruits, and vegetables. *The BRAT diet has been traditionally recommended but if used, should be used for only short periods of time as it is nutritionally incomplete (CDC, 2003). Avoid fatty foods and foods high in simple sugars (Behrman, Kliegman, & Jenson, 2004). When a child has diarrhea, dietary modification includes avoiding dairy products, because viral or bacterial infections can cause a transient lactase deficiency.*

Geriatric

- Monitor elderly clients for deficient fluid volume carefully, noting new onset of weakness, dizziness, and postural hypotension. *Older adults have a higher osmotic point for thirst sensation and a diminished sensitivity to thirst, relative to younger adults (Wotton, Crannitch, & Munt, 2008).*

- Evaluate the risk for dehydration using the Dehydration Risk Appraisal Checklist (Mentes, 2004).

- Check skin turgor of elderly client on the forehead, subclavian area, or inner thigh; also look for the presence of longitudinal furrows on the tongue and dry mucous membranes. *Elderly people commonly have decreased skin turgor from normal age-related loss of elasticity; therefore checking skin turgor on the arm is not reflective of fluid volume. The presence of longitudinal furrows or dry mucous membranes is a good indication of dehydration in the elderly (Wotton et al, 2008).*

- Encourage fluid intake by offering fluids regularly to cognitively impaired clients. **EB:** *A systematic review demonstrated that dehydration by overnight fluid restriction in both young and older subjects results in impaired alertness; in older individuals it also resulted in slower psychomotor processing speed and impaired memory performance (Ritz & Berrut, 2005).*

- Incorporate regular hydration into daily routines (e.g., extra glass of fluid with medication or social activities) (Wotton, Crannitch, & Munt, 2008). Consider use of a beverage cart and a hydration assistant to routinely offer increased beverages to clients in extended care. **EBN and EB:** *A nursing study demonstrated that institution of a beverage cart with a trained hydration assistant resulted in increased number of bowel movements, less use of laxatives, decreased number of falls, fewer urinary tract infections, respiratory infections, and skin breakdown (Robinson & Rosher, 2002). A study*

● = Independent   ▲ = Collaborative   **EBN** = Evidence-Based Nursing   **EB** = Evidence-Based

demonstrated that verbal prompting and offering preferred fluids resulted in increased fluid intake among nursing home residents (Simmons, Alessi & Schnelle, 2001).

- If client is identified as having chronic dehydration, flag the food tray to indicate to caregivers they should finish 75% to 100% of their food and fluids. *Elderly clients often have a combination of both malnutrition and fluid deficit (Mentes, 2004; Wotton, Crannitch & Munt, 2008).*
- Recognize that lower blood pressures and a higher BUN/creatinine ratio can be significant signs of dehydration in the elderly. **EBN:** *In this study, dehydrated older adults had significantly lower systolic and diastolic blood pressure and significantly higher BUN but similar creatinine levels compared to non-dehydrated adults (Bennett, Thomas, & Riegel, 2004).*
- Note the color of urine and compare against a urine color chart to monitor adequate fluid intake. **EBN:** *A research study on elderly veterans demonstrated that urine color correlated significantly with urine osmolality, serum sodium, and BUN/creatinine ratio (Wakefield et al, 2002).*
- Monitor elderly clients for excess fluid volume during the treatment of deficient fluid volume: listen to lung sounds, watch for edema, and note vital signs. *The elderly client has a decreased ability to adapt to rapid increases in intravascular volume and can quickly develop fluid overload.*

 ### Home Care

- Teach family members how to monitor output in the home (e.g., use of commode "hat" in the toilet, urinal, or bedpan, or use of catheter and closed drainage). Instruct them to monitor both intake and output.
- When weighing the client, use same scale each day. Be sure scale is on a flat, not cushioned, surface. Do not weigh the client with scale placed on any kind of rug.
- Teach family about complications of deficient fluid volume and when to call physician.
- If the client is receiving intravenous fluids, there must be a responsible caregiver in the home. Teach caregiver about administration of fluids, complications of IV administration (e.g., fluid volume overload, speed of medication reactions), and when to call for assistance. Assist caregiver with administration for as long as necessary to maintain client safety. *Administration of intravenous fluids in the home is a high-technology procedure and requires sufficient professional support to ensure safety of the client.*
- Identify an emergency plan, including when to call 911. *Some complications of deficient fluid volume cannot be reversed in the home and are life threatening. Clients progressing toward hypovolemic shock will need emergency care.*
- Support the family/client in a palliative care situation to decide if it is appropriate to intervene for deficient fluid volume or to allow the client to die without fluids. *Deficient fluid volume may be a symptom of impending death in terminally ill clients. There is no defined gold standard for hydrating dying clients, or allowing the client to die without fluids (Good et al, 2008; Schmidlin, 2008).*

 ### Client/Family Teaching and Discharge Planning

- Instruct the client to avoid rapid position changes, especially from supine to sitting or standing.
- Teach the client and family about appropriate diet and fluid intake.
- Teach the client and family how to measure and record intake and output accurately.
- Teach the client and family about measures instituted to treat hypovolemia and to prevent or treat fluid volume loss.
- Instruct the client and family about signs of deficient fluid volume that indicate they should contact health care provider.

⊖volve   See the EVOLVE website for Weblinks for client education resources.

REFERENCES

Armstrong LE: Hydration assessment techniques, *Nutr Rev* 63(6 Part 2): S40–S54, 2005.

Banks JB, Meadows S: Intravenous fluids for children with gastroenteritis, *Am Family Physician* 71(1):121, 2005.

Behrman RE, Kliegman RM, Jenson HB: *Nelson textbook of pediatrics*, ed 17, Philadelphia, 2004, WB Saunders.

Bennett JA, Thomas V, Riegel B: Unrecognized chronic dehydration in older adults: examining prevalence rate and risk factors, *J Gerontol Nurs* 30(11):22–28, 2004.

Boswell SA, Scalea TM: Sublingual capnometry: an alternative to gastric tonometry for the management of shock resuscitation, *AACN Clin Issues* 14(2):176, 2003.

• = Independent   ▲ = Collaborative   **EBN** = Evidence-Based Nursing   **EB** = Evidence-Based

Centers for Disease Control and Prevention: The management of acute diarrhea in children. 2003. www.cdc.gov/mmwr/preview/mmwrhtml/00018677.htm. Accessed May 21, 2009.

Dufault M, Davis B, Garman D et al: Translating best practices in assessing capillary refill, *Worldviews Evid Based Nurs* 5(1):36–44, 2008.

Farthing MJ: Oral rehydration: an evolving solution, *J Pediatr Gastroenterol Nutr* 34(Suppl 1):S64, 2002.

Fauci A, Braunwald E, Kasper D et al: *Harrison's principles of internal medicine*, ed 17, New York, 2008, McGraw-Hill.

Ferry M: Strategies for ensuring good hydration in the elderly, *Nutr Rev* 63(6 Part 2):S22–S29, 2005.

Good P, Cavenagh J, Mather Mark et al: Medically assisted hydration for adult palliative care patients, *Cochrane Database Syst Rev* (4): CD00075320, 2008.

Hahn S, Kim S, Garner P: Reduced osmolarity oral rehydration solution for treating dehydration caused by acute diarrhea in children, *Cochrane Database Syst Rev* ;(1):CD002847, 2002.

Kasper DL, Braunwald E, Hauser S, et al, editors: *Harrison's principles of internal medicine,* ed 16, New York, 2005, McGraw-Hill.

Mentes JC: *Hydration management.* Iowa City, 2004, University of Iowa Gerontological Nursing Interventions Research Center, Research Dissemination Core.

Ritz P, Berrut G: The importance of good hydration for day-to-day health, *Nutr Rev* 63(6 Part 2):S6–S13, 2005.

Robinson SB, Rosher RB: Can a beverage cart help improve hydration? *Geriatr Nurs* 23:4, 2002.

Scales K, Pilsworth J: The importance of fluid balance in clinical practice, *Nurs Stand* 22(47):50–57, 2008.

Schmidlin E: Artificial hydration: the role of the nurse in addressing patient and family needs. *Int J Pallit Nurs,* 14(10):485–489, 2008.

Sclater A, Kannayiram A: Orthostatic hypotension: a primary care primer for assessment and treatment, *Geriatrics* 59(8):22, 2004.

Shirreffs SM, Merson SJ, Fraser SM et al: The effects of fluid restriction on hydration status and subjective feelings in man, *Br J Nutr* 91(6):951, 2004.

Simmons SF, Alessi C, Schnelle JF: An intervention to increase fluid intake in nursing home residents: prompting and preference compliance, *J Am Geriatr Soc* 49(7):926, 2001.

Steiner MJ, DeWalt DA, Byerley JS: Is this child dehydrated? *JAMA* 291(22):2764, 2004.

Suhayda R, Walton JC: Preventing and managing dehydration, *Medsurg Nurs* 11(6):267, 2002.

Wakefield B: Fluid management guideline. In Ackley B, Ladwig G, Swan B: *Evidence-based nursing care guidelines: medical-surgical interventions,* Philadelphia, 2008, Mosby.

Wakefield B, Mentes J, Diggelmann L et al: Monitoring hydration status in elderly veterans, *West J Nurs Res* 24(2):132, 2002.

Wotton K, Crannitch K, Munt R: Prevalence, risk factors and strategies to prevent dehydration in older adults, *Contemp Nurse* 31(1):44–56, 2008.

Risk for deficient Fluid volume   *Betty J. Ackley, MSN, EdS, RN*

NANDA-I

Definition

At risk for experiencing vascular, cellular, or intracellular dehydration

Risk Factors

Deviations affecting access of fluids; deviations affecting intake of fluids; deviations affecting absorption of fluids; excessive losses through normal routes (e.g., diarrhea); extremes of age; extremes of weight; factors influencing fluid needs (e.g., hypermetabolic state); loss of fluid through abnormal routes (e.g., indwelling tubes); knowledge deficiency; medication (e.g., diuretics)

NOC, NIC, Client Outcomes, Nursing Interventions, Client/Family Teaching and Discharge Planning, *Rationales,* and References

Refer to care plans for **Deficient Fluid volume.**

⊖volve   See the EVOLVE website for Weblinks for client education resources.

Excess Fluid volume   *Betty J. Ackley MSN, EdS, RN*   ⊖volve

NANDA-I

Definition

Increased isotonic fluid retention

Defining Characteristics

Adventitious breath sounds; altered electrolytes; anasarca, anxiety, azotemia, blood pressure changes; change in mental status; changes in respiratory pattern, decreased hematocrit, decreased hemoglobin, dyspnea, edema, increased central venous pressure; intake exceeds output, jugular vein distension,

• = Independent   ▲ = Collaborative   **EBN** = Evidence-Based Nursing   **EB** = Evidence-Based

oliguria; orthopnea; pleural effusion; positive hepatojugular reflex; pulmonary artery pressure changes; pulmonary congestion; restlessness; specific gravity changes; S3 heart sound; weight gain over short period of time

Related Factors (r/t)

Compromised regulatory mechanism; excess fluid intake; excess sodium intake

 (Nursing Outcomes Classification)

Suggested NOC Outcomes

Electrolyte and Acid-Base Balance, Fluid Balance, Hydration

Example **NOC Outcome with Indicators**
Fluid Balance as evidenced by the following indicators: Peripheral edema/Neck vein distention/Adventitious breath sounds/Body weight increase (Rate each indicator of **Fluid Balance:** 1 = severe, 2 = substantial, 3 = moderate, 4 = mild, 5 = none [see Section I].)

Client Outcomes

Client Will (Specify Time Frame):

- Remain free of edema, effusion, anasarca
- Maintain body weight appropriate for the client
- Maintain clear lung sounds; no evidence of dyspnea or orthopnea
- Remain free of jugular vein distention, positive hepatojugular reflex, and gallop heart rhythm
- Maintain normal central venous pressure, pulmonary capillary wedge pressure, cardiac output, and vital signs
- Maintain urine output within 500 mL of intake with normal urine osmolality and specific gravity
- Explain actions that are needed to treat or prevent excess fluid volume including fluid and dietary restrictions, and medications
- Describe symptoms that indicate the need to consult with health care provider

NIC **(Nursing Interventions Classification)**

Suggested NIC Interventions

Fluid Management, Fluid Monitoring

Example **NIC Activities—Fluid Monitoring**
Weigh daily and monitor trends; Maintain accurate intake and output record

Nursing Interventions and *Rationales*

- Monitor location and extent of edema, use the 1+ to 4+ scale to quantify edema; also measure the legs using a millimeter tape in the same area at the same time each day. Note differences in measurement between extremities. *Generalized edema (e.g., in the upper extremities and eyelids) is associated with decreased oncotic pressure as a result of nephrotic syndrome. Heart failure and renal failure are usually associated with dependent edema because of increased hydrostatic pressure; dependent edema will cause swelling in the legs and feet of ambulatory clients (Fauci et al, 2008).*
- Monitor daily weight for sudden increases; use same scale and type of clothing at same time each day, preferably before breakfast. *Body weight changes reflect changes in body fluid volume.* **EB:** *A study demonstrated that body weight could safely be used to monitor for fluid overload when administering hyperhydration with high dose chemotherapy (Mank et al, 2003).*
- Monitor intake and output; note trends reflecting decreasing urine output in relation to fluid intake. *Accurately measuring intake and output is important for the client with fluid volume overload.*

• = Independent   ▲ = Collaborative   **EBN** = Evidence-Based Nursing   **EB** = Evidence-Based

EBN: *A study found that visual estimation of intake of fluid was inaccurate; instead, volumes should be measured (McConnell et al, 2007).*

- Monitor vital signs; note decreasing blood pressure, tachycardia, and tachypnea. Monitor for gallop rhythms. If signs of heart failure are present, see the care plan for **Decreased Cardiac output.** *Heart failure results in decreased cardiac output and decreased blood pressure. Tissue hypoxia stimulates increased heart and respiratory rates.*
- Listen to lung sounds for crackles, monitor respirations for effort, and determine the presence and severity of orthopnea. *Pulmonary edema results from excessive shifting of fluid from the vascular space into the pulmonary interstitial space and alveoli, resulting in dyspnea and orthopnea (Fauci et al, 2008).*
- Monitor serum and urine osmolality, serum sodium, BUN/creatinine ratio, and hematocrit for abnormalities. *These are all measures of concentration and will be altered with increased fluid volume (Fauci et al, 2008).*
- With head of bed elevated 30 to 45 degrees, monitor jugular veins for distention in the upright position; assess for positive hepatojugular reflex. *Increased intravascular volume results in jugular vein distention, even in a client in the upright position, and also a positive hepatojugular reflex (Fauci et al, 2008).*
- Monitor the client's behavior for restlessness, anxiety, or confusion; use safety precautions if symptoms are present. *When excess fluid volume compromises cardiac output, the client may experience cerebral tissue hypoxia, and the client may demonstrate restlessness and anxiety. When the excess fluid volume results in hyponatremia, symptoms such as agitation, irritability, inappropriate behavior, confusion, and seizures may occur (Fauci et al, 2008).*
- Monitor for the development of conditions that increase the client's risk for excess fluid volume, including heart failure, renal failure, and liver failure, all of which result in decreased glomerular filtration rate and fluid retention. Other causes are increased intake of oral or intravenous fluids in excess of the client's cardiac and renal reserve levels, and increased levels of antidiuretic hormone (Fauci et al, 2008). *Many clients with fluid overload have acute kidney disease, and fluid balance is an important indicator of outcomes, with increased morbidity and mortality in clients with fluid overload (Mehta, 2009).*
- ▲ Provide a restricted-sodium diet as appropriate if ordered. *Restricting the sodium in the diet will favor the renal excretion of excess fluid. Take care to avoid hyponatremia. Decreasing sodium can be just as important as restricting fluid intake with fluid overload (Fauci et al, 2008).*
- ▲ Monitor serum albumin level and provide protein intake as appropriate. *Serum albumin is the main contributor to serum oncotic pressure, which favors the movement of fluid from the interstitial space into the intravascular space. When serum albumin is low, peripheral edema may be severe.*
- ▲ Administer prescribed diuretics as appropriate; check blood pressure before administration to ensure is adequate. If IV administration of a diuretic, note and record urine output following the dose. **EB:** *Clinical practice guidelines on heart failure site that monitoring I&Os is useful for monitoring effects of diuretic therapy (Jessup et al, 2009).*
- Monitor for side effects of diuretic therapy: orthostatic hypotension (especially if the client is also receiving ACE inhibitors), hypovolemia and electrolyte imbalances (hypokalemia and hyponatremia). *Observe for hyperkalemia in clients receiving a potassium-sparing diuretic, especially with the concurrent administration of an ACE inhibitor (Fauci et al, 2008).*
- ▲ Implement fluid restriction as ordered, especially when serum sodium is low; include all routes of intake. Schedule fluids around the clock, and include the type of fluids preferred by the client. *Fluid restriction may decrease intravascular volume and myocardial workload. Overzealous fluid restriction should not be used because hypovolemia can worsen heart failure. Client involvement in planning will enhance participation in the necessary fluid restriction.*
- Maintain the rate of all IV infusions, carefully utilizing an IV pump. *This is done to prevent inadvertent exacerbation of excess fluid volume.*
- Turn clients with dependent edema frequently (i.e., at least every 2 hours). *Edematous tissue is vulnerable to ischemia and pressure ulcers (Casey, 2004).*
- Provide for scheduled rest periods. *Bed rest can induce diuresis related to diminished peripheral venous pooling, resulting in increased intravascular volume and glomerular filtration rate.*
- Promote a positive body image and good self-esteem. *Visible edema may alter the client's body image.* Refer to the care plan for **Disturbed Body image.**

• = Independent   ▲ = Collaborative   **EBN** = Evidence-Based Nursing   **EB** = Evidence-Based

▲ Consult with physician if signs and symptoms of excess fluid volume persist or worsen. *Because excess fluid volume can result in pulmonary edema, it must be treated promptly and aggressively (Fauci et al, 2008).*

Critically Ill

▲ Insert a foley catheter if ordered and measure urine output hourly. Notify physician if less than 30 mL/hr. *A decrease in urine output is seen with increasing severity of heart failure or decreased kidney, function (Fauci et al, 2008; Scales & Pilsworth, 2008).*

● Monitor central venous pressure, mean arterial pressure, pulmonary artery pressure, pulmonary capillary wedge pressure, and cardiac output/index; note and report trends indicating increasing or decreasing pressures over time. *Increased vascular volume with decreased cardiac contractility increases intravascular pressures, which are reflected in hemodynamic parameters. Over time, this increased pressure can result in uncompensated heart failure (Fauci et al, 2008).*

▲ Assist with continuous renal replacement therapy (CRRT) as ordered if the client is critically ill and excessive fluid must be removed. *CRRT is indicated for severe volume overload, refractory heart failure, oliguric renal failure, and possibly sepsis and multiorgan dysfunction syndrome (Dirkes & Hodge, 2007).*

Geriatric

● Recognize that the presence of fluid volume excess is particularly serious in the elderly. *Sodium and fluid overload is common in hospitalized elderly clients because of heart and kidney disease, and can result in increased morbidity and mortality (Allison & Lobo, 2004; Zarowitz & Lefkovitz, 2008). In clients receiving hemodialysis, fluid retention is associated with increased cardiovascular mortality (Kalantar-Zadeh et al, 2009).*

● Monitor electrolyte levels carefully, including sodium levels and potassium levels, with both increased and decreased levels possible. *Elderly are prone to electrolyte abnormalities because of failure of regulatory mechanisms associated with heart and kidney disease, plus the large number of medications that are taken that can affect electrolyte levels (Zarowitz & Lefkovitz, 2008). Many elderly clients are receiving selective serotonin reuptake inhibitors in treatment of depression, which can result in hyponatremia (Bowen, 2009).* Refer to the care plan for **Risk for Electrolyte imbalance.**

Home Care

● Assess client and family knowledge of disease process causing excess fluid volume.

▲ Teach about disease process and complications of excess fluid volume, including when to contact physician.

● Assess client and family knowledge and compliance with medical regimen, including medications, diet, rest, and exercise. Assist family with integrating restrictions into daily living. *Assistance with integration of cultural values, especially those related to foods, with medical regimen promotes compliance and decreased risk of complications.*

▲ Teach and reinforce knowledge of medications. Instruct the client not to use over-the-counter (OTC) medications (e.g., diet medications) without first consulting the physician.

▲ Instruct the client to make primary physician aware of medications ordered by other physicians.

● Identify emergency plan for rapidly developing or critical levels of excess fluid volume when diuresing is not safe at home. *When out of control, excess fluid volume can be life threatening.*

▲ Teach about signs and symptoms of both excess and deficient fluid volume and when to call physician. *Fluid volume balance can change rapidly with aggressive treatment.*

Client/Family Teaching and Discharge Planning

● Describe signs and symptoms of excess fluid volume and actions to take if they occur.

▲ Teach client on diuretics to weigh self daily in the morning, and notify the physician if there is a 3 pound or more change in weight (Karch, 2004). **EB:** *Clinical practice guidelines on heart failure suggest that daily weight monitoring leads to early recognition of excess fluid retention, which, when re-*

● = Independent   ▲ = Collaborative   **EBN** = Evidence-Based Nursing   **EB** = Evidence-Based

ported, can be offset with additional medication to avoid hospitalization from HF decompensation (Jessup et al, 2009).

▲ Teach the importance of fluid and sodium restrictions. Help the client and family to devise a schedule for intake of fluids throughout entire day. Refer to dietitian concerning implementation of low-sodium diet.

▲ Teach how to take diuretics correctly: take one dose in the morning and second dose (if taken) no later than 4 PM. Adjust potassium intake as appropriate for potassium-losing or potassium-sparing diuretics. Note the appearance of side effects such as weakness, dizziness, muscle cramps, numbness and tingling, confusion, hearing impairment, palpitations or irregular heartbeat, and postural hypotension.

• For the client undergoing hemodialysis, teach client the required restrictions in dietary electrolytes, protein and fluid. Spend time with the client to detect any factors that may interfere with the client's compliance with the fluid restriction or restrictive diet. **EBN:** *An educational program on fluid compliance of hemodialysis clients resulted in a decreased weight gain between dialysis treatments (Barnett et al, 2008).*

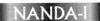 See the Evolve website for Weblinks for client education resources.

REFERENCES

Allison SP, Lobo DN: Fluid and electrolytes in the elderly, *Curr Opin Clin Nutr Metab Care* 7(1):27, 2004.

Barnett T, Li Yoong T, Pinikahana J et al: Fluid compliance among patients having hemodialysis: can an educational program make a difference? *J Adv Nurs* 61(3):300–306, 2008.

Bowen P: Use of selective serotonin reuptake inhibitors in the treatment of depression in older adults: identifying and managing potential risk for hyponatremia, *Geriatr Nurs* 30(2):85–89, 2009.

Casey G: Edema: causes, physiology and nursing management, *Nur Stand* 18(51):45, 2004.

Dirkes S, Hodge K: Continuous renal replacement therapy in the adult intensive care unit: history and current trends, *Crit Care Nurse* 27(2):61–6, 68–72, 74–80, 2007.

Fauci A, Brauwald E, Kasper DL, et al, editors: *Harrison's principles of internal medicine*, ed 17, New York, 2008, McGraw-Hill.

Jessup M, Abraham WT, Casey DE et al: 2009 focused update: ACCF/AHA guidelines for the diagnosis and management of heart failure in adults. content.onlinejacc.org. Accessed March 26, 2009.

Kalantar-Zadeh K, Regidor DL, Dovesdy CP et al: Fluid retention is associated with cardiovascular mortality in patients undergoing long-term hemodialysis, *Circulation* 119(5):671–679, 2009.

Karch AM. Practice errors. On the rebound: maintaining normal fluid intake is critical while on diuretics, *Am J Nurs* 104(10):73, 2004.

Mank A, Semin-Goossens A, Lelie J et al: Monitoring hyperhydration during high-dose chemotherapy: body weight or fluid balance? *Acta Haematol* 109(4):163, 2003.

McConnell JS et al: "About a cupful": a prospective study into accuracy of volume estimation by medical and nursing staff, *Accid Emerg Nurs* 15(2):101–105, 2007.

Mehta RL: Fluid balance and acute kidney injury: the missing link for predicting adverse outcomes? *Nat Clin Pract Nephrol*, 5(1):10–11, 2009.

Scales K, Pilsworth J: The importance of fluid balance in clinical practice, *Nurs Stand* 22(47):50–57, 2008.

Zarowitz B, Lefkovitz A: Recognition and treatment of hyperkalemia, *Geriatr Nurs* 29(5):333–339, 2008.

Risk for imbalanced Fluid volume   *Terri A. Foster RN, BSN, CNOR, and Betty J. Ackley, MSN, EdS, RN*

NANDA-I

Definition

At risk for a decrease, increase, or rapid shift from one to the other of intravascular, interstitial, and/or intracellular fluid (refers to body fluid loss, gain, or both)

Risk Factors

Major invasive procedures

NOC   (Nursing Outcomes Classification)

Suggested NOC Labels

Fluid Balance, Electrolyte and Acid-Base Balance, Hydration

• = Independent   ▲ = Collaborative   **EBN** = Evidence-Based Nursing   **EB** = Evidence-Based

---

Example NOC Outcome with Indicators

Maintains **Fluid Balance** as evidenced by the following indicators: BP/Peripheral pulses palpable/Skin turgor/Moist mucous membranes/Serum electrolytes/Hematocrit/Peripheral edema/Neck vein distention/Body weight stable/24–hour intake and output balanced/Urine specific gravity/Adventitious breath sounds (Rate each indicator of **Fluid Balance:** 1 = severely compromised, 2 = substantially compromised, 3 = moderately compromised, 4 = mildly compromised, 5 = not compromised [see Section I].)

Client Outcomes

- Lung sounds clear, respiratory rate 12 to 20, and free of dyspnea postoperatively
- Urine output greater than 30 mL/hr
- Blood pressure, pulse rate, temperature, and pulse oximetry within expected range
- Laboratory values within expected range
- Extremities and dependent areas free of edema
- Mental orientation unchanged from preoperative status

NIC   (Nursing Interventions Classification)

Suggested NIC Interventions

Autotransfusion, Bleeding Precautions, Bleeding Reduction: Wound, Electrolyte Management, Fluid Management, Fluid Monitoring, Hemodynamic Regulation, Hypervolemia Management, Hypovolemia Management, Intravenous Therapy, Invasive Hemodynamic Monitoring, Shock Management: Volume, Vital Signs Monitoring

---

Example NIC Activities—Fluid Management

Maintain accurate intake and output record; Monitor vital signs

---

Nursing Interventions and *Rationales*

Surgical Clients

- Monitor the surgical client's fluid balance. If there are symptoms of hypovolemia, please refer to the interventions in the care plan **Deficient Fluid volume.** If there are symptoms of hypervolemia, please refer to the interventions in the care plan **Excess Fluid volume.**

Preoperative

- Perform a preoperative assessment including a history to identify clients with increased risk for hemorrhage or hypovolemia. Those with increased risk include clients with recent traumatic injury, abnormal bleeding or clotting times, complicated renal/liver disease, diabetes, cardiovascular disease, major organ transplant, history of aspirin and/or NSAID use, anticoagulant therapy, or history of hemophilia, von Willebrand's disease, or disseminated intravascular coagulation. *Use of laxatives, preoperative dehydration, infection, abnormal drainage, or hemorrhage can lead to hypotension during anesthesia induction if not corrected preoperatively. NPO status preoperatively can lead to dehydration, and when combined with the stress of undergoing surgery can cause changes in the circulating volume and hydrostatic-oncotic pressure (vanWissen & Breton, 2004). Assessment of the client's use of herbal products is important as some herbs act as anticoagulants and could cause increased blood loss, and some herbs have diuretic or laxative effects (Edlund, 2003; Young et al, 2009)*
- Determine and document the client's mental status preoperatively. *This action is important so that changes in mental status in the postoperative period can be easily identified.*

Intraoperative

- Recognize that liberal fluid given intravenously preoperatively or during surgery is not needed unless there is an indicated fluid deficit. **EB:** *Evidence does not support fluid preloading and liberal intraoperative fluid use (Jacob, Chappell, & Rehm, 2007; Chappell et al, 2008). Increased crystalloid fluids given preoperatively or intraoperatively did not decrease surgical wound infections (Kabon et al, 2005). Weight of the client, fluid and electrolyte excess/deficit, insensible water loss, and gastrointestinal*

• = Independent   ▲ = Collaborative   **EBN** = Evidence-Based Nursing   **EB** = Evidence-Based

and renal loss are factors used to determine fluid replacement in clients undergoing a major surgical procedure (Hughes, 2004).

- Monitor for signs of intraoperative hypovolemia with symptoms of dry skin, dry mucous membranes, tachycardia, decreased urinary output, decreased central venous pressure, hypotension, increased pulse, and/or deep rapid respirations. *Hypovolemia can occur in the surgical client due to NPO status, hemorrhage, or third spacing (vanWissen & Breton, 2004). To ensure adequate hydration, it is important to provide replacement fluids during the postoperative period as needed (Hughes, 2004). Elevating the hypovolemic client's legs can aid venous return and cardiac output unless they also have severe oliguria (Phillips, 2004).* **EB:** *Evidence shows that fluid lost should be replaced. Fluid overload should be avoided (Brandstrup, 2006). Perioperative hypovolemia leads to poor organ perfusion (Lopes et al, 2007).*

- Monitor for signs of intraoperative third spacing. *Fluid can shift to the surgical site and produce edema due to the surgically induced inflammatory response. This fluid is temporarily unavailable and requires replacement to prevent hypovolemic shock (Hughes, 2004).* **EB:** *Evidence shows that predetermined algorithms for replacement of fluid due to third spacing and from diuresis is not necessary (Joshi, 2005).*

- Accurately measure blood loss intraoperatively. *Weighing sponges is a reliable means of estimating blood loss and gauging replacement needs (Rothrock, 2006).* **EB:** *Maximizing cardiac output as a result of optimizing fluid management leads to improved surgical outcomes (McFall, Woods, & Wakeling, 2004).*

- Recognize that IV solutions containing glucose should not be used routinely during surgery. **EB:** *Intraoperative fluid replacement should not routinely contain glucose because plasma cortisol increases during surgery and this in turn causes hyperglycemia (vanWissen & Breton, 2004).*

- Monitor for signs of intraoperative hypervolemia, with symptoms of dyspnea, coarse crackles, increased pulse and respirations, decreased urinary output, all of which could progress to pulmonary edema. *Surgical clients with preexisting chronic kidney or liver disease, or congestive heart failure may be prone to hypervolemia. Increased fluid intake, can potentially increase postoperative cardiac morbidity, predispose the client to pneumonia and respiratory failure, cause urinary retention due to increased excretory demands on the kidney and resultant diuresis, inhibition of gastrointestinal motility resulting in prolonged postoperative ileus, decreased tissue oxygenation resulting in poor wound healing and postoperative thrombosis formation due to coagulation being enhanced (Holte, Sharrock, & Kehlet, 2002).*

- In the critically ill surgical client with a pulmonary artery catheter, monitor pressures, especially wedge pressure. *Pulmonary artery pressures are helpful for determining fluid balance, especially in the cardiac or renal client, and can help to guide fluid administration and administration of vasoactive IV drips such as dopamine.* **EB:** *Use of the Starling curve in combination with central venous pressures or esophageal Doppler cardiac output measurements "optimizes" cardiac function by allowing better fluid regimens. Fluids must be individually titrated based on each client's changes in monitored variables (Mitchell et al, 2003).*

- Assess the client for signs and symptoms of hyponatremia: headache, anorexia, nausea and vomiting, diarrhea, tachycardia, general malaise, muscle cramps, weakness, lethargy, change in mental status, disorientation, seizures, and death. *Many pathologies can predispose the client to hyponatremia including adrenal insufficiency, brain tumor, cirrhosis, hypothyroidism, lung cancer, meningitis, renal disease, tuberculosis, use of complementary therapies, and head trauma (Young et al, 2009).*

- Monitor clients undergoing laparoscopic or hysteroscopic procedures for the development of hyponatremia, hypervolemia, and pulmonary edema when an irrigation fluid is used. *The procedure of hysteroscopy can be complicated by development of hyponatremia and hypervolemia (Estes & Maye, 2003). Local or spinal anesthesia can cause the client to develop symptoms of hyponatremia and hypervolemia sooner than with other anesthetics (Young et al, 2009).*

- Measure the irrigation fluid used during urological and gynecological procedures accurately. Watch for a volume deficit: the amount of irrigation used minus the amount of irrigation recovered via suction. *Absorption of large amounts of fluid can cause complications for the client (Young et al, 2009).*

- Monitor intraoperative intake and output. **EB:** *Low-molecular-weight fluids can cause fluid overload; therefore, it is mandatory that an accurate accounting of input and output be maintained (Gordon, 2003).*

● = Independent   ▲ = Collaborative   **EBN** = Evidence-Based Nursing   **EB** = Evidence-Based

- Monitor clients undergoing TURP (transurethral resection of the prostate) procedures for the development of hyponatremia, and hypervolemia with symptoms of TURP syndrome: headache, visual changes, agitation, lethargy, vomiting, muscle twitching, bradycardia, diminished pupillary reflexes, hypertension, and respiratory distress. *Considerable fluid absorption occurs during TURP procedures which can result in severe hyponatremia (Kukreja et al, 2002; Mutlu, Titiz, & Gogus, 2007).*
- Assess the client for fluid extravasation in and around the surgical area. *Fluid delivered under pressure, such as during an arthroscopic procedure, can result in fluid entering the tissues. Extraarticular fluid migration can occur with prolonged high flow rates and pressures and long procedures with low pressures. When using an automated fluid delivery system, follow manufacturer's recommendations for pump pressures (Young et al, 2009).*
- Assess the liposuction client for fluid and electrolyte imbalance. *Liposuction clients who receive large amounts of IV hydration both intraoperatively and postoperatively are at increased risk for fluid and electrolyte imbalance (Young et al, 2009)*
- Observe the surgical client for signs of hyperkalemia with symptoms of dysrhythmias, heart block, asystole, abdominal distention, and weakness. *Hyperkalemia can occur intraoperatively due to massive blood transfusions, tissue breakdown from surgery, shifting of potassium from the cells into the extracellular fluid, decreased potassium excretion due to renal failure or hypovolemia, crush injuries, or burns (Rothrock, 2006).*
- Observe surgical clients closely for signs of hypokalemia. *Hypokalemia commonly causes dysrhythmias. Stress and/or gastrointestinal fluid loss in surgical clients make them susceptible to hypokalemia.*
- Maintain the client's core temperature at normal levels. *Fluids used for distention can increase risk of hypothermia.* **EB:** *Research has shown that perioperative hypothermia can adversely affect the cardiopulmonary system. It is important to use warming devices as needed (Young et al, 2009).*

Postoperative

- Recognize that accurate postoperative assessment and fluid management should include not only traditional intake/output measurement, but also monitoring of the client's weight, lab values, and checks of peripheral pulses. *Measurement of intake/output may be of limited use for fluid balance determination because input could be much higher than output (vanWissen & Breton, 2004). Poor peripheral pulses are a good indication that blood volume is inadequate and volume deficit is indicated when the extremities are cool, cyanosed, and have poor capillary refill (vanWissen & Breton, 2004).* **EBN:** *In order to ensure adequate hydration of the client and safe nursing practice, it is necessary for postoperative fluid replacement to occur (Hughes, 2004).*

 Geriatric

- Be especially vigilant when monitoring vital signs and fluids in elderly surgical clients. *Fluid intake in the geriatric client should be at least 1500 mL. Some geriatric clients limit fluid intake due to fear of incontinence, inability to drink on their own, altered sensorium/cognition, or decreased thirst as a part of the aging process (Phillips, 2004). Older adults have a higher osmotic point for thirst sensation and a diminished sensitivity to thirst, relative to younger adults (Wotton, Crannitch, & Munt, 2008).* **EB:** *Geriatric clients have a higher risk of developing dehydration then younger clients (Ferry, 2005).*
- Assess elderly client preoperatively for symptoms of dehydration with symptoms of weakness, dizziness, dry mouth, sunken eyes and cheeks, concentrated urine, and decreased skin turgor on the forehead, sternum, or inner thigh. *Elderly people commonly have decreased skin turgor from normal age-related loss of elasticity; checking skin turgor on the arm is not reflective of fluid volume. The presence of longitudinal furrows or dry mucous membranes is a good indication of dehydration in the elderly (Wotton, Crannitch, & Munt, 2008). Dehydrated geriatric clients who are to undergo surgery should receive IV fluids preoperatively in an effort to prevent complications due to dehydration (Phillips, 2004).*
- Ensure that when food intake is reduced or limited, it is compensated with an increase in water/fluid intake. **EB:** *Food contains water, thus any reduction in food intake also involves a reduction in water intake (Ferry, 2005). Anorexia increases the risk of dehydration—the geriatric client is frequently anorexic (Ferry, 2005).*

- Note the color of urine and compare against a urine color chart to monitor adequate fluid intake. **EBN:** *A research study on elderly veterans demonstrated that urine color correlated significantly with urine osmolality, serum sodium, and BUN/creatinine ratio (Wakefield et al, 2002).*
- Monitor elderly clients for excess fluid volume during the treatment of deficient fluid volume: listen to lung sounds, watch for edema, and note vital signs. *The elderly client has a decreased ability to adapt to rapid increases in intravascular volume and can quickly develop fluid overload (Allison & Lobo, 2004).*

 Pediatric

- Assess the pediatric client's weight, length of NPO status, underlying illness, and the surgical procedure to be performed. *This information is used to determine appropriate fluid replacement (Aker, 2002).*
- Recognize that newborns require very little fluid replacement when undergoing major surgical procedures during the first few days of life. **EB:** *10 to 30 mL total may be all that is necessary for fluid replacement during an average surgical procedure involving a newborn (Phillips, 2004).*
- Monitor pediatric surgical clients closely for signs of fluid loss. *Small losses can be life-threatening to these clients (Kumar, 2001). Mild dehydration, although difficult to determine, often presents with dry mouth, malaise, and history of decreased urinary output. Moderate dehydration presents as loss of appetite, oliguria, and lethargy. Severe dehydration presents with tachycardia, mottled cool skin, capillary refill <5 seconds, anuria, and hypotension (Aker, 2002).*
- Administer fluids preoperatively until NPO status must be initiated, so that fluid deficit is decreased. **EB:** *Recommendations for pediatric NPO times have been revised to allow "clear" liquids up to 2 hours preoperatively for pediatric clients <6 months age and up to 3 hours preoperatively for pediatric clients 6 months and older (Aker, 2002).*

ⓔvolve See the Evolve website for Weblinks for client education resources.

REFERENCES

Aker J: Pediatric fluid management, *Curr Rev Pain* 24(7):73–84, 2002.

Allison SP, Lobo, DN: Fluid and electrolytes in the elderly, *Curr Opin Clin Nutr Metab Care* 7(1):27, 2004.

Brandstrup B: Fluid therapy for the surgical patient, *Best Pract Res Clin Anaesthesiol* 20(2):265–283, 2006.

Chappell D, Jacob M, Hofmann-Kiefer K et al: A rational approach to perioperative fluid management, *Anesthesiol* 109(4):723–740, 2008.

Edlund BJ: Fluid and electrolyte imbalances, *The Learning Scope* 5(15):17, 2003.

Estes CM, Maye JP: Severe intraoperative hyponatremia in a patient scheduled for elective hysteroscopy: a case report, *AANA J* 71(3):203–205, 2003.

Ferry M: Strategies for ensuring good hydration in the elderly, *Nutr Rev* 63(6):S22, 2005.

Gordon AG: Complications of hysteroscopy. 2003. www.gfmer.ch/Books/Endoscopy_book/Ch24_Complications_hyster.html. Accessed October 9, 2009.

Holte K, Sharrock NE, Kehlet H: Pathophysiology and clinical implications of perioperative fluid excess, *Br J Anaesth* 89(4):622–632, 2002.

Hughes E: Principles of post-operative patient care, *Nurs Stand* 19(5):43–51, 2004.

Jacob M, Chappell D, Rehm M: Clinical update: perioperative fluid management, *Lancet* 369(9578):1984–1986, 2007.

Joshi GP: Intraoperative fluid restriction improves outcome after major elective gastrointestinal surgery, *Anesth Analg* 101(2):601–605, 2005.

Kabon B, Akca O, Taguchi A et al: Supplemental intravenous crystalloid administration does not reduce the risk of surgical wound infection, *Anesth Analg* 101:1546–1553, 2005.

Kukreja RA, Desai MR, Sabnis RB et al: Fluid absorption during percutaneous nephrolithotomy: does it matter? *J Endourol* 16(4):221–224, 2002.

Kumar N: Monitoring fluids and electrolytes in the surgical patient. http://nursing.advanceweb.com/Article/Monitoring-Fluids-and-Electrolytes-in-the-Surgical-Patient.aspx, 2001. Accessed October 9, 2009.

Lopes MR, Oliveira MA, Oliveira V et al: Goal-directed fluid management based on pulse pressure variation monitoring during high risk surgery: a pilot randomized trial, *Crit Care* 11(5):R100, 2007.

McFall MR, Woods GA, Wakeling HG: The use of oesophageal Doppler cardiac output measurement to optimize fluid management during colorectal surgery (readers response to editor), *Eur J Anaesthesiol* 21(7):581, 2004.

Mitchell G, Hucker T, Venn R et al: Pathophysiology and clinical implications of perioperative fluid excess (reader comments to article published in 2002), *Br J Anaesth* 90(3):395, 2003.

Mutlu NM, Titiz APM, Gogus N: Hyponatremia and neurological manifestations of TURP syndrome, *Internet J Anesthesiol* 12(1):1–14, 2007.

Phillips N: *Berry & Kohn's operating room technique*, ed 10, St Louis, 2004, Mosby.

Rothrock J: *Alexander's care of the patient in surgery*, ed 13, St Louis, 2006, Mosby.

vanWissen K, Breton C: Perioperative influences on fluid distribution. *MedSurg Nurs* 13:5, 304–311, 2004.

Wakefield B, Mentes J, Diggelmann L et al: Monitoring hydration status in elderly veterans, *West J Nurs Res* 24(2):132, 2002.

Wotton K, Crannitch K, Munt R: Prevalence, risk factors and strategies to prevent dehydration in older adults, *Contemp Nurse* 31(1):44–56, 2008.

Young E, Sherrard-Jacob A, Knapp K et al: Perioperative fluid management, *AORN J* 89(1):167–178, 2009.

● = Independent ▲ = Collaborative **EBN** = Evidence-Based Nursing **EB** = Evidence-Based

Impaired Gas exchange   *Betty J. Ackley, MSN, EdS, RN*   ⊖volve

NANDA-I

Definition

Excess or deficit in oxygenation and/or carbon dioxide elimination at the alveolar-capillary membrane

Defining Characteristics

Abnormal arterial blood gases; abnormal arterial pH; abnormal breathing (e.g., rate, rhythm, depth); abnormal skin color (e.g., pale, dusky); confusion; cyanosis; decreased carbon dioxide; diaphoresis; dyspnea; headache upon awakening; hypercapnia; hypoxemia; hypoxia; irritability; nasal flaring; restlessness, somnolence; tachycardia; visual disturbances

Related Factors (r/t)

Ventilation-perfusion imbalance; alveolar-capillary membrane changes

NOC   **(Nursing Outcomes Classification)**

Suggested NOC Outcomes

Respiratory Status: Gas Exchange, Ventilation

Example **NOC** Outcome with Indicators
Achieves appropriate **Respiratory Status: Gas Exchange** as evidenced by the following indicators: Cognitive status/Partial pressure of oxygen/Partial pressure of carbon dioxide/Arterial pH/Oxygen saturation (Rate each indicator of **Respiratory Status:** 1 = severe deviation from normal range, 2 = substantial deviation from normal range, 3 = moderate deviation from normal range, 4 = mild deviation from normal range, 5 = no deviation from normal range [see Section I].)

Client Outcomes

Client Will (Specify Time Frame):

- Demonstrate improved ventilation and adequate oxygenation as evidenced by blood gas levels within normal parameters for that client
- Maintain clear lung fields and remain free of signs of respiratory distress
- Verbalize understanding of oxygen supplementation and other therapeutic interventions

NIC   **(Nursing Interventions Classification)**

Suggested NIC Interventions

Acid-Base Management, Airway Management

Example **NIC** Activities—Acid-Base Management
Monitor for symptoms of respiratory failure (e.g., low PaO_2 and elevated $PaCO_2$ levels and respiratory muscle fatigue); Monitor determinants of tissue oxygen delivery (e.g., PaO_2, SaO_2, and hemoglobin levels, and cardiac output) if available

Nursing Interventions and *Rationales*

- Monitor respiratory rate, depth, and ease of respiration. Watch for use of accessory muscles and nasal flaring. *Normal respiratory rate is 14 to 16 breaths/min in the adult (Bickley & Szilagyi, 2009).* **EBN:** *A study demonstrated that when the respiratory rate exceeds 30 breaths/min, along with other physiological measures, a significant cardiovascular or respiratory alteration exists (Considine, 2005; Hagle, 2008).*
- Auscultate breath sounds every 1 to 2 hours. The presence of crackles and wheezes may alert the nurse to airway obstruction, which may lead to or exacerbate existing hypoxia. *In severe exacerba-*

• = Independent   ▲ = Collaborative   **EBN** = Evidence-Based Nursing   **EB** = Evidence-Based

tions of chronic obstructive pulmonary disease (COPD), lung sounds may be diminished or distant with air trapping (Bickley & Szilagyi, 2009).

- Monitor the client's behavior and mental status for the onset of restlessness, agitation, confusion, and (in the late stages) extreme lethargy. *Changes in behavior and mental status can be early signs of impaired gas exchange (Simmons & Simmons, 2004). In the late stages the client becomes lethargic and somnolent.*

▲ Monitor oxygen saturation continuously using pulse oximetry. Note blood gas results as available. *An oxygen saturation of less than 90% (normal: 95% to 100%) or a partial pressure of oxygen of less than 80 mm Hg (normal: 80 to 100 mm Hg) indicates significant oxygenation problems (Clark, Giuliano, & Chen, 2006).*

- Observe for cyanosis of the skin; especially note color of the tongue and oral mucous membranes. *Central cyanosis of the tongue and oral mucosa is indicative of serious hypoxia and is a medical emergency. Peripheral cyanosis in the extremities may be due to activation of the central nervous system or exposure to cold and may or may not be serious (Bickley & Szilagyi, 2009).*

- Position clients in semi-Fowler's position, with an upright posture at 45 degrees if possible. **EB:** *Research done on clients on a ventilator demonstrated that being in a 45–degree upright position increased oxygenation and ventilation (Speelberg & Van Beers, 2003). Research on healthy subjects demonstrated that sitting upright resulted in higher tidal volumes and minute ventilation versus sitting in a slumped posture (Landers et al, 2003).*

- If the client has unilateral lung disease, alternate semi-Fowler's position in an upright posture with a lateral position (with 10– to 15–degree elevation and "good lung down" for 60 to 90 minutes). This method is contraindicated for clients with pulmonary abscess or hemorrhage or interstitial emphysema. *Gravity and hydrostatic pressure cause the dependent lung to become better ventilated and perfused, which increases oxygenation (Marklew, 2006).*

- If the client has bilateral lung disease, position the client in either semi-Fowler's or a side-lying position, which increases oxygenation as indicated by pulse oximetry (or, if the client has a pulmonary catheter, venous oxygen saturation).

▲ Turn the client every 2 hours. Monitor mixed venous oxygen saturation closely after turning. If it drops below 10% or fails to return to baseline promptly, turn the client back into the supine position and evaluate oxygen status. If the client does not tolerate turning, consider use of a kinetic bed that rotates the client from side to side in a turn of at least 40 degrees. **EBN:** *Use of the kinetic bed was shown to decrease development of atelectasis and ventilator associated pneumonia in critically ill clients (Ahrens et al, 2004).*

- If the client is acutely dyspneic, consider having the client lean forward over a bedside table, resting elbows on the table if tolerated. *Leaning forward can help decrease dyspnea, possibly because gastric pressure allows better contraction of the diaphragm (Langer et al, 2009). This is called the tripod position and is used during times of distress, including when walking, leaning forward on the walker.*

- Help the client deep breathe and perform controlled coughing. Have the client inhale deeply, hold the breath for several seconds, and cough two or three times with the mouth open while tightening the upper abdominal muscles as tolerated. *Controlled coughing uses the diaphragmatic muscles, which makes the cough more forceful and effective.* NOTE: If the client has excessive fluid in the respiratory system, see the interventions for **Ineffective Airway clearance**.

▲ Monitor the effects of sedation and analgesics on the client's respiratory pattern; use judiciously. *Both analgesics and medications that cause sedation can depress respiration at times. However, these medications can be very helpful for decreasing the sympathetic nervous system discharge that accompanies hypoxia.*

- Schedule nursing care to provide rest and minimize fatigue. *The hypoxic client has limited reserves; inappropriate activity can increase hypoxia.*

▲ Administer humidified oxygen through an appropriate device (e.g., nasal cannula or Venturi mask per the physician's order); aim for an oxygen (O_2) saturation level of 90% or above. Watch for onset of hypoventilation as evidenced by increased somnolence. *There is a fine line between ideal or excessive oxygen therapy; increasing somnolence is caused by retention of carbon dioxide (CO_2) leading to CO_2 narcosis (Simmons & Simmons, 2004; Wong & Elliott, 2009).*

- Assess nutritional status including serum albumin level and body mass index (BMI). *Weight loss in a client with COPD has a negative effect on the course of the disease; it can result in loss of muscle mass in the respiratory muscles, including the diaphragm, which can lead to respiratory failure (Celli & MacNee, 2004; Odencrants, Ehnfors, & Ehrenbert, 2008).*

- Assist the client to eat small meals frequently and use dietary supplements as necessary. For some clients, drinking 30 mL of a supplement such as Ensure or Pulmocare every hour while awake can be helpful.
- If the client is severely debilitated from chronic respiratory disease, consider the use of a wheeled walker to help in ambulation. **EB:** *Use of a wheeled walker has been shown to result in significant decrease in disability, hypoxemia, and breathlessness during a 6–minute walk test (Honeyman, Barr, & Stubbing, 1996).*
- ▲ Watch for signs of psychological distress including anxiety, agitation, and insomnia. Refer for counseling as needed. **EBN:** *One study demonstrated a clear association between hospitalization for COPD and psychological distress (Andenaes, Kalfoss, & Wahl, 2004).*
- ▲ Refer the COPD client to a pulmonary rehabilitation program. **EB:** *A Cochrane review demonstrated that pulmonary rehabilitation has been shown to relieve dyspnea and fatigue, help the clients deal with emotions, and enhance the clients' sense of control over the disease (Lacasse et al, 2006). Pulmonary rehabilitation is now considered a standard of care for the client with COPD (Nici et al, 2009).*

Critical Care

- ▲ If the client has adult respiratory distress syndrome with difficulty maintaining oxygenation, consider positioning the client prone with the upper thorax and pelvis supported, allowing the abdomen to protrude. Monitor oxygen saturation and turn back to supine position if desaturation occurs. **EBN and EB:** *Oxygenation levels have been shown to improve in the prone position, probably due to decreased shunting and better perfusion of the lungs (Vollman, 2004).* NOTE: If the client becomes ventilator dependent, see the care plan for **Impaired spontaneous Ventilation**.

Geriatric

- ▲ Use central nervous system (CNS) depressants carefully to avoid decreasing respiration rate. *An elderly client is prone to respiratory depression.*
- ▲ Maintain low-flow oxygen therapy. *An elderly client is susceptible to oxygen-induced respiratory depression.*

Home Care

- Work with the client to determine what strategies are most helpful during times of dyspnea. Educate and empower the client to self manage the disease associated with impaired gas exchange. **EBN and EB:** *A study found that use of oxygen, self-use of medication, and getting some fresh air were most helpful in dealing with dyspnea (Thomas, 2009). Evidence-based reviews have found that self-management offers COPD clients effective options for managing the illness, leading to more positive outcomes (Kaptein et al, 2008).*
- Assess the home environment for irritants that impair gas exchange. Help the client to adjust the home environment as necessary (e.g., install an air filter to decrease the level of dust).
- ▲ Refer the client to occupational therapy as necessary to assist the client in adaptation to the home and environment and in energy conservation.
- Assist the client with identifying and avoiding situations that exacerbate impairment of gas exchange (e.g., stress-related situations, exposure to pollution of any kind, proximity to noxious gas fumes such as chlorine bleach). *Irritants in the environment decrease the client's effectiveness in accessing oxygen during breathing.*
- Refer to GOLD and ACP-ASIM/ACCP guidelines for management of home care and indications of hospital admission criteria (Chojnowski, 2003).
- Instruct the client to keep the home temperature above 68° F (20° C) and to avoid cold weather. *Cold air temperatures cause constriction of the blood vessels, which impairs the client's ability to absorb oxygen.*

- Instruct the client to limit exposure to persons with respiratory infections. *Viruses, bacteria, and environmental pollutants are the main causes of exacerbations of COPD (Barnett, 2008).*
- Instruct the family in the complications of the disease and the importance of maintaining the medical regimen, including when to call a physician.
- ▲ Refer the client for home health aide services as necessary for assistance with activities of daily living. *Clients with decreased oxygenation have decreased energy to carry out personal and role-related activities.*
- When respiratory procedures are being implemented, explain equipment and procedures to family members, and provide needed emotional support. *Family members assuming responsibility for respiratory monitoring often find this stressful.*
- When electrically based equipment for respiratory support is being implemented, evaluate home environment for electrical safety, proper grounding, and so on. Ensure that notification is sent to the local utility company, the emergency medical team, and police and fire departments. *Notification is important to provide for priority service.*
- ▲ Assess family role changes and coping ability. Refer the client to medical social services as appropriate for assistance in adjusting to chronic illness. *Inability to maintain the level of social involvement experienced before illness leads to frustration and anger in the client and may create a threat to the family unit.*
- Support the family of the client with chronic illness. *Severely compromised respiratory functioning causes fear and anxiety in clients and their families. Reassurance from the nurse can be helpful.*

Client/Family Teaching and Discharge Planning

- Teach the client how to perform pursed-lip breathing and inspiratory muscle training, and how to use the tripod position. Have the client watch the pulse oximeter to note improvement in oxygenation with these breathing techniques. **EB:** *Studies have demonstrated that pursed-lip breathing was effective in decreasing breathlessness and improving respiratory function (Nield, Hoo, & Roper, 2007; Faager, Stahle, & Larsen, 2008). A systematic review found that inspiratory muscle training was effective in increasing endurance of the client and decreasing dyspnea (Langer et al, 2009).*
- Teach the client energy conservation techniques and the importance of alternating rest periods with activity. See nursing interventions for **Fatigue.**
- ▲ Teach the importance of not smoking. Refer to smoking cessation programs, and encourage clients who relapse to keep trying to quit. Ensure that client receives appropriate medications to support smoking cessation from the primary health care provider. **EB:** *A systemic review of research demonstrated that the combination of medications and an intensive, prolonged counseling program supporting smoking cessation were effective in promoting long-term abstinence from smoking (Fiore et al, 2008). A Cochrane review found that use of the medication varenicline (Chantix) increased the rate of smoking withdrawal two to three times more than smoking withdrawal without use of medications (Cahill, Stead, & Lancaster, 2008).*
- ▲ Instruct the family regarding home oxygen therapy if ordered (e.g., delivery system, liter flow, safety precautions). *Long-term oxygen therapy can improve survival, exercise ability, sleep and ability to think in hypoxemic clients. Client education improves compliance with prescribed use of oxygen (Celli & MacNee, 2004).*
- ▲ Teach the client the need to receive a yearly influenza vaccine. *Receiving a yearly influenza vaccine is helpful to prevent exacerbations of COPD (Black & McDonald, 2009).*
- Teach the client relaxation techniques to help reduce stress responses and panic attacks resulting from dyspnea. **EB:** *Relaxation therapy can help reduce dyspnea and anxiety (National Lung Health Education Program, 2007; Langer et al, 2009)*
- Teach the client to use music, along with a rest period, to decrease dyspnea and anxiety. **EBN:** *A study demonstrated that use of music along with a resting period were effective in relieving anxiety and exercise induced dyspnea in clients with COPD (Sidani et al, 2004).*

ⓔvolve   See the EVOLVE website for Weblinks for client education resources.

• = Independent   ▲ = Collaborative   **EBN** = Evidence-Based Nursing   **EB** = Evidence-Based

REFERENCES

Ahrens T, Kollef M, Stewart J et al: Effect of kinetic therapy on pulmonary complications, *Am J Crit Care* 13(5):376, 2004.

Andenaes R, Kalfoss MH, Wahl A: Psychological distress and quality of life in hospitalized patients with chronic obstructive pulmonary disease, *J Adv Nurs* 46(5):523, 2004.

Barnett M: Nursing management of chronic obstructive pulmonary disease, *Br J Nurs* 17(21):1314–1318, 2008.

Bickley LS, Szilagyi P: *Guide to physical examination*, ed 10, Philadelphia, 2009, Lippincott Williams & Wilkins.

Black PN, McDonald CF: Interventions to reduce the frequency of exacerbations of chronic obstructive pulmonary disease, *Postgrad Med J* 85(1001):141–147, 2009.

Cahill K, Stead LF, Lancaster T: Nicotine receptor partial agonists for smoking cessation, *Cochrane Database Syst Rev* (3):CD006103, 2008.

Celli BR, MacNee W, ATS/ERS Task Force: Standards for the diagnosis and treatment of patients with COPD: a summary of the ATS/ERS position paper, *Eur Respir J* 23(6):932, 2004.

Chojnowski D: "GOLD" standards for acute exacerbation in COPD, *Nurs Pract* 28(5):26, 2003.

Clark AP, Giuliano K, Chen HM: Pulse oximetry revisited: "but his O(2) sat was normal!", *Clin Nurse Spec* 20(6):268–272, 2006.

Considine J: The role of nurses in preventing adverse events related to respiratory dysfunction: literature review, *J Adv Nurs* 49(6):624–633, 2005.

Faager G, Ståhle A, Larsen FF: Influence of spontaneous pursed lips breathing on walking endurance and oxygen saturation in patients with moderate to severe chronic obstructive pulmonary disease, *Clin Rehabil* 22(8):675–683, 2008.

Fiore MC, Jaen CR, Baker TB et al: *Treating tobacco use and dependence clinical practice guideline, 2008 update*, Rockville MD: U.S. department of Health and Human Services, Public Health Service, 2008.

Hagle M: Vital signs monitoring. An EBP Guideline. In Ackley B, Ladwig, G, Swann BA et al, editors: *Evidence-based nursing care guidelines: medical-surgical interventions*, Philadelphia, 2008, Mosby.

Honeyman P, Barr P, Stubbing DG: Effect of a walking aid on disability, oxygenation, and breathlessness in patients with chronic airflow limitation, *J Cardiopulm Rehabil* 16(1):63–67, 1996.

Kaptein AA, Scharloo M, Fischer MJ et al: 50 years of psychological research on patients with COPD—road to ruin or highway to heaven? *Respir Med* 103:3–11, 2008.

Lacasse Y, Goldstein R, Lasserson TJ et al: Pulmonary rehabilitation for chronic obstructive pulmonary disease, *Cochrane Database Syst Rev* (4):CD003793, 2006.

Landers M, Barker G, Wallentine S et al: A comparison of tidal volume breathing frequency, and minute ventilation between two sitting postures in healthy adults, *Physiother Theory Pract* 19(2):109–119, 2003.

Langer D, Hendriks E, Burtin C et al: A clinical practice guideline for physiotherapists treating patients with chronic obstructive pulmonary disease based on a systematic review of available evidence. *Clinc Rehabil* 23(5):445–462, 2009.

Marklew A: Body positioning and its effect on oxygenation—a literature review, *Br Assoc Crit Care Nurs* 11(1):16–22, 2006.

National Lung Health Education Program: A breath of fresh air, *Consum Rep Hlth* 19(2):3–6, 2007.

Nici L, Raskin J, Rochester CL et al: Pulmonary rehabilitation: what we know and what we need to know, *J Cardiopulm Rehabil Prev* 29(3):141–151, 2009.

Nield MA, Hoo GWS, Roper JM: Efficacy of pursed-lips breathing: a breathing pattern retraining strategy for dyspnea reduction, *J Cardiopulm Rehabil Prev* 27(4):237–244, 2007.

Odencrants S, Ehnfors M, Ehrenbert A: Nutritional status and patient characteristics for hospitalized older patients with chronic obstructive pulmonary disease. *J Clin Nurs* 17(13):1771–1778, 2008.

Sidani S, Brooks D, Graydon J et al: Evaluating the effects of music on dyspnea and anxiety in patients with COPD: a process-outcome analysis, *Int Nurs Perspect* 4(1): 5–14, 2004.

Simmons P, Simmons M: Informed nursing practice: the administration of oxygen to patients with COPD, *Medsurg Nurs* 13(2):82–85, 2004.

Speelberg B, Van Beers F: Artificial ventilation in the semi-recumbent position improves oxygenation and gas exchange, *Chest* 124(4):S203, 2003.

Simmons P, Simmons M: Informed nursing practice: the administration of oxygen to patients with COPD, *Medsurg Nurs* 13(2):82–85, 2004

Thomas L: Effective dyspnea management strategies identified by elders with end-stage chronic obstructive pulmonary disease, *Appl Nurs Res* 22(2):79–85, 2009.

Vollman KM: Prone positioning in the patient who has acute respiratory distress syndrome: the art and science, *Crit Care Nurs Clin North Am* 16(3):319–336, 2004.

Wong M, Elliott M: The use of medical orders in acute care oxygen therapy, *Br J Nurs* 18(8):462–464, 2009.

Risk for unstable blood Glucose level   *Paula D. Hopper, MSN, RN*   ⊖volve

NANDA-I

Definition

Risk for variation of blood glucose/sugar levels from the normal range

Risk Factors

Deficient knowledge of diabetes management (e.g., action plan); developmental level; dietary intake; inadequate blood glucose monitoring; lack of acceptance of diagnosis; lack of adherence to diabetes management (e.g., action plan); lack of diabetes management; (e.g., action plan); medication management; mental health status; physical activity level; physical health status; pregnancy; rapid growth periods; stress; weight gain; weight loss

● = Independent   ▲ = Collaborative   **EBN** = Evidence-Based Nursing   **EB** = Evidence-Based

(Nursing Outcomes Classification)

Suggested NOC Outcome

Example NOC Outcome with Indicators
Blood Glucose Level as evidenced by the following indicators: Blood glucose/Glycosylated hemoglobin/Fructosamine/Urine glucose/Urine ketones (Rate the outcome and indicators of **Blood Glucose Level:** 1 = Severe deviation from normal range, 2 = substantial deviation from normal range, 3 = moderate deviation from normal range, 4 = mild deviation from normal range, 5 = no deviation from normal range [see Section I].)

Client Outcomes

Client Will (Specify Time Frame):

- Maintain A1C <7% (normal level 4% to 6%) (American Diabetes Association [ADA], 2009)
- Maintain goals higher than <7% in clients with a history of severe hypoglycemia or advanced diabetes complications (ADA, 2009)
- Maintain outpatient preprandial blood glucose between 70 and 130 mg/dL (ADA, 2009); consult primary care provider for client-specific goals
- Maintain outpatient postprandial glucose <180 mg/dL (ADA, 2009)
- In gestational diabetes, maintain preprandial blood glucose ≤95 mg/dL, 1-hour pc level ≤140 mg/dL, and 2-hour pc level ≤120 mg/dL (ADA, 2009)
- In critically ill hospitalized clients, maintain blood glucose between 140 and 180 mg/dL (Moghissi et al, 2009)
- In noncritically ill hospitalized clients, maintain pre-meal blood glucose values <140 mg/dL and random blood glucose values <180 mg/dL. Higher levels may be acceptable in terminally ill patients (Moghissi et al, 2009)
- Demonstrate how to accurately test blood glucose
- Identify self-care actions to take to maintain target glucose levels
- Identify self-care actions to take if blood glucose level is too low or too high
- Demonstrate correct administration of prescribed medications

NIC **(Nursing Interventions Classification)**

Suggested NIC Interventions

Hypoglycemia Management, Hyperglycemia Management

Example NIC Activities—Hypoglycemia Management
Monitor blood glucose levels, as indicated; Provide simple carbohydrate, as indicated

Nursing Interventions and *Rationales*

▲ Monitor blood glucose before meals and at bedtime. **EB:** *Clients using multiple insulin injections should do self-monitoring of blood glucose (SMBG) three or more times daily. SMBG is also useful as a guide to therapy in clients on less frequent injections (ADA, 2009).*

▲ Monitor blood glucose every 4 to 6 hours in clients who are NPO or who are continuously fed. *Testing every 4 to 6 hours is usually sufficient for determining correction insulin doses (ADA, 2009).*

▲ Monitor blood glucose hourly for clients on continuous insulin drips; may decrease to every 2 hours once stable. *Bedside monitoring can be done rapidly where therapeutic decisions are made (ADA, 2009).*

▲ Consider continuous glucose monitoring (CGM) in clients with type 1 diabetes on intensive insulin regimens. **EB:** *CGM use reduces time in hypo- and hyperglycemic ranges and may improve glycemic control. CGM monitors also have alarms to warn clients of high and low glucose levels (ADA, 2009).*

▲ Evaluate A1C level for glucose control over previous 2 to 3 months. *"All clients with diabetes admitted to the hospital should have an A1C obtained for discharge planning if the result of testing in the previous 2 to 3 months is not available" (ADA, 2009).*

• = Independent   ▲ = Collaborative   **EBN** = Evidence-Based Nursing   **EB** = Evidence-Based

- Consider postmeal blood glucose monitoring. *Postmeal monitoring may be necessary to achieve postmeal targets (ADA, 2009).*
- Evaluate blood glucose levels in hospitalized clients prior to administering oral hypoglycemic agents or insulin. *Adjust timing of medication appropriately with meal times. Inappropriately timed insulin can result in hypoglycemia (ADA, 2009).*
- Monitor for signs and symptoms of hypoglycemia. *Rapidly falling blood glucose can cause sympathetic symptoms such as anxiety, dizziness, diaphoresis, tachycardia, headache, tremor, or hunger. Confusion, irritability, lethargy, or behavior changes may signal low glucose in the central nervous system, which can lead to coma if not treated. Early recognition and treatment of falling glucose can prevent more severe hypoglycemia (Tomky, 2005).*
- Be alert to hypoglycemia in clients with or without diabetes who also have heart failure, renal or liver disease, malignancy, infection, sepsis, sudden reduction of corticosteroids, altered ability to self-report symptoms, altered nutritional intake, emesis, new NPO status, or altered consciousness. *Clients may develop hypoglycemia in relation to these conditions (ADA, 2009).*
- ▲ If client is experiencing signs and symptoms of hypoglycemia, test glucose and if result is below 70 mg/dL, administer 15 to 20 g glucose (½ cup fruit juice or regular [not diet] soda, 1 cup milk, 1 small piece of fruit, or 3 to 4 glucose tablets). Pure glucose is the preferred treatment, but any form of carbohydrate that contains glucose will suffice. Avoid treating with foods that contain fat. Repeat test in 15 minutes and repeat treatment if indicated. *"Hypoglycemia responds best to glucose-containing foods; added fat may slow the response" (ADA, 2009). "The use of nurse-driven hypoglycemia protocol for any BG levels <70 mg/dL can prevent deterioration of potentially mild events . . . to more severe events" (Moghissi et al, 2009).*
- ▲ Administer intravenous 50% dextrose or intramuscular glucagon according to agency protocol if client is hypoglycemic and is unable to take oral carbohydrate. *Intravenous (IV) bolus of 50% dextrose or intramuscular glucagon are alternatives to oral carbohydrate (Tomky, 2005).*
- Monitor for signs and symptoms of hyperglycemia, such as polydipsia, polyuria, and polyphagia. *Early recognition and treatment of hyperglycemia can prevent progression to ketoacidosis or hyperosmolar hyperglycemia (ADA, 2004).*
- ▲ Test urine for ketones during acute illness or stress, or when blood glucose levels are >300 mg/dL. *"The presence of ketones may indicate impending or even established ketoacidosis, a condition that requires immediate medical attention" (ADA, 2004).*
- ▲ If client is acutely ill, continue insulin and oral hypoglycemic agents and frequent monitoring. Ensure client is receiving adequate fluids and carbohydrates. **EB:** *"Acute illnesses can lead to the development of hyperglycemia and, in individuals with type 1 diabetes, ketoacidosis. During acute illnesses, with the usual increases in counterregulatory hormones, the need for insulin and oral glucose-lowering medications continues and often is increased. Testing plasma glucose and ketones, drinking adequate amounts of fluid, and ingesting carbohydrates, especially if plasma glucose is <100 mg/dL, are all important during acute illness. In adults, ingestion of 150 to 200 g carbohydrate daily (45–50 g every 3–4 h) should be sufficient to prevent starvation ketosis" (ADA, 2007).*
- ▲ Prime IV tubing with 20 mL IV diluted intravenous insulin solution before initiating insulin drip. *Glucose adsorbs to IV tubing; priming with 20 mL is enough to minimize this effect (Goldberg et al, 2006).*
- ▲ Evaluate client's medication regimen for medications that can alter blood glucose. *Some antipsychotic agents, diuretics, and glucocorticoids, among others, can cause hyperglycemia. Alcohol, aspirin, and beta blockers are among agents that can cause hypoglycemia (Diabetes in Control, 2005).*
- ▲ Refer client to dietitian for carbohydrate counting instruction. **EB:** *"Monitoring carbohydrate, whether by carbohydrate counting, exchanges, or experience-based estimation remains a key strategy in achieving glycemic control" (ADA, 2009).*
- ▲ Refer overweight clients to dietitian for weight loss counseling. **EB:** *"In overweight and obese insulin-resistant individuals, modest weight loss has been shown to improve insulin resistance" (ADA, 2009).*
- ▲ Refer client with prediabetes for diet and exercise counseling. **EBN:** *"Metaanalysis showed that exercise plus diet decreased incidence of type 2 diabetes and improved fasting glucose and triglyceride concentrations, blood pressure, body weight, body mass index, and waist circumference compared with standard recommendations" (Carrier, 2009).*

• = Independent   ▲ = Collaborative   **EBN** = Evidence-Based Nursing   **EB** = Evidence-Based

Geriatric

- Assess possible barriers to following nutrition recommendations: food preferences, ability to prepare meals, dentition, swallowing problems, decreased appetite or thirst sensation, use of taste-altering medications, limited finances, and social isolation. *An individual nutrition plan can minimize barriers in nutrition management and facilitate changes in eating behavior that will result in improved clinical outcomes, improved function, and enhanced quality of life (Suhl & Bonsignore, 2006).*
- Assess for age-related cognitive changes that can impair self-management of diabetes. **EB:** *Some studies suggest that deficits in cognitive functions are associated with poorer glycemic control (Awad, Gagnon, & Messier, 2004).*
- Assess for vision and dexterity impairments that may affect the older client's ability to accurately measure insulin doses. *Medication therapy can present a challenge due to possible visual and dexterity impairments (Haas, 2006).*
- Teach client and family caregiver to recognize signs and symptoms of hyperosmolar hyperglycemia. *"Adequate supervision and help from staff or family may prevent many of the admissions for HHS due to dehydration among elderly individuals who are unable to recognize or treat this evolving condition" (ADA, 2007).*
- Assist client to set up pill boxes or reminder system for taking medications. *Therapy may involve many medications and can become confusing (Haas, 2006).*

Pediatric

- Ensure that daycare or school personnel are trained in diabetes management and treatment of emergencies. *"Knowledgeable trained personnel are essential if the student is to avoid the immediate health risks of low blood glucose and to achieve the metabolic control required to decrease risks for later development of diabetes complications" (ADA, 2007).*
- Be aware that young children (<6 or 7 years) may not be aware of symptoms of hypoglycemia. *Counterregulatory mechanisms are immature and may not cause hypoglycemia symptoms; also, children may not recognize symptoms (ADA, 2007).*

Home Care

- ▲ Teach family how to use an emergency glucagon kit (if prescribed). *Severe hypoglycemia in which client is unable to take oral glucose should be treated with glucagon (ADA, 2009).*

Client Education and Discharge Planning

- Provide "survival skills" education for hospitalized clients, including information about: (1) diabetes and its treatment, (2) medication administration, (3) nutrition therapy, (4) self-monitoring of blood glucose, (5) symptoms and treatment of hypoglycemia, (6) basic foot care, and (7) follow-up appointments for in-depth training. *Clients need enough information to be safely discharged, and can then be followed up with outpatient instruction (Nettles, 2005).*
- Educate clients on self-monitoring of blood glucose. **EB:** *A systematic review found that self-monitoring of blood glucose is an effective tool in the self-management of glucose levels in clients using insulin therapy. Clients can use the glucose values to adjust their insulin doses. Clients with type 2 diabetes who are not using insulin can use glucose values to adjust diet and lifestyle (Welschen et al, 2005).*
- Evaluate clients' monitoring technique initially at regular intervals. *Accuracy of SMBG is instrument- and user-dependent (ADA, 2009).*
- ▲ Refer client to a diabetes treatment and teaching program (DTTP) for training in flexible intensive insulin therapy and dietary freedom. Most large hospitals or medical centers offer such programs. *Type 1 clients at risk for severe hypoglycemia or ketoacidosis experienced fewer incidents of severe hypoglycemia and ketoacidosis, fewer hospital days, and improved A1C after DTTP (Samann et al, 2006).*
- ▲ Refer client for Blood Glucose Awareness Training (BGAT) for instruction in detection, anticipation, avoidance, and treatment of extremes in blood glucose levels. **EB:** *BGAT has been shown to significantly reduce both hypoglycemia and hyperglycemia (Cox et al, 2006).*

• = Independent   ▲ = Collaborative   **EBN** = Evidence-Based Nursing   **EB** = Evidence-Based

- Teach client to maintain a blood glucose diary. *A diary can help clients learn to associate symptoms with actual glucose readings, as well as guide treatment (Cox, 2006).*
- Provide group-based training programs for instruction. **EB:** *Adults with type 2 diabetes who participate in group-based training programs have improved fasting blood glucose and A1C levels (Deakin et al, 2005).*
- Teach client the benefits of regular adherence to prescribed exercise regimen. **EB:** *A systematic review found that "exercise significantly improves glycemic control and reduces visceral adipose tissue and plasma triglycerides, but not plasma cholesterol, in people with type 2 diabetes, even without weight loss" (Thomas, Elliott, & Naughton, 2006).* **EB:** *At least 150 min/week of moderate intensity aerobic physical activity improves blood glucose control, helps with weight loss, reduces risk of CVD, and improves well-being (ADA, 2009).*
- Teach client with type 1 diabetes to avoid vigorous activity if ketones are present in urine or blood. *Exercise can worsen hyperglycemia and ketosis in people deprived of insulin for 12 to 48 hours (ADA, 2009).*
- Teach clients who are treated with insulin or insulin-stimulating oral agents to eat added carbohydrates prior to exercise if glucose levels are <100 mg/dL. *Physical activity can cause hypoglycemia; hypoglycemia is rare in clients who are not taking insulin or insulin-stimulating agents (ADA, 2009). Forty grams of glucose taken 15 minutes before exercise can prevent hypoglycemia in a client engaging in 60 minutes of moderate exercise (Dube et al, 2005).*
- Provide culturally appropriate diabetes health education. **EB:** *A systematic review found that health education "specifically tailored to the cultural needs of a target minority group" improved knowledge level and glucose control in clients with type 2 diabetes (Hawthorne et al, 2008).*
- Teach client that stopping insulin therapy can lead to hyperglycemic crisis (ketoacidosis or hyperosmolar hyperglycemia). Ensure client has resources to purchase insulin. *"Stopping insulin is a common precipitant of DKA in African Americans. . ." (ADA, 2004).*
- Educate client about the benefits of smoking cessation. **EB:** *"Smoking has been linked to worsening diabetes control and insulin resistance and may even induce diabetes" (Foy et al, 2005).*

⊖volve   See the Evolve website for Weblinks for client education resources.

REFERENCES

American Diabetes Association (ADA): 2004 Clinical Practice Recommendations, *Diabetes Care* 27(Suppl 1), 2004.

American Diabetes Association (ADA: 2007 Clinical Practice Recommendations, *Diabetes Care* 30(Suppl 1), 2007.

American Diabetes Association (ADA): 2009 Clinical Practice Recommendations, *Diabetes Care* 32(Suppl 1), 2009.

Awad N, Gagnon M, Messier C: The relationship between impaired glucose tolerance, type 2 diabetes, and cognitive function, *J Clin Exp Neuropsychol* 26(8):1044–80, 2004.

Carrier J: Review: exercise plus diet prevents type 2 diabetes, *Evid Based Nurs* 12(1):11, 2009.

Cox DJ, Gonder-Frederick L, Ritterband L et al: Blood glucose awareness training: what is it, where is it, and where is it going? *Diabetes Spectr* 19(1):43–49, 2006.

Deakin T, McShane CE, Cade JE et al: Group-based training for self-management strategies in people with type 2 diabetes mellitus, *Cochrane Database Syst Rev* (2):CD003417, 2005.

Diabetes in Control: Drugs that may affect glucose levels, *Diabetes in Control Newsletter*, Issue 246, February 9, 2005. www.diabetesincontrol.com/issues/issue246/drugs.pdf. Accessed June 8, 2009.

Dube M, Weisnagel S, Prodhomme D et al: Exercise and newer insulins: how much glucose supplement to avoid hypoglycemia? *Med Sci Sports Exerc* 37(8):1276–1282, 2005.

Foy CG, Bell RA, Farmer DF et al: Smoking and the incidence of diabetes amongst US adults: findings from the Insulin Resistance Atherosclerosis Study, *Diabetes Care* 28(1):2501–2507, 2005.

Goldberg PA, Kedves A, Walter K et al: "Waste not, want not": determining the optimal priming volume for intravenous insulin infusions, *Diabetes Technol Ther* 8(5):598–601, 2006.

Haas L: Caring for community-dwelling older adults with diabetes: perspectives from health care providers and caregivers, *Diabetes Spectr* 19(4):240–244, 2006.

Hawthorne K, Robles Y, Cannings-John R et al: Culturally appropriate health education for type 2 diabetes mellitus in ethnic minority groups, *Cochrane Database Syst Rev* (3):CD006424, 2008.

Moghissi ES, Korytkowski MT, DiNardo M et al: American Association of Clinical Endocrinologists and American Diabetes Association consensus statement on inpatient glycemic control, *Endocr Pract* 15(4):353–369, 2009.

Nettles A: Patient education in the hospital, *Diabetes Spectr* 18(1):44–48, 2005.

Samann A, Muhlhauser I, Bender R et al: Flexible intensive insulin therapy in adults with type 1 diabetes and high risk for severe hypoglycemia and diabetic ketoacidosis, *Diabetes Care* 29(10):2196–2199, 2006.

Suhl E, Bonsignore P: Diabetes self-management education for older adults: general principles and practical application, *Diabetes Spectr* 19(4):234–250, 2006.

Thomas DE, Elliott EJ, Naughton GA. Exercise for type 2 diabetes mellitus, *Cochrane Database Syst Rev* (3):CD002968, 2006.

Tomky D: Detection, prevention, and treatment of hypoglycemia in the hospital, *Diabetes Spectr* 18(1):39–44, 2005.

Welschen LMC, Bloemendal E, Nijpels G et al: Self-monitoring of blood glucose in patients with type 2 diabetes mellitus who are not using insulin, *Cochrane Database Syst Rev* (2):CD005060, 2005.

● = Independent   ▲ = Collaborative   **EBN** = Evidence-Based Nursing   **EB** = Evidence-Based

Grieving   *Gail B. Ladwig, MSN, RN, CHTP*

Definition

A normal, complex process that includes emotional, physical, spiritual, social, and intellectual responses and behaviors by which individuals, families, and communities incorporate an actual, anticipated, or perceived loss into their daily lives

Defining Characteristics

Alteration in activity level; alterations in dream patterns; alterations in immune function; alterations in neuroendocrine function; alteration in sleep patterns; anger; blame; detachment; despair; disorganization; experiencing relief; maintaining connection to the deceased; making meaning of the loss; pain; panic behavior; personal growth; psychological distress; suffering

Related Factors (r/t)

Anticipatory loss of significant object (e.g., possession, job, status, home, parts and processes of body); anticipatory loss of a significant other; death of a significant other; loss of significant object (e.g., possession, job, status, home, parts and processes of body)

NOC   (Nursing Outcomes Classification)

Suggested NOC Outcomes

Family Resiliency, Dignified Life Closure, Grief Resolution, Hope, Psychosocial Adjustment: Life Change

> ### Example NOC Outcome with Indicators
>
> **Grief Resolution** as evidenced by the following indicators: Resolves feelings about the loss/Verbalizes reality and acceptance of loss/Maintains living environment/Seeks social support: Rate the outcome and indicators of **Grief Resolution:** 1 = never demonstrated, 2 = rarely demonstrated, 3 = sometimes demonstrated, 4 = often demonstrated, 5 = consistently demonstrated [see Section I].)

Client/Family Outcomes

Client/Family Will (Specify Time Frame):

- Discuss meaning of the loss to his/her life and the functioning of the family
- Identify ways to support family members and articulate methods of support he or she requires from family and friends
- Utilize effective conflict management strategies
- Accept assistance in meeting the needs of the family from friends/extended family

NIC   (Nursing Interventions Classification)

Suggested NIC Interventions

Family Integrity Promotion, Dying Care, Emotional Support, Grief Work Facilitation: Perinatal Death, Hope Installation, Support System Enhancement

> ### Example NIC Activities—Grief Work Facilitation
>
> Identify the loss; Encourage expression of feelings about the loss; Assist to identify personal coping strategies; Identify sources of community support

Nursing Interventions and *Rationales*

- Concentrate on improving communication and providing an environment in which families can physically touch and care for their seriously ill loved one as much as possible. **EBN:** *Caregivers play*

 = Independent   ▲ = Collaborative   **EBN** = Evidence-Based Nursing   **EB** = Evidence-Based

an important role in the dying experience; these interventions have been identified in research studies as ways that improve the death experience for loved ones (Kruse, 2004). **EB:** *Communication within the family has been shown to be a major predictor of grief because it is an important component in the ability to share grief and express feelings about the loss in a supportive environment (Traylor et al, 2003).*

- Focus on enhancing the individual coping skills of the person's grieving to alleviate life problems and distressing symptoms. **EB:** *This study identified the uniqueness of the griever, recognized there are multiple factors that influence the grieving process (i.e., culture, personality, and gender), that most bereaved individuals use both cognitive and affective strategies in adapting to bereavement, and that bereaved individuals experience both internal and external pressures to grieve in particular ways (Doughty, 2009). This study suggests that men and women respond differently to bereavement groups and require interventions to address their particular needs (Maruyama & Atencio, 2008).*

- Provide interventions for bereaved persons that specifically attempt to enhance positive emotions. **EB:** *This study of 292 recently widowed men (39%) and women (61%) age 50 and over examined both the perceived importance of and actual experience of having positive emotions in their daily lives and how they might impact bereavement adjustments. Most of the bereaved spouses rated humor and happiness as being very important in their daily lives. Experiencing humor, laughter, and happiness was strongly associated with favorable bereavement adjustments (lower grief and depression) (Lund et al, 2008–2009).*

- Understand and support the family's expression of pain in its own way and in its own time. Encourage the family to create quiet and comfortable healing environments. **EBN:** *Especially when faced with traumatic grief, such as related to suicide or unexpected and/or violent death, intense emotional responses need to be accepted as appropriate and healthy responses to catastrophic loss (Kalischuk & Hayes, 2004).*

- Encourage the family to follow comforting grief rituals such as interacting with nature, lighting votive candles, saying a prayer, or whatever ritual brings spiritual comfort in dealing with the loss. *These traditional methods of grieving can help the family find meaning in the loss (Eisenhandler, 2004).*

- ▲ Refer the family members for spiritual counseling if desired. **EB:** *Getting in touch with their spirituality may help clients cope more effectively with the psychological and emotional effects of cancer. Researchers have found a striking correlation between good spiritual health and good physical health. Spiritual well-being may improve the quality of life in clients (Wess, 2007).*

- Help the family determine the best way and place to find social support. Encourage family members to continue to use supports for 1 to 2 years. **EB:** *Social support has been shown to help bereaved individuals as they reconstruct their lives and find new meaning in life (Hogan, Worden, & Schmidt, 2004). Web memorials may be one method of enabling family support across distance and time (Nager & deVries, 2004).*

- Identify available community resources, including bereavement groups at local hospitals and hospice centers. Volunteers who provide bereavement support can also be effective. **EB and EBN:** *Social support has been shown to help bereaved individuals as they reconstruct their lives and find new meaning in life (Hogan, Worden, & Schmidt, 2004). Web memorials may be one method of enabling family support across distance and time (Nager & deVries, 2004).* **EBN:** *Psychoeducational group activity and self-assessment caused suicide rates to decrease among elderly women in a Japanese culturally sensitive intervention study (Oyama et al, 2005).*

Pediatric/Parent

- Treat the child with respect, give him or her the opportunity to talk about concerns, and answer questions honestly. *Children know much more than many adults realize. They generally know if a parent or loved one is dying and/or the cause of death, even if they have not been told (Schuurman, 2002).*

- Listen to the child's expression of grief. *The best thing to help children is to listen to them with our ears, eyes, hearts, and souls and recognize that we do not have to have answers (Schuurman, 2002).*

- Consider giving the child a "memory bag" to have after experiencing a sudden death; contents include a teddy bear, a coloring book on working through grief for different ages, a journal for children to write in, and crayons. *The memory bags give children permission to grieve and feel the loss they experience so deeply (Foley, 2004).*

- Help parents recognize that the child does not have to be "fixed"; instead he or she needs support going through an experience of grieving just as adults do. *The role of the nurse, parent, and friends is to support and assist, not help a child "get over it" (Schuurman, 2002).*

▲ Refer grieving children and parents to a program to help facilitate grieving if desired, especially if the death was traumatic. **EB:** *Treatment for children and parents with grief associated with trauma helps decrease symptoms of posttraumatic stress disorder (PTSD) (Cohen, Mannarino, & Knudsen, 2004).* **EBN:** *A program desired for grieving children involving riding horses was shown to increase self-confidence and self-esteem (Glazer, Clark, & Stein, 2004).* **EB:** *This study supported the use of Orff-based music therapy interventions for bereaved children in a school-based grief program (Hilliard, 2007).*

- Help the adolescent determine sources of support and how to use them effectively. **EBN:** *In a study of adolescents dealing with the death of a loved one, the most important factors that helped adolescents cope with the grief were self-help and support from parents, relatives, and friends (Rask, Kaunonen, & Paunonen-Ilmonen, 2002).*

▲ Encourage parents to seek mental health services as needed, learn stress reduction, and take good care of their health. *The loss of a child for a mother results in an increased loss of life within 18 years either from disease or suicide (Lawson, 2003).* **EBN:** *A study analyzing the grief and coping of mothers who had lost children younger than 7 years found that the spouse, remaining children, grandparents, next of kin, friends, and colleagues were the main sources of support (Laakso & Paunonen-Ilmonen, 2002).* **EB:** *The death of a child is a traumatic event that can have long-term effects on the lives of parents (Rogers et al, 2008).*

Geriatric

- Monitor an older adult who has been treated for bereavement-related depression for relapse or recurrence. **EB:** *Loss of a significant other can trigger ineffective coping mechanisms that can require intervention from medication to hospitalization for behavior modification (Davies, 2001).*

▲ Use reminiscence therapy in conjunction with the expression of emotions. Refer to a reminiscence group if available. **EBN and EB:** *Two studies demonstrated that participation in a reminiscence group reduced symptoms of depression (Jones, 2003; Zauszniewski et al, 2004).*

- Provide support for the family when the loss is associated with dementia of the family member. **EB:** *In this study; 44 spouses and adult children who were caregivers of persons with Alzheimer's disease and related dementias (ADRD) scored high on the Marwit and Meuser Caregiver Grief Inventory. Coping strategies used by this group of caregivers included spiritual faith, social supports, and pets. Caregivers with high levels of grief may benefit from supportive interventions and interventions that facilitate building a supportive network (Sanders et al, 2008).*

Multicultural

- See interventions and rationales in care plans for **Complicated Grieving** and **Chronic Sorrow**.
- Assess the influence of cultural beliefs, norms, and values on the client's grief and mourning practices. **EBN:** *Grief and mourning practices may be based on cultural conventions (Clements et al, 2004).*
- Empathy may be especially important in caring for women with pregnancy loss who live in patrilineal cultures in which producing children is a critical role for women. *Use of narrative therapy may support in empowering mothers and assist them in moving forward (Hsu et al, 2003).*
- Validate the client's feelings regarding the loss. **EBN:** *Clients who were from an ethnic minority group were significantly more likely to report that interviews about death, dying, and bereavement were helpful (Emanuel et al, 2004). Storytelling was at the heart of every African American widow's description of her bereavement experience (Rodgers, 2004).*
- Teach clients to recognize grief responses. **EBN:** *Recognition of grief patterns allows clients to manage their responses more effectively and may prevent adverse outcomes to their physical and mental health (Van & Meleis, 2003).*

Home Care

NOTE: **Grieving** may be encountered as the client comes to terms with his or her own loss or death, or as the family reacts to the client's death.

- The interventions previously described may be adapted for home care use.
- Actively listen as the client grieves for his or her own death or for real or perceived loss. Normalize the client's expressions of grief for himself or herself. Demonstrate a caring and hopeful approach. **EBN:** *Caring for and with the client and projecting hopefulness have been shown to inspire hope in bereavement counseling (Cutcliffe, 2004).*
- ▲ Refer the client to medical social services as necessary for losses not related to death. *Support is helpful to grief work for all types of losses. Social workers can help the client plan for financial changes as a result of job losses and help with community referrals as appropriate.*
- ▲ Refer the bereaved to hospice bereavement programs. *Relief of the suffering of clients and families (physical, emotional, and spiritual) is the goal of hospice care (Krisman-Scott & McCorkle, 2002).*
- ▲ Refer the bereaved spouse to an Internet self-help group if desired. *Palliative home care resources include a number of available websites (Smith-Stoner & Oliver, 2003). An Internet-based self-help group can assist the bereaved spouse in coping, receiving support, developing a sense of family, sharing information, and helping others (Bacon, Condon, & Fernsler, 2000). Hospice provides interdisciplinary end-of-life care including the use of the Internet (McKay, 2008).*
- Assess caregiver reaction to bereavement issues and caregiver burden. Suggest preventive intervention for potential bereavement maladjustment if indicated. **EB:** *Bereavement maladjustment is more likely with caregivers who are older than 61 years, who perceive a substantial emotional burden, and who have been unable to continue working. Preventive interventions could reduce health and social costs (Rossi Ferrario et al, 2004).*
- Modify expectations of the family's response according to the degree of anticipation of the loved one's death. *If the loved one died at an old age or of a natural cause, the family most likely has anticipated the loss; the current reaction may be less than expected. If the loved one died of accidental or criminal causes, the grief reaction may be magnified. Grief may be prolonged, and a referral for supportive counseling is more likely to be needed.*
- ▲ After loss of a pregnancy, encourage the client and family to follow through on a counseling referral. **EBN and EB:** *Parents with a history of perinatal loss are at higher risk for depressive symptoms and pregnancy-specific anxiety during subsequent pregnancies, particularly before the third trimester. Nurses need to be alert to mothers' reactions during this trauma, as they often must overcome self-blame (Armstrong, 2002; Hsu et al, 2003).*

⊖volve   See the EVOLVE website for Weblinks for client education resources.

REFERENCES

Armstrong DS: Emotional distress and prenatal attachment in pregnancy after perinatal loss, *J Nurs Scholarsh* 34:339–345, 2002.

Bacon ES, Condon EH, Fernsler JI: Young widows' experience with an Internet self-help group, *J Psychosoc Nurs Ment Health Serv* 38(7):24–33, 2000.

Clements PT, DeRanieri JT, Vigil GJ et al: Life after death: grief therapy after the sudden traumatic death of a family member, *Perspect Psychiatr Care* 40(4):149–154, 2004.

Cohen JA, Mannarino AP, Knudsen K: Treating childhood traumatic grief: a pilot study, *J Am Acad Child Adolesc Psychiatry* 43(10):1225–1233, 2004.

Cutcliffe JR: The inspiration of hope in bereavement counseling, *Issues Ment Health Nurs* 25(2):165–190, 2004.

Davies B: Supporting families in palliative care. In Ferrell BF, Coyle N, editors: *Textbook of palliative care nursing*, New York, 2001, Oxford University.

Doughty EA: Investigating adaptive grieving styles: a Delphi study, *Death Stud* 33(5):462–480, 2009.

Eisenhandler SA: The arts of consolation: commemoration and folkways of faith, *Generations* 28(2):37, 2004.

Emanuel EJ, Fairclough DL, Wolfe P et al: Talking with terminally ill patients and their caregivers about death, dying, and bereavement: is it stressful? Is it helpful? *Arch Intern Med* 164(18):1999–2004, 2004.

Foley T: Encouraging the inclusion of children in grief after a sudden death: memory bags, *J Emerg Nurs* 30(4):341–342, 2004.

Glazer HR, Clark MD, Stein DS: The impact of hippotherapy on grieving children, *J Hospic Palliat Nurs* 6(3):171–175, 2004.

Hilliard RE: The effects of Orff-based music therapy and social work groups on childhood grief symptoms and behaviors, *J Music Ther* 44(2):123–138, 2007.

Hogan N, Worden JW, Schmidt L: An empirical study of the proposed complicated grief disorder criteria, *Omega (Westport)* 48(3):263–277, 2004.

Hsu MT, Tseng YF, Banks J et al: Interpretations of stillbirth, *J Adv Nurs* 47(4):408–416, 2003.

Jones ED: Reminiscence therapy for older women with depression. Effects of nursing intervention classification in assisted-living long-term care, *J Gerontol Nurs* 29(7):26–33, 2003.

Kalischuk R, Hayes V: Grieving, mourning, and healing following youth suicide: a focus on health and well-being in families, *Omega (Westport)* 48(1):45–67, 2004.

Krisman-Scott MA, McCorkle R: The tapestry of hospice, *Holist Nurs Pract* 16(2):32–39, 2002.

• = Independent   ▲ = Collaborative   **EBN** = Evidence-Based Nursing   **EB** = Evidence-Based

Kruse B: The meaning of letting go: the lived experience for caregivers of persons at the end of life, *J Hospice Palliat Nurs* 6(4):215–222, 2004.

Laakso H, Paunonen-Ilmonen M: Mothers' experience of social support following the death of a child, *J Clin Nurs* 11(2):176–185, 2002.

Lawson W: Grieving mothers suffer early deaths, *Psychol Today* 36(3):18, 2003.

Lund D, Utz R, Caserta M et al: Humor, laughter & happiness in the daily lives of recently bereaved spouses, *Omega (Westport)* 58(2):87–105, 2008–2009.

Maruyama NC, Atencio CV: Evaluating a bereavement support group, *Palliat Support Care,* 6(1):43–49, 2008.

McKay B: Internet resources for hospice and bereavement, *Med Ref Serv Q* 27(2):199–210, 2008.

Nager E, deVries B: Memorializing on the World Wide Web: patterns of grief and attachment in adult daughters of deceased mothers, *Death Stud* 49(1):43–56, 2004.

Oyama H, Watanabe N, Ono Y et al: Community-based suicide prevention through group activity for the elderly successfully reduced the high suicide rate for females, *Psychiatr Clin Neurosci* 59(3):337–344, 2005.

Rask K, Kaunonen M, Paunonen-Ilmonen M: Adolescent coping with grief after the death of a loved one, *Int J Nurs Pract* 8(3):137–142, 2002.

Rodgers LS: Meaning of bereavement among older African American widows, *Geriatr Nurs* 25(1):10–16, 2004.

Rogers CH, Floyd FJ, Seltzer MM et al: Long-term effects of the death of a child on parents' adjustment in midlife, *J Fam Psychol* 22(2):203–211, 2008.

Rossi Ferrario S, Cardillo V, Vicario F et al: Advanced cancer at home: caregiving and bereavement, *Palliative Med* 18:129–136, 2004.

Sanders S, Ott CH, Kelber ST et al: The experience of high levels of grief in caregivers of persons with Alzheimer's disease and related dementia, *Death Stud* 32(6):495–523, 2008.

Schuurman DL: *The club no one wants to join: a dozen lessons I've learned from grieving children and adolescents,* Centre for Grief Education, 2002. www.grief.org.au/child_support.html. Accessed March 7, 2005.

Smith-Stoner M, Oliver M: Ten palliative home care resources, *Home Healthc Nurs* 21(11):731–733, 2003.

Traylor E, Hayslip B, Kaminski P et al: Relationships between grief and family system characteristics: a cross lagged longitudinal analysis, *Death Stud* 27:575–601, 2003.

Van P, Meleis AI: Coping with grief after involuntary pregnancy loss: perspectives of African American women, *J Obstet Gynecol Neonatal Nurs* 32(1):28–39, 2003.

Wess M: Bringing hope and healing to grieving patients with cancer, *J Am Osteopath Assoc* 107(12 Suppl 7):ES41–ES47, 2007.

Zauszniewski JA, Eggenschwiler K, Preechawong S et al: Focused reflection reminiscence group for elders: implementation and evaluation, *Appl Gerontol* 23(4):429, 2004.

Complicated Grieving   *Gail B. Ladwig, MSN, RN, CHTP*

NANDA-I

Definition

A disorder that occurs after the death of a significant other in which the experience of distress accompanying bereavement fails to follow normative expectations and manifests in functional impairment

Defining Characteristics

Decreased functioning in life roles; decreased sense of well-being; depression; experiencing somatic symptoms of the deceased; fatigue; grief avoidance; longing for the deceased; low levels of intimacy; persistent emotional distress; preoccupation with thoughts of the deceased; rumination; searching for the deceased; self-blame; separation distress; traumatic distress; verbalizes anxiety; verbalizes distressful feelings about the deceased; verbalizes feeling dazed; verbalizes feeling empty; verbalizes feeling in shock; verbalizes feeling stunned; verbalizes feelings of anger; verbalizes feelings of detachment from others; verbalizes feelings of disbelief; verbalizes feelings of mistrust; verbalizes lack of acceptance of the death; verbalizes persistent painful memories; verbalizes self-blame; yearning

Related Factors (r/t)

Death of a significant other; emotional instability; lack of social support; sudden death of a significant other

NOC   (Nursing Outcomes Classification)

Suggested NOC Outcomes

Anxiety Level, Coping, Depression, Grief Resolution, Mood Equilibrium, Personal Well-Being, Psychosocial Adjustment: Life Change, Sleep

Example NOC Outcome with Indicators
See care plan for **Grieving**.

Client Outcomes

Client Will (Specify Time Frame):

- Express appropriate feelings of guilt, fear, anger, or sadness
- Identify somatic distress associated with grief (e.g., anxiety, changes in appetite, insomnia, nightmares, loss of libido, decreased energy, altered activity levels)
- Seek support in dealing with grief-associated issues
- Identify personal strengths and effective coping strategies
- Function at a normal developmental level and begin to successfully and increasingly perform activities of daily living

 NIC   **(Nursing Interventions Classification)**

Suggested NIC Interventions

Grief Work Facilitation, Grief Work Facilitation: Perinatal Death, Guilt Work Facilitation, Hope Installation

Example NIC Activities—Grief Work Facilitation

See care plan for **Grieving**.

Nursing Interventions and *Rationales*

- Assess the client's state of grieving. Use a tool such as the Texas Revised Inventory of Grief (TRIG), Pathological Grief Items (PGI), Impact of Events Scale (IES), Hogan Grief Reaction Checklist (HGRC), Beck Depression Inventory (BDI-II), Hamilton Rating Scale for Depression or Social Adjustment Scale—Self Report (SAS-SR). **EBN and EB:** *It is important to differentiate between depression and complicated grief because they can be easily confused (Hogan, Worden, & Schmidt, 2004; Matthews & Marwit, 2004). These standardized tools have been shown to measure grief symptoms effectively and may help differentiate depression from complicated grief (Hogan, Worden, & Schmidt, 2004).*
- ▲ Assess caregivers, particularly younger caregivers, for pessimistic thinking and additional stressful life events and refer for appropriate support. **EB:** *The study found that those under 60 years old had higher levels of complicated grief pre-death than caregivers 60 and older. There was a significant correlation with levels of complicated grief and pessimistic thinking and severity of stressful life events (Tomarken et al, 2008).*
- Develop a trusting relationship with the client by using presence and therapeutic communication techniques. **EB:** *Communication style and relationship with health care providers were significant themes that influenced hope in women diagnosed with ovarian cancer (Reb, 2007).*
- ▲ Determine whether the client is experiencing depression, suicidal tendencies, or other emotional disorders. Refer the client for counseling or therapy as appropriate. **EB:** *Counseling, including the use of relaxation therapy, desensitization, cognitive-behavioral therapy, biofeedback, and/or traditional psychotherapy, has been shown to be supportive (Matthews & Marwit, 2004). Cognitive-behavioral therapy can be helpful for traumatic grief (Matthews & Marwit, 2004).*
- Identify problems of eating and sleeping; ensure that basic human needs are being met. **EB:** *Bereaved individuals, regardless of whether they have counseling for grief resolution, have a moderate risk for poor nutrition (Johnson, 2002).*
- Educate the client and his or her support systems that grief resolution is not a sequential process and that the positive outcome of grief resolution is the integration of the deceased into the ongoing life of the griever. **EB:** *Expectation that the griever will in some way "get over" or "get past" the grief is no longer seen as valid; continued involvement with the deceased regularly occurs (Matthews & Marwit, 2004).*
- See the interventions and rationales in the care plans for **Grieving** and **Chronic Sorrow**.

 Pediatric/Parent

- If client is an adolescent exposed to a peer's suicide, watch for symptoms of traumatic grief as well as PTSD, which include numbness, preoccupation with the deceased, functional impairment, and

• = Independent   ▲ = Collaborative   **EBN** = Evidence-Based Nursing   **EB** = Evidence-Based

poor adjustment to the loss. **EB:** *Adolescents in this situation are at high risk for depression, anxiety disorder, substance abuse, conduct disorder, and attention deficit–hyperactivity disorder (Melhem et al, 2004).*

- See the interventions and rationales in the care plans for **Grieving** and **Chronic Sorrow**.

Geriatric

- See the interventions and rationales in the care plans for **Grieving** and **Chronic Sorrow**.

Multicultural

- Assess for the influence of cultural beliefs, norms, and values on the client's grief and mourning practices. **EBN:** *Cubans may observe a wake service the day after the announcement of the death. Extreme care is taken to notify relatives and significant others to announce the death. Finding out about the death later adds to a feeling of estrangement and defeat. Cuban wake and funeral services are dictated by the religious identity and economic status of the deceased. Catholics traditionally have a priest present at the wake that provides a short prayer service. Jewish practices depend on orthodox, conservative, or reformed traditions and are primarily solemn expressions of grief for 7 days, with burial in a wooden coffin the day after death (Franco & Wilson, 2008).* **EBN:** *When an Amish person is near death, it is extremely useful to have the client in a private room to allow as many visitors as can comfortably stand. The visitors sing softly to the client to make the journey to their God more peaceful. Death is not feared but is rather a solemn and profound event in the life of a person. Amish persons tend to prefer to die at home without the interference of institutional rules (Helmuth & Schwartz, 2008).* **EBN:** *Many of the beliefs and practices about death are so woven into the fabric of Vietnamese life that it is difficult to separate them into either religious or cultural concepts. An important aspect of filial piety and family loyalty is an obligation that extends beyond death: observing the anniversary day of the death, gathering at the family home and altar, and cleaning the ancestral tombs. For Buddhists, there typically are special observances, usually with elaborate rites at 100 days, and 1 and 2 years after the death (Stauffer, 2008).*
- Encourage discussion of the grief process. **EBN:** *Clients who were from an ethnic minority group were significantly more likely to report that interviews about death, dying, and bereavement were helpful (Cherry & Giger, 2008).* **EBN:** *While Afghans grieve expressively and strongly over the death of a loved one, death is seen as the beginning of a new and better life. Close family members gather together to mourn at specified intervals for 40 days or related to the number of children (Lipson, Askaryar, & Omidian, 2008).* **EB:** *In this study African Americans reported higher levels of complicated grief symptoms than Caucasians, especially when they spent less time speaking to others about their loss experience (Laurie & Neimeyer, 2008).*
- Identify whether the client had been notified of the health status of the deceased and was able to be present during illness and death. **EBN:** *Not being present during terminal illness and death can disrupt the grieving process (Franco & Wilson, 2008).*
- See the interventions and rationales in the care plan for **Grieving**.

Home Care

- Provide support via the Internet. **EB:** *Bereaved parents and individuals bereaved by the sudden, unexpected, or violent death of a loved one are at high risk for developing complicated grief. In this study an Internet-based intervention led to a significant reduction in symptoms of complicated grief and depression at posttreatment (Wagner & Maercker, 2008).* **EB:** *Results of this study of an Internet bereavement support group indicate that the reduction in symptoms of complicated grief observed at posttreatment was maintained at 1.5–year follow-up (Wagner & Maercker, 2007).*
- See the interventions and rationales in the care plan for **Grieving** and **Chronic Sorrow**.

⊖volve   See the EVOLVE website for Weblinks for client education resources.

REFERENCES

Cherry B, Giger J: African-Americans. In Giger J, Davidhizar RE, editors: *Transcultural nursing: assessment and intervention,* ed 5, St Louis, 2008, Mosby.

Franco M, Wilson T: Cuban Americans. In Giger J, Davidhizar RE, editors: *Transcultural nursing: assessment and intervention,* ed 5, St Louis, 2008, Mosby.

Helmuth M, Schwartz K: Amish. In Giger J, Davidhizar RE, editors: *Transcultural nursing: assessment and intervention,* ed 5, St Louis, 2008, Mosby.

Hogan NS, Worden JW, Schmidt LA: An empirical study of the proposed complicated grief disorder criteria, *Omega* 48(3):263–277, 2004.

Johnson CS: Nutritional considerations for bereavement and coping with grief, *J Nutr Health Aging* 6(3):171, 2002.

Laurie A, Neimeyer RA: African Americans in bereavement: grief as a function of ethnicity, *Omega (Westport)* 57(2):173–193, 2008.

Lipson J, Askaryar R, Omidian P: Afghans and Afghan Americans. In Giger J, Davidhizar RE, editors: *Transcultural nursing: assessment and intervention,* ed 5, St Louis, 2008, Mosby.

Matthews L, Marwit S: Complicated grief and the trend toward cognitive-behavioral therapy, *Death Stud* 28:849–863, 2004.

Melhem NM, Day N, Shear MK et al: Traumatic grief among adolescents exposed to a peer's suicide, *Am J Psychiatry* 161(8):1411, 2004.

Reb A: Transforming the death sentence: elements of hope in women with advanced ovarian cancer, *Oncol Nurs Forum* 34(6):E70–E81, 2007.

Stauffer R: Vietnamese. In Giger J, Davidhizar RE, editors: *Transcultural nursing: assessment and intervention,* ed 5, St Louis, 2008, Mosby.

Tomarken A, Holland J, Schachter S et al: Factors of complicated grief pre-death in caregivers of cancer patients, *Psychooncol* 17(2):105–111, 2008.

Wagner B, Maercker A: A 1.5–year follow-up of an Internet-based intervention for complicated grief, *J Trauma Stress* 20(4):625–629, 2007.

Wagner B, Maercker A: An Internet-based cognitive-behavioral preventive intervention for complicated grief: a pilot study, *G Ital Med Lav Ergon* 30(3 Suppl B):B47–B53, 2008.

Risk for complicated Grieving *Betty J. Ackley, MSN, EdS, RN*

NANDA-I

Definition

At risk for a disorder that occurs after the death of a significant other in which the experience of distress accompanying bereavement fails to follow normative expectations and manifests in functional impairment

Risk Factors

Death of a significant other; emotional instability; lack of social support

NOC, NIC, Client Outcomes, Nursing Interventions, *Rationales*, and References

Refer to care plan for **Complicated Grieving**.

Delayed Growth and development *Dena L. Jarog, DNP, RN, CCNS* ⊖volve

NANDA-I

Definition

Deviations from age-group norms

Defining Characteristics

Altered physical growth; decreased response time; delay in performing skills typical of age group; difficulty in performing skills typical of age group; inability to perform self-care activities appropriate for age; inability to perform self-control activities appropriate for age; flat affect; listlessness

Related Factors (r/t)

Effects of physical disability; environmental deficiencies; inadequate caretaking; inconsistent responsiveness; indifference; multiple caretakers; prescribed dependence; separation from significant others; stimulation deficiencies

• = Independent   ▲ = Collaborative   **EBN** = Evidence-Based Nursing   **EB** = Evidence-Based

(Nursing Outcomes Classification)

Suggested NOC Outcomes

Child Development: 1 Month, 2 Months, 4 Months, 6 Months, 12 Months, 2 Years, 3 Years, 4 Years, 5 Years, Middle Childhood, Adolescence, Development: Late Adulthood, Middle Adulthood, Young Adulthood, Growth, Physical Aging, Physical Maturation: Female, Male

Example **NOC Outcome** with Indicators
Child Development—Middle Childhood as evidenced by the following indicators: Plays in groups; Follows safety rules; Expresses increasingly complex thoughts; Performs in school to level of ability (Rate the outcome and indicators of **Child Development—Middle Childhood:** 1 = never demonstrated, 2 = rarely demonstrated, 3 = sometimes demonstrated, 4 = often demonstrated, 5 = consistently demonstrated [see Section I].)

Client Outcomes

Client/Parents/Primary Caregiver Will (Specify Time Frame):

- Describe realistic, age-appropriate patterns of growth and development
- Promote activities and interactions that support age-related developmental tasks
- Display consistent, sustained achievement of age-appropriate behaviors (social, interpersonal, and/or cognitive) and/or motor skills
- Achieve realistic developmental and/or growth milestones based on existing abilities, extent of disability, and functional age
- Attain steady gains in growth patterns

 (Nursing Interventions Classification)

Suggested NIC Interventions

Developmental Enhancement: Adolescent, Child, Nutrition Therapy, Nutritional Monitoring

Example **NIC Activities—Developmental Enhancement: Adolescent, Child**
Promote personal hygiene and grooming (Adolescent); Facilitate integration of child with peers (Child); Build a trusting relationship (Both)

Nursing Interventions and *Rationales*

 Pregnancy/Pediatric

- Counsel women who smoke to quit smoking prior to conception if possible and to avoid smoking and secondhand smoke while pregnant. **EB:** *In prospective studies, environmental tobacco smoke exposure was associated with a 33–g reduction in mean birth weight, and in retrospective studies a 40–g reduction in mean birth weight (Bee et al, 2008).* **EB:** *Smoking during pregnancy is a well-established determinant of fetal growth and risk of low birth weight. Maternal smoking in pregnancy may influence the development of the fetal respiratory system (Jaakkola & Gissler, 2004).*
- To determine risk for or actual deviations in normal development, consider the use of a screening tool. **EB:** *The early detection of developmental and behavioral problems in children is crucial for early intervention. Among the many tests that can be employed for this purpose, the DENVER II and the Alberta Infant Motor Scale are the most often used. Also, the Movement Assessment of Infants is starting to be used. Two other tests are recommended in the literature due to their high sensibility and specificity: the Test of Infant Motor Performance and the General Movements (Santos, Araújo, & Porto, 2008).*
- Regularly compare height and weight measurements for the child or adolescent with established age-appropriate norms and previous measurements. **EB:** *The revised growth charts provide an improved tool for evaluating the growth of children in clinical and research settings (CDC, 2007).*

● = Independent   ▲ = Collaborative   **EBN** = Evidence-Based Nursing   **EB** = Evidence-Based

- Provide opportunities for mother-infant skin-to-skin contact (kangaroo care) for preterm infants. **EB:** *Preterm babies exposed to skin-to-skin contact showed a better mental development and better results in motor tests. It also improves thermal care (Thukral et al, 2008).*
- Provide meaningful stimulation for hospitalized infants and children. **EB:** *There is good evidence that infants progress toward matching the development of their full-term counterparts earlier if they receive appropriate intervention (Mahoney & Cohen, 2005).*
- Provide normal sleep wake times for clients to promote growth and development. **EBN:** *The great amount of sleep, especially in the neonatal period (term or preterm), suggests that sleep is important for brain development and synaptic plasticity during early life (Bertelle et al, 2007).*
- ▲ Engage the child in appropriate play activities. Refer the child to a Child Life Therapist or recreational therapist (if available) for supplemental strategies. **EBN:** *Play is a very important part of children's lives, and heighten the importance of integrating therapeutic play as an essential component of holistic and quality nursing care (Li & Lopez, 2008).*

Multicultural

- Assess the influence of cultural beliefs, norms, and values on the client's perceptions of child development. **EBN:** *What the client considers normal and abnormal child development may be based on cultural perceptions (Leininger & McFarland, 2002; Giger & Davidhizar, 2008).*
- Assess and identify for possible environmental conditions, which may be a contributing factor to altered growth and development. **EB:** *Insecticide exposures were widespread among minority women in New York City during pregnancy, and high levels were associated with lower birth weight and length (Whyatt et al, 2004).*
- Acknowledge racial and ethnic differences at the onset of care. **EBN:** *Acknowledgment of race and ethnicity issues enhances communication, establishes rapport, and promotes treatment outcomes (Ludwick & Silva, 2000; D'Avanzo & Naegle, 2001).*
- Provide information on the effects of environmental risk exposure on growth and development. **EB:** *Minority children with prenatal environmental tobacco smoke exposure were twice as likely to be classified as significantly cognitively delayed when compared with unexposed children (Rauh et al, 2004). Data suggest that environmental exposure may lead to delayed growth and pubertal development in African American and Mexican American girls (Shevell et al, 2003).*

Home Care

- The interventions previously described may be adapted for home care use.
- Assess whether exposure to violence is contributing to developmental problems. **EB:** *Children and young people may be significantly affected by living with domestic violence, and impact can endure even after measures have been taken to secure their safety (Holt, Buckley, & Whelan, 2008).*
- ▲ Refer premature neonates for follow-up home care and assessment of functional performance. **EBN:** *Functional performance is a useful clinical measure to understand how well preterm children perform age-expected daily activities as well as the family burden of preterm sequelae (Sullivan & Msall, 2007).*
- ▲ If possible, refer the family to a program of animal-assisted therapy. **EB:** *AAT helps the client by diminishing anxiety, stress, and pain. Positive changes have been reported in blood pressure, mobility, and muscular strength. Human contact with animals, including visual attention, has a "substantial calming effect" on the heart rate and blood pressure (Hastings et al, 2008).*

Client/Family Teaching and Discharge Planning

- Encourage parents to take infants and children for routine health visits to the family physician or pediatrician. *Family physicians play a major role in the early recognition and referral of children with developmental delays or mental retardation. Once the physician has recognized a possible developmental problem, she or he can help determine whether neurological, audiological, or ophthalmological evaluations or rehabilitative services are needed (Moeschler & Shevell, 2006).*
- Encourage parents of children with language delays to approach their physician during regular visits regarding the delay. **EB:** *Language delay (LD) at 2 years proved to represent a sensitive marker*

• = Independent ▲ = Collaborative **EBN** = Evidence-Based Nursing **EB** = Evidence-Based

for different developmental problems. Adequate early intervention requires a clear distinction between specific expressive or receptive-expressive LD and LD associated with other neurodevelopmental problems (Buschmann et al, 2008).

- Provide parents and/or caregivers realistic expectations for attainment of growth and development milestones. Clarify expectations and correct misconceptions. **EBN:** *Learning about the growth and developmental differences between children with congenital heart defects and normal children may help parents of the former to detect problems associated with delayed growth and development earlier (Chen, Li, & Wang, 2004).*

- Instruct the client regarding appropriate baby equipment and the importance of buying new equipment rather than used. **EB:** *190 auctions contained or were suspected to contain a recalled children's item from a target list. Most of the recalled items were listed for sale from addresses within the United States, with sellers from Canada, Australia, Great Britain, and Ireland also represented. On average, six bids were placed on each recalled item, with 70% of auctions eventuating in a sale (Brown, Kirschman, & Smith, 2007).*

- Elicit the involvement of parents and caregivers in social support groups and parenting classes. *Postnatal services that included parenting classes had a positive impact on children's health and supported developmental development (Miller, 2006). Women in particular geographical areas can use asynchronous mail systems to share information with and obtain support from other mothers. Cohort-based electronic communication could be particularly important in rural areas where travel is restricted for women and access to professional support is limited (Hall & Irvine, 2009).*

- Assess whether parents may benefit from Internet/electronic support groups. **EBN:** *The majority of participants in an Internet parent support group not only obtained what they sought, but found more than expected in terms of insight and people to trust. The strongest outcome factor related to satisfaction was improved caregiver-child relationship, and nearly 90% of the sample suggested participating in an Internet parent support group as soon as possible. Nurses may want to consider Internet parent support groups as an adjunct for social support in this population (Baum, 2004).*

⊖volve   See the EVOLVE website for Weblinks for client education resources.

REFERENCES

Baum LS: Internet parent support groups for primary caregivers of a child with special health care needs, *Pediatr Nurs* 30(5):381–388, 401, 2004.

Bee JL, Smyth A, Britton J et al: Environmental tobacco smoke and fetal health: systematic review and meta-analysis, *Arch Dis Child Fetal Neonatal Ed* 93(5):F351–361, 2008.

Bertelle V, Sevestre A, Laou-Hap K et al: Sleep in the Neonatal Intensive Care Unit, *J Perinat Neonat Nurs* 21(2):140–148, 2007.

Brown Kirschman K, Smith GA: Resale of recalled children's products online: an examination of the world's largest yard sale, *Inj Prev* 13(4):228–231, 2007.

Buschmann A, Jooss B, Rupp A et al: Children with developmental language delay at 24 months of age: results of a diagnostic work-up, *Dev Med Child Neurol* 50(3):223–229, 2008.

Centers for Disease Control and Prevention (CDC): *National Center for Health Statistics clinical growth charts,* 2007, www.cdc.gov/nchs/about/major/nhanes/growthcharts/clinical_charts.htm. Accessed February 28, 2007.

Chen C, Li C, Wang J: Growth and development of children with congenital heart disease, *J Adv Nurs* 47(3):260–269, 2004.

D'Avanzo CE, Naegle MA: Developing culturally informed strategies for substance-related interventions. In Naegle MA, D'Avanzo CE, editors: *Addictions and substance abuse: strategies for advanced practice nursing,* St Louis, 2001, Mosby.

Giger JN, Davidhizar RE: *Transcultural nursing: assessment and intervention,* ed 4, St Louis, 2008, Mosby.

Hall W, Irvine V: E-communication among mothers of infants and toddlers in a community-based cohort: a content analysis, *J Adv Nurs* 65(1):175–183, 2009.

Hastings T, Burris A, Hunt J et al: Pet therapy: a healing solution, *J Burn Care Res* 29(6):874–876, 2008.

Holt S, Buckley H, Whelan S: The impact of exposure to domestic violence on children and young people: a review of the literature, *Child Abuse Negl* 32(8):797–810, 2008.

Jaakkola JJ, Gissler M: Maternal smoking in pregnancy, fetal development, and childhood asthma, *Am J Public Health* 94(1):136–140, 2004.

Leininger MM, McFarland MR: *Transcultural nursing: concepts, theories, research and practices,* ed 3, New York, 2002, McGraw-Hill.

Li HC, Lopez V: Effectiveness and appropriateness of therapeutic play intervention in preparing children for surgery: a randomized controlled trial study, *J Spec Pediatr Nurs* 13(2):63–73, 2008.

Ludwick R, Silva M: Nursing around the world: cultural values and ethical conflicts, *NursingWorld,* August 14, 2000, www.nursingworld.org/ojin/ethicol/ethics_4.htm. Accessed June 19, 2003.

Mahoney MC, Cohen, MI: Effectiveness of developmental intervention in the neonatal intensive care unit: implications for neonatal physical therapy, *Pediatr Phys Ther* 17(3):194–208, 2005.

Miller K: Interventions for child health and parenting practices, *Am Fam Physician* 74(12):2112–2113, 2006.

Moeschler J, Shevell M: American Academy of Pediatrics Committee on Genetics: clinical genetic evaluation of the child with mental retardation or developmental delays, *Pediatrics* 117(6):2304–2316, 2006.

Rauh VA, Whyatt RM, Garfinkel R et al: Developmental effects of exposure to environmental tobacco smoke and material hardship among inner-city children, *Neurotoxicol Teratol* 26(3):373–385, 2004.

Santos RS, Araújo AP, Porto MA: Early diagnosis of abnormal development of preterm newborns: assessment instruments, *J Pediatr* 84(4):289–299, 2008.

Shevell M, Ashwal S, Donley D et al: Practice parameter: evaluation of the child with global developmental delay: report of the Quality Standards Subcommittee of the American Academy of Neurology

● = Independent   ▲ = Collaborative   **EBN** = Evidence-Based Nursing   **EB** = Evidence-Based

and The Practice Committee of the Child Neurology Society, *Neurology* 60(3):367–380, 2003.

Sullivan MC, Msall ME: Functional performance of preterm children at age 4, *J Pediatr Nurs* 22(4):297–309, 2007.

Thukral A, Chawla D, Agarwal R et al: Kangaroo mother care—an alternative to conventional care, *Indian J Pediatr* 75(5):497–503, 2008.

Whyatt RM, Rauh V, Barr DB et al: Prenatal insecticide exposures and birth weight and length among an urban minority cohort, *Environ Health Perspect* 112(10):1125, 2004.

Risk for disproportionate Growth   *Dena L. Jarog, DNP, RN, CCNS*

NANDA-I

Definition

At risk for growth above the 97th percentile or below the 3rd percentile for age, crossing two percentile channels

Risk Factors

Caregiver

Abuse; learning difficulties (mental handicap); mental illness; or severe learning disability

Environmental

Deprivation; lead poisoning; natural disasters; poverty; teratogen; violence

Individual

Anorexia; caregiver's maladaptive feeding behaviors; chronic illness; individual maladaptive feeding behaviors; infection; insatiable appetite; prematurity; malnutrition; substance abuse

Prenatal

Congenital disorders; genetic disorders; maternal infection; maternal nutrition; multiple gestation; teratogen exposure; substance abuse: substance use

NOC   (Nursing Outcomes Classification)

Suggested NOC Outcomes

Body Image, Child Development: 1 Month, 2 Months, 4 Months, 6 Months, 12 Months, 2 Years, 3 Years, 4 Years, 5 Years, Middle Childhood, Adolescence, Growth, Knowledge: Infant Care, Preconception Maternal Health, Pregnancy, Physical Maturation: Female, Male, Weight: Body Mass

Example NOC Outcome with Indicators
Growth as evidenced by the following indicators: Weight percentile for sex/Weight percentile for age/Weight percentile for height/Length/height percentile for age/Length/height percentile for sex (Rate the outcome and indicators of **Growth:** 1 = severe deviation from normal range, 2 = substantial deviation from normal range, 3 = moderate deviation from normal range, 4 = mild deviation from normal range, 5 = no deviation from normal range [see Section I].)

Client Outcomes

Client/Parents/Primary Caregiver Will (Specify Time Frame):

- State information related to possible teratogenic agents
- Identify components of healthy nutrition that will promote growth
- Maintain or improve weight to be within a healthy range for age and sex

NIC   (Nursing Interventions Classification)

Suggested NIC Interventions

Eating Disorders Management, Weight Gain/Loss Assistance, Weight Management, Nutrition Therapy, Nutrition Management, Teaching: Infant Nutrition, Toddler Nutrition

• = Independent   ▲ = Collaborative   **EBN** = Evidence-Based Nursing   **EB** = Evidence-Based

Example NIC Activities—Nutrition Management
Determine, in collaboration with dietician as appropriate, number of calories and type of nutrients needed to meet nutrition requirements; Ensure that diet includes foods high in fiber content to prevent constipation; Weigh patient at appropriate intervals

Nursing Interventions and *Rationales*

Preconception/Pregnancy

- Counsel women who smoke to quit smoking prior to conception if possible and to avoid smoking and secondhand smoke while pregnant. **EB:** *In prospective studies, environmental tobacco smoke exposure was associated with a 33-g reduction in mean birth weight, and in retrospective studies a 40-g reduction in mean birth weight (Bee et al, 2008).*
- Assess alcohol consumption of pregnant women and advise those that drink alcohol to discontinue all use of alcohol through the pregnancy. **EB:** *Current research suggests that alcohol intake of seven or more standard drinks (one standard drink = 13.6 grams of absolute alcohol) per week during pregnancy places the fetus at significant risk for the negative effects of ethanol. Effects of alcohol on the fetus are influenced not only by the amount of alcohol consumed, but by the pattern of alcohol (binge drinking versus daily consumption of alcohol), exposure threshold amounts of alcohol in the blood as well as the timing of exposure during gestation (Stade et al, 2009).*
- Assess and limit exposure to all drugs (prescription, "recreational," and over the counter) and give the mother information on known teratogenic agents. **EB:** *According to the National Research Council, 3% of all birth defects and developmental disabilities are caused by environmental exposures. No drug can be considered safe during pregnancy. It should be emphasized that any drug has the potential to cause a birth defect, so no listing of known teratogens is ever complete (Florida Birth Defects Registry, 2009).*
- All women of childbearing age who are capable of becoming pregnant should take 400 mcg of folic acid daily. **EB:** *Periconceptional use of folic acid reduces the incidence of neural tube defects. Up to 70% of neural tube defects could be prevented if all women who can become pregnant consumed 400 mcg of folic acid from at least 1 month before conception through the first trimester of pregnancy (Florida Birth Defects Registry, 2009).*
- ▲ Promote a team approach toward preconception and pregnancy glucose control for women with diabetes. **EB:** *Offspring of women with diabetes mellitus type 1 or type 2 have a two- to fourfold increased risk of birth defects. Available data suggest that excellent preconception and first-trimester glucose control in the mother can greatly reduce, if not eliminate, this risk. Fetal morbidity may still be high in the second and third trimesters if gestational diabetes is not under good control. Programs with a team approach have been the most successful (Florida Birth Defects Registry, 2009).*
- ▲ Advise women with mental health disorders to seek appropriate counseling prior to pregnancy. **EB:** *Well-characterized risks are associated with valproate, carbamazepine, lamotrigine, and lithium (Nguyen, Sharma, & McIntyre, 2009).*

Pediatric

- Consider regular breast milk and protein-fortified breast milk for low birth weight infants in the neonatal intensive care unit. **EB:** *Observational studies, and metaanalyses of trials comparing feeding with formula milk versus donor breast milk, suggest that feeding with breast milk has major nonnutrient advantages for preterm or low birth weight infants (Henderson, Anthony & McGuire, 2007). In an earlier study it was concluded that protein-enriched breast milk enables low birth weight infants requiring especially intensive care to attain growth at discharge comparable to that of healthier infants not given enriched milk (Funkquist et al, 2006).*
- Provide tube feedings per physician's orders when appropriate for clients with neuromuscular impairment. **EB:** *Malnutrition and gastrointestinal disorders are common in children with cerebral palsy. On the other hand, improved nutritional status seems to have a positive effect on motor function in these children (Bekem et al, 2008).*
- Provide for adequate nutrition and nutritional monitoring in clients with medical disorders requiring chronic medication and those with developmental delay. **EB:** *One study found a high*

prevalence of overweight children who had developmental delay. Many factors can contribute to over- weight issues in this population including sedentary lifestyle and medications with weight gain as a side effect (De, Small, & Baur, 2008). Drugs such as antidepressants used to treat certain medical disorders can cause weight gain while others can cause weight loss (American Dietetic Association, 2003).

- Adequate intake of vitamin D is set at 400 IU/day by the National Academy of Sciences. Because adequate sunlight exposure is difficult to determine, a supplement of 400 IU/day is recommended for the following groups to prevent rickets and vitamin D deficiency in healthy infants and children:
    - All breastfed infants unless they are weaned to at least 500 mL/day of vitamin D–fortified formula or milk
    - All non-breastfed infants who are ingesting less than 500 mL/day of vitamin D–fortified formula or milk
    - Children and adolescents who do not receive regular sunlight exposure, do not ingest at least 500 mL/day of vitamin D–fortified milk, or do not take a daily multivitamin supplement containing at least 400 IU of vitamin D

    EB: *It is now recommended that all infants and children, including adolescents, have a minimum daily intake of 400 IU of vitamin D beginning soon after birth. New evidence supports a potential role for vitamin D in maintaining innate immunity and preventing diseases such as diabetes and cancer (Wagner & Greer, 2008).*

- Provide adequate nutrition to clients with active intestinal inflammation. **EB:** *Nutrition plays a role in inflammatory bowel disease (IBD) primarily in prevention and treatment of malnutrition and growth failure. Furthermore, in Crohn disease (CD), nutrition can induce remission, maintain remission, and prevent relapse. Malnutrition is common in IBD and the mechanisms involved include decreased food intake, malabsorption, increased nutrient loss, increased energy requirements, and drug–nutrient interactions (Shamir, 2009).*

Multicultural

- Assess the influence of cultural beliefs, norms, values, and expectations on parents' perceptions of normal growth and development. **EBN:** *One Mexican American pediatrician reported that the primary complaint of his Mexican American parents is that their children do not eat enough despite being obviously overweight (Garcia, 2004). Nutrition education efforts targeting Latino mothers of young children can be culturally reframed to identify positive eating behaviors rather than focusing on a child's weight (Crawford et al, 2004).*
- Assess for the influence of acculturation. **EB:** *Acculturation to the United States is a risk factor for obesity-related behaviors among Asian American and Hispanic adolescents (Unger et al, 2004).*
- Assess whether the parents are concerned about the amount of food eaten. **EBN:** *Some cultures may add semisolid food within the first month of life because of concerns that the infant is not getting enough to eat and the perception that "big is healthy" (Higgins, 2000).*
- Assess the influence of family support on patterns of nutritional intake. **EBN:** *Women are the keepers and transmitters of culture in families. Female family members can play a dominant role in how children and infants are fed (Cesario, 2001).*
- Negotiate with clients regarding which aspects of healthy nutrition can be modified while still honoring cultural beliefs. **EBN:** *Give and take with clients will lead to culturally congruent care (Leininger & McFarland, 2002).*
- Encourage parental efforts at increasing physical activity and decreasing dietary fat for their children. **EB:** *Physical activity and dietary fat consumption were inversely related among African American girls (Thompson et al, 2004). Interventions to increase physical activity among preadolescent African American girls may benefit from a parental component to encourage support and self-efficacy for daughters' physical activity (Adkins et al, 2004).*
- Encourage limiting television viewing to <2 hours/day for children and discourage the consumption of sweetened soft drinks. **EB:** *Longer hours of child television viewing and higher soft drink intake was associated with the occurrence of overweight for Hispanic children (Giammattei et al, 2003; Ariza et al, 2004).*

Home Care

- The interventions previously described may be adapted for home care use.
- Assess parental perception of their child's weight. **EBN:** *If parents do not recognize their child as at risk for overweight, or overweight, they cannot intervene to diminish the risk factors for pediatric obesity and its related complications (Doolen, Alpert, & Miller, 2009).*
- Assess family meal planning and family participation in meal time activities such as eating together at a scheduled time. **EB:** *Lifestyle assessment is an opportunity to identify potential targets for prevention and increase families' self-awareness of current behaviors (Daniels et al, 2009).*

 Client/Family Teaching and Discharge Planning

- Educate families and children about providing healthy meals and healthy eating to improve learning ability. **EB:** *Using standardized tests, results of one study suggest that a nutritional education program can improve academic performance measured by achievement of specific mathematics and English education standards (Shilts et al, 2009).*

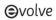 See the EVOLVE website for Weblinks for client education resources.

REFERENCES

Adkins S, Sherwood NE, Story M et al: Physical activity among African-American girls: the role of parents and the home environment, *Obes Res* (suppl 12):38S-S45, 2004.

American Dietetic Association: Position of the American Dietetic Association integration of medical nutrition therapy and pharmacotherapy, *J Am Diet Assoc* 103(10):1363–1370, 2003.

Ariza AJ, Chen EH, Binns HJ et al: Risk factors for overweight in five- to six-year-old Hispanic-American children: a pilot study, *J Urban Health* 81(1):150–161, 2004.

Bee JL, Smyth A, Britton J et al: Environmental tobacco smoke and fetal health: systematic review and meta-analysis, *Arch Dis Child Fetal Neonatal Ed* 93(5):F351–F361, 2008.

Bekem O, Unalp A, Uran N et al: Effect of nutritional support in children with spastic quadriplegia, *Pediatr Neurol* 39:330–334, 2008.

Cesario S: Care of the Native American woman: strategies for practice, education, and research, *J Gynecol Neonat Nurs* 30(1):13, 2001.

Crawford PB, Gosliner W, Anderson C et al: Counseling Latina mothers of preschool children about weight issues: suggestions for a new framework, *J Am Diet Assoc* 104(3):387–394, 2004.

Daniels SR, Jacobson MS, McCrindle BW et al: American Heart Association Childhood Obesity Research Summit: executive summary, *Circulation* 119(15):2114–2123, 2009.

De S, Small J, Baur LA: Overweight and obesity among children with developmental disabilities, *J Intellect Devel Disabil* 33(1):43–47, 2008.

Doolen J, Alpert PT, Miller SK: Parental disconnect between perceived and actual weight status of children: a metasynthesis of the current research. *J Am Acad Nurse Pract* 21:160–166, 2009.

Florida Birth Defects Registry: *Prevention strategies index: strategies to prevent birth defects: limit all drug exposures (prescriptions, "recreational," and over-the-counter.* www.fbdr.org. Accessed April 1, 2009.

Funkquist EL, Tuvemo T, Jonsson B et al: Growth and breastfeeding among low birth weight infants fed with or without protein enrichment of human milk, *Ups J Med Sci* 111(1):97–108, 2006.

Garcia RS: No come nada, *Health Aff* 23(2):215–219, 2004.

Giammattei J, Blix G, Marshak HH et al: Television watching and soft drink consumption: associations with obesity in 11– to 13–year-old schoolchildren, *Arch Pediatr Adolesc Med* 157(9):882–886, 2003.

Henderson G, Anthony MY, McGuire W: Formula milk versus maternal breast milk for feeding preterm or low birth weight infants, *Cochrane Database Syst Rev* (4):CD002972, 2007.

Higgins B: Puerto Rican cultural beliefs: influence on infant feeding practices in western New York, *J Transcult Nurs* 11(1):19, 2000.

Leininger MM, McFarland MR: *Transcultural nursing: concepts, theories, research and practices,* ed 3, New York, 2002, McGraw-Hill.

Nguyen HT, Sharma V, McIntyre RS: Teratogenesis associated with antibipolar agents, *Adv Ther* 26(3):281–294, 2009.

Shamir R: Nutritional aspects in inflammatory bowel disease, *J Pediatr Gastroenterol Nutr* 48:S86–S88, 2009.

Shilts MK, Lamp C, Horowitz M et al: Pilot study: EatFit impacts sixth graders' academic performance on achievement of mathematics and english education standards, *J Nutr Educ Behav* 41(2):127–131, 2009.

Stade BC, Bailey C, Dzendoletas D et al: Psychological and/or educational interventions for reducing prenatal alcohol consumption in pregnant women and women planning pregnancy, *Cochrane Database Syst Rev* (2):CD004228, 2009.

Thompson D, Jago R, Baranowski T et al: Covariability in diet and physical activity in African-American girls, *Obes Res* 12(suppl):46S-S54, 2004.

Unger JB, Reynolds K, Shakib S et al: Acculturation, physical activity, and fast-food consumption among Asian-American and Hispanic adolescents, *J Community Health* 29(6):467–481, 2004.

Wagner CL, Greer FR: Prevention of rickets and vitamin D deficiency in infants, children, and adolescents, *Pediatrics* 122(5):1142–1152, 2008.

Ineffective Health maintenance   *Kathaleen C. Bloom, PhD, CNM, and Barbara J. Olinzock, RN, EdD*

Definition

Inability to identify, manage, and/or seek out help to maintain health

• = Independent   ▲ = Collaborative   **EBN** = Evidence-Based Nursing   **EB** = Evidence-Based

Defining Characteristics

Demonstrated lack of adaptive behaviors to environmental changes; demonstrated lack of knowledge about basic health practices; lack of expressed interest in improving health behaviors; history of lack of health-seeking behavior; inability to take responsibility for meeting basic health practices; impairment of personal support systems

Related Factors (r/t)

Cognitive impairment; complicated grieving; deficient communication skills; diminished fine motor skills; diminished gross motor skills; inability to make appropriate judgments; ineffective family coping; ineffective individual coping; insufficient resources (e.g., equipment, finances); lack of fine motor skills; lack of gross motor skills; perceptual impairment; spiritual distress; unachieved developmental tasks

NOC (Nursing Outcomes Classification)

Suggested NOC Outcomes

Health Beliefs: Perceived Resources, Health-Promoting Behavior, Health-Seeking Behavior

Example **NOC Outcome with Indicators**
Health-Seeking Behavior as evidenced by the following indicators: Completes health-related tasks/Performs self-screening/Obtains assistance from health professionals when indicated (Rate the outcome and indicators of **Health-Seeking Behavior:** 1 = never demonstrated, 2 = rarely demonstrated, 3 = sometimes demonstrated, 4 = often demonstrated, 5 = consistently demonstrated [see Section I].)

Client Outcomes

Client Will (Specify Time Frame):

- Discuss fear of or blocks to implementing health regimen
- Follow mutually agreed on health care maintenance plan
- Meet goals for health care maintenance

NIC (Nursing Interventions Classification)

Suggested NIC Interventions

Health Education, Health System Guidance, Support System Enhancement

Example **NIC Activities—Health Education**
Prioritize identified learner needs based on client preference, skills of nurse, resources available, and likelihood of successful goal attainment; Emphasize immediate or short-term positive health benefits to be received by positive lifestyle behaviors, rather than long-term benefits or negative effects of noncompliance

Nursing Interventions and *Rationales*

- Assess the client's feelings, values, and reasons for not following the prescribed plan of care. See Related Factors. **EBN:** *Assessment of an individual's preferences for participation in decision making will allow for enlisting involvement in decision making at the preferred level (Florin, Ehrenberg, & Ehnfor, 2006).*
- Assess for family patterns, economic issues, and cultural patterns that influence compliance with a given medical regimen. **EB:** *The family's reaction to the diagnosis and cultural, spiritual beliefs and norms have a significant influence on adherence to the treatment regimen (Zivin & Kales, 2008). There are marked differences in use of health care services among different cultural groups (Uiters et al, 2006).*
- Help the client to choose a healthy lifestyle and to have appropriate diagnostic screening tests. **EBN:** *Healthy lifestyle measures, such as exercising regularly, maintaining a healthy weight, not smoking, and limiting alcohol intake, help reduce the risk of cancer and other chronic illnesses (Holmes, 2006).*

 = Independent ▲ = Collaborative **EBN** = Evidence-Based Nursing **EB** = Evidence-Based

- Assist the client in reducing stress. **EB:** *Individuals with high perceived stress are significantly more likely to be nonadherent with treatment regimens. This happens with individuals with high blood pressure (Proulx et al, 2007), clients who are opioid-dependent (Hyman et al, 2007), and clients who have had an organ transplant (Achille et al, 2006; Kerkar et al, 2006).*

- Help the client determine how to manage complex medication schedules (e.g., HIV/AIDS regimens or polypharmacy). **EBN:** *Simplifying treatment regimens and tailoring them to individual lifestyles encourages adherence to treatment (Battaglioli-Denero, 2007). Components of successful self-management of medications include establishing habits, adjusting routines, tracking, simplifying, and managing costs (Swanlund et al, 2008).*

- Identify complementary healing modalities, such as herbal remedies, acupuncture, healing touch, yoga, or cultural shamans that the client uses in addition to or instead of the prescribed allopathic regimen. **EB:** *Use of complementary healing modalities among clients with chronic disease is relatively high, ranging from 41% in clients with diabetes to 59.6% in clients with arthritis. Less than 30% of users of complementary healing modalities share this information with their health care provider (Saydah & Eberhardt, 2006).*

- ▲ Refer the client to appropriate services as needed. **EB:** *When appropriate referrals are missed or delayed, clients often experience poor outcomes, including complications, psychological distress, and hospital readmissions (Bowles et al, 2008; Lebecque et al, 2009).*

- Identify support groups related to the disease process. **EB:** *Individuals who attend support groups demonstrate improved disease management and enhanced quality of life (Schulz et al, 2008).*

- Use technology such as text messaging to remind clients of scheduled appointments. **EB:** *"No show" rates are reduced when appointment reminders are sent as text messages to clients' mobile telephones (Koshy, Car, & Majeed, 2008).*

Geriatric

- Assess the client's perception of health. **EB:** *Perceived ill health in older clients is associated with lower self-care ability and sense of control (Söderhamn, Bachrach-Lindström, & Ek, 2008).*

- Assist client to identify both life- and health-related goals. **EB:** *Older individuals endorse health goals and disease management that is congruent with their life goals (Morrow et al, 2008).*

- Provide information that supports informed decision making. **EBN:** *Encouraging independence and enhancing social networks can enhance client autonomy (Hwang et al, 2006; Matsui & Capezuti, 2008).*

- Discuss with the client and support person realistic goals for changes in health maintenance. **EB:** *Shared decision making, including the setting of realistic goals, may improve outcomes (Corser et al, 2007).* **EBN:** *This study demonstrates that the Modified Caregiver Strain Index can be given to family members of older adults. This helps to determine the level of stress/burden and the consequences on the caregiver's overall health. Often the caregiver is an older adult as well. The index can act as a guide to select interventions that will help the older adult but also reduce caregiver strain and improve the lives of both (Onega, 2008).*

- Educate the client about the symptoms of life-threatening illness, such as myocardial infarction (MI), and the need for timeliness in seeking care. **EBN:** *Women, especially those of advanced age, wait longer before seeking treatment for signs and symptoms of acute MI (Higginson, 2008).*

Multicultural

- Assess influence of cultural beliefs, norms, and values on the client's ability to modify health behavior. **EB:** *Awareness of the cultural importance of family and social relationships, symbolic and social meanings of food, and the spiritual dimensions of disease are key in encouraging self-management of disease (Finucane & McMullen, 2008).*

- Assess the effect of fatalism on the client's ability to modify health behavior. **EBN:** *Chinese women may not request (or may refuse) analgesics after an injury because of their fear of side effects and the belief that pain is inevitable after a traumatic event and should be borne without analgesia (Wong & Chan, 2008).*

- Assess for use of and reasons for not using health services. **EBN:** *Compared with Caucasians, women of color had later initiation of prenatal care and fewer prenatal visits overall (Park, Vincent, &*

Hastings-Tolsma, 2007). Language and cultural barriers were identified as barriers to utilization of mental health services for Latino children (Lopez, Bergren, & Painter, 2008).

- Clarify culturally-related health beliefs and practices. **EB:** *Language, culture, and ethnicity influence the choice of a health care provider as well as health management strategies (Wang, Rosenberg, & Lo, 2008). Use of trained medical interpreters and familiarity with folk illness beliefs treatments positively affects the client's health outcomes (Brotanek, Seeley, & Flores, 2008).*
- Provide culturally targeted education and health care services. **EB:** *A culturally sensitive diabetes education program produced improvement in HbA1c, fasting plasma glucose, cholesterol/HDL ratio, and HDL in Hispanic clients (Metghalchi et al, 2008).*

Home Care

- The interventions described previously may be adapted for home care use.
- ▲ Provide nurse-led case management. **EBN:** *A home care service model utilizing nurse-led case management facilitates access to services and resources and has a positive impact on the clients' functional ability (Morales-Asencio et al, 2008).*
- Include a health-promotion focus for the client with disabilities, with the goals of reducing secondary conditions (e.g., obesity, hypertension, pressure sores), maintaining functional independence, providing opportunities for leisure and enjoyment, and enhancing overall quality of life. **EB:** *People with disabilities who participate in a planned health promotion program report improved self-efficacy, increased health behavior, reduced limitations from secondary conditions, decreased number of unhealthy days, and decreased need for health care (Ravesloot et al, 2006; Robinson-Whelen et al, 2006).*
- Encourage a regular routine for health-related behaviors. **EBN:** *Individuals who establish a regular routine for exercise are more likely to be compliant over time than those who use an ad hoc approach to exercise (Hines, Seng, & Messer, 2007).*
- Provide support and individual training for caregivers before the client is discharged from the hospital. **EBN:** *Caregivers are very interested in receiving instruction and hands-on practice of procedures they would need to perform at home. They report increased confidence in their ability to provide such care and to help their loved ones manage symptoms at home (Hendrix & Ray, 2006).*
- Assist client to develop confidence in ability to manage the health condition. **EB:** *Self-management education targeted at self-efficacy improves physiologic outcomes, enhances coping techniques, and reduces health care use (Wade, Michaud, & Brown, 2006).*
- Consider a written contract with the client to follow the agreed-upon health care regimen. Written agreements reinforce the verbal agreement and serve as a reference. **EB:** *Written agreement between health care providers and clients may promote adherence (Bosch-Capblanch et al, 2007).*
- Using self-care management precepts, instruct the client about possible situations to which he or she may need to respond; include the use of role playing. Instruct in generating hypotheses from available evidence rather than solely from experience. **EBN:** *Interventions that focus on increasing self-awareness of cues relative to health increase the client's ability to recognize and respond to changes in symptoms and health status (Hernandez, Hume, & Rodger, 2008).*

Client/Family Teaching and Discharge Planning

- Provide the family with website addresses where information can be obtained from the Internet. (Most libraries have Internet access with printing capabilities.) **EB:** *Internet/video-delivered interventions are successful in increasing physical activity and fruit and vegetable intake in adolescents (Mauriello et al, 2007). One third of older adults perform online searches for information about their own health or health care (Flynn, Smith, & Freese, 2006).*
- ▲ Develop collaborative multidisciplinary partnerships. **EBN:** *Multidisciplinary and multifactorial interventions are likely to be more effective in achieving desired outcomes (Norlund, Ropponen, & Alexanderson, 2009).*
- Tailor both the information provided and the method of delivery of information to the specific client and/or family. **EBN:** *Client-centered educational interventions that focus on individualization have a positive impact on the client's sense of well-being and optimism that therapy will be effective (Radwin, Cabral, & Wilkes, 2009).*

● = Independent   ▲ = Collaborative   **EBN** = Evidence-Based Nursing   **EB** = Evidence-Based

- Obtain or design educational material that is appropriate for the client; use pictures if possible. **EB:** *The use of materials tailored to the individual has a stronger effect than the use of standard materials (Kroeze, Werkman, & Brug, 2006). Inclusion of pictures in written materials increases attention, recall, and comprehension. Use of pictures can change adherence to health instructions, but emotional response to pictures affects whether they increase or decrease target behaviors (Houts et al, 2006).*
- Teach the client about the symptoms associated with discontinuation of medications, such as a selective serotonin reuptake inhibitor (SSRI). **EB:** *Educate client about SSRI discontinuation syndrome, which may include lightheadedness, dizziness, headaches, GI disturbances, diaphoresis, lethargy, vivid dreams, and flu-like symptoms. A 3– to 4–week graded dosage tapering is encouraged with short-acting SSRIs to avoid this syndrome (Schatzberg et al, 2006).*
- Explain nonthreatening aspects before introducing more anxiety-producing information regarding possible side effects of the disease or medical regimen. **EBN:** *Anxiety often interferes with concentration and the ability to understand (Stephenson, 2006).*
- Treat tobacco use as a chronic problem. Tailor the smoking cessation program to the individual. Consider mixed groups of current and past smokers. **EB:** *Flexible smoking cessation programs that are tailored to the individual's culture and life situation and offer support to a range of smokers are perceived by participants as both beneficial and valued (Ritchie, Schulz, & Bryce, 2007).*

⊖volve   See the EVOLVE website for Weblinks for client education resources.

REFERENCES

Achille MA, Ouellette A, Fournier S et al: Impact of stress, distress and feelings of indebtedness on adherence to immunosuppressants following kidney transplantation, *Clin Transplant* 20(3):301–306, 2006.

Battaglioli-Denero AM: Strategies for improving patient adherence to therapy and long-term patient outcomes, *J Assoc Nurses AIDS Care* 18(Suppl 1):S17–S22, 2007.

Bosch-Capblanch X, Abba K, Prictor M et al: Contracts between patients and healthcare practitioners for improving patients' adherence to treatment, prevention and health promotion activities, *Cochrane Database Syst Rev* (2):CD004808, 2007.

Bowles KH, Ratcliffe SJ, Holmes JH et al: Post-acute referral decisions made by multidisciplinary experts compared to hospital clinicians and the patients' 12–week outcomes, *Med Care* 46(2):158–166, 2008.

Brotanek JM, Seeley CE, Flores G: The importance of cultural competency in general pediatrics. *Curr Opin Pediatr* 20(6):711–718, 2008.

Corser W, Holmes-Rovner M, Lein C et al: A shared decision-making primary care intervention for type 2 diabetes, *Diabetes Educ* 33(4):700–708, 2007.

Finucane ML, McMullen CK: Making diabetes self-management education culturally relevant for Filipino Americans in Hawaii, *Diabetes Educ* 34(5):841–853, 2008.

Florin J, Ehrenberg A, Ehnfor M: Patient participation in clinical decision-making in nursing: a comparative study of nurses' and patients' perceptions, *J Clin Nurs* 15(12):1498–1508, 2006.

Flynn KE, Smith MA, Freese J: When do older adults turn to the Internet for health information? Findings from the Wisconsin Longitudinal Study, *J Gen Intern Med* 21(12):1295–1301, 2006.

Hendrix C, Ray C: Informal caregiver training on home care and cancer symptom management prior to hospital discharge: a feasibility study, *Oncol Nurs Forum* 33(4):793–798, 2006.

Hernandez CA, Hume MR, Rodger NW: Evaluation of a self-awareness intervention for adults with type 1 diabetes and hypoglycemia unawareness, *Can J Nurs Res* 40(3):38–56, 2008.

Higginson R: Women's help-seeking behaviour at the onset of myocardial infarction, *Br J Nurs* 17(1):10–14, 2008.

Hines SH, Seng JS, Messer KL: Adherence to a behavioral program to prevent incontinence, *West J Nurs Res* 29(1):36–56, 2007.

Holmes S: Nutrition and the prevention of cancer, *J Fam Health Care* 16(2):43–46, 2006.

Houts PS, Doak CC, Doak LG et al: The role of pictures in improving health communication: a review of research on attention, comprehension, recall, and adherence, *Patient Educ Couns* 61(2):173–190, 2006.

Hwang HL, Lin HS, Tung YL et al: Correlates of perceived autonomy among elders in a senior citizen home: a cross-sectional survey, *Int J Nurs Stud* 43(4):429–437, 2006.

Hyman SM, Fox H, Hong KI et al: Stress and drug-cue-induced craving in opioid-dependent individuals in naltrexone treatment, *Exp Clin Psychopharmacol* 15(2):134–143, 2007.

Kerkar N, Annunziato RA, Foley L et al: Prospective analysis of nonadherence in autoimmune hepatitis: a common problem, *J Pediatr Gastroenterol Nutr* 43(5):629–634, 2006.

Koshy E, Car J, Majeed A: Effectiveness of mobile-phone short message service (SMS) reminders for ophthalmology outpatient appointments: observational study, *BMC Ophthalmol* 8:9, 2008.

Kroeze W, Werkman A, Brug J: A systematic review of randomized trials on the effectiveness of computer-tailored education on physical activity and dietary behaviors, *Ann Behav Med* 31(3):205–223, 2006.

Lebecque P, Leonard A, De Boeck K et al: Early referral to cystic fibrosis specialist centre impacts on respiratory outcome, *J Cyst Fibros* 8(1):26–30, 2009.

Lopez C, Bergren MD, Painter SG: Latino disparities in child mental health services. *J Child Adolesc Psychiatr Nurs* 21(3):137–145, 2008.

Matsui M, Capezuti E: Perceived autonomy and self-care resources among senior center users, *Geriatr Nurs* 29(2):141–147, 2008.

Mauriello LM, Sherman KJ, Driskell MM et al: Using interactive behavior change technology to intervene on physical activity and nutrition with adolescents, *Adolesc Med State Art Rev* 18(2):383–99, xiii, 2007.

Metghalchi S, Rivera M, Beeson L et al: Improved clinical outcomes using a culturally sensitive diabetes education program in a Hispanic population, *Diabetes Educ* 34(4):698–706, 2008.

Morales-Asencio JM, Gonzalo-Jiménez E, Martin-Santos FJ et al: Effectiveness of a nurse-led case management home care model in primary health care. A quasi-experimental, controlled, multi-centre study, *BMC Health Serv Res* 8:193, 2008.

Morrow AS, Haidet P, Skinner J et al: Integrating diabetes self-management with the health goals of older adults: a qualitative exploration, *Patient Educ Couns* 72(3):418–423, 2008.

• = Independent   ▲ = Collaborative   **EBN** = Evidence-Based Nursing   **EB** = Evidence-Based

Norlund A, Ropponen A, Alexanderson K: Multidisciplinary interventions: review of studies of return to work after rehabilitation for low back pain, *J Rehabil Med* 41(3):115–121, 2009.

Onega L: Helping those who help others: the Modified Caregiver Strain Index, *Am J Nurs* 108(9):62–69, 2008.

Park JH, Vincent D, Hastings-Tolsma M: Disparity in prenatal care among women of colour in the USA, *Midwifery* 23(1):28–37, 2007.

Proulx M, Leduc N, Vandelac L et al: Social context, the struggle with uncertainty, and subjective risk as meaning-rich constructs for explaining HBP noncompliance, *Patient Educ Couns* 68(1):98–106, 2007.

Radwin LE, Cabral HJ, Wilkes G: Relationships between patient-centered cancer nursing interventions and desired health outcomes in the context of the health care system, *Res Nurs Health* 32(1):4–17, 2009.

Ravesloot CH, Seekins T, Cahill T et al: Health promotion for people with disabilities: development and evaluation of the Living Well with a Disability program, *Health Educ Res* 22(4):522–531, 2006.

Ritchie D, Schulz S, Bryce A: One size fits all? A process evaluation—the turn of the 'story' in smoking cessation. *Public Health* 121(5):341–318, 2007.

Robinson-Whelen S, Hughes RB, Taylor HB et al: Improving the health and health behaviors of women aging with physical disabilities: a peer-led health promotion program, *Womens Health Issues* 16(6):334–345, 2006.

Saydah SH, Eberhardt MS: Use of complementary and alternative medicine among adults with chronic diseases: United States 2002, *J Altern Complement Med* 12(8):805–812, 2006.

Schatzberg AF, Blier P, Delgado PL et al: Antidepressant discontinuation syndrome: consensus panel recommendations for clinical management and additional research, *J Clin Psychiatry* 67(Suppl 4):27–30, 2006.

Schulz U, Pischke CR, Weidner G et al: Social support group attendance is related to blood pressure, health behaviours, and quality of life in the Multicenter Lifestyle Demonstration Project, *Psychol Health Med* 3(4):423–437, 2008.

Söderhamn U, Bachrach-Lindström M, Ek AC: Self-care ability and sense of coherence in older nutritional at-risk patients, *Eur J Clin Nutr* 62(1):96–103, 2008.

Stephenson PL: Before the teaching begins: managing patient anxiety prior to providing education, *Clin J Oncol Nurs* 10(2):241–245, 2006.

Swanlund SL, Scherck KA, Metcalfe SA et al: Keys to successful self-management of medications, *Nurs Sci Q* 21(3):238–246, 2008.

Uiters E, Deville WL, Foets M et al: Use of health care services by ethnic minorities in The Netherlands: do patterns differ? *Eur J Public Health* 16(4):388–393, 2006.

Wade SL, Michaud L, Brown TM: Putting the pieces together: preliminary efficacy of a family problem-solving intervention for children with traumatic brain injury, *J Head Trauma Rehabil* 21(1):57–67, 2006.

Wang L, Rosenberg M, Lo L: Ethnicity and utilization of family physicians: a case study of Mainland Chinese immigrants in Toronto, Canada, *Soc Sci Med* 67(9):1410–1422, 2008.

Wong EM, Chan SW: The pain experience and beliefs of Chinese patients who have sustained a traumatic limb fracture, *Int Emerg Nurs* 16(2):80–87, 2008.

Zivin K, Kales HC: Adherence to depression treatment in older adults: a narrative review, *Drugs Aging* 25(7):559–571, 2008.

Ineffective self Health management   *Dawn Fairlie, ANP, FNP, GNP, DNS(c)*   ⊖volve

Definition

Pattern of regulating and integrating into daily living a therapeutic regime for treatment of illness and its sequelae that is unsatisfactory for meeting specific health goals

Defining Characteristics

Failure to include treatment regimens in daily living; failure to take action to reduce risk factors; makes choices in daily living ineffective for meeting health goals; verbalizes desire to manage the illness; verbalizes difficulty with prescribed regimens

Related Factors (r/t)

Complexity of health care system; complexity of therapeutic regimen; decisional conflicts; economic difficulties; excessive demands made (e.g., individual, family); family conflict; family patterns of health care; inadequate number of cues to action; knowledge deficit; regimen; perceived barriers; powerlessness; perceived seriousness; perceived susceptibility; perceived benefits; social support deficit

NOC   (Nursing Outcomes Classification)

Suggested NOC Outcomes

Knowledge: Disease Process, Knowledge: Treatment Regimen, Participation in Health Care Decisions

Example **NOC** Outcome with Indicators
Knowledge: Treatment Regimen as evidenced by the following indicator: Description of prescribed medication, activity, exercise, and specific disease process (Rate the outcome and indicators of **Knowledge: Treatment Regimen: 1** = no knowledge, **2** = limited knowledge, **3** = moderate knowledge, **4** = substantial knowledge, **5** = extensive knowledge [see Section I].)

● = Independent   ▲ = Collaborative   **EBN** = Evidence-Based Nursing   **EB** = Evidence-Based

Client Outcomes

Client Will (Specify Time Frame):

- Describe daily food and fluid intake that meets therapeutic goals
- Describe activity/exercise patterns that meet therapeutic goals
- Describe scheduling of medications that meets therapeutic goals
- Verbalize ability to manage therapeutic regimens
- Collaborate with health providers to decide on a therapeutic regimen that is congruent with health goals and lifestyle

 (Nursing Interventions Classification)

Suggested NIC Interventions

Health System Guidance, Learning Facilitation, Learning Readiness Enhancement

Example **NIC** Activities—Learning Facilitation
Present the information in a stimulating manner; Encourage the patient's active participation

Nursing Interventions and *Rationales*

NOTE: This diagnosis does not have the same meaning as the diagnosis **Noncompliance.** This diagnosis is made with the client, so if the client does not agree with the diagnosis, it should not be made. The emphasis is on helping the client direct his or her own life and health, not on the client's compliance with the provider's instructions.

- Establish a collaborative partnership with the client for purposes of meeting health-related goals. **EBN:** *Nurse-client partnerships reflect nursing models for practice (Farrell, Wicks, & Martin, 2004; Pellatt, 2004), and this approach differs from a traditional health care model in which the provider assumes authoritative and paternalistic approaches to care (Pellatt, 2004). At least one study showed that the professionals' perceptions of partnership behaviors were actually paternalistic behaviors (Pellatt, 2004).*
- Listen to the person's story about his or her illness self-management. **EB:** *In a study of the meaning of active participation in self-management from the perspective of 16 participants aged 30 to 81 years, client participation was found to be more complex than expected. Implications of the study were that physicians and other providers may be able to influence the person's illness story positively by recognizing their part in the illness story (Haidet, Kroll, & Sharf, 2006).*
- Explore the meaning of the person's illness experience and identify uncertainties and needs through open-ended questions. **EB:** *Even though providers agree that self-management is the ideal approach to client care, studies show significant discrepancies between providers' and clients' views. Providers talk about self-management but may still expect compliance (Rogers et al, 2005).*
- Help the client identify the "self" in self-management; show respect for the client's self-determination. **EBN:** *In a qualitative study with 24 older adults with asthma, three self-management models were developed that reflected data from the participants (Koch, Jenkin, & Kralik, 2004). Even the participants interpreted self-management as medical management and were mainly talking about compliance and adherence. Self-management means that the person uses self-determination to adapt medical and nursing recommendations for their own lives and personal needs (Farrell, Wicks, & Martin, 2004).*
- Help the client enhance self-efficacy or confidence in his or her own ability to manage the illness. **EBN:** *In a pilot study using a quasiexperimental pretest/posttest design with 48 persons recruited from two clinics, specific self-management strategies to improve self-efficacy were associated with significant improvements in self-efficacy and self-management behaviors (Farrell, Wicks, & Martin, 2004). A review of the literature indicates that enhancement of self-efficacy was important to achieve optimal self-management (Sol et al, 2005).*
- Involve family members in knowledge development, planning for self-management, and shared decision making. **EBN:** *Family support was one of two predictors of positive self-management strategies in a study of 53 women with type 2 diabetes (Whittemore, Melkus, & Grey, 2005). In a review of research related to self-management, family management was found to be integral to self-management (Grey, Knafl, & McCorkle, 2006).*

● = Independent   ▲ = Collaborative   **EBN** = Evidence-Based Nursing   **EB** = Evidence-Based

- Review factors of the Health Belief Model (individual perceptions of seriousness and susceptibility, demographic and other modifying factors, and perceived benefits and barriers) with the client. **EBN:** *Studies using the Health Belief Model support the view that individual perceptions and a variety of modifying factors affect the likelihood of changing health behaviors (Pender, Murdaugh, & Parsons, 2006). In a study of 52 post–myocardial infarction clients, following a physical activity regimen was associated with health motivation, whereas following professional advice on smoking cessation was associated with self-efficacy (Leong, Molassiotis, & Marsh, 2004).*

- Use various formats to provide information about the therapeutic regimen, including group education, brochures, videotapes, written instructions, computer-based programs, and telephone contact. **EB and EBN:** *In a 5-year study at Stanford University of more than 1000 clients with chronic illnesses, self-management education was effective in achieving positive outcomes (Lorig et al, 2006; Stanford University, 2007). In a systematic review of controlled clinical trials of clients with diabetes, it was determined that group-based training for self-management had many positive effects (Deakin et al, 2005). In a study of two groups of adults (n = 16) with dyspnea, the results of Internet-based support on outcomes were tested. Most subjects reported that the Internet-based program increased their access to information and resources for managing their dyspnea (Nguyen et al, 2005). A telephone survey with 781 persons was found to yield reliable and valid data on self-management and other variables (Baker et al, 2005).*

- Help the client identify and modify barriers to effective self-management. **EB:** *In a random sample of 446 people with diabetes and focus groups with subgroups of six to 12 persons, it was found that many barriers exist to self-management (Vijan et al, 2005). Cost was the most commonly identified barrier. Other barriers were moderation in diet, medication therapies, need for small portion sizes, difficulties communicating with providers, and staying on a rigid schedule. In a cross-sectional study of 993 diabetic clients in the Veterans Association system, pain was identified as a significant barrier to diabetes self-management (Krein et al, 2005). In a study of 24 adults diagnosed with diabetes, the respondents identified the barrier of lack of knowledge and understanding of the diet and its relation to the illness (Nagelkerk, Reick, & Meengs, 2006). A study of 46 overweight and obese adults participating in a behavioral weight loss program concluded that weight bias may interfere with overweight and obese treatment-seeking adults' ability to achieve optimal health (Carels et al, 2009).*

- Help the client self-manage his or her own health through teaching about strategies for changing habits such as overeating, sedentary lifestyle, and smoking. **EB:** *Self-management education helps achieve positive health outcomes such as reductions in glycosylated hemoglobin levels and systolic blood pressure as well as fewer asthmatic attacks (Warsi et al, 2004; Govil et al, 2009).*

- Develop a contract with the client to maintain motivation for changes in behavior. **EBN:** *The nursing intervention of client contracting provides a concrete means of keeping track of actions to meet health-related goals (Bulechek, Butcher, & Dochterman, 2008).*

- Help the client maintain consistency in therapeutic regimen management for optimal results. **EBN:** *With clients on hemodialysis, self-management activities varied tremendously (Curtin et al, 2004).*

- Review how to contact health providers as needed to address issues and concerns regarding self-management. **EBN:** *The partnership process includes continued contact as changes occur; people with chronic illnesses need to know how to obtain interventions that are needed in the future (Pellatt, 2004).*

- Implement organizational changes to facilitate shared decision making for self-management of chronic illnesses. **EB:** *With the goal of shared decision making and instructions on how to accomplish this goal, providers still approach client care as if compliance were the goal. Organizational structures and patterns were found to contribute to the difficulty of adopting a client-centered self-management approach (Rogers et al, 2005).*

- Use focus groups to evaluate the implementation of self-management programs. **EBN:** *The focus group format facilitated identification and understanding of themes that were important to self-management (Benavides-Vaello et al, 2004; Vijan et al, 2005). Themes identified were health maintenance, barriers to self-management, self-awareness, familial support, folk remedies, and confidence to manage diabetes (Benavides-Vaello et al, 2004). In a larger study with quantitative and qualitative components, cost, portion size, and family support were found to be major issues of concern (Vijan et al, 2005).*

- Refer to the care plan **Ineffective family Therapeutic regimen management.**

• = Independent   ▲ = Collaborative   **EBN** = Evidence-Based Nursing   **EB** = Evidence-Based

Geriatric

- Identify the reasons for actions that are not therapeutic and discuss alternatives. **EBN:** *Many possible reasons exist for actions that do not meet therapeutic goals. Fatigue and pain can have profound effects on the ability to perform therapeutic actions (Krein et al, 2005). Perceptions may differ according to diseases. In a longitudinal study of 7991 middle-age and older adults, those who did not take medications as prescribed because the medications were too costly were 50% more likely to have adverse events such as heart attacks (Heisler, 2004).*

Multicultural

- Provide support for self-management throughout the process of care. **EB:** *In a survey of 956 people in 17 locations throughout the country, respondents' perceptions of provider support for self-management were found to be significantly related to better self-management. African Americans constituted 34% of the sample; Hispanics constituted 14% (Greene & Yedidia, 2005).*
- Assess the influence of cultural beliefs, norms, and values on the individual's perceptions of the therapeutic regimen. **EBN:** *Cultural beliefs and values may be individual or group related. One study of 186 low-income African Americans (n = 100) and whites (n = 86) found no substantial differences in self-management between groups. Yet, in other studies, African Americans, Latinos born in the United States, and Latinos born in Mexico were less likely to follow dietary recommendations (Sharma et al, 2004). A recent study showed that Hispanic psychiatric outpatients experienced akathisia as an increase in nervousness. Addressing this issue, as well as using anxiolytics and low doses of antipsychotics when beginning treatment, led to an improvement in medication taking (Opler et al, 2004).*
- Discuss all strategies with the client in the context of the client's culture. **EBN:** *Research studies involving culture, health behaviors, and self-management show that culture significantly affects decision making for meeting therapeutic goals and is related to self-management strategies (Degazon, 2006; Grey, Knafl, & McCorkle, 2006).*
- Provide health information that is consistent with the health literacy of clients. **EB:** *Individuals with marginal or inadequate functional health literacy have difficulty reading, understanding, and interpreting most written health texts and instructions. In addition, clients with marginal or inadequate health literacy scores are more likely to misunderstand directions for health care (Georges, Bolton, & Bennett, 2004).*
- Determine that health information is culturally relevant. **EB:** *A study of breast health information needs of women from minority ethnic groups found that health care professionals' lack of understanding about cultural beliefs, values, and knowledge, together with racial stereotyping and misconceptions about cancer in minority ethnic groups, posed challenges to information dissemination (Watts et al, 2004).*
- Assess for barriers that may interfere with client follow-up of treatment recommendations. **EB:** *Optimal follow-up of treatment regimen is often compounded by variables such as cost, availability of services, and convenience of accessing care. Knowledge of barriers to seeking health care is important when developing interventions to address self-management of therapeutic regimens (Unzueta et al, 2004).*
- Use electronic monitoring to improve management of medications. **EB:** *A recent study showed that the use of electronic monitors had a positive effect on medication taking for minority women (Robbins et al, 2004).*
- Validate the client's feelings regarding the ability to manage his or her own care and the impact on current lifestyle. **EB:** *A recent study elicited the expectations of treatment in 93 hypertensive African American clients (Ogedegbe, Mancuso, & Allegrante, 2004). Client expectations of treatment could serve as the basis for client education and counseling about hypertension and its management in this client population.*

Home Care

- Prepare and instruct clients and family members in the use of a medication box. Set up an appropriate schedule for filling of the medication box, and post medication times and doses in an accessible area (e.g., attached by a magnet to the refrigerator). *Improved self-management of therapeutic regimen is increased through the use of cues and supports that help clients remember to take medications.*

• = Independent ▲ = Collaborative **EBN** = Evidence-Based Nursing **EB** = Evidence-Based

- Monitor self-management of the medical regimen. **EBN:** *In elderly clients with diabetes mellitus living alone, home visits (both daily and weekly) were associated with reductions in fasting blood sugar, postmeal blood sugar, and hemoglobin A1c (Huang et al, 2004).*
- ▲ Refer to health care professionals for questions and self-care management **EBN:** *A study demonstrated that nurses monitoring medication regimens and appropriate referrals for medication review helped increase clients' knowledge of medications and appropriate use of aids to self-management (Griffiths et al, 2004).* **EBN:** *Enhanced nursing case management may both improve self-care and reduce emotional distress for clients with diabetes (Stuckey et al, 2009).*

Client/Family Teaching and Discharge Planning

- Identify what the client and/or family know and adjust teaching accordingly. *Teach the client and family about all aspects of the therapeutic regimen, providing as much knowledge as the client and family will accept, in a culturally congruent manner.*
- Teach ways to adjust ADLs for inclusion of therapeutic regimens.
- Teach safety in taking medications.
- Teach the client to act as a self-advocate with health providers who prescribe therapeutic regimens.

℮volve   See the EVOLVE website for Weblinks for client education resources.

REFERENCES

Baker DW, Brown J, Chan KS et al: A telephone survey to measure communication, education, self-management, and health status for patients with heart failure: the improving chronic illness care evaluations (ICICE), *J Card Failure* 11(1):36–42, 2005.

Benavides-Vaello S, Garcia AA, Brown SA et al: Using focus group to plan and evaluate diabetes self-management interventions for Mexican Americans, *Diabetes Educ* 30(2):238–256, 2004.

Bulechek GM, Butcher HK, Dochterman JM: *Nursing interventions classification (NIC),* ed 4, St Louis, 2008, Mosby.

Carels RA, Young KM, Wott CB et al: Weight bias and weight loss treatment outcomes in treatment seeking adults, *Ann Behav Med* 37(3):350–355, 2009.

Curtin RB, Sitter DCB, Schatell D et al: Self-management, knowledge, and functioning and well being of patients on hemodialysis, *Neph Nurs J* 31(4):378–386, 2004.

Deakin T, McShane CE, Cade JE et al: Group-based training for self management strategies in people with type 2 diabetes mellitus, *Cochrane Database Sys Rev* (2):CD003417, 2005.

Degazon C: Cultural influences in nursing in community health. In Stanhope M, Lancaster J, editors: *Foundations of nursing in the community: community-oriented practice,* ed 2, St Louis, 2006, Mosby.

Farrell K, Wicks MN, Martin JC: Chronic disease self management improved with enhanced self efficacy, *Clin Nurs Res* 13(4):289–308, 2004.

Georges CA, Bolton LB, Bennett C: Functional health literacy: an issue in African-American and other ethnic and racial communities, *J Natl Black Nurses Assoc* 15(1):1–4, 2004.

Govil SR, Weidner G, Merritt-Worden T et al: Socioeconomic status and improvements in lifestyle, coronary risk factors, and quality of life: the Multisite Cardiac Lifestyle Intervention Program, *Am J Public Health* 99(7):1263–1270, 2009.

Greene J, Yedidia MJ: Provider behaviors contributing to patient self-management of chronic illness among underserved populations, *J Health Care Poor Underserved* 16:808–824, 2005.

Grey M, Knafl K, McCorkle R: A framework for the study of self- and family management of chronic conditions, *Nurs Outlook* 54:278–286, 2006.

Griffiths R, Johnson M, Piper M et al: A nursing intervention for the quality use of medicines by elderly community clients, *Intl J Nurs Pract* 10(4):166, 2004.

Haidet P, Kroll TL, Sharf BF: The complexity of patient participation: lessons learned from patients' illness narratives, *Patient Educ Couns* 62:323–329, 2006.

Heisler M: The health effects of restricting prescription medication use because of cost, *Med Care* 42(7):626–634, 2004.

Huang CL, Wu SC, Jeng CY et al: The efficacy of a home-based nursing program in diabetic control of elderly people with diabetes mellitus living alone, *Publ Health Nurse* 21(1):49, 2004.

Koch T, Jenkin P, Kralik D: Chronic illness self management: locating the "self," *J Adv Nurs* 48:484–492, 2004.

Krein SL, Heisler M, Piette JD et al: The effect of chronic pain on diabetes patients' self-management, *Diabetes Care* 28(1):65–70, 2005.

Leong J, Molassiotis A, Marsh H: Adherence to health recommendations after a cardiac rehabilitation programme in post-myocardial infarction patients: the role of heath beliefs, locus of control and psychological status, *Clin Effectiveness Nurs* 8(1):26–38, 2004.

Lorig KR, Ritter PL, Laurent DD et al: Internet-based chronic disease self management: a randomized trial, *Med Care* 44:964–971, 2006.

Nagelkerk J, Reick K, Meengs L: Perceived barriers and effective strategies to diabetes self-management, *J Adv Nurs* 54:151–158, 2006.

Nguyen HQ, Carrieri-Kohlman V, Rankin SH et al: Is Internet-based support for dyspnea self-management in patients with chronic obstructive pulmonary disease possible? Results of a pilot study, *Heart Lung* 34(1):51–62, 2005.

Ogedegbe G, Mancuso CA, Allegrante JP: Expectations of blood pressure management in hypertensive African-American patients: a qualitative study, *J Natl Med Assoc* 96(4):442–449, 2004.

Opler LA, Ramirez PM, Dominguez LM et al: Rethinking medication prescribing practices in an inner-city Hispanic mental health clinic, *J Psychiatr Pract* 10(2):134–140, 2004.

Pellatt GC: Patient-professional partnership in spinal cord injury rehabilitation, *Br J Nurs* 13(16):948–953, 2004.

Pender NJ, Murdaugh CL, Parsons MA: *Health promotion in nursing practice,* ed 5, Upper Saddle River, NJ, 2006, Prentice Hall.

Robbins B, Rausch KJ, Garcia RI et al: Multicultural medication adherence: a comparative study, *J Gerontol Nurs* 30(7):25–32, 2004.

Rogers A, Kennedy A, Nelson E et al: Uncovering the limits of patient centeredness: implementing a self management trail for chronic illness, *Qual Health Res* 15(2):224–239, 2005.

Sharma S, Murphy SP, Wilkens LR et al: Adherence to the food guide pyramid recommendations among African Americans and Latinos: results from the Multiethnic Cohort, *J Am Diet Assoc* 104(12):1873–1877, 2004.

Sol BGM, Van Der Biji JJ, Banga JD et al: Vascular risk management through nurse-led self management programs, *J Vasc Nurs* 23(1):20–24, 2005.

Stanford University, Department of Medicine: *Educational materials,* http://patienteducation.stanford.edu/internet/. Accessed April 25, 2007.

Stuckey HL, Dellasega C, Graber NJ et al: Diabetes nurse case management and motivational interviewing for change (DYNAMIC): study design and baseline characteristics in the Chronic Care Model for type 2 diabetes, *Contemp Clin Trials* 30(4):366–374, 2009.

Unzueta M, Globe D, Wu J et al: Los Angeles Latino Eye Study Group. Compliance with recommendations for follow-up care in Latinos: the Los Angeles Latino Eye Study, *Ethn Dis* 14(2):285–291, 2004.

Vijan S, Stuart, NS, Fitzgerald JT et al: Barriers to following dietary recommendations in type 2 diabetes, *Diabet Med* 22(1):32–38, 2005.

Warsi A, Wang PS, LaValley MP et al: Self management education programs in chronic disease, *Arch Intern Med* 164:1641–1649, 2004.

Watts T, Merrell J, Murphy F et al: Breast health information needs of women from minority ethnic groups, *J Adv Nurs* 47(5):526–535, 2004.

Whittemore R, Melkus GD, Grey M: Metabolic control, self management and psychosocial adjustment in women with type 2 diabetes, *J Clin Nurs* 14(2):195–204, 2005.

Impaired Home maintenance

Kathaleen C. Bloom, PhD, CNM, and Barbara J. Olinzock, RN, EdD

Definition

Inability to independently maintain a safe, growth-promoting immediate environment

Defining Characteristics

Objective

Disorderly surroundings; inappropriate household temperature; insufficient clothes; insufficient linen; lack of clothes; lack of linen; lack of necessary equipment; offensive odors; overtaxed family members; presence of vermin; repeated unhygienic disorders; repeated unhygienic infections; unavailable cooking equipment; unclean surroundings

Subjective

Household members describe financial crises; household members describe outstanding debts; household members express difficulty in maintaining their home in a comfortable fashion; household members request assistance with home maintenance

Related Factors (r/t)

Deficient knowledge; disease; inadequate support systems; injury; impaired functioning; insufficient family organization; insufficient family planning; insufficient finances; lack of role modeling; unfamiliarity with neighborhood resources

 (Nursing Outcomes Classification)

Suggested NOC Outcomes

Safe Home Environment, Self-Care Assistance: Instrumental Activities of Daily Living (IADLs)

Example NOC Outcome with Indicators
Safe Home Environment as evidenced by the following indicators: Elimination of rodents and insects/Smoke detector maintenance/Provision of assistive devices in accessible location/Elimination of tobacco smoke (Rate the outcome and indicators of **Safe Home Environment:** 1 = not adequate, 2 = slightly adequate, 3 = moderately adequate, 4 = substantially adequate, 5 = totally adequate [see Section I].)

• = Independent   ▲ = Collaborative   **EBN** = Evidence-Based Nursing   **EB** = Evidence-Based

Client Outcomes

Client Will (Specify Time Frame):
- Maintain a healthy home environment
- Use community resources to assist with home care needs

NIC   (Nursing Interventions Classification)

Suggested NIC Intervention

Home Maintenance Assistance

Example NIC Activities—Home Maintenance Assistance
Involve client/family in deciding home maintenance requirements; Provide information on how to make home environment safe and clean; Help family use social support network

Nursing Interventions and *Rationales*

- Assess the concerns of family members, especially the primary caregiver, about long-term home care. **EBN:** *Caregivers express frustration with health care providers' lack of awareness of circumstances at home (Salin & Åstedt-Kurki, 2007). Poor family support increases the risk of adverse outcomes for caregivers (Etters, Goodall, & Harrison, 2008).*
- ▲ Consider a pre-discharge home assessment referral to determine the need for accessibility and safety-related environmental changes. **EB:** *Pre-discharge home assessments reveal a significant number of environmental changes that are necessary, including the need for equipment changes, home modifications and furniture changes (Harris, James, & Snow, 2008).*
- Use an assessment tool to identify environmental safety hazards in the home. **EB:** *Use of assessment tools such as the Cougar Home Safety Assessment provide structure in the identification of key environmental hazards in the home (Fisher et al, 2007).*
- Establish a plan of care with the client and family based on the client's needs and the caregiver's capabilities. **EBN:** *Collaborative identification of health-related concerns, goals, determination of ways to enhance facilitators of change and overcome barriers and obstacles is effective in engaging the family in home care that is feasible for the particular family's situation (Tyler & Horner, 2008).*
- Assist family members to develop realistic expectations of themselves in the performance of their caregiving roles. **EB:** *Interventions for caregivers of people with dementia positively affect client and caregiver general mental health as well as caregiver burden and distress (Smits et al, 2007; Signe & Elmstahl, 2008).*
- Set up a system of relief for the main caregiver in the home, and plan for sharing of household duties. **EBN:** *Respite care provides decreased burden and improved quality of life for the caregiver (Mason, Weatherly, & Spilsbury, 2007; Salin, Kaunonen, & Astedt-Kurki, 2009).*
- ▲ Initiate referral to community agencies as needed, including housekeeping services, Meals on Wheels (MOW), wheelchair-compatible transportation services, and oxygen therapy services. **EBN:** *MOW programs improve dietary intake of recipients (Roy & Payette, 2006).*
- ▲ Obtain adaptive equipment and telemedical equipment, as appropriate, to help family members continue to maintain the home environment. **EB:** *The provision of adaptive equipment, implementation of environmental modifications and in-home telemonitoring and education keeps persons with chronic illnesses out of inpatient facilities without increasing the cost of care (Bendixen et al, 2009).*
- Ask the family to identify support people. **EB:** *Mothers' abilities to safeguard their children against injury are influenced by many contextual factors, including relationships with neighbors and trust in community services (Olsen et al, 2008).*

Geriatric

- All of the previously mentioned interventions are applicable for the geriatric population.
- Explore community resources to assist with home maintenance (e.g., senior centers, Department of Aging, hospital case managers, the Internet, or church parish nurse). **EB:** *Older adults often attempt to do home maintenance and repairs themselves due to lack of awareness of available services*

• = Independent   ▲ = Collaborative   **EBN** = Evidence-Based Nursing   **EB** = Evidence-Based

and their fears related to personal safety, or being overcharged or sold services they do not need (Ashby, Ozanne-Smith, & Fox, 2007).

- Provide assistive technology devices: barrier-free environment (home modification), daily living aids, mobility aids, seating and positioning devices, and sensory aids. **EB:** *Accessibility problems in the home affect both life satisfaction and perceived health of community-dwelling older adults (Iwarsson, Horstmann, & Slaug, 2007). Proper use of technology can help "aging in place" (Chu & Chen, 2006).*
- See the care plans for **Risk for Injury** and **Risk for Falls.**

Multicultural

- Acknowledge the stresses unique to racial/ethnic communities. *Minority adults who moved to low-poverty neighborhoods were less likely to be exposed to violence and disorder, experience health problems, abuse alcohol, and receive cash assistance (Fauth, Leventhal, & Brooks-Gunn, 2008).*

Home Care

- The previously mentioned interventions incorporate these resources.
- ▲ Refer clients with mental illness and medical conditions to in-home behavioral health case management. *Clients in this program receive integrated medical and mental health services (Theis, Kozlowski, & Behrens, 2006).*
- ▲ Consider referral for new home safety technologies as they become available. *Technologies designed for functional monitoring, safety monitoring, physiological monitoring, cognitive support, sensory aids, monitoring security, and increasing social interaction are currently being investigated (Demiris & Hensel, 2008; Martin et al, 2008).*
- See care plans **Contamination** and **Risk for Contamination.**

Client/Family Teaching and Discharge Planning

- Teach the caregiver the need to set aside some personal time every day to meet his or her own needs. **EBN:** *Family needs and need for relief are important (Smits et al, 2007).*
- Identify support groups within the community to assist families in the caregiver role. **EBN:** *A nurse-led support group may have a positive effect on the well-being of spouses of stroke clients (Franzén-Dahlin et al, 2008). Caregivers who receive support services that include information, advice, and social support are more likely to be satisfied with the care (Savard et al, 2006).*
- Provide counseling and support for clients and for caregivers of clients. **EBN:** *Individual counseling and support including risk assessment, education, and referrals decreases lighting and other hazards related to falls in the home (Wyman et al, 2007). Clients whose spouses had counseling and support experienced a decrease in the rate of nursing home placement. Improvements in caregivers' satisfaction with social support, response to client behavior problems, and symptoms of depression were observed (Mittelman et al, 2006).*
- Focus teaching on environmental hazards identified in the nursing assessment. Areas may include, but are not limited to:
    - ▪ **Home Safety.** Identify the need for and use of common safety devices in the home. **EB:** *Environmental hazards were found in all homes of community-dwelling older adults assessed, with a range of 4 to 17 hazards found (Wyman et al, 2007). More than 50% of homes assessed did not have functional carbon monoxide detectors, fire extinguishers, or smoke detectors (Fisher et al, 2007).*
    - ▪ **Biologic and Chemical Contaminants.** Assess for and reduce the presence of allergens, contaminants, and pollutants in the home. **EB:** *Biologic and chemical sensitizers including dust mites, mold, tobacco smoke, and pollen are implicated in the exacerbation of chronic conditions such as asthma (Nambu et al, 2008; Dixon et al, 2009). Combining use of protective bedding covers, improved cleaning practices, and parental education produces reduction in asthma triggers and improved health outcomes (Wu & Takaro, 2007).*
    - ▪ **Food Safety.** Instruct client to avoid microbial food-borne illness by regularly washing hands, food contact surfaces, and fruits and vegetables. Meat and poultry should not be washed or rinsed.

Separate raw, cooked, and ready-to-eat foods while shopping, preparing, or storing foods. Cook foods to a safe temperature to kill microorganisms. Chill (refrigerate) perishable food promptly and defrost foods properly. Avoid raw (unpasteurized) milk or any products made from unpasteurized milk, raw or partially cooked eggs, foods containing raw eggs, raw or undercooked meat and poultry, unpasteurized juices, and raw sprouts. *The Dietary Guidelines for Americans 2005 contains additional recommendations for specific populations (USDHHS, 2005).*

- ■ **Environmental Stressors.** Assist clients and families with decision making regarding potential conflicts in home maintenance priorities, given financial constraints. **EB:** *Many families encounter conflicts prioritizing the allocation of scarce financial resources among the regulation of heating and cooling, provision of adequate food, and access to and use of health care services (Cook et al, 2008).*

- • Teach clients to prevent exposure that could result in adverse health effects from disturbed mold. Avoid areas where mold contamination is obvious; use environmental controls; use personal protective equipment; and keep hands, skin, and clothing clean and free from mold-contaminated dust. *Extensive water damage after major hurricanes and floods increases the likelihood of mold contamination in buildings. These measures help to limit exposure to mold and help to prevent mold-related health effects (Brandt et al, 2006).*

- • See care plans **Contamination, Risk for Contamination, Risk for Falls, Risk for Infection,** and **Risk for Injury.**

Ⓔvolve   See the EVOLVE website for Weblinks for client education resources.

REFERENCES

Ashby K, Ozanne-Smith J, Fox B: Investigating the over-representation of older persons in do-it-yourself home maintenance injury and barriers to prevention, *Inj Prev* 13(5):328–333, 2007.

Bendixen RM, Levy CE, Olive ES et al: Cost effectiveness of a telerehabilitation program to support chronically ill and disabled elders in their homes, *Telemed J E Health*, 15(1):31–38, 2009.

Brandt M, Brown C, Burkhart J et al: Mold prevention strategies and possible health effects in the aftermath of hurricanes and major floods, *MMWR Recomm Rep* 55(RR-8):1–27, 2006.

Chu HT, Chen MH: Assistive technology devices for the elderly at home [in Chinese], *Hu Li Za Zhi* 53(5):20–27, 2006.

Cook JT, Frank DA, Casey PH et al: A brief indicator of household energy security: associations with food security, child health, and child development in US infants and toddlers, *Pediatrics* 122(4):e867–e875, 2008.

Demiris G, Hensel BK: Technologies for an aging society: a systematic review of "smart home" applications, *Yearb Med Inform* 33–40, 2008.

Dixon SL, Fowler C, Harris J et al: An examination of interventions to reduce respiratory health and injury hazards in homes of low-income families, *Environ Res* 109(1):123–130, 2009.

Etters L, Goodall D, Harrison BE: Caregiver burden among dementia patient caregivers: a review of the literature, *Am Acad Nurse Pract* 20(8):423–428, 2008.

Fauth RC, Leventhal T, Brooks-Gunn J: Seven years later: effects of a neighborhood mobility program on poor Black and Latino adults' well-being, *J Health Soc Behav* 49(2):119–30, 2008.

Fisher GS, Baker A, Koval D et al: A field test of the Cougar Home Safety Assessment (version 2.0) in the homes of older persons living alone, *Aust Occup Ther J* 54(2):124–130, 2007.

Franzén-Dahlin A, Larson J, Murray V et al: A randomized controlled trial evaluating the effect of a support and education programme for spouses of people affected by stroke, *Clin Rehabil* 22(8):722–730, 2008.

Harris S, James E, Snow P: Predischarge occupational therapy home assessment visits: towards an evidence base, *Aust Occup Ther J* 55(2):85–95, 2008.

Iwarsson S, Horstmann V, Slaug B: Housing matters in very old age—yet differently due to ADL dependence level differences, *Scand J Occup Ther* 14(1):3–15, 2007.

Martin S, Kelly G, Kernohan WG et al: Smart home technologies for health and social care support, *Cochrane Database Syst Rev* (4): CD006412, 2008.

Mason A, Weatherly H, Spilsbury K: A systematic review of the effectiveness and cost-effectiveness of different models of community-based respite care for frail older people and their carers, *Health Technol Assess* 11(15):1–157, iii, 2007.

Mittelman MS, Haley WE, Clay OJ et al: Improving caregiver well-being delays nursing home placement of patients with Alzheimer disease, *Neurology* 67(9):1592–1599, 2006.

Nambu M, Shirai H, Sakaguchi M et al: The effect of dust mite-free pillow on clinical course of asthma and IgE level—a randomized, double-blind, controlled study, *Pediatr Asthma Allergy Immunol* 21(3):137–143, 2008.

Olsen L, Bottorff JL, Raina P et al: An ethnography of low-income mothers' safeguarding efforts, *J Safety Res* 39(6):609–616, 2008.

Roy MA, Payette H: Meals-on-wheels improves energy and nutrient intake in a frail free-living elderly population, *J Nutr Health Aging* 10(6):554–560, 2006.

Salin S, Åstedt-Kurki P: Women's views of caring for family members: use of respite care, *J Gerontol Nurs* 33(9):37–45, 2007.

Salin S, Kaunonen M, Åstedt-Kurki P: Informal carers of older family members: how they manage and what support they receive from respite care, *J Clin Nurs* 18(4):492–501, 2009.

Savard J, Leduc N, Lebel P et al: Caregiver satisfaction with support services: influence of different types of services, *J Aging Health* 18(1):3–27, 2006.

Signe A, Elmståhl S: Psychosocial intervention for family caregivers of people with dementia reduces caregiver's burden: development and effect after 6 and 12 months, *Scand J Caring Sci* 22(1):98–109, 2008.

Smits CH, de Lange J, Dröes RM et al: Effects of combined intervention programmes for people with dementia living at home and their caregivers: a systematic review, *Int J Geriatr Psychiatry* 22(12):1181–1193, 2007.

• = Independent   ▲ = Collaborative   **EBN** = Evidence-Based Nursing   **EB** = Evidence-Based

Theis GA, Kozlowski D, Behrens J: In-home behavioral health case management: an integrated model for high-risk populations, *Case Manager* 17(6):60–65, 68, 2006.

Tyler DO, Horner SD: Collaborating with low-income families and their overweight children to improve weight-related behaviors: an intervention process evaluation, *Spec Pediatr Nurs* 13(4):263–274, 2008.

U.S. Department of Health and Human Services and U.S. Department of Agriculture: *Dietary guidelines for Americans 2005*, 6th edition, Washington, DC, 2005, U.S. Government Printing Office.

Wu F, Takaro TK: Childhood asthma and environmental interventions, *Environ Health Perspect* 115(6):971–975, 2007.

Wyman JF, Croghan CF, Nachreiner NM et al: Effectiveness of education and individualized counseling in reducing environmental hazards in the homes of community-dwelling older women, *J AM Geriatr Soc* 55(10):1548–1556, 2007.

Readiness for enhanced Hope   *Marie Giordano, RN, MS*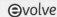

Definition

A pattern of expectations and desires that is sufficient for mobilizing energy on one's own behalf and can be strengthened

Defining Characteristics

Expresses desire to enhance ability to set achievable goals; expresses desire to enhance belief in possibilities; expresses desire to enhance congruency of expectations with desires; expresses desire to enhance hope; expresses desire to enhance interconnectedness with others; expresses desire to enhance problem solving to meet goals; expresses desire to enhance sense of meaning to life; expresses desire to enhance spirituality

NOC   (Nursing Outcomes Classification)

Suggested NOC Outcomes

Hope, Quality of Life

Example NOC Outcome with Indicators
Hope as evidenced by the following indicators: Expresses expectation of a positive future/Expresses faith/Expresses meaning in life/Exhibits a zest for life/Sets goals (Rate the outcome and indicators of **Hope** as: 1 = never demonstrated, 2 = rarely demonstrated, 3 = sometimes demonstrated, 4 = often demonstrated, 5 = consistently demonstrated [see Section I].)

Client Outcomes

Client Will (Specify Time Frame):

- Describe values, expectations, and meanings
- Set achievable goals that are consistent with values
- Design strategies to achieve goals
- Express belief in possibilities

NIC   (Nursing Interventions Classification)

Suggested NIC Interventions

Emotional Support, Hope Instillation, Presence, Support System Enhancement

Example NIC Activities—Hope Instillation
Assist patient and family to identify areas of hope in life; Demonstrate hope by recognizing the patient's intrinsic worth; Encourage therapeutic relationships; Help the person expand spiritual self

Nursing Interventions and *Rationales*

- Develop an open and caring relationship that enables the client to discuss hope. **EBN:** *Hope and well-being were strongly related in a study of 130 older adults. The authors concluded that nurses need to foster hope in a variety of ways, with development of an open and caring relationship being the first step (Davis, 2005).*
- Screen the client for hope using a valid and reliable instrument as indicated. **EBN:** *The Herth Hope Index (HHIndex) was developed and tested for use in screening for hope in clinical settings (Herth 1992; Rustoen et al, 2005). Use of the HHIndex to compare the hope of 93 clients hospitalized with heart failure and 441 healthy control subjects showed that hope does not relate to disease; those with CHF had higher levels of hope than the random group of healthy community-dwelling persons (Rustoen et al, 2005). Findings in this study indicate that the HHIndex is a reliable measure of hope in adolescents and young adults with cancer (Phillips-Salimi et al, 2007).*
- Focus on the positive aspects of hope, rather than the prevention of hopelessness. **EBN:** *Numerous studies conducted during development of the health promotion model show that promotion differs from prevention and requires a positive rather than negative approach (Pender, Murdaugh, & Parsons, 2006).*
- Provide emotional support. **EBN:** *A qualitative longitudinal study of the meaning of hope with 10 persons who had had acute spinal cord injury one year previous showed that emotional and motivational strategies were important to promote hope and that hope is a powerful experience for health (Lohne & Severinsson, 2006).*
- Promote the client's awareness of the existential meanings in life events. **EB:** *In an undergraduate population (n = 191), research findings strongly supported that existential meanings, both explicit and implicit, were related to decreased depressive symptoms and increased levels of hope measured with two different instruments (Mascaro & Rosen, 2005).*
- Help the person to identify his or her desires and expectations. **EBN:** *Future orientation was one type of hope identified in a study of the nature of hope in chronically ill hospitalized clients (Kim et al, 2006). A review of 13 studies that looked at cancer prognosis and disease trajectory, focused on the effects of knowing. Having increased control over end-of-life planning was seen as giving them enhanced hope (Innes & Payne, 2009).*
- Use a family-oriented approach when discussing hope. **EB:** *Including the family may facilitate the family's hope to be similar to the client's hope. In a study of 40 clients with cancer and 45 family members, the level of hope in family members was significantly lower than the clients (p <.005) (Benzein & Berg, 2005).*
- Review internal and external resources to enhance hope. **EB:** *In a study of 1041 medical records over a 2–year period, higher levels of hope were associated with decreased likelihood of having or developing a disease (Richman et al, 2005).* **EBN:** *In a concept analysis of hope, based on a review of 17 research studies of terminally ill clients, the ten attributes of hope were identified as "positive expectation, positive qualities, spirituality, goals, comfort, help/caring, interpersonal relationships, control, legacy, and life review"(Johnson, 2007).*
- Identify spiritual beliefs and practices. **EBN:** *In a cross-sectional correlational study with 130 adults aged 60 to 89, spirituality was identified as a mediator of hope and well-being (N = .52, p <.001) (Davis, 2005). In Weil's (2000) study, hope was related to spiritual beliefs and other factors. Spiritual beliefs and practices are associated with higher levels of existential meaning, which is related to hope (Mascaro & Rosen, 2005). Hope is a spiritual need, as identified in a study of 683 individuals (Flannelly, Galek, & Flannelly, 2006).*
- Assist the person to consider possible adaptations to changes. **EBN:** *A grounded theory study of 41 women looked at refocusing hope after having a diagnosis of fetal abnormality identified by ultrasound. It identified four phases they experienced as "assume normal", "shock", "gaining meaning" and "rebuilding." It showed that they maintained hope by attaching their hopes to reality and adapting to changes as needed (Lalor, Begley, & Galavan, 2009).*

 Home Care

- The above interventions may be adapted for home care use.

• = Independent   ▲ = Collaborative   **EBN** = Evidence-Based Nursing   **EB** = Evidence-Based

Client/Family Teaching and Discharge Planning

- Assess client and family hope prior to teaching. **EBN:** *The degree and type of client and family hope may differ from each other, which may interfere with learning and use of knowledge for problem solving (Benzein & Berg, 2005).*
- Incorporate client and family goal setting with teaching content. **EBN:** *Realistic goal setting fosters and supports hope (Lalor, Begley, & Galavan, 2009).*
- Provide information to the client and family regarding all aspects of the client's health condition. **EBN:** *Accurate and complete information sharing empowers, which is more likely to support hope than the perceptions that might occur without accurate and complete information (Forbat et al, 2009; Lalor, Begley, & Galavan, 2009).*

evolve   See the EVOLVE website for Weblinks for client education resources.

REFERENCES

Benzein EG, Berg AC: The level of and relation between hope, hopelessness and fatigue in patients and family members in palliative care, *Palliat Med* 19:234–240, 2005.

Davis B: Mediators of the relationship between hope and well-being in older adults, *Clin Nurs Res,* 14(3):253–272, 2005.

Flannelly KJ, Galek K, Flannelly LT: A test of the factor structure of the patient spiritual needs assessment scale, *Holist Nurs Pract* 20(4):187–190, 2006.

Forbat L, Maguire R, McCann L et al: The use of technology in cancer care: applying Foucault's ideas to explore the changing dynamics of power in health care, *J Adv Nurs* 65(2):306–315, 2009.

Herth K: Abbreviated instrument to measure hope: development and psychometric evaluation, *J Adv Nurs,* 17:1251–1259, 1992.

Innes P, Payne S: Advanced cancer patients' prognostic information preferences: a review, *Pall Med,* 23(1):29–39, 2009.

Johnson S: Hope in terminal illness: an evolutionary concept analysis, *Int J Palliat Nurs* 13(9):451–459, 2007.

Kim DS, Kim HS, Schwartz-Barcott D et al: The nature of hope in hospitalized chronically ill patients, *Int J Nurs Stud* 43(5):547–556, 2006.

Lalor J, Begley CM, Galavan E: Recasting hope: a process of adaptation following fetal anomaly diagnosis, *Soc Sci Med* 68(3):362–372, 2009.

Lohne V, Severinsson E: The power of hope: patient's experiences of hope a year after spinal cord injury, *J Clin Nurs* 15(3):315–323, 2006.

Mascaro N, Rosen DH: Existential meanings' role in the enhancement of hope and prevention of depressive symptoms, *J Pers* 73(4):985–1013, 2005.

Pender NJ, Murdaugh CL, Parsons MA: *Health promotion in nursing practice,* ed 5, Stamford CT, 2006, Appleton & Lange.

Phillips-Salimi CR, Haase JE, Kintner EK et al: Psychometric properties of the Herth Hope Index in adolescents and young adults with cancer, *J Nurs Measurement* 15(1):3–23, 2007.

Richman LS, Kubzansky L, Maselko J et al: Positive emotion and health: going beyond the negative, *Health Psychol* 24(4):422–429, 2005.

Rustoen T, Howie J, Eidsmo I et al: Hope in patients hospitalized with heart failure, *Am J Crit Care* 14(5):417–425, 2005.

Weil CM: Exploring hope in patients with end stage renal disease on chronic hemodialysis, *Nephrol Nurs J* 27(2):219–224, 2000.

Hopelessness   *Wendy Duggleby, PhD*   evolve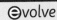

NANDA-I

Definition

Subjective state in which an individual sees limited or no alternatives or personal choices available and is unable to mobilize energy on own behalf

Defining Characteristics

Closing eyes; decreased affect; decreased appetite; decreased response to stimuli; decreased verbalization; lack of initiative; lack of involvement in care; passivity; shrugging in response to speaker; sleep pattern disturbance; turning away from speaker; verbal cues (e.g., despondent content, "I can't," sighing)

Related Factors (r/t)

Abandonment; deteriorating physiological condition; lost belief in spiritual power; lost belief in transcendent values; long-term stress; prolonged activity restriction creating isolation

NOC   **(Nursing Outcomes Classification)**

Suggested NOC Outcomes

Decision Making, Hope, Mood Equilibrium, Nutritional Status: Food and Fluid Intake, Quality of Life, Sleep

 • = Independent   ▲ = Collaborative   **EBN** = Evidence-Based Nursing   **EB** = Evidence-Based

---

Example NOC Outcome with Indicators

Has a presence of **Hope** as evidenced by the following indicators: Expresses expectation of a positive future/Expresses faith/Expresses will to live (Rate the outcome and indicators of **Hope:** 1 = never demonstrated, 2 = rarely demonstrated, 3 = sometimes demonstrated, 4 = often demonstrated, 5 = consistently demonstrated [see Section I].)

Client Outcomes

Client Will (Specify Time Frame):

- Verbalize feelings, participate in care
- Make positive statements (e.g., "I can" or "I will try")
- Set goals
- Make eye contact, focus on speaker
- Maintain appropriate appetite for age and physical health
- Sleep appropriate length of time for age and physical health
- Express concern for another
- Initiate activity

 (Nursing Interventions Classification)

Suggested NIC Intervention

Hope Inspiration

Example NIC Activities—Hope Inspiration

Assist patient/family to identify areas of hope in life; Demonstrate hope by recognizing client's intrinsic worth and viewing patient's illness as only one facet of the individual; Expand the patient's repertoire of coping mechanisms

Nursing Interventions and *Rationales*

▲ Monitor and document the potential for suicide. (Refer the client for appropriate treatment if a potential for suicide is identified.) Refer to the care plan **Risk for Suicide** for specific interventions. **EB:** *Hopelessness is a major risk factor for suicide (McMillan et al, 2007).*

▲ Monitor potential for depression. (Refer the client for appropriate treatment if depression is identified.) **EB:** *Hopelessness is a potential predictor for depressive symptoms for breast cancer clients (Brothers & Andersen, 2008).* **EB:** *Treatment of depression significantly decreased hopelessness in older adults (Saghafi, Brown, & Butters, 2007).*

- Monitor family caregivers for symptoms of hopelessness. **EB:** *Caregivers of advanced cancer clients are at risk for experiencing hopelessness (Mystakidou et al, 2007a).* **EBN:** *Parents of children with cancer are at risk for hopelessness (Bayat, Erdem, & Kuzucu, 2008).* **EB:** *Caregivers of persons with dementia were more hopeless than non-caregivers (Bandera, Pawlowski, & Goncalves, 2007).*

- Determine appropriate approaches based on the underlying condition or situation that is contributing to feelings of hopelessness. **EB:** *Understanding the source of the hopelessness such as negative life events, will indicate the approaches that may be most beneficial to the person (Toussaint et al, 2008).* **EBN:** *Women with advanced breast cancer and their families and men with prostate cancer and their families benefit from specific strategies of intervention (Northouse, Kershaw, & Mood, 2005; Northouse et al, 2007).*

- Assess for pain and respond with appropriate measures for pain relief. **EB:** *Pain that interferes with mood and enjoyment in life results in feelings of hopelessness for clients with advanced cancer (Mystakidou et al, 2007b).*

- Facilitate access to resources to support spiritual well-being. **EB:** *Low spiritual well-being is a risk factor for hopelessness (Arnette et al, 2007; Rodin, Lo, & Mikulincer, 2009).* **EB:** *Strategies to enhance spiritual well-being may decrease hopelessness (Toussaint et al, 2008).*

- Assist the client in looking at alternatives and setting goals that are important to him or her. *Use of the nurse's knowledge along with the client's experience within the context of a supportive relationship stimulates an unfolding of possibilities (Kylma, 2005).* **EBN:** *When health professionals work with men*

• = Independent   ▲ = Collaborative   **EBN** = Evidence-Based Nursing   **EB** = Evidence-Based

with prostate cancer and their family caregivers, they should help them replace avoidant coping strategies (Northouse et al, 2007).

- Discussion of hope may be helpful in increasing hope. *Entering into discussion of hope may be helpful in increasing hope (Cutcliff & Koehn, 2007).* **EBN:** *Health-promoting conversations about hope and suffering with couples in palliative care has potential for improving hope (Benzein & Savemant, 2008).*
- Provide accurate information. **EBN:** *Accurate information allows the redefining and transforming of hope (Duggleby & Wright, 2005; Duggleby et al, 2009).* **EB:** *Educational interventions may decrease hopelessness related to the threat of breast cancer in young women (Fry & Prentice-Dunn, 2006).*
- Encourage decision making and problem solving. **EBN:** *Hopelessness may be an outgrowth of a perceived loss of control and/or self-efficacy. As changes occur, the nurse interacts with the client to evaluate their impact on life goals and assists in making adaptations that support hopefulness and decrease hopelessness (Kylma, 2005).* **EB:** *Problem-solving therapy decreased depression and suicide in adolescents and young adults (Eskin, Ertekin, & Demir, 2007).*
- Spend one-on-one time with the client. Use empathy; try to understand what the client is saying and communicate this understanding to the client to create a nonjudgmental trusting environment to develop therapeutic relationships with the client. *The therapeutic relationship is an essential component of interventions to address hopelessness (Koehn & Cutcliff, 2007).* **EBN:** *Establishing new relationships and control over events within them is constructive within the context of nurturing hopefulness (Kylma, 2005).*
- Teach alternative coping strategies such as physical activity. **EBN:** *As the number of minutes of exercise increased, hopelessness decreased in prison inmates (Cashin, Potter, & Butler, 2008).* **EB:** *In college students, physical activity each week was associated with decreased feelings of hopelessness (Taliaferro, Rienzo, & Pigg, 2008).*
- Review the client's strengths and resources with the client. **EBN:** *Working with the client to identify positive experiences, resources and personal strengths facilitates the development of hopefulness (Kylma, 2005).*
- Involve family and significant others in the plan of care. **EB:** *The levels of depressive symptoms in children was associated with depressive symptoms of their parents (Abela et al, 2006).* **EBN:** *Social support decreased hopelessness and anxiety in parents of children with cancer (Bayat, Erdem, & Kuzucu, 2008).*
- For additional interventions, see the care plans for **Readiness for enhanced Hope**, **Spiritual distress**, **Readiness for enhanced Spiritual well-being**, and **Disturbed Sleep pattern**.

Geriatric

- Previous interventions may be adapted for geriatric clients.
- ▲ If depression is suspected; confer with the primary physician regarding referral for mental health services. *Studies with the elderly confirm that suicidal thoughts are strongly associated with the presence of depressive disorder (Thompsell, 2009).*
- Take threats of self-harm or suicide seriously. *Suicide is preventable and ranks among the top causes of death in the United States among those over age 65. Upon detecting clues that the older person is thinking about suicide, the risk should be considered serious and evaluation should occur promptly (Valente, 2008).*
- Use reminiscence and life-review therapies to identify past coping skills. *Older people in residential facilities benefit from this therapy (Wang, 2004). Life review produced a positive outcome when used with individuals with right hemisphere cerebral vascular accidents (Davis, 2004).*
- Encourage visits from children. *Social relationships foster hopefulness (Duggleby, 2001).*
- Position the client by a window, take the client outside, or encourage such activities as gardening (if ability allows). *Using nature can help older people expand their perspectives, connect with strength, and expand their coping strategies, while gaining a wider sense of acceptance and completion in life (Berger, 2009).*
- Provide esthetic forms of expression, such as dance, music, literature, and pictures. **EBN:** *Aesthetic experiences are related to feelings of timelessness and spacelessness, and serve as sources of gratification (Wikstrom, 2004).*

• = Independent   ▲ = Collaborative   **EBN** = Evidence-Based Nursing   **EB** = Evidence-Based

Multicultural

- Assess for the influence of cultural beliefs, norms, and values on the client's feelings of hopelessness. **EBN:** *The client's expressions of hopelessness may be based on cultural perceptions (Leininger & McFarland, 2002).* **EB:** *Perceived racism is associated with higher levels of hopelessness for African American boys (Nyborg & Curry, 2003). The interrelationship between contextual risk factors, rational choice theory, and opportunity cost provide a model to explain why African Americans die at a disproportionately higher rate from cardiovascular-related diseases (Appel, Giger, & Davidhizar, 2005).*
- Assess the effect of fatalism on the client's expression of hopelessness. **EBN:** *Fatalistic perspectives, which involve the belief that one cannot control one's own fate, may influence health behaviors in some Asian, African American, and Latino populations (Chen, 2001).*
- ▲ Assess for depression and refer to appropriate services. **EBN:** *Older Taiwanese American adults with depressive symptoms report hopelessness as a symptom (Suen & Tusaie, 2004). The severity of depression in African Americans and Latinos may be predicted by feelings of hopelessness (Myers et al, 2002).*
- Encourage spirituality as a source of support for hopelessness. **EBN:** *African Americans and Latinos may identify spirituality, religiousness, prayer, and church-based approaches as coping resources (Samuel-Hodge et al, 2000).* **EBN:** *Spiritual beliefs, the role of prayer, and the role of family in caregiving were predominant aspects in the end-of-life experience in Mexican Americans. There is a need to focus on the role of religious institutions in Mexican American culture, where spirituality and religion are strong influences in the life experience (Johnston, 2007).*

 Home Care

- Previously mentioned interventions may be adapted for home care use.
- ▲ Assess for isolation within the family unit. Encourage the client to participate in family activities. If the client cannot participate, encourage him or her to be in the same area and watch family activities. Refer for telephone support. *Hope is facilitated by meaningful interpersonal relationships (Koehn & Cutcliff, 2007).* **EB:** *Clients show significant improvements in depression and positive affect during the 16 weeks of telephone-administered treatment (Mohr, Hart, & Julian, 2005).*
- Reminisce with the client about his or her life. **EBN:** *The process of remembering past activities helps find meaning and purpose in life and inspires hope (Duggleby & Wright, 2005).* **EB:** *Older people in residential facilities benefit from life review (Chin, 2007).*
- Identify areas in which the client can have control. *Allow the client to set achievable goals in these areas. Assist the client when necessary to negotiate desirable outcomes.* **EBN:** *Mobilization of resources to promote self-efficacy promotes hope (Kylma, 2005).*
- If illness precipitated the hopelessness, discuss knowledge of and previous experience with the disease. *Help the client to identify past coping strengths.* **EBN:** *Knowledge of the disease and previous positive coping experience with the illness provide hope for the future (Duggleby & Wright, 2005).*
- ▲ Provide plant or pet therapy if possible. **EBN:** *Caring for pets or plants helps to find meaning and purpose and foster hope (Holtslander & Duggleby, 2009).* **EB:** *Pet therapy has been reported to have a positive effect on psychological well-being (Colombo et al, 2006).*

 Client/Family Teaching and Discharge Planning

- Provide information regarding the client's condition, treatment plan, and progress. **EBN:** *Clear, direct communication of the potential of an intervention to overcome a threat along with honest discussion of negative aspects fosters hope for clients and their families (Duggleby & Wright, 2005; Holtslander et al, 2005).*
- Teach family caregivers skills to provide care in the home. **EBN:** *Family caregivers find hope in giving skilled care to their family members (Duggleby et al, 2009).* **EBN:** *A psychoeducational program preparing family caregivers for caring for a dying relative a home increased their feeling of caregiving competence and rewards (Hudson et al, 2008).*
- Provide positive reinforcement, praise, and acknowledgment of the challenges of caregiving to family members. **EBN:** *Positive comments and praise foster hope in family caregivers (Holtslander et al, 2005).*

• = Independent   ▲ = Collaborative   **EBN** = Evidence-Based Nursing   **EB** = Evidence-Based

▲ Refer the client to self-help groups, such as I Can Cope and Make Today Count. **EBN:** *Self-help and/or professionally led curriculum-based support programs for families are effective in reducing stress and facilitating coping and hope (Northouse et al, 2007).*

ⓔvolve   See the EVOLVE website for Weblinks for client education resources.

REFERENCES

Abela JR, Skitch SA, Adams P et al: The timing of parent and child depression: a hopelessness theory perspective, *J Clin Child Adolesc Psychol* 35(2):253–263, 2006.

Appel SJ, Giger JN, Davidhizar RE: Opportunity cost: the impact of contextual risk factors on the cardiovascular health of low-income rural southern African American women, *J Cardiovasc Nurs* 20:315–324, 2005.

Arnette NC, Mascaro N, Santana MC et al: Enhancing spiritual well-being among suicidal African American female survivors of intimate partner violence, *J Clin Psychol* 63(10):909–924, 2007.

Bandera DR, Pawlowski J, Goncalves TR: Psychological distress in Brazilian caregivers of relatives with dementia, *Aging Ment Health* 11(1):14–19, 2007.

Bayat M, Erdem E, Kuzucu EG: Depression, anxiety, hopelessness and social support levels of the parents of children with cancer, *J Pediatr Oncol Nurs* 25:247–253, 2008.

Benzein EV, Savemant BI: Health-promoting conversation about hope and suffering with couples in palliative care, *Int J Palliat Nurs* 14(9):409–445, 2008.

Berger R: Being in nature: an innovative framework for incorporating nature in therapy with older adults, *J Holist Nurs* 27(1):45–50, 2009.

Brothers BM, Andersen BL: Hopelessness as a predictor of depressive symptoms for breast cancer patients coping with recurrence, *Psychooncol* 18(3):267–275, 2008.

Cashin A, Potter E, Butler T: The relationship between exercise and hopelessness in prison, *J Psychiatr Ment Health Nurs* 15:66–71, 2008.

Chen YC: Chinese values, health and nursing, *J Adv Nurs* 36(2):270, 2001.

Chin A: Clinical effects of reminiscence therapy in older adults: a meta-analysis of controlled trials, *Hong Kong J Occupat Ther* 17(1):10–22, 2007.

Colombo G, Dello Buono M, Smania K et al: Pet therapy and institutionalized elderly: a study on 144 cognitively unimpaired subjects, *Arch Gerontol Geriatr* 42(2):207–216, 2006.

Cutcliff JR, Koehn CV: Hope and interpersonal psychiatric/mental health nursing: a systematic review of the literature—part two, *J Psychiatr Ment Health Nurs* 14:141–147, 2007.

Davis MC: Life review therapy as an intervention to manage depression and enhance life satisfaction in individuals with right hemisphere cerebral vascular accidents, *Issues Ment Health Nurs* 25(5):503–515, 2004.

Duggleby W: Hope at the end of life, *J Hospice Palliat Nurs* 3(2):51, 2001.

Duggleby W, Williams A, Wright K et al: Renewing everyday hope: the hope experience of family caregivers of persons with dementia, *Issues Ment Health Nurs* 30(8):514–521, 2009.

Duggleby W, Wright K: Transforming hope: how elderly palliative patients live with hope, *Can J Nurs Res* 37:2, 70–84, 2005.

Eskin M, Ertekin K, Demir H: Efficacy of a problem-solving therapy for depression and suicide potential in adolescents and young adults, *Cogn Ther Res* 32(2):227–245, 2007.

Fry RB, Prentice-Dunn S: Effects of psychosocial intervention on breast self-examination attitudes and behaviors, *Health Educ Res* 21:2, 287–295, 2006.

Holtslander L, Duggleby W: The hope experience of older bereaved women who cared for a spouse with terminal cancer, *Qual Health Res* 19:388–400, 2009.

Holtslander L, Duggleby W, Willams A et al: The experience of hope for informal caregivers of palliative patients, *J Palliat Care* 21(4):285–291, 2005.

Hudson P, Quinn K, Kristjanson L et al: Evaluation of a psycho-educational group program for family caregivers in home-based palliative care, *Palliat Med* 22:270–280, 2008.

Johnston R: *Religions in society,* ed 7, Upper Saddle River NJ, 2007, Pearson Prentice Hall.

Koehn CV, Cutcliff JR: Hope and interpersonal psychiatric/mental health nursing: a systematic review of the literature-part one, *J Psychiatr Ment Health Nurs* 14:134–140, 2007.

Kylma J: Despair and hopelessness in the context of HIV: a meta-synthesis on qualitative research findings, *J Clin Nurs* 14:813–821, 2005.

Leininger MM, McFarland MR: *Transcultural nursing: concepts, theories, research and practices,* ed 3, New York, 2002, McGraw-Hill.

McMillan D, Gilbody S, Beresford E et al: Can we predict suicide and non-fatal self-harm with the Beck Hopelessness Scale? A meta-analysis, *Psychol Med* 37:769–778, 2007.

Mohr D, Hart S, Julian L: Telephone administered psychotherapy for depression, *Arch Gen Psychiatry* 62(9):1007–1014, 2005.

Myers HF, Lesser I, Rodriguez N et al: Ethnic differences in clinical presentation of depression in adult women, *Cultur Divers Ethnic Minor Psychol* 8(2):138–156, 2002.

Mystakidou K, Tsilika E, Parpa E et al: Caregivers of advanced cancer patients: feelings of hopelessness and depression, *Cancer Nurs* 30(5):412–418, 2007a.

Mystakidou K, Tsilika E, Parpa E et al: Exploring the relationships between depression, hopelessness, cognitive status, pain and spirituality in patients with advanced cancer, *Arch Psychiatr Nurs* 21(3):150–161, 2007b.

Northouse L, Kershaw T, Mood DW: Effects of a family intervention on the quality of life of women with recurrent breast cancer and their members, *Psychooncol* 14(6):478–491, 2005.

Northouse L, Mood DW, Schafenacker A et al: Randomized clinical trial of a family intervention for prostate cancer patients and their spouses, *Cancer* 110:2809–2811, 2007.

Nyborg VM, Curry JF: The impact of perceived racism: psychological symptoms among African American boys, *J Clin Child Adolesc Psychol* 32(2):258–266, 2003.

Rodin G, Lo C, Mikulincer M: Pathways to distress: the multiple determinants of depression, hopelessness and the desire for hastened death in metastatic cancer patients, *Soc Sci Med* 68(3):562–569, 2009.

Saghafi R, Brown C, Butters MA: Predicting 6–week treatment response to excitalpropram pharmacotherapy in late-life major depressive disorder. *Int J Geriatr Psychiatry* 22:1141–1146, 2007.

Samuel-Hodge CD, Headen SW, Skelly AH et al: Influences on day-to-day self-management of type 2 diabetes among African American women: spirituality, the multi-caregiver role, and other social context factors, *Diabetes Care* 23(7):928, 2000.

Suen LJ, Tusaie K: Is somatization a significant depressive symptom in older Taiwanese Americans? *Geriatr Nurs* 25(3):157–163, 2004.

Taliaferro LS, Rienzo BA, Pigg M: Associations between physical activity and reduced rates of hopelessness, depression and suicidal behavior among college students, *J Am Coll Health* 57(4):427–425, 2008.

Thompsell A: Self-harm and suicide-related behaviour in the elderly, *Nurs Resid Care* 11(2):84, 86–87, 2009.

● = Independent   ▲ = Collaborative   **EBN** = Evidence-Based Nursing   **EB** = Evidence-Based

Toussaint L, Williams DR, Musick MA et al: Why forgiveness may protect against depression: Hopelessness as an explanatory mechanism, *Pers Ment Health* 2:89–103, 2008.

Valente S: Suicide risk in elderly patients, *Nurse Pract* 33(8):34–40, 2008.

Wang J: The comparative effectiveness among institutionalized and non-institutionalized elderly people in Taiwan of reminiscence therapy as a psychological measure, *J Nurs Res* 12(3):237–244, 2004.

Wikstrom B: Older adults and the arts: the importance of aesthetic forms of expression in later life, *J Gerontol Nurs* 30(9):30–36, 2004.

Hyperthermia   *Betty J. Ackley, MSN, EdS, RN*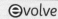

NANDA-I

Definition

Body temperature elevated above normal range

NOTE: Elevated body temperature can be either fever or hyperthermia. Fever is a regulated rise in the core body temperature or variation in the temperature set-point, as part of the host defense (Henker & Carlson, 2007). Hyperthermia is an unregulated rise in body temperature which is seen with heat illness, neurological disorders, neuroleptic malignant syndrome, or malignant hyperthermia, often with the temperature above 104° F (40° C). Hyperthermia is **not** adaptive and should be treated as a medical emergency.

Defining Characteristics

Flushed skin; increase in body temperature above normal range; tachycardia; tachypnea; warm to touch; seizures in children

Related Factors (r/t)

Anesthesia; decreased perspiration; dehydration; exposure to hot environment; inappropriate clothing; increased metabolic rate; illness; medications; trauma; vigorous activity

NOC   (Nursing Outcomes Classification)

Suggested NOC Outcomes

Thermoregulation, Thermoregulation: Newborn

Example NOC Outcome with Indicators
Thermoregulation as evidenced by the following indicators: Increased skin temperature/Decreased skin temperature/Skin color changes/Dehydration/Hyperthermia (Rate the outcome and indicators of **Thermoregulation**: 1 = severe, 2 = substantial, 3 = moderate, 4 = mild, 5 = none [see Section I].)

Client Outcomes

Client Will (Specify Time Frame):

- Maintain oral temperature within adaptive levels (less than 104° F, 40° C)
- Remain free of complications of malignant hypertension (MH)
- Remain free of dehydration

NIC   (Nursing Interventions Classification)

Suggested NIC Interventions

Fever Treatment, Malignant Hyperthermia Precautions, Temperature Regulation

Example NIC Activities—Fever Treatment
Institute a continuous core temperature monitoring device as appropriate; Monitor for decreasing levels of consciousness

Nursing Interventions and *Rationales*

- Measure and record a febrile client's temperature using an oral or rectal thermometer every 1–4 hours depending on severity of the fever or whenever a change in condition occurs (e.g., chills, change in

• = Independent   ▲ = Collaborative   **EBN** = Evidence-Based Nursing   **EB** = Evidence-Based

mental status). If client is critically ill, use an indwelling method of temperature measurement. **EBN and EB:** *Oral temperature measurement provides a more accurate temperature than tympanic measurement, axillary measurement, or use of a chemical dot thermometer (Hill, 2004; Fallis, Hamelin, & Wang, 2006; Devrim et al, 2007; Frommelt, Ott, & Hays, 2008). Research has demonstrated the accuracy of temperature measurement from most accurate to least accurate: Intravascular, esophageal, bladder thermistor, rectal, oral, tympanic membrane. Axillary, temporal artery, and chemical dot thermometers are less accurate and should be avoided in caring for the critically ill adult client (O'Grady et al, 2008).*

• Use the same site and method (device) for temperature measurement for a given client so that temperature trends are assessed accurately; record site of temperature measurement. **EBN and EB:** *There are significant differences in temperature depending on the site (oral, rectal, axillary, or temporal artery (Devrim et al, 2007; Frommelt, Ott, & Hays, 2008; O'Grady et al, 2008).*

▲ Notify the physician of temperature according to institutional standards or written orders, or when temperature reaches 100.5° F (38.3° C) and above (O'Grady et al, 2008). Also notify the physician of the presence of a change in mental status. *A change in mental status may indicate the onset of septic shock (Kleinpell & Ahrens, 2008).*

▲ Work with the physician to help determine the cause of the temperature increase, which will often help direct appropriate treatment. Collect stat cultures before beginning antibiotic therapy (O'Grady et al, 2008), and ensure that needed imaging studies are performed quickly. *It is generally more important to treat the underlying cause of the temperature increase than treat the symptom of fever (Henker & Carlson, 2007; Dellinger et al, 2008).*

▲ Administer antipyretic medication per physician orders, when the cause of the temperature is not adaptive (neurological, heat stroke, critically ill client), when infection-induced fever is greater than 38.3° C, and when the client cannot tolerate the increase in metabolic demand, such as the acutely ill client. *Elimination of fever will interfere with its enhancement of the immune response, but temperature elevation is accompanied by an increase in oxygen consumption and metabolic rate that may not be tolerated by the acutely ill client (Henker & Carlson, 2007).* **EB:** *A systematic review of three studies found little evidence to support the administration of antipyretics for fever (Hudgings et al, 2004).*

▲ Assess fluid loss and facilitate oral intake or administer intravenous fluids as ordered to accomplish fluid replacement. *Increased metabolic rate and diaphoresis associated with fever cause loss of body fluids (Heckenberg, 2008).* Refer to the care plan for **Deficient Fluid volume.**

• Use external cooling measures carefully such as tepid water baths, or removal of blankets and clothing for fever management; these measures cause shivering, which will increase the temperature. *If the client's temperature drops in response to rapid external cooling measures, shivering often results, which leads to significantly increased oxygen consumption and cardiorespiratory effort (Henker & Carlson, 2007).*

▲ Recognize that a hypothermia blanket use is indicated for temperature reduction if the client's fever is above 104° F (39.5° C) and cannot be controlled with antipyretics, or if a high body temperature is related to a disorder of temperature regulation (Henker & Carlson, 2007).

▲ When using a cooling blanket, choose a convective airflow system if possible, and set the temperature regulator to 1° to 2° F (0.6° to 1.1° C) below the client's current temperature. *Use cooling blanket temperatures closer to body temperature because this will help prevent shivering and skin breakdown, and it is more comfortable (Henker & Carlson, 2007). Shivering results in aerobic muscle activity with up to a 200% increase in metabolic rate, and increased oxygen, glucose use, heart rate, and blood pressure, and is poorly tolerated by clients who are weak, anemic, or at risk for myocardial ischemia (Henker & Carlson, 2007).* **EBN:** *Airflow blankets were more effective than water-cooling blankets (Loke, Chan, & Chan, 2005).*

▲ Use a nonsteroidal antipyretic (e.g., acetaminophen) as ordered instead of or in conjunction with a cooling blanket to improve fever reduction and decrease the duration of cooling blanket use. **EB:** *Although external cooling and use of antipyretics were equally effective in decreasing body temperature in critically ill clients, there was an increase in energy expenditure with the use of the external cooling versus a decrease of energy expenditure with the use of an antipyretic (Gozzoli et al, 2004).*

Malignant Hyperthermia

▲ If the client has just received general anesthesia, especially halothane or succinylcholine, recognize that the hyperthermia may be caused by malignant hyperthermia, and require immediate treatment

• = Independent   ▲ = Collaborative   **EBN** = Evidence-Based Nursing   **EB** = Evidence-Based

to prevent death. *Malignant hyperthermia is often a fatal disease and must be treated promptly. As more surgeries are done in ambulatory surgery centers, it is important that the medication dantrolene be stocked for rapid administration as ordered (AORN, 2008; DeJohn, 2008).*

▲ If the client has malignant hyperthermia, recognize that the treatment is administration of dantrolene stat, along with antiarrhythmics, and continued support of the cardiovascular system. *Dantrolene helps decrease the increased muscle activity associated with MH and can be life-saving (Fauci, Braunwald, & Kasper, 2008).*

 Pediatric

• For routine measurement of temperature, use an electronic thermometer in the axilla in infants under the age of 4 weeks; for a child up to 5 years of age, use an electronic thermometer in the axilla, or an infrared tympanic thermometer. **EBN:** *Oral and rectal routes should not be used routinely to measure the temperature of infants to children of 5 years of age (National Collaborating Centre for Women's and Children's Health, 2007; Xue, 2008).*

• Assess risk factors of malignant hyperthermia as this has an increased prevalence in the pediatric population. *The administration of inhalation anesthesia and succinylcholine is common in this age group. Risk assessment includes a personal or family history of anesthesia-related complications or death (Hommertzheim & Steinke, 2006).*

▲ Administer dantrolene and oxygen as ordered if malignant hyperthermia is present. *Dantrolene and oxygen should administered as treatment of malignant hyperthermia (Barone, Pablo, & Barone, 2004).*

• Use cool sponging (not cold sponging), fanning, and decreased clothing to bring down the temperature. **EBN:** *Excessive cooling using cold water can initiate shivering, which increases metabolic demand and is uncomfortable (Xue, 2008).*

▲ Do not give the child aspirin to decrease fever; use acetaminophen or NSAIDs as ordered. *Aspirin should not be used for children because of possibility of Reyes syndrome (Xue, 2008).*

 Geriatric

• Recognize that an increase in oral temperature above their baseline temperature should be considered a fever in the elderly. *Febrile response to infection was found to be reduced with increasing age, and baseline temperatures were generally lower in older clients (Barakzai & Fraser, 2008; Heckenberg, 2008).*

• Recognize that rectal temperature may be more accurate to diagnose fever in elderly clients. Use nursing judgment to determine if rectal temperature measurement is acceptable to the client, especially a client with mental changes or dementia. **EBN:** *Rectal thermometry identified fevers in elderly clients that were missed by the oral and tympanic routes (Varney et al, 2002).*

• Assess for other signs and symptoms of infection in addition to or in the absence of fever in the elderly. Suspect infection when there has been a decline in function, including new or increased confusion, incontinence, falling, decreased mobility, or failure to cooperate. *The elderly characteristically have different symptoms of infection, including nonspecific complaints, development of confusion, behavior changes, and fewer coughs and less fever (Barakzai & Fraser, 2008).*

▲ Help the client seek medical attention immediately if fever is present. To diagnose the fever source, assess for possible precipitating factors, including changes in medication, environmental changes, and recent medical interventions or infectious exposures. *The elderly are more susceptible to environmentally and medication-induced hyperthermia, due to the greater incidence of underlying chronic medical conditions that impair thermal regulation or prevent removal from a hot environment (Glazer, 2005).*

• In hot weather, encourage elderly clients to drink eight glasses of fluid per day (within their cardiac and renal reserves) regardless of whether they are thirsty. Assess for the need for and presence of fans or air conditioning; also appropriate clothing. *The elderly are more susceptible to a hot environment than are younger adults because of a decreased sensitivity to heat, decreased sweat gland function, decreased thirst, and decreased mobility (Glazer, 2005).*

▲ In hot weather, monitor the elderly client for signs of heat stroke: temperature of 100° F (37.8° C) to 102° F (38.9° C), orthostatic blood pressure drop, weakness, restlessness, mental status changes, faint-

---

ness, thirst, nausea, and vomiting. If signs are present, move the client to a cool place, have the client lie down, give sips of water, check orthostatic blood pressure, spray with lukewarm water, cool with a fan, and seek medical assistance immediately. *The elderly are predisposed to heat exhaustion and should be watched carefully for its occurrence; if it is present, it should be treated promptly (Glazer, 2005).*

 Home Care

- Some of the interventions described previously may be adapted for home care use.
- Determine whether the client or family has a functioning thermometer, and know how to use it. Please refer to the interventions above on taking a temperature. Teach the client and family about the immune-enhancing effects of fever under 104° F (40° C), as long as the client is not critically ill. *Elimination of fever will interfere with its enhancement of the immune response, but also temperature elevation is accompanied by an increase in oxygen consumption and metabolic rate which may not be tolerated by the acutely ill client (Henker & Carlson, 2007).*
- ▲ Teach the client to use ordered antipyretic medications safely, when needed for comfort or to decrease metabolic effects of fever. *Medications for fever can cause organ damage when taken in large doses. Aspirin should not be used for children because of possibility of Reye's syndrome (Rutledge, 2004; Xue, 2008).* Please refer to care plan **Risk for impaired Liver function.**
- Help the client and caregivers prevent and monitor for heat stroke/hyperthermia during times of high outdoor temperatures. *Preventive measures include minimizing time spent outdoors, use of air conditioning or fans, increasing fluid intake, and taking frequent rest periods (Glazer, 2005).*
- To prevent heat-related injury in athletes, laborers, and military personnel, instruct them to acclimate gradually to the higher temperatures, increase fluid intake, wear vapor-permeable clothing, and take frequent rests (Glazer, 2005).
- In the event of temperature elevation above the adaptive range, institute measures to decrease temperature (e.g., get the client out of the sun and into a cool place, remove excess clothing, have the client drink fluids, spray the client with lukewarm water, and fan with cool air). Initiate emergency transport. *Hyperthermia is an acute and possibly life-threatening situation (Glazer, 2005).*

 Client/Family Teaching and Discharge Planning

- ▲ Teach that infection-induced fever generally enhances the immune system, so the client can participate in the decision of whether to treat the fever. If treatment is chosen, instruct in the use of antipyretics as ordered (Heckenberg, 2008).
- Teach the client that shivering with infection-induced fever has detrimental effects and that activities that can cause shivering (e.g., lowering of room temperature, ice packs) should be avoided. *External cooling measures can result in shivering and discomfort (Henker & Carlson, 2007).*
- Instruct to increase fluids to prevent heat-induced hyperthermia and dehydration in the presence of fever. *Liberal fluid intake replaces fluid lost through perspiration and respiration (Heckenberg, 2008).*
- Teach the client to stay in a cooler environment during periods of excessive outdoor heat or humidity. If the client does go out, instruct him or her to avoid vigorous physical activity, wear lightweight, loose-fitting clothing, and wear a hat to minimize sun exposure. *Such methods reduce exposure to high environmental temperatures, which can cause heat stroke and hyperthermia (Pennsylvania Medical Society, 2007).*

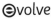 See the Evolve website for Weblinks for client education resources.

REFERENCES

AORN: *Malignant hyperthermia guideline. Perioperative standards and recommended practices,* Denver, 2008, AORN.

Barakzai MD, Fraser D: Assessment of infection in older adults: signs and symptoms in four body systems, *J Gerontol Nurs* 34(1):7–13, 2008.

Barone CP, Pablo CS, Barone GW: Post-anesthetic care in the critical care unit, *Crit Care Nurs* 24(1):38–45, 2004.

DeJohn P: Be prepared: malignant hyperthermia, *OR Manager* 24(6):26–27, 2008.

Dellinger RP, Levy MM, Carlet JM et al: Surviving sepsis campaign: international guidelines for management of severe sepsis and septic shock: 2008, *Intens Care Med* 34(1):17–61, 2008.

Devrim I, Kara A, Ceyhan M et al: Measurement accuracy of fever by tympanic and axillary thermometry, *Pediatr Emerg Care* 23(1):16–19, 2007.

Fallis WM, Hamelin K, Wang X: A multimethod approach to evaluate chemical dot thermometers for oral temperature measurement, *J Nurs Meas* 14(3):151–161, 2006.

• = Independent ▲ = Collaborative **EBN** = Evidence-Based Nursing **EB** = Evidence-Based

Fauci A, Braunwald E, Kasper D: *Harrison's principles of internal medicine,* ed 17, New York, 2008, McGraw Hill.

Fremont-Rideout Health Group launches groundbreaking programs for the treatment of shock, *Blood Weekly* Dec 20:466, 2007.

Fremont-Rideout Health Group launches groundbreaking programs for the treatment of shock, *Blood Weekly* Dec 20:466, 2007. www.newsrx.com/article.php?articleID=811425. Accessed on October 28, 2009.

Frommelt T, Ott C, Hays V: Accuracy of different devices to measure temperature, *Medsurg Nurs* 17(3):171–177, 2008.

Glazer JL. Management of heatstroke and heat exhaustion, *Am Fam Physician* 71(11):2133–2141, 2005.

Gozzoli V, Treggiari MM, Kleger GR et al: Randomized trial of the effect of antipyresis by metamizol, propacetamol or external cooling on metabolism, hemodynamics and inflammatory response, *Intens Care Med* 30(3):401, 2004.

Heckenberg G: *Febrile response: management.* Evidence summaries—Joanna Briggs Institute, July 28, 2008.

Henker R, Carlson KK: Fever: applying research to bedside practice, *AACN Adv Crit Care* 18(1):76–87, 2007.

Hill PD: *A comparison of tympanic and oral temperature readings in adults* [dissertation], Gonzaga University, Washington (UMI No. 1420518), 2004.

Holtzclaw BJ: Shivering in acutely ill vulnerable populations, *AACN Clin Issues* 15(2):267–279, 2004.

Hommertzheim R, Steinke EE: Malignant hyperthermia—the perioperative nurse's role, *AORN J* 83(1):149–168, 2006.

Hudgings L, Kelsberg G, Safranek S et al: Do antipyretics prolong febrile illness? *J Fam Pract* 53(1):57–58, 61, 2004.

Kleinpell RM, Ahrens T: Shock prevention. In Ackley BJ, Ladwig GB, Swan BA et al: *Evidence-based nursing care guidelines: medical-surgical interventions,* Philadelphia, 2008, Mosby.

Loke AY, Chan HC, Chan TM: Comparing the effectiveness of two types of cooling blankets for febrile patients, *Nurs Crit Care* 10(5):247–254, 2005.

National Collaborating Centre for Women's and Children's Health (UK): *Feverish illness in children: assessment and initial management in children younger than 5 years.* National Institute for Health and Clinical Excellence (NICE), Clinical Guideline 47. London, 2007, ROCG Press.

O'Grady NP, Barie PS, Bartlett JG et al: Guidelines for evaluation of new fever in critically ill adult patients: 2008 update from the American College of Critical Care Medicine and the Infectious Diseases Society of America, *Crit Care Med* 36(4):1330–1349, 2008.

Pennsylvania Medical Society: Keep a cool head on hot, humid days to avoid heat stroke, *Obesity, Fitness & Wellness Week* Jul 7, 2007:305, 2007.

Rutledge D. *Fever management. Evidence-based care sheets,* CINAHL Information Services, Dec 16, CINAHL AN: 5000000295, 2004.

Varney SM, Manthey DE, Culpepper VE et al: A comparison of oral, tympanic, and rectal temperature measurement in the elderly, *J Emerg Med* 22:153, 2002.

Xue, Y: *Febrile response: management,* Joanna Briggs Institute. May 5, 2008.

Hypothermia   *Betty J. Ackley, MSN, EdS, RN*

NANDA-I

Definition

Body temperature below normal range

Defining Characteristics

Body temperature below normal range; cool skin; cyanotic nail beds; hypertension; pallor; piloerection; shivering; slow capillary refill; tachycardia

Related Factors (r/t)

Aging; consumption of alcohol; damage to hypothalamus; decreased ability to shiver; decreased metabolic rate; evaporation from skin in cool environment; exposure to cool environment; illness; inactivity; inadequate clothing; malnutrition; medications; trauma

NOC   (Nursing Outcomes Classification)

Suggested NOC Outcomes

Thermoregulation, Thermoregulation: Newborn

Example NOC Outcome with Indicators
Thermoregulation as evidenced by the following indicators: Increased skin temperature/Decreased skin temperature/Skin color changes/Dehydration/Hypothermia (Rate the outcome and indicators of **Thermoregulation**: 1 = severe, 2 = substantial, 3 = moderate, 4 = mild, 5 = none [see Section I].)

Client Outcomes

Client Will (Specify Time Frame):

• Maintain body temperature within normal range

● = Independent   ▲ = Collaborative   **EBN** = Evidence-Based Nursing   **EB** = Evidence-Based

- Identify risk factors of hypothermia
- State measures to prevent hypothermia
- Identify symptoms of hypothermia and actions to take when hypothermia is present

NIC   (Nursing Interventions Classification)

Suggested NIC Interventions

Hypothermia Treatment, Temperature Regulation, Temperature Regulation: Intraoperative, Vital Signs Monitoring

Example NIC Activities—Temperature Regulation
Institute use of a continuous core temperature–monitoring device, as appropriate; Promote adequate fluid and nutritional intake

Nursing Interventions and *Rationales*

- Remove the client from the cause of the hypothermic episode (e.g., cold environment, cold or wet clothing). Ensure that the client is in a warm environment. *The goal is to eliminate the causative or contributing factor and begin the warming process (Day, 2006; Lasater, 2008).*
- Watch the client for signs of hypothermia: shivering, slurred speech, clumsy movements, fatigue, confusion. *As hypothermia progresses, the skin becomes pale, numb, and waxy. Muscles are tense, fatigue and weakness progress, and there can be a gradual loss of consciousness with loss of a pulse and breathing (Day, 2006).*
- Cover the client with warm blankets and apply a covering to the head and neck to conserve body heat. *Layering of dry clothing, including wearing a hat, can be effective in warming a client with mild hypothermia (Day, 2006), and the goal is also to prevent any further heat loss (Fauci, Braunwald, & Kasper, 2008).*
- ▲ Take the temperature at least hourly; if more than mild hypothermia is present (temperature lower than 95° F [35° C]), use a continuous temperature-monitoring device, preferably two of them, one in the rectum, the other in the esophagus (Fauci, Braunwald, & Kasper, 2008).
- ▲ Measure and record the client's temperature using an oral or rectal thermometer every 1 to 4 hours depending on severity of the hypothermia or whenever a change in condition occurs (e.g., chills, change in mental status). If client is critically ill, use an indwelling method of temperature measurement. **EBN and EB:** *Oral temperature measurement provides a more accurate temperature than tympanic measurement, axillary measurement, or use of a chemical dot thermometer (Hill, 2004; Fallis, Hamelin, & Wang, 2006; Devrim et al, 2007; Frommelt, Ott, & Hays, 2008). Research has demonstrated the accuracy of temperature measurement from most accurate to least accurate: intravascular, esophageal, bladder thermistor, rectal, oral, tympanic membrane. Axillary, temporal artery, and chemical dot thermometers are less accurate and should be avoided in caring for the critically ill adult client (O'Grady et al, 2008).*
- Use the same site and method (device) for temperature measurement for a given client so that temperature trends are assessed accurately and record site of temperature measurement. **EBN and EB:** *There are significant differences in temperature depending on the site (oral, rectal, axillary, or temporal artery) (Devrim et al, 2007; Frommelt, Ott, & Hays, 2008; O'Grady et al, 2008).*
- ▲ Use a pulmonary artery catheter–temperature measuring device if available; if not, consider using a bladder catheter that measures temperature. **EBN:** *Measurement of the pulmonary artery temperature is considered the gold standard in assessing core body temperature. If a pulmonary artery catheter is not appropriate for the client, temperature measurement with a temperature-sensitive indwelling urinary catheter can be effective and provide a reliable indication of core temperature (Fallis, 2002).*
- ▲ Administer oxygen as ordered. *Oxygenation is hampered by the change in the oxyhemaglobin curve caused by hypothermia (Fauci, Braunwald, & Kasper, 2008).*
- Monitor the client's vital signs every hour and as appropriate. Note changes associated with hypothermia, such as initially increased pulse rate, respiratory rate, and blood pressure with mild hypothermia, and then decreased pulse rate, respiratory rate, and blood pressure with moderate to severe hypothermia. *With mild hypothermia, there is activation of the sympathetic nervous system, which can increase the values of vital signs. As hypothermia progresses, decreased circulating volume*

• = Independent   ▲ = Collaborative   **EBN** = Evidence-Based Nursing   **EB** = Evidence-Based

develops, which results in decreased cardiac output and depressed oxygen delivery. Hypoxia, metabolic acidosis, and intrinsic irritability of a cold myocardium result in various dysrhythmias (Ruffolo, 2002; Day, 2006).

▲ Attach electrodes and a cardiac monitor. Watch for dysrhythmias. *With hypothermia the client is prone to dysrhythmias because of the cold myocardium; dysrhythmias may include atrial fibrillation, ventricular fibrillation, or asystole (McCullough & Arora, 2004; Day, 2006).*

▲ Monitor for signs of coagulopathy (e.g., oozing of blood from any open areas or from intravascular catheter sites or mucous membranes). Also note results of clotting studies as available. *Coagulopathy is a common occurrence during hypothermia in trauma clients (McCullough & Arora, 2004).*

• For mild hypothermia (core temperature of 90° to 95° F [32.2° to 35° C]), rewarm client passively:
  ▪ Set room temperature to 70° to 75° F (21° to 24° C).
  ▪ Keep the client dry; remove any damp or wet clothing.
  ▪ Layer clothing and blankets and cover the client's head; use insulated metallic blankets.
  ▪ Offer warm fluids; avoid alcohol or caffeine.

For mild hypothermia, allow the client to rewarm at his or her own pace. Heat is regained through the body's ability to generate heat (Lasater, 2008). Passive rewarming is not encouraged for clients with temperatures lower than 82.4° F (28° C) because it is a slow process and may increase the risk of cardiac arrest in these circumstances (McCullough & Arora, 2004).

▲ For moderate hypothermia (core temperature 82.4° to 90° F [28° to 32.2° C]) use active external rewarming methods. The rewarming rate should not exceed 1.8° F (1° C) per hour. Methods include the following (Fauci, Braunwald, & Kasper, 2008):
  ▪ Forced-air warming blankets
  ▪ Carbon-fiber blanket

▲ For severe hypothermia (core temperature below 82.4° F [28° C]) use active core-rewarming techniques as ordered (Lasater, 2008):
  ▪ Recognize that extracorporeal blood rewarming methods, such as coronary artery bypass, are most effective
  ▪ Use of an intravascular temperature modulation device (Fauci, Braunwald, & Kasper, 2008; Lasater, 2008)
  ▪ Use of heated and humidified oxygen through the ventilator as ordered
  ▪ Administering heated intravenous (IV) fluids at prescribed temperature
  ▪ Performing peritoneal lavage or bladder irrigations as ordered

Severe hypothermia is associated with acidosis, coma, ventricular fibrillation, apnea, thrombocytopenia, platelet dysfunction, impaired clotting, and increased mortality in trauma clients and requires prompt core body rewarming (McCullough & Arora, 2004; Lasater, 2008).

• Rewarm clients slowly, generally at a rate of 1° C every hour. *Slow rewarming helps prevent a phenomena entitled "afterdrop," where cold, hyperkalemic blood from the periphery returns to the heart, resulting in a biochemical injury leading to dysrhythmias and severe hypotension (Lasater, 2008).*

• Check blood pressure frequently when rewarming; watch for hypotension. *As the body warms, formerly vasoconstricted vessels dilate, which results in hypotension (Day, 2006).*

▲ Administer IV fluids, using a rapid infuser IV fluid warmer as ordered. *Fluids are often needed to maintain adequate fluid volume. If the client develops untreated fluid depletion, hypotension with decreased cardiac output and acute renal failure can result. A rapid infuser warmer is needed to keep IV fluids warmed sufficiently to be effective in raising the body temperature (Fauci, Braunwald, & Kasper, 2008).*

• Determine the factors leading to the hypothermic episode; see Related Factors. *It is important to assess risk factors and precipitating events to prevent another incident of hypothermia and to direct treatment (Day, 2006).*

▲ Request a social service referral to help the client obtain the heat, shelter, and food needed to maintain body temperature. *A preventive approach that includes adequate food and fluid intake, shelter, heat, and clothing decreases the risk of hypothermia (Fauci, Braunwald, & Kasper, 2008).*

▲ Encourage proper nutrition and hydration. Request a referral to a dietitian to identify appropriate dietary needs. *Insufficient calorie and fluid intake predispose the client to hypothermia, especially the elderly (Fauci, Braunwald, & Kasper, 2008).*

• = Independent   ▲ = Collaborative   **EBN** = Evidence-Based Nursing   **EB** = Evidence-Based

Pediatric

- Recognize that pediatric clients have a decreased ability to adapt to temperature extremes. Take the following actions to maintain body temperature in the infant/child:
  - Keep the head covered.
  - Use blankets to keep the client warm.
  - Keep the client covered during procedures, transport, and diagnostic testing.
  - Keep the room temperature at 72° F (22.2° C).

  The combination of a relatively smaller body surface area, smaller body fluid volume, less well-developed temperature control mechanisms, and smaller amount of protective body fat limits the infant's and child's ability to maintain normal temperatures (Hockenberry, 2005).
- ▲ For the preterm or low-birth-weight newborn, use specially designed bags, skin-to-skin care, and transwarmer mattresses to keep preterm infants warm. **EB:** *These methods can help keep the vulnerable newborn warm in the delivery room, yet there is a need for more studies in this area (McCall et al, 2005).*

Geriatric

- Assess neurological signs frequently, watching for confusion and decreased level of consciousness. *Older adults are less likely to shiver or complain of feeling cold. Early signs of hypothermia are subtle (McCullough & Arora, 2004).*
- Recognize that the elderly can develop indoor hypothermia from air conditioning or ice baths. *Clients present with vague complaints of mental and/or other skill deterioration (McCullough & Arora, 2004).*
- Recognize that the elderly often wear socks and sweaters to protect themselves from feeling cold, even in warmer weather.

Home Care

NOTE: Hypothermia is not a symptom that appears in the normal course of home care. When it occurs, it is a clinical emergency and the client/family should access emergency medical services immediately.

- Some of the interventions described earlier may be adapted for home care use.
- Before a medical crisis occurs, confirm that the client or family has a thermometer and can read it. Instruct as needed. Verify that the thermometer registers accurately.
- Instruct the client or family to take the temperature when the client displays cyanosis, pallor, or shivering.
- ▲ Monitor temperature every hour, as noted previously. If the temperature of the client begins dropping below the normal range, apply layers of clothing or blankets, or adjust environmental heat to the comfort level. Do not overheat. Contact a physician. *Passive rewarming is the only method of rewarming that is appropriate for home care under normal circumstances.*
- ▲ If temperature continues to drop, activate the emergency system and notify a physician. *Hypothermia is a clinically acute condition that cannot be managed safely in the home.*
- ▲ If the client is in hospice care or is terminally ill, follow advance directives, client wishes, and the physician's orders. Keep the client free of pain. *The goal of terminal care is to provide dignity and comfort during the dying process.*

Client/Family Teaching and Discharge Planning

- Teach the client and family signs of hypothermia and the method of taking the temperature (age-appropriate).
- Teach the client methods to prevent hypothermia: wearing adequate clothing, including a hat and mittens; heating the environment to a minimum of 68° F (20° C); and ingesting adequate food and fluid. *Simple measures such as layering clothes, wearing a hat, and avoiding extremes in temperature prevent significant heat loss (Elliott, 2004; McLafferty, Farley, & Hendry, 2009).*

• = Independent ▲ = Collaborative **EBN** = Evidence-Based Nursing **EB** = Evidence-Based

▲ Teach the client and family about medications such as sedatives, opioids, and anxiolytics that predispose the client to hypothermia (as appropriate). *If the client has had hypothermia in the past, using alternative medications is an option if there is no contraindication (Elliott, 2004).*

⊖volve See the EVOLVE website for Weblinks for client education resources.

REFERENCES

Day MP: Hypothermia: a hazard for all seasons, *Nursing* 36(12):36–47, 2006.

Devrim I, Kara A, Ceyhan M et al: Measurement accuracy of fever by tympanic and axillary thermometry, *Pediatr Emerg Care* 23(1):16–19, 2007.

Elliott F: You'd better watch out, *Occup Health Saf* 73(11):76, 2004.

Fallis WM: Monitoring urinary bladder temperature in the intensive care unit: state of the science, *Am J Crit Care* 11(1):38, 2002.

Fallis WM, Hamelin K, Wang X: A multimethod approach to evaluate chemical dot thermometers for oral temperature measurement, *J Nurs Meas* 14(3):151–161, 2006.

Fauci A, Braunwald E, Kasper D: *Harrison's principles of internal medicine*, ed 17, New York, 2008, McGraw Hill.

Frommelt T, Ott C, Hays V: Accuracy of different devices to measure temperature, *Medsurg Nurs* 17(3):171–177, 2008.

Hill PD: *A comparison of tympanic and oral temperature readings in adults* [dissertation], Gonzaga University, Washington (UMI No. 1420518), 2004.

Hockenberry MJ: *Wong's essentials of pediatric nursing*, ed 7, St Louis, 2005, Mosby.

Lasater M: Treatment of severe hypothermia with intravascular temperature modulation, *Crit Care Nurse* 28(6):24–31, 2008.

McCall E, Alderdice F, Halliday H et al: Interventions to prevent hypothermia at birth in preterm and/or low birth weight babies, *Cochrane Database Syst Rev* (1):CD004210, 2005.

McCullough L, Arora S: Diagnosis and treatment of hypothermia, *Am Fam Physician* 70(12):2325, 2004.

McLafferty E, Farley A, Hendry C: Prevention of hypothermia, *Nurs Older People* 21(4):34–38, 2009.

O'Grady NP, Barie PS, Bartlett JG et al: Guidelines for evaluation of new fever in critically ill adult patients: 2008 update from the American College of Critical Care Medicine and the Infectious Diseases Society of America, *Crit Care Med* 36(4):1330–1349, 2008.

Ruffolo DC: Hypothermia in trauma: the cold, hard facts, *RN* 65(2):46, 2002.

Disturbed personal Identity
Patricia Ferreira, RN, MSN, Michelangelo Juvenale, BSc, MSc, PhD, and Gail B. Ladwig, MSN, RN, CHTP

NANDA-I

Definition

Inability to maintain an integrated and complete perception of self**

Defining Characteristics

Contradictory personal traits; delusional description of self; disturbed body image; disturbed relationships; feelings of emptiness; feelings of strangeness; fluctuating feelings about self; gender confusion; ineffective coping; ineffective role performance; unable to distinguish between inner and outer stimuli; uncertainty about goals; uncertainty about cultural values (e.g., beliefs, religion, and moral questions); uncertainty about ideological values (e.g., beliefs, religion, and moral questions)

Related Factors (r/t)

Cult indoctrination; cultural discontinuity; discrimination or prejudice; dysfunctional family processes; ingestion of toxic chemicals; inhalation of toxic chemicals; low self-esteem; manic states; multiple personality disorder; organic brain syndromes; psychiatric disorders (e.g., psychosis, depression, dissociative disorder); situational crisis; social role change; stages of growth; stages of development; use of psychoactive drugs

---

**Identity can be defined by the sum of characteristics by which a person is recognized by self and others (Dirckx, 2001); identity emerged as the core category through the process of linking among categories (Parvizy, Ahmadi, & Nasrabad, 2008); the conscious person realizes himself as a whole person, which gives his/her life leading and purpose (Stuart & Laraia, 2005). According to Marjo Piironen and Liisa Timonen (International Conference: Issues of Identity in and across Cultures and Professional Worlds, Rome, 26 October 2007), "the concept of identity in itself refers to self-image or self-concept. Identity is not a stable or permanent perception of one's self-image but changes in time and place and is constructed in social interaction in everyday life. Identity can also be studied as a group image or a group concept. Diana Petkova (2005) refers to individual (personal) and collective (group) identities as main concepts, whereas social and cultural identities are regarded as subconcepts. According to Petkova identity can be divided into two main groups: individual (personal) identity and collective (group) identity. Both of these categories can further be divided into two subcategories: social and cultural identities."

• = Independent ▲ = Collaborative **EBN** = Evidence-Based Nursing **EB** = Evidence-Based

(Nursing Outcomes Classification)

Suggested NOC Outcomes

Anxiety Self-Control, Abuse Recovery (Emotional, physical, sexual), Body Image, Decision-Making, Distorted Thought Self-Control, Identity, Self-Mutilation/Self-Restraint, Suicide

Example NOC Outcome with Indicators
Identity as evidenced by the following indicators: Verbalizes affirmations of personal identity/Exhibits congruent verbal and nonverbal behavior about self/Differentiates self from environment and other human beings. (Rate each indicator of **Identity** as follows: 1 = never demonstrated, 2 = rarely demonstrated, 3 = sometimes demonstrated, 4 = often demonstrated, 5 = consistently demonstrated [see Section I].)

Client Outcomes

Client Will (Specify Time Frame):

- Demonstrate new purposes for life
- Show interests in surroundings
- Perform self-care and self-control activities appropriate for age
- Acknowledge personal strengths
- Engage in interpersonal relationships

 (Nursing Interventions Classification)

Suggested NIC Interventions

Decision-Making Support, Mutual Goal Setting, Self-Awareness Enhancement, Self-Esteem Enhancement, Sexual Counseling, Substance Use Prevention

Example NIC Activities—Self-Esteem Enhancement
Monitor client's statements of self-worth; Encourage client to identify strengths

Nursing Interventions and *Rationales*

- Assess and support family strengths of commitment, appreciation, and affection towards each other, positive communication, time together, a sense of spiritual well-being, and the ability to cope with stress and crisis. **EBN:** *With the family-strengths approach, nurses help families cope by defining their visions and hopes for the future instead of looking at what factors contribute to family problems (Sittner, Brage, & Defrain, 2007).*
- ▲ Assess for suicidal idea and make appropriate referral for clients with schizophrenia and bipolar disorder. **EB:** *Suicide is a major cause of death among clients with schizophrenia. Research indicates that at least 5% to 13% of schizophrenic clients die by suicide (Pompili et al, 2007).* **EB:** *Bipolar clients with rapid-cycling—a course modifier of bipolar disorder that often implicates a poor prognosis—are more likely to attempt suicide (Garcia-Amador et al, 2009). Rapid-cycling clients are defined as those suffering from four or more episodes per year (Goodwin et al, 2008).*
- ▲ Assess women with mood disorders for reproductive and metabolic disorders and make appropriate referrals for treatment. **EB:** *Women with mood disorders, especially bipolar disorder (BD), have been shown to have high rates of reproductive and metabolic dysfunction. Many of the psychotropic medications used in the treatment of BD are associated with weight gain, insulin resistance, and dyslipidemia. These metabolic side effects further compound the neuroendocrine system dysregulation in women with BD (Kenna, Jiang, & Rasgon, 2009).*
- ▲ Assess and make appropriate referrals for clients with obesity and depression. **EB:** *The marked alteration of body weight (and appetite) is one of the most frequent of the nine symptoms of major depressive episodes, and these symptoms occur during recurrent episodes of depression with a remarkably high consequence (Rihmer et al, 2008).*

• = Independent   ▲ = Collaborative   **EBN** = Evidence-Based Nursing   **EB** = Evidence-Based

▲ Assess lymphocyte counts and make appropriate referrals for clients with bulimia nervosa (BN), who may present with psychopathological variables associated with psychological instability (depression, hostility, impulsivity, self-defeating personality traits, and borderline personality symptoms). **EB:** *In this study of clients with BN and psychological instability, hostility was negatively correlated with the number of helper T-cells (CD4+). These results support the idea that hostility, as an expression of disturbed interpersonal relationships, could play a role as a modulator of immune activity in clients with BN (Vaz-Leal et al, 2007).*

• Use empathetic communication and encourage the client and family to verbalize fears, express emotions, and set goals. Be present for clients physically or by telephone. **EBN:** *This study of social support by telephone demonstrated that therapeutic, presence facilitated outcomes that included problem solving, adaptive behavior change, and diminished distress (Finfgeld-Connett, 2005). Presence involves knowing the uniqueness of the person, listening intently, and mutually defining changes in the provision of confident caring (Caldwell et al, 2005).*

• Empower the client to set realistic goals and to engage in problem solving. **EBN:** *This case study assesses how individuals who have had a stroke use continued problem solving and goal setting. It demonstrates that health care workers need to empower individuals to make decisions about their care so the individuals can achieve life satisfaction (Western, 2007).*

• Encourage expression of positive thoughts and emotions. **EB:** *This is a technique that may help clients with bipolar diagnosis to cope with their illness (Straughan, 2007).*

• Encourage the client to use spiritual coping mechanisms such as faith and prayer. **EBN:** *Prayer is a powerful way of coping and is practiced by all Western religions and several Eastern traditions (Mohr, 2006). Spirituality inspired hope among caregivers of stroke clients (Pierce et al, 2008).*

• Help the clients with serious and chronic conditions such as depression, cancer diagnosis, and chemotherapy treatment to maintain social support networks or assist in building new ones. **EBN:** *Health care providers can encourage social support networks to help clients cope with the negative aspects of cancer and chemotherapy (Mattioli, Repinski, & Chappy, 2008).* **EB:** *Decades of research have shown that individuals with more social ties have better health outcomes and lower mortality rates across many illnesses and diseases (Voils et al, 2007).*

▲ Refer women facing diagnostic and curative breast cancer surgery for psychosocial support. **EB:** *Psychological distress is a central experience for women facing diagnostic and curative breast cancer surgery. Psychosocial interventions are recommended for both groups (Schnur et al, 2008).*

▲ Refer for cognitive behavioral therapy (CBT). **EBN:** *CBT approaches in adult acute inpatient settings can help clients to cope by facilitating client-caregiver engagement and improving hope-inspiring interventions to reduce distress (Forsyth et al, 2008).*

▲ Refer clients with borderline personality disorder (BPD) and dual-diagnosed BPD and substance-dependent female clients for dialetical behavior therapy (DBT) and psychoanalytic-oriented day-hospital therapy. **EB:** *Dialectical behavior therapy (DBT) included treatment components such as prioritizing a hierarchy of target behaviors, telephone coaching, group skills training, behavioral skill training, contingency management, cognitive modification, exposure to emotional cues, reflection, empathy, and acceptance. DBT seemed to be helpful on a wide range of outcomes, such as admission to hospital or incarceration in prison. Psychoanalytic-oriented day-hospital therapy also seemed to decrease admission and use of prescribed medication and to increase social improvement and social adjustment (Binks et al, 2006). Two randomized controlled trials in 59 clients, female only, with BPD and substance abuse provided the best evidence-based data for the effectiveness of DBT. For dual-focus schema therapy, a single randomized controlled trial indicated a curative effect in a small group of clients with personality disorder and substance dependence (Kienast & Foerster, 2008).*

• Refer to the care plans for **Readiness for enhanced Communication** and **Readiness for enhanced Spiritual well-being**.

Pediatric

• Encourage exercise for children and adolescents to promote positive self-esteem, to enhance coping, and to prevent behavioral and psychological problems. **EBN:** *Physical activity helped to decrease depression and anxiety and to increase coping skills in adolescents (Beauchemin & Manns, 2008).*

▲ Refer children, adolescents, and their parents—and relatives occasionally—in eating disorder prevention programs. **EB:** *The impact of prevention programs for eating disorders in children and adolescents is not clear, although none of the pooled comparisons indicated evidence of harm. From a research perspective, the idea of "thresholds" for identifying young people at risk of developing eating disorders has been raised, and denial of concern or denial of illness represents a further issue complicating early identification in relation to eating disorder symptoms (Pratt & Woolfenden, 2009; Shaw, Stice, & Becker, 2009).*

• Provide gifted children with low self-esteem with appropriate support. **EB:** *Gifted children in this study manifested a lack of self-esteem, and in particular a lack of academic self-esteem, coupled with depressive symptoms (Bénony et al, 2007).*

• Suggest that parents with children diagnosed with cancer use computer-mediated support groups to exchange messages with other parents. **EBN:** *Using computer technology for support was particularly useful for this dispersed group with limited time, helping to decrease depression and anxiety in fathers and mothers (Bragadóttir, 2008).*

 ## Geriatric

• Consider the use of telephone support for caregivers of family members with dementia. **EBN and EB:** *Family caregivers can be helped through a variety of social support mechanisms including telephone support (Chang et al, 2004; Belle et al, 2006).*

• Encourage clients to discuss "life history." *Use life history–based interventions, and self-esteem and life-satisfaction questionnaires, to develop "ways of reaffirming a generative identity," sustaining elements for this therapy, to stimulate a hope in their own families' future (Coleman & Podolskij, 2007).*

▲ Refer the older client to self-help support groups, such as the "Red Hat Society" for older women. **EB:** *A leisure-focused group (Red Hat Society) helped the members to cope with stressors associated with the challenges and losses of old age (Hutchinson et al, 2008).*

▲ Refer the client with Alzheimer's disease who is terminally ill to hospice. **EB:** *The National Institute of Clinical Excellence (NICE) and the National Council for Palliative Care (NCPC) have highlighted the importance of palliative care for people with dementia (Chatterjee, 2008).*

 ## Multicultural

• Assess an individuals' sociocultural background in teaching self-management and self-regulation as a means of supporting hope and coping with a diagnosis of type 2 diabetes. **EBN:** *Findings obtained from the themes of this study illustrated that self-management of clients with diabetes is highly related to their own sociocultural environment and experiences (Lin et al, 2008).*

• Encourage spirituality as a source of support for coping. **EBN:** *Many African Americans and Latinos identify spirituality, religiousness, prayer, and church-based approaches as coping resources (Abrums, 2004; Coon et al, 2004; Weaver & Flannelly, 2004).*

• Refer to care plan for **Ineffective Coping**.

 ## Home Care

• The interventions described previously may be adapted for home care use.

• Provide an Internet-based health coach to encourage self-management for clients with chronic conditions such as depression, impaired mobility, and chronic pain. **EBN:** *Clients who have higher self-efficacy and participate actively in their care have better disease management. Client–provider Internet portals offer a new venue for empowering and engaging clients in better management of chronic conditions (Allen et al, 2008).*

▲ Refer the client to mutual health support groups. *Participating in mutual health support groups led to enhanced coping by improving psychological and social functioning (Pistrang, Barker, & Humphreys, 2008).*

▲ Refer the client for a behavioral program that teaches coping skills via "Lifeskills" workshop and/or video. **EB:** *Commercially available, facilitator- or self-administered behavioral training products can have significant beneficial effects on psychosocial well-being in a healthy community sample (Kirby et al, 2006).*

• = Independent   ▲ = Collaborative   **EBN** = Evidence-Based Nursing   **EB** = Evidence-Based

▲ Refer prostate cancer clients and their spouses to family programs that include family-based interventions of communication, hope, coping, uncertainty, and symptom management. **EBN:** *Men with prostate cancer and their spouses reported positive outcomes from a family intervention that offered them information and support (Northouse et al, 2007).*

▲ Refer combat veterans and service members directly involved in combat as well as those providing support to combatants, including nurses for mental health services. **EBN:** *Early identification and treatment of mental health problems may decrease the psychosocial impact of combat and thus prevent progression to more chronic and severe psychopathology such as depression and posttraumatic stress disorder (PTSD) (Gaylord, 2006; Jones et al, 2008).* **EB:** *Combat duty in Iraq was associated with high utilization of mental health services and attrition from military service after deployment (Hoge, Auchterlonie, & Milliken, 2006).*

Client/Family Teaching and Discharge Planning

▲ Teach the client about available community resources (e.g., therapists, ministers, counselors, self-help groups, family-education groups). **EB:** *Families need assistance in coping with health changes (Pickett-Schenk et al, 2008).*

▲ Teach coping skills to family caregivers of cancer clients. **EBN:** *A coping-skills intervention was effective in improving caregiver quality of life, and reducing burdens related to client's symptoms and caregiver's tasks, compared with hospice care alone or hospice plus emotional support (McMillan et al, 2006).*

▲ Teach caregivers the COPE intervention (creativity, optimism, planning, expert information) to assist with symptom management. **EBN:** *Symptom distress, a measure that encompasses client suffering along with intensity, was significantly decreased in the group in which caregivers were trained to better manage client symptoms (McMillan & Small, 2007).*

ⓔvolve   See the EVOLVE website for Weblinks for client education resources.

REFERENCES

Refer to **Ineffective Coping** for additional references.

Abrums M: Faith and feminism: how African American women from a storefront church resist oppression in healthcare, *Adv Nurs Science* 27(3):187–201, 2004.

Allen MB, Iezzoni I, Huang A et al: Improving patient-clinician communication about chronic conditions: description of an Internet-based nurse e-coach intervention, *Nurs Res* 57(2):107, 2008.

Beauchemin J, Manns J: Walking talking therapy, *Ment Health Today* 34:2, 2008.

Belle S, Burgio L, Burns R et al: Enhancing the quality of life of dementia caregivers from different ethnic or racial groups: a randomized, controlled trial, *Ann Intern Med* 145(10):727–738, 2006.

Bénony H, Van Der Elst D, Chahraoui K et al: Link between depression and academic self-esteem in gifted children, *Encephale* 33(1):11–20, 2007.

Binks C, Fenton M, McCarthy L et al: Psychological therapies for people with borderline personality disorder, *Cochrane Database Syst Rev* (1): CD005652, 2006.

Bragadóttir H: Computer-mediated support group intervention for parents, *J Nurs Scholarsh* 40(1):32–39, 2008.

Caldwell B, Doyle M, Morris M et al: Presencing: channeling therapeutic effectiveness with the mentally ill in a state psychiatric hospital, *Issues Ment Health Nurs* 26:853–871, 2005.

Chang BL, Nitta S, Carter PA et al: Technology innovations. Perceived helpfulness of telephone calls: providing support for care-givers of family members with dementia, *J Gerontol Nurs* 30(9):14–21, 2004.

Chatterjee J: End-of-life care for patients with dementia, *Nurs Older People* 20(2):29–35, 2008.

Coleman PG, Podolskij A: Identity loss and recovery in the life stories of Soviet World War II veterans, *Gerontologist*, 47(1):52–60, 2007.

Coon DW, Rubert M, Solano N et al: Well-being, appraisal, and coping in Latina and Caucasian female dementia caregivers: findings from the REACH study, *Aging Ment Health* 8(4):330–345, 2004.

Dirckx, JH (Editor). *Stedman's concise medical dictionary for the health professions*, Philadelphia, 2001, Lippincott Williams and Wilkins.

Finfgeld-Connett D: Telephone social support or nursing presence? Analysis of a nursing intervention, *Qual Health Res* 15(1):19–29, 2005.

Forsyth A, Weddle R, Drummond A et al: Implementing cognitive behaviour therapy skills in adult acute inpatient settings, *Ment Health Pract* 11(5):24–28, 2008.

Garcia-Amador M, Colom F, Valenti M et al: Suicide risk in rapid cycling bipolar patients, *J Affect Disord* 117(1–2):74–78, 2009.

Gaylord KM: The psychosocial effects of combat: the frequently unseen injury, *Crit Care Nurs Clin North Am* 18(3):349–357, 2006.

Goodwin GM, Anderson I, Arango C et al: ECNP consensus meeting. Bipolar depression. Nice (France), March 2007, *Eur Neuropsychopharmacol* 18(7):535–549, 2008.

Hoge CW, Auchterlonie JL, Milliken CS: Mental health problems, use of mental health services, and attrition from military service after returning from deployment to Iraq or Afghanistan, *JAMA* 295(9): 1023–1032, 2006.

Hutchinson SL, Yarnal CM, Staffordson J et al: Beyond fun and friendship: the Red Hat Society as a coping resource for older women, *Ageing Soc* 28(7):979–1000, 2008.

Jones DE, Perkins K, Cook JH et al: Intensive coping skills training to reduce anxiety and depression for forward-deployed troops, *Military Medicine* 173(3):241–247, 2008.

Kenna HA, Jiang B, Rasgon NL: Reproductive and metabolic abnormalities associated with bipolar disorder and its treatment, *Harv Rev Psychiatry* 17(2):138–146, 2009.

● = Independent   ▲ = Collaborative   **EBN** = Evidence-Based Nursing   **EB** = Evidence-Based

Kienast T, Foerster J: Psychotherapy of personality disorders and concomitant substance dependence, *Curr Opin Psychiatry* 21(6):619–624, 2008.

Kirby ED, Williams VP, Hocking MC et al: Psychosocial benefits of three formats of a standardized behavioral stress management program, *Psychosom Med* 68(6):816–823, 2006.

Lin C, Anderson R, Hagerty B et al: Diabetes self-management experience: a focus group study of Taiwanese patients with type 2 diabetes, *J Clin Nurs* 17(5a):34, 2008.

Mattioli JL, Repinski R, Chappy SL: The meaning of hope and social support in patients receiving chemotherapy, *Oncol Nurs Forum* 35(5):822–829, 2008.

McMillan SC, Small BJ: Using the COPE intervention for family caregivers to improve symptoms of hospice homecare patients: a clinical trial, *Oncol Nurs Forum* 34(2):313–321, 2007.

McMillan SC, Small BJ, Weitzner M et al: Impact of coping skills intervention with family caregivers of hospice patients with cancer: a randomized clinical trial, *Cancer* 106(1):214–222, 2006.

Mohr WK: Spiritual issues in psychiatric care, *Perspect Psychiatr Care* 42(3):174–183, 2006.

Northouse LL, Mood DW, Schafenacker A et al: Randomized clinical trial of a family intervention for prostate cancer patients and their spouses, *Cancer* 110(12):2809–2818, 2007.

Parvizy S, Ahmadi F, Nasrabad AN: An identity-based model for adolescent health in the Islamic Republic of Iran: a qualitative study, *East Mediterr Health J* 14(4):869–879, 2008.

Petkova D: Cultural identity in a pluralistic world, *in* Cultural identity in an intercultural context, University of Jyväskylä, 2005.

Pickett-Schenk SA, Lippincott RC, Bennett C et al: Improving knowledge about mental illness through family-led education: the journey of hope, *Psychiatr Serv* 59(1):49, 2008.

Pierce L, Steiner V, Havens H et al: spirituality expressed by caregivers of stroke survivors, *West J Nurs Res* 30(5):606, 2008.

Piironen M, Timonen L: *International conference: issues of identity in and across cultures and professional worlds*, Rome, 26 October 2007.

Pistrang N, Barker C, Humphreys K: Mutual help groups for mental health problems: a review of effectiveness studies, *Am J Community Psychol* 42(1–2):110–122, 2008.

Pompili M, Amador XF, Girardi P et al: Suicide risk in schizophrenia: learning from the past to change the future, *Ann Gen Psychiatry* 6(6):10, 2007.

Pratt BM, Woolfenden S: Interventions for preventing eating disorders in children and adolescents, *Cochrane Database Syst Rev* (2): CD002891, 2009.

Rihmer Z, Purebl G, Faludi G et al: Association of obesity and depression, *Neuropsychopharmacol*, 10(4):183–189, 2008.

Schnur JB, Montgomery GH, Hallquist MN et al: Anticipatory psychological distress in women scheduled for diagnostic and curative breast cancer surgery, *Int J Behav Med* 15(1):21, 2008.

Shaw H, Stice E, Becker CB: Preventing eating disorders, *Child Adolesc Psychiatr Clin N Am* 18(1):199–207, 2009.

Sittner B, Brage HD, Defrain JJ: Using the concept of family strengths to enhance nursing care, *MCN Am J Mat Child Nurs* 32(6):353, 2007.

Straughan H: Learning to cope together, *Ment Health Today* 34:6, 2007.

Stuart GW, Laraia MT: *Principles and practice of psychiatric nursing*, ed 8, Orlando, 2005, Mosby.

Vaz-Leal FJ, Rodríguez-Santos L, Melero MJ et al: Hostility and helper T-cells in patients with bulimia nervosa, *Eat Weight Disord* 12(2):83–90, 2007.

Voils CI, Allaire JC, Olsen MK et al: Five-year trajectories of social networks and social support in older adults with major depression, *Int Psychogeriatr* 19(6):1110–1125, 2007.

Weaver AJ, Flannelly KJ: The role of religion/spirituality for cancer patients and their caregivers, *South Med J* 97(12):1210–1214, 2004.

Western H: Altered living: coping, hope and quality of life after stroke, *BJN* 16(20):1266, 2007.

Readiness for enhanced Immunization status   ⊖volve

Susan Mee, RN, PhD, CPNP, and Kathleen Karsten, MS, RN, BC

NANDA-I

Definition

A pattern of conforming to local, national, and/or international standards of immunization to prevent infectious disease(s) that is sufficient to protect a person, family, or community and can be strengthened

Defining Characteristics

Expresses desire to enhance: behavior to prevent infectious disease; identification of possible problems associated with immunizations; identification of providers of immunizations; immunization status; knowledge of immunization standards; recordkeeping of immunizations

NOC   (Nursing Outcomes Classification)

Suggested NOC Outcomes

Health-Seeking Behavior, Immune status, Immunization Behavior, Knowledge: Infection Management

• = Independent   ▲ = Collaborative   **EBN** = Evidence-Based Nursing   **EB** = Evidence-Based

---

Example NOC Outcomes with Indicators

Immunization Behavior as evidenced by the following indicators: Acknowledges disease risk without immunization/Brings updated immunization card to each visit/Obtains immunizations recommended for age by the AAP or USPHS/Describes relief measures for vaccine side effects/Reports any adverse reactions/Confirms date of next immunization/Identifies community resources for immunization (Rate the outcome and indicators of **Immunization Behavior**: 1 = never demonstrated, 2 = rarely demonstrated, 3 = sometimes demonstrated, 4 = often demonstrated, 5 = consistently demonstrated [see Section I].)

Client Outcomes

Client/Caregiver Will (Specify Time Frame):

- Review appropriate recommended immunization schedule with provider
- Ask questions about the benefits and risks of immunizations
- Ask questions regarding the risks of choosing not to be immunized
- Accurately respond to provider's questions related to pertinent information regarding individual health status as it relates to contraindications for individual vaccines
- Inform provider of the health status of close contacts and household members
- Evidence understanding of the risks and benefits of individual immunization decisions
- Evidence understanding of the benefits of community immunization
- Communicate decisions about immunization decision to provider in relation to personal preferences, values, and goals
- Communicate to provider ongoing personal record of immunization
- Evidence understanding of the client's responsibility to maintain an accurate record of immunization

NIC (Nursing Interventions Classification)

Suggested NIC Interventions

Decision-Making Support, Immunization/Vaccination Management, Mutual Goal Setting

Example NIC Activities—Immunization/Vaccination Management

Teach parent(s) recommended immunizations necessary for children, their route of medication administration, reasons and benefits of use, adverse reactions, and side effects schedule; Identify latest recommendations regarding use of immunizations; Provide and update diary for recording date and type of immunizations

Nursing Interventions and *Rationales*

Psychosocial

- Assess barriers to immunization:
  - Anxiety related to injection/parenteral pharmacologic therapy. **EBN:** *Fear of needles is a reported barrier to immunization (Mayo & Cobler, 2004).*
  - Anxiety related to immunization side effects. **EBN:** *For many parents or caregivers, the number, the strange-sounding names, the combinations of different vaccines, and the schedule of due dates can create considerable confusion and may contribute to nonadherence to the immunization schedule (Baker, Wilson, & Legwand, 2007).*
  - Knowledge of risk associated with disease. **EB:** *There is a general lack of awareness among parents and adolescents about the risk and severity of infectious diseases and the need for immunizations (Lehmann & Benson, 2009).*
  - Cost of health care. **EB:** *Minorities report lesser self-rated general health and a higher cost barrier to health care, particularly in Hispanic communities. Removing barriers to health care is an important aspect of health promotion and disease prevention (Liao et al, 2004). Programs to improve health insurance coverage and having a usual source of medical care positively impact age-appropriate immunization status (Dombroswki, Lantz, & Freed, 2004).*
- Assess client-provider relationship. **EBN:** *The most common source of information about vaccinations were found to be physicians and nurses. This finding was not unexpected because health care*

● = Independent ▲ = Collaborative **EBN** = Evidence-Based Nursing **EB** = Evidence-Based

professionals are seen as trustworthy and reliable sources of information (Baker, Wilson, & Legwand, 2007). **EB:** *Clients who report trusting their health care provider have higher immunization rates (Norwalk et al, 2005).*

- Assess client/caregiver level of participation in decision-making process. **EB:** *It is important to note that trust in the child's health care provider is reported as a key factor in a parent's immunization decision making; written materials may aid the provider in discussions with the parent (Gust et al, 2009).*
- Assess sources of information client has previously turned to. **EB:** *Lack of knowledge, fear of vaccine side effects, and misinformation perpetuated by antivaccine media contribute to low vaccination rates and vaccine refusal (Kimmel et al, 2007).*
- Assist client/caregiver to find appropriate educational resources. **EBN:** *Vaccine risk/benefit information needs to be communicated as simply as possible (Davis et al, 2006).* **EB:** *Vaccine Information Statements (VISs) are information sheets produced by the Centers for Disease Control and Prevention (CDC) that explain to vaccine recipients, their parents, or their legal representatives both the benefits and risks of a vaccine, and are required to be handed out whenever (before each dose) certain vaccines are given (CDC, 2007).*
- Assess cultural or religious beliefs that may relate to either the decision-making process or specific immunizations such as for sexually transmitted diseases. **EB:** *There is considerable dissension among parents in relation to attitude toward vaccination for sexually transmitted diseases (STDs). Public health policy makers, legislators, and school boards need to be sensitive to the concerns and rights of parents/caregivers regarding the potential mandate of immunization for STDs (Liddon et al, 2005).*

Physiological

- Perform comprehensive interview to elicit information regarding the client's susceptibility to adverse reactions to specific vaccines according to the manufacturer guidelines.
- Identify clients for whom a specific vaccine is contraindicated. **EBN:** *Client's perception of vaccine-related adverse effects and related allergy account for a proportion of vaccine refusal (Mayo & Cobler, 2004).*
- ▲ Report potential or actual adverse effects. **EB:** *Surveillance for adverse effects is important, and in some instances, mandated (Kretsinger et al, 2006).*
- Inform client/caregiver of the vaccine-specific risks to both women of childbearing age and the fetus. **EBN:** *Women's reproductive health overlaps with epidemiology of vaccine-preventable disease or physiological aspects of immunization (Schmidt, Kroger, & Roy, 2004).*
- Discuss pregnancy planning with appropriate clients considering immunization. **EBN:** *Women's reproductive health overlaps with epidemiology of vaccine-preventable disease or physiological aspects of immunization. Prevention of vaccine-preventable disease is a critical element of women's health promotion (Schmidt, Kroger, & Roy, 2004).*
- Identify high-risk individuals for specific vaccine-preventable diseases. **EBN:** *A metaanalysis of nursing-sensitive interventions targeted to improve nursing-sensitive client outcomes recommends clients with cancer and their household contact receive annual influenza immunization (Zitella et al, 2006).* **EB:** *Determination of altered immunocompetence is important to the vaccine provider because the incidence or severity of certain vaccine-preventable diseases is higher in persons with altered immunocompetence (CDC, 2007).*
- Identify high-risk groups for specific vaccine-preventable disease. **EB:** *Serologic and survey data indicate that U.S. adults are undervaccinated against tetanus and diptheria, and that rates of coverage decline with increasing age (Kretsinger et al, 2006).* **EB:** *In a study of female day care center educators, 10.2% presented as rubella seronegative. Women who are in contact with young children should be concerned due to the risk for infection and resultant congenital rubella syndrome (Gyorkos et al, 2005). Health care workers are a vulnerable population who benefit from influenza vaccination directly and indirectly by providing secondary benefit to health care facility consumers. In a study of 26,261 Mayo Clinic employees, influenza vaccination compliance improved via the Peer Vaccination Program, which provided incentives and made raffles available only to vaccinated employees, offered vaccination during grand rounds, and provided e-mail encouragement (CDC, 2005).*
- Identify high-risk populations for specific vaccine-preventable disease. **EBN:** *More than 50% of sexually active women are exposed to at least one HPV type in their lifetime, and prophylactic vaccines are likely to be of value as a primary prevention strategy (Keam & Harper, 2008).* **EBN:** *Nurses*

● = Independent   ▲ = Collaborative   **EBN** = Evidence-Based Nursing   **EB** = Evidence-Based

engaged in both disaster planning and disaster interventions need to be proactive in emergency administration of vaccines such as tetanus (Walton, 2006). Vaccination rates for populations at high risk for hepatitis B virus (HBV) remain low (Willis et al, 2005).

- Assess client's recent travel history and future travel plans. **EB:** *The CDC has isolated the H1N1 virus, and vaccines are being made to protect against the 2009 H1N1 virus (www.cdc.gov/h1n1flu/ vaccination/general.htm, Nov 17, 2009, accessed Dec 13, 2009).* **EB:** *Communicable diseases that are currently not endemic in the United States persist among travelers, often resulting in delayed recognition and notification of public health authorities (CDC, 2007).*
- Identify vulnerable populations and marginalized populations. **EB:** *Residents of minority communities bear greater risk for disease; substantial variation in the use of preventive services among different minority populations provide opportunities for health interventions (Liao et al, 2004). High-risk groups for HBV include men having sex with men, risk behaviors such as IV drug use, and multiple sex partners (Willis et al, 2005).*
- Tailor educational programs specific to these marginalized and vulnerable populations. **EB:** *In a study of 432 men having sex with men (MSM), researchers concluded that health education intervention that address perceived susceptibility and severity are likely to improve vaccination status. This study recommended interventions specific to influencing perceived susceptibility as a preferred intervention (deWit et al, 2005).*
- Adopt recommendations made by national and international professional groups advocating the use of Immunization Central Registries and standing orders. **EBN:** *Adaptation of multimodal interventions targeted to improve immunization rates resulted in 97% compliance rate for 12-month-old children and 87% compliance rate for immunization standards for 24-month-old children. Recommendations include electronic medical records, phone calls, postcards and letters to clients, staff education, and client record surveillance (Parve, 2004).* **EB:** *Strategies to enhance immunization status include standing orders, computerized record reminders, chart reminders, performance feedback, home visits, mailed/telephone reminders, expanded access in clinical settings, client education, personal health records (Ahmed et al, 2004; Committee on Practice and Ambulatory Medicine, 2006; CDC, 2007).*
- Support access to health care that enables clients to access well-preventive care on a walk-in basis during times that are consistent with client schedules. **EBN:** *Comprehensive efforts to identify population-specific barriers to access and targeted interventions to address barriers is effective in improving immunization rates (Parve, 2004).* **EB:** *Lack of transportation, geographical isolation, and inconvenient clinic hours were identified as barriers to successful immunization among low-income rural families (Thomas, Kohli, & King 2004).*

 ## Multicultural

- Assess cultural beliefs and practices that may have an impact on the educational and decision-making process specific to immunization as well as vaccine-specific illness. **EB:** *Variation exists both between and within cultural affiliations with respect to health beliefs and health seeking behaviors. In a study of Chinese Americans in New York City, Ma et al (2006) reports differences between attitudes and behavior of younger versus older members of the Chinese American community with respect to screening behavior, immunization acceptance, and willingness to discuss HPV with their health care provider.*
- Actively listen and be sensitive to how communication is shared culturally. **EB:** *Cultural sensitivity is the foundation of community outreach (Stauffer, 2008).*
- Employ culturally sensitive educational strategies to maximize the individual, family, or community response. **EBN:** *Every participant expressed the view that the immunization encounter should be conducted in the language with which the mother was most comfortable. It was also important that printed educational materials or consent forms are in the preferred language of the mother (Keller, 2008).*

 ## Home Care

- Above interventions may be adapted for home care use.
- Develop clinical practice guidelines that include shared decision making. **EBN:** *The quality of the interaction between nurse and parent/caregiver at the time of administering immunizations is crucial for maintaining an ongoing immunization schedule (Plumridge, Goodyear-Smith, & Ross, 2009).*

• = Independent   ▲ = Collaborative   **EBN** = Evidence-Based Nursing   **EB** = Evidence-Based

- Implement home care strategies that will enhance decision making and ability to maintain current immunization status. **EB:** *Provider-initiated phone calls to clients/caregivers, reminder postcards, and letters are effective strategies to improve immunization status (Norwalk et al, 2005).*
- Implement mechanisms to contact the client/caregiver at appropriate intervals with reminder literature or phone contact. **EB:** *The use of reminder postcards and/or employer-provided tool kits may enhance immunization status. The cost-benefit of these strategies should be regularly monitored to improve outcomes and make effective use of health resources (Ahmed et al, 2004).*

Client/Family Teaching and Discharge Planning

- Before teaching, evaluate the client preference for involvement with the decision-making process.
- Use community-based and school-based interventions to teach school-age children and thereby provide vicarious education to the family. **EBN:** *Every participant expressed the view that the immunization encounter should be conducted in the language with which the mother was most comfortable. It was also important that printed educational materials or consent forms are in the preferred language of the mother (Keller, 2008).* **EB:** *School-based curricula are effective in increasing immunization knowledge, enhancing positive attitude toward immunization, and improving health-promotion behavior with respect to immunization (Glik et al, 2004).*
- Develop curricula and media that enhance immunization education. **EB:** *Only through direct dialogue with parents and by using available resources can health care providers prevent acceptance of media reports and information from nonauthoritative Internet sites as scientific fact (Kroger et al, 2006).*
- Employ media and curricula in office waiting rooms. **EBN:** *Using handouts, videos, and discussions throughout an office visit can enhance vaccine education and address the various learning needs of parents/guardians (Tenrreiro, 2005).* **EB:** *Clients benefit when waiting room time is utilized as an educational opportunity (CDC, 2007).*
- Develop and distribute client log books that provide recordkeeping and foster ownership of the responsibility of current immunization status. **EB:** *An electronic health record-based clinical alert intervention was associated with increases in captured opportunities for vaccination and significant improvements in immunization rate (Fiks et al, 2007).* **EB:** *Client/caregiver personal health records improve immunization rates (CDC, 2007).*

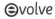 See the EVOLVE website for Weblinks for client education resources.

REFERENCES

Ahmed F, Friedman C, Franks A et al: Effect of the frequency of delivery of reminders and an influenza tool kit on increasing influenza vaccination rates among adults with high-risk conditions, *Am J Manag Care* 10(10):698–712, 2004.

Baker L, Wilson F, Legwand C: Mother's knowledge and information needs relating to childhood immunizations, *Issues in Comprehensive Pediatric Nursing*, 30:39–53, 2007.

Centers for Disease Control and Prevention (CDC): Interventions to increase influenza vaccination of health-care workers—California and Minnesota, *MMWR Morb Mortal Wkly Rep* 54(8):196–199, 2005.

Centers for Disease Control and Prevention (CDC): Measles among adults associated with adoption of children in China—California, Missouri, and Washington, July-August 2006, *MMWR Morb Mortal Wkly Rep* 56(7):144–146, 2007.

Centers for Disease Control and Prevention (CDC): Strategies for increasing adult vaccination rates. www.cdc.gov/vaccines/programs/iis/default.htm. Accessed on April 20, 2007.

Committee on Practice and Ambulatory Medicine: Immunization information systems, *Pediatrics* 118(3):1293–1295, 2006.

Davis T, Frederickson D, Kennan E et al: Vaccine risk/benefit communication: effect of an educational package for public health nurses, *Health Education & Behavior*, 33:767–801, 2006.

deWit JBF, Vet R, Schitten M et al: Social-cognitive determinants of vaccination behavior against hepatitis B: an assessment among men who have sex with men, *Prev Med* 40(6):795–802, 2005.

Dombrowski KJ, Lantz PM, Freed GL: Role of health insurance and a usual source of medical care in age appropriate vaccination, *Am J Public Health*, 94(6):960–966, 2004.

Fiks A, Grundmeier R, Biggs L et al: Impact of clinical alerts within an electronic health record on routine childhood immunization in an urban pediatric population, *Pediatrics*, 120(4):707–714, 2007.

Glik D, Macpherson F, Todd W et al: Impact of an immunization education program on middle school adolescents, *Am J Health Behav* 28(6):487–497, 2004.

Gust D, Kennedy A, Weber D et al: Parents questioning immunization: evaluation of an intervention, *American Journal of Health Behavior* 33(3):287–298, 2009.

Gyorkos TW, Beliveau C, Rahme E et al: High rubella seronegativity in daycare educators, *Clin Invest Med* 28(3):105–111, 2005.

Keam S, Harper D: Human papillomavirus type 16 and 18 Vaccine, *Drugs*, 68(3):359–372, 2008.

Keller T: Mexican American parent's perceptions of culturally congruent interpersonal processes of care during childhood immunization episodes—a pilot study, *Online Journal of Rural Nursing and Health Care*, 8(2):33–41, 2008.

Kimmel SR, Burns I, Wolfe RM et al: Addressing immunization barriers, benefits and risks, *J Fam Pract* 56(2):561–569, 2007.

Kretsinger K, Broder KR, Cortese MM et al: Preventing tetanus, diphtheria, and pertussis among adults: use of tetanus toxoid, reduced diphtheria toxoid and acellular pertussis vaccine recommendations of the Advisory Committee on Immunization Practices (ACIP) and recommendation of ACIP, supported by the Healthcare Infection Control Practices Advisory Committee (HICPAC), for use of Tdap among health-care personnel, *MMWR Recomm Rep* 55(RR-17):1–37, 2006.

Kroger A, Atkinson W, Marcse E et al: General recommendations on immunization, recommendations of the Advisory Committee on Immunization Practices (ACIP), Centers for Disease Control and Prevention (CDC): *MMWR Morb Mortal Wkly Rep* 55(RR-15):1–46, 2006.

Lehmann C, Benson P: Vaccine adherence in adolescents, *Clin Pediatr* 48(8):801–811, 2009.

Liao Y, Tucker P, Okoro CA et al: REACH 2010 Surveillance for Health Status in Minority Communities—United States, 2001–2002, *MMWR Surveill Summ* 53(6):1–36, 2004.

Liddon N, Pulley L, Cocherham WC et al: Parents'/guardians' willingness to vaccinate their children against genital herpes, *J Adolesc Health* 37(3):187–193, 2005.

Ma G, Shive S, Toubbeh J et al: Risk perceptions, barriers, benefits and self-efficacy of hepatitis B screening and vaccination among Chinese immigrants, *Int J Health Educ* 9:141–153, 2006.

Mayo AM, Cobler S: Flu vaccines and patient decision making: what we need to know, *J Am Acad Nurse Pract* 16(9):402–410, 2004.

Norwalk MP, Lin CJ, Zimmerman RK et al: Tailored interventions to introduce influenza vaccine among 6–23 month old children at inner city health centers, *Am J Manag Care* 11:717–724, 2005.

Parve J: Remove vaccination barriers for children 12–24 months, *Nurse Pract* 29(4):35–38, 2004.

Plumridge E, Goodyear-Smith F, Ross J: Nurse and parent partnership during children's vaccinations: a conversation analysis, *J Adv Nurs* 65(6):1187–1194, 2009.

Schmidt JV, Kroger AT, Roy SL: Vaccines in women, *J Women's Health* 13(3):249–257, 2004.

Stauffer R: Vietnamese American. In Giger JN, Davidhizar R, editors: *Transcultural nursing: assessment and intervention,* St Louis, 2008, Mosby.

Tenrreiro K: Time-efficient strategies to ensure vaccine risk/benefit communication, *Journal of Pediatric Nursing,* 20(6):469–476, 2005.

Thomas M, Kohli V, King D: Barriers to childhood immunization: findings from a needs assessment study, *Home Health Care Services Quarterly,* 23(2):19–32, 2004.

U.S. Department of Health and Human Services: Healthy People 2010, ed 2, (2 vols), Washington DC, 2000, U.S. Government Printing Office.

Walton F: One nurse can make a big difference, *Aust Nurs J* 14(2):15, 2006.

Willis BC, Ndiaye SM, Hopkins DP et al: Improving influenza, pneumococcal polysaccharide, and hepatitis B vaccination coverage among adults aged <65 years at high risk: a report on recommendations of the Task Force on Community Preventive Services, *MMWR Recomm Rep* 54(RR-5):1–11, 2005.

Zitella LJ, Friese CR, Hauser J et al: Putting evidence into practice: prevention of infection, *Clin J Oncol Nurs* 10:739–750, 2006.

Functional urinary Incontinence   *Mikel Gray, PhD, CUNP, CCCN, FAANP, FAAN*

 NANDA-I

Definition

Inability of usually continent person to reach toilet in time to avoid unintentional loss of urine (NANDA-I, 2009)

Impairment or loss of continence due to functional deficits, including altered mobility, dexterity, or cognition, or environmental barriers (Gray, 2007)

Defining Characteristics

Although functional limitations (impaired mobility, dexterity, and cognition) are risk factors for urinary incontinence (UI) (Hunskaar et al, 2005; Jenkins & Fultz, 2005), the nature of their relationship is complex and only partly understood. For example, impaired cognition associated with Alzheimer's-type dementia leads to detrusor overactivity (Rosenberg, Griffiths, & Resnick, 2005). Whether or not detrusor overactivity leads to UI (either urge UI or UI without sensory awareness) depends on multiple factors, including mobility and the severity of cognitive impairment, among other factors. Thus, while functional impairment exacerbates the severity of urinary incontinence, the underlying factors that contribute to these functional limitations themselves also contribute to abnormal lower urinary tract function and impaired continence.

Related Factors (r/t)

Cognitive disorders (delirium, dementia, severe, or profound retardation); neuromuscular limitations impairing mobility or dexterity; environmental barriers to toileting

NOTE: Defining Characteristics and Related Factors adapted from the work of NANDA-I.

• = Independent   ▲ = Collaborative   **EBN** = Evidence-Based Nursing   **EB** = Evidence-Based

(Nursing Outcomes Classification)

Suggested NOC Outcomes

Urinary Continence, Urinary Elimination

Example **NOC Outcome with Indicators**
Urinary Continence as evidenced by the following indicators: Recognizes urge to void/Responds to urge in timely manner/Voids in appropriate receptacle/Underclothing remains dry during day/Underclothing or bedding remains dry during night (Rate the outcome and indicators of **Urinary Continence:** 1 = never demonstrated, 2 = rarely demonstrated, 3 = sometimes demonstrated, 4 = often demonstrated, 5 = consistently demonstrated [see Section I].)

Client Outcomes

Client Will (Specify Time Frame):

- Eliminate or reduce incontinent episodes
- Eliminate or overcome environmental barriers to toileting
- Use adaptive equipment to reduce or eliminate incontinence related to impaired mobility or dexterity
- Use portable urinary collection devices or urine containment devices when access to the toilet is not feasible

 (Nursing Interventions Classification)

Suggested NIC Interventions

Urinary Habit Training, Urinary Incontinence Care

Example **NIC Activities—Urinary Habit Training**
Keep a continence-specification record for 3 days to establish voiding pattern; Establish interval for toileting of preferably not less than 2 hours

Nursing Interventions and *Rationales*

- Perform a history-taking and physical assessment focusing on bothersome lower urinary tract symptoms, cognitive status, functional status (particularly physical mobility and dexterity), frequency and severity of leakage episodes, and alleviating and aggravating factors. *The history provides clues to the causes, the severity of the condition, and its management (Vickerman, 2002).*
- ▲ Consult with the client and family, the client's physician, and other health care professionals concerning treatment of incontinence in the elderly client undergoing detailed geriatric evaluation.
- Teach the client, the client's care providers, or the family to complete a voiding diary (bladder log) by recording voiding frequency, the frequency of urinary incontinent episodes, and their association with urgency (a sudden and strong desire to urinate that is difficult to defer) over a 3- to 7-day period. An electronic voiding diary may be kept whenever feasible. In addition to these parameters, the client may be asked to record voided volume and fluid intake. *The voiding diary provides a more objective record of lower urinary tract function than the oral history, and it often provides a modest therapeutic effect by alerting the client to factors that promote urinary incontinence episodes (Sampselle, 2003). An electronic voiding diary provides an efficient and possibly more accurate method for documenting these parameters (Quinn, Goka, & Richardson, 2003).*
- Assess the client for potentially reversible or modifiable causes of acute/transient urinary incontinence (e.g., urinary tract infection; atrophic urethritis; constipation or impaction; use of sedatives or narcotics, antidepressants or psychotropic medications interfering with efficient detrusor contractions, parasympatholytics, or alpha-adrenergic antagonists; polyuria caused by uncontrolled diabetes mellitus or insipidus). *Transient or acute incontinence may be relieved or eliminated by treating the underlying cause (Reilly, 2002).*
- ▲ Consult with the physician about discontinuing antimuscarinic medications in clients receiving cholinesterase reuptake inhibitors for Alzheimer's type dementia. *Retrospective clinical evidence*

● = Independent   ▲ = Collaborative   **EBN** = Evidence-Based Nursing   **EB** = Evidence-Based

suggests that clients receiving both cholinesterase reuptake inhibitors and antimuscarinics experience more rapid functional decline than do clients taking cholinesterase reuptake inhibitors alone (Sink et al, 2008).

- Assess the client in an acute care or rehabilitation facility for risk factors for functional incontinence. **EBN:** *Risk factors include confusion, use of a wheelchair or assistive device for walking, and dependence on others for ambulation prior to admission (Palmer et al, 2002).*

- Assess the client for coexisting or premorbid urinary incontinence. *A history of previous incidences of urinary incontinence predicts a higher risk for persistent urinary leakage and poorer functional outcomes.*

- Assess clients, regardless of frailty or age, residing in a long-term care facility for UI. **EB:** *UI significantly impairs quality of life, even among frail, and functionally or cognitively impaired elders residing in a nursing home (Dubeau, Simon, & Morris, 2006).*

- Assess the home, acute care, or long-term care environment for accessibility to toileting facilities, paying particular attention to the following:
  - Distance of the toilet from the bed, chair, and living quarters
  - Characteristics of the bed, including presence of side rails and distance of the bed from the floor
  - Characteristics of the pathway to the toilet, including barriers such as stairs, loose rugs on the floor, and inadequate lighting
  - Characteristics of the bathroom, including patterns of use, lighting, height of the toilet from the floor, presence of handrails to assist transfers to the toilet, and breadth of the door and its accessibility for a wheelchair, walker, or other assistive device

  Functional continence requires access to a toilet; environmental barriers blocking this access can produce functional incontinence (Chadwick, 2005).

- Assess the client for mobility, including the ability to rise from chair and bed, transfer to the toilet, and ambulate, and the need for physical assistive devices such as a cane, walker, or wheelchair. *Functional continence requires the ability to gain access to a toilet facility, either independently or with the assistance of devices to increase mobility.*

- ▲ Assess the client for dexterity, including the ability to manipulate buttons, hooks, snaps, loop and pile closures, and zippers as needed to remove clothing. Consult a physical or occupational therapist to promote optimal toilet access as indicated. *Functional continence requires the ability to remove clothing to urinate (Lekan-Rutledge, 2004).*

- Assess the functional and cognitive status using a tool such as the Mini Mental Status Examination for the elderly client with functional incontinence. *Limitations in both cognition and functional status affect the severity and management of functional urinary incontinence (Ouslander et al, 2001). Functional continence requires sufficient mental acuity to respond to sensory input from a filling urinary bladder by locating the toilet, moving to it, and emptying the bladder.* **EB:** *In a cohort of nondisabled elderly people, those with severe white matter changes (dementia) were found to have more urinary urge incontinence (Poggesi et al, 2008).*

- Remove environmental barriers to toileting in the acute care, long-term care, or home setting. Assist the client in removing loose rugs from the floor and improving lighting in hallways and bathrooms. *Functional continence requires ready access to a bathroom (Lekan-Rutledge, 2004).*

- Provide an appropriate, safe urinary receptacle such as a three-in-one commode, female or male hand-held urinal, no-spill urinal, or containment device when toileting access is limited by immobility or environmental barriers. *These receptacles provide access to a substitute toilet and enhance the potential for functional continence.*

- ▲ Help the client with limited mobility to obtain evaluation by a physical therapist and to obtain assistive devices as indicated; assist the client in selecting shoes with a nonskid sole to maximize traction when arising from a chair and transferring to the toilet. *A physical therapist is an important member of the interdisciplinary team needed to manage urinary incontinence in the client with functional impairments.*

- Assist the client in altering the wardrobe to maximize toileting access. Select loose-fitting clothing with stretch waistbands rather than buttoned or zippered waist; minimize buttons, snaps, and multilayered clothing; and substitute a loop-and-pile closure or other easily loosened systems for buttons, hooks, and zippers in existing clothing.

- Begin a prompted voiding program or patterned urge response toileting program for the elderly client in the home or a long-term care facility who has functional incontinence and dementia:
  - Determine the frequency of current urination using an alarm system or check-and-change device.
  - Record urinary elimination and incontinent patterns in a bladder log to use as a baseline for assessment and evaluation of treatment efficacy.
  - Begin a prompted toileting program based on the results of this program; toileting frequency may vary from every 1.5 to 2 hours to every 4 hours.
  - Praise the client when toileting occurs with prompting.
  - Refrain from any socialization when incontinent episodes occur; change the client and make her or him comfortable.

  EBN: *Prompted voiding or patterned urge response toileting executed during waking hours has been shown to markedly reduce or eliminate functional incontinence in selected clients in long-term care facilities and in the community setting (Engberg et al, 2002). Based on a systematic review of 14 clinical trials, prompted voiding has been shown to improve daytime incontinence and the percentage of appropriate toileting episodes in clients with dementia and functional incontinence (Fink et al, 2008).*

Geriatric

- Institute aggressive continence management programs for the cognitively intact, community-dwelling client in consultation with the client and family. *Uncontrolled incontinence can lead to institutionalization of an elderly person who prefers to remain in a home care setting.*
- Monitor the elderly client in a long-term care facility, acute care facility, or home for dehydration. *Dehydration can exacerbate urine loss, produce acute confusion, and increase the risk of morbidity and mortality, particularly in the frail elderly client.*

Home Care

- The interventions described previously may be adapted for home care use.
- Assess current strategies used to reduce urinary incontinence, including limitation of fluid intake, restriction of bladder irritants, prompted or scheduled toileting, and use of containment devices. *Many elderly clients and care providers use a variety of self-management techniques to control urinary incontinence, such as fluid limitation, avoidance of social contacts, and use of absorptive materials, that may or may not be effective for reducing urinary leakage or beneficial to general health (Johnson, 2000).*
- Encourage a mind-set and program of self-care management. **EBN:** *Addressing self-care activities through exercise, diet, fluid intake, and use of protective devices helps the client to exercise control over incontinence (Leenerts, Teel, & Pendleton, 2002).*
- Implement a bladder-training program, including self-monitoring activities (e.g., reducing caffeine intake, adjusting amount and timing of fluid intake, decreasing long voiding intervals while awake, instituting dietary changes to promote bowel regularity); bladder training; and pelvic muscle exercise. **EBN:** *In women age 55 years or older with involuntary urine loss associated with stress, urge, or mixed incontinence, clients responded to the aforementioned interventions with a 61% decrease in the severity of urinary incontinence at 2 years after intervention. Self-monitoring and bladder training accounted for most of the improvement (Dougherty et al, 2002).*
- For a memory-impaired elderly client, implement an individualized, scheduled toileting program (on a schedule developed in consultation with the caregiver, approximately every 2 hours, with toileting reminders provided and existing patterns incorporated, such as toileting before or after meals). **EBN:** *Functional incontinence in memory-impaired elderly clients decrease significantly with the described intervention. The client must be able to cooperate (Jirovec & Templin, 2001).*
- Teach the family the general principles of bladder health, including avoidance of bladder irritants, adequate fluid intake, and a routine schedule of toileting. (Refer to the care plan for **Impaired Urinary elimination**.)
- Teach prompted voiding to the family and client for the client with mild to moderate dementia (refer to previous description).

- Inspect the perineal and perianal skin for evidence of incontinence-associated dermatitis, including inflammation, vesicles in skin exposed to urinary leakage, and especially skin folds or denudation of the skin, particularly when incontinence is managed by absorptive pads or containment briefs. *Urinary incontinence, particularly when combined with fecal incontinence or use of absorptive pads or adult containment briefs, increases the risk of incontinence-associated dermatitis (Gray et al, 2007).* **EBN:** *In the acute care setting, 20% of clients with urinary and/or fecal incontinence were found to have perineal or perigenital skin damage, and 18% were found to have evidence of secondary cutaneous candidiasis (Junkin & Selekof, 2007).*
- Begin a preventive skin care regimen for all clients with urinary and/or fecal incontinence and treat clients with incontinence-associated dermatitis or related skin damage.
- Advise the client about the advantages of using disposable or reusable insert pads, pad-pant systems, or replacement briefs specifically designed for urinary incontinence (or double urinary and fecal incontinence) as indicated. *Many absorptive products used by community-dwelling elders are not designed to absorb urine, prevent odor, and protect the perineal skin. Disposable or reusable absorptive devices specifically designed to contain urine or double incontinence are more effective than household products, particularly in cases of moderate to severe incontinence (Shirran & Brazelli, 2000).*
- Assist the family with arranging care in a way that allows the client to participate in family or favorite activities without embarrassment. Elicit discussion of the client's concerns about the social or emotional burden of incontinence. **EBN and EB:** *Careful planning can allow the dignity and integrity of family patterns to be retained. Urinary incontinence has a demonstrated influence on subjective well-being and quality of life, with depression, loneliness, or sadness possible (Fultz & Herzog, 2001). Discussing emotional concerns helps the client to develop a sense of control over incontinence (Leenerts, Teel, & Pendleton, 2002).*
- ▲ Refer to occupational therapy for help in obtaining assistive devices and adapting the home for optimal toilet accessibility.
- ▲ Consider the use of an indwelling catheter for continuous drainage in the client who is both homebound and bed-bound and is receiving palliative or end-of-life care (requires a physician's order). *An indwelling catheter may increase client comfort, ease care provider burden, and prevent urinary incontinence in bed-bound clients receiving end-of-life (palliative) care (Gray & Campbell, 2001).*
- ▲ When an indwelling urinary catheter is in place, follow prescribed maintenance protocols for managing the catheter, replacing the catheter, drainage bag, perineal skin, and urethral meatus. Teach infection control measures adapted to the home care setting. *Proper care reduces the risk of catheter-associated urinary tract infection.*
- Assist the client in adapting to the catheter. Encourage discussion of the client's response to the catheter. **EBN:** *Clients living with a catheter are often keenly aware of its presence; adaptation is served by normalizing the experience. Instruction could include the fact that the client will be more aware of some sensations and sounds (e.g., urine sloshing in the bag, the weight of the bag, pressure or pain when urine flow has been altered). Rehearsing emptying of the bag when away from home will support resumption of activities. Discussion of the client's response will assist him or her in dealing with embarrassment or frustration (Wilde, 2002).*

Client/Family Teaching and Discharge Planning

- Work with the client, family, and their extended support systems to assist with needed changes in the environment and wardrobe, and other alterations required to maximize toileting access.
- Work with the client and family to establish a reasonable and manageable prompted voiding program using environmental and verbal cues to remind caregivers of voiding intervals, such as television programs, meals, and bedtime.
- Teach the family to use an alarm system for toileting or to carry out a check-and-change program and to maintain an accurate log of voiding and incontinence episodes.

⊖volve   See the EVOLVE website for Weblinks for client education resources.

● = Independent   ▲ = Collaborative   **EBN** = Evidence-Based Nursing   **EB** = Evidence-Based

REFERENCES

Chadwick V: Assessment of functional incontinence in disabled living centers, *Nurs Times* 101(2):65–67, 2005.

Dougherty MC, Dwyer JW, Pendergast JF et al: A randomized trial of behavioral management for continence with older rural women, *Res Nurs Health* 25:3, 2002.

Dubeau CE, Simon SE, Morris JN: The effect of urinary incontinence on quality of life in older nursing home residents, *J Am Geriatr Soc* 54(9):1325–1333, 2006.

Engberg S, Sereika SM, McDowell BJ et al: Effectiveness of prompted voiding in treating urinary incontinence in cognitively impaired homebound older adults, *J Wound Ostomy Continence Nurs* 29(5):252–265, 2002.

Fink HA. Taylor BC. Tacklind JW et al: Treatment interventions in nursing home residents with urinary incontinence: a systematic review of randomized trials. *Mayo Clinic Proceedings* 83(12):1332–1343, 2008.

Fultz NH, Herzog AR: Self-reported social and emotional impact of urinary incontinence, *J Am Geriatr Soc* 49:892, 2001.

Gray M, Bliss DZ, Doughty DB et al: Incontinence-associated dermatitis: a consensus, *J Wound Ostomy Continence Nurs* 24(1):45–56, 2007.

Gray M, Campbell F: Urinary tract disorders. In Ferrell B, Coyle N, editors: *Textbook of palliative nursing*, Oxford, England, 2001, Oxford University Press.

Hunskaar S et al: *Epidemiology of urinary (UI) and fecal (FI) incontinence and pelvic organ prolapse (POP) 3rd International Consultation on Incontinence*, ed 3, Plymouth, England, 2005, Health Publication, Plymbridge Distributors.

Jenkins KR, Fultz NH: Functional impairment as a risk factor for urinary incontinence among older Americans, *Neurourol Urodyn* 24(1): 51–55, 2005.

Jirovec MM, Templin T: Predicting success using individualized scheduled toileting for memory-impaired elders at home, *Res Nurs Health* 24:1, 2001.

Johnson ST: From incontinence to confidence, *Am J Nurs* 100(2):69, 2000.

Junkin J, Selekof J: Prevalence of incontinence and associated skin injury in an acute care population, *J Wound Ostomy Continence Nurs* 34(3), 260–269, 2007.

Leenerts MH, Teel CS, Pendleton MK: Building a model of self-care for health promotion in aging, *J Nurs Sch* 34:355, 2002.

Lekan-Rutledge D: Urinary incontinence strategies for frail elderly women, *Urol Nurs* 24(4):281–302, 2004.

Ouslander JG, Greendale GA, Uman G et al: Effects of oral estrogen and progestin on the lower urinary tract among female nursing home residents, *J Am Geriatr Soc* 49(6):803–807, 2001.

Palmer MH, Baumgarten M, Langenberg P et al: Risk factors for hospital acquired incontinence in elderly female hip fracture patients, *J Gerontol A Biol Sci Med Sci* 57(10):M672, 2002.

Poggesi A, Pracucci G, Chabriat H et al: Urinary complaints in non-disabled elderly people with age-related white matter changes: the Leukoaraiosis and DISability (LADIS) Study, *J Am Geriatr Soc* 56(9):1638–1643, 2008.

Quinn P, Goka J, Richardson H: Assessment of an electronic daily diary in patients with overactive bladder, *BJU Int* 91(7):647–652, 2003.

Reilly N: Assessment and management of acute or transient urinary incontinence. In Doughty D, editor: *Urinary and fecal incontinence: nursing management*, ed 2, St Louis, 2002, Mosby.

Rosenberg LJ, Griffiths DJ, Resnick NM: Factors that distinguish continent from incontinent older adults with detrusor overactivity, *J Urol* 174(5):1868–1872, 2005.

Sampselle CM: Bladder matters. Teaching women to use a voiding diary: what "mind over bladder" can accomplish, *Am Nurs* 103(11):62–64, 2003.

Shirran E, Brazelli M: Absorbent products for the containment of urinary and/or fecal incontinence, *Cochrane Database Syst Rev* (2): CD0011406, 2000.

Sink KM, Thomas J 3rd, Xu H et al: Dual use of bladder anticholinergics and cholinesterase inhibitors: long-term functional and cognitive outcomes, *J Am Geriatr Soc* 56(5):847–853, 2008.

Vickerman J: Thorough assessment of functional incontinence, *Nurs Times* 98(28):58, 2002.

Wilde MH: Urine flowing: a phenomenological study of living with a urinary catheter, *Res Nurs Health* 25:14, 2002.

Overflow urinary Incontinence   *Mikel Gray, PhD, CUNP, CCCN, FAANP, FAAN*

NANDA-I

Definition

Involuntary loss of urine associated with overdistention of the bladder

Defining Characteristics

Bladder distention; high postvoid residual volume; nocturia; observed involuntary leakage of small volumes of urine; reports involuntary leakage of small volumes of urine

Related Factors (r/t)

Bladder outlet obstruction; detrusor external sphincter dyssynergia; poor detrusor contraction strength; fecal impaction; severe pelvic prolapse; side effects of medications with anticholinergic actions; side effects of calcium channel blockers; side effects of medication with alpha-adrenergic agonistic effects; urethral obstruction

NOC, NIC, Client Outcomes, Nursing Interventions, Client/Family Teaching and Discharge Planning, *Rationales,* and References

Refer to care plans for **Urinary retention.**

• = Independent   ▲ = Collaborative   **EBN** = Evidence-Based Nursing   **EB** = Evidence-Based

Reflex urinary Incontinence   *Mikel Gray, PhD, CUNP, CCCN, FAANP, FAAN*

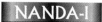 **NANDA-I**

Definition

Involuntary loss of urine at somewhat predictable intervals when a specific bladder volume is reached (NANDA-I, 2009). Involuntary loss of urine caused by a defect in the spinal cord between the nerve roots at or below the first cervical segment and those above the second sacral segment. Urine elimination occurs at unpredictable intervals; micturition may be elicited by tactile stimuli, including stroking of inner thigh or perineum (Gray, 2006).

Defining Characteristics

Urinary incontinence caused by neurogenic detrusor overactivity; disruption of spinal pathways leads to absent or diminished awareness of the desire to void or the occurrence of an overactive detrusor contraction; incomplete bladder emptying caused by dyssynergia of striated sphincter mechanism, which produces functional outlet obstruction of bladder; reflex urinary incontinence may be associated with sweating and acute elevation in blood pressure and pulse rate in clients with spinal cord injury. Refer to the care plan for **Autonomic dysreflexia**.

Related Factors (r/t)

Paralyzing spinal disorder affecting spinal segments C1 to S2

 NOC   **(Nursing Outcomes Classification)**

Suggested NOC Outcomes

Urinary Continence, Urinary Elimination

Example **NOC** Outcome with Indicators
Urinary Continence as evidenced by the following indicators: Urine leakage between voidings/Urinary tract infection/Wets clothing during day/Wets clothing or bedding during night (Rate the outcome and indicators of **Urinary Continence:** 1 = consistently demonstrated, 2 = often demonstrated, 3 = sometimes demonstrated, 4 = rarely demonstrated, 5 = never demonstrated [see Section I].)

Client Outcomes

Client Will (Specify Time Frame):

- Follow prescribed schedule for bladder evacuation
- Demonstrate successful use of triggering techniques to stimulate voiding
- Have intact perineal skin
- Remain clear of symptomatic urinary tract infection
- Demonstrate how to apply containment device or insert indwelling catheter or be able to provide caregiver with instructions for performing these procedures
- Demonstrate awareness of risk of autonomic dysreflexia, its prevention, and management

NIC   **(Nursing Interventions Classification)**

Suggested NIC Interventions

Urinary Catheterization: Intermittent, Urinary Elimination Management, Urinary Incontinence Care

Example **NIC** Activities—**Urinary Elimination Management**
Monitor urinary elimination including frequency, consistency, odor, volume, and color as appropriate; Teach patient signs and symptoms of urinary tract infection

• = Independent   ▲ = Collaborative   **EBN** = Evidence-Based Nursing   **EB** = Evidence-Based

Nursing Interventions and *Rationales*

▲ Assess the client's neurological status, including the type of neurological disorder, the functional level of neurological impairment, its completeness (effect on motor and sensory function), and the ability to perform bladder management tasks, including intermittent catheterization, application of a condom catheter, and so on. *Knowledge of single, well-circumscribed neurological lesion level strongly correlates with bladder function. This correlation is weaker in clients with multilevel cord trauma due to secondary bleeding or swelling (Weld, Graney, & Dmochowski, 2000).*

• Knowledge of functional impairments related to a spinal cord injury, including upper extremity function, is essential because it determines the client's ability to manage the bladder by self-catheterization (Gray, 2006).

• Inspect the perineal and perigenital skin for signs of incontinence-associated dermatitis and pressure ulcers. *Urinary and fecal incontinence associated with neurogenic bladder and bowel dysfunction in the client with a paralyzing disorder increases the risk of incontinence-associated dermatitis and pressure ulceration, particularly when a urine containment device such as an adult containment brief or condom catheter is used (Gray et al, 2007; Junkin & Selekof, 2007).*

• Complete a bladder log to determine the pattern of urine elimination, incontinence episodes, and current bladder management program. *The bladder log provides an objective record of urine elimination that confirms the accuracy of the historical report, and a baseline for assessment and evaluation of treatment efficacy (Gray, 2006).*

▲ Consult with the physician concerning current bladder function and the potential of the bladder to produce upper urinary tract distress (hydronephrosis, vesicoureteral reflux, febrile urinary tract infection, or compromised renal function). **EBN:** *Reflex incontinence is typically accompanied by detrusor striated sphincter dyssynergia, which increases the risk of upper urinary tract distress (Gray et al, 1991; Weld et al, 2000).*

▲ Determine a bladder management program in consultation with the client, family, and rehabilitation team. **EBN:** *The bladder management program profoundly affects the client and significant others; it is determined by holistic assessment that addresses the potential of the bladder to create upper urinary tract distress, the potential for incontinence and related complications, client and family preference, and the perceived impact of the bladder management program on the client's lifestyle (Gray, Rayome, & Anson 1995; Merenda & Hickey, 2005).*

▲ In consultation with the rehabilitation team, counsel the client and family concerning the merits and potential risks associated with each possible bladder management program, including spontaneous voiding, intermittent self-catheterization, reflex voiding with condom catheter containment, and indwelling catheterization. *All bladder management programs carry some risk of urinary incontinence or serious urinary system complications (Wyndaele, Madersbacher, & Kovindha, 2001).* **EBN:** *Spontaneous voiding and intermittent catheterization carry greater risk of urine loss than condom catheter containment or indwelling catheter, but these latter strategies carry higher risk for serious urinary system complications when evaluated over a period of years. Long-term indwelling catheterization carries the greatest risk for serious urologic complications (Gray, Rayome, & Anson, 1995; Saint et al, 2006).*

• Teach the client with reflex incontinence to consume an adequate amount of fluids on a daily basis (approximately 30 mL/kg of body weight). *Dehydration exacerbates urine loss and increases the risk of related complications, including constipation and urinary tract infection. Increasing fluid intake has also been associated with a diminished risk for bladder cancer, which is particularly important for the client managed by long-term indwelling catheterization (Gray & Krissovich, 2003).*

▲ Teach the client with reflex urinary incontinence that is managed by spontaneous voiding to self-administer an alpha-adrenergic blocking medication as directed and to recognize and manage potential side effects. *Clients who spontaneously urinate may take an alpha-adrenergic blocking drug to reduce urethral resistance during voiding (Linsenmeyer, Horton, & Benevento, 2002).*

▲ Begin intermittent catheterization using a modified clean or sterile technique based on facility policies. *Modified clean intermittent catheterization may be used in an inpatient setting with appropriate staff and client education.*

▲ Teach intermittent catheterization as the client approaches discharge as directed. Instruct the client and at least one family member, spouse, or partner in the performance of catheterization using clean technique. Teach the client with quadriplegia how to instruct others to perform this

• = Independent   ▲ = Collaborative   **EBN** = Evidence-Based Nursing   **EB** = Evidence-Based

procedure. **EBN:** *Intermittent catheterization is a safe and effective bladder management strategy for persons with reflex urinary incontinence. Inclusion of a family member, spouse, or significant other is particularly helpful for the client with limited upper extremity dexterity and reflex urinary incontinence (Woodbury, Hayes, & Askes, 2008). Intermittent catheterization among children with spinal cord injuries and reflex urinary incontinence is safe and effective (Generao et al, 2004).*

▲ Teach the client managed by intermittent catheterization to self-administer antispasmodic (parasympatholytic) medications as directed, and to recognize and manage potential side effects. *Antimuscarinic medications enhance catheterized volumes and reduce the frequency of incontinence episodes in persons with reflex incontinence owing to spinal cord injury or multiple sclerosis (Ethans et al, 2004; Verpoorten & Buyse, 2008).*

▲ Consult with the physician and occupational therapist concerning the use of a neuroprosthesis or other device designed to improve hand use for the quadriplegic client with partial hand function. *Use of a neuroprosthetic device designed to improve hand function increases clients' independence when performing multiple functions, including bladder management (Creasey et al, 2000).*

• For a male client with reflex incontinence who cannot manage the condition effectively with spontaneous voiding, does not choose to perform intermittent catheterization, or cannot perform catheterization, teach the client and his family to obtain, select, and apply an external collective device and urinary drainage system. Assist the client and family to choose a product that adheres to the glans penis or penile shaft without allowing seepage of urine onto surrounding skin or clothing, and one that avoids provoking hypersensitivity reactions on the skin, and includes a urinary drainage reservoir that is easily concealed under the clothing and does not cause irritation to the skin of the thigh. *Multiple components of the external collection device affect the product's ability to contain urinary leakage, protect underlying skin, and preserve the client's dignity (Gray, 2006; Wells, 2008).*

• Teach the client who uses an external collection device to remove the device, inspect the skin, cleanse the penis thoroughly, and reapply a new device daily or every other day. *Urinary tract infections develop in up to 50% of users of condom catheters, especially with prolonged use of the catheter or a tight fitted condom catheter (Dingwall, 2008).*

• Teach the client whose incontinence is managed by a condom catheter to routinely inspect the skin with each catheter change for evidence of lesions caused by pressure from the containment device or by exposure to urine. *Skin breakdown is a common complication associated with routine use of the condom catheter (Wells, 2008).*

• Teach the client managed by intermittent or indwelling catheter to recognize signs of significant urinary tract infection and to seek care promptly when these signs occur. The signs of significant infection are the following:
  ▪ Discomfort over the bladder or during urination
  ▪ Acute onset of urinary incontinence
  ▪ Fever
  ▪ Markedly increased spasticity of muscles below the level of the spinal lesion
  ▪ Malaise, lethargy
  ▪ Hematuria
  ▪ Autonomic dysreflexia (hyperreflexia)

• Recognize that intermittent catheterization is typically associated with asymptomatic bacteriuria, and the indwelling catheter is routinely associated with asymptomatic colonization. *Antibiotic treatment of asymptomatic bacteriuria has not proven helpful (Morton et al, 2002; Murphy & Lampert, 2003), but prompt management of significant infection is necessary to prevent urosepsis or related complications (Siroky, 2002).*

 Geriatric

▲ If difficulties are encountered in client teaching, refer the elderly client to a nurse who specializes in care of the aging client with urinary incontinence.

 Home Care

• The interventions described previously may be adapted for home care use.

- Teach the client what the complications of reflex incontinence are and when to report changes to a physician or primary nurse. *Early detection allows for rapid diagnosis and treatment before irreversible damage to the renal parenchyma occurs (Burns, Rivas, & Ditunno, 2001).*
▲ If the client is taught intermittent self-catheterization, arrange for contingency care in the event that the client is unable to perform self-catheterization. *Although self-catheterization has proved to be an effective and safe bladder management strategy, acute illness or surgery may render the client unable to perform self-catheterization and temporarily reliant on others to carry out this critical task.*
- Assess and instruct the client and family in care of the catheter and supplies in the home.
- Encourage a mind-set and program of self-care management. **EBN:** *Addressing self-care activities through exercise, diet, fluid intake, and protective devices helps the client to exercise control over incontinence (Leenerts, Teel, & Pendleton, 2002). Encouraging self-care may reduce the substantial careprovider burden affecting a significant proportion of spouse, partner, or familial care providers (Post, Bloemen, & de Witte, 2005).*
- Assist the family with arranging care in a way that allows the client to participate in family or favorite activities without embarrassment. Elicit discussion of the client's concerns about the social or emotional burden of incontinence. **EBN and EB:** *Careful planning can help the client retain dignity and maintain the integrity of family patterns. Urinary incontinence has a demonstrated influence on subjective well-being and quality of life, with depression, loneliness, or sadness possible (Fultz & Herzog, 2001). Discussing emotional concerns helps the client to develop a sense of control over incontinence (Leenerts, Teel, & Pendleton, 2002).*
- If medications are ordered, instruct the family or caregivers and the client in medication administration, use, and side effects. *Adherence to a medication regimen increases its chances of success and decreases the risk of losing the regimen as an option for care when other alternatives are unacceptable.*

Client/Family Teaching and Discharge Planning

- Teach the client with a spinal injury the signs of autonomic dysreflexia, its relationship to bladder fullness, and management of the condition. Refer to the care plan for **Autonomic dysreflexia**.
- Teach the client and several significant others the techniques of intermittent catheterization, indwelling catheter care and removal, or condom catheter management as appropriate.
- Teach the client and family techniques to clean catheters used for intermittent catheterization, including washing with soap and water and allowing to air dry, and using microwave cleaning techniques.

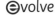 See the EVOLVE website Weblinks for client education resources.

REFERENCES

Burns AS, Rivas DA, Ditunno JF: The management of neurogenic bladder and sexual dysfunction after spinal cord injury, *Spine* 26(Suppl 24):S129, 2001.

Creasey GH, Kilgore KL, Brown-Triolo DL et al: Reduction of costs of disability using neuroprostheses, *Assist Technol* 12(1):67, 2000.

Dingwall L: Promoting social continence using incontinence management products, *Br J Nurs* 17(9):S12–S19, 2008.

Ethans KD, Nance PW, Bard RJ et al: Efficacy and safety of tolterodine in people with neurogenic detrusor overactivity, *J Spinal Cord Med* 27(3):214–218, 2004.

Fultz NH, Herzog AR: Self-reported social and emotional impact of urinary incontinence, *J Am Geriatr Soc* 49:892, 2001.

Generao SE, Dall'era JP, Stone AR et al: Spinal cord injury in children: long-term urodynamic and urological outcomes, *J Urol* 172(3):1092–1094, 2004.

Gray M: Reflex urinary incontinence. In Doughty DB, editor: *Urinary and fecal incontinence: nursing management*, ed 3, St Louis, 2006, Mosby.

Gray M, Bliss DZ, Doughty DB et al: Incontinence-associated dermatitis: a consensus, *J Wound Ostomy Continence Nurs* 24(1):45–56, 2007.

Gray M, Krissovich M: Does fluid intake influence the risk for urinary incontinence, urinary tract infection and bladder cancer? *J Wound Ostomy Continence Nurs* 30(3):126–131, 2003.

Gray M, Rayome RG, Anson C: Incontinence and clean intermittent catheterization following spinal cord injury, *Clin Nurs Res* 4:6, 1995.

Gray ML et al: Urethral pressure gradient in the prediction of upper urinary tract distress following spinal cord injury, *J Am Paraplegia Soc* 14:105, 1991.

Junkin J, Selekof J: Prevalence of incontinence and associated skin injury in an acute care population, *J Wound Ostomy Continence Nurs* 34(3):260–269, 2007.

Leenerts MH, Teel CS, Pendleton MK: Building a model of self-care for health promotion in aging, *J Nurs Scholarsh* 34:355, 2002.

Linsenmeyer TA, Horton J, Benevento J: Impact of alpha$_1$-blockers in men with spinal cord injury and upper tract stasis, *J Spinal Cord Med* 25(2):124, 2002.

Merenda LA. Hickey K: Key elements of bladder and bowel management for children with spinal cord injuries, *Sci Nursing* 22(1):8–14, 2005.

Morton SC, Shekelle PG, Adams JL et al: Antimicrobial prophylaxis for urinary tract infection in persons with spinal cord dysfunction, *Arch Phys Med Rehabil* 83(1):129, 2002.

Murphy DP, Lampert V: Current implications of drug resistance in spinal cord injury, *Am J Phys Med Rehabil* 82(1):72, 2003.

Post MW, Bloemen J, de Witte LP: Burden of support for partners of persons with spinal cord injuries, *Spinal Cord* 43(5):311–319, 2005.

Saint S, Kaufman SR, Rogers MA et al: Condom versus indwelling urinary catheters: a randomized trial, *J Am Geriatr Soc* 54(7):1055–1061, 2006.

Siroky MB: Pathogenesis of bacteriuria and infection in the spinal cord injured patient, *Am J Med* 113(suppl 1A):67S, 2002.

Verpoorten C, Buyse GM: The neurogenic bladder: medical treatment, *Pediatr Nephrol* 23(5):717–725, 2008.

Weld KJ, Graney MJ, Dmochowski RR: Clinical significance of detrusor sphincter dyssynergia in patients with post traumatic spinal cord injury, *Urology* 56:565, 2000.

Weld KJ, Wall BM, Mangold TA et al: Influences on renal function in chronic spinal cord injured patients, *J Urol* 164(5):1490, 2000.

Wells M: Managing urinary incontinence with BIODERM external continence device, *BJN* 17(9):524, 526–529, 2008.

Woodbury MG, Hayes KC, Askes HK: Intermittent catheterization practices following spinal cord injury: a national survey, *Can J Urol* 15(3):4065–4071, 2008.

Wyndaele JJ, Madersbacher H, Kovindha A: Conservative treatment of the neuropathic bladder in spinal cord injured patients, *Spinal Cord* 39(6):294, 2001.

Stress urinary Incontinence   *Mikel Gray, PhD, CUNP, CCCN, FAANP, FAAN*   ⊖volve

Definition

Sudden leakage of urine with activities that increase intraabdominal pressure

Defining Characteristics

Observed urine loss with physical exertion (sign of stress incontinence); reported loss of urine associated with physical exertion or activity (symptom of stress incontinence); urine loss associated with increased abdominal pressure (urodynamic stress urinary incontinence) (Abrams et al, 2002)

Related Factors (r/t)

Urethral hypermobility/pelvic organ prolapse (genetic factors/familial predisposition, multiple vaginal deliveries, delivery of infant large for gestational age, forceps-assisted or breech delivery, obesity, changes in estrogen levels at climacteric, extensive abdominopelvic, or pelvic surgery); urethral sphincter mechanism incompetence (multiple urethral suspensions in women, radical prostatectomy in men, uncommon complication of transurethral prostatectomy or cryosurgery of prostate, spinal lesion affecting sacral segments 2 to 4 or cauda equina, pelvic fracture)

NOTE: Defining Characteristics and Related Factors adapted from the work of NANDA-I.

 (Nursing Outcomes Classification)

Suggested NOC Outcomes

Urinary Continence, Urinary Elimination

> **Example NOC Outcome with Indicators**
>
> **Urinary Continence** as evidenced by the following indicators: Experiences no urine loss with physical activity or exertion, coughing, sneezing, or other maneuvers that precipitously raise abdominal pressure/Voids in appropriate receptacle/Able to move to toilet after strong desire to urinate is perceived/Underclothing remains dry during day/Underclothing or bedding remains dry during night (Rate the outcome and indicators of **Urinary Continence:** 1 = never demonstrated, 2 = rarely demonstrated, 3 = sometimes demonstrated, 4 = often demonstrated, 5 = consistently demonstrated [see Section I].)

Client Outcomes

Client Will (Specify Time Frame):

• Report fewer stress incontinence episodes and/or a decrease in the severity of urine loss
• Experience reduction in grams of urine loss measured objectively by a pad test
• Experience reduction in frequency of urinary incontinence episodes as recorded on voiding diary (bladder log)
• Identify containment devices that assist in management of stress incontinence

• = Independent   ▲ = Collaborative   **EBN** = Evidence-Based Nursing   **EB** = Evidence-Based

NIC   (Nursing Interventions Classification)

Suggested NIC Intervention

Pelvic Muscle Exercises, Urinary Incontinence Care

Example NIC Activities—Urinary Incontinence Care
Explain etiology of problem and rationale for actions; Modify clothing and environment to provide easy access to toilet

Nursing Interventions and *Rationales*

- Take a focused history addressing duration of urinary leakage and related lower urinary tract symptoms, including daytime voiding frequency, urgency, frequency of nocturia, frequency of urinary leakage, and factors provoking urine loss, focusing on the differential diagnosis of stress, urge or mixed stress and urge urinary symptoms. Consider using a symptom questionnaire that elicits relevant lower urinary tract symptoms and provides differentiation between stress and urge incontinence symptoms. *Some interventions used to treat stress and urge urinary incontinence are the same (such as pelvic floor muscle training), but some differ (such as pharmacotherapy). Over 23 validated symptom questionnaires have been developed for the evaluation of urinary and fecal incontinence (Avery et al, 2007).* **EBN:** *A questionnaire has been developed that is specifically designed to enable the clinician to differentiate between stress and urge incontinence based on symptom report (Brown et al, 2006).*

- Perform a focused physical assessment, including inspection of the perineal skin, vaginal examination to determine hypoestrogenic changes in the mucosa, pelvic examination to determine the presence of vaginal wall prolapse and uterine prolapse, and to reproduce the sign of stress urinary incontinence. **EBN:** *There is limited evidence supporting the diagnostic value of the physical examination in the diagnosis of urinary incontinence and differential diagnosis of stress versus urge incontinence in elderly women (van Gerwen & Lagro-Janssen, 2006).*

- Inspect the perineal skin for evidence of incontinence-associated dermatitis, including inflammation, vesicles in skin exposed to urinary leakage, and especially skin folds or denudation of the skin, particularly when incontinence is managed by absorptive pads or containment briefs. *Urinary incontinence, particularly when combined with fecal incontinence or use of absorptive pads or adult containment briefs, increases the risk of incontinence-associated dermatitis (Gray et al, 2007).* **EBN:** *20% of 608 clients with urinary and/or fecal incontinence in the acute care setting were found to have perineal or perigenital skin damage; 18% were found to have evidence of secondary cutaneous candidiasis (Junkin & Selekof, 2007).*

- Attempt to reproduce the sign of stress urinary incontinence by asking the client to perform Valsalva maneuver or to cough while observing the urethral meatus for urine loss. **EBN:** *Urine loss, the sign of stress urinary incontinence, can be reproduced by asking the client to perform provocative maneuvers (cough or perform Valsalva maneuver) during physical examination. Mild to moderate stress urinary incontinence can be reproduced by asking the client to perform these maneuvers while standing and holding a paper towel in front of the urethral meatus. Urine loss volumes of less than 1 mL can be detected using this technique (Neumann et al, 2004). Among clients with moderately severe to severe cases associated with urethral sphincter mechanism incompetence, the sign of stress urinary incontinence can be elicited even when the client is lying in a supine position and has as little as 10 mL of urine in the bladder vesicle. Nevertheless, it is strongly recommended that the client be tested in both supine and upright positions and with a moderately filled bladder (Walter, Thornton, & Steele, 2004).*

- ▲ Perform a focused pelvic examination, including visual inspection of the vaginal mucosa, observation of urethral hypermobility and related pelvic floor descent (prolapse), and digital assessment of pelvic floor muscle strength. **EBN:** *Digital assessment of pelvic muscle strength is completed by asking the female client to contract the pelvic floor muscles after placing one to two gloved fingers in the vaginal vault. Pelvic floor muscle strength can be similarly evaluated in men during the digital rectal examination. There is mixed evidence concerning the relationship of a digital assessment of pelvic floor muscle strength with dynamic manometric measurements, but it remains a well-accepted technique for determining the overall strength of the pelvic floor muscles and the client's ability to identify, contract, and relax this muscle group (Isherwood & Rane, 2000; Morin et al, 2004).*

● = Independent   ▲ = Collaborative   **EBN** = Evidence-Based Nursing   **EB** = Evidence-Based

- Determine the client's current use of containment devices; evaluate the devices for their ability to adequately contain urine loss, protect clothing, and control odor. Assist the client in identifying containment devices specifically designed to contain urinary leakage. *Clients, particularly women, tend to select feminine hygiene pads for urine containment. These pads are not that useful in containing urine.*
- Teach the client to complete a voiding diary (bladder log) by recording voiding frequency, the frequency of urinary incontinent episodes, and their association with urgency (a sudden and strong desire to urinate that is difficult to defer) over a 3- to 7-day period. An electronic voiding diary may be kept whenever feasible. In addition to these parameters, the client may be asked to record voided volume and fluid intake. *The voiding diary provides a more objective record of lower urinary tract function than the oral history, and it often provides a modest therapeutic effect by alerting the client to factors that promote urinary incontinence episodes (Sampselle, 2003). An electronic voiding diary provides an efficient and possibly more accurate method for documenting these parameters (Quinn, Goka, & Richardson, 2003).*
- ▲ With the client and in close consultation with the physician, review treatment options, including behavioral management; drug therapy; use of a pessary, vaginal device, or urethral insert; and surgery. Outline their potential benefits, efficacy, and side effects. *Multiple treatments have been used to manage stress incontinence; behavioral management options should be offered initially (Doughty & Burns, 2006).*
- Assess the client's pelvic muscle strength immediately prior to initiating pelvic floor muscle training using pressure manometry, a digital evaluation technique, or urine stop test. **EBN:** *A baseline of pelvic muscle strength is needed for initial assessment and for evaluation of treatment efficacy. Digital vaginal examination, a urine stream interruption test, or measurement of pelvic floor muscle contraction strength by a fluid-filled balloon are valid and reliable techniques for assessing pelvic floor muscle strength and contractile function (Brink et al, 1992; Sampselle & DeLancey, 1992).*
- Begin a pelvic floor muscle training program. *Pelvic floor muscle training is effective in the treatment of stress and mixed urinary incontinence (Hay-Smith et al, 2008).*
- Teach the client undergoing pelvic muscle training to identify, contract, and relax the pelvic floor muscles without contracting distant muscle groups (e.g., abdominal muscles) using tactile, audible, or visual biofeedback techniques. *Existing evidence suggests that incorporation of biofeedback enhances the efficacy of pelvic floor muscle training (Gray & David, 2005).*
- Incorporate principles of exercise physiology into a pelvic muscle training program using the following strategies:
  - Begin a graded exercise program, usually starting with 5 to 10 repetitions and advancing gradually to no more than 35 to 50 repetitions every day or every other day based on baseline and ongoing evaluation of maximal strength and endurance.
  - Continue exercise sessions over a period of 3 to 6 months.
  - Integrate muscle training into activities of daily living.
  - Assess progress every 2 weeks during the first month and every 4 to 6 weeks thereafter.

  Pelvic muscle training alleviates or cures stress incontinence using a combination of techniques, including biofeedback and strength training (Hay-Smith et al, 2008; Shamliyan et al, 2008).
- Alternatively, female clients may be taught pelvic muscle training using weighted vaginal cones. **EBN:** *Weighted vaginal cones help women increase pelvic floor muscle tone and function and alleviate stress urinary incontinence (Laycock et al, 2001). The efficacy of weighted cones may be comparable to that achieved by pelvic muscle training, but more comparative studies are needed before a definitive conclusion can be reached (Herbison, Plevnik, & Mantle, 2002).*
- ▲ Begin transvaginal or transrectal electrical stimulation therapy in selected persons with stress incontinence in consultation with the client and physician. *Electrical stimulation alleviates stress incontinence in selected clients (Wein, 2005).*
- Teach the principles of bladder training to women with stress urinary incontinence:
  - Assist the client in completing a voiding diary over a period of a minimum of 3 days or up to 7 days.
  - Review the results with the client, determining typical voiding frequency and establishing goals for voiding frequency.
  - Using baseline voiding frequency, as determined by the diary, teach the client to urinate by the clock when awake, typically every 30 to 120 minutes.

● = Independent   ▲ = Collaborative   **EBN** = Evidence-Based Nursing   **EB** = Evidence-Based

- ■ Encourage adherence to the program with timing devices, as well as verbal encouragement and support, and address individual reasons for schedule interruption.
- ■ Gradually increase the time between urinations to the negotiated goal. Time intervals between voiding are typically increased in increments of 15 to 30 minutes for clients with a baseline frequency of less than every 60 minutes and increments of 25 to 30 minutes for clients with a baseline frequency of more than every 60 minutes.

Bladder training reduces the frequency and severity of urinary leakage in women with stress incontinence, urge incontinence, and mixed incontinence. The results of bladder training in ambulatory, community-dwelling women is comparable to that achieved through pelvic floor muscle training (Milne, 2008).

- • Teach the client to self-administer duloxetine and imipramine as directed, and to monitor for adverse side effects. *There are no prescriptive drugs approved for use in stress urinary incontinence in the United States. Nevertheless, several agents are sometimes prescribed to highly selected clients with stress urinary incontinence. They include duloxetine (Schagen van Leeuwen et al, 2008) and imipramine (Andersson, 2000).*
- • Teach the client to self-administer topical (vaginal) estrogens as directed, and to monitor for adverse side effects. *Although existing evidence suggests that topical (vaginal) estrogens are most effective for urgency and urge incontinence, they are sometimes prescribed for women with stress urinary incontinence associated with symptomatic urogenital atrophy (Jackson & Fihn, 2009).*
- ▲ Refer the female client with stress urinary incontinence and pelvic organ prolapse who wishes to employ a pessary to manage stress incontinence to a nurse specialist or gynecologist with expertise in the placement and maintenance of these devices. *Placement of an appropriately sized dish pessary resolved stress urinary incontinence in 60% of a group of 95 women (Noblett, McKinney & Lane, 2008). When fitted by an individual with adequate expertise, approximately 90% of bothersome symptoms associated with pelvic organ prolapse and 50% of lower urinary tract symptoms resolved, although occult stress urinary incontinence is uncovered in approximately 21% (Clemons et al, 2004).*
- • Discuss potentially reversible or controllable risk factors with the client with stress incontinence and assist the client to formulate a strategy to alleviate or eliminate these conditions. *Although research supports a strong familial predisposition to stress incontinence among women, other risk factors associated with the condition, including obesity (Richter et al, 2005; Mishra et al, 2008) and chronic coughing from smoking (Richter et al, 2005), are reversible.*
- • Provide information about support resources such as the National Foundation for Continence or The Simon Foundation for Continence.
- ▲ Refer the client with persistent stress incontinence to a continence service, physician, or nurse who specializes in the management of this condition.

Geriatric

- • Evaluate the elderly client's functional and cognitive status to determine the effect of functional limitations on the frequency and severity of urine loss and on plans for management.

Home Care

- • The interventions described previously may be adapted for home care use.
- • Elicit discussion of the client's concerns about the social or emotional burden of stress incontinence. **EBN and EB:** *Urinary incontinence has a demonstrated influence on subjective well-being and quality of life, with depression, loneliness, or sadness possible (Fultz & Herzog, 2001). Discussing emotional concerns helps the client to develop a sense of control over incontinence (Leenerts, Teel, & Pendleton, 2002).*
- • Encourage a mindset and program of self-care management. **EBN:** *Addressing self-care activities through exercise, diet, fluid intake, and protective devices helps the client to exercise control over incontinence (Leenerts, Teel, & Pendleton, 2002).*
- • Implement a bladder-training program, including self-monitoring activities (reducing caffeine intake, adjusting amount and timing of fluid intake, decreasing long voiding intervals while awake, making dietary changes to promote bowel regularity), bladder training, and pelvic muscle exercise. **EBN:** *Women age 55 years or older with involuntary urine loss associated with stress, urge, or mixed*

● = Independent   ▲ = Collaborative   **EBN** = Evidence-Based Nursing   **EB** = Evidence-Based

incontinence, responded to the aforementioned interventions with a 61% decrease in the severity of urinary incontinence at 2 years after intervention. Self-monitoring and bladder training accounted for most of the improvement (Dougherty et al, 2002).

▲ Consider the use of an indwelling catheter for continuous drainage in the client with severe stress urinary incontinence who is homebound, bed-bound, and receiving palliative or end-of-life care (requires a physician's order). *An indwelling catheter may increase client comfort, ease caregiver burden, and prevent urinary incontinence in bed-bound clients receiving end-of-life care.*

▲ When an indwelling catheter is in place, follow the prescribed maintenance protocols for managing the catheter, drainage bag, and perineal skin and urethral meatus. Teach infection control measures adapted to the home care setting. *Proper care reduces the risk of catheter-associated urinary tract infection.*

• Assist the client in adapting to the catheter. Encourage discussion of the client's response to the catheter. **EBN:** *Clients living with a catheter are keenly aware of its presence; adaptation is served by normalizing the experience. Rehearsing emptying of the bag when away from home will support resumption of activities. Discussion of the client's response will help him or her to deal with embarrassment or frustration (Wilde, 2002).*

• Begin a program of pelvic muscle training in the homebound elderly client who is motivated to adhere to the program and has adequate cognitive function to understand and follow instructions. **EBN:** *Homebound elders are capable of completing a program of pelvic muscle training and achieving clinically relevant relief from stress and urge urinary incontinence.*

 ### Client/Family Teaching and Discharge Planning

• Teach the client to perform pelvic muscle exercise using an audiotape or videotape if indicated.
• Teach the client the importance of avoiding dehydration and instruct the client to consume fluid at the rate of 30 mL/kg of body weight daily (0.5 ounce/pound/day).
• Teach the client the importance of avoiding constipation by a combination of adequate fluid intake, adequate intake of dietary fiber, and exercise.
▲ Teach the client to apply and remove support devices such as a urethral insert.
• Teach the client to select and apply urine containment devices.

Ⓔvolve   See the EVOLVE website for Weblinks for client education resources.

REFERENCES

Abrams P, Cardozo L, Fall M et al: The standardization of terminology of lower urinary tract function: report from the Standardisation Sub-committee of the International Continence Society, *Am J Obstet Gynecol* 187(1):116, 2002.

Andersson KE: Drug therapy for urinary incontinence, *Best Pract Res Clin Obstet Gynecol* 14(2):291, 2000.

Avery KN, Bosch JL, Gotoh M et al: Questionnaires to assess urinary and anal incontinence: review and recommendations, *J Urol* 177(1):39–49, 2007.

Brink CA et al: Pelvic muscle exercise for elderly incontinence women. In Funk SG et al, editors: *Key aspects of elder care: managing falls, incontinence and cognitive impairment,* New York, 1992, Springer.

Brown JS, Bradley CS, Subak LL et al: Diagnostic Aspects of Incontinence Study (DAISy) Research Group. The sensitivity and specificity of a simple test to distinguish between urge and stress urinary incontinence, *Ann Intern Med* 144(10):715–723, 2006.

Clemons JL, Aguilar VC, Tillinghast TA et al: Patient satisfaction and changes in prolapse and urinary symptoms in women who were fitted successfully with a pessary for pelvic organ prolapse, *Am Obstet Gynecol* 190(4):1025–1029, 2004.

Doughty DB, Burns PA: Pathology and management of stress incontinence. In Doughty DB, editor: *Urinary and fecal incontinence: nursing management,* ed 3, St Louis, 2006, Elsevier/Mosby.

Dougherty MC, Dwyer JW, Pendergast JF et al: A randomized trial of behavioral management for continence with older rural women, *Res Nurs Health* 25:3, 2002.

Fultz NH, Herzog AR: Self-reported social and emotional impact of urinary incontinence, *J Am Geriatr Soc* 49:892, 2001.

Gray M, Bliss DZ, Doughty DB et al: Incontinence-associated dermatitis: a consensus, *J Wound Ostomy Continence Nurs* 24(1):45–56, 2007.

Gray M, David DJ: Does biofeedback improve the efficacy of pelvic floor muscle training for urinary incontinence or overactive bladder dysfunction in women? *J Wound Ostomy Cont Nurs* 32(4):222–225, 2005.

Hay-Smith J, Mørkved S, Fairbrother KA et al: Pelvic floor muscle training for prevention and treatment of urinary and faecal incontinence in antenatal and postnatal women. *Cochrane Database Syst Rev* (4):D007471, 2008.

Herbison P, Plevnik S, Mantle J: Weighted vaginal cones for urinary incontinence, *Cochrane Database Syst Rev* (2):CD002114, 2002.

Isherwood PJ, Rane A: Comparative assessment of pelvic floor strength using a perineometer and digital examination, *BJOG* 107(8):1007–1011, 2000.

Jackson SL, Fihn SD: Exogenous estrogen and urinary incontinence, *Journal of Urology* 181(5):1989–1991, 2009.

• = Independent   ▲ = Collaborative   **EBN** = Evidence-Based Nursing   **EB** = Evidence-Based

Junkin J, Selekof J: Prevalence of incontinence and associated skin injury in an acute care population, *J Wound Ostomy Continence Nurs* 34(3):260–269, 2007.

Laycock J, Brown J, Cusack C et al: Pelvic floor reeducation for stress incontinence: comparing three methods, *Br J Community Nurs* 6(5):230, 2001.

Leenerts MH, Teel CS, Pendleton MK: Building a model of self-care for health promotion in aging, *J Nurs Scholarsh* 34:355, 2002.

Milne J: Bladder training, guideline. In Ackley B, Ladwig G, Swan BA, Tucker S, editors: *Evidence-based nursing care guidelines*, Philadelphia, 2008, Mosby.

Mishra GD, Hardy R, Cardozo L et al: Body weight through adult life and risk of urinary incontinence in middle-aged women: results from a British prospective cohort, *Int J Obesity* 32(9):1415–1422, 2008.

Morin M, Dumoulin C, Bourbonnais D et al: Pelvic floor maximal strength using vaginal digital assessment compared to dynamometric measurements, *Neurourol Urodyn* 23(4):336–341, 2004.

Neumann P, Blizzard L, Grimmer K et al: Expanded paper towel test: an objective test of urine loss for stress incontinence, *Neurourol Urodyn* 23(7):649–655, 2004.

Noblett KL, McKinney A, Lane FL: Effects of the incontinence dish pessary on urethral support and urodynamic parameters, *American Journal of Obstetrics & Gynecology* 198(5):592.e1–5, 2008.

Quinn P, Goka J, Richardson H: Assessment of an electronic daily diary in patients with overactive bladder, *BJU Int* 91(7):647–652, 2003.

Richter HE, Burgio KL, Brubaker L et al: Urinary Incontinence Treatment Network. Factors associated with incontinence frequency in a surgical cohort of stress incontinent women, *Am J Obst Gynecol* 193(6):2088–2093, 2005.

Sampselle CM: Bladder matters. Teaching women to use a voiding diary, *Am J Nurs* 103(11):62–64, 2003.

Sampselle CM, DeLancey JOL: The urine stream interruption test and pelvic muscle function, *Nurs Res* 41:73, 1992.

Schagen van Leeuwen JH, Lange RR, Jonasson AF et al: Efficacy and safety of duloxetine in elderly women with stress urinary incontinence or stress-predominant mixed urinary incontinence, *Maturitas* 60(2):138–147, 2008.

Shamliyan TA, Kane RL, Wyman J et al: Systematic review: randomized, controlled trials of nonsurgical treatments for urinary incontinence in women, *Ann Intern Med* 148(6):459–473, 2008.

van Gerwen M, Lagro-Janssen AL: [Diagnostic value of patient history and physical examination in elderly patients with urinary incontinence; a literature review], *Ned Tijdschr Geneesk* 150(32):1771–1775, 2006 [article in Dutch].

Walter AJ, Thornton JA, Steele AC: Further characterization of the supine empty stress test for predicting low Valsalva leak point pressures, *Int Urogynecol J* 15(5):298–301, 2004.

Wein AJ: Transvaginal electrical stimulation in the treatment of urinary incontinence, *J Urol* 174(3):1007, 2005.

Wilde MH: Urine flowing: a phenomenological study of living with a urinary catheter, *Res Nurs Health* 25:14, 2002.

Urge urinary Incontinence Mikel Gray, PhD, CUNP, CCCN, FAANP, FAAN ⊖volve

NANDA-I

Definition

Involuntary passage of urine occurring soon after a strong sense of urgency to void

Urge incontinence is defined within the context of overactive bladder syndrome. The overactive bladder is characterized by bothersome urgency (a sudden and strong desire to urinate that is not easily deferred) (Abrams et al, 2002). Overactive bladder is typically associated with frequent daytime voiding and nocturia, and approximately 37% will experience urge urinary incontinence (Stewart et al, 2003).

Defining Characteristics

Diurnal urinary frequency (voiding more than once every 2 hours while awake); nocturia (awakening three or more times per night to urinate); voiding more than eight times within a 24-hour period as recorded on a voiding diary (bladder log); bothersome urgency (a sudden and strong desire to urinate that is not easily deferred); symptom of urge incontinence (urine loss associated with desire to urinate); enuresis (involuntary passage of urine while asleep).

Related Factors (r/t)

Neurological disorders (brain disorders, including cerebrovascular accident, brain tumor, normal pressure hydrocephalus, traumatic brain injury); inflammation of bladder (calculi; tumor, including transitional cell carcinoma and carcinoma in situ; inflammatory lesions of the bladder; urinary tract infection); bladder outlet obstruction (see **Urinary retention**); stress urinary incontinence (mixed urinary incontinence; these conditions often coexist but relationship between them remains unclear); idiopathic causes (associated factors include depression, sleep apnea [Kemmer et al, 2009; Lowerstein et al, 2008], and obesity [Mishra et al, 2008].

NOTE: Defining Characteristics and Related Factors adapted from the work of NANDA-I.

• = Independent   ▲ = Collaborative   **EBN** = Evidence-Based Nursing   **EB** = Evidence-Based

(Nursing Outcomes Classification)

Suggested NOC Outcomes

Tissue Integrity: Skin and Mucous Membranes, Urinary Continence, Urinary Elimination

Example **NOC Outcome with Indicators**
Urinary Continence as evidenced by the following indicators: Responds in timely manner to urge/Voids in appropriate receptacle/Has adequate time to reach toilet between urge and evacuation of urine/Underclothing remains dry during day/Underclothing or bedding remains dry during night (Rate the outcome and indicators of **Urinary Continence**: 1 = never demonstrated, 2 = rarely demonstrated, 3 = sometimes demonstrated, 4 = often demonstrated, 5 = consistently demonstrated [see Section I].)

Client Outcomes

Client Will (Specify Time Frame):

• Report relief from urge urinary incontinence or a decrease in the frequency of incontinent episodes
• Identify containment devices that assist in the management of urge urinary incontinence

 (Nursing Interventions Classification)

Suggested NIC Interventions

Urinary Habit Training, Urinary Incontinence Care

Example **NIC Activities—Urinary Habit Training**
Keep a continence specification record for 3 days to establish voiding pattern; Establish interval for toileting of preferably not less than 2 hours

Nursing Interventions and *Rationales*

• Take a nursing history focusing on duration of urinary incontinence, diurnal frequency, nocturia, severity of symptoms, and alleviating and aggravating factors. *A focused history helps determine the cause of urinary incontinence and guides its subsequent management.* **EBN:** *Querying the client about the isolated symptom of urge incontinence shows a poor correlation with a diagnosis of detrusor over-activity incontinence. However, the agreement between urodynamic testing and the clinical diagnosis obtained by the history rises sharply when the client reports three symptoms: diurnal frequency, urge-related urine loss, and nocturia (Gray et al, 2001).*

▲ In close consultation with a physician or advanced practice nurse, consider administering a symptom questionnaire that elicits relevant lower urinary tract symptoms and differentiates stress and urge incontinence symptoms. *Some interventions used to treat stress and urge urinary incontinence are the same (such as pelvic floor muscle training) but some differ (such as pharmacotherapy). Over 23 validated symptom questionnaires have been developed for the evaluation of urinary and fecal incontinence (Avery et al, 2007).* **EBN:** *Several questionnaires have been developed that are specifically designed to enable the clinician differentiate between stress and urge incontinence based on symptom report (Brown et al, 2006).*

▲ Perform a focused physical assessment, including inspection of the perineal skin, vaginal examination to determine hypoestrogenic changes in the mucosa, pelvic examination to determine the presence of severe vaginal wall prolapse, and to reproduce the sign of stress urinary incontinence. **EBN:** *There is limited evidence supporting the diagnostic value of the physical examination in the diagnosis of urinary incontinence and differential diagnosis of stress versus urge incontinence in elderly women (van Gerwen & Lagro-Janssen, 2006).*

• Inspect the perineal and perianal skin for evidence of incontinence-associated dermatitis, including inflammation, vesicles in skin exposed to urinary leakage, and especially skin folds or denudation of the skin, particularly when incontinence is managed by absorptive pads or containment briefs. *Urinary incontinence, particularly when combined with fecal incontinence or use of absorptive*

• = Independent   ▲ = Collaborative   **EBN** = Evidence-Based Nursing   **EB** = Evidence-Based

pads or adult containment briefs, increases the risk of incontinence-associated dermatitis (Gray et al, 2007). **EBN:** *20% of clients with urinary and/or fecal incontinence in the acute care setting were found to have perineal or perigenital skin damage; 18% were found to have evidence of secondary cutaneous candidiasis (Junkin & Selekof, 2007).*

▲ Perform a focused pelvic examination including visual inspection of the vaginal mucosa, observation of urethral hypermobility and related pelvic floor descent (prolapse), and digital assessment of pelvic floor muscle strength. Refer the woman with severe vaginal wall prolapse (descent to or beyond the introitus) to a female urologist or urogynecologist. *Severe pelvic organ prolapse complicates the management of urge urinary incontinence and predisposes the female client to urinary retention (Romanzi, 2002). In addition, limited evidence suggests that surgical repair of pelvic organ prolapse may relieve overactive bladder symptoms including urge urinary incontinence in some women (Digesu et al, 2007). Baseline of pelvic muscle strength is needed for initial assessment and for evaluation of treatment efficacy. It also provides an opportunity for the nurse to determine whether the client is able to identify, isolate, contract, and relax the pelvic floor muscles.*

▲ Complete a urinalysis, examining for the presence of nitrites, leukocytes, glucose, or hemoglobin (red blood cells). *The presence of nitrites and leukocytes raises a suspicion of urinary tract infection, the presence of glucosuria raises the risk of undiagnosed or poorly controlled diabetes mellitus, and the presence of red blood cells in the absence of signs of infection raises a suspicion of a bladder tumor. Each condition may produce urgency and urinary incontinence mimicking overactive bladder syndrome and associated urinary incontinence (Fourcroy, 2001).*

• Teach the client to complete a voiding diary (bladder log) by recording voiding frequency, the frequency of urinary incontinent episodes and their association with urgency (a sudden and strong desire to urinate that is difficult to defer) over a 3- to 7-day period. An electronic voiding diary may be kept whenever feasible. In addition to these parameters, the client may be asked to record voided volume and fluid intake. *The voiding diary provides a more objective record of lower urinary tract function than the oral history, and it often provides a modest therapeutic effect by alerting the client to factors that promote urinary incontinence episodes (Sampselle, 2003). A voiding diary provides an important supplement to the oral history, research reveals that clients tend to overestimate voiding frequency when asked to recall voiding behavior (Stav, Dwyer, & Rosamilia, 2009). An electronic voiding diary provides an efficient and possibly more accurate method for documenting these parameters (Quinn, Goka, & Richardson, 2003).*

▲ Review all medications the client is receiving, paying particular attention to sedatives, opioid analgesics, diuretics, antidepressants, psychotropic drugs, and cholinergics. Consult the physician or nurse practitioner about altering or eliminating these medications if they are suspected of affecting incontinence. *The side effects of multiple medications may produce or exacerbate urge incontinence (Fourcroy, 2001).*

• Assess the client for urinary retention (see the care plan for **Urinary retention**).

• Assess the client for functional limitations (environmental barriers, limited mobility or dexterity, impaired cognitive function; refer to the care plan for **Functional urinary Incontinence**). **EBN:** *Du Moulin et al (2008) analyzed a group of 2866 clients receiving home care and found that functional impairment (poor mobility) was associated with an increased likelihood of urinary incontinence.*

▲ Consult the physician concerning diabetic management or pharmacotherapy for urinary tract infection when indicated. *In specific cases, urgency and an increased risk of urge incontinence may be related to bacteriuria or urinary tract infection (Rodhe et al, 2008) or polyuria from undiagnosed or poorly managed diabetes mellitus.*

▲ Assess for signs and symptoms of atrophic vaginal changes in the perimenopausal or postmenopausal woman, including vaginal dryness, tenderness to touch, mucosal dryness, friability, and discomfort with gentle palpation. Specifically query the woman with atrophic vaginitis concerning associated lower urinary tract symptoms (usually voiding frequency, urgency, and dysuria). Refer the woman with atrophic vaginal changes and bothersome lower urinary tract symptoms to a gynecologist, urologist, or women's health nurse practitioner for further evaluation and management. *The relationship between atrophic vaginitis and urge incontinence risk remains unclear. However, a study has shown that oral estrogen replacement increases the risk of urinary incontinence in postmenopausal women (Hendrix et al, 2005). Topical or intravaginal estrogen, particularly rings or tablets, provide an alternative for relieving bothersome symptoms associated with atrophic vaginitis and associated lower urinary tract symptoms (Crandall, 2002). In addition, systematic reviews of existing*

• = Independent ▲ = Collaborative **EBN** = Evidence-Based Nursing **EB** = Evidence-Based

evidence suggest that local hormone replacement therapy may reduce the risk of urinary tract infection in elderly women (Crandall, 2002; Rozenberg et al, 2004).

- Teach the principles of bladder training to women with urge urinary incontinence.
  - Assist the client in completing a voiding diary over a period of a minimum of 3 days or up to 7 days.
  - Review the results with the client, determining typical voiding frequency and establishing goals for voiding frequency.
  - Using baseline voiding frequency, as determined by the diary, teach the client to urinate by the clock when awake, typically every 30 to 120 minutes.
  - Encourage adherence to the program with timing devices and verbal encouragement and support, and address individual reasons for schedule interruption.
  - Gradually increase the time between urinations to the negotiated goal. Time intervals between voiding are typically increased in increments of 15 to 30 minutes for clients with a baseline frequency of less than every 60 minutes and increments of 25 to 30 minutes for clients with a baseline frequency of more than every 60 minutes.

  EBN: *Bladder training reduces the frequency and severity of urinary leakage in women with urge, stress, or mixed urinary incontinence. Research suggests that the results of bladder training in ambulatory, community-dwelling women is comparable to that achieved through pelvic floor muscle rehabilitation (Theofrastous et al, 2002; Milne, 2008). Bladder training has also been shown to augment the efficacy of pharmacotherapy for clients with urge urinary incontinence (Mattiasson et al, 2003; Song et al, 2006).*

- Review with the client the types of beverages consumed, focusing on the intake of caffeine, which is associated with a transient effect on lower urinary tract symptoms. Advise all clients to reduce or eliminate intake caffeinated beverages or over-the-counter medications of dietary aids containing caffeine. *Caffeine acts as a smooth muscle stimulant, increasing voiding frequency, urgency, and urge urinary incontinence episodes among those with this condition. Reducing the intake of caffeine alleviates these lower urinary tract symptoms (Gray, 2001; Kincade et al, 2007).*

- Review with the client the volume of fluids consumed and gradually adjust the fluid intake to meet the Adequate Intake recommendation of 3 L for the 19- to 30-year-old male and 2.2 L for the 19- to 30-year-old female. Water balance studies suggest that adult men require 2.5 L/day (Institute of Medicine, 2004). *Dehydration is postulated to exacerbate the symptoms of urgency, and excessive fluid intake increases voided volume and urinary frequency (Fitzgerald & Brubaker, 2003). Increasing fluid intake in women with urinary incontinence may reduce the risk of urinary tract infection without increasing the frequency or severity of urine loss (Dougherty et al, 2002).*

- Instruct in techniques of urge suppression. Teach the client to identify, isolate, contract, and relax the pelvic floor muscles. When a strong or precipitous urge to urinate is perceived, teach the client to avoid running to the toilet. Instead, she or he should perform repeated, rapid pelvic muscle contractions until the urge is relieved. Relief is followed by micturition within 5 to 15 minutes, using non-hurried movements when locating a toilet and voiding. **EB:** *Randomized controlled trials comparing urge suppression techniques to pharmacotherapy or bladder training have shown it to be an effective method for reducing urge urinary incontinence episodes (Burgio, 2002).*

▲ Begin transvaginal or transrectal electrical stimulation using a low-frequency current (5 to 20 Hz) in consultation with the physician. *Electrical stimulation is an effective treatment for some women with urge incontinence (Wein, 2005).*

▲ Begin posterior tibial nerve stimulation in consultation with the physician. **EB:** *Limited evidence suggests that posterior tibial nerve stimulation alleviates idiopathic and neurogenic detrusor overactivity and associated lower urinary tract symptoms including urge urinary incontinence (Kabay et al, 2009).*

▲ Teach the client to self-administer antimuscarinic (anticholinergic) drugs as directed. Teach dosage and administration of the medication and the importance of combining pharmacotherapy with scheduled voiding, adequate fluid intake, restriction of bladder irritants, and urge suppression techniques. *Antimuscarinic drugs increase bladder capacity, reduce the frequency of incontinence episodes, and diminish voiding frequency. However, they do not cure bladder dysfunction or reduce the time between perception of a strong urge and onset of an overactive detrusor contraction. The efficacy of pharmacotherapy for urge incontinence and overactive bladder dysfunction is enhanced when combined with behavioral interventions (Burgio, 2002; Song et al, 2006).*

• = Independent   ▲ = Collaborative   **EBN** = Evidence-Based Nursing   **EB** = Evidence-Based

- Assist the client in selecting, obtaining, and applying a containment device for urine loss as indicated.
- Provide the client with information about incontinence support groups such as the National Association for Continence and the Simon Foundation for Continence. *Self-help groups provide social support and a forum for sharing strategies for the management of all types of urinary incontinence (Irwin, 2000).*

Geriatric

- Assess the functional and cognitive status of the elderly client with urge incontinence. *Functional limitations affect the severity and management of urge urinary incontinence (Ouslander et al, 2002).*
- Plan care in long-term or acute care facilities based on knowledge of the elderly client's established voiding patterns, paying particular attention to patterns of nocturia.
- Carefully monitor the elderly client for potential adverse effects of antispasmodic medications, including a severely dry mouth interfering with the use of dentures, eating, or speaking, or confusion, nightmares, constipation, mydriasis, or heat intolerance.

Home Care

- The interventions described previously may be adapted for home care use.
- Teach the importance of avoiding dehydration or excessive fluid consumption and the paradoxical relationship between dehydration and symptoms of urgency.
- Teach the family and client to identify and correct environmental barriers to toileting within the home.
- Encourage a mind-set and program of self-care management. **EBN:** *Addressing self-care activities through exercise, diet, fluid intake, and protective devices helps the client to exercise control over incontinence (Leenerts, Teel, & Pendleton, 2002).*
- Implement a bladder-training program as appropriate, including self-monitoring activities (reducing caffeine intake, adjusting amount and timing of fluid intake, decreasing long voiding intervals while awake, making dietary changes to promote bowel regularity), bladder training, and pelvic muscle exercise. **EBN:** *In one study of women age 55 years or older with involuntary urine loss associated with stress, urge, or mixed incontinence, clients responded to the aforementioned interventions with a 61% decrease in the severity of urinary incontinence at 2 years after intervention. Self-monitoring and bladder training accounted for most of the improvement (Dougherty et al, 2002).*
- Help the client and family to identify and correct environmental barriers to toileting within the home.

Client/Family Teaching and Discharge Planning

- Teach the client and family to recognize foods and beverages that are likely to irritate the bladder.
- Teach the family and client to recognize and manage side effects of antispasmodic medications used to treat urge incontinence.
- Help the client and family to recognize and manage side effect of anticholinergic medications used to manage irritative lower urinary tract symptoms.

ⓔvolve   See the EVOLVE website for Weblinks for client education resources.

REFERENCES

Abrams P, Cardozo L, Fall M et al: The standardisation of terminology of lower urinary tract function: report from the Standardization Sub-committee of the International Continence Society, *Am J Obstet Gynecol* 187(1):116–126, 2002.

Avery KN, Bosch JL, Gotoh M et al: Questionnaires to assess urinary and anal incontinence: review and recommendations, *J Urol* 177(1):39–49, 2007.

Brown JS, Bradley CS, Subak LL et al: The sensitivity and specificity of a simple test to distinguish between urge and stress urinary inconti-

nence. Diagnostic Aspects of Incontinence Study (DAISy) Research Group, *Ann Intern Med* 144(10):715–723, 2006.

Burgio KL: Influence of behavior modification on overactive bladder, *Urology* 60(5 Suppl 1):S72, 2002.

Burgio KL, Locher JL, Goode PS: Combined behavioral and drug therapy for urge incontinence in older women, *J Am Geriatr Soc* 48(4):370, 2000.

Crandall C: Vaginal estrogen preparations: a review of safety and efficacy for vaginal atrophy, *J Womens Health* 11(10):857–877, 2002.

● = Independent   ▲ = Collaborative   **EBN** = Evidence-Based Nursing   **EB** = Evidence-Based

Digesu GA, Salvatore S, Chaliha C et al: Do overactive bladder symptoms improve after repair of anterior vaginal wall prolapse? *Int Urogynecol J* 18(12):1439–1443, 2007.

Dougherty MC, Dwyer JW, Pendergast JF et al: A randomized trial of behavioral management for continence with older rural women, *Res Nurs Health* 25(1):3, 2002.

Du Moulin MF, Hamers JP, Ambergen AW et al: Prevalence of urinary incontinence among community-dwelling adults receiving home care, *Res Nurs Health* 31(6):604–612, 2008.

Fitzgerald MP, Brubaker L: Variability of 24-hour voiding diary variables among asymptomatic women, *J Urol* 169(1):207, 2003.

Fjorback MV, van Rey FS, van der Pal F et al: Acute urodynamic effects of posterior tibial nerve stimulation on neurogenic detrusor overactivity in patients with MS, *Eur Urol* 51(2):464–472, 2007.

Fourcroy JL: Overactive bladder: a practical overview of diagnosis and treatment, *Adv Nurse Practit* 9(3):59, 2001.

Gray M: Caffeine and urinary incontinence, *J Wound Ostomy Continence Nurs* 28:66, 2001.

Gray M: Urinary retention: management in the acute care setting, Part 2, *Am J Nurs* 100:36, 2000.

Gray M, Bliss DZ, Doughty DB et al: Incontinence-associated dermatitis: a consensus, *J Wound Ostomy Continence Nurs* 24(1):45–56, 2007.

Gray M, McClain R, Peruggia M et al: A model for predicting motor urge urinary incontinence, *Nurs Res* 50:116, 2001.

Hendrix SL, Cochrane BB, Nygaard IE et al: Effects of estrogen with and without progestin on urinary incontinence, *JAMA* 293(8):935–948, 2005.

Institute of Medicine: Food and Nutrition Board: *Dietary reference intakes for water, potassium, sodium chloride and sulfate,* Washington DC, 2004, The National Academies Press.

Irwin B: User support groups in continence care, *Nurs Times* 96(Suppl 31):S24, 2000.

Junkin J, Selekof J: Prevalence of incontinence and associated skin injury in an acute care population, *J Wound Ostomy Continence Nurs* 34(3):260–269, 2007.

Kabay SC, Kabay S, Yucel M et al: Acute urodynamic effects of percutaneous posterior tibial nerve stimulation on neurogenic detrusor overactivity in patients with Parkinson's disease, *Neurourol Urodyn* 28(1):62–67, 2009.

Kemmer H, Mathes AM, Dilk O et al: Obstructive sleep apnea syndrome is associated with overactive bladder and urgency incontinence in men, *Sleep* 32(2):271–275, 2009.

Kincade JE, Dougherty MC, Carlson JR et al: Factors related to urinary incontinence in community-dwelling women, *Urol Nurs* 27(4):307–317, 2007.

Leenerts MH, Teel CS, Pendleton MK: Building a model of self-care for health promotion in aging, *J Nurs Scholarsh* 34(4):355–361, 2002.

Lowenstein L, Kenton K, Brubaker L et al: The relationship between obstructive sleep apnea, nocturia, and daytime overactive bladder syndrome in women, *Am J Obstet Gynecol* 198(5):598:e1–5, 2008.

Mattiasson A, Blaakaer J, Hoye K et al: Simplified bladder training augments the effectiveness of tolterodine in patients with an overactive bladder. Tolterodine Scandinavian Study Group, *BJU Int* 91(1):54–60, 2003.

Milne J: Bladder training, guideline. In Ackley B, Ladwig G, Swan BA, Tucker S, editors: *Evidence-based nursing care guidelines,* Philadelphia, 2008, Mosby.

Mishra GD, Hardy R, Cardozo L et al: Body weight through adult life and risk of urinary incontinence in middle-aged women: results from a British prospective cohort, *International Journal of Obesity* 32(9):1415–1422, 2008.

Ouslander JG, Greendale GA, Uman G et al: Effects of oral estrogen and progestin on the lower urinary tract among female nursing home residents, *J Am Geriatr Soc* 49(6):803–807, 2001.

Quinn P, Goka J, Richardson H: Assessment of an electronic daily diary in patients with overactive bladder, *BJU Int* 91(7):647–652, 2003.

Rodhe N, Englund L, Molstad S et al: Bacteriuria is associated with urge urinary incontinence in older women, *Scand J Primary Health Care* 26(1):35–39, 2008.

Romanzi LJ: Management of the urethral outlet in patients with severe prolapse, *Curr Opin Urol* 12(4):339–344, 2002.

Rozenberg S, Pastijn A, Gevers R et al: Estrogen therapy in older patients with recurrent urinary tract infections: a review, *Int J Fertil Womens Med* 49(2):71–74, 2004.

Sampselle CM: Teaching women to use a voiding diary, *Am J Nurs* 103(11):62–64, 2003.

Song C, Park JT, Heo KO et al: Effects of bladder training and/or tolterodine in female patients with overactive bladder syndrome: a prospective, randomized study, *J Korean Med Sci* 21(6):1060–1063, 2006.

Stav K, Dwyer PL, Rosamilia A: Women overestimate daytime urinary frequency: the importance of the bladder diary, *Journal of Urology* 181(5):2176–2180, 2009.

Stewart WF, Van Rooyen JB, Cundiff GW et al: Prevalence and burden of overactive bladder in the United States, *World J Urol* 20(6):327–336, 2003.

Theofrastous JP, Wyman JF, Bump RC et al: Effects of pelvic floor muscle training on strength and predictors of response in the treatment of urinary incontinence, *Neurourol Urodyn* 21(5):486–490, 2002.

van Gerwen M, Lagro-Janssen AL: [Diagnostic value of patient history and physical examination in elderly patients with urinary incontinence; a literature review], *Ned Tijdsch Geneesk* 150(32):1771–1775, 2006 [article in Dutch].

Wein AJ: Transvaginal electrical stimulation in the treatment of urinary incontinence, *J Urol* 174(3):1007, 2005.

Risk for urge urinary Incontinence
Mikel Gray, PhD, CUNP, CCCN, FAANP, FAAN, and Betty J. Ackley, MSN, EdS, RN

NANDA-I

Definition

At risk for involuntary loss of urine associated with a sudden, strong sensation of urinary urgency

Risk Factors

Effects of alcohol; effects of caffeine; effects of medications; detrusor hyperreflexia (e.g., from cystitis, urethritis, tumors, renal calculi, central nervous system disorders above pontine micturition center); impaired bladder contractility; involuntary sphincter relaxation; ineffective toileting habits; small bladder capacity

• = Independent   ▲ = Collaborative   **EBN** = Evidence-Based Nursing   **EB** = Evidence-Based

NOC, NIC, Client Outcomes, Nursing Interventions, Client/Family Teaching and Discharge Planning, *Rationales,* and References

Refer to care plans for **Urge urinary Incontinence.**

Disorganized Infant behavior   *Mary A. DeWys, BS, RN, and Peg Padnos, AB, BSN, RN*

 NANDA-I

Definition

Disintegrated physiological and neurobehavioral responses of infant to the environment

Defining Characteristics

Attention-Interaction System

Abnormal response to sensory stimuli (e.g., difficult to soothe, inability to sustain alert status)

Motor System

Altered primitive reflexes; changes to motor tone; finger splaying; fisting; hands to face; hyperextension of extremities; jittery; startles; tremors; twitches; uncoordinated movement

Physiological

Arrhythmias; bradycardia; desaturation; feeding intolerances; skin color changes; tachycardia; time-out signals (e.g., gaze, grasp, hiccough, cough, sneeze, sigh, slack, jaw, open mouth, tongue thrust)

Regulatory Problems

Inability to inhibit startle; irritability

State-Organization System

Active-awake (fussy, worried gaze); diffuse sleep; irritable crying; quiet-awake (staring, gaze aversion); state-oscillation

Related Factors (r/t)

Caregiver

Cue knowledge deficit; cue misreading; environmental stimulation contribution

Environmental

Lack of containment within environment; physical environment inappropriateness; sensory deprivation; sensory inappropriateness; sensory overstimulation

Individual

Gestational age; illness; immature neurological system; postconceptual age

Postnatal

Feeding intolerance; invasive procedures; malnutrition; motor problems; oral problems; pain; prematurity

Prenatal

Congenital disorders; genetic disorders; teratogenic exposure

NOC (Nursing Outcomes Classification)

Suggested NOC Outcomes

Child Development, Neurological Status, Preterm Infant Organization, Sleep, Thermoregulation: Newborn

• = Independent   ▲ = Collaborative   **EBN** = Evidence-Based Nursing   **EB** = Evidence-Based

---

Example NOC Outcome with Indicators

Preterm Infant Organization as evidenced by the following indicators: O_2 saturation >85%/Thermoregulation/ Feeding tolerance/Self-consolability/Quiet-alert/Attentiveness to stimuli/Responsive to stimuli (Rate the outcome and indicators of **Preterm Infant Organization:** 1 = severely compromised, 2 = substantially compromised, 3 = moderately compromised, 4 = mildly compromised, 5 = not compromised [see Section 1].)

Client Outcomes

Client Will (Specify Time Frame):

Infant/Child
- Display physiologic/autonomic stability: cardiorespiratory, visceral, neurofunctional
- Display organized motor system (Wyngarden, DeWys, & Padnos, 1999)
- Display signs of state organization: ability to maintain organized sleep and awake states (Wyngarden, DeWys, & Padnos, 1999)
- Demonstrate progress toward effective self-regulation (Wyngarden, DeWys, & Padnos, 1999)
- Display clear behavior cues that communicate approach/engagement and stress/avoidance (Wyngarden, DeWys, & Padnos, 1999)
- Demonstrate ability to engage in positive interactive experiences with parent(s)
- Demonstrate ability to process, organize, and respond to sensory information in an adaptive way

Parent/Significant Other
- Recognize infant/child behaviors as a unique way of communicating needs
- Recognize infant behaviors used to communicate stress/avoidance and approach/engagement
- Recognize and support infant/child's coping behaviors used to self-regulate
- Read and respond to infant/child behavior cues in a way that facilitates autonomic/physiologic, motor, and state organization
- Recognize how the personal style of interactions can positively or negatively affect the infant/child's responses
- Recognize that following the infant's lead will help in fostering effective interactions
- Identify appropriate positioning and handling techniques that will enhance normal motor development and prevent positioning acquired abnormalities (Wyngarden, DeWys, & Padnos, 1999)
- Promote infant/child's attention capabilities to orient to visual and auditory input (Wyngarden, DeWys, & Padnos, 1999)
- Engage in pleasurable parent/infant/child interactions that encourage bonding and attachment (Wyngarden, DeWys, & Padnos, 1999)
- Structure and modify the environment in response to infant/child's behavioral, personal, nurturing, medical, and sensory needs (Wyngarden, DeWys, & Padnos, 1999)
- Identify available community resources that provide early intervention services, emotional support, community health nursing, and parenting classes (Wyngarden, DeWys, & Padnos, 1999)

NIC   (Nursing Interventions Classification)

Suggested NIC Interventions

Developmental Care, Infant, Positioning, Sleep Enhancement

Example NIC Activities—Developmental Care

Teach parents to recognize infant states and cues and in planning care responsive to infant cues and states

Nursing Interventions and *Rationales*

- Identify infant/child's behavioral organization as unique way of communicating in five sub-systems of functioning (i.e., physiologic/autonomic, motor, state, self-regulatory, attention-interactional). The Assessment of Preterm Infants' Behavior (APIB) is a newborn neurobehavioral assessment appropriate for preterm, at risk, and full-term newborns, from birth to 1 month after expected due date. *The APIB is based in ethological-evolutionary thought and focuses on the assessment of mutually interacting behavioral subsystems in simultaneous interaction with the environment (Als et al, 2005).*

● = Independent   ▲ = Collaborative   **EBN** = Evidence-Based Nursing   **EB** = Evidence-Based

- Provide individualized developmental care for low-birth-weight, preterm infants that positively influences neurodevelopmental functioning and reduces the severity of medical illness. **EB:** *Positive outcomes include earlier transition to full oral feedings; younger discharge age; reduced hospital charges; improved weight, length, and head circumference; and lower family stress (Als et al, 2003).*
- Identify appropriate positioning and handling techniques that enhance normal development and motor organization and prevent position-acquired abnormalities. *Developmentally correct positioning (e.g., positioning in flexion, frequent positioning changes, using comforting physical containment as appropriate, giving opportunities for sucking and finger grasping) has been shown to be effective in providing comfort, decreasing stress, conserving energy, enhancing sleep, and facilitating normal development of the preterm infant (Sweeney & Gutierrez, 2002; Aita & Snider, 2003).* **EB:** *Prone positioning may improve quality of sleep and respiratory function and decrease stress for ventilated preterm infants (Chang, Anderson, & Lin, 2002; see also Monterosso, Kristjanson, & Cole, 2002).*
- Demonstrate ways to facilitate state organization and control. *Pacing type, intensity, and timing of stimulation according to infant state and behavior cues is critical to facilitating state organization (Fajardo et al, 1990).* **EBN:** *Effective developmental handling during caregiving has been shown to promote behavioral state organization (Becker, Brazy & Grunwald, 1997).*
- Support the infant's need for uninterrupted sleep periods. Consider swaddling in supine position for sleep. *This study showed that, when infants between 6 and 16 weeks of age sleep swaddled and supine, they sleep longer, spend more time in NREM sleep, and awake less spontaneously than when not swaddled (Franco et al, 2005).*
- Cluster care whenever possible, allowing for longer periods of uninterrupted sleep. *Introduce one intervention at a time and observe infant cues, taking care not to overstimulate (Als et al, 1994).*
- Structure and organize the environment. *A developmental care approach designed to reduce environmental stress and facilitate motor and sleep-wake organization may result in improved behavioral organization during the preterm period (Als et al, 1994; Buehler et al, 1995; Als, 1998).*
- Identify and support the infant/child's use of self-regulatory/consoling behaviors needed for mastering the environment. **EBN:** *When providing infant stimulation, it can be helpful to modify developmental interventions based on physiologic and behavioral cues (Burns et al, 1994).*
- Recognize behavior used to communicate stress/avoidance and approach/engagement. *The ability to read and interpret infant/child behavior provides a framework for responding contingently, that is, in a way that communicates the infant/child's importance and ability to affect the environment (Als et al, 2005). When mothers evaluated their caregiving from birth through their infant's first year of life, they said that their most frequent source of confidence and competence came from their infant's contentedness of mood and soothability (Pridham, Chin-Yu, & Brown, 2001).*
- Correlate stress/disorganized behaviors to internal factors (e.g., pain, hunger, discomfort) and/or external factors (e.g., lights, noise, handling). *Noise is one of the common stressors in hospital intensive care units (ICUs), resulting in sensory overload that has the potential to alter development adversely (DePaul & Chambers, 1995; Elander & Hellstrom, 1995). Intrauterine cocaine exposure can result in disorganized behavior patterns of infants (DeWys & McComish-Fry, 1992). Provide ongoing support during and after procedures (e.g., heel stick); stay with infant throughout recovery period (VandenBerg, 1999).*
- Provide opportunities for physical closeness, loving touch, massage, cuddling, skin-to-skin (kangaroo care), and rocking. *Infant massage improves physical growth, fosters behavioral changes and decreases infant stress. It reinforces attachment and interactions between babies and parents. (Chang, Sung, & Tseng, 2007).* **EBN and EB:** *Parents have been found to be more sensitive and to show more positive affect when participating in skin-to-skin "kangaroo" care (Feldman et al, 2002). Infants who have had kangaroo care have been found to benefit with cardiorespiratory stabilization, improved oxygenation, improved thermoregulation, increased weight gain, earlier breastfeeding, less crying, increased quiet sleep, and decreased length of stay (Chwo et al, 2002).*
- Provide opportunities for parent/caregiver to engage in positive parent-infant interactions. *Engagement and disengagement are infant cues signaling responses to internal and external stimuli (Blackburn, 1978). The parent/caregiver becomes the mediator between infant and environment (Blackburn, 1983).*

• = Independent   ▲ = Collaborative   **EBN** = Evidence-Based Nursing   **EB** = Evidence-Based

- Encourage parents' competence by affirming their strengths and capabilities when caring for their infants. **EBN:** *New neonatal intensive care unit (NICU) mothers who participated in one parent-to-parent support program had less anxiety during the first four months postdischarge than the comparison group; at twelve months postdischarge, self-esteem was found to have increased, and mothers also had better maternal-infant relationships and more nurturing home environments (Roman et al, 1995). Parents must be supported and welcomed as active collaborators in their infant's care (Lawhon, 2002).*
- Identify and support infant/child's attention capabilities. *In organized quiet-alert states, infants are able to focus their attention and interact with their environment in a purposeful way. It is important to give the baby opportunities to attend to sensory input, but not at the cost of behavioral disorganization (Burns et al, 1994).* **EBN:** *A study of state organization of very low birth weight infants demonstrated the positive effects of developmental handling and recognized that alertness may be promoted without physiological and behavioral disorganization (Becker, Brazy & Grunwald, 1997).*
- Provide pleasurable experiences (i.e., visual, auditory, tactile, vestibular, proprioceptive) that enhance development of sensory pathways. *Healthy 33- to 34-week postconceptual age infants who received 15 minutes of auditory, visual, tactile, and vestibular stimulation each day were found to have improved state modulation and better ability to maintain quiet-alert state, resulting in enhanced parent-infant interactions and feedings (White-Traut et al, 1993). Observe how the infant responds to different sensations and modify as appropriate. Promote behavioral organization, positive patterns of maternal-infant interactions, and conserve energy for growth (Burns et al, 1994).*
- ▲ Provide information or refer to community based follow-up programs for preterm/at-risk infants and their families. *Seamless communication between NICU staff and community agencies enhances parent's feelings of confidence during the difficult transition from NICU discharge to home (Sherman, Aylward, & Shoemaker, 2009).*

Multicultural

- Assess for the influence of cultural beliefs, norms, and values on the family's perceptions of infant/child behavior. **EBN:** *What the family considers normal infant/child behavior may be based on cultural perceptions (Guarnaccia, 1998; Leininger & McFarland, 2002).* **EBN:** *The theory of hot and cold espoused by many Mexican Americans have symbolic significance for the nature and process of reproduction and for the relationship between mother and child (Giger & Davidhizar, 2008). Beliefs related to the phenomena of communication, time, space, social organization, environmental control, and biological variations can all influence the family's perceptions of infant/child behavior (Giger & Davidhizar, 2008).*
- Use a neutral, indirect style when addressing areas where improvement is needed (such as a need for verbal or oral stimulation) when working with Native American clients. **EBN:** *Using indirect statements such as "Other mothers have tried..." or "I had a client who tried 'X' and it seemed to work very well" will assist in avoiding resentment from the parent (Seideman et al, 1996).*
- Use therapeutic communication techniques that emphasize acceptance, offer the self, validate the client's concerns, and convey respect when discussing the infant/child behavior. **EBN:** *Validation is a therapeutic communication technique that lets the client know that the nurse has heard and understands what was said, and it promotes the nurse-client relationship (Heineken, 1998).*

Client/Family Teaching and Discharge Planning

- Assist family's support systems in recognizing and responding to infant's unique behavioral cues. *Demonstrating and modeling appropriate interactional skills is an integral component of family education and will improve family-infant interactions (McGrath & Conliffe-Torres, 1996).*
- Provide information on techniques to promote sleep for infants. *Education on sleep enhancement appears to increase infant sleep (Gagnon & Bryanton, 2009).*
- Nurture parents so that they in turn can nurture their infant/child. *The most difficult and overlooked aspects of care of the high risk neonate is effective, timely, and compassionate information delivery to parents and family by the medical staff (Sherman, Aylward, & Shoemaker, 2009).*
- Have knowledge of community early intervention services and follow-up programs for preterm and at-risk infants and families (Akers et al, 2007).

• = Independent   ▲ = Collaborative   **EBN** = Evidence-Based Nursing   **EB** = Evidence-Based

Home Care

- The above interventions may be adapted for home care use.
- Educate families in preparing home environment. *Patterns of sound, light, and caregiving tasks should minimize stress, conserve energy, and protect the developing neonate from inappropriate environmental stimuli (VandenBerg, 1999; Akers et al, 2007).*
- Prepare families for realistic challenges of caring for preterm and at-risk infants prior to discharge. Areas include corrected versus chronological age, feeding skills, poor endurance/easy fatigability, shorter sleep-wake cycles, decreased alertness and increased fussiness, overstimulation, and so forth. *Help parents identify their infant's characteristics, developmental capabilities and limitations, along with interventions that will support optimal growth and development. Facilitate creation of a support network that will help parents ease the transition from NICU to home (VandenBerg, 1999).*
- Encourage families to teach friends/visitors to recognize and respond to infant's unique behavioral cues. *It is important for families to feel comfortable obtaining support from their regular support systems; therefore, supportive persons need to be taught how to interact in the environment in a way that supports both the family and the infant (Als et al, 2005).*
- Provide information about community resources, developmental follow-up services, and parent-to-parent support programs. *Parents benefit from knowledge of their infant's autonomic sensitivity, lower sensory threshold, potential difficulties with self-calming, and more tentative ability to orient and attend to environmental and social stimuli. Additional anticipatory guidance should include knowledge about prevention of overstimulation and exhaustion of these more sensitive infants (Mouradian, Als, & Coster, 2000).*

evolve   See the EVOLVE website for Weblinks for client education resources.

REFERENCES

Aita M, Snider L: The art of developmental care in the NICU: a concept analysis, *J Adv Nurs* 41(3):223, 2003.

Akers AL et al: InReach: connecting NICU infants and their parents with community early intervention services, *Zero to Three* 27(3), 2007.

Als H: Developmental care in the newborn intensive care unit, *Curr Opin Pediatr* 10:138, 1998.

Als H, Butler S, Kosta S et al: The Assessment of Preterm Infants' Behavior (APIB): furthering the understanding and measurement of neurodevelopmental competence in preterm and full-term infants, *Ment Retard Dev Disabil Res Rev* 11(1):94–102, 2005.

Als H, Gilkerson L, Duffy FH et al: A three-center, randomized, controlled trial of individualized developmental care for very low birth weight preterm infants: medical, neurodevelopmental, parenting, and caregiving effects, *J Dev Behav Pediatr* 24(6):399–408, 2003.

Als H, Lawhon G, Duffy FH et al: Individualized developmental care for the very low-birth-weight preterm infant: medical and neurofunctional effects, *JAMA* 272(11):853–858, 1994.

Becker PT, Brazy JE, Grunwald PC: Behavioral state organization of very low birth weight infants: effects of developmental handling during caregiving, *Infant Behav Dev* 20(4):503, 1997.

Blackburn S: Fostering behavior development of high-risk infants, *J Obst Gynecol Neonatal Nurs* 12:76–86, 1983.

Blackburn S: State related behaviors and individual differences. In Barnard KE, editor: *Nursing child assessment satellite training: learning resource manual,* Seattle, 1978, University of Washington.

Buehler D, Als H, Duffy FH et al: Effectiveness of individualized developmental care for low-risk preterm infants: behavioral and electrophysiologic evidence, *Pediatrics* 96(5):923–932, 1995.

Burns K, Cunningham M, White-Traut R et al: Infant stimulation: modification of an intervention based on physiologic and behavioral cues, *J Obstet Gynecol Neonatal Nurs* 23(7):581–589, 1994.

Chang S, Sung H, Tseng C: Application of infant massage in community nursing (Chinese), *Tzu Chi Nursing Journal* 6(6):73–79, 2007.

Chang Y, Anderson G, Lin C: Effects of prone and supine positions on sleep state and stress responses in mechanically ventilated preterm infants during the first postnatal week, *J Adv Nurs* 40(2):161, 2002.

Chwo M, Anderson GC, Good M et al: A randomized controlled trial of early kangaroo care for preterm infants: effects on temperature, weight, behavior, and acuity, *J Nurs Res* 10(2):129–142, 2002.

DePaul D, Chambers SE: Environmental noise in the neonatal intensive care unit: implications for nursing practice, *J Perinatal Neonatal Nurs* 8:71, 1995.

DeWys M, McComish-Fry J: *Infants states and cues: facilitating effective parent-infant interactions.* In *Caring for infants: a resource manual for caring for infant trainers,* East Lansing MI, 1992, Michigan State University Board of Trustees.

Elander G, Hellstrom G: Reduction of noise levels in intensive care units for infants: evaluation of an intervention program, *Heart Lung* 24:376, 1995.

Fajardo B, Browning M, Fisher D et al: Effect of nursery environment on state regulation in very-low-birth-weight premature infants, *Infant Behav Dev* 13:287–303, 1990.

Feldman R, Eidelman AI, Sirota L et al: Comparison of skin-to-skin (kangaroo) and traditional care: parenting outcomes and preterm infant development, *Pediatrics* 110(1 Pt 1):16–26, 2002.

Franco P, Seret N, Van Hees J et al: Influence of swaddling on sleep and arousal characteristics of healthy infants, *Pediatrics* 115(5):1307–1311, 2005.

Gagnon AJ, Bryanton J: Postnatal parental education for optimizing infant general health and parent-infant relationships, *Cochrane Database Syst Rev* 2009(1) CD004068.

Giger J, Davidhizar R: *Transcultural nursing: assessment and intervention,* St Louis, 2008, Mosby.

Guarnaccia PJ: Multicultural experiences of family caregiving: a study of African American, European American, and Hispanic American families, *New Direct Ment Health Serv* (77):45–61, 1998.

Heineken J: Patient silence is not necessarily client satisfaction: communication in home care nursing, *Home Healthc Nurse* 16(2):115, 1998.

Lawhon G: Facilitation of parenting the premature infant within the newborn intensive care unit, *J Perinatal Neonatal Nurs* 16(1):71, 2002.

Leininger MM, McFarland MR: *Transcultural nursing: concepts, theories, research and practices,* ed 3, New York, 2002, McGraw-Hill.

McGrath J, Conliffe-Torres S: Integrating family-centered developmental assessment and intervention into routine care in the neonatal intensive care unit, *Nurs Clin North Am* 31(2):367, 1996.

Monterosso L, Kristjanson L, Cole J: Neuromotor development and the physiologic effects of positioning in very low birth weight infants, *J Obstet Gynecol Neonatal Nurs* 31(2):128, 2002.

Mouradian LE, Als H, Coster WJ: Neurobehavioral functioning of healthy preterm infants of varying gestational ages, *J Dev Behav Pediatr*, 21(6):408–427, 2000.

Pridham K, Chin-Yu CY, Brown R: Mothers' evaluation of their caregiving for premature and full-term infants through the first: contributing factors, *Res Nurs Health* 24(3):157–169, 2001.

Roman LA, Lindsey JK, Boger RP et al: Parent-to-parent support initiated in the neonatal intensive care unit, *Res Nurs Health* 18(5):385–394, 1995.

Seideman RY, Jacobson S, Primeaux M et al: Assessing American Indian families, *MCN Am J Matern Child Nurs* 21(6):274, 1996.

Sherman MP, Aylward GP, Shoemaker CT: *Follow-up of the NICU patient.* updated July 1, 2009 at http://emedicine.medscape.com/article/977318–overview, accessed October 28, 2009.

Sweeney J, Gutierrez T: Musculoskeletal implications of preterm infant positioning in the NICU, *J Perinatal Neonatal Nurs* 16(1):58, 2002.

VandenBerg KA: What to tell parents about the developmental needs of their baby at discharge, *Neonatal Netw* 18(1):57, 1999.

White-Traut R, Nelson MN, Silvestri JM et al: Patterns of physiological and behavioral response of intermediate care preterm infants to intervention, *Pediatr Nurs* 19(6):625–629, 1993.

Wyngarden K, DeWys M, Padnos P: *Learnings from the field: the impact of using two new nursing diagnoses, organized infant behavior and disorganized infant behavior* (abstract), Classification of Nursing Diagnoses: Proceedings of the Thirteenth Conference, NANDA, 1999.

Risk for disorganized Infant behavior   *Betty J. Ackley, MSN, EdS, RN*

NANDA-I

Definition

Risk for alteration in integrating and modulation of the physiological and behavioral systems of functioning (i.e., autonomic, motor, state, organizational, self-regulatory, and attentional-interactional systems)

Risk Factors

Environmental overstimulation; invasive procedures; lack of containment within environment; motor problems; oral problems; pain; painful procedures; prematurity

NOC, NIC, Client Outcomes, Nursing Interventions, Client/Family Teaching and Discharge Planning, *Rationales,* and References

Refer to **Disorganized Infant behavior.**

Readiness for enhanced organized Infant behavior   *Betty J. Ackley, MSN, EdS, RN*

NANDA-I

Definition

A pattern of modulation of the physiological and behavioral systems of functioning (i.e., autonomic, motor, state-organization, self-regulatory, and attentional-interactional systems) in an infant who is satisfactory but can be improved

Defining Characteristics

Definite sleep-wake states; response to stimuli (e.g., visual, auditory); stable physiologic measures; use of some self-regulatory behaviors

NOC, NIC, Client Outcomes, Nursing Interventions, Client/Family Teaching and Discharge Planning, *Rationales,* and References

Refer to care plans for **Disorganized Infant behavior** and **Risk for disorganized Infant behavior.**

Risk for Infection   *Ruth M. Curchoe, RN, MSN, CIC*   ⊖volve

NANDA-I

Definition

At increased risk for being invaded by pathogenic organisms

Risk Factors

Chronic disease; inadequate acquired immunity; inadequate primary defenses (broken skin, traumatized tissue, decrease in ciliary action, stasis of body fluids, change in pH secretions, altered peristalsis); inadequate secondary defenses (decreased hemoglobin, leukopenia, suppressed inflammatory response); increased environmental exposure to pathogens; immunosuppression; invasive procedures; insufficient knowledge to avoid exposure to pathogens; malnutrition; pharmaceutical agents (e.g., immunosuppressants); premature rupture of amniotic membranes; prolonged rupture of amniotic membranes; trauma; tissue destruction

NOC   (Nursing Outcomes Classification)

Suggested NOC Outcomes

Immune Status, Knowledge: Infection Management, Risk Control, Risk Detection

Example NOC Outcome with Indicators
Immune Status as evidenced by the following indicators: Recurrent infections not present/Skin and mucosa integrity/ Gastrointestinal (GI), Respiratory, Genitourinary (GU) function/Weight and body temperature in expected range (Rate the outcome and indicators of **Immune Status:** 1 = severely compromised, 2 = substantially compromised, 3 = moderately compromised, 4 = mildly compromised, 5 = not compromised [see Section I].)

Client Outcomes

Client Will (Specify Time Frame):

- Remain free from symptoms of infection
- State symptoms of infection of which to be aware
- Demonstrate appropriate care of infection-prone site
- Maintain white blood cell count and differential within normal limits
- Demonstrate appropriate hygienic measures such as handwashing, oral care, and perineal care

NIC   (Nursing Interventions Classification)

Suggested NIC Interventions

Immunization/Vaccination Management, Infection Control, Infection Protection

Example NIC Activities—Infection Protection and Control
Wash hands before and after each patient care activity; Ensure aseptic handling of all intravenous lines; Ensure appropriate wound care technique; Teach patient and family members how to avoid infections; Teach patient and family members proper hand hygiene technique

Nursing Interventions and *Rationales*

- Consider targeted surveillance for methicillin-resistant *Staphylococcus aureus* (MRSA) (screen clients at risk for MRSA on admission). *Targeted surveillance for MRSA colonization was cost-effective and provided substantial benefits by reducing the rate of health care–acquired MRSA infections in a community hospital system (West et al, 2006). Active surveillance for MRSA has been identified as an important tool for the control of MRSA spread in many health care settings (Weber et al, 2007).*

• = Independent   ▲ = Collaborative   **EBN** = Evidence-Based Nursing   **EB** = Evidence-Based

▲ Observe and report signs of infection such as redness, warmth, discharge, and increased body temperature. **EB:** *Prospective surveillance study for health care acquired infection on hematology-oncology units should include fever of unknown origin as the single most common and clinically important entity (Engelhart et al, 2002).*

▲ Assess temperature of neutropenic clients; report a single temperature of greater than (100.5° F). *Fever is often the first sign of an infection (NCCN, 2006).*

• Oral or tympanic thermometers may be used to assess temperature in adults and infants. **EBN:** *The use of tympanic thermometers in addition to oral thermometers in obtaining temperatures is supported (Gilbert, Barton, & Counsell, 2002; Mains, 2008). Tympanic membrane temperature recordings in healthy preterm neonates are safe, accurate, easy, and comfortable for the baby (Bailey & Rose, 2001).*

• The chemical (Tempa-DOT) thermometer may be used with intensive care unit (ICU) clients. *This study demonstrated the accuracy of the chemical thermometer but the pulmonary artery catheter remains the "gold standard" (Farnell et al, 2005).*

▲ Note and report laboratory values (e.g., white blood cell count and differential, serum protein, serum albumin, and cultures). **EB:** *The white blood cell count and the automated absolute neutrophil count are better diagnostic tests for adults and most children (Cornbleet, 2002).*

• Assess skin for color, moisture, texture, and turgor (elasticity). Keep accurate, ongoing documentation of changes. *The skin is the body's first line of defense in protecting the body from infection (NCCN, 2006).*

• Carefully wash and pat dry skin, including skinfold areas. Use hydration and moisturization on all at-risk surfaces. **EBN:** *Atopic dermatitis is a common, chronic skin condition that can be managed in most clients by prescribing avoidance measures, good skin care, antihistamines, and conservative topical medications (Mack, 2004). Refer to care plan for **Risk for impaired Skin integrity**.*

• Monitor weight loss, leaving 25% or more of food uneaten at most meals. **EBN:** *This study demonstrated the above criteria as significant predictors of protein calorie malnutrition (Crogan, Corbett & Short, 2002). Refer to care plan **Readiness for enhanced Nutrition** for additional interventions.*

• Use strategies to prevent health care–acquired pneumonia (HCAP) (CDC, 2004): assess lung sounds, and sputum color and characteristics; use sterile water rather than tap water for mouth care of immunosuppressed clients; use sterile technique when suctioning; suction secretions above tracheal tube before suctioning; drain accumulated condensation in ventilator tubing into a fluid trap or other collection device before repositioning the client; assess patency and placement of nasogastric tubes; elevate the client's head to 30 degrees or higher to prevent gastric reflux of organisms in the lung. **EB:** *Ventilator-associated pneumonia is the most common health care–acquired infection seen in the intensive care unit (Hunter, 2006).*

• Encourage fluid intake. *Fluid intake helps thin secretions and replace fluid lost during fever (CDC, 2004).*

• Use appropriate "hand hygiene" (i.e., handwashing or use of alcohol-based hand rubs). **EBN:** *Meticulous infection prevention precautions are required to prevent health care–associated infection, with particular attention to hand hygiene and standard precautions (CDC, 2002; Gould, 2004). In this study a lower rate of MRSA was linked to good hand hygiene (Mears et al, 2009).*

• When using an alcohol-based hand rub, apply product to palm of one hand and rub hands together, covering all surfaces of hands and fingers, until hands are dry. Note that the volume needed to reduce the number of bacteria on hands varies by product. **EB:** *By introducing the use of hand rubbing with an alcoholic solution, there was significant improved hand-cleansing compliance (Girou & Oppein, 2001).*

• Follow standard precautions and wear gloves during any contact with blood, mucous membranes, nonintact skin, or any body substance except sweat. Use goggles, powder-free gloves, and gowns when appropriate. Standard Precautions apply to all clients. You must assume all clients are carrying blood-borne pathogens (CDC, 2007). **EBN:** *Research has shown that several postsurgical complications can occur when powder particles from surgical and exam gloves fall into an open incision or are accidentally placed in the body with an instrument on which the particles have attached themselves (Same-Day Surgery, 2004).*

• Follow transmission-based precautions for airborne-, droplet-, and contact-transmitted microorganisms:

▪ **Airborne:** Isolate the client in a room with monitored negative air pressure, with the room door closed and the client remaining in the room. Always wear appropriate respiratory protection

• = Independent   ▲ = Collaborative   **EBN** = Evidence-Based Nursing   **EB** = Evidence-Based

when you enter the room. Limit the movement and transport of the client from the room to essential purposes only. Have the client wear a surgical mask during transport *(CDC, 2005)*.

- ■ **Droplet:** Keep the client in a private room, if possible. If not possible, maintain a spatial separation of 3 feet from other beds or visitors. The door may remain open. Wear a surgical mask when you must come within 3 feet of the client. Some hospitals may choose to implement a mask requirement for droplet precautions for anyone entering the room. Limit transport to essential purposes and have the client wear a mask if possible.
- ■ **Contact:** Place the client in a private room if possible or with someone (cohorting) who has an active infection from the same microorganism. Wear clean, nonsterile gloves when entering the room. When providing care, change gloves after contact with any infective material such as wound drainage. Remove the gloves and clean your hands before leaving the room and take care not to touch any potentially infectious items or surfaces on the way out. Wear a gown if you anticipate your clothing may have substantial contact with the client or other potentially infectious items. Remove the gown before leaving the room. Limit transport of the client to essential purposes and take care that the client does not contact other environmental surfaces along the way. Dedicate the use of noncritical client care equipment to a single client. If use of common equipment is unavoidable, adequately clean and disinfect equipment before use with other clients.

Standard Precautions are based on the likely routes of transmission of pathogens. The second tier of the new CDC guidelines is Transmission-Based Precautions. This replaces many old categories of isolation precautions and disease-specific precautions with three simpler sets of precautions. These three sets of precautions are designed to prevent airborne transmission, droplet transmission, and contact transmission (CDC, 2007).

- Use alternatives to indwelling catheters whenever possible (external catheters, incontinence pads, bladder control techniques). Sterile technique must be used when inserting urinary catheters. **EB:** *Urinary tract infections (UTIs) account for almost half of all health care–associated infection (HAI), and a significant number of these infections are related to the insertion of urinary catheters (Bissett, 2005; Saint et al, 2008).*
- If a urinary catheter is necessary, follow catheter management practices: All indwelling catheters should be connected to a sterile, closed drainage system (i.e., not broken), except for good clinical reasons. Cleanse the perineum and meatus twice daily using soap and water. *Health care–acquired UTIs account for up to 40% of all hospital-acquired infections, with 80% of these associated with the use of urinary catheters (Hampton, 2004).*
- Use evidence-based practices and educate personnel in care of peripheral catheters: use aseptic technique for insertion and care, label insertion sites and all tubing with date and time of insertion, inspect every 8 hours for signs of infection, record, and report. **EB:** *This study demonstrated that an education-based intervention that uses evidence-based practices can be successfully implemented in a diverse group of medical and surgical units and reduce catheter-associated bloodstream infection rates (Warren et al, 2006).* **EBN:** *Care in selection of site and catheter is important. The shortest catheter and smallest size should be used when possible. Accommodate the need to replace catheters before they occlude (Schmid, 2000).*
- Use sterile technique wherever there is a loss of skin integrity. **EB:** *An extensive literature search revealed that sterile gloves should be used for postoperative wound dressing changes (St. Clair & Larrabee, 2002).*
- Use clean gloves for all high-risk hospitalized clients. **EB:** *This study demonstrated the effectiveness of using clean gloves to prevent cross-contamination of all multi-drug resistant health care–acquired pathogens (Safdar et al, 2006).*
- Ensure the client's appropriate hygienic care with handwashing; bathing; oral care; and hair, nail, and perineal care performed by either the nurse or the client. *Daily showers or baths can help to reduce the number of bacteria on the client's skin. The oral cavity is a common site for infection (Coughlan & Healy, 2008).*
- Recommend responsible use of antibiotics; use antibiotics sparingly. *Widespread use of certain antibiotics, particularly third-generation cephalosporins, has been shown to foster development of generalized beta-lactam resistance in previously susceptible bacterial populations (Tillotson, Blondeau, & Carroll, 2007).* **EB:** *The reduction of endometritis by two thirds to three quarters and a decrease in wound infections justify a policy of recommending prophylactic antibiotics to women undergoing elective or nonelective cesarean section (Smaill & Hofmeyr, 2002; CDC, 2007).*

• = Independent   ▲ = Collaborative   **EBN** = Evidence-Based Nursing   **EB** = Evidence-Based

- Carefully screen and treat women with infertility who may have female genital tuberculosis. **EB:** *Female genital tuberculosis is a symptomless disease inadvertently uncovered during investigation for infertility (Aliyu, Aliyu, & Salihu, 2004).*

Pediatric

NOTE: Many of the above interventions are appropriate for the pediatric client.
- Follow meticulous hand hygiene when working with premature infants. **EB:** *Cross-transmission through transient hand carriage of a health care worker appeared to be the probable route of transmission in NICU (Milisavljevic et al, 2004; Borghesi & Stronati, 2008).*
- Cluster nursing procedures to decrease number of contacts with infants allowing time for appropriate hand hygiene. **EBN:** *Enhancement of minimal handling and clustering of nursing procedures reduced the total client contact episodes, which could help to overcome the major barrier of time constraints (Lam, Lee, & Lau, 2004).*
- Avoid the prophylactic use of topical cream in premature infants. **EB:** *Prophylactic application of topical ointment increases the risk of coagulase negative staphylococcal infection and any health care–acquired infection. A trend toward increased risk of any bacterial infection was noted in infants prophylactically treated (Conner, Soll, & Edwards, 2004).*
- Encourage early enteral feeding with human milk. *Enhances immune defenses of infant (Borghesi & Stronati, 2008).*
- Monitor recurrent antibiotic use in infants. Instruct parents on appropriate indicators for medical visits and on the influence of breastfeeding and day care at home for avoiding increased need for antibiotics. **EB:** *Families who sought frequent antibiotic therapy for infants with fever or cold had a low threshold for seeking medical help. Breastfeeding and care at home was found to decrease medical visits for antibiotics (Louhi-Pirkanniemi, 2004).*

Geriatric

- Suspect pneumonia when the client has symptoms of lethargy or confusion. **EB:** *Many elderly persons do not have the classic symptoms of community acquired pneumonia; instead, they may present with confusion, lethargy, tachypnea, anorexia, or abdominal pain (Patel & Criner, 2003).*
- Most clients develop HCAP by either aspirating contaminated substances or inhaling airborne particles. Refer to care plan for **Risk for Aspiration**.
- Carefully screen elderly women with symptoms of urinary tract infections for salmonella. **EB:** *Salmonellosis is a major cause of gastroenteritis in the United States and can lead to septicemia and other extraintestinal illness, including urinary tract infections (Sivapalasingam et al, 2004).*
- ▲ Observe and report if the client has a low-grade temperature or new onset of confusion. Use an electronic axillary thermometer. **EBN:** *Those caring for elderly clients must be alerted to the potential presence of infection when even low-grade temperature elevations appear for short periods (Holtzclaw, 2003). In the majority of acute confusion in the elderly, the etiology was multifactorial infections and dehydration as the most common causes (Cacchione et al, 2003). The electronic axillary thermometer is safe and accurate for geriatric clients (Giantin et al, 2008).*
- ▲ Recommend that the geriatric client receive an annual influenza immunization and one-time pneumococcal vaccine. **EB:** *Immunization against influenza is an effective intervention that reduces serologically confirmed cases by between 60% and 70% (Hull et al, 2002). Oseltamivir prophylaxis was very effective in protecting nursing home residents from influenza-like illnesses and in halting an outbreak of influenza B (Parker, Loewen, & Skowronski, 2001).*
- Recognize that chronically ill geriatric clients, particularly those with depression, have an increased susceptibility to infection; practice meticulous care of all invasive sites. *Depression has been noted as a risk factor for lethal infectious disease in disabled older adults, with reduced reactivity in humoral and cellular immunity (Shinkawa et al, 2002). A successful infection prevention program can provide the foundation for expanding performance improvement throughout the long-term care facility (Stevenson & Loeb, 2004).*

Home Care

- Some of the above interventions may be adapted for home care use.
- Assess and treat wounds in the home. **EBN:** *Wound treatment in the community, when combined with comprehensive nursing assessment, can be effective while reducing costs (Carville, 2004).*
- Review standards for surveillance of infections in home care. *Home care has expanded in the United States, but infection surveillance, prevention, and control have lagged behind. In this article, it is recommended that infectious disease control principles form the basis of training for home care providers to assess infection risk and develop prevention strategies (Rhinehart, 2001).*
- Maintain strong infection-prevention policies. *Strong guidelines are important to avoid infection in the home setting, especially addressing such issues as storage and use of irrigation solutions and supplies (Friedman, 2003).*
- ▲ Monitor for the occurrence of infectious exacerbation of chronic obstructive pulmonary disease (COPD); refer to physician for treatment. *Atypical* Haemophilus influenzae, Streptococcus pneumoniae, *and* Moraxella *can cause exacerbation of COPD (Sheikh & Sethi, 2001).*
- ▲ Refer for nutritional evaluation; implement dietary changes to support recovery and address antibiotic side effects. *Overgrowth of* Clostridium difficile *can cause abdominal pain, fever, and diarrhea. Inclusion of probiotics in the diet can counteract antibiotic-associated diarrhea (Vogelzang, 2001).*

 Client/Family Teaching and Discharge Planning

- Teach the client risk factors contributing to surgical wound infection (e.g., smoking, and higher body mass index). **EB:** *These are some of the factors associated with risk of surgical wound infection (Reilly, 2002).*
- Teach the client and family the symptoms of infection that should be promptly reported to a primary medical caregiver (e.g., redness, warmth, swelling, tenderness or pain, new onset of drainage or change in drainage from wound, increase in body temperature). **EB:** *Two thirds of wound infections occur after discharge (Reid et al, 2002).*
- Encourage high-risk persons, including health care workers, to get vaccinated (CDC, 2008).
- Influenza: Teach frequent hand hygiene, limited contact with sick person, use of masks by caregiver and sick person, and keeping sick person in the "sick room." *Respiratory droplets from sneezing or coughing spread the influenza virus, and the virus can live on items for days (Allen, 2006).*
- Assess whether the client and family know how to read a thermometer; provide instructions if necessary. Chemical dot thermometers are easy to use and decrease risk of infection. Clients need to know that the instructions should be followed carefully and that electronic thermometers may be the best choice for accuracy. *Single-use clinical thermometers provide a safe alternative to the traditional mercury in glass thermometers for routine temperature taking (MacQueen, 2001).*

ⓔvolve   See the EVOLVE website for Weblinks for client education resources.

REFERENCES

Aliyu MH, Aliyu SH, Salihu HM: Female genital tuberculosis: a global review, *Int J Fertil Womens Med* 49(3):123–136, 2004.

Allen P: Home care fact sheet: influenza, *Pediatric Nurs* 32(6):573–576, 2006.

Bailey J, Rose P: Axillary and tympanic membrane temperature recording in the preterm neonate: a comparative study, *J Adv Nurs* 34(4):465–471, 2001.

Bissett L: Reducing the risk of catheter-related urinary tract infection, *Nurs Times* 101(12):64–65, 2005.

Borghesi A, Stronati M: Strategies for the prevention of hospital-acquired infections in the neonatal intensive care unit, *J Hosp Infect*, 68(4):293–300, 2008.

Cacchione PZ, Culp K, Laing J et al: Clinical profile of acute confusion in the long-term care setting, *Clin Nurs Res* 12(2):145–158, 2003.

Carville K: A report on the effectiveness of comprehensive wound assessment and documentation in the community, *Prim Intent* 12(1):41, 2004.

Centers for Disease Control and Prevention: Guideline for hand hygiene in health-care settings. Recommendations of the Healthcare Infection Control Practices Advisory Committee and the HICPAC/SHEA/APIC/IDSA Hand Hygiene Task Force, *MMWR: Recomm Rep* 51 (RR-16):1–45, 2002.

Centers for Disease Control and Prevention, Healthcare Infection Control Practices Advisory Committee: Guidelines for preventing health-care-associated pneumonia, 2003 recommendations of the CDC and the Healthcare Infection Control Practices Advisory Committee, *Respir Care* 49(8):926–939, 2004.

Centers for Disease Control and Prevention: Guidelines for preventing the transmission of *Mycobacterium tuberculosis* in health-care settings, 2005, *MMWR Recomm Rep* 54(RR-17):1–141, 2005.

Centers for Disease Control and Prevention: Prevention and control of influenza: Recommendations of the Advisory Committee on Immunization Practices (ACIP), 2008, *MMWR Recomm Rep* 57(RR-7):1–60, 2008.

• = Independent   ▲ = Collaborative   **EBN** = Evidence-Based Nursing   **EB** = Evidence-Based

Centers for Disease Control and Prevention, Healthcare Infection Control Practices Advisory Committee: 2007 guideline for isolation precautions: Preventing transmission of infectious agents in healthcare settings, www.cdc.gov/ncidad/dh9p/pdf/guidelines/isolation2007.pdf. Accessed Dec 14, 2009.

Conner JM, Soll RF, Edwards WH: Topical ointment for preventing infection in preterm infants, *Cochrane Database Syst Rev* (1): CD001150, 2004.

Cornbleet PJ: Clinical utility of the band count, *Clin Lab Med* 22(1):101, 2002.

Coughlan M, Healy C: Nursing care, education and support for patients with neutropenia, *Nurs Stand* 22(46):35–41, 2008.

Crogan NL, Corbett CF, Short RA: The minimum data set: predicting malnutrition in newly admitted nursing home residents, *Clin Nurs Res* 11(3):341, 2002.

Engelhart S, Glasmacher A, Exner M et al: Surveillance for health care acquired infections and fever of unknown origin among adult hematology-oncology patients, *Infect Control Hosp Epidemiol* 23(5):244, 2002.

Farnell S, Maxwell L, Tan S et al: Temperature measurement: comparison of non-invasive methods used in adult critical care, *J Clin Nurs* 14(5):632–639, 2005.

Friedman MM: Infection control update for home care and hospice organizations, *Home Healthc Nurse* 21(11):753, 2003.

Giantin V, Toffanello ED, Enzi G et al: Reliability of body temperature measurements in hospitalised older patients, *J Clin Nurs*, 17(11):1518–1525, 2008.

Gilbert M, Barton AJ, Counsell CM: Comparison of oral and tympanic temperatures in adult surgical patients, *Appl Nurs Res* 15(1):42, 2002.

Girou E, Oppein F: Handwashing compliance in a French university hospital: new perspective with the introduction of hand-rubbing with a waterless alcohol-based solution, *J Hosp Infect* 48(Suppl A): S55, 2001.

Gould D: Systematic observation of hand decontamination, *Nurs Stand* 18(47):39–44, 2004.

Hampton S: Nursing management of urinary tract infections for catheterized patients, *Br J Nurs* 13(20):1180–1184, 2004.

Holtzclaw BJ: Use of thermoregulatory principles in patient care: fever management, *Online J Clin Innovat* 5(5):1–23, 2003.

Hull S, Hagdrup N, Hart B et al: Boosting uptake of influenza immunization: a randomized controlled trial of telephone appointing in general practice, *Br J Gen Pract* 52(482):710, 2002.

Hunter JD: Ventilator associated pneumonia, *Postgrad Med J*, 82(965): 172–178, 2006.

Lam BC, Lee J, Lau YL: Hand hygiene practices in a neonatal intensive care unit: a multimodal intervention and impact on health care acquired infection, *Pediatrics* 114(5):e565–e571, 2004.

Louhi-Pirkanniemi K: Recurrent antibiotic use in a small child and the effects on the family, *Scand J Prim Health Care* 22(1):16, 2004.

Mack S: Atopic dermatitis: an overview for the nurse practitioner, *J Am Acad Nurse Pract* 16(10):451–454, 2004.

MacQueen S: Clinical benefits of 3M Tempa Dot thermometer in paediatric setting, *Br J Nurs* 10(1):55–58, 2001.

Mains JA: Measuring temperature, *Nursing Standard.* 22(39):44–47, 2008.

Mears A, White A, Cookson B et al: Healthcare-associated infection in acute hospitals: which interventions are effective? J Hosp Infect, 71(4):307–313, 2009.

Milisavljevic V, Wu F, Larson E et al: Molecular epidemiology of *Serratia marcescens* outbreaks in two neonatal intensive care units, *Infect Control Hosp Epidemiol* 25(9):719–721, 2004.

NCCN (National Comprehensive Cancer Network): Fever and Neutropenia Treatment Guidelines for Patients with Cancer—Version II/ March 2006, *NCCN (National Cancer Comprehensive Network).* www.nccn.org/patients/patient_gls/_english/_fever_and _neutropenia/1_introduction.asp. Accessed Feb 26, 2007.

Parker R, Loewen N, Skowronski D: Experience with oseltamivir in the control of a nursing home influenza B outbreak, *Can Commun Dis Rep* 27(5):37, 2001.

Patel N, Criner G: Community-acquired pneumonia in the elderly: update on treatment strategies, *Consultant* 43(6):689–690, 692, 695–697, 2003.

Reid R, Simcock JW, Chisholm L et al: Postdischarge clean wound infections: incidence underestimated and risk factors overemphasized, *ANZ J Surg* 72(5):339, 2002.

Reilly J: Evidence-based surgical wound care on surgical wound infection, *Br J Nurs* 11(Suppl 16):S4, 2002.

Rhinehart E: Infection control in home care, *Emerg Infect Dis* 7(2):208–211, 2001.

Safdar N, Marx J, Meyer N et al: Effectiveness of preemptive barrier precautions in controlling health care acquired colonization and infection by methicillin-resistant Staphylococcus aureus in a burn unit, *Am J Infect Control* 34(8):476–483, 2006.

Saint S et al: Preventing hospital-acquired urinary tract infection in the United States: a national study, *CID* 46(2):243–250, 2008.

Same-Day Surgery: Powdered gloves increase surgical complication risk: adhesions, granulomas, decreased resistance linked, 28(5):54–55, 2004.

Schmid MW: Risks and complications of peripherally and centrally inserted intravenous catheters, *Crit Care Nurs Clin North Am* 12(2):165, 2000.

Sheikh S, Sethi S: Management of infectious exacerbation of COPD, *Home Health Care Consult* 8(5):21, 2001.

Shinkawa M, Nakayama K, Hirai H et al: Depression and immunoreactivity in disabled older adults, *J Am Geriatr Soc* 50:198, 2002.

Sivapalasingam S, Hoekstra RM, McQuiston JR et al: Salmonella bacteriuria: an increasing entity in elderly women in the United States, *Epidemiol Infect* 132(5):897–902, 2004.

Smaill FM, Hofmeyr GJ: Antibiotic prophylaxis for cesarean section. *Cochrane Database Syst Rev* (3):CD000933, 2002.

St Clair K, Larrabee JH: Clean versus sterile gloves: which to use for postoperative dressing changes? *Outcomes Manag* 6(1):17, 2002.

Stevenson KB, Loeb M: Topics in long-term care. Performance improvement in the long-term-care setting: building on the foundation of infection control, *Infect Control Hosp Epidemiol* 25(1):72–79, 2004.

Tillotson GS, Blondeau JM, Carroll J: Hospital-based strategies to reduce antibiotic resistance: are they valid in the community setting, *Expert review of anti-infective therapy*, 5(1):53–59, 2007.

Vogelzang JL: Nutrition in home care. Nonfunctional gut? Try a probiotic food, *Home Healthc Nurse* 19:467, 2001.

Warren D, Cosgrove S, Diekema D et al: A multicenter intervention to prevent catheter-associated bloodstream infections, *Infect Control Hosp Epidemiol* 27(7):662–669, 2006.

Weber SG, Huang SS, Oriola S et al: Legislative mandates for use of active surveillance cultures to screen for methicillin-resistant *Staphylococcus aureus* and vancomycin-resisteant enterococci: position statement from the Joint SHEA and APIC Task Force, *American Journal of Infection Control* 35(2):73–85, 2007.

West TE, Guerry C, Hiott M et al: Effect of targeted surveillance for control of methicillin-resistant Staphylococcus aureus in a community hospital system, *Infect Control Hosp Epidemiol* 27(3):233–238, 2006.

● = Independent   ▲ = Collaborative   **EBN** = Evidence-Based Nursing   **EB** = Evidence-Based

Risk for Injury   *Amy Brown, APRN, MSN*

NANDA-I

Definition

At risk of injury as a result of the interaction of environmental conditions interacting with the individual's adaptive and defensive resources

NOTE: This nursing diagnosis overlaps with other diagnoses such as **Risk for Falls, Risk for Trauma, Risk for Poisoning, Risk for Suffocation, Risk for Aspiration**, and if the client is at risk of bleeding, **Ineffective Protection.** Refer to care plans for these diagnoses if appropriate.

Risk Factors

External

Biological (e.g., immunization level of community, microorganism); chemical (e.g., poisons, pollutants, drugs, pharmaceutical agents, alcohol, nicotine, preservatives, cosmetics, dyes); human (e.g., nosocomial agents; staffing patterns; cognitive, affective, psychomotor factors); mode of transport; nutritional (e.g., vitamins, food types); physical (e.g., design, structure, and arrangement of community, building, and/or equipment)

Internal

Abnormal blood profile (leukocytosis/leucopenia, altered clotting factors, thrombocytopenia, sickle cell, thalassemia, decreased hemoglobin); biochemical dysfunction; developmental age (physiological, psychosocial); effector dysfunction; immune-autoimmune dysfunction; integrative dysfunction; malnutrition; physical (e.g., broken skin, altered mobility); psychological (affective orientation); sensory dysfunction; tissue hypoxia

NOC   (Nursing Outcomes Classification)

Suggested NOC Outcomes

Personal Safety Behavior, Risk Control, Safe Home Environment, Knowledge: Fall Prevention

Example NOC Outcome with Indicators
Risk Control as evidenced by the following indicators: Monitors environmental risk factors/Develops effective risk control strategies/Follows selected risk control strategies (Rate the outcome and indicators of **Risk Control:** 1 = never demonstrated, 2 = rarely demonstrated, 3 = sometimes demonstrated, 4 = often demonstrated, 5 = consistently demonstrated [see Section I].)

Client Outcomes

Client Will (Specify Time Frame):

- Remain free of injuries
- Explain methods to prevent injuries

NIC   (Nursing Interventions Classification)

Suggested NIC Interventions

Health Education, Environmental Management, Fall Prevention

Example NIC Activities—Health Education
Identify internal or external factors that may enhance or reduce motivation for healthy behavior; Determine current health knowledge and lifestyle behaviors of individual, family, or target group

Nursing Interventions and *Rationales*

- Prevent iatrogenic harm to the hospitalized client by following the 2009 National Patient Safety goals:

Accuracy of Patient Identification

- Use at least two methods (e.g., client's name and medical record number or birth date) to identify the client before administering medications, blood products, treatments, or procedures.
- Prior to beginning any invasive or surgical procedure, have a final verification to confirm the correct client, the correct procedure, and the correct site for the procedure using active communication techniques.

Effectiveness of Communication Among Care Staff

- When taking verbal or telephone orders, the orders should be written down and then read back for verification to the individual giving the order.
- Standardize use of abbreviations, acronyms, symbols, and dose designations that are used in the institution.
- Make sure of timeliness of reporting and taking action of critical test results and values.
- Utilize a standardized approach of "handing off" communications, including opportunities to ask and answer questions.

Medication Safety

- Standardize and limit the number of drug concentrations utilized by the institution (e.g., concentrations of medications such as morphine in patient-controlled analgesia [PCA] pumps).
- Label all medications and medication containers (e.g., syringes, medication cups, or other solutions on or off the surgical field).
- Identify all of the client's current medications upon admission to a health care facility, and ensure that all health care staff have access to the information.
- Reconcile all medication at discharge, and provide list to the client.
- Improve the effectiveness of alarm systems in the clinical area.
- Standardize a list of medications that look alike or sound alike. This list needs to be updated yearly.
- Identify and take extra care with clients who are on blood-thinning medications.

Infection Control

- Reduce the risk of infections by following Centers for Disease Control and Prevention (CDC) hand hygiene guidelines.
- Clients who obtain injuries or die from infectious disease must be documented.
- Utilize proven guidelines to prevent infections that are difficult to treat.
- Utilize proven guidelines to prevent infection of the blood.
- Utilize safe practices to treat the surgical site of the client.

Fall Prevention

- Evaluate all clients for fall risk and take appropriate actions to prevent falls.

Patient Involvement in Care

- Educate the client and family on how to recognize and report complaints about safety issues.

Identify Patients with Safety Risks

- Identify which clients are at risk for harming themselves.

Identify Patients Who Are Susceptible to Changes in Health Status

- Educate staff on how to recognize changes in client condition, how to respond quickly, and how to alert specially trained staff to intervene if needed.
- Prevent errors in surgery.
- Standardize steps to educate staff so documents for surgery are ready prior to surgery.

- ▪ Educate staff to mark the body part scheduled for surgery and engage the client in this process as well.

  These actions have been shown to increase client safety and are required actions for accreditation by the Joint Commission (2009).

- • See care plan for **Risk for Falls.**
- ▲ Avoid use of restraints if at all possible. Restraint-free is now the standard of care for hospitals and long-term care facilities. Obtain a physician's order if restraints are necessary. *The use of restraints has been associated with serious injuries, including rhabdomyolysis, brachial plexus injury, neuropathy, dysrhythmias, as well as strangulation, traumatic brain injuries, and all the consequences of immobility (Capezuti, 2004; Park & Tang, 2007).* **EBN and EB:** *A current research study has shown a significant reduction in falls in a group that use quarter bedrails as a restraint versus a group that were using bedrails times four as a restraint (Capezuti et al, 2007).*
- • In place of restraints, use the following:
  - ▪ Well-staffed and educated nursing personnel with frequent client contact
  - ▪ Continuity of care with familiar staff
  - ▪ Nursing units designed to care for clients with cognitive or functional impairments
  - ▪ Avoiding use of IVs or tubes that are susceptible to being removed
  - ▪ Alarm systems with ankle, above-the-knee, or wrist sensors
  - ▪ Bed or wheelchair alarms
  - ▪ Increased observation of the client
  - ▪ Providing exercise to diffuse and deflect client behavior
  - ▪ Low or very low height beds
  - ▪ Border-defining pillow/mattress to remind the client to stay in bed
  - ▪ Mobility exercise to strength muscles and steady gait
  - ▪ Floor mats and transfer poles for client safety

  These alternatives to restraints can be helpful to prevent falls (Capezuti et al, 2007; Park & Tang, 2007).
- • For an agitated client, consider providing individualized music of the client's choice. **EB:** *Irish et al (2006) found a significant reduction in agitation with Alzheimer's clients while playing background music. A quasiexperimental study showed a significant reduction in overall agitation and physical nonaggressive behaviors (Sung, Chang, & Abbey, 2006).*
- • Review drug profile for potential side effects that may increase risk of injury. **EB:** *Confused clients receiving benzodiazepines were significantly more likely to fall that those clients that were not confused or receiving benzodiazepines (Vassallo et al, 2006). Clients' fall rates were directly related to the number of psychotropic medications they were receiving (Cooper et al 2007).*
- • Use one quarter– to one half–length side rails only, and maintain bed in a low position. Ensure that wheels are locked on bed and commode. Keep dim light in room at night. **EBN:** *Use of full side rails can result in the client climbing over the rails, leading with the head, and sustaining a head injury. Side rails with widely spaced vertical bars and side rails not situated flush with the mattress have been associated with asphyxiation deaths because of rail and in bed entrapment and should not be used (Capezuti et al, 2007).*
- • If the client has a new onset of confusion (delirium), refer to the care plan for **Acute Confusion.** If the client has chronic confusion, see the care plan for **Chronic Confusion.**
- • Ask family to stay with the client to prevent the client from accidentally falling or pulling out tubes. *Geriatric clients with chronic conditions and activity limitations had higher rates of fall injuries compared with older adults without chronic conditions (Schiller, Bramarow, & Dey, 2007).*
- • Remove all possible hazards in environment such as razors, medications, and matches.
- • Place an injury-prone client in a room that is near the nurse's station. **EB:** *A pilot study has shown a slight decrease in fall rates due to the nurse's ability to check on the client more frequently and react to call lights more quickly by placing the client closer to the nurse's station (Nazarko, 2007).*
- • Help clients sit in a stable chair with armrests. Avoid use of wheelchairs and geri-chairs except for transportation as needed. *Clients are likely to fall when left in a wheelchair or geri-chair because they may stand up without locking the wheels or removing the footrests.*
- ▲ Refer to physical therapy for strengthening exercises and gait training to increase mobility. **EB:** *A metaanalysis conducted on utilizing individualized exercise training regimen with clients at risk for*

---

falls, showed a 14% decrease in falls with that population (Hill-Westmoreland & Gruber-Baldini, 2005).

▲ For the agitated psychotic client, use nonphysical forms of behavior management, such as verbal intervention or show of force. If medication is required, use oral medications if at all possible. **EBN:** *The nurse should encourage strict schedules in the client's activities of daily living. The nurse should communicate with the client in a calm and encouraging voice and use distraction with activities that the client enjoys. The likelihood of multiple medications being prescribed to psychiatric population, the nurse should be aware of drug interactions, half lives, and preferred route of administration (Sharer, 2008).*

Pediatric

- Teach parents the need for close supervision of all young children playing near water, including washing machines. **EB:** *Children can be harmed by washing machines by the wringer mechanism, also by hot water, and by drowning (Warner, Kenney, & Rice, 2003).*
- If child has epilepsy, recommend showers instead of tub baths, and no unsupervised swimming is ever allowed. *Most drowning accidents involving children are preventable if basic safety measures are taken (Bolte, 2000).*
- Assess the client's social economic status. **EB:** *Pediatric clients living in poverty are at higher risk for injury (Shenassa, Stubbendick, & Brown, 2004).*
- Never leave young children unsupervised around cooking areas. **EB:** *Some identified hazards to young children include burns and scalds, water temperatures set at greater than 54° C, kettles or appliances with dangling wires, or no stove guards to prevent a child from grabbing pots (Leblanc et al, 2006).*
- Teach parents and children the need to maintain safety for the exercising child, including wearing helmets when biking and using breakaway bases for baseball. *A parent's use of helmets appears to affect a child's use (Martin, 2002).* **EB:** *Use of breakaway bases was shown to reduce the number of injuries in baseball and softball by 96% (Janda, Bir, & Kedroske, 2001).*
- Teach both parents and children the need for gun safety. *There are a number of programs available to teach gun safety, including Eddie the Eagle Gun Safe Program, Straight Talk about Risks (STAR), Steps to Prevent Firearm Injury in the Home, and the Emergency Nurses Association Gun Safety Program (Howard, 2001).*

Geriatric

- Encourage the client to wear glasses and hearing aids and to use walking aids when ambulating.
- If the client experiences dizziness because of orthostatic hypotension when getting up, teach methods to decrease dizziness, such as rising slowly, remaining seated several minutes before standing, flexing feet upward several times while sitting, sitting down immediately if feeling dizzy, and trying to have someone present when standing. *If orthostatic hypotension is present and there is minimal change in the heart rate, most likely the baroreceptors are not working to maintain blood pressure on arising. This is common in the elderly and can be from cardiovascular disease, neurological disease, or a medication effect (Sclater & Alagiakrishnan, 2004).*
- Discourage driving at night. *A decline in depth perception, slower recovery from glare, and night blindness are common in the elderly and make night driving a difficult and unsafe task.*

Multicultural

- Acknowledge racial/ethnic differences at the onset of care. **EBN:** *Acknowledgment of race/ethnicity issues will enhance communication, establish rapport, and promote treatment outcomes (D'Avanzo et al, 2001). A recent study found that burns, guns, drowning, and being pierced/cut appeared to be particularly important mechanisms of injury for Hispanic children (Karr, Rivara, & Cummings, 2005). Death by violence has increased significantly among Alaska Natives, who have a suicide rate, frequently related to alcohol and self-inflicted gunshot wounds, three times that of the general U.S. population (National Center for Health Statistics, 2008).*

● = Independent ▲ = Collaborative **EBN** = Evidence-Based Nursing **EB** = Evidence-Based

- Assess for the influence of cultural beliefs, norms, and values on the client's perceptions of risk for injury. **EBN:** *What the client considers risky behavior may be based on cultural perceptions (Giger & Davidhizar, 2008). Young African American, and Hispanic pregnant women are at higher risk for trauma in pregnancy and are most likely to benefit from primary trauma prevention efforts (Ikossi et al, 2005). African Americans, American Indians, and Alaska Natives were identified as high-risk groups who engaged in the following risky traffic-related behavior: not wearing seatbelts, not using child safety seats, not wearing bicycle or motorcycle helmets, driving after drinking, driving while fatigued or distracted, speeding, running red lights, and aggressive driving (Schlundt, Warren, & Miller, 2004).*
- Assess whether exposure to community violence is contributing to risk for injury. **EBN:** *Exposure to community violence has been associated with increases in aggressive behavior and depression (Balter & Tamis-LeMonda, 2006). Minority students, especially African American and Hispanic students in lower grades, may participate in and may more often be victims of school violence (Wright & Fitzpatrick, 2004).*
- Use culturally relevant injury prevention programs whenever possible.
- Validate the client's feelings and concerns related to environmental risks. **EBN:** *Ethnic minority families were less likely to engage in some safety practices and have less access to information regarding the availability and fitting of safety equipment (Mulvaney & Kendrick, 2004). Injuries were identified as the third leading cause of death among Hispanics and the leading cause for those Hispanic individuals 1 to 44 years of age (Mallonee, 2003).*

Home Care/Client/Family Teaching and Discharge Planning

- See **Risk for Trauma** for interventions and rationales.

evolve See the EVOLVE website for Weblinks for client education resources.

REFERENCES

Balter L, Tamis-LeMonda C: *Child psychology: a handbook of contemporary issues,* New York, 2006, Psychology Press.

Bolte R: Drowning: a preventable cause of death, *Patient Care* 34(7):129, 2000.

Capezuti E: Minimizing the use of restrictive devices in dementia patients at risk for falling, *Nurs Clin North Am* 39:625, 2004.

Capezuti E, Wagner L, Brush B et al: Consequences of an intervention to reduce restrictive side rail use in nursing homes, *J Am Geriatr Soc* 55:334–341, 2007.

Cooper J, Freeman M, Cook D et al: Assessment of psychotropic and psychoactive drug loads and falls in nursing facility residents, *Consult Pharm* 22:483–489, 2007.

D'Avanzo CE et al: Developing culturally informed strategies for substance-related interventions. In Naegle MA, D'Avanzo CE, editors: *Addictions and substance abuse: strategies for advanced practice nursing,* St Louis, 2001, Mosby.

Giger J, Davidhizar R: *Transcultural nursing: assessment and intervention,* St Louis, 2008, Mosby.

Hill-Westmoreland E, Gruber-Baldini A: Falls documentation in nursing homes: agreement between the minimum data set and chart abstractions of medical and nursing documentation, *J Am Geriatr Soc* 53(2):268–273, 2005.

Howard PK: An overview of a few well-known national children's gun safety programs and ENA's newly developed program, *J Emerg Nurs* 27(5):485, 2001.

Ikossi DG, Lazar AA, Morabito D et al: Profile of mothers at risk: an analysis of injury and pregnancy loss in 1,195 trauma patients, *J Am Col Surg* 200(1):49–56, 2005.

Irish M, Cunningham C, Walsh J et al: Investigating the enhancing effect of music on autobiographical memory in mild Alzheimer's disease, *Dement Geriatr Cogn Disord* 22(1):108–120, 2006.

Janda DH, Bir C, Kedroske B: A comparison of standard versus breakaway bases: an analysis of a preventative intervention for softball and baseball foot and ankle injuries, *Foot Ankle Int* 22:810, 2001.

Joint Commission 2009 National Patient Safety Goals. www.jointcommission.org/PatientSafety/NationalPatientSafetyGoals/07_npsg_facts.htm. Accessed March 15, 2009.

Karr CJ, Rivara FP, Cummings P: Severe injury among Hispanic and non-Hispanic white children in Washington state, *Public Health Rep* 120(1):19–24, 2005.

Leblanc J, Pless I, King W et al: Home safety measures and the risk of unintentional injury among young children: a multi-centre case control study, *Can Med Assoc J* 175(8):883–887, 2006.

Mallonee S: Injuries among Hispanics in the United States: implications for research, *J Transcult Nurs* 14(3):217–226, 2003.

Martin S: Everyone should wear a helmet, *Can Med Assoc J* 167(11):1282, 2002.

Mulvaney C, Kendrick D: Engagement in safety practices to prevent home injuries in preschool children among white and non-white ethnic minority families, *Inj Prev* 10(6):375, 2004.

National Center for Health Statistics: *Health: United States, 2002 with urban and rural chartbook,* Washington DC, 2008, U.S. Government Printing Office.

Nazarko L: Reducing the risk of falls in the care home, *Nurs Residential Care* 9(11):524–526, 2007.

Park M, Tang JH: Changing the practice of physical restraint use in acute care, *J Gerontol Nurs* 33(2):9–16, 2007.

Schiller J, Bramarow E, Dey A: Fall injury episodes among noninstitutionalized older adults, United States 2001–2003, *Adv Data* 392:1–16, 2007.

Schlundt D, Warren R, Miller S: Reducing unintentional injuries on the nation's highways: a literature review, *J Health Care Poor Underserved* 15(1):76–98, 2004.

Sclater A, Alagiakrishnan K: Orthostatic hypotension. A primary care primer for assessment and treatment, *Geriatrics* 59(8):22, 2004.

Sharer, J: Tackling sundowning in a patient with Alzheimer's disease, *Medsurg Nursing* 17(1):27–29, 2008.

Shenassa ED, Stubbendick A, Brown MJ: Social disparities in housing and related pediatric injury: a multilevel study, *Am J Public Health* 94(4):633, 2004.

Sung H, Chang A, Abbey J: The effects of preferred music on agitation of older people with dementia in Taiwan, *Int J Geriatr Psychiatry* 21:999–1000, 2006.

Vassallo M, Vignaraja R, Sharma J et al: Tranquiliser use as a risk factor for falls in hospital patients, *Int J Clin Pract* 60(5):549–552, 2006.

Warner BL, Kenney BD, Rice M: Washing machine related injuries in children: a continuing threat, *Injury Prev* 9(4):357, 2003.

Wright D, Fitzpatrick K: Psychosocial correlates of substance use behaviors among African American youth, *Adolescence*, 39(156):653–667, 2004.

Risk for perioperative positioning Injury   *Terri A. Foster, RN, BSN, CNOR*

NANDA-I

Definition

At risk for inadvertent anatomical and physical changes as a result of positioning or equipment used during an invasive/surgical procedure

Risk Factors

Disorientation; edema; emaciation; immobilization; muscle weakness; obesity; sensory/perceptual disturbances due to anesthesia (NANDA-I, 2009).

High pressure for short periods of time and low pressure for extended periods of time are risk factors for tissue injury (AORN, 2008).

NOC   (Nursing Outcomes Classification)

Suggested NOC Outcomes

Circulation Status, Immobility Consequences: Physiological, Joint Movement, Neurological Status, Respiratory Status, Risk Control, Sensory Function, Skeletal Function, Tissue Integrity: Skin and Mucous Membranes, Tissue Perfusion: Peripheral

---

Example NOC Outcome with Indicators

Tissue Perfusion: Peripheral as evidenced by the following indicators: Peripheral edema/Localized extremity pain/Skin breakdown/Muscle cramps/Peripheral pulses/Numbness/Tingling/Necrosis (Rate the outcome and indicators of **Tissue Perfusion: Peripheral:** 1 = severe, 2 = substantial, 3 = moderate, 4 = mild, 5 = none [see Section I].)

Client Outcomes

Client Will (Specify Time Frame):

• Demonstrate unchanged skin condition, with exception of the incision, throughout the perioperative experience
• Demonstrate resolution of redness of the skin at points of pressure within 30 minutes after pressure is eliminated
• Will remain injury-free related to surgical positioning, including intact skin and absence of pain and/or numbness associated with surgical positioning
• Demonstrate unchanged or improved physical mobility from preoperative status
• Demonstrate unchanged or improved cardiovascular and respiratory status from preoperative status
• Demonstrate unchanged or improved peripheral sensory integrity from preoperative status
• Maintain sense of privacy and dignity

● = Independent   ▲ = Collaborative   **EBN** = Evidence-Based Nursing   **EB** = Evidence-Based

NIC   (Nursing Interventions Classification)

Suggested NIC Interventions

Circulatory Precautions, Fall Prevention, Neurological Monitoring, Peripheral Sensation Management, Positioning: Intraoperative, Pressure Ulcer Prevention, Risk Identification, Skin Surveillance, Surgical Precautions

Example NIC Activities—Positioning: Intraoperative

Use an adequate number of personnel to transfer patient; Maintain client's proper body alignment

Nursing Interventions and *Rationales*

General Interventions for Any Surgical Client

- Recognize that there is a new accountability for perioperative nurses in the need to maintain skin integrity. **EB:** *As a result of research and evidence-based practice, all nurses have been mandated to manage skin integrity—this includes perioperative RN's—it is difficult to ignore this mandate (Brazen, 2007).*

Prevention of Pressure Ulcers

- Identify clients at risk for pressure ulcer development so that cost-effective, evidence-based preventive measures can be instituted. **EB:** *All surgical clients are at risk for pressure ulcer development. A literature review showed that most pressure ulcers occur within several days after surgery, and this delay in presentation can contribute to the surgery being overlooked as the trigger event (Sewchuk, Padula, & Osborne, 2006). One study stated that all surgical clients are at moderate to severe risk for pressure ulcer development (Price et al, 2005).*
- Recognize that clients undergoing cardiac surgical procedures are at increased risk of developing a pressure ulcer, especially below the waist or in the occiput area. **EB:** *In one study, 52.9% of all pressure ulcers occurred on the heels, and most of these clients underwent cardiac surgery (26 out of 37) (Sewchuk, Padula, & Osborne, 2006).*
- Use pressure-reducing devices and pressure-relieving mattresses as necessary to prevent ulcer formation. **EB:** *A randomized controlled study showed that using a viscoelastic polymer pad reduced pressure ulcer development by half in comparison to using a standard OR mattress. Research studies have shown the following: pressure ulcer occurrence decreases with the use of a fluid pressure-reducing mattress along with comprehensive staff education (Sewchuk, Padula, & Osborne, 2006). The standard 2–inch thick operating room (OR) table mattress significantly contributes to the development of pressure ulcers (Scott-Williams, 2006). Up to 38% of surgical clients developed pressure ulcers when using a standard OR mattress versus 7% when using a pressure-relieving mattress (Scott-Williams, 2006).*
- Recognize that extended pressure on the scalp can cause localized alopecia postoperatively. **EB:** *Research shows that the likelihood of alopecia developing can be reduced if the head is repositioned every 30 minutes (Steris, 2004).*
- Avoid using rolled towels and bolsters made using towels, sheets, etc., as they tend to produce high and inconsistent pressures (Goodman, 2006). Special positioning devices are available for use that redistribute pressure.
- Avoid covering positioning devices as the material used to cover the device reduces the effectiveness of the positioning device (Goodman, 2006; St Arnaud & Paquin, 2008).
- Recognize that the nurse must demonstrate knowledge of not only the equipment, but also anatomy and the application of physiological principles in order to properly position the client. **EBN:** *Pre-planning ensures that the correct positioning devices are available and in good working condition, and that appropriate numbers of personnel are available to position the client safely and appropriately (AORN, 2008).*
- A preoperative assessment should be completed to identify physical alterations that may require addition precautions for procedure-specific positioning, to identify specific procedural positioning needs, type of anesthesia, etc. (AORN, 2008).

• = Independent   ▲ = Collaborative   **EBN** = Evidence-Based Nursing   **EB** = Evidence-Based

- Monitor pressure being applied to the client intraoperatively by staff, equipment, and/or instruments. An adequate clearance of 2 to 3 inches should be maintained in order to protect feet and protuberant parts from over bed tables, mayo stands, and frames (Phillips, 2007). **EB:** *Injury due to retraction and manipulation of tissue has been observed during pelvic procedures (femoral nerve injuries) as well as during hip surgery (sciatic nerve injuries), and head straps can cause facial nerve injury if too tight (Phillips, 2007).*
- Pad all bony prominences. **EB:** *Pressure over bony prominences causes blood vessel compression, which in turn diminishes the flow of oxygen and nutrients to the area, which eventually results in cell death (Goodman, 2006).*
- Recognize that reddened areas or areas injured by pressure should not be massaged. **EB:** *One research study showed that pressure ulcer incidence was reduced 38% in non-massaged versus massaged areas (Goodman, 2006).*
- Implement measures to prevent inadvertent hypothermia. *Anesthesia can compromise perfusion by causing hypotension and hypothermia. When coupled with the client being immobile on a noncompliant surface for an extended time period, increases vulnerability for pressure ulcer development during surgery (St-Arnaud & Paquin, 2008).*

Positioning the Perioperative Client

- Ensure that linens on the OR table are free of wrinkles. *Folds and creases in linen can cause pressure on the skin (Phillips, 2007).*
- Lock the OR table, cart, or bed and stabilize the mattress before transfer/positioning of the client. *Clients should be monitored when on the OR table, at all times.* **EBN:** *Studies showed that a lack of clear communication about who should be watching the client has contributed to falls (AORN, 2008).*
- Lift rather than pull or slide the client when positioning to reduce the incidence of skin injury from shearing and/or friction (Phillips, 2007). **EBN:** *Sliding or pulling the client can cause shearing force and/or friction (AORN, 2008).*
- Ensure that appropriate numbers of personnel are present to assist in positioning the client. *Use of transfer devices and adequate staff, when moving/positioning clients, decreases frictional forces, tissue bruising, and pressure injury (Scott-Williams, 2006).* **EBN:** *A minimum of two people should assist an awake client to transfer from a cart/bed to the OR table: one person on the stretcher side to assist the client onto the OR table and a second person on the far side of the OR table to prevent the client from falling off the table (Phillips, 2007). A minimum of four persons are necessary when transferring/ positioning an anesthetized, unconscious, obese, or weak client (Evans, 2005; Phillips, 2007).*
- Recognize that optimally, clients (especially those with limited range of motion/mobility) should be asked to position themselves under the nurse's guidance before induction of anesthesia so that he or she can verify that a position of comfort has been obtained.
- Ensure nerves are protected by positioning extremities carefully. *Improperly positioned arms, hands, shoulders, legs, or feet can lead to serious injury or paralysis (OR Insider, 2006).*
- Avoid hyperextension of joints. **EB:** *Hyperextension of joints can cause postoperative pain and permanent injury to extremities (Phillips, 2007).*
- Use slow and smooth movements during position of clients. **EB:** *Slow movements allow the body time to adjust to circulatory and respiratory changes, and also allow the staff to have better control of the client's body (Phillips, 2007).*
- Place a pillow under the back of the knees to relieve lower back pressure. **EB:** *Flexing hips and knees aids in keeping the client in correct position and protects common peroneal & tibial nerves. Pillows placed directly in the popliteal space can injure the peroneal and tibial nerves (St. Armand & Paquin, 2008).*
- Reassess the client after positioning and periodically during the procedure for maintenance of proper alignment and skin integrity. **EBN:** *Changes in position can expose or injure body parts (e.g., shearing, friction, compression) that were originally protected and the safety strap can shift and apply increased pressure (AORN, 2008).*
- Monitor intraocular pressure when client is in prone or knee-chest position. **EB:** *Compression and perioperative central retinal artery occlusion can occur with pressure to the eyes (Price et al, 2005).*
- Position hips in proper alignment with knees flexed. Unaligned hips can cause pressure to the low back and hip joints. *When strained, hips are prone to lumbar plexus damage (Millsap, 2006).*

● = Independent   ▲ = Collaborative   **EBN** = Evidence-Based Nursing   **EB** = Evidence-Based

- Position the arms extended on armboards so that they do not extend beyond a 90–degree angle. Do not position arms at sides unless surgically necessary. **EB:** *Positioning at a <90–degree angle decreases the risk of a stretching injury to the brachial plexus and possible compression or occlusion injury to the subclavian and axillary arteries. When positioning arms at sides is necessary, place the arms beneath the sheet and bring the sheet over the top of the arm and then tuck the sheet beneath the mattress, so the arm can't fall off the mattress and hang over the metal edge of the table, where it is exposed to being leaned against by the surgical team (AORN, 2008).*
- Prevent pooling of preparative solutions, blood, irrigation, urine, and feces. *Moisture can predispose the client to pressure ulcer development.*
- Keep the client appropriately covered during the procedure. *Reducing unnecessary exposure provides privacy and dignity for the client during positioning and also helps in the prevention of hypothermia (Phillips, 2007; AORN, 2008).*
- If the client is positioned in Trendelenburg/Reverse Trendelenburg or with the head of the bed raised/lowered, every attempt should be made to lift the client for several seconds, prior to prepping and draping, to allow the skin to realign itself. *When raising/lowering the head of the bed or placing the client in Trendelenburg/Reverse Trendelenburg position, gravity can cause the skeleton to be pulled, which in turn can lead to tearing, folding, and/or stretching of tissue (Rothrock, 2007).*
- Recognize that clients positioned in lithotomy position, should be kept in this position for as short a time as possible. **EB:** *One research review suggests that the client's legs be removed from lithotomy positioning devices every 2 hours if the procedure is expected to last 4 hours or longer (AORN, 2008).*
- Position the client's legs parallel and uncrossed. *Crossing of the client's ankles and legs creates occlusive pressure on blood vessels and nerves that can lead to pressure necrosis and also place the client at risk for development of a deep vein thrombosis (Phillips, 2007).*
- Maintain normal body alignment. *Misalignment, flexion, extension, and rotation may cause muscle and nerve damage, as well as airway interference; pressure on the carotid sinus can cause arrhythmias; and restricted venous outflow can occur with extreme rotation of the head (St Arnaud & Paquin, 2008).*
- When applying body supports and restraint straps (safety belt), apply loosely and secure over waist or mid-thigh at least 2 inches above knees, avoiding bony prominences by placing a blanket between the strap and the client. **EB:** *Belts, positioned directly over the knees cause compression of the peroneal nerve against the fibula (St. Armand & Paquin 2008).*
- Check equipment to verify it is in good working order and is used according to manufacturer's instructions. **EB:** *Equipment that is working properly leads to client safety and aids in improved exposure of the surgical site (AORN, 2008). Many beds have a weight limit for safe use; therefore, it is necessary to check the equipment to ensure that it will tolerate the client's weight (Phillips, 2007).* **EBN:** *A research review of 16 incident reports found that 63% involved using positioning equipment with specific weight limits on clients above the specified weight limit (AORN, 2008).*
- Assess the client's skin integrity immediately postoperatively. **EB:** *Assess and document postoperative skin/tissue integrity focusing on areas with constant pressure during the procedure and limb function for nerve damage (St. Arnaud & Paquin, 2008).*
- Remove client jewelry before surgery because it can cause pressure injury, become entangled in bedding, or catch on equipment during transfer (AORN, 2008).
- Recognize that complete, concise, accurate documentation of client assessment and use of positioning devices is imperative. For information on specific positioning—Supine, Prone, Lateral, Lithotomy, Trendelenburg, Reverse Trendelenburg—please refer to Phillips NF: *Berry & Kohn's operating room technique,* ed 11, Philadelphia, 2007, Mosby.

Ⓔvolve   See the EVOLVE website for Weblinks for client education resources.

REFERENCES

AORN: Recommended practices for positioning the patient in the perioperative practice setting. In *AORN Standards and Recommended Practices for Perioperative Nursing,* Denver, 2008, The Association of Perioperative Registered Nurses.

Brazen L: OR RNs lead the way in managing surgical patients' skin integrity. Nurse.com CE. Course=NW0022b. www.nurse.com/ce. Accessed March 19, 2007.

Evans G: Time out: patient positioning a safety essential, *OR Today* 36–37, 2005.

Goodman T: Positioning: a patient safety initiative, *Infect Control Today* Sep:53, 2003. Millsap CC: Pay attention to patient positioning! *RN* 69(1):59–63, 2006.

Millsap CC: Pay attention to patient positioning! *RN* 69(1):59–63, 2006.

● = Independent   ▲ = Collaborative   **EBN** = Evidence-Based Nursing   **EB** = Evidence-Based

OR Insider (supplement to Nursing Management): Preventing intracoperative positioning injuries. *Nurs Manage* 37(7, Supplement OR Insider), pp 9–10, 2006.

Phillips NF: *Berry and Kohn's operating room technique, positioning the patient*, ed 11, Philadelphia, 2007, Mosby.

Price MC, Whitney JD, King CA et al: Development of a risk assessment tool for intraoperative pressure ulcer. *JWOCN* 32(1):19–30, 2005.

Rothrock J: *Alexander's care of the patient in surgery*, ed 13, St Louis, 2007, Mosby.

Scott-Williams S: Prevent patient positioning problems, *Outpatient Surgery Magazine* 7(12), 2006.

Sewchuk D, Padula C, Osborne E: Prevention and early diction of pressure ulcers in patients undergoing cardiac surgery, *AORN J* 84(1):75–96, 2006.

St. Arnaud D, Paquin MJ: Safe positioning for the neurosurgical patient. *AORN J* 87(6):1156–1168, 2008.

Steris: Intraoperative patient positioning. It's more than just comfort. Study Guide 2004. www.steris.com. Accessed January 9, 2009.

Insomnia

⊖volve

Judith A. Floyd, PhD, RN, FAAN, Jean D. Humphries, PhD(c), RN, and Elizabeth S. Jenuwine, PhD, MLIS

NANDA-I

Definition

Frequent complaints of disruption in amount and quality of sleep that impairs functioning

Defining Characteristics

Observed changes in affect; observed lack of energy; increased work/school absenteeism; client reports changes in mood; client reports decreased health status; client reports decreased quality of life; client reports difficulty concentrating; client reports difficulty falling asleep; client reports difficulty staying asleep; client reports dissatisfaction with sleep (current); client reports increased accidents; client reports lack of energy; client reports nonrestorative sleep; client reports sleep disturbances that produce next-day consequences; client reports waking up too early

Related Factors (r/t)

Activity pattern (e.g., timing, amount); anxiety; depression; environmental factors (e.g., ambient noise, daylight/darkness exposure, ambient temperature/humidity, unfamiliar setting); fear; gender-related hormonal shifts; grief; inadequate sleep hygiene (current); intake of stimulants; intake of alcohol; impairment of normal sleep pattern (e.g., travel, shift work); interrupted sleep; medications; parental responsibilities; physical discomfort (e.g., body temperature, pain, shortness of breath, cough, gastroesophageal reflux, nausea, incontinence/urgency); stress (e.g., ruminative pre-sleep pattern)

NOC (Nursing Outcomes Classification)

Suggested NOC Outcomes

Comfort Level, Pain Level, Personal Well-Being, Psychosocial Adjustment: Life Change, Quality of Life, Rest, Sleep

Example NOC Outcome with Indicators
Sleep as evidenced by the following indicators: Hours of sleep/Sleep pattern/Sleep quality/Sleep efficiency/Feels rejuvenated after sleep/Sleeps consistently through the night (Rate the outcome and indicators of **Sleep:** 1 = severely compromised, 2 = substantially compromised, 3 = moderately compromised, 4 = mildly compromised, 5 = not compromised [see Section I].)

Client Outcomes

Client Will (Specify Time Frame):

- Wake up less frequently during night
- Awaken refreshed and not be fatigued during day
- Fall asleep without difficulty
- Verbalize plan to implement sleep promoting routines

● = Independent   ▲ = Collaborative   **EBN** = Evidence-Based Nursing   **EB** = Evidence-Based

(Nursing Interventions Classification)

Suggested NIC Intervention

Sleep Enhancement

Example NIC Activities—Sleep Enhancement
Monitor/record patient's sleep pattern and number of sleep hours; Encourage patient to establish a bedtime routine to facilitate transition from wakefulness to sleep

Nursing Interventions and *Rationales*

- Obtain a sleep history including bedtime routines, sleep patterns, use of medications and stimulants, and use of complementary/alternative medical practices. *Assessment of sleep behavior and patterns is an important part of any health status examination (Lee & Ward, 2005; Mastin et al, 2006; Humphries, 2008).*
- From the history assess the degree and chronic nature of insomnia. For clients with chronic insomnia, evaluate interventions listed. *Adults can be considered to have insomnia if their daytime tiredness and sleepiness is accompanied by one or more or the following several nights/week: (a) inability to initiate sleep within 30 minutes; (b) awakening during the night with inability to reinitiate sleep within 30 minutes; and/or (c) sleeping less than 6 hours/night; insomnia is considered chronic if it continues beyond 6 weeks (Ohayon & Reynolds, 2009).*
- Avoid negative associations with ability to sleep. *Fear of not sleeping can interfere with sleep initiation and maintenance (Stepanski & Wyatt, 2003).*
- Have client arise from bed to participate in calming activities whenever anxious about failure to fall asleep. **EBN:** *Restricting use of bed to sleeping promotes sleep initiation (Wang et al, 2005).*
- Avoid a focus on the clock and subsequent worry about sleep time lost to sleeplessness. **EBN:** *Controlling negative stimuli promotes sleep initiation (Wang et al, 2005).*
- Focus on positive aspects of life. **EB:** *Subjects' focus on gratitude was related to other positive pre-sleep cognitions, shorter times to fall asleep, longer nighttime sleep, and better daytime function (Wood et al, 2009).*
- Assist clients with chronic insomnia to select nights for sleeping pill use if discontinuance of sleeping pills is not feasible. **EB:** *An effective early phase of treatment for chronic insomnia included use of sleeping pills 2 to 3 nights per week while subjects simultaneously learned cognitive-behavioral strategies for relaxing the mind and body prior to sleep and during the night (Morin et al, 2009).*
- Consider use of full-emersion baths or foot-baths in the evening. **EBN:** *A systematic review showed that passive heating by use of warm baths relaxed sleepers and increased deep sleep in the elderly (Liao, 2002).* **EB:** *Small manipulations of core body and skin temperature have been found to affect sleep onset in adults including normal older sleepers and elderly insomniacs (Raymann & VanSomeren, 2008).*
- ▲ Assess level of pain and use available pharmacological and nonpharmacological approaches to pain management. Provide pain relief shortly before bedtime and position client comfortably for sleep. *Chronic pain leads to chronic sleep disruption and sleep disruption increases the perception of pain (Stiefel & Stagno, 2004; Roehrs & Roth, 2005).* **EB:** *Duration of sleep is related to next day pain in general population of men and women (Smith et al, 2007; Edwards et al, 2008).*
- Assess level of anxiety. If the client is anxious, use relaxation techniques. (See further Nursing Interventions and Rationales for **Anxiety.**) **EBN and EB:** *A systematic review shows the use of relaxation techniques to promote sleep in people with chronic insomnia has been shown to be effective (Wang et al, 2005).*
- ▲ Assess for signs of depression: depressed mood state, statements of hopelessness, poor appetite. Refer for counseling as appropriate. *Many symptoms associated with sleep disruption arise from central nervous system hyperarousal in the depressed client (Sateia, 2009).* **EBN:** *Several metaanalyses have found that undiagnosed depressive disorders sometimes account for what is presumed to be normal age-related sleep change (Floyd, 2002).*
- ▲ Assess for signs of sleep apnea and restless leg syndrome; if present, refer to an accredited sleep clinic for evaluation. *If the client is waking frequently during the night, other primary sleep disorders*

● = Independent   ▲ = Collaborative   **EBN** = Evidence-Based Nursing   **EB** = Evidence-Based

may be the cause (Cole & Richards, 2007; Cuellar, Strumpf, & Ratcliff, 2007). **EBN:** *Several meta-analyses have found that undiagnosed sleep disorders sometimes account for what is presumed to be normal age-related sleep change (Floyd, 2002).*

▲ Assess for signs of drug use/abuse including prescription, OTC, illicit, and social drugs (e.g., alcohol, caffeine); suggest lifestyle change and refer for addiction counseling as appropriate. *Stimulants and mood alternators can greatly disrupt the circadian rhythm of sleep and waking and disrupt sleep (Templin et al, 2006).*

• Supplement other interventions with teaching about sleep and sleep promotion. (See further Nursing Interventions and Rationales for **Readiness for enhanced Sleep.**) **EB:** *A systematic review found that sleep education alone is not an effective treatment for chronic insomnia (McCurry et al, 2007).*

Geriatric

• Assessments for pain, anxiety, depression, sleep apnea, restless leg syndrome, and substance use/abuse are especially important in the elderly if they report sleep problems because insomnia is often secondary to these conditions (Sateia, 2009).
• Interventions discussed above may be used with geriatric clients.
• In addition see the Geriatric Section of Nursing Interventions and Rationales for **Readiness for enhanced Sleep.**

Home Care

• Assessments and interventions may be adapted for use in home care.
• In addition, see the Home Care Section of Nursing Interventions and Rationales for **Readiness for enhanced Sleep.**

Client/Family Teaching and Discharge Planning

• Teach family about normal sleep and promote adoption of behaviors that enhance it. See Nursing Interventions and Rationales for **Readiness for enhanced Sleep.**
• Teach family about sleep deprivation and how to avoid it. See Nursing Interventions and Rationales for **Sleep deprivation.**
• Advise family of importance of not disrupting sleep of others unnecessarily. See Nursing Interventions and Rationales for **Disturbed Sleep pattern.**
• Help family differentiate insomnia from sleep interruptions and sleep deprivation; they may cause interruptions and deprivation, but they do not cause the client's insomnia, i.e., inability to initiate and maintain normal sleep.

⊖volve   See the EVOLVE website for Weblinks for client education resources.

REFERENCES

Cole C, Richards K: Sleep disruption in older adults. Harmful and by no means inevitable, it should be assessed and treated, *Am J Nurs* 107(5):40, 2007.

Cuellar NG, Strumpf NE, Ratcliff SJ: Symptoms of restless legs syndrome in older adults: outcomes on sleep quality, sleepiness, fatigue, depression, and quality of life, *J Am Geriatr Soc* 55(9):1387–1392, 2007.

Edwards RR, Almeida DM, Klick B et al: Duration of sleep contributes to next-day pain report in the general population, *Pain* 137(1):202–207, 2008.

Floyd JA: Sleep and aging, *Nurs Clin North Am* 37(4):719, 2002.

Humphries JD: Sleep disruption in hospitalized adults, *Medsurg Nurs* 17(6):391, 2008.

Lee KA, Ward TM: Critical components of a sleep assessment for clinical practice, *Issues Ment Health Nurs* 26:739, 2005.

Liao WC: Effects of passive body heating on body temperature and sleep regulation in the elderly: a systematic review, *Int J Nurs Stud* 39(8):803, 2002.

Mastin DF et al: Assessment of sleep hygiene using the sleep hygiene index, *J Behav Med* 29(3):223, 2006.

McCurry SM et al: Evidence-based psychological treatments for insomnia in older adults, *Psychol Aging* 22(1):18, 2007.

Morin CM et al: Cognitive behavioral therapy, singly and combined with medication, for persistent insomnia: a randomized controlled trial, *JAMA* 301(19):2005, 2009.

Ohayon MM, Reynolds CF: Epidemiological and clinical relevance of insomnia diagnosis algorithms according to the OSM-IV and the International Classification of Sleep Disorders (ICSD), *Sleep Med* 10(7):952, 2009.

Raymann RJ, VanSomeren EJ: Diminished capability to recognize the optimal temperature for sleep initiation may contribute to poor sleep in elderly people, *Sleep* 31(9):1301, 2008.

Roehrs T, Roth T: Sleep and pain: interaction of two vital functions, *Semin Neurol* 25(1):106, 2005.

• = Independent   ▲ = Collaborative   **EBN** = Evidence-Based Nursing   **EB** = Evidence-Based

Stiefel F, Stagno D: Management of insomnia in patients with chronic pain conditions, *CNS Drugs* 18(5):285, 2004.

Sateia MJ: Update on sleep and psychiatric disorders, *Chest* 135(5):1370, 2009.

Smith MT et al: The effects of sleep deprivation on pain inhabitation and spontaneous pain in women, *Sleep* 30(4):494, 2007.

Stepanski E, Wyatt J: Use of sleep hygiene in the treatment of insomnia, *Sleep Med Rev* 7(3):215, 2003.

Templin D et al: Screening for substance use patterns among patients referred for a variety of sleep complaints, *Am J Drug Alcohol Abuse* 32(1):111, 2006.

Wang et al: Cognitive behavioural therapy for primary insomnia: a systematic review, *J Adv Nurs* 50(5):553, 2005.

Wood et al: Gratitude influences sleep through the mechanism of pre-sleep cognitions, *J Psychosom Res* 66(1):43, 2009.

Decreased Intracranial adaptive capacity   *Laura H. McIlvoy, PhD, RN, CCRN, CNRN*   ⊖volve

NANDA-I

Definition

Intracranial fluid dynamic mechanisms that normally compensate for increases in intracranial volumes are compromised, resulting in repeated disproportionate increases in intracranial pressure (ICP) in response to a variety of noxious and nonnoxious stimuli

Defining Characteristics

Baseline ICP greater than 10 mm Hg; disproportionate increases in ICP following a single environmental or nursing maneuver stimulus; repeated increases in ICP of greater than 10 mm Hg for more than 5 minutes following any of a variety of external stimuli; volume-pressure response test variation (volume-pressure ratio of 2, pressure-volume index of less than 10); wide-amplitude ICP waveform (Kirkness, Burr & Cain, 2006)

Related Factors (r/t)

Brain injuries: decreased cerebral perfusion less than or equal to 50 to 60 mm Hg; sustained increase in ICP greater than 10 to 15 mm Hg; systemic hypotension with intracranial hypertension

NOC   (Nursing Outcomes Classification)

Suggested NOC Outcomes

Neurological Status, Neurological Status: Consciousness

Example NOC Outcome with Indicators
Neurological Status as evidenced by the following indicators: Consciousness/Intracranial pressure/Vital signs/Central motor control/Cranial sensory-motor function/Spinal sensory-motor function (Rate the outcome and indicators of **Neurological Status:** 1 = severely compromised, 2 = substantially compromised, 3 = moderately compromised, 4 = mildly compromised, 5 = not compromised [see Section I].)

Client Outcomes

Client Will (Specify Time Frame):

- Experience fewer than five episodes of disproportionate increases in intracranial pressure (DIICP) in 24 hours
- Have neurological status changes that are not triggered by episodes of DIICP
- Have cerebral perfusion pressure (CPP) remaining greater than 60 to 70 mm Hg in adults

NIC   (Nursing Interventions Classification)

Suggested NIC Interventions

Cerebral Edema Management, Cerebral Perfusion Promotion, Intracranial Pressure (ICP) Monitoring, Neurological Monitoring

• = Independent   ▲ = Collaborative   **EBN** = Evidence-Based Nursing   **EB** = Evidence-Based

| **Example NIC Activities—Cerebral Edema Management** |
| Monitor for confusion, changes in mentation, complaints of dizziness, syncope; Allow ICP to return to baseline between nursing activities |

Nursing Interventions and *Rationales*

▲ To assess ICP and CPP effectively:

■ Maintain and display ICP and CPP continuously. ICP data guide therapy and predict outcome. *The only way to determine CPP is to continuously monitor ICP and blood pressure (CPP = MAP − ICP). Continuous monitoring of CPP improves odds of survival at hospital discharge in clients with traumatic brain injury (TBI).* **EBN:** *An elevated P2 component of ICP waveform has been shown not to be a diagnostic criteria of decreased intracranial adaptive capacity (Kirkness, Burr, & Cain, 2006; Brain Trauma Foundation et al, 2007; Fan et al, 2008).*

■ Maintain ICP <20 mm Hg and CPP >60 mm Hg. *The Guidelines for the Management of Severe Brain Injury established the treatment threshold for ICP as >20 mm Hg. These guidelines also state CPP should be maintained at a minimum of 60 mm Hg (Brain Trauma Foundation et al, 2007).*

■ Monitor neurological status frequently using the Glasgow Coma Scale (GCS), noting changes in eye opening, motor response to painful stimuli, and awareness of self, time, and place. *The GCS is the most widely used tool to assess level of consciousness in neurologically injured clients. A decrease of 2 points in a GCS score without identifiable cause (administration of sedation, narcotics, or anesthetic agents) should be reported to the physician (McNett, 2007).*

■ Monitor brain temperature. *Hyperthermia is prevalent in clients with acute brain injury, contributes to increased length of stays, and has been strongly associated with poor outcomes in severe TBI. Brain temperature has been found higher than core temperatures in all published studies. In the absence of brain temperature monitoring, the likelihood of detecting a brain fever is limited (McIlvoy, 2007).*

■ Monitor brain tissue oxygen (PbtO$_2$). **EB:** *Low brain PbtO$_2$ has been significantly correlated with poor outcomes and increased mortality in clients with severe TBI (Vespa, 2006).*

▲ To prevent harmful increases in ICP:

■ Elevate head of bed at least 30 degrees with head in midline position. **EBN:** *Elevating the head of the bed to 30 degrees or greater allows for increased venous drainage that decreases ICP. However, if client is suffering acute stroke, CPP may be compromised with head elevation (Fan, 2004; Murphy et al, 2004, Wojner-Alexandrov et al, 2005; Blissitt, Mitchell, & Newell, 2006; Schulz-Stubner & Thiex, 2006).*

■ Administer sedation per collaborative protocol. **EB:** *Propofol infusions, compared with morphine sulfate infusions, lower ICP; decrease need for paralytic agents, benzodiazepines, pentobarbital, and cerebrospinal fluid (CSF) drainage; and improve outcomes in terms of disability and mortality at 6 months. ICP was higher and CPP lower with endotracheal suctioning among clients who were inadequately sedated compared to clients who were well sedated with propofol. There was no difference in outcome among severe TBI clients sedated with propofol or medazolam (Gemma et al, 2002; Ghori et al, 2007).*

■ Administer pain medication per collaborative protocol. *Propofol in combination with narcotics prevents elevations of ICP in TBI clients. Narcotics do not adversely affect ICP in postcraniotomy clients (Englehard et al, 2004).*

■ Maintain glycemic control per collaborative protocol. **EB:** *Glucose levels exceeding 170 mg/dL during the first 5 days of a severe TBI correlate with prolonged hospital stays and increased mortality. Severe TBI clients treated with insulin therapy to maintain glucose levels less than 110 mg/dL had lower ICP's than a control group treated with insulin only when glucose levels exceeded 220 mg/dL (Jeremitski, Omert, & Dunham, 2005; VanBeek, Schoonheydt, & Becx, 2005).*

■ Maintain normothermia. *Elevation in brain temperature is associated with a rise in ICP. However, antipyretics and external cooling methods are only 40% effective in reducing fever in neurologically injured clients. Research into effective fever management continues (Ogden, Mayer, & Connolly, 2005; McIlvoy, 2007).*

● = Independent ▲ = Collaborative **EBN** = Evidence-Based Nursing **EB** = Evidence-Based

- Maintain optimal oxygenation and ventilation, applying positive end expiratory pressure (PEEP) as needed and avoiding hyperventilation. *Hypoxia causes increased mortality and morbidity in neurologically injured clients. It must be scrupulously avoided or corrected immediately.* **EB:** *PEEP markedly improves gas exchange by increasing pulmonary volumes and is an effective treatment for refractory hypoxemia. PEEP levels of 10 cm H_2O have been found to produce no significant changes in ICP, especially when combined with head of bed elevation of 30 degrees. PEEP levels of 15 cm H_2O produced a significant increase in ICP in one study but did not approach intracranial hypertension. Hyperventilation, especially in the absence of intracranial hypertension, has been found to worsen outcomes in TBI clients and should be avoided, especially in the first 24 hours postinjury (Huynh et al, 2002; Videtta et al, 2002; Brain Trauma Foundation et al, 2007).*
- Limit endotracheal suction passes to two in order to limit ICP increases. Premedicate clients with adequate sedation, opiates, and/or neuromuscular blocking agents to prevent coughing and associated increases in ICP. **EBN and EB:** *Suctioning is known to increase ICP and CPP. In well-sedated or paralyzed clients, these elevations in ICP are attenuated. Particular care must be taken in suctioning clients with spiking ICP patterns, as increases in ICP may be cumulative with each suction pass (Kerr et al, 2001; Gemma et al, 2002).*

▲ To prevent harmful decreases in CPP:
- Maintain euvolemia. **EB:** *Infusing intravenous fluids to sustain normal circulating volume helps maintain normal cerebral blood flow. A fluid balance lower than 594 mL is associated with poor outcomes in traumatic brain injury (Bullock, Chestnut, & Clifton, 2001).*
- Maintain head of bed flat or less than 30 degrees in acute stroke clients. **EB:** *Both mean blood flow velocity in the middle cerebral artery and CPP are increased with lowering head position from 30 degrees to 0 degrees in both ischemic and hemorrhagic stroke clients (Schwarz et al, 2002; Wojner-Alexandrov et al, 2005).*

▲ To treat sustained intracranial hypertension (ICP >20 mm Hg):
- Remove or loosen rigid cervical collars. **EB:** *Most TBI clients are maintained in a rigid cervical collar until cervical spines are clear or as a treatment for cervical injury. Loosening or removing these collars allows for unrestricted venous drainage that lowers ICP (Hunt, Hallworth, & Smith, 2001; Mobbs, Stoodley, & Fuller, 2002).*
- Administer a bolus dose of mannitol and/or hypertonic saline per collaborative protocol. **EB:** *Mannitol is recommended for control of raised ICP after a severe brain injury. Mannitol provides an immediate plasma expanding effect that reduces blood viscosity and increases cerebral blood flow. Five to fifteen minutes later, the osmotic diuretic effect occurs with eventual decrease of cerebral edema. Infusion of hypertonic saline also produces immediate volume expansion and provides an osmotic effect. Initial studies demonstrate that hypertonic saline may decrease ICP more effectively than mannitol with the effect lasting longer. However, the optimal concentration and dosage is unknown (Vialet et al, 2003; Murphy et al, 2004; Battison et al, 2005; Brain Trauma Foundation et al, 2007; Lin et al, 2008).*
- Drain CSF from an intraventricular catheter system per collaborative protocol. **EBN:** *A withdrawal of 3 mL of CSF decreases ICP by 10.1% sustained for 10 minute. CSF drainage has been found to be as effective as mannitol in severe TBI (Kerr et al, 2001; Kinoshita et al, 2006).*
- Administer barbiturates per collaborative protocol. **EB:** *Barbiturates decrease ICP but are associated with clinically significant hypotension that produces detrimental decreases in MAP and CPP. They should only be used in clients that are hemodynamically stable and monitored closely for decreases in blood pressure. Recent studies have shown that barbiturates given for intractable intracranial hypertension increase $PbtO_2$ levels in approximately 70% of clients (Brain Trauma Foundation et al, 2007; Chen et al, 2008; Thorat et al, 2008).*
- Induce moderate hypothermia (32° to 35° C) per collaborative protocol. **EB:** *Reducing body/brain temperatures has been effective in reducing ICP in both traumatic and ischemic brain injuries. A recent metaanalysis suggests that hypothermia maintained for 48 hours reduces mortality and results in favorable neurological outcomes, but only in clients who do not receive barbiturates. The odds of clients developing pneumonia with hypothermia are nearly double those of normothermia. The optimal degree of hypothermia and the timing of induction are under investigation, though it is known that rapid rewarming can increase ICP (Tokutomi et al, 2003; Peterson et al, 2008).*

• = Independent   ▲ = Collaborative   **EBN** = Evidence-Based Nursing   **EB** = Evidence-Based

▲ To treat decreased CPP (sustained CPP <60 mm Hg):
- Administer norepinephrine to raise MAP per collaborative protocol. **EB:** *Vasopressors are frequently used to maintain adequate MAP in support of cerebral perfusion. Norepinephrine is effective in raising MAP and CPP, and may be more effective than dopamine (Johnston et al, 2004; Steiner et al, 2004).*
- Administer hypertonic saline per collaborative protocol. **EB:** *Infusions of hypertonic saline have been found to raise CPP while decreasing ICP (Bentsen et al, 2004; Al-Rawl et al, 2005).*

Ⓔvolve   See the EVOLVE website for Weblinks for client education resources.

REFERENCES

Al-Rawl P, Zygun D, Tseng M et al: Cerebral blood flow augmentation in patients with severe subarachnoid haemorrhage, *Acta Neurchir Suppl* 95:123–127, 2005.

Battison C, Andrews P, Graham C et al: Randomized, controlled trial on the effect of a 20% mannitol solution and a 7.5% saline/6% dextran solution on increased intracranial pressure after brain injury, *Crit Care Med* 33(11):196–202, 2005.

Bentsen G, Breivik H, Lundar T et al: Predictable reduction of intracranial hypertension with hypertonic saline hydroxyethyl starch: a prospective clinical trial in critically ill patients with subarachnoid haemorrhage, *Acta Anaesthesiol Scand* 48(9):1089–1095, 2004.

Blissitt P, Mitchell P, Newell D et al: Cerebrovascular dynamics with head-of-bed elevation in patients with mild or moderate vasospasm after aneurysmal subarachnoid hemorrhage, Amer J Crit Care 15(2):206–210, 2006.

Brain Trauma Foundation, American Association of Neurological Surgeons, and Congress of Neurological Surgeons, Joint Section on Neurotrauma and Critical Care, AANS/CNS: Guidelines for the management of severe traumatic brain injury, ed 3, *J Neurotrauma*, 24(Suppl 1):S1–S106, 2007.

Bullock R, Chestnut R, Clifton G: Management and prognosis of severe traumatic brain injury, *J Neurotrauma* 17(6&7):451–627, 2001.

Chen H, Malhutra N, Oddo M et al: Barbiturate infusion for intractable intracranial hypertension and its effect on brain oxygenation, *Neurosurgery* 63(5):880–887, 2008.

Englehard K, Reeker W, Kochs E et al: Effect of remifentanil on intracranial pressure and cerebral blood flow velocity in patients with head trauma, *Acta Anaesthesiol Scand* 48(4):396–399, 2004.

Fan J: Effect of backrest position on intracranial pressure and cerebral perfusion pressure in individuals with brain injury: a systematic review, *J Neurosci Nurs* 36(5):278–288, 2004.

Fan J, Kirkness C, Vicini P et al: Intracranial pressure waveform morphology and intracranial adaptive capacity, *Amer J Crit Care* 17(6):545–554, 2008.

Gemma M, Tommasino C, Cerri M et al: Intracranial effects of endotracheal suctioning in the acute phase of head injury, *J Neurosurg Anesthesiol* 14(1):50–54, 2002.

Ghori K, Harmon D, Elashaal A et al: Effect of midazolam versus propofol sedation on markers of neurological injury and outcome after isolated head injury: a pilot study, *Critical Care & Resuscitation* 9(2):166–171, 2007.

Hunt K, Hallworth S, Smith M: The effects of rigid collar placement on intracranial and cerebral perfusion pressures, *Anaesthesia* 56(6):511–513, 2001.

Huynh T, Messer M, Sing R et al: Positive end-expiratory pressure alters intracranial and cerebral perfusion pressure in severe traumatic brain injury, *J Trauma* 53(3):488–493, 2002.

Jeremitski E, Omert L, Dunham C: The impact of hyperglycemia in patients with severe brain injury, *J Tra-Inj, Inf, & Crit Care* 58(1):47–60, 2005.

Johnston J, Steiner L, Chatfield D et al: Effect of cerebral perfusion pressure augmentation with dopamine and norepinephrine on global

and focal brain oxygenation after traumatic brain injury, *Inten Care Med* 30(5):791–797 2004.

Kelly D, Goodale D, Williams J et al: Propofol in the treatment of moderate and severe head injury: a randomized prospective double-blinded pilot trial, *J Neurosurgery* 90(6):1042–1052, 1999.

Kenoshita K, Sakurai A, Utagawa T et al: Importance of CPP management using cerebrospinal drainage in severe TBI, *Acta Neurochirurgia* 96(Suppl):S37–S39, 2006.

Kerr M, Weber B, Sereika S et al: Dose response to cerebrospinal fluid drainage on cerebral perfusion in traumatic brain-injured adults, *Neurosurg Focus* 11(4):E1, 2001.

Kirkness C, Burr R, Cain K: Effect of continuous display of cerebral perfusion pressure on outcomes in patients with traumatic brain injury, *Am J Crit Care* 15(6):600–610, 2006.

Lin K, Chou C, Chang W et al: The early response of mannitol infusion in TBI, *Acta Neurologica Taiwanica* 17(1):26–32, 2008.

Mcilvoy LH: Impact of brain temperature and core temperature on ICP and CPP, *J Neurosci Nurs* 39(6):324–331, 2007.

McNett M: A review of the predictive ability of Glasgow Coma Scale scores in head-injured patients, *J Neurosci Nurs* 39(2):68–75, 2007.

Mobbs R, Stoodley M, Fuller J: Effect of cervical hard collar on intracranial pressure after head injury, *ANZ J Surg* 72(6):389–391, 2002.

Murphy N, Auzinger G, Bernel W et al: The effect of hypertonic sodium chloride on intracranial pressure in patients with acute liver failure, *Hepatology* 39(2):464–470, 2004.

O'Donnell J, Lorber B: Use and effectiveness of hypothermia blankets for febrile patients in the intensive care unit, *Clin Infect Dis* 24:1208–1213, 1997.

Ogden A, Mayer S, Connolly E: Hyperosmolar agents in neurosurgical practice: the evolving role of hypertonic saline, *Neurosurgery* 57(2):207–215, 2005.

Peterson K, Carson S, Carnea N et al: Hypothermia treatment for TBI: a systematic review and meta-analysis, *J Neurotrauma* 25:62–71, 2008.

Rauch ME et al: Validation of risk factors for the nursing diagnosis decreased intracranial adaptive capacity, *J Neurosci Nurs* 22(3):173–178, 1990.

Roberts I: Barbiturates for acute traumatic brain injury, *Cochrane Database Syst Rev* (2):CD000033, 2000.

Rossi S, Zanier E, Mauri I et al: Brain temperature, core temperature, and intracranial pressure in acute cerebral damage, *J Neurol Neurosurg Psychiatr* 71(4):448–454, 2001.

Schulz-Stubner S, Thiex R: Raising the head-of-bed by 30 degrees reduces ICP and improves CPP without compromising cardiac output in euvolemic patients with traumatic brain injury and subarachnoid hemorrhage: a practice audit, *Eur J Anaesthesiol* 23:177–180, 2006.

Schwarz S, Georgiadis D, Aschoff A et al: Effects of induced hypertension on intracranial pressure and flow velocities of the middle cerebral arteries in patients with large hemispheric stroke, *Stroke* 33(4):998–1004, 2002.

Steiner L, Johnson A, Czosnyka M et al: Direct comparison of cerebrovascular effects of norepinephrine and dopamine in head-injured patients, *Crit Care Med* 32(4):1049–1054, 2004.

● = Independent   ▲ = Collaborative   **EBN** = Evidence-Based Nursing   **EB** = Evidence-Based

Thorat J, Wang E, Leek et al: Barbiturate therapy for patients with re-fractory intracranial hypertension following severe TBI: its effects on tissue oxygenation, brain temperature, and autoregulation, *J Clin Neurosciences* 15(2):143–148, 2008.Tokutomi T, Morimoto K, Miyagi T et al: Optimal temperature for the management of severe traumatic brain injury: Effect of hypothermia on intracranial pressure, systemic and intracranial hemodynamics, and metabolism, *Neurosurgery* 52(1):102–111, 2003.

VanBeek J, Schoonheydt K, Becx P: Insulin therapy protects the central and peripheral nervous system of intensive care patients, *Neurology* 64:1348–1353, 2005.

Vespa P: Brain tissue oxygen monitoring: a measure of supply and demand, *Crit Care Med* 35(6):1850–1852, 2006.

Vialet R, Albanese J, Thomachot L et al: Isovolume hypertonic solutes (sodium chloride and mannitol) in the treatment of refractory post-traumatic intracranial hypertension: 2 mL/kg 7.5% saline is more effective than 2 ml/kg 20% mannitol, *Crit Care Med* 31(6):1683–1687, 2003.

Videtta W, Villarejo F, Cohen M et al: Effects of positive end-expiratory pressure on intracranial pressure and cerebral perfusion pressure, *Acta Neurochir Suppl* 81:93–97, 2002.

Wojner-Alexandrov A, Gerami Z, Chernyshev O et al: Heads down: flat positioning improves blood flow velocity in acute ischemic stroke, *Neurology* 64:1354–2357, 2005.

Neonatal Jaundice   *David Wilson, MS, RNC*   ⊖volve

NANDA-I

Definition

The yellow orange tint of the neonate's skin and mucous membranes that occurs after 24 hours of life as a result of unconjugated bilirubin in the circulation

Defining Characteristics

Abnormal blood profile (hemolysis; total serum bilirubin >2 mg/dL; inherited disorder; total serum bilirubin in high-risk range on age in hour-specific nomogram); abnormal skin bruising; yellow-orange skin; yellow sclera

Related Factors (r/t)

Abnormal weight loss (>7% to 8% in breastfeeding newborn; 15% in term infant); feeding pattern not well established; infant experiences difficulty making transition to extrauterine life; neonate age 1 to 7 days; stool (meconium) passage delayed

NOC   (Nursing Outcomes Classification)

Suggested NOC Outcomes

Breastfeeding Establishment: Infant, Breastfeeding Maintenance, Bowel Elimination; Parent: Knowledge: Parenting/Infant Care, Risk Detection/Control

Example NOC Outcome with Indicators
Breastfeeding Establishment: Infant as evidenced by the following indicators: Proper alignment and latch-on/Proper areolar grasp/Proper areolar compression/Correct suck and tongue placement/Audible swallow/Minimum eight feedings per day/Urinations per day appropriate for age/Weight gain appropriate for age (Rate the outcome and indicators of **Breastfeeding Establishment: Infant:** 1 = not adequate, 2 = slightly adequate, 3 = moderately adequate, 4 = substantially adequate, 5 = totally adequate [see Section I].)

Client Outcomes

Client (Infant) Will (Specify Time Frame):

- Establish effective feeding pattern (breast or bottle)
- Receive bilirubin assessment and screening within the first week of life to detect increasing levels of serum bilirubin
- Receive appropriate therapy to enhance indirect bilirubin excretion
- Receive nursing assessments to determine risk for severity of jaundice
- Maintain hydration: moist buccal membranes, 4 to 6 wet diapers in 24 hours period, weight loss no greater than 8% of birth weight
- Evacuate stool within 48 hours of birth, and pass 3 to 4 stools per 24 hours by Day 4 of life

● = Independent   ▲ = Collaborative   **EBN** = Evidence-Based Nursing   **EB** = Evidence-Based

Client (Parent[s]) Will (Specify Time Frame):

- Receive information on neonatal jaundice prior to discharge from birth hospital
- Verbalize understanding of physical signs of jaundice prior to discharge
- Verbalize signs requiring immediate health practitioner notification: sleepy infant who does not awaken easily for feedings, fewer than 4 to 6 wet diapers in 24 hour period, fewer than 3 to 4 stools in 24 hours by Day 4, breastfeeds fewer than 8 times per day
- Demonstrate ability to operate home phototherapy unit if prescribed

NIC   (Nursing Interventions Classification)

Suggested NIC Interventions

Parent Education: Infant, Phototherapy: Neonate

Example NIC Activities—Phototherapy: Neonate
Review maternal and infant history for risk factors for hyperbilirubinemia (e.g., Rh or ABO incompatibility, polycythemia, sepsis, prematurity, malpresentation); Observe for signs of jaundice

Nursing Interventions and *Rationales*

- Evaluate maternal and delivery history for risk factors for neonatal jaundice (RhD, ABO, G6PD deficiency, direct Coombs). *Assessment of maternal and neonatal risk factors which may cause jaundice is important in the detection of neonatal jaundice (Cohen, 2006).*
- Perform neonatal gestational age assessment once the newborn has had an initial period of interaction with mother and father. **EB:** *Gestational age assessment is important to determine potential risk factors in the neonatal population. Infants who are born late preterm (34 to 36⁶⁄₇ weeks at birth) are at significantly increased risk for problems related to hyperbilirubinemia, feeding problems, and hospital readmission (Sarici et al, 2004; Hillman, 2007; Smith, Donze, & Schuller, 2007).*
- Encourage breastfeeding within the first hour of the neonate's life. **EB:** *Early feedings increase neonatal intestinal activity, and infant begins establishing intestinal flora; in addition, early breastfeeding promotes enhanced maternal confidence in breastfeeding (Blackburn, 2007; Alex & Gallant, 2008).*
- Encourage skin-to-skin mother-newborn contact shortly after delivery. *Early skin-to-skin mother-baby contact helps promote maternal confidence in nurturing abilities (Alex & Gallant, 2008).*
- Assess infant's skin color at birth and every 8 hours thereafter until birth hospital discharge for the appearance of jaundice. *Initial and ongoing neonatal skin assessment is important in the detection of jaundice (Schwoebel & Gennaro, 2006). Jaundice is visible when bilirubin levels reach 5 to 7 mg/dL (Blackburn, 2007), and is reported to first appear on the face and head, then slowly advance to the trunk, arms, and lower extremities (Cohen, 2006). Skin color alone is not a reliable assessment for neonatal jaundice, therefore it is important that such assessments be supported with empiric serum bilirubin measurements or transcutaneous bilirubin measurements when jaundice is suspected (American Academy of Pediatrics, 2004).*
- Encourage and assist mother with frequent breastfeeding (at least 8 to 12 times per day in the first week of life). *Frequent breastfeeding stimulates neonatal gut motility and enhances stooling, thus decreasing intestinal reabsorption of bilirubin; in addition, frequent breastfeeding stimulates breast milk production (Blackburn, 2007). Exclusive breastfeeding is recommended for neonatal feedings yet is associated with the development of hyperbilirubinemia, not directly as a result of the feeding substrate but perhaps due to decreased caloric intake in the first week of life and a substance in breast milk that may interfere with bilirubin excretion (Blackburn, 2007; Alex & Gallant, 2008).*
- Assist parents with bottle feeding neonate. *Adequate caloric intake is essential for the promotion of stooling and the subsequent elimination of bilirubin from the intestine. Parents are assisted in feeding the neonate to ensure adequate growth and development (Blackburn, 2007; Hockenberry & Wilson, 2009).*
- Avoid feeding supplements such as water, dextrose water, or any other milk substitutes in breastfeeding neonate. **EB:** *Supplements may act to decrease the effective establishment of breastfeeding (American Academy of Pediatrics, 2004; Blackburn, 2007).*
- Assess neonate's stooling pattern in first 48 hours of life. *Delayed stooling may indicate inadequate breast milk intake and may further increase reabsorption of bilirubin from neonate's intestine (Blackburn, 2007).*

• = Independent   ▲ = Collaborative   **EBN** = Evidence-Based Nursing   **EB** = Evidence-Based

▲ Collect and evaluate laboratory blood specimens as prescribed. *Because visual assessments of skin color alone are inadequate to determine rising levels of bilirubin, serum bilirubin measurement may be gathered to evaluate risk for pathology (Schwoebel & Gennaro, 2006). The purpose in monitoring, evaluating, and implementing treatment in moderate to severe cases of neonatal hyperbilirubinemia is to prevent neonatal encephalopathy, an acute central nervous system bilirubin toxicity that is related to the amount of unbound (indirect) bilirubin. Kernicterus describes the yellow staining of brain cells and subsequent necrosis that occurs secondary to exposure to high levels of unconjugated (indirect) bilirubin; kernicterus involves long-term, permanent central nervous system changes (American Academy of Pediatrics, 2004; Blackburn, 2007).*

▲ Monitor transcutaneous bilirubin level in jaundiced neonate per unit protocol or at least once every 8 hours. *Noninvasive bilirubin monitoring is a safe and effective means for monitoring bilirubin levels and determining risk for increasing serum bilirubin levels (American Academy of Pediatrics, 2004).*

• Perform hour-specific total serum bilirubin risk assessment prior to newborn's birth center discharge and document results of same. **EB:** *The use of an hour-specific nomogram for designation of risk in healthy, late preterm and term infants, as well as clinical risk factors, may be used to determine the relative risk of rapidly increasing bilirubin levels requiring medical intervention such as phototherapy (American Academy of Pediatrics, 2004; Bhutani et al, 2006).*

• Monitor newborn for signs of inadequate breast milk or formula intake: dry oral mucous membranes, fewer than 4 to 6 wet diapers per 24 hours, no stool in 24 hours, body weight loss greater than 7% to 8% in breastfeeding infant. *Inadequate intake of breast milk in the neonatal period has been identified as a risk factor for the development of hyperbilirubinemia (Alex & Gallant, 2008).*

• Assist mother with breastfeeding and assess latch-on. *Successful breastfeeding in the first few weeks of life is associated with decreased levels of serum bilirubin (Blackburn, 2007).*

• Encourage alternate methods for providing expressed breast milk if maternal health status is compromised (use of expressed breast milk) and assist mother with collection of breast milk via use of breast pump or hand expression. *Alternate feeding methods for the ingestion of breast milk may be used to enhance milk intake necessary to promote stooling and enhance bilirubin excretion (Alex & Gallant, 2008).*

• Encourage father's participation in newborn care by changing diapers, helping position newborn for breastfeeding, and holding newborn while mother rests. Weigh newborn daily. *Daily weights assist in the detection of excess weight loss, which is often indicative of inadequate caloric intake (Alex & Gallant, 2008).*

▲ When ordered, place seminude infant (diaper only) under prescribed amount of phototherapy lights. **EB:** *Phototherapy is the primary therapy used to treat mild to moderate neonatal indirect (unconjugated) hyperbilirubinemia; phototherapy enhances indirect bilirubin excretion. In order for phototherapy to be effective the infant must have a large skin surface area exposed to the light source (Stokowski, 2006; Blackburn, 2007).*

• Protect infant's eyes from phototherapy light source with eye shields. Remove eye shields periodically when infant is removed from light source for feeding and parent-infant interaction. *Retinal damage may occur from light exposure (Stokowski, 2006; Blackburn, 2007).*

• Monitor infant's hydration status, fluid intake, skin status, and body temperature while undergoing phototherapy. *Transient side effects of phototherapy include increased body temperature, increased insensible water loss, increased gastrointestinal water loss (loose stools), lethargy, irritability, and poor feeding. There is no evidence that removing the infant for parent-infant interaction during feedings and for brief caregiving activities prevents the effectiveness of phototherapy when the infant has mild to moderate hyperbilirubinemia (Blackburn, 2007).*

▲ Collect and evaluate laboratory blood specimens (total serum bilirubin) while infant is undergoing phototherapy. *Transcutaneous bilirubin measurements do not provide an adequate estimate of serum bilirubin level and are not effective once phototherapy has been initiated (American Academy of Pediatrics, 2004).*

• Encourage continuation of breastfeeding and infant care activities such as changing diapers while infant is being treated with phototherapy; phototherapy may be interrupted for breastfeeding. **EB:** *In most cases breastfeeding is not interrupted for phototherapy; the benefits of breastfeeding exceed any potential harm (American Academy of Pediatrics, 2004). If the infant's oral intake with breastfeeding is inadequate, the American Academy of Pediatrics (2004) recommends supplementation with expressed breast milk or formula.*

• Provide emotional support for parent(s) of infant undergoing phototherapy. *Separation of the infant from the mother for phototherapy disrupts parent-infant interaction, and may promote parental stress and decrease the effective establishment of breastfeeding (Blackburn, 2007).*

Multicultural

• Assess infants of Chinese ethnicity for early rising bilirubin levels, especially when breastfeeding. **EB:** *Studies have shown Chinese and other Asian newborns to have higher peak serum bilirubin levels than Caucasian and African American newborns (Blackburn, 2007; Huang et al, 2009).*
• Encourage early and exclusive breastfeeding among Chinese and other Asian newborns. *Early and exclusive breastfeeding may serve to increase elimination of bilirubin in stool (Blackburn, 2007).*
• Assess Chinese and other Asian newborns suspected of being jaundiced with a serum bilirubin level or transcutaneous monitor. *Skin color alone is not a reliable assessment for neonatal jaundice, therefore it is important that such assessments be supported with empiric serum bilirubin measurements or transcutaneous bilirubin measurements when jaundice is suspected (American Academy of Pediatrics, 2004).*

Client/Family Teaching and Discharge Planning

• Teach the breastfeeding mother and support persons about the appearance of jaundice (yellow or orange color of skin) after birth center discharge, and provide health care resource telephone number for parents to call for concerns related to newborn's care. **EB:** *Follow-up for evaluation of jaundice and feeding is recommended by the American Academy of Pediatrics (2004).*
• Teach parents regarding the signs of inadequate milk intake: fewer than 3 to 4 stools by Day 4, fewer than 4 to 6 wet diapers in 24 hours, and dry oral mucous membranes; additional danger signs include a sleepy baby that does not awaken for breastfeeding, or appears lethargic (decreased activity level from usual newborn pattern). *Providing information about jaundice and effective breastfeeding may serve to decrease risk factors associated with increasing bilirubin levels (Alex & Gallant, 2008).*
• Teach parents to avoid placing infant in sunlight at home to treat jaundice. *Exposure of the neonate to sunlight is not safe (American Academy of Pediatrics, 2004).*
▲ Teach the parent(s) about the importance of medical follow up in the first several days of life for the evaluation of jaundice. *Because of earlier postpartum hospital discharge, follow-up visits in the first several days of life are important for the evaluation of breastfeeding, stooling and voiding pattern (hydration), and jaundice (American Academy of Pediatrics, 2004).*
• Teach parents about the use of phototherapy (hospital or home, as prescribed), the proper use of the phototherapy equipment, feedings, and assessment of hydration, body temperature, skin status, and urine and stool output. *Information is provided to the parents of the infant undergoing phototherapy to prevent misinformation about the condition and treatment of same, and to decrease parental anxiety and stress (Hockenberry & Wilson, 2009).*

ⓔvolve   See the EVOLVE website for Weblinks for client education resources.

References

Alex M, Gallant DP: Toward understanding the connections between infant jaundice and infant feeding, *J Pediatr Nurs* 23(6):429–438, 2008.

American Academy of Pediatrics: Management of hyperbilirubinemia in the newborn infant 35 or more weeks of gestation, *Pediatrics* 114(1):297–316, 2004.

Bhutani VK, Johnson LH, Schwoebel A et al: A systems approach for neonatal hyperbilirubinemia in term and near-term newborns, *J Obstet Gynecol Neonatal Nurs* 35(4):444–455, 2006.

Blackburn ST: *Maternal, fetal, & neonatal physiology: a clinical perspective,* ed 3, St Louis, 2007, Elsevier.

Cohen SM: Jaundice in the full-term newborn, *Pediatr Nurs* 32(3):202–207, 2006.

Hillman N: Hyperbilirubinemia in the late preterm infant, *Newb Infant Nurs Rev* 7(2):91–94, 2007.

Hockenberry MJ, Wilson D: *Wong's essentials of pediatric nursing,* ed 8, St. Louis, 2009, Elsevier.

Huang A, Tai BC, Wong LY et al: Differential risk for early breastfeeding jaundice in a multi-ethnic Asian cohort, *Ann Acad Med Singapore* 38(3):217–224, 2009.

Sarici SU, Serdar MA, Korkmaz A et al: Incidence, course, and prediction of hyperbilirubinemia in near-term and term newborns, *Pediatrics* 113(4):775–780, 2004.

• = Independent   ▲ = Collaborative   **EBN** = Evidence-Based Nursing   **EB** = Evidence-Based

Schwoebel A, Gennaro S: A systems approach for neonatal hyperbilirubinemia in term and near-term newborns, *J Obstet Gynecol Neonatal Nurs* 35(4):444–455, 2006.

Smith JR, Donze A, Schuller L: An evidence-based review of hyperbilirubinemia in the late preterm infant, with implications for practice management, follow-up, and breastfeeding support, *Neonatal Netw* 26(6):395–405, 2007.

Stokowski LA: Fundamentals of phototherapy for neonatal jaundice, *Adv Neonatal Care* 6(6):303–312, 2006.

Deficient Knowledge (specify)   *Barbara J. Olinzock, RN, EdD, and Kathaleen C. Bloom, PhD, CNM* ⊖volve

NANDA-I

Definition

Absence or deficiency of cognitive information related to a specific topic

Defining Characteristics

Exaggerated behaviors; inaccurate follow-through of instruction; inaccurate performance of test; inappropriate behaviors (e.g., hysterical, hostile, agitated, apathetic); verbalization of the problem

Related Factors (r/t)

Cognitive limitation; information misinterpretation; lack of exposure; lack of interest in learning; lack of recall; unfamiliarity with information resources

NOC   (Nursing Outcomes Classification)

Suggested NOC Outcomes

Knowledge: Diet, Disease Process, Energy Conservation, Health Behavior, Health Resources, Infection Management, Medication, Personal Safety, Prescribed Activity, Substance Use Control, Treatment Procedure(s), Treatment Regimen

Example NOC Outcome with Indicators
Knowledge: Health Behavior as evidenced by the following indicators: Healthy nutritional practices/Benefits of activity and exercise/Safe use of prescription and nonprescription medication (Rate the outcome and indicators of **Knowledge: Health Behavior:** 1 = no knowledge, 2 = limited knowledge, 3 = moderate knowledge, 4 = substantial knowledge, 5 = extensive knowledge [see Section I].)

Client Outcomes

Client Will (Specify Time Frame):

- Explain disease state, recognize need for medications, and understand treatments
- Describe the rationale for therapy/treatment options
- Incorporate knowledge of health regimen into lifestyle
- State confidence in one's ability to manage health situation and remain in control of life
- Demonstrate how to perform health-related procedure(s) satisfactorily
- List resources that can be used for more information or support after discharge

NIC   (Nursing Interventions Classification)

Suggested NIC Interventions

Teaching: Disease Process, Individual, Learning Facilitation

Example NIC Activities—Teaching: Disease Process
Discuss therapy/treatment options; Describe rationale behind management/therapy/treatment recommendations

Nursing Interventions and *Rationales*

- Consider the client's ability and readiness to learn (e.g., mental acuity, ability to see or hear, existing pain, emotional readiness, motivation, and previous knowledge) when teaching clients. **EB:** *Each*

• = Independent   ▲ = Collaborative   **EBN** = Evidence-Based Nursing   **EB** = Evidence-Based

client is unique, and client motivation, beliefs, and expectations will influence learning (Price, 2008). **EBN:** *Learning readiness changes over time based upon situational, physical, and emotional challenges. The nurse assumes the role of authority, guide, motivator, mentor, and consultant depending on the learning readiness of the client (Olinzock, 2008).*

- Assess personal context and meaning of illness (e.g., perceived change in lifestyle, financial concerns, cultural patterns, and lack of acceptance by peers or coworkers). **EB:** *Improved symptom management and client satisfaction were noted as a result of interventions that focused on the needs of the client and the meaning and perspective of their illness (Hörnsten et al, 2008).*
- Monitor how clients process information over time. **EBN:** *Clients are unique in how they process information. Some clients will be more uncertain than others and may need more educational intervention over time (Suhonen, Valimaki, & Leino-Kilpi, 2008).*
- Use individualized approaches that support client priorities, preferences, and choice. **EBN:** *Individualized educational interventions have a positive effect on client outcomes (Suhonen, Valimaki, & Leino-Kilpi, 2008).*
- Engage client as a partner in the educational process. **EBN:** *A nursing approach that is collaborative and that uses encouragement and support to increase self-efficacy resulted in client satisfaction, empowerment, and confidence (Hannula, Kaunonen, & Tarkka, 2008).* **EB:** *Low literacy clients who were active and participated in the development of educational materials became more involved in the process of learning (Seligman et al, 2007).*
- Provide information to support self-efficacy, self-regulation, and self-management. **EB:** *Knowledge of disease management alone does not directly result in behavioral change. Enhancing self-efficacy and confidence in one's ability to problem-solve and make decisions should be included in self-management education (Effing et al, 2007).*
- Assess the client's literacy skill when using written information. **EBN:** *Health care professionals may overestimate reading and comprehension levels of their clients. Education for those with low literacy should be as least threatening as possible (Schaefer, 2008).* **EB:** *Multiple educational strategies including picture, digital, and telephone follow-up have proven effective in reducing complications in those with chronic conditions (DeWalt et al, 2006: Hoffmann & McKenna, 2006).*
- Provide visual aids to enhance learning. **EB:** *Visual aids such as pictures and simple word captions have proven to be effective when used to highlight important information, especially when working with clients with low literacy (Houts et al, 2006).*
- Consider coordinated, multifaceted methods of disbursing information. **EB:** *Coordinated efforts using a combination of written and verbal information, regular review, and a written action plan have proven beneficial for self-care behavioral change (Glazier et al, 2006; Sheard & Garrud, 2006).*
- Use coaching methods such as telephone follow-up to reinforce learning. **EBN:** *Coaching clients using telephone follow-up by expert nurses and allied health care professionals has proven effective in improving symptom management, increasing self-efficacy, and increasing client satisfaction (Francis, Feyer, & Smith, 2007).*
- Help the client appropriate follow-up resources for continuing information and support. **EBN:** *Advocating for client's participation using a community-based case management program has demonstrated improved clinical and financial outcomes for clients with complex chronic conditions (Chow et al, 2008).*
- Consider using a problem-solving group educational program. **EB:** *Group care that uses a discovery and problem-solving approach and tailors learning to individual information needs has proven more effective than standard one-to-one teaching in empowering individuals (Deakin et al, 2006).* **EB:** *More intensive one-to-one attention may be needed for socially disadvantaged populations (Glazier et al, 2006).*
- Use computer- and Web-based methods as appropriate. **EB:** *Information disbursed as an interactive Web-based method contributed to a greater behavioral changes, increased participation, and self-efficacy. However, the effectiveness for specific populations such as disadvantaged populations is unclear (Murray et al, 2005).*
- Use teaching methods that reinforce learning and allow adequate time for mastery of content. **EB:** *Teaching strategies that focus on repetition, simplifying content, and stating rationale for the "why" of learning enhances adherence (Price, 2008).* **EB:** *Offering more than one educational session and longer face-to-face contact have been implicated in positive outcomes especially for clients with low literacy (DeWalt et al, 2006; Schaefer, 2008).*

• = Independent ▲ = Collaborative **EBN** = Evidence-Based Nursing **EB** = Evidence-Based

- Use outreach and community educational intervention as appropriate. **EB:** *Using support groups including community and lay educators may be helpful particularly for disadvantaged populations (Glazier et al, 2006).*

Pediatric

- Use family-centered approaches when teaching children and adolescents. *Parents expressed a need to negotiate and participate with health care providers about decisions regarding the care of their children (Corlett & Twylcross, 2006).*
- Use educational strategies that are interactive and engaging for younger children and toddlers. *Information transfer that is highly individualized and interactive is recommended (McPherson et al, 2006).*
- Provide a developmentally appropriate environment when addressing the health education needs of adolescents. **EB:** *Select communication strategies that are developmentally appropriate when providing information to children and adolescents and that take into consideration the uniqueness of the young person's physical condition, cognitive ability, perceived needs, and preferences (Ranmal, Prictor, & Scott, 2008).*

Geriatric

- Involve older clients in setting their own goals and participating in the decision-making process. **EBN:** *Allowing senior clients to set goals that are meaningful to them and are realistic have demonstrated positive clinical outcomes (Davis & White, 2008).*
- Adapt the teaching process for the physical constraints of the aging process (e.g., speak clearly, use a variety of audio-visual-psychomotor methods, provide examples, and allow time for the client to repeat and review). **EBN:** *Adults are capable of learning at any age. Age modifies but does not inhibit learning (Zurakowski, Taylor, & Bradway, 2006).*
- Ensure that the client uses necessary reading aids (e.g., eyeglasses, magnifying lenses, large-print text) or hearing aids. **EBN:** *Visual and hearing deficits require amplification or clarification of sensory input (Zurakowski, Taylor, & Bradway, 2006).* **EBN:** *Educating the older adult about health care information is affected by cognitive decline associated with the aging process. Use of cognitive resources: sensory input, processing speed, working memory, and inhibition must be assessed to assist the older adult in learning. The nurse must understand these resources to choose effective teaching strategies to use with older adults (Cutilli, 2008).*
- Use printed material, videotapes, lists, diagrams. *Methods that clients can refer to at another time are recommended (Zurakowski, Taylor, & Bradway, 2006).*
- Repeat and reinforce information during several brief sessions. **EBN:** *Brief sessions focus attention on essential information. Older clients benefit from repeated follow-up sessions (Zurakowski, Taylor, & Bradway, 2006).*
- Discuss healthy lifestyle changes that promote wellness for the older adult. **EBN:** *Greater efforts must be made both to improve preventive health care and enhance quality-of-life interventions for older people (Nakasato & Carnes, 2006).*
- Offer opportunities for practice of psychomotor skills. **EBN:** *Older adults indicate a preference for hands-on learning. They learn with hands on and through rehearsal when taught psychomotor skills (Zurakowski, Taylor, & Bradway, 2006).*
- ▲ Refer elderly clients for postdischarge follow-up as they transition from hospital to home in regards to their treatment and medication regimens. *Extended follow-up and social support may prevent relapses and readmissions in older, vulnerable clients (Cumbler, Carter, & Kutner, 2008).*
- Consider using technology, including interactive computer programs and other creative interventions, to dispense health education to older adults. **EB:** *Older adults will use technology based upon a decision-making process of costs versus benefits regardless of previous positive or negative experiences (Melenhorst, Rogers, & Bouwhuis, 2006). Group support made available through interactive E-health programs may be helpful in dispersing information and providing social support (Marziali, 2009). Creativity interventions have been shown to positively affect mental and physiological health indicators. Use of creative interventions, such as art, poetry, and writing are useful interventions to help an older adult learn. Recent research indicates that creative interventions help to stimulate cognitive abilities in older adults (Flood & Phillips, 2007).*

• = Independent   ▲ = Collaborative   **EBN** = Evidence-Based Nursing   **EB** = Evidence-Based

Multicultural

- Acknowledge racial/ethnic differences at the onset of care. **EBN:** *Show respect, acknowledge racial ethnic/differences, show sensitivity and self-awareness to enhance communication and rapport, and promote treatment outcomes (Rust et al, 2006).*
- Assess for the influence of cultural beliefs, norms, and values on the client's knowledge base. **EBN:** *Illness beliefs guide health behavior (Russell, 2006).*
- Provide written health care information to clients with limited English proficiency in their native language. **EB:** *Clients with limited English proficiency were unable to understand routinely dispensed medication instructions written in English (Fernander et al, 2006).*
- Assess for cultural/ethnic self-care practices. **EBN:** *Folk and home remedies may interact with medications and treatment (Russell, 2006).*
- Use teaching methods that are culturally sensitive and support client customs, values, and lifestyle. **EB:** *Educational programs that focus on the cultural context and not disease symptoms alone have proven to be more effective than generic education programs (Bailey et al, 2009; Brown et al, 2007).*
- Be aware of the potential influence of medical interpreters in information sharing and decision making and of the possible difficulties for clients when using medical interpreters. *Different categories of interpreters (e.g., trained, untrained, professional) may influence how information is shared (Hsieh, 2006).*

Home Care

- All of the previously mentioned interventions are applicable to the home setting.
- Assess the client/family learning needs, information needs, and current level of knowledge. **EB:** *Caregivers express a need for having their informational needs met (Van Heugten et al, 2006).*
- Monitor the appropriateness of using telehome health care as a teaching method for families. *While clients report satisfaction with telehome health methods, they also express that they do not want to lose the personal contact (Bowles & Baugh, 2007).*
- Encourage family and peer support. **EB:** *A partner-guided protocol that included integrated education and training of clients and partners improved symptom management. There was also significant improvement in self-efficacy and caregiver strain (Keefe, Somers, & Martire, 2008).*
- Assess for specific areas of learning that have the potential for strong emotional responses by the client or family/caregiver. **EBN:** *Attending to physical care and failing to assess for distress in clients and family caregivers can impact health outcomes and quality of life (Madden, 2006).*

⊖volve   See the EVOLVE website for Weblinks for client education resources.

REFERENCES

Bailey EJ, Cates CJ, Kruske SG et al: Culture-specific programs for children and adults from minority groups who have asthma. *Cochrane Database Syst Rev* (1):CD006580, 2009.

Bowles KH, Baugh AC: Applying research to optimize telehomecare, *J Cardiovasc Nurs* 22(1):5–15, 2007.

Brown A, Blozis S, Kouzekanani K et al: Health beliefs of Mexican Americans with type 2 diabetes: the Starr County border health initiative, *Diabetes Educ* 33(2):300–308, 2007.

Chow, SK, Wong, FK, Chan TM et al: Community nursing services for postdischarge chronically ill patients, *J Clin Nurs* 17(7B):260–271, 2008.

Corlett J, Twylcross A: Negotiation of parental roles within family-centered care: a review of the research, *J Clin Nurs* 15(10):1308–1316, 2006.

Cumbler E, Carter, J, Kutner, J: Failure at the transition of care: challenges in the discharge of the vulnerable elderly patient, *J Hosp Med* 3(4):349–352, 2008.

Cutilli C: Teaching the geriatric patient: making the most of "cognitive resources" and "gains", *Orthop Nurs* 27(3):195–200, 2008.

Davis GC, White TL: A goal attainment pain management program for older adults with arthritis, *Pain Manag Nurs* 9(4):171–179, 2008.

Deakin TA, Cade JE, Williams R et al: Structured patient education: the diabetes X-PERT Programme makes a difference, *Diab Med* 23(9):944–954, 2006.

DeWalt DA, Malone RM, Bryant ME et al: A heart failure self-management program for patients with literacy levels: a randomized, controlled trial, *BMC Health Serv Res* 6:30, 2006.

Effing T, Monninkhoff EM, van der Valk PD et al: Self-management education for patients with chronic obstructive pulmonary disease, *Cochrane Database Syst Rev* (4):CD002990, 2007.

Fernander AF, Patten CA, Schroeder DR et al: Characteristics of six-month tobacco use outcomes of black patients seeking smoking cessation intervention, *J Health Care Poor Underserved* 17(2):413–424, 2006.

Flood M, Phillips K: Creativity in older adults: a plethora of possibilities, *Issues Ment Health Nurs* 28(4):389–411, 2007.

Francis CF, Feyer AM, Smith BJ: Implementing chronic disease self-management in community settings: lessons from Australian demonstration projects, *Aust Health Rev* 31(4):499–509, 2007.

Glazier RH, Bajcar J, Kennie R et al: A systematic review of interventions to improve diabetes care in socially disadvantaged populations, *Diabetes Care* 29(7):1675–1688, 2006.

• = Independent   ▲ = Collaborative   **EBN** = Evidence-Based Nursing   **EB** = Evidence-Based

Hannula L, Kaunonen M, Tarkka MT: A systematic review of professional support interventions for breastfeeding, *J Clin Nurs* 17(9): 1132–1143, 2008.

Hoffmann T, McKenna K: Analysis of stroke patients' and carers' reading ability and the content and design of written materials: recommendations for improving stroke information, *Patient Educ Couns* 60(3): 286–293, 2006.

Hörnsten A, Stenlund H, Lundman B et al: Improvements in HbA1c remain after 5 years—a follow-up of an educational intervention focusing on patients' personal understandings of type 2 diabetes, *Diabetes Res Clin Pract* 81(1):50–55, 2008.

Houts PS, Doak CC, Doak LG et al: The role of pictures in improving health communication: a review of research on attention, comprehension, recall, and adherence, *Patient Educ Couns* 61(2):173–190, 2006.

Hsieh E: Understanding medical interpreters' reconceptualizing bilingual health communications, *Health Comm* 20(2):177–186, 2006.

Keefe FJ, Somers TJ, Martire LM: Psychologic interventions and lifestyle modifications for arthritis pain management, *Rheum Dis Clin N Am* 34(2):352–368, 2008.

Madden J: The problem of distress in patients with cancer: more effective assessment, *Clin J Oncol Nurs* 10(5):615–619, 2006.

Marziali E: E-health program for patients with chronic disease, *Telemed J E Health* 15(2):176–181, 2009.

McPherson AC, Glazebrook C, Forster D et al: A randomized, controlled trial of an interactive educational computer package for children with asthma, *Pediatrics* 117(4):1046–1054, 2006.

Melenhorst AS, Rogers WA, Bouwhuis DG: Older adults' motivated choice for technological innovation: evidence for benefit-driven selectivity, *Psycho Aging* 21(1):190–195, 2006.

Murray E, Burns J, See TS et al: Interactive health communication applications for people with chronic disease, *Cochrane Database Syst Rev* (4):CD004274, 2005.

Nakasato YR, Carnes BA: Health promotion in older adults: promoting successful aging in primary care settings, *Geriatrics* 61(4):27–31, 2006.

Olinzock BJ: Enhancing the learning of patients with SCI: a patient education tool, *Sci Nurs* 25(2):10–20, 2008.

Price PE: Education, psychology and compliance, *Diabetes Metab Res Rev* 24(Supp 1):S101–S105, 2008.

Ranmal R, Prictor M, Scott JT: Interventions for improving communication with children and adolescents about their cancer, *Cochrane Database Syst Rev* (4):CD002969, 2008.

Russell S: An overview of adult learning processes, *Urol Nurs* 26(5):349–352, 2006.

Rust G, Kondwani K, Martinez R et al: A crash-course in cultural competence, *Ethn Dis* 16(2 Suppl 3):S3–S29–S36, 2006.

Schaefer CT: Integrated review of health literacy interventions, *Orthop Nurs* 27(5):302–308, 2008.

Seligman HK, Wallace AS, DeWalt DA et al: Facilitating behavior change with low-literacy patient education materials, *Am J Health Behav* 31(Suppl 1):S69–S78, 2007.

Sheard C, Garrud P: Evaluation of generic patient information: effects on health outcomes, knowledge and satisfaction, *Patient Educ Couns* 61(1):43–47, 2006.

Suhonen R, Valimaki M, Leino-Kilpi H: A review of outcomes of individualised nursing interventions on adult patients, *J Clin Nurs* 17(7): 843–860, 2008.

Van Heugten C, Visser-Meily A, Post M et al: Care for carers of stroke patients: evidence-based clinical practice guidelines, *J Rehabil Med* 38(3):153–158, 2006.

Zurakowski T, Taylor M, Bradway C: Effective teaching strategies for the older adult with urologic concerns, *Urol Nurs* 6(5):355–360, 2006.

Readiness for enhanced Knowledge
Barbara J. Olinzock, RN, EdD, and Kathaleen C. Bloom, PhD, CNM

NANDA-I

Definition

The presence or acquisition of cognitive information related to a specific topic is sufficient for meeting health-related goals and can be strengthened

Defining Characteristics

Behaviors congruent with expressed knowledge; explains knowledge of the topic; expresses an interest in learning; describes previous experiences pertaining to the topic

NOC (Nursing Outcomes Classification)

Suggested NOC Outcome

Knowledge: Health Promotion

Example NOC Outcome with Indicators
Knowledge: Health Promotion as evidenced by the following indicator: Behaviors that promote health/Reputable health care resources (Rate the outcome and indicators of **Knowledge: Health Promotion:** 1 = no knowledge, 2 = limited knowledge, 3 = moderate knowledge, 4 = substantial knowledge, 5 = extensive knowledge [see Section I].)

Client Outcomes

Client Will (Specify Time Frame):

- Meet personal health-related goals
- Explain how to incorporate new health regimen into lifestyle
- List sources to obtain information

NIC	(Nursing Interventions Classification)

Suggested NIC Interventions

Health Education, Health System Guidance

> **Example NIC Activities—Health Education**
>
> Prioritize identified learner needs based on client preference, skills of nurse, resources available, and likelihood of successful goal attainment

Nursing Interventions and *Rationales*

- ▲ Include clients as members of the health care team in mutual goal setting when providing education. **EBN:** *Involving individuals in setting goals that are relevant and meaningful to them is an important component of supporting client participation (Davis & White, 2008).*
- Use open-ended questions and encourage two-way communication. **EBN:** *Intervention strategies that use interpersonal communication, including an open-ended interview process versus a structured didactic approach, are recommended (Timmins, 2006).*
- Support client priorities, preferences, and choice. **EBN:** *Adult learning theories and models support the use of choice with self-directed, autonomous learners (Olinzock, 2008). Clients will express preferences about information needs and the when, how, and from whom they want to learn (Russell, 2006).*
- Use strategies to promote client motivation and sustain learning. **EBN:** *The use of motivational and disease management interventions has demonstrated promise for improved adherence and lifestyle change (Dusing, 2008).*
- Provide information to support self-efficacy, self-regulation, and self-management. **EB:** *Educational programs based upon empowerment and client participation, have demonstrated effectiveness (Suhonen & Leino-Kilpi, 2006).*
- Use a consultative, interactive teaching approach. **EBN:** *A consultative role is especially recommended for self-directed and motivated learners (Olinzock, 2008).* **EB:** *A targeted approach using consultation consisting of coaching, educational materials, and effective feedback and communication is believed to support client participation (Haywood, Marshall, & Fitzpatrick, 2006).*
- Seek teachable moments to encourage health promotion. **EB:** *Providers are encouraged to use teachable moments to offer information on health promotion and prevention behaviors such as healthy nutrition, exercise, and weight management (Demark-Wahnefried et al, 2008).*
- Use interactive and Web-based methods as appropriate. *Internet and Web-based interventions that are interactive such as self-care assessments and peer support are useful in supporting lifestyle changes (Kerr et al, 2008).*
- Individualize health education interventions. **EB:** *Interventions such as individualized computer use, brochures, and teaching sessions tailored to the learning needs of clients have demonstrated positive effects on risk reduction and lifestyle changes (Jones et al, 2006).*
- Facilitate individualized proactive planning with clients before visits to their health care provider. **EBN:** *A pre-visit questionnaire facilitates individualized proactive planning before a health care visit (Glynne-Jones et al, 2006).*
- Provide appropriate health care information and screening for clients with physical disabilities. **EB:** *Health promotion activities for clients with disabilities have been proven to contribute significantly to quality of life (Ennis et al, 2006).*
- Encourage group and peer support as appropriate to enhance learning. **EB:** *Peer support has proven instrumental in enhancing client knowledge, skills, and confidence (Harvey et al, 2008; Hoey et al, 2008).*

• = Independent   ▲ = Collaborative   **EBN** = Evidence-Based Nursing   **EB** = Evidence-Based

- Use a combination of teaching methods. **EB:** *The use of intensive, multiple modalities in lifestyle modification programs such as structured sessions in conjunction with "hands on" and creative activities is associated with a positive effect on health knowledge and on lifestyle changes (Gallegos, Ovalle-Berumen, & Gomez-Meza, 2006).*
- Reinforce learning through educational follow-up. **EBN:** *Longer periods of participation over time and consistent structured education programs have resulted in symptom management and risk reduction (Snethen, Broome, & Cashin, 2006).*
- Refer to care plan for **Deficient Knowledge.**

 Pediatric

- Consider the delivery of alternative settings for teaching parents of children with chronic conditions. **EBN:** *Programs and initiatives such as the Healthy Learning Model are effective in teaching children with chronic conditions self-care management in a school environment (Erickson et al, 2006).*
- Use educational strategies that are interactive and engaging for younger children and toddlers. *Information transfer that is highly individualized and interactive is recommended (McPherson et al, 2006).*
- Provide a developmentally appropriate environment when addressing the health education needs of adolescents. *Developmentally targeted educational materials are considered essential in educating adolescents about the prevention of sexually transmitted diseases (Kollar & Kahn, 2008).*
- Refer to **Deficient Knowledge** care plan.

 Geriatric and Multicultural

- Refer to **Deficient Knowledge** care plan.

 Home Care

- Consider high-tech options for delivery of home-based instruction. *Positive outcomes are reported in the use of telehome care, but clients prefer to continue with some amount of personal contact (Bowles & Baugh, 2007).*

evolve   See the EVOLVE website for Weblinks for client education resources.

REFERENCES

Bowles KH, Baugh AC: Applying research to optimize telehomecare, *J Cardiovasc Nurs* 22(1):5–15, 2007.

Davis GC, White TL: A goal attainment pain management program for older adults with arthritis, *Pain Manag Nurs* 9(4):171–179, 2008.

Demark-Wahnefried W, Rock CL Patrick K et al: Lifestyle interventions to reduce cancer risk and improve outcomes, *Am Fam Physician* 77(11):1573–1578, 2008.

Dusing R: Overcoming barriers to effective blood pressure control in patients with hypertension, *Curr Med Res Opin* 22(8):1545–1553, 2008.

Ennis M, Thain J, Boggild M et al: A randomized controlled trial of a health promotion education programme for people with multiple sclerosis, *Clin Rehabil* 20(9):783–792, 2006.

Erickson CD, Splett PL, Mullett, SS et al: The healthy learner model for student chronic condition management—part 1, *J Sch Nurs* 22(6): 319–329, 2006.

Gallegos EC, Ovalle-Berumen F, Gomez-Meza MV: Metabolic control of adults with type 2 diabetes mellitus through education and counseling, *J Nurs Scholarsh* 38(4):344–351, 2006.

Glynne-Jones R, Ostler P, Lumley-Graybow S et al: Can I look at my list? An evaluation of a "prompt sheet" within an oncology outpatient clinic, *Clin Oncol (R Coll Radiol)* 18(5):395–400, 2006.

Harvey PW, Petkov JN, Misan G et al: Self-management support and training for patients with chronic and complex conditions improves health-related behaviour and health outcomes, *Aust Health Rev* 32(2):330–338, 2008.

Haywood K, Marshall S, Fitzpatrick R: Patient participation in the consultation process: a structured review of intervention strategies, *Patient Educ Couns* 63(1–2):12–23, 2006.

Hoey LM, Ieropoli SC, White VM et al: Systematic review of peer-support programs for people with cancer, *Patient Educ Couns* 70(3): 315–337, 2008.

Jones RB, Pearson J, Cawsey AJ et al: Effect of different forms of information produced for cancer patients on their use of the information, social support, and anxiety: randomized trial, *BMJ* 332(7547):942–948, 2006.

Kerr J, Patrick K, Norman G et al: Randomized control trial of a behavioral intervention for overweight women: impact on depressive symptoms, *Depress Anxiety* 25(7):555–558, 2008.

• = Independent   ▲ = Collaborative   **EBN** = Evidence-Based Nursing   **EB** = Evidence-Based

Kollar LM, Kahn JA: Education about human papillomavirus and human papillomavirus vaccines in adolescents, *Curr Opin Obstet Gynecol*, 20(5):479–483, 2008.

McPherson AC, Glazebrook C, Forster D et al: A randomized, controlled trial of an interactive educational computer package for children with asthma, *Pediatrics* 117(4):1046–1054, 2006.

Olinzock BJ: Enhancing the learning of patients with SCI: a patient education tool, *SCI Nurs* 25(1):10–20, 2008.

Russell S: An overview of adult learning processes, *Urol Nurs* 26(5):349–352, 370, 2006.

Snethen JA, Broome ME, Cashin SE: Effective weight loss for overweight children: a meta-analysis of intervention studies, *Pediatr Nurs* 21(1):45–56, 2006.

Suhonen R, Leino-Kilpi H: Adult surgical patients and the information provided to them by nurses: a literature review, *Patient Educ Couns* 61(1):5–15, 2006.

Timmins F: Exploring the concept of information need, *Int J Nurs Pract* 12(6):375–381, 2006.

Sedentary Lifestyle   *Sherry H. Pomeroy, PhD, RN*

NANDA-I

Definition

Reports a habit of life that is characterized by a low physical activity level

Defining Characteristics

Chooses a daily routine lacking physical exercise; demonstrates physical deconditioning; verbalizes preference for activities low in physical activity

Related Factors (r/t)

Deficient knowledge of health benefits of physical exercise; lack of training for accomplishment of physical exercise; lack of resources (time, money, companionship, facilities); lack of motivation; lack of interest

NOC   (Nursing Outcomes Classification)

Suggested NOC Outcomes

Ambulation, Activity Tolerance, Endurance

Example **NOC** Outcome with Indicators
Ambulation as evidenced by the following indicators: Walks with effective gait/Walks at moderate pace/Walks up and down steps/Walks moderate distance (Rate the outcome and indicators of **Ambulation**: 1 = severely compromised, 2 = substantially compromised, 3 = moderately compromised, 4 = mildly compromised, 5 = not compromised [See Section I].)

Client Outcomes

Client Will (Specify Time Frame):

- Increase moderate-intensity aerobic or physical activity to 2 hours and 30 minutes (150 minutes), such as 30 minutes 5 or more days of the week, OR 1 hour and 15 minutes (75 minutes) a week of vigorous-intensity aerobic physical activity, OR an equivalent combination of moderate- and vigorous-intensity aerobic physical activity; aerobic activity should be performed in episodes of at least 10 minutes, preferably spread throughout the week
- Increase physical activity to minimum of 10,000 steps per day
- Increase muscle-strengthening activities that involve all major muscle groups (legs, hips, back, chest, abdomen, shoulders, and arms) performed on 2 or more days per week
- Meet mutually defined goals of increased *physical activity*
- Verbalize feeling of increased strength and ability to move

NIC   (Nursing Interventions Classification)

Suggested NIC Interventions

Exercise Therapy: Ambulation, Joint Mobility, Positioning

● = Independent   ▲ = Collaborative   **EBN** = Evidence-Based Nursing   **EB** = Evidence-Based

Example NIC Activities—Exercise Therapy: Ambulation
Assist the client to use footwear that facilitates walking and prevents injury; Instruct in availability of assistive devices, if appropriate

Nursing Interventions and *Rationales*

- Observe the client for cause of sedentary lifestyle. Determine whether cause is physical or psychological. *Some clients choose not to move because of physical pain, or psychological factors such as an inability to cope, fear, or depression.* See care plans for **Ineffective Coping** or **Hopelessness**.
- ▲ Assess for reasons why the client would be unable to participate in a physical activity or exercise program; refer for evaluation by a primary care practitioner as needed.
- Use the Outcome Expectation for Exercise Scale (Resnick, Zimmerman, & Orwig, 2001) to determine client's self-efficacy expectations and outcomes expectations toward exercise. **EBN:** *Findings suggested that to optimize exercise in post–hip fracture older women, self-efficacy and outcome expectations for exercise should be assessed, and that health care providers, friends, and families are critical to encouraging the client by reinforcing the positive benefits of exercise post–hip fracture (Resnick et al, 2007a).*
- Recommend the client enter an exercise program with a friend. **EBN:** *A study of rural women's motivators to adopting a walking program found that a combination of group- and individual-walking activities improved satisfaction and adherence to a walking program, while family responsibilities were a barrier (Perry, Rosenfeld, & Kendall, 2008).*
- Recommend the client begin a walking program using the following criteria:
  - Obtain a pedometer by purchase or from community/public health resources
  - Determine common times when brisk walking for at least 10–minute-intervals can be incorporated into usual lifestyle
  - Set incremental goal of walking a minimum of 10,000 steps per day (approximately 5 miles per day) (Tudor-Locke et al, 2008)
  - Toward end of day, if does not have required number of steps, go for a walk indoors or outdoors until reach designated goal of 10,000 steps per day

  EB: *Use of a pedometer resulted in two times the usual amount of activity and weight loss in overweight adults (VanWormer, 2004). Middle-aged women, who walked more than usual had lower body mass index (BMI), and if walked 10,000 plus steps per day were in the normal range for BMI (Thompson, Rakow, & Perdue, 2004).* **EBN:** *A study of midlife women aged 40 to 65 years who participated in a 24-week, home-based walking program (four times per week for 30 minutes) showed that 64% of participants adhered to the prescribed walks 6 months after the end of the intervention phase (Wilbur et al, 2006). African American women who participated in an enhanced behavioral-strategies walking intervention that used group workshops and tailored phone calls had significantly higher adherence and improved waist circumference and fitness (Wilbur et al, 2008).*
- Recommend client begin muscle strengthening activities for additional health benefits of increased bone strength and muscular fitness.
  - Encourage prescriptive resistance exercise of each major muscle group (hips, thighs, legs, back, chest, shoulders, and abdomen) using free weights, bands, stair climbing, or machines 2 to 3 days per week. Involve the major muscle groups for 10 to 15 repetitions each. Intensity should be between moderate (5 to 6) and vigorous (7 to 8) on a scale of 0 to 10 (ACSM, 2010).
  - Recommend progressive resistance training protocols using concentric, eccentric, and isometric muscle actions. Perform bilateral and unilateral single and multiple joint exercises. Optimize exercise intensity by working large before small muscle groups, multiple joint exercises before single-joint exercises, and higher intensity before lower intensity exercises (ACSM, 2009b).

  EB: *After a 12–week aquatic program compared to a non-exercise control group, statistically significant improvements in hip flexibility, strength, and aerobic fitness were reported; however, there was no effect on pain or physical functioning (Wang et al, 2007). A systematic review of 14 randomized controlled trials found a decrease in visceral adipose tissues, significant increased insulin response, and decreased plasma triglycerides (Thomas, Elliott, & Naughton, 2006). After 8 weeks of high-resistance muscle strength exercise and low-resistance exercise for persons with osteoarthritis, there was significant improvement in both groups for pain, function, walking time, and muscle torque (Jan et al, 2008).*

● = Independent   ▲ = Collaborative   **EBN** = Evidence-Based Nursing   **EB** = Evidence-Based

Pediatric

- Encourage child to increase the amount of walking done per day; if child is willing, ask him or her to wear a pedometer to measure number of steps. **EB:** *A study demonstrated that the recommended number of steps per day to have a healthy body composition for the 6– to 12–year-old is 12,000 for a girl and 15,000 for a boy (Tudor-Locke et al, 2004).*
- Recommend the child decrease television viewing, watching movies, and playing video games. Ask parents to limit television to 1 to 2 hours per day maximum (Calamaro & Faith, 2004). **EB:** *A study demonstrated that girls who watched more TV had a higher BMI and percentage of body fat (Davison, Downs, & Birch, 2006).*
- Encourage the adolescent to increase exercise to feel better. **EBN:** *Adolescents had positive feeling states once they began to exercise (Robbins et al, 2004).*

Geriatric

- Assess ability to move using the Get Up and Go test. *Ask the client to rise from a sitting position, walk 10 feet, turn, and return to the chair to sit. Performance on this screening examination demonstrates the client's mobility and ability to leave the house safely (Robertson & Montagnini, 2004).*
- Recommend the client begin a regular exercise program, even if generally active. *Walking is an effective exercise in the elderly (Resnick, 2009).* **EB:** *A research program demonstrated that people who exercise with a defined program had greater functional capacity or reserve than clients who had an active lifestyle, but no defined exercise program (Wellbery, 2005).*
- ▲ Refer the client to physical therapy for resistance exercise training as able including abdominal crunch, leg press, leg extension, leg curl, calf press, and more. **EB:** *When clients in an extended care facility were put on a strength-, balance-, and endurance-training program, the clients' balance and mobility improved significantly (Rydwik, Kerstin, & Akner, 2005). A Cochrane review found that progressive resistance-strength training for physical disability in older clients resulted in increased strength and positive improvements in some limitations (Liu & Latham, 2009).*
- Use the WALC Intervention (Walk; Address pain, fear, fatigue during exercise; Learn about exercise; Cue by self-modeling) to improve exercise adherence in the older adult. **EBN:** *The WALC Intervention resulted in more exercise and had greater self-efficacy expectations regarding exercise (Resnick, 2002). Self-efficacy consistently predicted more exercise behavior in a group of elderly women after surgery for a fractured hip (Resnick et al, 2007b).*
- Recommend the client begin a tai chi practice. **EB:** *A study demonstrated that tai chi resulted in increased function and quality of life for clients with osteoarthritis of the knee (Lee et al, 2009). Another study demonstrated that clients performing tai chi had better balance (Wong et al, 2009).*
- If client is scheduled for an elective surgery that will result in admission into the intensive care unit (ICU) and immobility, or recovery from a knee replacement, initiate a prehabilitation program that includes a warm-up, aerobic strength, flexibility, and functional task work. **EB:** *Aerobic training along with strength and interval training is effective and results in fewer postoperative complications, shorter postoperative stays, and reduced functional disabilities (Carli & Zavorsky, 2005).*

Home Care

- The above interventions may be adapted for home care use.
- ▲ Assess home environment for factors that create barriers to mobility. Refer to physical and occupational therapy services if needed to assist the client in restructuring home environment and daily living patterns.

Client/Family Teaching and Discharge Planning

- Work with the client using the transtheoretical model of behavior change and determine if the client is in the precontemplation, contemplation, preparation, action, or maintenance stage of behavior change for physical activity/exercise. *The transtheoretical model of behavior change can be very useful for nurses to utilize to increase exercise behavior utilizing-stage appropriate interventions (Burbank, Reibe, & Padula, 2002).*

- Provide appropriate strategies to support change to exercising based on stage of change. **EBN:** *In a behavioral validity study that examined validity evidence for physical activity stage of change across nine studies, physical activity stage of change was found to be behaviorally valid, evidenced by self-reported exercise, physical activity, pedometers, sedentary behaviors, and physical functioning. Physical fitness and weight indicators were not related to physical activity stage of change (Hellsten et al, 2008).*
- Recommend the client use the Exercise Assessment and Screening for You (EASY) tool to help determine appropriate exercise for the elderly client. *This tool is available online at: www.easyforyou .info (Resnick, 2009).*

⊖volve   See the EVOLVE website for Weblinks for client education resources.

REFERENCES

American College of Sports Medicine (ACSM): Exercise and physical activity for older adults, *Med Sci Sports Exerc* 41(7):1510–1530, 2009a.

American College of Sports Medicine: Progression models in resistance training for healthy adults, *Med Sci Sports Exerc*, 41(3):687–708, 2009b.

American College of Sports Medicine: *American College of Sports Medicine's guidelines for exercise testing and prescription,* ed 8, Philadelphia, 2010 Wolters Kluwer/Lippincott Williams & Wilkins.

Burbank PM, Reibe D, Padula CA: Exercise and older adults: changing behavior with the transtheoretical model, *Orthop Nurs* 21(4):51–61, 2002.

Calamaro CJ, Faith MS: Preventing childhood overweight, *Nutr Today* 39(5):194, 2004.

Carli F, Zavorsky GS: Optimizing functional exercise capacity in the elderly surgical population, *Curr Opin Clin Nutr Metab Care* 8(1):23, 2005.

Davison KK, Downs DS, Birch LL: Pathways linking perceived athletic competence and parental support at age 9 years to girls' physical activity at age 11 years, *Res Q Exerc Sport* 77(1):23–31, 2006.

Hellsten LA, Nigg C, Norman G et al: Accumulation of behavioral validation evidence for physical activity stage of change, *Health Psychol* 27(1 Suppl):S543–S553, 2008.

Jan MH, Lin JJ, Liau JJ et al: Investigation of clinical effects of high and low resistance training for patients with knee osteoarthritis: a randomized controlled trial, *Phys Ther* 88(4):427–436, 2008.

Lee HJ, Park HJ, Chae Y et al: Tai Chi Qigong for the quality of life of patients with knee osteoarthritis: a pilot, randomized, waiting list controlled trial, *Clin Rehabil* 23(6):504–511, 2009.

Liu CJ, Latham NK: Progressive resistance strength training for improving physical function in older adults, *Cochrane Database Syst Rev* (3): CD002759, 2009.

Perry CK, Rosenfeld AG, Kendall J: Rural women walking for health, *West J Nurs Res* 30(3):295–316, 2008.

Physical Activity Guidelines Advisory Committee. *Physical activity guidelines advisory committee report,* 2008. Washington DC: U.S. Department of Health and Human Services, 2008. Retrieved from Centers for Disease Control and Prevention (CDC) www.health.gov/paguidelines/.

U.S. Department of Health and Human Services (USDHHS): *2008 physical activity guidelines for Americans,* www.health.gov/paguidelines/ guidelines/default.aspx. Accessed October 29, 2009.

Resnick B: Testing the effect of the WALC intervention on exercise adherence in older adults, *J Gerontol Nurs,* 28(6):40, 2002.

Resnick B: Promoting exercise for older adults, *J Am Acad Nurse Pract* 21(2):77–78, 2009.

Resnick B, Zimmerman S, Orwig D: Model testing for reliability and validity of the outcome expectations for exercise scale, *Nurs Res* 50(5): 293, 2001.

Resnick B, Luisi D, Vogel A: Testing the Senior Exercise Self-Efficacy Project (SESEP) for use with urban dwelling minority older adults. *Public Health Nursing* 25(3), 221–234, 2008.

Resnick B, Orwig D, D'Adamo C et al: Factors that influence exercise activity among women post hip fracture participating in the Exercise Plus Program, *Clin Interv Aging* 2(3):413–427, 2007a.

Resnick B, Orwig D, Hawkes W et al: The relationship between psychosocial state and exercise behavior of older women 2 months after hip fracture, *Rehabil Nurs* 32(4):139–149, 2007b.

Robbins LB, Pis MB, Pender NJ et al: Exercise self-efficacy, enjoyment, and feeling states among adolescents, *West J Nurs Res* 26(7):716, 2004.

Robertson RG, Montagnini M: Geriatric failure to thrive, *Am Fam Physician* 70(2):343, 2004.

Rydwik E, Kerstin F, Akner G: Physical training in institutionalized elderly people with multiple diagnoses—a controlled pilot study, *Arch Gerontol Geriatr* 40(1):29, 2005.

Thomas D, Elliott EJ, Naughton GA: Exercise for type 2 diabetes mellitus, *Cochrane Database Syst Rev* (3):CD002968, 2006.

Thompson DL, Rakow J, Perdue SM: Relationship between accumulated walking and body composition in middle-aged women, *Med Sci Sports Exerc* 36(5):911, 2004.

Tudor-Locke C, Pangrazi RP, Corbin CB et al: BMI-referenced standards for recommended pedometer-determined steps/day in children, *Prev Med* 38(6):857, 2004.

Tudor-Locke C, Hatano Y, Pangrazi RP et al: Revisiting "how many steps are enough?" *Med Sci Sports Exerc* 40(7 Suppl):S537–S543, 2008.

VanWormer JJ: Pedometers and brief e-counseling: increasing physical activity for overweight adults *J Appl Behav Anal* 37(3):421, 2004.

Wang T, Belza B, Elaine Thompson F et al: Effects of aquatic exercise on flexibility, strength and aerobic fitness in adults with osteoarthritis of the hip or knee, *J Adv Nurs* 57(2):141–152, 2007.

Wellbery C: Physical function and levels of activity in the elderly, *Am Family Physician* 71(3):557, 2005.

Wilbur J, McDevitt J, Wang E et al: Recruitment of African American women to a walking program: eligibility, ineligibility, and attrition during screening, *Res Nurs Health* 29(3):176–189, 2006.

Wilbur J, McDevitt JH, Wang E et al: Outcomes of a home-based walking program for African-American women, *Am J Health Prom* 22(5): 307–317, 2008.

Wong AM, Pei YC, Lan C et al: Is Tai Chi Chuan effective in improving lower limb response time to prevent backward falls in the elderly? *Age* 31(2):163–170, 2009.

● = Independent   ▲ = Collaborative   **EBN** = Evidence-Based Nursing   **EB** = Evidence-Based

Risk for impaired Liver function

Nancy Albright Beyer, RN, CEN, MS, and Betty J. Ackley, MSN, EdS, RN

⊖volve

Definition

At risk for a decrease in liver function that may compromise health

Risk Factors

Hepatotoxic medications (e.g., acetaminophen, statins); HIV co-infection; substance abuse (e.g., alcohol, cocaine); viral infection (e.g., hepatitis A, B, C, E, Epstein-Barr)

 (Nursing Outcomes Classification)

Suggested NOC Outcome

Knowledge: Health Behavior

Example NOC Outcome with Indicators
Knowledge: Health Behavior as evidenced by the following indicators: Safe use of prescription drugs/Adverse health effects of alcohol misuse/Adverse health effects of recreational drug use/Healthy nutritional practices/Self-screening techniques (Rate the outcome and indicators of **Knowledge: Health Behavior:** 1 = no knowledge, 2 = limited knowledge, 3 = moderate knowledge, 4 = substantial knowledge, 5 = extensive knowledge [see Section I].)

Client Outcomes

Client Will (Specify Time Frame):

- State the upper limit of the amount of acetaminophen can safely take per day
- Have normal liver enzymes, serum and urinary bilirubin levels, white blood cell count (WBC), red blood cell count (RBC)
- Be free of jaundice, pruritus, bruising, petechiae, gastrointestinal bleeding, hemorrhage
- Have coagulation studies within normal limits
- Report abdominal girth of normal dimensions
- Be oriented to time, place, and person
- Be able to eat frequent small meals per day without nausea and/or vomiting
- State rationale for seeking medical attention for gallbladder/biliary disease
- If alcohol abuse is factor, state relationship between abuse and worsening gastrointestinal and liver disease
- Be free of cardiovascular and/or renal compromise: fluid retention, peripheral edema, ascites, decreased urinary output, changes in serum blood urea nitrogen (BUN) and creatinine levels
- Be free of abdominal tenderness/pain and have normal-colored stool

NIC **(Nursing Interventions Classification)**

Suggested NIC Interventions

Teaching: Disease Process, Substance Use Treatment

Example NIC Activities—Teaching Disease Process
Appraise the client's current level of knowledge related to specific disease process; Discuss lifestyle changes that may be required to prevent future complications and/or control the disease process

Nursing Interventions and *Rationales*

- Watch for signs of liver dysfunction including: jaundice of the eyes or skin, pruritus, gastrointestinal bleeding, coagulopathy, infections, increasing abdominal girth, fluid overload, shortness of breath, mental status changes, changes in the color of the stool, changes in urinary function con-

• = Independent   ▲ = Collaborative   **EBN** = Evidence-Based Nursing   **EB** = Evidence-Based

current with increased serum and urinary bilirubin levels *These are symptoms and laboratory results associated with liver disorders (Whiteman & McCormick, 2005; McKinley, 2009).*

▲ Evaluate liver function tests. *Standard liver panels include the serum enzymes aspartate transaminase (AST), alanine transaminase (ALT), alkaline phosphatase, and g-glutamyltransferase; total, direct, and indirect serum bilirubin; and serum albumin. The ALT is thought to be the most cost-effective screening test for identifying metabolic or drug-induced hepatic injury, but like other liver function tests, it is of limited use in predicting degree of inflammation and of no use in estimating severity of fibrosis.* **EB:** *A platelet count of less than 160,000 per mm³ has a sensitivity of 80% for detecting cirrhosis in clients with chronic hepatitis C (Heidelbaugh & Bruderly, 2006).*

▲ Evaluate coagulation studies such as international normalized ratio (INR), prothrombin time (PT), and partial thromboplastin time (PTT), especially with bleeding of the mouth or gums. *Prolonged prothrombin time and decreased production of clotting factors can result in bleeding (Whiteman & McCormick, 2005).*

• Monitor for signs of hemorrhage, especially in the upper GI tract, as it is the most frequent site. *Synthesis of coagulation factors II, V, VII, IX, and X are affected with liver impairment (Tripodi, Chantarangkul, & Mannucci, 2008).*

▲ Monitor for signs and symptoms of electrolyte and acid-base imbalances, especially hyperkalemia, hypoglycemia, and metabolic acidosis. *The cause of these imbalances are nutritional deficits, nausea and vomiting, fluid losses/shifts, and renal complications. Hypoglycemia is caused by loss of glycogen stores in the liver from damaged cells and decreased serum concentrations of glucose, insulin, and growth hormones (Kee, Paulanka, & Purnell, 2004).*

• Instruct client about possibility of a liver biopsy if he or she has other symptoms of possible liver problems, such as abnormal liver function tests, bleeding, jaundice, and nutritional deficits. *Liver biopsy is not necessary for diagnosis but is helpful for grading the severity of disease and staging the degree of fibrosis and permanent architectural damage (Wolfe, 2005; Luxon, 2006).* **EB:** *It is also useful for evaluation of effectiveness of treatments (Karamshi, 2008; Zeng et al, 2008).*

▲ Determine the total amount of acetaminophen the client is taking per day and administer medications for an overdose as ordered. The amount of acetaminophen ingested should not exceed 4 g per day as a limit (Deglin & Vallerand, 2008; McKinley, 2009). *It is common for clients to take multiple pain medications, all containing acetaminophen (Cohen, 2006). Acetaminophen overdose is the leading cause of liver failure in the United States (HealthFacts, 2006; Perkins, 2006).* **EB:** *Charcoal and N-acetylcysteine are the usual treatments of acetaminophen overdose. At times liver transplantation is needed (Brok, Buckley, & Gluud, 2006).*

▲ Evaluate the serum acetaminophen-protein adducts in the client with possible liver failure from excessive intake of acetaminophen. **EB:** *This diagnostic test was helpful in determining if liver failure is associated with acetaminophen toxicity (Davern, James, & Hinson, 2006).*

▲ If the client is an alcoholic, refer to a cessation program. *It is essential the client stop drinking as soon as possible to allow the liver to heal. Alcoholism is associated with malnutrition, which is harmful to the liver (DiCecco & Francisco-Ziller, 2006). Alcoholism is also associated with formation of proteins called cytokines, which cause inflammation and resultant damage to the liver (Jeong & Gao, 2008). It has been noted that serum levels of AST, ALT, total bilirubin, prothrombin time, and red blood cells, once elevated, may return to normal within 4 weeks of cessation of alcohol (Zeng et al, 2008).* See care plan for **Ineffective Denial** and **Dysfunctional Family processes.**

• Provide frequent smaller meals for easier digestion. Provide diet with optimal carbohydrates, proteins, and fats. Proteins can be increased as client can tolerate, and serum protein, albumin levels, and bilirubin levels indicate improved liver function. Provide essential vitamins and minerals. Consult with a registered dietician to discuss best nutritional support. *Improved nutrition will help the client with liver dysfunction regain strength and increase activity (McKinley, 2009). For those patients showing signs of fatty liver involvement, sound nutritional support can reduce the severity and also mitigate the already existing secondary malnutrition (Zeng et al, 2008).*

• Recognize that severe malnutrition may result in acute liver failure, which is reversible with improved nutrition. *Severe malnutrition from anorexia nervosa resulted in liver disease in two young females (De Caprio et al, 2006).*

• Review medical history with the client, recognizing that obesity and type-2 diabetes along with hypertriglyceridemia and polycystic ovarian syndrome are major risk factors in the development

of liver disease, specifically nonalcoholic fatty liver disease (NAFLD). *Rapid weight loss is also a risk (Fitzgerald, 2007).*
- Encourage vaccinations for hepatitis A and B for all ages. *Hepatitis A can affect anyone in the United States. Vaccination can prevent hepatitis A and B, which at times can cause liver failure (Rein et al, 2007; CDC, 2008; CDC, 2009).*
- Measure abdominal girth if individual presents with abdominal distention and pain. *Increasing abdominal distention and pain are signs of impending portal hypertension with presence of fluid shifts resulting in ascites (Whiteman & McCormick, 2005).*
- Assess for tenderness and/or pain level in the right upper quadrant. *Tenderness in this area is a symptom of biliary, liver, and/or pancreatic problems (Wilson & Giddens, 2005).*
- Recognize that new onset of symptoms of liver dysfunction such as jaundice, fatigue, and nausea may be caused by infection with hepatitis C (Wolfe, 2005).
- Observe for signs and symptoms of mental status changes such as confusion from encephalopathy. Assess ammonia level if mental changes occur (Sargent, 2007).

 Pediatric

- Encourage vaccinations for hepatitis A and B for all ages. *Hepatitis A can affect anyone in the United States. Vaccination can prevent hepatitis A and B, which at times can cause liver failure. Children should be vaccinated between ages 12 months to 23 months for hepatitis A (Rein et al, 2007; CDC, 2008).*
- Recognize that children can develop fatty liver disease, which can result in liver failure. Most children are asymptomatic, but others complain of malaise, fatigue, or vague recurrent abdominal pain (Lerret & Skelton, 2008). **EBN:** *Risk factors for fatty liver disease include obesity, insulin resistance, elevated ALT, low HDL cholesterol levels, and hypertriglyceridemia. The diagnosis is made by liver biopsy, and the mainstay of treatment is weight loss (Sharp, Santos, & Cruz, 2009).*
- ▲ During a well-baby visit, assess for signs of potential liver problems. Observe for prolonged jaundice, pale stools, and urine that is anything other than colorless. Consult with physician to order a split bilirubin as needed. *"Prolonged jaundice is defined as jaundice that persists past two weeks of age in a term infant and beyond three weeks of age in a preterm infant." With the lab test, if the conjugated fraction is greater than 20% of the total (conjugated hyperbilirubinemia), referral and further work-up are necessary (Tizzard & Yiannouzis, 2008).*
- Teach about healthy lifestyle modifications with sound nutrition and physical exercise to reduce obesity. *Nonalcoholic fatty liver disease (NAFLD) is becoming prevalent in the pediatric population in direct correlation with the emergence of childhood obesity as a significant pediatric health problem (Lerret & Skelton, 2008).*

 Geriatric

- The interventions above are appropriate for the elderly. *Liver disease in the elderly varies little from liver disease in younger people (Zaw & Joglekar, 2005).*

 Home Care

- Encourage rest, optimal nutrition (high carbohydrates, sufficient protein, essential vitamins and minerals) during initial inflammatory processes of the liver.
- Watch for liver dysfunction in the client receiving long-term parenteral nutrition. *There can be multiple causes of liver disease in this client population including hepatoxic medications, infections, other chronic conditions, preexisting liver disease, and sometimes the parenteral formula (Hamilton & Austin, 2006).*

 Client/Family Teaching and Discharge Planning

- Teach the client and family to examine all medications the client is taking, looking for acetaminophen as an ingredient, and reinforce the 4 gm upper limit of intake of acetaminophen to protect liver function (Deglin & Vallerand, 2008; McKinley, 2009).

● = Independent   ▲ = Collaborative   **EBN** = Evidence-Based Nursing   **EB** = Evidence-Based

- For the caregiver and client with hepatitis A, B, and C, teach the need for careful handwashing, use of gloves, and other precautions to prevent spread of any of these diseases.
- Teach avoidance of high-risk behaviors that cause hepatitis and ways to avoid those behaviors.
- Educate clients and their caregivers about treatment options and interventions for hepatitis.
- Teach client and family to report signs and symptoms that may indicate further complications including increased abdominal girth, bleeding, bruising, petechiae, jaundice, pruritus, confusion, rapid weight gain or weight loss (fluid overload versus anorexia and nausea/vomiting), and shortness of breath (McKinley, 2009).

⊖volve   See the EVOLVE website for Weblinks for client education resources.

REFERENCES

Brok J, Buckley N, Gluud C: Interventions for paracetamol (acetaminophen) overdose, *Cochrane Database Syst Rev* (2):CD003328, 2006.

CDC: *Viral hepatitis A*, 2008. www.cdc.gov/hepatitis/HAV/HAVfaq.htm. Accessed on May 3, 2009.

CDC: *Viral hepatitis B*, 2009. www.cdc.gov/hepatitis/HBV.htm. Accessed on May 3, 2009.

Cohen MR: Medication errors. Acetaminophen toxicity: undercover agent, *Nursing* 36(7):15, 2006.

Davern TJ II, James LP, Hinson JA: Measurement of serum acetaminophen-protein adducts in patients with acute liver failure, *Gastroenterol* 130(3):687–694, 2006.

De Caprio C, Alfano A, Senatore I et al: Severe acute liver damage in anorexia nervosa: two case reports, *Nutrition* 22(5):572–575, 2006.

Deglin JH, Vallerand AH: Acetaminophen clinical teaching. In Deglin JH, Vallerand AH, editors: *Davis's drug guide for nurses,* ed 11, Philadelphia, 2008, F.A. Davis.

DiCecco SR, Francisco-Ziller N: Nutrition in alcoholic liver disease, *Nutr Clin Pract* 21(3):245–254, 2006.

Fitzgerald MA: Nonalcoholic fatty liver disease, *Nurse Pract* 32(2):24–25, 2007.

Hamilton C, Austin T: Liver disease in long-term parenteral nutrition, *Supp Line* 28(1):16–18, 2006.

Heidelbaugh JJ, Bruderly M: Cirrhosis and chronic liver failure: part I. diagnosis and evaluation, *Am Fam Physician* 74(5):756–763, 2006.

Jeong WI, Gao B: Innate immunity and alcoholic liver fibrosis, *J Gastroenerol Hepatol* 23(supp l1):S112–S118, 2008.

Karamshi M: Performing a percutaneous liver biopsy in parenchymal liver diseases, *Br J Nurs* 17(12):746–752, 2008.

Kee JL, Paulanka BJ, Purnell L: *Fluids and electrolytes with clinical applications,* ed 7, Cincinnati, 2004, Delmar Publishers.

Lerret SM, Skelton JA: Pediatric nonalcoholic fatty liver disease, *Gastroenterol Nurs* 31(2):115–119, 2008.

Luxon BA: Symposium on liver disease. Noninvasive tests for liver fibrosis, *Postgrad Med* 119(3):8–13, 2006.

McKinley M: Acute liver failure, *Nursing* 39(3):38–45, 2009.

Perkins JD: Acetaminophen sets records in the United States: number 1 analgesic and number 1 cause of acute liver failure, *Liver Transpl* 12(4):682–683, 2006.

Rein DB, Hicks KA, Wirth KE et al: Cost-effectiveness of routine childhood vaccination for hepatitis A in the United States, *Pediatrics* 119(1):e12–e21, 2007.

Sargent S: Hepatic nursing. Pathophysiology and management of hepatic encephalopathy, *Br J Nurs* 16(6):335–339, 2007.

Sharp DB, Santos LA, Cruz ML: Fatty liver in adolescents on the U.S.-Mexico border, *J Am Acad Nurse Pract* 21(4):225–230, 2009.

Tizzard S, Yiannouzis K: Yellow alert! How to identify neonatal liver disease, *J Fam Health Care* 18(3):98–100, 2008.

Tripodi A, Chantarangkul V, Mannucci PM: The international normalized ratio to prioritize patients for liver transplantation: problems and possible solutions, *J Thromb Haemos* 6(2):243–248, 2008.

[no author]:Overdose of acetaminophen, aka Tylenol, the leading cause of liver failure in the U.S., *HealthFacts* 31(4):6, 2006.

Wilson SF, Giddens JF: *Health assessment for nursing practice,* ed 3, St Louis, 2005, Mosby.

Whiteman K, McCormick C: When your patient is in liver failure, *Nursing* 35(4):58–63, 2005.

Wolfe G: Hepatitis C: laboratory tests to be done before the diagnosis can be made, *Lippincotts Case Manag* 10(2):115–117, 2005.

Zaw K, Joglekar M: Liver disease and the elderly, *Geriatr Med* 35(5):33–39, 2005.

Zeng MD, Li YM, Chen CW et al: Guidelines for the diagnosis and treatment of alcoholic liver disease, *J Digest Dis* 9(2):113–116, 2008.

Risk for Loneliness   *Mary T. Shoemaker, RN, MSN, SANE*

NANDA-I

Definition

At risk for experiencing discomfort associated with a desire or need for more contact with others

Risk Factors

Affectional deprivation; cathectic deprivation; physical isolation; social isolation

NOC   (Nursing Outcomes Classification)

Suggested NOC Outcomes

Loneliness Severity, Social Interaction Skills, Social Involvement, Social Support

• = Independent   ▲ = Collaborative   **EBN** = Evidence-Based Nursing   **EB** = Evidence-Based

Example NOC Outcome with Indicators
Loneliness Severity as evidenced by the following indicators: Sense of social isolation/Difficulty in establishing contact with others (Rate the outcome and indicators of **Loneliness Severity:** 1 = severe, 2 = substantial, 3 = moderate, 4 = mild, 5 = none [see Section I].)

Client Outcomes

Client Will (Specify Time Frame):

- Maintain one or more meaningful relationships (growth-enhancing versus codependent or abusive in nature)—relationships allowing self-disclosure—and demonstrate a balance between emotional dependence and independence
- Participate in ongoing positive and relevant social activities and interactions that are personally meaningful
- Demonstrate positive use of time alone when socialization is not possible

NIC (Nursing Interventions Classification)

Suggested NIC Interventions

Family Integrity Promotion, Socialization Enhancement, Visitation Facilitation

Example NIC Activities—Socialization Enhancement
Encourage enhanced involvement in already established relationships; Help client increase awareness of strengths and limitations in communicating with others

Nursing Interventions and *Rationales*

- Assess the client's perception of loneliness. (Is the person alone by choice, or do others impose the aloneness?) **EBN:** *Among persons with severe mental illness, more than half identify problems with loneliness and social isolation (Perese & Wolf, 2005).* Refer to care plan for **Social isolation**.
- Assess the client's ability and/or inability to meet physical, psychosocial, spiritual, and financial needs and how unmet needs further challenge the ability to be socially integrated. NOTE: See care plan for **Disturbed Body image** if loneliness is associated with chronic illness afflictions (i.e., MS, skin disturbance, etc.). **EBN:** *Clients' perception of general health, symptoms, and social support influences health status outcome (Beal & Stuifbergen, 2007).*
- ▲ Assess the bereaved client who is alone for suicide and make appropriate referrals. *Bereaved persons are at excess risk of suicidal ideation compared to nonbereaved people. Heightened suicidal ideation in bereavement is associated with loneliness and severe depressive symptoms (Stroebe, Stroebe & Abakoumkin, 2005).* Refer to care plan for **Risk for Suicide**.
- ▲ Assess the client who is alone for substance abuse and make appropriate referrals. *Women who abused substances in this study reported negative feelings of boredom and loneliness (Harris, Fallot, & Berley, 2005).*
- Evaluate the client's desire for social interaction in relation to actual social interaction. Art may enhance an understanding of loneliness. **EBN:** *The use of art as a medium for evaluating loneliness and its levels can promote positive interaction as well as increased self-esteem in clients (Blomqvist, Pitkälä, & Routasalo, 2007).*
- Use active listening skills. Establish therapeutic relationship and spend time with the client. **EBN:** *Presence and caring communication are important (Sundin, Jansson, & Norberg, 2002; Savage et al, 2006).*
- ▲ Assist the client with identifying loneliness as a feeling and the causes related to loneliness; make appropriate referrals. **EBN:** *This study demonstrated that providing care for chronic conditions of the homeless at a nurse-managed clinic has the potential to improve health and reduce use of the emergency department (Savage et al, 2006).*
- Explore ways to increase the client's support system and participation in groups and organizations. **EBN:** *Psychosocial group intervention on loneliness and social support in Japanese women with breast cancer demonstrated significantly lower scores for loneliness (Fukui et al, 2003).*

• = Independent ▲ = Collaborative **EBN** = Evidence-Based Nursing **EB** = Evidence-Based

- Encourage the client to be involved in meaningful social relationships and provide support of one's personal attributes. **EBN:** *Both self-respect and other people's respect for one's own personal values have been shown to be important for self-esteem and quality of life (Drageset et al, 2009).*
- Encourage the client to develop closeness in at least one relationship. **EB:** *Dependence and independence should be balanced in healthy relationships. The development of a balanced level of emotional dependence and the ability for self-disclosure is important for end-of-life issues (Rokach, 2007).*

Adolescents

- Assess the client's social support system. **EBN:** *Use a social support tool or validated assessment tool if possible (e.g., Personal Lifestyle Questionnaire [PLQ]) (Mahon, Yarcheski, & Yarcheski, 2003).*
- Evaluate the family stability of younger and middle adolescent clients, and advocate and encourage healthy, growth-producing relationships with family and support systems. **EB:** *This study showed a fear of intimacy and loneliness among adolescents who were taught during childhood not to trust strangers (Terrell, Terrell, & Von Drashek, 2000).* **EBN:** *Predictors (gender, depression, shyness, and self-esteem), and additional predictors (social support, social anxiety, maternal expressiveness, and paternal expressiveness) emerged as predictors of loneliness, in this study of loneliness in adolescents (Mahon et al, 2006).*
- Evaluate peer relationships. **EB:** *Peer relations appear to be the best predictors of adolescent loneliness (Uruk & Demir, 2003).*
- Encourage social support for clients with visual impairments. **EB:** *Personal networks and social support for Dutch adolescents with visual impairments indicate that social support, especially the support of peers, is important to adolescents with visual impairments (Kef, 2002).*
- For older adolescents, encourage close relationships with peers and involvement with groups and organizations. **EBN:** *A positive relationship with friends and parents promotes psychological well-being in adolescents and reduces malaise. Loneliness can be a risk for the adolescent's well-being (Corsano, Majorano, & Champretavy, 2006).*
- Consider use of pets to cope with loneliness. **EBN:** *Homeless youths identified pets as companions that provide unconditional love and decrease feelings of loneliness (Rew, 2000).* **EBN:** *Equine-facilitated psychotherapy is a little-known experiential intervention that offers the opportunity to achieve healing (Vidrine, Owen-Smith, & Faulkner, 2002).*

Geriatric

- Assess the client's adaptive sensory functions or any other health deviations that may limit or decrease his or her ability to interact with others. **EB:** *Greater loneliness was found to be associated with an increased probability of having a coronary condition, as were low levels of both emotional support and companionship (Bergland & Kirkevold, 2006).*
- Assess caregivers for Alzheimer's disease clients for depression related to loneliness. **EBN:** *Loneliness was significantly related to depression of husbands, wives, and daughters providing care for Alzheimer's disease family members (Beeson et al, 2000).*
- Identify community support systems specific to elderly populations who are living in a nursing home. **EBN:** *Aging is often accompanied by significant losses of family members and other social support. Residents of a nursing facility show that social relationships with other residents were a strong predictor of decreased depression and loneliness (Lee, Lee, & Woo, 2005).*
- When relocation is necessary for the elderly, evaluate relocation stress as a contributing factor to loneliness. **EBN:** *Participants reported that isolation and loneliness increased when clients are relocated from one living arrangement to another (Walker, Curry, & Hogstel, 2007).*
- Encourage support by friends and family when the decision to stop driving must be made. **EBN:** *Adequate support from family and friends was critical to the maintenance of driving cessation (Johnson, 2008).*
- Provide opportunities for indoor gardening for those who enjoy gardening. **EBN:** *Indoor gardening enhances socialization, activities of daily living (ADLs), and perceptions of loneliness in elderly nursing home residents (Brown et al, 2004).*
- Provide activities that are pleasurable to the client. *Older people who have activities they enjoy are not as lonely (Walker, Curry, & Hogstel, 2007). The specific behaviors in this study that were found to ameliorate loneliness included utilizing friends and family as an emotional resource, engaging in eating*

and drinking rituals as a means of maintaining social contacts, and spending time constructively by reading and gardening (Pettigrew & Roberts, 2008).

- Refer to the care plan for **Social isolation** for additional interventions.

Multicultural

- Refer to the care plan for **Social isolation**.

Home Care

▲ Above interventions may be adapted for home care use. Assess for depression with the lonely elderly client and make appropriate referrals. **EBN:** *Findings have related loneliness in older adults to mental health problems, especially depression (McInnis & White, 2001).*

- If the client is experiencing somatic complaints, evaluate client complaints to ensure physical needs are being met, and then identify relationship between somatic complaints and loneliness. **EBN:** *Three factors have been found to increase levels of loneliness among elderly individuals residing in a nursing home: lack of intimate relationships, increased dependency, and loss (Hicks, 2000).*

- Identify alternatives to being alone (e.g., telephone contact, Internet). **EBN:** *Social support can be provided by telephone to low-income pregnant women who may have little or no social support and feel alienated in a clinical setting (Bullock, Browning, & Geden, 2002).*

- Consider using computers and the Internet to alleviate or reduce loneliness and social isolation. **EBN:** *Residents age 65 years and older who were living alone used the computer to combat loneliness (Clark, 2002). Internet use was found to decrease loneliness and depression significantly, while perceived social support and self-esteem increased significantly (Shaw & Gant, 2002). Among Internet users there were trends toward less loneliness and less depression (White et al, 2002).*

- Refer to the care plan for **Social isolation**.

Client/Family Teaching and Discharge Planning

- Encourage positive use of solitude to prevent loneliness (e.g., reading, listening to music, enjoying nature and art). *Solitude may be positive or negative depending on personal and situational factors (Long et al, 2003).*

- Include the family in all client-teaching activities, and give them accurate information regarding the illness severity. **EBN:** *By listening to residents and family members, nurses can improve life for residents and dignify them as individuals (Iwasiw et al, 2003).*

- Give family members something to do such as holding a hand, applying lotion, or assisting with feeding. **EB:** *Perceived family support was predictive of reduced loneliness in this study of women with HIV (Serovich et al, 2001).*

- Encourage family members to express caring by telling the client where they will be and sending messages when they cannot be present. **EBN:** *If people could spare a smile or a word for others who might be perceived as lonely, such a small gesture might just make the day of a lonely person a little less of an ordeal (Killeen, 1998). Loneliness can be alleviated and made less painful. This can only be achieved by increasing humankind's awareness of this distressing condition that all people endure sometime during their lives (Killeen, 1998).*

- Provide appropriate education for clients and their support persons about hepatitis C transmission and treatment. *Clients with hepatitis C often face significant social problems, ranging from social isolation, living alone, and familial stress. Data from this study suggest that educational interventions targeting support persons of clients and their relatives and friends about the disease, the risk factors for its spread, and about potential consequence and the stressors may lessen or alleviate the social strains clients with hepatitis C experience (Blasiole et al, 2006).*

- Refer to the care plan for **Social isolation** for additional interventions.

⊖volve   See the EVOLVE website for World Wide Web resources for client education.

• = Independent   ▲ = Collaborative   **EBN** = Evidence-Based Nursing   **EB** = Evidence-Based

REFERENCES

Beal C, Stuifbergen A: Loneliness in women with multiple sclerosis, *Rehabil Nurs* 32(4):165–171, 2007.

Beeson R, Horton-Deutsch S, Farran C et al: Loneliness and depression in caregivers of persons with Alzheimer's disease or related disorders, *Issues Ment Health Nurs* 21(8):779–806, 2000.

Bergland A, Kirkevold M: Thriving in nursing homes in Norway: contributing aspects described by residents, *Int J Nurs Stud* 43(6):681–691, 2006.

Blasiole JA, Shinkunas L, Labrecque DR et al: Mental and physical symptoms associated with lower social support for patients with hepatitis C, *World J Gastroenterol* 12(29):4665–4672, 2006.

Blomqvist L, Pitkälä K, Routasalo P: Images of loneliness: using art as an educational method in professional training, *J Contin Educ Nurs* 38(2):89–93, 2007.

Brown VM, Allen AC, Dwozan M et al: Indoor gardening and older adults: effects on socialization, activities of daily living, and loneliness, *J Gerontol Nurs* 30(10):34–42, 2004.

Bullock LF, Browning C, Geden E: Telephone social support for low-income pregnant women, *J Obstet Gynecol Neonatal Nurs* 31(6):658–664, 2002.

Clark DJ: Older adults living through and with their computers, *Comput Inform Nurs* 20(3):117–124, 2002.

Corsano P, Majorano M, Champretavy L: Psychological well-being in adolescence: the contribution of interpersonal relations and experience of being alone, *Adolescence* 41(162):341–353, 2006.

Drageset J, Eide GE, Nygaard HA et al: The impact of social support and sense of coherence on health-related quality of life among nursing home residents—a questionnaire survey in Bergen, Norway, *Int J Nurs Stud* 46(1):65–75, 2009.

Fukui S, Koike M, Ooba A et al: The effect of a psychosocial group intervention on loneliness and social support for Japanese women with primary breast cancer, *Oncol Nurs Forum* 30(5):823–830, 2003.

Harris M, Fallot RD, Berley RW: Qualitative interviews on substance abuse relapse and prevention among female trauma survivors, *Psychiatr Serv* 56(10):1292–1296, 2005.

Hicks TJ Jr: What is your life like now? Loneliness and elderly individuals residing in nursing homes, *J Gerontol Nurs* 26(8):15–19, 2000.

Iwasiw C, Goldenberg D, Bol N et al: Resident and family perspectives. The first year in a long-term care facility, *J Gerontol Nurs* 29(1):45–54, 2003.

Johnson JE.: Informal social support networks and the maintenance of voluntary driving cessation by older rural women, *J Community Health Nurs* 25(2):65–72, 2008.

Kef S: Psychosocial adjustment and the meaning of social support for visually impaired adolescents, *J Vis Impair Blind* 96(1):22, 2002.

Killeen C: Loneliness: an epidemic in modern society, *J Adv Nurs* 28(4):762–770, 1998.

Lee LY, Lee DT, Woo J: Predictors of satisfaction among cognitively intact nursing home residents in Hong Kong, *Res Nurs Health* 28(5):376–387, 2005.

Long CR, Seburn M, Averill JR, et al: Solitude experiences: varieties, settings, and individual differences, *Pers Soc Psychol Bull* 29(5):578–583, 2003.

Mahon NE, Yarcheski A, Yarcheski TJ et al: A meta-analytic study of predictors for loneliness during adolescence, *Nurs Res* 55(5):308–315, 2006.

Mahon NE, Yarcheski T, Yarcheski A: The revised Personal Lifestyle Questionnaire for early adolescents, *West J Nurs Res* 25(5):533–547, 2003.

McInnis GJ, White JH: A phenomenological exploration of loneliness in the older adult, *Arch Psychiatr Nurs* 15(3):128–139, 2001.

Perese EF, Wolf M: Combating loneliness among persons with severe mental illness: social network interventions' characteristics, effectiveness, and applicability, *Issues Ment Health Nurs* 26(6):591–609, 2005.

Pettigrew S, Roberts M: Addressing loneliness in later life, *Aging Ment Health* 12(3):302–309, 2008.

Rew L: Friends and pets as companions: strategies for coping with loneliness among homeless youth, *J Child Adolesc Psychiatr Nurs* 13(3):125–132, 2000.

Rokach A: Coping with loneliness among the terminally ill, *Soc Indic Res* 82(3):487–503, 2007.

Savage CL, Lindsell CJ, Gillespie GL et al: Health care needs of homeless adults at a nurse-managed clinic, *J Community Health Nurs* 23(4):225–234, 2006.

Serovich JM, Kimberly JA, Mosack KE et al: The role of family and friend social support in reducing emotional distress among HIV-positive women, *AIDS Care* 13(3):335–341, 2001.

Shaw LH, Gant LM: In defense of the Internet: the relationship between Internet communication and depression, loneliness, self-esteem, and perceived social support, *Cyberpsychol Behav* 5(2):157–171, 2002.

Stroebe M, Stroebe W, Abakoumkin G: The broken heart: suicidal ideation in bereavement, *Am J Psychiatry* 162(11):2178–2180, 2005.

Sundin K, Jansson L, Norberg A: Understanding between care providers and patients with stroke and aphasia: a phenomenological hermeneutic inquiry, *Nurs Inq* 9(2):93–103, 2002.

Terrell F, Terrell IS, Von Drashek SR: Loneliness and fear of intimacy among adolescents who were taught not to trust strangers during childhood, *Adolescence* 35(140):611–617, 2000.

Uruk AC, Demir A: The role of peers and families in predicting the loneliness level of adolescents, *J Psychol* 137(2):179–193, 2003.

Vidrine M, Owen-Smith P, Faulkner P: Equine-facilitated group psychotherapy: applications for therapeutic vaulting, *Issues Ment Health Nurs* 23(6):587–603, 2002.

Walker C, Curry LC, Hogstel M: Relocation stress syndrome in older adults transitioning from home to a long-term care facility: myth or reality? *J Psychosoc Nurs Ment Health Serv* 45(1):38–45, 2007.

White H, McConnell E, Clipp E et al: A randomized controlled trial of the psychosocial impact of providing Internet training and access to older adults, *Aging Ment Health* 6(3):213–221, 2002.

M

Risk for disturbed Maternal/Fetal dyad   *Sheri Holmes, RNC, MSN, CNS-C*

NANDA-I

Definition

At risk for disruption of the symbiotic maternal/fetal dyad as a result of comorbid or pregnancy-related conditions

• = Independent   ▲ = Collaborative   **EBN** = Evidence-Based Nursing   **EB** = Evidence-Based

Risk Factors

Complications of pregnancy (e.g., premature rupture of membranes, placenta previa or abruption, late prenatal care, multiple gestation, malnutrition); compromised O_2 transport (e.g., anemia, cardiac disease, asthma, hypertension, seizures, premature labor, hemorrhage); impaired glucose metabolism (e.g., diabetes, steroid use); physical abuse; substance abuse (e.g., tobacco, alcohol, drugs); treatment-related side effects (e.g., medications, surgery, chemotherapy)

 (Nursing Outcomes Classification)

Suggested NOC Outcomes

Fetal Status: Antepartum, Intrapartum, Maternal Status: Antepartum, Intrapartum, Depression Level, Diabetes Self-Management, Family Resiliency, Knowledge: Hypertension Management, Substance Use Control, Nausea & Vomiting Severity, Social Support, Spiritual Support

> **Example NOC Outcome with Indicators**
>
> **Maternal Status: Antepartum** as evidenced by the following indicators: Emotional attachment to fetus/Coping with discomforts of pregnancy/Mood lability/Blood pressure/Blood glucose/Hemoglobin (Rate each indicator of **Maternal Status: Antepartum**: 1 = severe deviation from normal range, 2 = substantial deviation from normal range, 3 = moderate deviation from normal range, 4 = mild deviation from normal range, 5 = no deviation from normal range [see Section I].)

Client Outcomes

Client Will (Specify Time Frame):

• Cope with discomforts of high-risk pregnancy

 (Nursing Interventions Classification)

Suggested NIC Interventions

High Risk Pregnancy Care, Intrapartal Care: High Risk Delivery

> **Example NIC Activities—High Risk Pregnancy Care**
>
> Determine the presence of medical factors that are related to poor pregnancy outcome (e.g., diabetes, hypertension, lupus erythmatosus, herpes, hepatitis, HIV, and epilepsy); Provide educational materials that address the risk factors and usual surveillance tests and procedures

Nursing Interventions and *Rationales*

• Standardize internal and external transport forms using SBAR format (situation, background, assessment, recommendation) to provide safe and efficient transport of a high-risk pregnant client. *Using a standardized form throughout the hospital system decreases the risk of errors, miscommunications, and omissions (Edwards & Woodward, 2008; Guise & Lowe, 2008).*

▲ Arrange for psychotherapeutic support when woman expresses intense fear related to high-risk pregnancy and fetal outcomes. **EB:** *Women with comorbid conditions, such as diabetes or epilepsy, may express intense fear that need to be addressed to ameliorate negative consequences to the woman and her family (Turner et al, 2008).*

• Screen all antepartum clients for depression using a tool that evaluates the biopsychosocial-spiritual dimensions in a culturally sensitive way. **EB and EBN:** *Assessing depression during the antepartum period identifies risks and resources that can be modified to further support the mental health of pregnant women, particularly in women of color (Dunn, Handley, & Shelton, 2007; Jesse & Swanson, 2007; Nguyen, Clark, & Ruiz, 2007).*

• Offer flexible visiting hours, private space for families, and nursing support for management of family stressors when a woman is hospitalized with a high-risk pregnancy. **EBN:** *In qualitative studies of women hospitalized for complications of pregnancy, accommodating individual family needs was recommended, such as flexible visiting hours and private space for family visits, and nursing support*

• = Independent   ▲ = Collaborative   **EBN** = Evidence-Based Nursing   **EB** = Evidence-Based

for management of family stressors, including identifying family strengths, such as spirituality (Handley & Stanton, 2006; Price et al, 2007; Richter, Parkes, & Chaw-Kant, 2007).

- Identify pregnant women at risk for eating disorders by asking them about prolonged periods of amenorrhea and a history of restricted food intake or avoidance of certain foods. **EB:** *Incidence of having a diagnosable eating disorder is 3% with up to 15% for subclinical eating disorders. Interventions to establish healthy eating habits while pregnant can reduce the incidence of low birth weight, smaller head circumference, and dysmaturity (Kouba et al, 2005; Chizawsky & Newton, 2006).*
- Focus on the abilities of a woman with disabilities by encouraging her to identify her support system, resources, and needs for modification of her environment. *Concern for safety and limitations for self-care for a woman with physical disabilities can lead nurses to question her desire to bear children and her ability to safely parent. Nurses need to seek knowledge about the physical disabilities their clients have and to provide holistic care to them (Smeltzer, 2007).*
- Recognize patterns of physical abuse in all pregnant and postpartum women, regardless of age, race, and socioeconomic status. **EB and EBN:** *Studies of women have shown a pattern of abuse despite level of socioeconomic status. The major site of physical abuse during pregnancy is the torso, rather than the head and neck, which are the major sites in nonpregnant women. Recognition of physical injury patterns for assault could aid in better detection of all women experiencing violence (Certain, Mueller, & Jagodzinki, 2008; Nannini et al, 2008).*
- Perform accurate blood pressure readings at each client's clinic encounter. **EB:** *Women who have a history of chronic hypertension and are at risk for preeclampsia (e.g., family history, over 40 years old, first pregnancy, multiple gestation) need to be identified to decrease risk for inadequate placental perfusion or a multisystem shutdown. Choose the correct equipment, prepare the client, and record the measurements accurately to identify women at risk for hypertension (Pickering et al, 2005; Peters, 2008).*
- Educate pregnant women about the importance of safe food handling and cooking to reduce foodborne illness such as hepatitis E, toxoplasmosis, and listeriosis. *Pregnant women have a higher incidence of contracting listerosis than the general public. Deli meats, soft cheeses, and meat spreads should be avoided (Moos, 2006; Bazaco, Albrecht, & Malek, 2008).*

evolve   See the EVOLVE website for Weblinks for client education resources.

REFERENCES

Bazaco M, Albrecht S, Malek A: Preventing foodbourne infection in pregnant women and infants, *Nurs Womens Health* 12(1):46–55, 2008.

Certain H, Mueller M, Jagodzinski T: Domestic abuse during the previous year in a sample of postpartum women, *J Obstet Gynecol Neonatal Nurs* 37(1)35–41, 2008.

Chizawsky L, Newton M: Eating disorders: identification and treatment in obstetrical patients, *AWHONN Lifelines*, 10(6):482–488, 2006.

Dunn LL, Handley MC, Shelton MM: Spiritual wellbeing, anxiety, and depression in antepartal women on bedrest, *Issues Ment Health Nurs* 28:1235–1246, 2007.

Edwards C, Woodward E: SBAR for maternal transports: going the extra mile, *Nurs Womens Health* 12(6):515–520, 2008.

Guise J, Lowe N: Do you speak SBAR? [editorial], *J Obstet Gynecol Neonatal Nurs* 35(3):313–314, 2008.

Handley M, Stanton M: Evidence-based case management in a high-risk pregnancy: a case study, *Lippincotts Case Manag* 11(5):240–246, 2006.

Jesse DE, Swanson MS: Risks and resources associated with antepartum risk for depression among rural southern women, *Nurs Res* 56(6):378–386, 2007.

Kouba S, Hällström T, Lindholm C et al: Pregnancy and neonatal outcomes in women with eating disorders, *Obstet Gynecol* 105(2):255–260, 2005.

Moos M-K: Listeriosis: how nurses can prevent the preventable, *AWHONN Lifelines* 10(6):498–501, 2006.

Nannini A, Lazar J, Berg C et al: Physical injuries reported on hospital visits for assault during the pregnancy-associated period, *Nurs Res* 57(3):144–149, 2008.

Nguyen HT, Clark M, Ruiz RJ: Effects of acculturation on the reporting of depressive symptoms among Hispanic pregnant women, *Nurs Res* 56(3):217–223, 2007.

Peters R: High blood pressure in pregnancy, *Nurs Womens Health* 12(5):410–421, 2008.

Pickering T, Hall J, Appel L et al: Recommendations for blood pressure measurement in humans and experimental animals part 1: blood pressure measurement in humans: a statement for professionals from the subcommittee of professional and public education of the American Heart Association Council on High Blood Pressure Research, *Hypertension* 46(6):437–445, 2005.

Price S, Lake M, Breen G et al: The spiritual experience of high-risk pregnancy, *J Obstet Gynecol Neonatal Nurs* 36(1):63–70, 2007.

Richter M, Parkes C, Chaw-Kant J: Listening to the voices of hospitalized high-risk antepartum patients, *J Obstet Gynecol Neonatal Nurs* 36(4):313–318, 2007.

Smeltzer S: Pregnancy in women with physical disabilities, *J Obstet Gynecol Neonatal Nurs* 36(1):88–96, 2007.

Turner K, Piazzini A, Franza A et al: Do women with epilepsy have more fear of childbirth during pregnancy compared with women without epilepsy? A case-control study, *Birth* 35(2):147–151, 2008.

• = Independent   ▲ = Collaborative   **EBN** = Evidence-Based Nursing   **EB** = Evidence-Based

Impaired Memory   *Graham J. McDougall Jr., PhD, RN, FAAN*   ⊖volve

Definition

Inability to remember or recall bits of information or behavioral skills; impaired memory may be attributed to pathophysiological or situational causes that are either temporary or permanent

Defining Characteristics

Experience of forgetting; forgets to perform a behavior at a scheduled time; inability to determine if a behavior was performed; inability to learn new information; inability to learn new skills; inability to perform a previously learned skill; inability to recall events; inability to recall factual information; inability to retain new information; inability to retain new skills

Related Factors (r/t)

Anemia; decreased cardiac output; excessive environmental disturbances; fluid and electrolyte imbalance; hypoxia; neurological disturbances

NOC   (Nursing Outcomes Classification)

Suggested NOC Outcomes

Cognitive Orientation, Memory, Neurological Status: Consciousness

Example NOC Outcome with Indicators
Memory as evidenced by the following indicators: Recalls immediate information accurately/Recalls recent information accurately/Recalls remote information accurately (Rate each indicator of **Memory:** 1 = severely compromised, 2 = substantially compromised, 3 = moderately compromised, 4 = mildly compromised, 5 = not compromised [see Section I].)

Client Outcomes

Client Will (Specify Time Frame):

- Demonstrate use of techniques to help with memory loss
- State has improved memory for everyday concerns

NIC   (Nursing Interventions Classification)

Suggested NIC Interventions

Memory Training, Realistic Appraisal of Memory

Example NIC Activities—Memory Training
Stimulate memory by repeating patient's last expressed thought, as appropriate; Provide opportunity to use memory for recent events, such as questioning patient about a recent outing; Give examples of external memory strategies, e.g., calendar

Nursing Interventions and *Rationales*

▲ Assess overall cognitive function and memory. The emphasis of the assessment is everyday memory, the day-to-day operations of memory in real-world ordinary situations. Use an assessment tool such as the Mini-Mental State Examination (MMSE). *The MMSE can help determine whether the client has cognitive impairment, memory loss, or delirium and needs to be referred for further evaluation and treatment (Britton & Russell, 2007; Federman et al, 2009).*

▲ Assess for memory complaints because memory loss may be the earliest manifestation of mild cognitive impairment (MCI). *An MCI diagnosis includes the five criteria of cognitive complaints not normal for the age of the individual, no dementia, cognitive decline, memory impairment, and essentially normal functional activities (McDougall et al, 2007).*

• = Independent   ▲ = Collaborative   **EBN** = Evidence-Based Nursing   **EB** = Evidence-Based

▲ Determine whether onset of memory loss is gradual or sudden. If memory loss is sudden, refer the client to a physician or neuropsychologist for evaluation. *Acute onset of memory loss may be associated with neurological disease, medication effect, electrolyte disturbances, hypoxia, hypothyroidism, mental illness, or many other physiological factors (Mosconi, Pupi, & De Leon, 2008).*

● Determine amount and pattern of alcohol intake. *Alcohol intake has been associated with blackouts; clients may function but not remember their actions. Long-term alcohol use causes Korsakoff's syndrome with associated memory loss; however, moderate consumption of alcohol may be health promoting (Kopelman et al, 2009). Both infrequent and long-term use of marijuana and other illicit substances are associated with impaired memory and may become more of a concern to evaluate with the aging of the baby boomers (Yücel et al, 2007).*

▲ Note the client's current medications and intake of any mind-altering substances such as benzodiazepines, ecstasy, marijuana, cocaine, or glucocorticoids. *Benzodiazepines, oxybutynin, amitriptyline, fluoxetine, and diphenhydramine can produce memory loss for events that occur after taking the medication; information is not stored in long-term memory (Barton et al, 2008).* **EB:** *Glucocorticoid therapy may cause a decrease in memory function that is usually reversible once a person is off the medications (de Quervain & Margraf, 2008). By inhibiting memory retrieval, cortisol may weaken the traumatic memory trace, and thus reduce symptoms even beyond the treatment period. This type of treatment has been useful in posttraumatic stress disorder and social phobias.*

● Note the client's current level of stress. Ask if there has been a recent traumatic event. *Posttraumatic stress and anxiety-inducing general life factors may induce memory problems. Stress or elevated cortisol levels temporarily blocks memory retrieval (van Stegeren, 2009; Wolf, 2009).*

▲ If stress is associated with memory loss, refer to a stress reduction clinic. *If not available, suggest that the client meditate, receive massages, and participate in moderate physical activity, all of which may promote stress reduction and reduce anxiety and depression (Loizzo, 2007).*

● Encourage the client to develop an aerobic exercise program. **EB:** *A systematic review demonstrated that strength training and aerobic exercise had a positive effect on the immune system (Haaland et al, 2008).*

● Determine the client's sleep patterns. If insufficient, refer to care plan for **Disturbed Sleep pattern.** **EB:** *Studies demonstrate that memory consolidation is enhanced by sleep (Stickgold & Walker, 2007).*

▲ Determine the client's blood sugar levels. *If they are elevated, refer to physician for treatment and encourage healthy diet and exercise to improve memory. Elevated blood sugar levels were associated with impaired memory (Watson & Craft, 2006).*

▲ If signs of depression such as weight loss, insomnia, or sad affect are evident, refer the client for psychotherapy. *Depression can result in source memory errors, in which case the client is not sure if he or she did something or just thought about doing it (Gohier et al, 2008).*

▲ Perform a nutritional assessment. If nutritional status is marginal, confer with a dietitian and primary care practitioner to evaluate whether the client needs supplementation with foods or vitamins. Teach the client the need to eat a healthy diet with adequate intake of whole grains, fruits, and vegetables to decrease cerebrovascular infarcts. *Moderate, long-term deficiencies of nutrients may lead to loss of memory, which may be preventable or diminished through diet (Shukitt-Hale, Lau, & Joseph, 2008). Adequate levels of vitamin E may help protect memory (Bourre, 2006).* **EB:** *A large study demonstrated that people who ate daily quantities of fruits and vegetables had decreased incidence of ischemic strokes (He, Nowson, & MacGregor, 2006).*

▲ Question the client about cholesterol level. If it is high, refer to physician or dietitian for help in lowering. Encourage the client to eat a healthy diet, avoiding saturated fats and trans-fatty acids. **EB:** *A systematic review of observational studies found that individuals who were prescribed statin medications to reduce total cholesterol had a lowered risk of developing dementia (Panza et al, 2006).*

● Suggest clients use cues, including alarm watches, electronic organizers, calendars, lists, or pocket computers, to trigger certain actions at designated times. *Cues and external cognitive strategies can help remind clients of certain actions, particularly for future intentions known as prospective memory (Kliegel, Jäger, & Phillips, 2008).*

▲ Encourage the client to use external memory devices, such as a calendar for appointments; keep reminder lists; place a string around finger or rubber band around wrist as reminders; or enlist someone else to remind him or her of important events. **EBN:** *Using reminders can serve as cues for memory-impaired clients (Insel & Cole, 2005).*

● = Independent   ▲ = Collaborative   **EBN** = Evidence-Based Nursing   **EB** = Evidence-Based

- Help the client set up a medication box that reminds the client to take medication at needed times; assist the client with refilling the box at intervals if necessary. *Medication boxes are effective because clients will know whether medication has been taken when corresponding compartments are empty.*

- If safety is an issue with certain activities (e.g., the client forgets to turn off stove after use or forgets emergency telephone numbers), suggest alternatives such as using a microwave or whistling tea-kettle for heating water and programming emergency numbers in telephone so that they are readily available.

- ▲ Refer the client to a memory clinic (if available), a neuropsychologist, or an occupational therapist. *Memory clinics can help the client learn ways to improve memory. Clinics may be more effective if work is done in groups because of increased support, reinforcement, and motivation (Hutchison et al, 2006).*

- For clients with memory impairments associated with dementia, see care plan for **Chronic Confusion.**

Geriatric

- Assess for signs of depression. *Depression is the most important affective variable for memory loss in the older adult (Potter & Steffens, 2007).* **EB:** *Cognitive impairment is not an inevitable consequence of aging, even in very old age (Steffens, 2008).*

- ▲ Evaluate all medications that the client is taking to determine whether they are causing the memory loss. *Many medications, both prescription and over the counter, may cause memory loss in the elderly, including anticholinergics, H2–receptor antagonists, beta-blockers, digitalis, benzodiazepines, barbiturates, and even mild opiates (Lowenthal et al, 2007).*

- Evaluate all herbal and/or nutraceutical products that the individual might be using to improve their memory function. For example, products that claim to enhance some aspect of cognitive function, such as attention, concentration, or memory are readily accessible in local pharmacies and food markets. *The individual may read the products' names, which use some "cognitive terminology," and assume there will be an intended cognitive benefit. The ingredients contained in the product may not be known outside of the homeopathic field. The treatment efficacy is often contradictory because products are recommended for purposes other than cognitive or memory loss. And, because the manufacturers of the product have usually conducted the research on individual products, it is not clear how to evaluate the stated benefits (McDougall, Austin-Wells, & Zimmerman, 2005).*

- Recommend that elderly clients maintain a positive attitude and active involvement with the world around them and that they maintain good nutrition. **EB:** *Evidence from the Nun Study indicated that it is possible to maintain cognitive function until extreme old age if elderly persons maintain active involvement with their environment and are able to avoid having vascular disease with infarction of brain tissue (Tyas et al, 2007).*

- Encourage the elderly to believe in themselves and to work to improve their memory. *Negative attitudes and belief may decrease motivation and impair everyday memory function Research has shown that there is formation of new neurons in the brain, a process called neurogenesis, throughout the life span, and stimulation of the brain is necessary for this formation (McDougall, 2009).* **EB:** *Elderly clients may be able to improve their memory function up to 50% if they use appropriate strategies and invest the energy and time (Ball et al, 2002).*

- ▲ Refer the client to a memory class that focuses on helping older adults learn memory strategies. **EBN and EB:** *Research has demonstrated that classes that focus on memory strategies could improve memory (McDougall, 2009). In memory impairment associated with strokes, there is insufficient evidence to determine if memory training is effective (Vance et al, 2007). The group of individuals with traumatic brain injury who received spaced-retrieval training delivered over the telephone produced significantly more treatment goal mastery, strategy use, and maintenance than didactic instruction in use of memory strategies. However, both treatments produced improvements in everyday memory function (Bourgeois et al, 2007).*

- Help family label items such as the bathroom or sock drawer to increase recall. *A supportive environment that includes orientation can help increase the client's awareness (Vance & Farr, 2007).*

• = Independent   ▲ = Collaborative   **EBN** = Evidence-Based Nursing   **EB** = Evidence-Based

Multicultural

- Assess for the influence of cultural beliefs, norms, and values on the family or caregiver's understanding of impaired memory. *A national survey in the United States found that there were large misconceptions in knowledge, awareness, and beliefs about Alzheimer's disease among different ethnic and racial groups (Connell, Scott Roberts, & McLaughlin, 2007).*
- Use bias-free instruments when assessing memory in the culturally diverse client. **EBN:** *Use of the Mini-Mental State Exam (MMSE) has significant differential item functioning when translated into Spanish (Ramirez et al, 2006).*
- Inform the client's family or caregiver of meaning of and reasons for common behavior observed in the client with impaired memory. *An understanding of impaired memory behavior will enable the client family/caregiver to provide the client with a safe environment.*
- Attempt to validate family members' feelings regarding the impact of the client's behavior on family lifestyle.

Home Care

- Above interventions may be adapted for home care use.
- Assess the client's need for outside assistance with recall of treatment, medications, and willingness/ability of family to provide needed support. *During initial phase of home care, increased frequency of visits may be necessary to compensate for the client's inability to recall treatment or medications. Counting of medications may be needed to determine if the client is following medication regimen. Telephone calls from family/friends may help to remind the client of treatment schedule.*
- Identify a checking-in support system (e.g., Lifeline or significant others). *Checking in ensures the client's safety.*
- Keep furniture placement and household patterns consistent. *Change increases risk of impaired memory and decreased functioning.*

Client/Family Teaching and Discharge Planning

- When teaching the client, determine what the client knows about memory techniques and build on that knowledge. *New material is organized in terms of what knowledge already exists, and efficient teaching should attempt to take advantage of what is already known in order to graft on new material (Sorrell, 2008).*
- When teaching a skill to the client, set up a series of practice attempts that will enhance motivation. Begin with simple tasks so that the client can be positively reinforced and progress to more difficult concepts. *Distributed practice with correct recall attempts can be a very effective teaching strategy. Widely distribute practice over time if possible (Koestner et al, 2008).*
- Teach clients to use memory techniques such as concentrating and attending, repeating information, making mental associations, and placing items in strategic places so that they will not be forgotten. *These methods increase recall of information the client thinks is important. The internal methods of increasing memory can be effective, especially if used along with external methods such as calendars, lists, and other methods (McDougall, 2009).*

 See the EVOLVE website for Weblinks for client education resources.

REFERENCES

Ball K, Berch DB, Helmers KF et al: Effects of cognitive training interventions with older adults: a randomized controlled trial, *JAMA* 288(18):2271–2281, 2002.

Barton C, Sklenicka J, Sayegh P et al: Contraindicated medication use among patients in a memory disorders clinic, *Am J Geriatr Pharmacother* 6(3):147–152, 2008.

Britton A, Russell R: Multidisciplinary team interventions for delirium in patients with chronic cognitive impairment, *Cochrane Database Syst Rev* (2):CD000395, 2007.

Bourgeois MS, Lenius K, Turkstra L et al: The effects of cognitive teletherapy on reported everyday memory behaviours of persons with chronic traumatic brain injury, *Brain Inj* 21(12):1245–1257, 2007.

Bourre JM: Effects of nutrients (in food) on the structure and function of the nervous system: update on dietary requirements for brain. Part 1: micronutrients, *J Nutr Health Aging* 10(5):377–385, 2006.

Connell CM, Scott Roberts J, McLaughlin SJ: Public opinion about Alzheimer disease among blacks, Hispanics, and whites: results from a national survey, *Alzheimer Dis Assoc Disord* 21(3):232–240, 2007.

de Quervain DJ, Margraf J: Glucocorticoids for the treatment of post-traumatic stress disorder and phobias: a novel therapeutic approach, *Eur J Pharmacol* 583(2–3):365–371, 2008.

Federman AD, Sano M, Wolf MS et al: Health literacy and cognitive performance in older adults, *J Am Geriatr Soc* 57(8):1475–1480, 2009.

Gohier B, Ferracci L, Surguladze SA et al: Cognitive inhibition and working memory in unipolar depression, *J Affect Disord* 116(1–2):100–105, 2008.

Haaland DA, Sabljic TF, Baribeau DA et al: Is regular exercise a friend or foe of the aging immune system? A systematic review, *Clin J Sport Med* 18(6):539–548, 2008.

He FJ, Nowson CA, MacGregor GA: Fruit and vegetable consumption and stroke: meta-analysis of cohort studies, *Lancet* 367(9507):320–326, 2006.

Hutchison LC, Jones SK, West DS et al: Assessment of medication management by community-living elderly persons with two standardized assessment tools: a cross-sectional study, *Am J Geriatr Pharmacother* 4(2):144–153, 2006.

Insel KC, Cole L: Individualizing memory strategies to improve medication adherence, *Appl Nurs Res* 18(4):199–204, 2005.

Kliegel M, Jäger T, Phillips LH: Adult age differences in event-based prospective memory: a meta-analysis on the role of focal versus nonfocal cues, *Psychol Aging* 23(1):203–208, 2008.

Koestner R, Otis N, Powers TA et al: Autonomous motivation, controlled motivation, and goal progress, *J Pers* 76(5):1201–1230, 2008.

Kopelman MD, Thomson AD, Guerrini I et al: The Korsakoff syndrome: clinical aspects, psychology and treatment, *Alcohol Alcohol* 44(2):148–154, 2009.

Loizzo JJ: Optimizing learning and quality of life throughout the lifespan: a global framework for research and application, *Ann N Y Acad Sci* Sep 28, 2007, Epub ahead of print.

Lowenthal DT, Paran E, Burgos L et al: General characteristics of treatable, reversible, and untreatable dementias, *Am J Geriatr Cardiol* 16(3):136–142, 2007.

McDougall GJ: A framework for cognitive interventions targeting everyday memory performance and memory self-efficacy, *Fam Community Health* 32(1 Suppl):S15–S26, 2009.

McDougall GJ, Austin-Wells V, Zimmerman T: Utility of nutraceutical products marketed for cognitive and memory enhancement, *J Hol Nur* 23:415, 2005.

McDougall GJ Jr, Vaughan PW, Acee TW et al: Memory performance and mild cognitive impairment in black and white community elders, *Ethn Dis* 17(2):381–388, 2007.

Mosconi L, Pupi A, De Leon MJ: Brain glucose hypometabolism and oxidative stress in preclinical Alzheimer's disease, *Ann N Y Acad Sci* 1147:180–195, 2008.

Panza F, Solfrizzi V, Colacicco AM et al: Cerebrovascular disease in the elderly: lipoprotein metabolism and cognitive decline, *Aging Clin Exp Res* 18(2):144–148, 2006.

Potter GG, Steffens DC: Contribution of depression to cognitive impairment and dementia in older adults, *Neurologist* 13(3):105–117, 2007.

Ramirez M, Teresi JA, Holmes D et al: Differential item functioning (DIF) and the Mini-Mental State Examination (MMSE). Overview, sample, and issues of translation, *Med Care* 44(11 Suppl 3):S95–S106, 2006.

Shukitt-Hale B, Lau FC, Joseph JA: Berry fruit supplementation and the aging brain, *J Agric Food Chem* 56(3):636–641, 2008.

Sorrell JM: Remembering: forget about forgetting and train your brain instead, *J Psychosoc Nurs Ment Health Serv* 46(9):25–27, 2008.

Steffens DC: Separating mood disturbance from mild cognitive impairment in geriatric depression, *Int Rev Psychiatry* 20(4):374–381, 2008.

Stickgold R, Walker MP: Sleep-dependent memory consolidation and re-consolidation, *Sleep Med* 8(4):331–343, 2007.

Tyas SL, Snowdon DA, Desrosiers MF et al: Healthy ageing in the Nun Study: definition and neuropathologic correlates, *Age Ageing* 36(6):650–655, 2007.

Vance DE, Farr KF: Spaced Retrieval for enhancing memory: implications for nursing practice and research, *J Gerontol Nurs* 33(9):46–52, 2007.

Vance DE, Ball KK, Moore BS et al: Cognitive remediation therapies for older adults: implications for nursing practice and research, *J Neurosci Nurs* 39(4):226–231, 2007.

van Stegeren AH: Imaging stress effects on memory: a review of neuroimaging studies, *Can J Psychiatry* 54(1):16–27, 2009.

Watson GS, Craft S: Insulin resistance, inflammation, and cognition in Alzheimer's Disease: lessons for multiple sclerosis, *J Neurol Sci* 245(1–2):21–33, 2006.

Wolf OT: Stress and memory in humans: twelve years of progress? *Brain Res* 1293:142–54, 2009.

Yücel M, Lubman DI, Solowij N et al: Understanding drug addiction: a neuropsychological perspective, *Aust N Z J Psychiatry* 41(12):957–968, 2007.

Impaired bed Mobility   *Brenda Emick-Herring, RN, MSN, CRRN*

NANDA-I

Definition

Limitation of independent movement from one bed position to another

Defining Characteristics

Impaired ability to move from supine to sitting; to move from sitting to supine; to move from supine to prone; to move from prone to supine; to move from supine to long sitting; to move from long sitting to supine; to "scoot" or reposition self in bed; to turn from side to side

Related Factors (r/t)

Cognitive impairment; deconditioning; deficient knowledge; environmental constraints (i.e., bed size, bed type, treatment equipment, restraints); insufficient muscle strength; musculoskeletal impairment; neuromuscular impairment; obesity; pain; sedating medications. NOTE: specify level of independence using a standardized functional scale

● = Independent   ▲ = Collaborative   **EBN** = Evidence-Based Nursing   **EB** = Evidence-Based

(Nursing Outcomes Classification)

Suggested NOC Outcomes

Mobility, Self-Care: Activities of Daily Living (ADLs)

Example **NOC Outcome with Indicators**
Mobility as evidenced by the following indicators: Body positioning performance/Gait/Joint movement (Rate the outcome and indicators of **Mobility:** 1 = severely compromised, 2 = substantially compromised, 3 = moderately compromised, 4 = mildly compromised, 5 = not compromised [see Section I].)

Client Outcomes

Client Will (Specify Time Frame):

- Demonstrate optimal independence in positioning, exercising, and performing functional activities in bed
- Demonstrate ability to direct others on how to do bed positioning, exercising, and functional activities

 (Nursing Interventions Classification)

Suggested NIC Intervention

Bed Rest Care

Example **NIC Activities—Bed Rest Care**
Position in proper body alignment; Teach bed exercises, as appropriate

Nursing Interventions and *Rationales*

- Critically think/set priorities to use the most therapeutic bed positions based on client's history, risk profile, preventative needs; realize positioning for one condition may negatively affect another. *Conditions such as dyspnea, chest injury, pressure ulcer, pain, spinal cord or head injury, fractures, and amputation warrant certain bed positions to prevent complications (Gallimore, 2005).*
- Assess client's risk for aspiration; if present elevate height of bed (HOB) to 30°, especially when feeding. *Maintaining a sitting position with and after meals can help decrease aspiration pneumonia (Guy & Smith, 2009).*
- Raise HOB 30° for clients with acute increased intracranial pressure (ICP) and brain injury. Refer to care plan for **Decreased Intracranial adaptive capacity.**
- ▲ Consult physician for HOB elevation of clients with acute stroke and monitor their response. Refer to care plan for **Decreased Intracranial adaptive capacity.**
- Raise HOB as close to 45° as possible for critically ill, ventilated clients to prevent pneumonia (this height may place clients at higher risk for pressure ulcers). *Elevating the HOB decreases regurgitation and risk of aspiration of gastric contents.* **EB:** *Researchers reviewed random controlled trials/reviews of prevention of ventilator-associated pneumonia (VAP), and their recommendations included elevating HOB to 45° (Muscedere et al, 2008).*
- Assist client to sit as upright as possible during meals/ingestion of pills if dysphagic. Refer to care plan for **Impaired Swallowing.** *Sitting helps prevent aspiration of food, liquids, and pills (Flannery & Pugh, 2004; Gavin-Dreschnack, 2004).*
- Periodically sit client as upright as tolerated in bed and dangle client, if vital signs/oxygen saturation levels remain stable. *Being vertical reduces the work of the heart and improves circulation/lung ventilation/strength and stimulates reflexes and awareness of surroundings.* **EB:** *Sitting inpatients with community-acquired pneumonia 20 minutes the first day with progressive mobilization thereafter shortened the length of stay by one day (Mundy et al, 2003).*
- Maintain HOB at lowest elevation that is medically possible to prevent pressure ulcers; check sacrum often. *Sacral shearing risk is high when HOB is above 30°; skin may stick to linen if clients slide down, causing skin to pull away from underlying muscle tissue/bone (WOCN, 2003).*

● = Independent   ▲ = Collaborative   **EBN** = Evidence-Based Nursing   **EB** = Evidence-Based

- Trial prone positioning for clients with acute respiratory distress syndrome (ARDS), acute lung injury (ALI), and amputation and monitor their tolerance/response. *Prone positioning may improve oxygenation; it allows hip extension and thus prevents flexor contractions in amputated lower extremities.* **EBN:** *Systematic review of the literature demonstrated that a large portion of clients with ARDS who were turned prone had improved oxygenation patterns (Vollman, 2004; Essat, 2005; Voggenreiter et al, 2005). EB: In a review, subjects with ARDS or ALI on prone kinetic therapy had increased improvement in PaO_2/FiO_2 ratios, lower mortality, and "less pulmonary-related mortality" than those on supine kinetic therapy (Davis et al, 2007).*

- Assess client's risk for falls using a valid tool, establish individualized fall prevention strategies, and perform post fall–assessment to further refine fall-prevention interventions. **EBN:** *Fall assessment tools help identify clients at high risk so early prevention and protection measures can be implemented (Morse, 2006). A cohort study showed a fall program, using the Morse Scale to identify high-risk clients, reduced multiple falls (Schwendimann et al, 2006). A validation study demonstrated that a post fall–assessment tool identified causes of falls and guided future prevention interventions (Gray-Miceli et al, 2006).*

- Lock bed brakes, use low rise beds at lowest position with floor mats next to them, avoid use of side rails, and apply personal exit alarms on confused clients. *Such interventions help prevent falls and reduce injury if fall occurs. Low rise beds sit about 14" above the floor, so reduce the distance of a fall (Lyons, 2004).* **EB:** *Bowers and colleagues' (2008) study results suggested a 25% chance of serious head injury with feet-first falls from about 3' onto a tiled floor surface, and that use of an appropriately sized mat (15 cm beyond head/foot boards) significantly reduced risk. Mats seemed to provide "a protective effect" for the pelvis during head-first falls and for the thorax during feet-first falls. Kelly et al (2002), in a descriptive study, reported that the NOC WATCH personal alarms decreased falls.*

- ▲ Avoid use of bedrails and restraints unless ordered by physician. *Tan and others (2005) analyzed incident report data on falls and reported more serious injuries occurred in restrained elders.*

- Place call light, bedside table, and telephone within reach of clients. *Clients won't fall out of bed reaching for needed items (Gray-Miceli, 2008).*

- Use a formalized screening tool to identify persons at high risk for thromboembolism (DVT). *Early detection of high risk prompts early initiation of prophylaxis (Hums & Blostein, 2006).*

- ▲ Implement thromboembolism prophylaxis/treatment as ordered (e.g., anticoagulants, antiembolic stockings, elastic leg wraps, sequential compression devices, feet/ankle exercises, and hydration). *Anticoagulants prevent blood clots; mechanical devices/exercises prevent venous stasis (Anderson & Spencer, 2003).* Refer to care plan for **Ineffective peripheral tissue Perfusion.**

- Use a formal tool to assess for risk of pressure ulcers. *Braden and Norton scales are valid tools along with nursing judgment to assess for risk of pressure ulcer (WOCN, 2003).*

- Implement the following interventions to prevent pressure ulcers and complications of immobility:
  - Position joints/limbs in neutral alignment and safely pad pressure points/body parts needing support preoperatively/intraoperatively. *This prevents pressure ulcers, trauma, nerve injury, and restricted blood flow to immobile and strapped body parts during surgery (Murphy, 2004).*
  - Turn (logroll) clients at high risk for pressure/shear/friction frequently (Salcido, 2006). **EBN:** *Turn clients **at least** every 2 to 4 hours on pressure-reducing mattress/every 2 hours if on standard foam mattress (WOCN, 2003).*
  - Use static/dynamic bed surfaces and assess for "bottoming out" under susceptible bony areas (body sinks into mattress, thus the recommended 1 inch between mattress/bones is absent). Refer to care plan for **Risk for impaired Skin integrity.**
  - Place positioning devices such as pillows/foam between bony prominences (knees, etc.). Place pillows lengthwise under calves to relieve heel pressure *except* after total knee replacement (WOCN, 2003).
  - Implement a 2–hour on/off schedule for heel protector boots or high-top tennis shoes with socks underneath on clients with paralyzed feet, and check condition of heels when removed. **EBN:** *A study found that use of a specialized boot resulted in reduction of heel ulcers (Brainard & Ortiz, 2007).*
  - Strictly maintain leg abduction in persons with a surgical hip pinning or replacement by placing an abductor splint/pillow between legs. *Abduction stabilizes new prosthesis in the hip joint (Olson, 2008).*

- Use devices such as trapeze, friction-reducing slide sheets, mechanical lateral transfer aids, and ceiling-mounted or floor lifts to move (rather than drag) dependent/obese persons in bed. *Devices prevent musculoskeletal injuries in staff and protect clients' skin against friction and shear (WOCN, 2003; Nelson & Baptiste, 2006).* **EBN:** *Nelson et al (2006) demonstrated a significant improvement in two areas of job satisfaction: reduced staff musculoskeletal injuries, and facility cost savings after a multifaceted ergonomics program was implemented for client-handling activities.* **EB:** *Ronald et al (2002) analyzed injury reports 3 years before and 1.5 years after installation of ceiling-mounted lifts; results showed a significant reduction of staff musculoskeletal injuries when transferring/lifting clients.*

- Apply elbow pads to comatose/restrained clients and to those who use elbows to prop/scoot up in bed; apply nocturnal elbow splint as ordered if ulnar nerve palsy exists or if painful elbow with paresthesia in ulnar side of fourth/fifth fingers develops. *Prolonged compression or flexion puts pressure on the ulnar nerve, causing neuropathy/nerve damage; pads prevent this. Elbow splints provide joint extension (Szabo & Kwak, 2007).* NOTE: *An enclosure bed for agitated clients may alleviate restraints, thus preventing arm abrasions, nerve damage, and pain.*

- Explain importance of exhaling versus holding one's breath (Valsalva maneuver) and straining during bed activities. *Exhaling* with movement *prevents increased intraabdominal and intrathoracic pressure which elevates blood pressure and impairs myocardial/cerebral perfusion (Weimer & Zadeh, 2009).*

- Reassess pain level, especially before movement/exercising, and accept clients' pain rating and level they think is appropriate for comfort, then administer analgesics based on rating (Pasero & McCaffery, 2004). *It is a client's right for pain assessment/intervention. Systematic ongoing pain assessment/documentation provides sound, client-focused direction for acute/chronic pain management (Berry et al, 2006).*

- Use special beds/equipment to move bariatric (very obese) clients, such as mattress overlay, sliding/roller board, trapeze, stirrup, and pulley attached to overhead traction system (holds one leg up during pericare). *This reduces skin shear and frictional burn plus decreases resistance for staff to overcome when repositioning obese clients (Dionne, 2005).*

- Place bariatric clients in free-standing or ceiling-mounted lifts with padded slings while changing bed linen. *Less manual lifting reduces staff musculoskeletal injuries (Logan, 2008).*

- Place bariatric beds along a corner wall. *Helps keep bed from moving during repositioning.*

- Logroll and tilt dependent bariatric clients (avoid full side-lying position) in bariatric beds with side rails up until familiar with client's ability to help turn in bed. *If client starts to slide out of bed in full side-lying position, it is difficult for staff to stop the motion (Dionne, 2005).*

- Identify/modify hospital beds with large gaps between bedrail/mattress that create an entrapment hazard. Ensure mattresses fit the bed; instill gap fillers/rail inserts, then monitor effectiveness. *Entrapment can be life threatening (Powell-Cope, Baptiste, & Nelson, 2005).*

Exercise

- Perform passive range of motion (ROM) of three repetitions, at least twice a day, to immobile joints (Nursing, 2007).

- Perform ROM slowly/rhythmically. Do not range beyond point of pain. Range only to point of resistance in those with loss of sensation/mentation. *Fast, jerky ROM increases pain/tone. Slow, rhythmical movements relax/lengthen spastic muscles so they can be ranged further.* NOTE: *This is not the case with rigidity, as in Parkinson's disease.*

- Range/move a hemiplegic arm with the shoulder slightly externally rotated (hand up). *Spasticity prevents normal gliding movements of shoulder thus soft tissue gets pinched between bones, causing pain. External rotation prevents this (de Jong, Nieuwboer, & Aufdem Kampe, 2006).*

- ▲ Emphasize client's practice of exercises taught them by therapists (muscle setting, strengthening, contraction against resistance, and weight lifting). *Exercises/weight lifting helps maintain muscle tone/strength/lengthening.* **EB:** *Results from a literature review of various stretching techniques of the hamstring indicated increased ROM after stretching (Decoster et al, 2005). In a study with clients on bed rest, results indicated resistive exercises prevented tendon structure stiffness in knee extensors (Kubo et al, 2004).*

• = Independent   ▲ = Collaborative   **EBN** = Evidence-Based Nursing   **EB** = Evidence-Based

Bed Positioning

- Incorporate the following measures to promote normal tone and prevent complications in clients with neurological impairment.
  - Use a flat head pillow when clients are supine. Use a small pillow behind the head and/or between shoulder blades if neck extension occurs. *Prevents contractures of the cervical spine and abnormal tone of the neck (Potter & Perry, 2009).*
  - Lay a sandbag under the pillow along one or both sides of the head to help prevent lateral neck rotation when clients are supine, and one thick pillow under the head when they are side-lying. *Lateral head flexion and rotation, if allowed, may occlude the internal jugular vein, thus preventing cerebral venous outflow, which can increase ICP (Gallimore, 2005).*
  - Abduct the shoulders of persons with high paraplegia or quadriplegia horizontally to 90 degrees briefly two to three times a day while supine. *Promotes full upper extremity range of motion in spinal cord–injured/diseased clients.*
  - Position a hemiplegic shoulder fairly close to the client's body. *Too much abduction increases spasticity around the scapula, inhibits normal gliding movements, and pinches soft tissue, causing pain (Hoeman, Lizner, & Alverzo, 2008).*
- ▲ Elevate paralyzed forearm(s) on a pillow when supine and apply Isotoner gloves; elevate edematous legs on a pillow and apply elastic wraps and compression garments as ordered. *Lymph fluid collects in dependent hands/legs, causing venous insufficiency and limited motion; elevation/gravity/ROM prevents lymphedema especially if history of venous insufficiency (Kelly, 2007).*
- Tilt hemiplegics onto both unaffected/affected sides with the affected shoulder slightly forward (move/lift the affected shoulder, *not* the forearm/hand. *Weight bearing on and placement of the affected shoulder slightly forward reduces tone. Moving the affected shoulder versus the wrist or hand prevents shoulder pain (Hoeman, Liszner, & Alverzo, 2008).*
- ▲ Apply resting wrist and hand splints. Strictly adhere to on/off orders. Routinely check underlying skin for signs of pressure/poor circulation. *Devices maintain hands/wrists in neutral alignment and/or immobilize inflamed joints as a means of controlling pain (Hoeman, Liszner, & Alverzo, 2008).*
- ▲ Range weak/paralyzed ankle joints before applying foot splints, boots, or high-top tennis shoes on rotation schedule recommended by the physical therapist; routinely assess underlying skin for signs of pressure. *This helps prevent foot drop, spasticity, and joint contractures (Hoeman, Liszner, & Alverzo, 2008).*
- ▲ Components of normal bed mobility include rolling, bridging, scooting, long sitting, and sitting upright. Activity starts with the client supine, flat in bed and promotes normal movements which are bilateral, segmental, well-timed, and involve set positions such as weight bearing and trunk centering. Refer to physician therapist (PT) for individualized instructions/strategies.

Geriatric

- Assess caregivers' strength, health history, and cognitive status to predict ability/risk for assisting bed-bound clients at home. Explore alternatives if risk is too high. *Caregivers are often frail elders with chronic health problems who cannot physically help loved ones.* Refer to care plan for **Caregiver role strain.**
- Assess the client's stamina and energy level during bed activities/exercises; if limited, spread out activities and allow rest breaks. *Elders may have fatigue and poor energy reserves due to cardiopulmonary impairments (McAnaw, 2001).*

Home Care

- ▲ Utilize nurse case managers, care coordinators, or social workers to assess support systems and identify need for durable medical equipment, assistive technology, and home health services. *Professional advocates can help clients understand coverage issues and locate resources (Berry & Ignash, 2003).* **EBN:** *A systematic review of research indicated access to health/social services was problematic and that care referrals was a priority for transitional care of elders (Naylor, 2002).*
- Encourage use of the client's bed unless contraindicated. Raise HOB with commercial blocks or grooved-out pieces of wood under legs; set bed against walls in a corner. *Emotionally, persons may*

benefit from sleeping in their own bed with their partner. Blocks/walls help secure the bed for persons who need to be elevated during sleep.

- Suggest home modifications and rearranging rooms/furniture to meet sleeping/toileting/living needs on one level. *Such conversions enhance accessibility, safety, and functioning and are less taxing and costly than home additions or institutionalization (McCullagh, 2006).*
- Stress psychological/physical benefits of clients being as self-sufficient as possible with bed mobility/cares even though it may be time-consuming. *Allowing independence and autonomy may help prevent disuse syndromes and feelings of helplessness and low self-esteem.*
- Offer emotional support and help client identify usual coping responses to help with adjustment and loss issues. *The home environment may trigger the reality of lost function and disability.*
- Discuss support systems available for caregivers to help them cope. *Please refer to care plan for* **Caregiver role strain.**
- ▲ In the presence of medical disorders, institute case management for the frail elderly to support continued independent living.
- Refer to the Home Care interventions of the care plan for **Impaired physical Mobility.**

Client/Family Teaching and Discharge Planning

- Use various sensory modalities to teach client/caregivers correct ROM, exercises, positioning, self-care activities, and use of devices. *Readiness and learning styles vary but may be enhanced with visual/auditory/tactile/cognitive stimulus as described below.*
  - ■ Provide visual information such as demonstrations, sketches, instructional videos, written directions/schedules, notes. *Written information reinforced family learning of techniques for discharge (Ignatavicius & Workman, 2006).* **EB:** *A Cochrane review about communicating cares and health issues before discharge to home recommended written and verbal information (Johnson, Sandford, & Tyndall, 2003).*
  - ■ Provide auditory information such as verbal instructions, recorded audiotapes, timers, reading aloud written directions, and self-talk during activities.
  - ■ Use tactile stimulation such as motor task practice/repetition, return demonstrations, note taking, manual guidance, or staff's hand-on-client's hand technique.
- Schedule time with family/caregivers for education and practice. Suggest they come prepared with questions and wear comfortable, safe clothing/shoes. *Motor practice provides opportunity for learning; repetition helps memory retention.*
- Implement safe approaches for caregivers/home care staff and reinforce adequate number of people and handling equipment (friction pads, slide boards, lifts, etc.) during bed mobility, exercise, toileting, and bathing. *Risk of injury is high because home care staff and caregivers often work alone, without mechanical aids, and in crowded spaces, especially in bathrooms, as commode/shower chairs are less stable and clients are wet or need clothing to be removed (Long, 2008).*
- Coordinate bariatric equipment for home use before discharge including a weight-rated bed, a wheelchair or mobility device (scooter) and lift device; doorways may need to be widened, floors reinforced, and ramps may need to be added for safety (Logan, 2008).

ⓔvolve   See the EVOLVE website for Weblinks for client education resources.

REFERENCES

Anderson FA, Spencer FA: Risk factors for venous thromboembolism, *Circulation* 107(23 Suppl 1):I9–I16, 2003.

Berry BE, Ignash S: Assistive technology: providing independence for individuals with disabilities, *Rehabil Nurs* 28(1):6–14, 2003.

Berry PH, Covington ED, Dahl J et al: *Pain: Current understanding of assessment, management, and treatment.* Reston VA, 2006, National Pharmaceutical Council.

Bowers B, Lloyd J, Lee W: Biomechanical evaluation of injury severity associated with patient falls from bed, *Rehabil Nurs* 33(6):253–259, 2008.

Brainard N, Ortiz L: Simple low cost intervention saves VA hospital thousands through reduction in heel injury. Poster presented at Institute for Healthcare Improvement, Orlando, FL, December 2007.

Davis JW, Lemaster DM, Moore EC et al: Prone ventilation in trauma or surgical patients with acute lung injury and adult respiratory distress syndrome: is it beneficial? *J Trauma* 62(5):1201–1206, 2007.

Decoster LC, Cleland J, Altieri C et al: The effects of hamstring stretching on range of motion: A systematic literature review, *J Orthop Sports Phys Ther* 35(6):377–387, 2005.

de Jong LD, Nieuwboer A, Aufdemkampe G: Contracture preventive positioning of the hemiplegic arm in subacute stroke patients: a pilot randomized controlled trial, *Clin Rehabil* 20:656–667, 2006.

Dionne M: Watch your back, *Rehabil Manag* 18(6):30, 32–33, 2005.

Essat Z: Prone positioning in patients with acute respiratory distress syndrome, *Nurs Stand* 20(9):52–55, 2005.

● = Independent ▲ = Collaborative **EBN** = Evidence-Based Nursing **EB** = Evidence-Based

Flannery J, Pugh SB: Stroke rehabilitation. In Flannery J, editor: *Rehabilitation nursing secrets,* St Louis, 2004, Mosby.

Gallimore GH: Positioning critically ill patients in hospital, *Nurs Stand* 19(42):56–66, 2005.

Gavin-Dreschnack D: Effects of wheelchair posture on patient safety, *Rehabil Nurs* 29(6):221–226, 2004.

Gray-Miceli DL: Fall prevention. In Ackley BJ, Ladwig GB, Swan BA et al, editors: *Evidence-based nursing care guidelines,* St Louis, 2008, Mosby.

Gray-Miceli DL, Strumpf NE, Johnson J et al: Psychometric properties of the Post-Fall Index, *Clin Nurs Res* 15(3):157–176, 2006.

Hoeman SP, Liszner L, Alverzo J: Functional mobility with activities of daily living. In Hoeman SP, editor: *Rehabilitation nursing: prevention, intervention & outcomes,* ed 4, St Louis, 2008, Mosby.

Hums W, Blostein P: A comparative approach to deep vein thrombosis risk assessment, *J Trauma Nurs* 13(1):28–30, 2006.

Ignatavicius DD, Workman ML (Editors). *Medical-surgical nursing: Critical thinking for collaborative care,* ed 5, Philadelphia, 2006, Saunders.

Johnson A, Sandford J, Tyndall J: Written and verbal information versus verbal information only for patients being discharged from acute hospital settings to home, *Cochrane Database Syst Rev* (4):CD003716, 2003.

Kelly DG: Vascular, lymphatic, and integumentary disorders. In O'Sullivan SB, Schmitz TJ , editors: *Physical rehabilitation,* ed 5, Philadelphia, 2007, F.A. Davis.

Kelly KE, Phillips CL, Cain KC et al: Evaluation of a nonintrusive monitor to reduce falls in nursing home patients, *J Am Med Dir Assoc* 3(6):377–382, 2002.

Kubo K, Akima H, Ushiyama J et al: Effects of resistance training during bed rest on the viscoelastic properties of tendon structures in the lower limb, *Scand J Med Sci Sports* 14(5):296–302, 2004.

Logan C: Substantial solutions: creating safe and sensitive care pathways for bariatric patients, *Rehabil Manag,* 21(5):23–25, 2008.

Long F: Safe lift strategy, *Rehabil manage* 21(6):28–30, 2008.

Lyons SS: *Fall prevention for older adults,* University of Iowa Gerontological Nursing Interventions Research Center, Research Dissemination Core. Iowa City IA: Feb, 2004.

McAnaw MB: Normal changes with aging. In Maas ML et al, editors: *Nursing care of older adults: diagnoses, outcomes and interventions,* St Louis, 2001, Mosby.

McCullagh MC: Home modification: how to help patients make their homes safer and more accessible as their abilities change, *Am J Nurs* 106(10):54–64, 2006.

Morse, JM: The safety of safety research: the case of patient fall research, *Can J Nurs Res* 38(2):74, 2006.

Mundy LM, Leet TL, Darst K et al: Early mobilization of patients hospitalized with community-acquired pneumonia, *Chest* 124(3):883–889, 2003.

Murphy EK: Negligence cases concerning positioning injuries, *AORN J* 80(2):311–314, 2004.

Muscedere J, Dodek P, Keenan S et al: Comprehensive evidence-based clinical practice guidelines for ventilator-associated pneumonia: prevention, *J Crit Care* 23(1):126–137, 2008.

Naylor MD: Transitional care of older adults, *Annu Rev Nurs Res* 20: 127–147, 2002.

Nelson A, Baptiste AS: Evidence-based practices for safe patient handling and movement, *Orthop Nurs* 25(6):366–379, 2006.

Nelson A, Matz M, Chen F et al: Development and evaluation of a multifaceted ergonomics program to prevent injuries associated with patient handling tasks, *Int J Nurs Stud* 43:717–733, 2006.

Nursing: Performing passive range-of-motion exercises, *Nursing,* 36(3): 50–51, 2007.

Olson RS: Muscle and skeletal function. In SP Hoeman editor: *Rehabilitation nursing: prevention, intervention, & outcomes,* ed 4, St Louis, 2008, Mosby.

Pasero C, McCaffery M: Comfort-function goals: A way to establish accountability for pain relief, *Am J Nurs* 104(9):77–78, 81, 2004.

Potter PA, Perry AG: *Fundamentals of nursing,* ed 7, St Louis, Mosby, 2009.

Powell-Cope G, Baptiste AS, Nelson A: Modification of bed systems and use of accessories to reduce the risk of hospital-bed entrapment, *Rehabil Nurs* 30(1):9–17, 2005.

Ronald LA, Yassi A, Spiegel J et al: Effectiveness of installing overhead ceiling lifts. Reducing musculoskeletal injuries in an extended care hospital unit, *AAOHN J* 50(3):120–127, 2002.

Salcido R: Patient turning schedules: why and how often? *Adv Skin Wound Care* 17(4 pt 1):156, 2006.

Schwendimann R, Milisen K, Buhler H et al: Fall prevention in a Swiss acute care hospital setting: Reducing multiple falls, *J Gerontol Nurs* 32(3):13–22, 2006.

Smith LH. Preventing aspiration: a common and dangerous problem for patients with cancer. *Clin J Oncol Nurs* 13(1):105–108, 2009.

Szabo RM, Kwak C: Natural history and conservative management of cubital tunnel syndrome, *Hand Clin* 23:311–318, 2007.

Tan KM, Austin B, Shaughnassy M et al: Falls in acute care hospital and their relationship to restraint use, *Ir J Med Sci* 174(3):28–31, 2005.

Voggenreiter G, Aufmkolk M, Stiletto R et al: Prone positioning improves oxygenation in post-traumatic lung injury-A prospective randomized trial, *J Trauma* 59(2):333–341, 2005.

Vollman, KM: Prone positioning in the patient who has acute respiratory distress syndrome: the art and science, *Crit Care Nurs Clin North Am* 16(3):319–336, 2004.

Weimer LH, Zadeh P: Neurological aspects of syncope and orthostatic intolerance, *Med Clin North Am* 93:427–449, 2009.

Wound, Ostomy, and Continence Nurses Society (WOCN): *Guideline for prevention and management of pressure ulcers* (WOCN clinical practice guideline, no 2), Glenview IL, 2003.

Impaired physical Mobility   ⊝volve

Sherry H. Pomeroy, PhD, RN, and Brenda Emick-Herring, RN, MSN, CRRN

NANDA-I

Definition

A limitation in independent, purposeful physical movement of the body or of one or more extremities

● = Independent   ▲ = Collaborative   **EBN** = Evidence-Based Nursing   **EB** = Evidence-Based

Defining Characteristics

Decreased reaction time; difficulty turning; engages in substitutions for movement (e.g., increased attention to other's activity, controlling behavior, focus on pre-illness disability/activity); exertional dyspnea; gait changes; jerky movements; limited ability to perform gross motor skills; limited ability to perform fine motor skills; limited range of motion; movement-induced tremor; postural instability; slowed movement; uncoordinated movements

Related Factors (r/t)

Activity intolerance; altered cellular metabolism; anxiety; body mass index above 75th age-appropriate percentile; cognitive impairment; contractures; cultural beliefs regarding age-appropriate activity; deconditioning; decreased endurance; depressive mood state; decreased muscle control; decreased muscle mass; decreased muscle strength; deficient knowledge regarding value of physical activity; developmental delay; discomfort; disuse; joint stiffness; lack of environmental supports (e.g., physical or social); limited cardiovascular endurance; loss of integrity of bone structures; malnutrition; medications; musculoskeletal impairment; neuromuscular impairment; pain; prescribed movement restrictions; reluctance to initiate movement; sedentary lifestyle; sensoriperceptual impairments

Suggested functional level classifications include the following:

0—Completely independent
1—Requires use of equipment or device
2—Requires help from another person for assistance, supervision, or teaching
3—Requires help from another person and equipment device
4—Dependent (does not participate in activity)

 (Nursing Outcomes Classification)

Suggested NOC Outcomes

Ambulation, Ambulation: Wheelchair, Mobility, Self-Care: Activities of Daily Living (ADLs), Instrumental Activities of Daily Living (IADLs), Transfer Performance

Example NOC Outcome with Indicators
Ambulation as evidenced by the following indicators: Walks with effective gait/Walks at moderate pace/Walks up and down steps/Walks moderate distance (Rate the outcome and indicators of **Ambulation**: 1 = severely compromised, 2 = substantially compromised, 3 = moderately compromised, 4 = mildly compromised, 5 = not compromised [see Section I].)

Client Outcomes

Client Will (Specify Time Frame):

- Increase moderate-intensity aerobic or physical activity to 2 hours and 30 minutes (150 minutes), such as 30 minutes 5 or more days of the week, OR 1 hour and 15 minutes (75 minutes) a week of vigorous-intensity aerobic physical activity, OR an equivalent combination of moderate- and vigorous-intensity aerobic physical activity. Aerobic activity should be performed in episodes of at least 10 minutes, preferably spread throughout the week.
- Increase physical activity to minimum of 7500 to 10,000 steps per day (Tudor-Locke et al, 2008).
- Increase muscle-strengthening activities that involve all major muscle groups (legs, hips, back, chest, abdomen, shoulders, and arms) performed on 2 or more days per week.
- Meet mutually defined goals of increased physical activity and ambulation.
- Verbalize feeling of increased strength and ability to move.
- Verbalize less fear of falling and pain with physical activity.
- Demonstrate use of adaptive equipment (e.g., wheelchairs, walkers, weighted walking vests) to increase mobility.

• = Independent   ▲ = Collaborative   **EBN** = Evidence-Based Nursing   **EB** = Evidence-Based

NIC (Nursing Interventions Classification)

Suggested NIC Interventions

Exercise Therapy: Ambulation, Joint Mobility, Positioning

Example NIC Activities—Exercise Therapy: Ambulation
Assist the client to use footwear that facilitates walking and prevents injury; Instruct in availability of assistive devices, if appropriate

Nursing Interventions and *Rationales*

NOTE: Adults with disabilities should follow the adult guidelines; however, if not possible these persons should be as physically active as their abilities allow and avoid inactivity (Physical Activity Guidelines: U.S. Department of Health & Human Services, 2008). Use "start low and go slow" approach for intensity and duration of physical activity if client highly deconditioned, functionally limited, or has chronic conditions affecting performance of physical tasks. When progressing client's activities, use an individualized and tailored approach based on client's tolerance and preferences (ACSM, 2010).

- Screen for mobility skills in the following order: (1) bed mobility; (2) supported and unsupported sitting; (3) transition movements such as sit to stand, sitting down, and transfers; and (4) standing and walking activities. Use a tool such as the Assessment Criteria and Care Plan for Safe Patient Handling and Movement (Sedlak et al, 2009). *Assess for quality of movement, ability to walk and move, gait pattern, ADL function, presence of spasticity, activity tolerance, and activity order (Kneafsey, 2007).*

- Screen for additional measures of physical function to assess strength of muscle groups including: unassisted leg stand, use of a balance platform, elbow flexion and knee extension strength, grip strength, timed chair stands, and the 6-minute walk. **EBN:** *The nursing assessment should include factors related to mobility problems (e.g., ability to walk and move), with nursing goals and interventions developed to promote maximum mobility (Kneafsey, 2007). The abilities of the client should be assessed to determine how best to facilitate movement and protect the nurse from harm (Curb et al, 2006; Nelson et al, 2006).*

- Assess the client for cause of impaired mobility. Determine whether cause is physical, psychological, or motivational. *Some clients choose not to move because of psychological factors such as fear of falling or pain; an inability to cope; or depression.* Refer to care plans for **Risk for Falls, Acute** or **Chronic Pain, Ineffective Coping,** or **Hopelessness.**

- Use the Outcome Expectation for Exercise Scale (Resnick, Zimmerman, & Orwig, 2001) to determine client's self-efficacy expectations and outcomes expectations toward exercise. **EBN:** *Findings suggested that to optimize mobility and exercise in post–hip fracture older women self-efficacy and outcome expectations for exercise should be assessed. The impact of fear of falling was greater 1 year post–hip fracture suggesting, efforts to address fear should be ongoing long after the hip fracture occurs (Resnick et al, 2007).* **EBN:** *Use a fear of falling assessment, e.g., 1 item fear of falling question, Falls Efficacy Scale, or Mobility Efficacy Scale (Messecar, 2008).*

- Monitor and record the client's ability to tolerate activity and use all four extremities; note pulse rate, blood pressure, dyspnea, and skin color before and after activity. Refer to the care plan for **Activity intolerance. EB:** *Use valid and reliable screening procedures and tools to assess the client's preparticipaton in exercise health screening and risk stratification for exercise testing (low, moderate, or high risk) (ACSM, 2010).*

- ▲ Before activity, observe for and, if possible, treat pain with massage, heat pack to affected area, or medication. Ensure that the client is not oversedated. *Pain limits mobility and is often exacerbated by movement.*

- ▲ Consult with physical therapist for further evaluation, strength training, gait training, and development of a mobility plan. **EBN:** *A review of interventions to enhance mobility found that prescribing a regimen of regular physical activity that includes both aerobic exercise and muscle strengthening activities is beneficial to minimizing impaired mobility; use exercise diary or log to improve adherence to mobility enhancement recommendations. Develop mobility enhancement programs that are specific to gender, ethnicity, and are culturally appropriate (Yeom, Keller, & Fleury, 2009).*

• = Independent   ▲ = Collaborative   **EBN** = Evidence-Based Nursing   **EB** = Evidence-Based

- Obtain any assistive devices needed for activity, such as gait belt, weighted vest, walker, cane, crutches, or wheelchair, before the activity begins. *Assistive devices can help increase mobility (Yeom, Keller, & Fleury, 2009).*
- If the client is immobile, perform passive ROM exercises at least twice a day unless contraindicated; repeat each maneuver three times. *Inactivity rapidly contributes to muscle shortening and changes in periarticular and cartilaginous joint structure. The formation of contractures starts after 8 hours of immobility (Fletcher, 2005).*
- ▲ If the client is immobile, consult with physician for a safety evaluation before beginning an exercise program; if program is approved, begin with the following exercises:
  - Active ROM exercises using both upper and lower extremities (e.g., flexing and extending at ankles, knees, hips)
  - Chin-ups and pull-ups using a trapeze in bed (may be contraindicated in clients with cardiac conditions)
  - Strengthening exercises such as gluteal or quadriceps sitting exercises
  These exercises help reverse weakening and atrophy of muscles (Fauci et al, 2008).
- If client is immobile, consider use of a transfer chair. *Utilizing a transfer chair where the client is pulled onto a flat surface and then seated upright in the chair can help previously immobile clients get out of bed (Nelson et al, 2003).* **EBN:** *Critical care clients are high risk for complications related to immobility such as ventilator-associated pneumonia (VAP), atelectasis, and long-lasting functional limitations; therefore, once hemodynamically stable use progressive mobilization to dangle legs, sit in a chair, stand and bear weight, and walk. Use rotation therapy (kinetic and continuous lateral) to reduce risk of VAP for clients on mechanical ventilation (Rauen et al, 2008).* **EBN:** *A review of mobility interventions to improve outcomes in clients with prolonged mechanical ventilation found whole body physical therapy, arm exercise, electrical stimulation, and inspiratory muscle training could improve outcomes but provided minimal evidence of how to translate into critical care practice (Choi, Tasota, & Hoffman, 2008).*
- Help the client achieve mobility and start walking as soon as possible if not contraindicated. **EB:** *Early mobilization for acute limb injuries generally resulted in improved function, less pain, and earlier return to work and sports (Ebell, 2005).* **EBN:** *Early ambulation prevents complications such as deep vein thrombosis and improves level of independence with assistive devices (Radawiec et al, 2009).*
- Use a gait-walking belt when ambulating the client. *Gait belts help improve the caregiver's grasp, reducing the incidence of injuries (Nelson et al, 2003).*
- ▲ Apply any ordered brace before mobilizing the client. *Braces support and stabilize a body part, allowing increased mobility.*
- Initiate a "No Lift" policy where appropriate assistive devices are utilized for manual lifting. **EBN:** *A "No Lift" policy along with other measures such as the "Back Injury Resource Nurses" and an algorithm on safe client handling resulted in decreased workers' compensation expenses with reduced lost and modified work days, along with nurse and client satisfaction (Nelson et al, 2006).*
- Increase independence in ADLs, encouraging self-efficacy and discouraging helplessness as the client gets stronger. *Providing unnecessary assistance with transfers and bathing activities may promote dependence and a loss of mobility.*
- ▲ If the client has osteoarthritis, or rheumatoid arthritis, ask for a referral to a physical therapist to begin an exercise program that includes aerobic exercise, resistance exercise and gentle stretching. **EB:** *Exercise has been shown to be beneficial in both kinds of arthritis (Westby & Li, 2006).*
- ▲ If client has had a cerebrovascular accident (CVA) with hemiparesis, consider use of constraint-induced movement therapy (CIMT), where the functional extremity is purposely constrained and the client is forced to use the involved extremity. *Constraint therapy is estimated to benefit about half of the total CVA population (Barker, 2005).* **EB:** *The plasticity of the brain allows the brain to rewire and reroute neural connections to take up the work of the injured area of the brain. Constraint therapy was effective with improved motor function and health-related quality of life (Wu et al, 2007).*
- If the client has had a CVA, recognize that balance is likely impaired, and protect from falling. **EB:** *Clients did not have normal balance after therapy, even if only a mild CVA (Garland, Ivanova, & Mochizuki, 2007). An RCT of clients with hemiparesis post-CVA for 6 months resulted in improved center of pressure and displacement under sensory conditions after an 8–week, task-oriented balance and mobility exercise program (Bayouk, Boucher, & Lerous, 2006). A study of exercise and health-related quality*

of life (HRQoL)concluded that a regular exercise group with self-initiated training improved HRQoL more than an intensive exercise group with scheduled training, and motor function, balance, walking ability, and independence in ADL affected perceived HRQoL (Langhammer, Stanghelle, & Lindmark, 2008).

- If the client does not feed or groom self, sit side-by-side with the client, put your hand over the client's hand, support the client's elbow with your other hand, and help the client feed self; use the same technique to help the client comb hair. **EBN:** *The effectiveness of a restorative care intervention on nursing home resident outcomes included significant improvements in the Tinetti Mobility Score and the subscores for gait and balance, as well as improved walking bathing, and stair climbing (Resnick et al, 2009).*

 Geriatric

- Assess ability to move using the "Get Up and Go" test. Ask the client to rise from a sitting position, walk 10 feet, turn, and return to the chair to sit. *Performance on this screening exam demonstrates the client's mobility and ability to leave the house safely (Robertson & Montagnini, 2004).*
- Help the mostly immobile client achieve mobility as soon as possible, depending on physical condition. *In the elderly, mobility impairment can predict increased mortality and dependence; however, this can be prevented by physical exercise (Hirvensalo, Rantanen, & Heikkinen, 2000; Fletcher, 2005).*
- Use the Outcome Expectation for Exercise Scale to determine client's self-efficacy expectations and outcomes expectations toward exercise. **EBN:** *The client's self-efficacy expectations and outcome expectations for exercise will greatly influence his or her willingness to exercise. If the individual has a low outcome, interventions can be implemented to strengthen the expectations and hopefully improve exercise behavior (Resnick, Zimmerman, & Orwig, 2001).*
- For a client who is mostly immobile, minimize cardiovascular deconditioning by positioning the client in the upright position several times daily. *The hazards of bed rest in the elderly are multiple, serious, quick to develop, and slow to reverse. Deconditioning of the cardiovascular system occurs within days and involves fluid shifts, fluid loss, decreased cardiac output, decreased peak oxygen uptake, and increased resting heart rate (Fletcher, 2005; Fauci et al, 2008).* **EB:** *Studies indicate that to prevent the functional decline of older clients that often results from restricted activity during hospitalization, an exercise program designed to educate clients about remaining mobile during their stay and to provide assistance in walking is beneficial. Screening procedures often identify clients who can benefit from physical therapy (Tucker & Molsberger, 2004).*
- ▲ Refer the client to physical therapy for resistance exercise training as able, including abdominal crunch, leg press, leg extension, leg curl, calf press, and more. **EB:** *Six months of resistance exercise for the elderly greatly increased their aerobic capacity, possibly from increased skeletal muscle strength (Vincent et al, 2002). When clients in an extended care facility were put on a strength, balance, and endurance training program, the client's balance and mobility improved significantly (Rydwik, Kerstin, & Akner, 2005).*
- Use the WALC Intervention (Walk; Address pain, fear, fatigue during exercise; Learn about exercise; Cue by self-modeling) to improve exercise adherence in the older adult. **EBN:** *The WALC Intervention resulted in more exercise and had greater self-efficacy expectations regarding exercise (Resnick, Orwig, & Magaziner, 2002).*
- If client is scheduled for an elective surgery that will result in admission into ICU and immobility, or recovery from a knee replacement, initiate a prehabilitation program that includes a warm-up, aerobic strength, flexibility, and functional task work. **EBN and EB:** *By increasing the functional capacity of the individual prior to the stressor of inactivity, the predictable declines in physical activity can be prevented or alleviated (Topp et al, 2002). Clients who performed strength activities preoperatively walked significantly greater distances postoperatively after total hip replacement (Whitney & Parkman, 2002). Aerobic training along with strength and interval training was effective in fewer postoperative complications, shorter postoperative stays, and reduced functional disabilities (Carli & Zavorsky, 2005).*
- ▲ Evaluate the client for signs of depression (flat affect, insomnia, anorexia, frequent somatic complaints) or cognitive impairment (use Mini-Mental State Exam [MMSE]). Refer for treatment or counseling as needed. *Depression and decreased cognition in the elderly correlate with decreased levels of functional ability (Fletcher, 2005).*

● = Independent   ▲ = Collaborative   **EBN** = Evidence-Based Nursing   **EB** = Evidence-Based

- Watch for orthostatic hypotension when mobilizing elderly clients. Have the client dangle at the side of the bed with legs hanging over the edge of the bed, flex and extend feet several times after sitting up, then stand up slowly with someone holding the client. If client becomes light headed or dizzy, return them to bed immediately. *Postural hypotension is very common in the elderly (Krecinic et al, 2009).*
- Do not routinely assist with transfers or bathing activities unless necessary. *The nursing staff may contribute to impaired mobility by helping too much. Encourage client independence (Fauci et al, 2008).*
- Use gestures and nonverbal cues when helping clients move if they are anxious or have difficulty understanding and following verbal instructions. *Nonverbal gestures are part of a universal language that can be understood when the client is having difficulty with communication.*
- Recognize that wheelchairs are not a good mobility device and often serve as a mobility restraint.
- Ensure that chairs fit clients. Chair seat should be 3 inches above the height of the knee. Provide a raised toilet seat if needed. *Raising the height of a chair can dramatically improve the ability of many older clients to stand up. Low, deep, soft seats with armrests that are far apart reduce a person's ability to get up and down without help.*
- If the client is mainly immobile, provide opportunities for socialization and sensory stimulation (e.g., television and visits). Refer to the care plan for **Deficient Diversional activity.**
- Recognize that immobility and a lack of social support and sensory input may result in confusion or depression in the elderly (Fletcher, 2005). Refer to nursing interventions for **Acute Confusion** or **Hopelessness** as appropriate.

 Home Care

- The above interventions may be adapted for home care use.
- ▲ Begin discharge planning as soon as possible with case manager or social worker and client/caregivers to assess need for home support systems, assistive devices, and community or home health services.
- ▲ Assess home environment for factors that create barriers to physical mobility. Refer to occupational therapy services if needed to assist the client in restructuring home environment and daily living patterns.
- ▲ Refer to home health aide services to support the client and family through changing levels of mobility. Reinforce need to promote independence in mobility as tolerated. *Providing unnecessary assistance with transfers and bathing activities may promote dependence and a loss of mobility (Fletcher, 2005).*
- ▲ Refer to physical therapy for gait training, strengthening, and balance training. *Physical therapists can provide direct interventions as well as assess need for assistive devices (e.g., cane, walker).* **EB:** *An outpatient group exercise intervention (2x/week for 5 weeks) for people with impaired mobility resulted in significantly better balance, sit to stand, and gait as compared to a no-intervention control group; however, strength did not improve (Sherrington et al, 2008).*
- Discuss with client and caregiver the possibility of a service dog to support the more immobile client. **EB:** *Service dogs can pull wheelchairs, find keys, open the door, bring the telephone, and more. Use of service dogs was found to increase socialization, increase self-esteem, and give peace of mind to caregivers (Rintala et al, 2005).*
- Assess skin condition at every visit. Establish a skin care program that enhances circulation and maximizes position changes. *Impaired mobility decreases circulation to dependent areas. Decreased circulation and shearing place the client at risk for skin breakdown.*
- Once the client is able to walk independently, suggest the client enter an exercise program, or walk with a friend. **EBN:** *Findings from a study of exercise behavior found that friends have the strongest influence to keep on an exercise program, more than family members or experts (Resnick, Orwig, & Magaziner, 2002).* **EBN:** *Nurse practitioners providing primary care should prescribe regular physical activity to minimize progressive impaired mobility. Clients should be instructed to use exercise logs or diary to improve adherence to the mobility enhancement prescription (Yeom, Keller, & Fleury, 2009).*
- Provide support to the client and family/caregivers during long-term impaired mobility. *Long-term impaired mobility may necessitate role changes within the family and precipitate caregiver stress.* Refer to the care plan for **Caregiver role strain.**

• = Independent ▲ = Collaborative **EBN** = Evidence-Based Nursing **EB** = Evidence-Based

▲ Institute care navigation/case management and transitional care management of frail elderly to support continued independent living.

Client/Family Teaching and Discharge Planning

- Teach the client progressive mobilization (e.g., dangle legs, get out of bed slowly when transferring from the bed to the chair).
- Teach the client relaxation techniques such as deep breathing and stretching to use during activity.
- Teach the client to use assistive devices such as a cane, a walker, or crutches to increase mobility.
- Teach family members and caregivers to work with clients actively during self-care activities utilizing a restorative care philosophy for eating, bathing, grooming, dressing, and transferring to restore the client to maximum function and independence (Resnick et al, 2009).
- Work with the client using self-efficacy interventions using single or multiple methods. Teach client and family members to assess fear of falling and develop strategies to mitigate its effect on mobility progression. **EBN:** *Use of self-efficacy based interventions resulted in increased exercise (Resnick et al, 2007).*
- Work with the client using the Transtheoretical model of behavior change and determine if the client is in the precontemplation, contemplation, preparation, action, or maintenance stage of behavior change for physical activity/exercise. Provide appropriate strategies to support change to exercising based on **stage** of change. **EBN:** *In a study that examined validity of evidence for physical activity stage of change across nine studies, physical activity stage of change was found to be behaviorally valid evidenced by self-reported exercise, physical activity, pedometers, sedentary behaviors, and physical functioning. Physical fitness and weight indicators were not related to physical activity stage of change. (Hellsten et al, 2008).*

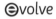 See the EVOLVE website for Weblinks for client education resources.

REFERENCES

American College of Sports Medicine (ACSM): Exercise and physical activity for older adults, *Med Sci Sports Exerc* 41(7):1510–1530, 2009.

ACSM: *American College of Sports Medicine's guidelines for exercise testing and prescription,* ed 8, Philadelphia, 2010, Lippincott Williams & Wilkins.

Barker E: New hope for stroke patients, *RN* 68(2):38–42, 2005.

Bayouk JF, Boucher JP, Lcrous A: Balance training following stroke: effects of task-oriented exercises with and without altered sensory input, *Int J Rehabil Res* 29(1):51–59, 2006.

Carli F, Zavorsky GS: Optimizing functional exercise capacity in the elderly surgical population, *Curr Opin Clin Nutr Metab Care* 8(1): 23–32, 2005.

Choi J, Tasota FJ, Hoffmann LA: Mobility interventions to improve outcomes in patients undergoing prolonged mechanical ventilation: a review of the literature, *Biol Res Nurs* 10(1):21–33, 2008.

Curb JD, Ceria-Ulep CD, Rodriguez BL et al: Performance-based measures of physical function for high-function populations, *J of Am Geriatr Soc* 54(5):737–742, 2006.

Ebell M: Early mobilization better for acute limb injuries, *Am Family Physician* 71(4):776, 2005.

Fauci A, Braunwald E, Kasper DL et al, editors: *Harrison's principles of internal medicine,* ed 17, New York, 2008, McGraw-Hill.

Fletcher K: Immobility: geriatric self-learning module, *Medsurg Nurs* 14(1):35, 2005.

Garland SJ, Ivanova TD, Mochizuki G: Recovery of standing balance and health-related quality of life after mild or moderately severe stroke, *Arc Phys Med Rehabil* 88(2):218–227, 2007.

Hellsten LA, Nigg C, Norman G et al: Accumulation of behavioral validation evidence for physical activity stage of change, *Health Psychol* 27(1 Suppl):543–553, 2008.

Hirvensalo M, Rantanen T, Heikkinen E: Mobility difficulties and physical activity as predictors of mortality and loss of independence in the community-living older population, *J Am Geriatr Soc* 48(5):493–498, 2000.

Kneafsey R: A systematic review of nursing contributions to mobility rehabilitation: examining the quality and content of the evidence, *J Clin Nurs* 16(11c):325–340, 2007.

Krecinic T, Mattace-Raso F, Van Der Velde N et al: Orthostatic hypotension in older persons: a diagnostic algorithm, *J Nutr Health Aging* 13(6):572–575, 2009.

Langhammer B, Stanghelle JK, Lindmark B: Exercise and health-related quality of life during the first year following acute stroke: a randomized controlled trial, *Brain Inj* 22(2):135–145, 2008.

Messecar DC: Review: several interventions reduce fear of falling in older people living in the community, *Evid Based Nurs* 11(1):21, 2008.

Nelson A, Matz M, Chen F et al: Development and evaluation of a multifaceted ergonomics program to prevent injuries associated with patient handling tasks, *Int J Nurs Stud* 43(6):717–733, 2006.

Nelson A, Owen B, Lloyd JD et al: Safe patient handling movement, *Am J Nurs* 103(3):32–40, 2003.

Physical Activity Guidelines Advisory Committee: *Physical activity guidelines advisory committee report,* 2008. Washington DC: U.S. Department of Health and Human Services, 2008. Retrieved from Centers for Disease Control and Prevention (CDC) www.health.gov/paguidelines/.

Physical Activity Guidelines for Americans (2008). U.S. Department of Health and Human Services, 2008. Retrieved from Centers for Disease Control and Prevention (CDC) www.health.gov/paguidelines/guidelines/default.aspx.

Radawiec SM, Howe C, Gonzalez CM et al: Safe ambulation of an orthopaedic patient, *Orthop Nurs* 28(2):24–27, 2009.

• = Independent   ▲ = Collaborative   **EBN** = Evidence-Based Nursing   **EB** = Evidence-Based

Rauen CA, Chulay M, Bridges E et al: Seven evidence-based practice habits: putting some sacred cows out to pasture, *Crit Care Nurse* 28(2):98–113, 2008.

Resnick B, Gruber-Baldini AL, Zimmerman S et al: Nursing home resident outcomes from the Res-Care Intervention, *J Am Geriatr Soc* 57(7):1156–1165, 2009.

Resnick B, Orwig D, D'Adamo C et al: Factors that influence exercise activity among women post hip fracture participating in the Exercise Plus Program, *Clin Int Aging* 2(3):413–427, 2007.

Resnick B, Orwig D, Magaziner J: The effect of social support on exercise behavior in older adults, *Clin Nurs Res* 11(1):52, 2002.

Resnick B, Zimmerman S, Orwig D: Model testing for reliability and validity of the outcome expectations for exercise scale, *Nurs Res* 50:5, 2001.

Rintala DH et al: The effects of service dogs on the lives of persons with mobility impairments: a pre-post study design, *Sci Psychosoc Process* 18(4):236–249, 2005.

Robertson RG, Montagnini M: Geriatric failure to thrive, *Am Family Physician*, 70(2):343, 2004.

Rydwik E, Kerstin F, Akner G: Physical training in institutionalized elderly people with multiple diagnoses—a controlled pilot study, *Arch Gerontol Geriatr* 40(1):29, 2005.

Sedlak CA, Doheny MO, Nelson A et al: Development of the National Association of Orthopaedic Nurses Guidance Statement on safe patient handling and movement in the orthopaedic setting, *Orthop Nurs* 28(25):52–58, 2009.

Sherrington C, Pamphlett PI, Jacka JA et al: Group exercise can improve participant's mobility in an outpatient rehabilitation setting: a randomized controlled trial, *Clin Rehabil* 22(6):493–502, 2008.

Topp, R, Ditmyer M, King K et al: The effect of bedrest and potential of prehabilitation on patients in the intensive care unit, *AACN Clin Issues* 13(2):263–276, 2002.

Tucker D, Molsberger S: Walking for wellness: a collaborative program to maintain mobility in hospitalized older adults, *Geriatr Nurs* 25(4): 242–245, 2004.

Tudor-Locke C, Hatano Y, Pangrazi RP et al: Revisiting "how many steps are enough?" *Med Sci Sports Exerc* 40(7 Suppl):S537–S543, 2008.

Vincent KR, Braith RW, Feldman RA et al: Improved cardiorespiratory endurance following 6 months of resistance exercise in elderly men and women, *Arch Intern Med* 162:673–678, 2002.

Westby MD, Li L: Physical therapy and exercise for arthritis: do they work? *Geriatr Aging* 9(9):624–630, 2006.

Whitney JA, Parkman S: Preoperative physical activity, anesthesia, and analgesia: effects on early postoperative walking after total hip replacement, *Appl Nurs Res* 15:1, 2002.

Wu CY Chen CL, Tsai WC et al. A randomized controlled trial of modified constraint-induced movement therapy for elderly stroke survivors: changes in motor impairment, daily functioning, and quality of life, *Arch Phys Med Rehabil* 88(3):273–278, 2007.

Yeom HA, Keller C, Fleury J: Interventions for promoting mobility in community-dwelling older adults, *J Am Acad Nurse Pract* 21(2):95–100, 2009.

Impaired wheelchair Mobility   *Brenda Emick-Herring, RN, MSN, CRRN*

NANDA-I

Definition

Limitation of independent operation of wheelchair within environment

Defining Characteristics

Impaired ability to operate: manual or power wheelchair on curbs; manual or power wheelchair on even surface; manual or power wheelchair on an uneven surface; manual or powered wheelchair on an incline; manual or powered wheelchair on a decline

Related Factors (r/t)

Cognitive impairment; deconditioning; deficient knowledge; depressed mood; environmental constraints (e.g., stairs, inclines, uneven surfaces, unsafe obstacles, distances, lack of assistive devices or person, wheelchair type); impaired vision; insufficient muscle strength; limited endurance; musculoskeletal impairment (e.g., contractures); neuromuscular impairment; obesity; pain

NOC   (Nursing Outcomes Classification)

Suggested NOC Outcome

Ambulation: Wheelchair

Example NOC Outcome with Indicators
Ambulation: Wheelchair as evidenced by the following indicators: Propels wheelchair safely/Transfers to and from wheelchair/Maneuvers curbs, doorways, ramps (Rate the outcome and indicators of **Ambulation: Wheelchair:** 1 = severely compromised, 2 = substantially compromised, 3 = moderately compromised, 4 = mildly compromised, 5 = not compromised [see Section I].)

 • = Independent   ▲ = Collaborative   **EBN** = Evidence-Based Nursing   **EB** = Evidence-Based

Client Outcomes

Client Will (Specify Time Frame):

- Demonstrate independence in operating and moving a wheelchair or other device with wheels
- Demonstrate the ability to direct others in operating and moving a wheelchair or other device
- Demonstrate therapeutic positioning, pressure relief, and safety principles while operating and moving wheelchair or other device equipped with wheels

NIC (Nursing Interventions Classification)

Suggested NIC Interventions

Exercise Therapy: Muscle Control, Positioning: Wheelchair

Example NIC Activities—Positioning: Wheelchair
Select the appropriate wheelchair for the client: standard adult, semi-reclining, fully reclining, amputees; Monitor for client's inability to maintain correct posture in wheelchair

Nursing Interventions and *Rationales*

- Assist client to put on and take off equipment (e.g., braces, orthoses, abdominal binders) in bed. *Provide stabilization and alignment; abdominal binder prevents postural hypotension and increases vital capacity (for hemodynamic stability, binder must be put on and taken off in bed).*
- Inspect skin where orthoses, braces, and other equipment rested, once they are removed. *Early detection of pressure allows for early pressure relief strategy implementation (WOCN, 2003).*
- ▲ Obtain referrals for physical and occupational therapy, or wheelchair seating clinic. *Individualized wheelchair seating system fits client abilities and provides postural alignment, comfort, and reduced pressure (Gavin-Dreschnack, 2004). The correct seating system allows client to propel chair safely and use the hands. Correct seating allows function and prevents slouching/leaning/sliding down, which all can cause deformity, discomfort, and overuse of physical restraints (Cox, 2004).* **EB:** *Results of a randomized clinical trial showed elderly residents in individualized compared to standard wheelchairs benefited in functions such as better/faster propulsion, increased forward reach and/or increased satisfaction or quality of life (Trefler et al, 2004). Reduced pain/discomfort occurred with individualized seating interventions according to Samuelsson et al (2001). Rader, Jones, & Miller (2000) via an intervention study found individualized seating systems improved posture/function in elderly residents.*
- Keep the right cushion and wheelchair with the right client (Gavin-Dreschnack, 2004). *Cushions lessen shock, pressure, vibration, pain, and fatigue (Cooper et al, 2000; Paleg, 2002).*
- Recognize that use of properly contoured, specialized cushions/supports and repositioning help prevent sitting-acquired pressure ulcers (Cooper et al, 2000; Paleg, 2002; WOCN, 2003). *Allows immobile clients to remain seated longer and distributes body mass, thus lowering peak pressure over bones.* **EBN and EB:** *A randomized clinical trial studied elders at risk for pressure ulcers by pressure mapping and measuring the peak pressure index of subjects placed on standard 3–inch foam cushions compared to two common pressure-reducing cushions; results demonstrated those with high-peak pressure indexes using foam cushions acquired more pressure ulcers than the pressure reducing cushions (Brienza, 2009).*
- Intervene to maintain continence, nutrition, and hydration. *Helps prevent pressure ulcers; continence or use of absorbent diapers keeps cushions dry. Some wheelchair cushions have moisture-wicking characteristics (Smith, 2008).*
- ▲ Obtain physical therapist (PT), occupational therapist (OT), or wheelchair clinic referral for cushion reevaluation if signs of pressure emerge. *Professionals assess, problem-solve, and perform pressure mapping to evaluate where peak pressures are and to objectively compare pressures on various cushions (Smith, 2008).* **EB:** *A pilot study indicated high buttock-cushion interface pressure was associated with pressure ulcers (Brienza et al, 2001). Pressure mapping is a reliable means of evaluating interface pressures (Stinson, Porter-Armstrong, & Eakin, 2003).*
- Emphasize importance of weight shifts every 15 minutes with safety belts in place (leaning forward/laterally) for about 2 minutes for clients with paralysis with trunk control. *This prevents capillary occlusion/force on skin over bony areas (Minkel, 2000).* **EB:** *Coggrave & Rose (2003) demon-*

• = Independent   ▲ = Collaborative   **EBN** = Evidence-Based Nursing   **EB** = Evidence-Based

strated that pressure relief for 1 minute 51 seconds raised transcutaneous oxygen tension enough to unload pressure while sitting.

- Remind paralyzed clients without trunk control to tilt back to at least 45 to 65 degrees when in specialized tilting power wheelchairs; or, if in manual chairs, they should be manually tilted back a few minutes every 15 minutes (Minkel, 2000). *Position changes relieve pressure.* **EBN:** *When wheelchairs of two quadriplegics were tilted back to 45 degrees or more, pressure at the ischial tuberosities decreased significantly (Pellow, 1999).*
- Activate passive standing position of wheelchair or, if applicable, manually stand client or use a sit-to-stand lift with sling for a few minutes. *This removes tissue pressure over bony prominences to help prevent pressure ulcers (WOCN, 2003; Baptiste et al, 2008).*
- Place both feet on floor when clients are passively sitting in a wheelchair. *Less pressure exists on sacral/buttock tissue sitting upright with feet on the floor than on foot rests (Rader, Jones, & Miller, 1999).*
- Routinely assess client's sitting posture and frequently reposition him/her into sound alignment. **EBN and EB:** *Nelson et al (2003) recommended safe techniques to reposition clients during chair sitting based on evidence and a positioning algorithm. A study demonstrated nursing personnel could reliably use the Resident Ergonomic Assessment Profile for Seating to assess posture of persons in their wheelchair (Gavin-Dreschnack et al, 2009).*
- Sit dysphagic clients as upright as possible in individualized wheelchair versus geri-chair when eating. *When fed in this position, there is less risk of aspiration (Gavin-Dreschnack, 2004).*
- Place client's feet securely on foot rests and fasten seat belts across the top of the thighs before propelling the wheelchair. *This prevents foot injuries and helps stabilize and hold the pelvis in place.* **EB:** *Use of seat belts and appropriately adjusted leg rests likely improves control and safety of occupants of electric wheelchairs going up various inclines (Corfman et al, 2003).*
- Implement use of friction-coated projection hand rims and leather gloves for clients to propel manual wheelchairs. *Friction-coated projection rims are less invasive and slippery than aluminum rims; gloves absorb forces of propulsion and help prevent nerve damage/carpal tunnel.*
- Manually guide or explain to push forward on both wheel rims to move ahead, push the right rim to turn left and vice versa, and pull backward on both wheel rims to back up.
- Recommend that clients back wheelchairs into an elevator. If entering face first, instruct them to turn chair around to face the elevator doors. *Clients can see the control panel, floor monitor display, and doors opening and can exit wheeling forward.*
- Reinforce principle of descending a curb backward ("popping a wheelie") if balance, trunk control, strength, and timing are adequate. *Backward descent carries less risk of clients losing control and falling forward out of wheelchair.*
- Ascend curbs in a forward position by popping a wheelie or having aid tilt chair back, place front wheels over curb, and roll chair up. If surface is muddy or sandy, ascend backwards. *Front casters will not roll on soft surfaces; a backward approach requires less energy and prevents getting stuck or falling forward.*
- During assisted wheelies, helper must hold wheelchair until all four wheels are back on the ground and client has control of wheelchair. *Releasing one's grip too soon may alter client's balance and cause injury.*
- ▲ Follow therapist's recommendations for how clients should propel manual wheelchairs to prevent upper extremity pain and joint degeneration. *Overuse and repetitive strain is common especially in those with spinal cord injury (Cooper, Cooper, & Boninger, 2004; Consortium for Spinal Cord Medicine, 2005).*
  - Stress that clients maintain normal versus extra weight. *Minimizes force and work of upper extremities during repetitive wheeling (Consortium for Spinal Cord Medicine, 2005).*
  - Reinforce use of long/smooth strokes to limit high force on the pushrim, and let the hand "naturally drift down" when letting go of the pushrim (Koontz & Boninger, 2003).
  - Remind clients to press with length of arm (not elbows) during repositioning and weight shifts; apply elbow pads and nocturnal splints as ordered. *Helps prevent nerve damage and tendonitis (Szabo & Kwak, 2007).*
  - Inform clients that ultra-lightweight, pushrim-activated, power-assisted, or electric wheelchairs may be more therapeutic than manual ones. *The arms are overworked during propulsion, transfers, and upper dressing and thus are at risk for painful syndromes (Minkel, 2000).*

● = Independent ▲ = Collaborative **EBN** = Evidence-Based Nursing **EB** = Evidence-Based

- Help clients transition from a manual to a powered wheelchair/scooter if progressive disability occurs. **EB:** *Powered mobility devices positively affected subject's roles, occupational performance, interests, independence, and self-esteem (Buning, Angelo, & Schmeler, 2001).*
- ▲ Reduce floor clutter and establish safety rules for drivers of electric/power mobility devices; make referrals to PT or OT for driver reevaluations if accidents occur or client's health deteriorates. *Safe driving prevents injury to client, pedestrians, and property.* **EB:** *A study identified risks related to power mobility devices and solutions to reduce risks to improve safety (Mortenson et al, 2005).*
- Request and receive client's permission before moving unoccupied wheelchair in room or out to hallway. *Chronic wheelchair users may view chair as part of their identity and independence and may become stressed if it's not readily available (Cox, 2004; Gavin-Dreschnack, 2004).*
- Reinforce compensatory strategies for unilateral neglect and agnosia (visual scanning, self-talk, self-questioning as to what could be wrong) as clients propel wheelchair through doorways and around obstacles. *Too often nurses physically move wheelchair or obstacle instead of cueing client to detect and solve problems.* Refer to care plan for **Unilateral Neglect.**
- Offer support to help clients cope with issues related to physical disability. *Depression and anxiety may occur with physical loss.* **EBN:** *Wheelchair users had frustration with barriers, accessibility, independence issues, and societal attitudes toward people with disabilities (Pierce, 1998).*
- Provide information on support group and Internet resource options. *Loss, chronic illness, and injury often trigger serious emotional responses (Purk, 2004).* **EB:** *A Cochrane review of interactive computer applications in persons with chronic disease found benefits such as increased knowledge, social support, and self-efficacy (Murray et al, 2005).* **EBN:** *Caregivers used and benefited from an Internet site that offered stroke education, support, and group discussion (Pierce, Steiner & Govoni, 2004). Support group members attended meetings to meet others with the same diagnosis/issues and to obtain information; married couples also attended for socialization (Purk, 2004).*
- Provide information about advocacy, accessibility, assistive technology, and issues under the Americans with Disabilities Act. *Creates the potential for greater accessibility/independence (Berry & Ignash, 2003).*
- ▲ Make social service or wheelchair clinic referral to educate clients on financial coverage/regulations of third-party payers and Health Care Financing Association for wheelchairs. *It's wise to recognize cost, advantages, and durability of different wheelchair models before purchasing one.*
- Suggest that clients test-drive wheelchairs and try out cushions/postural supports before purchasing them. *Equipment is expensive, and different models have different advantages and disadvantages.*

 Geriatric

- Avoid using restraints on fidgeting clients who slide down in a wheelchair; rather, assess for deformities, spinal curvatures, abnormal tone, discomfort, and limited joint range. *Elders may move to get comfortable or do a task that inadvertently results in poor posture and sliding (Rader, Jones, & Miller, 1999); special seating system aids posture/comfort (Minkel, 2001; Taylor, 2003).* **EB:** *There's no clinical evidence that restraints prevent falls (AGS Panel on Falls in Older Persons, 2001).*
- Ensure proper seat depth/leg positioning and use custom foot rests (not elevated leg rests) to prevent elders from sliding down in wheelchairs. *Tight hamstrings and a posterior pelvic tilt are common in elders and may pull pelvis toward front of chair; special leg/foot rests are needed (Gavin-Dreschnack, 2004).* **EB:** *Trained research staff conducted studies on wheelchair use and exercise. Time-measured studies indicated increase in independence with locomotion and toileting when activity was conducted on a regular basis (Ouslander et al, 2005).*
- ▲ Assess for side effects of medications and potential need for dosage readjustments to increase wheelchair tolerance. *Medications can cause orthostatic hypotension, dizziness, and altered cardiac output (Fauci et al, 2008).* **EB:** *Study review/metaanalysis showed a "weak association" between digoxin, type IA antiarrhythmics, and diuretics and falling elders; taking three to four or more meds increased recurrent fall rates (Leipzig, Cumming, & Tinetti, 1999).*
- Allow client to propel wheelchair independently at his or her own speed. *Elders may move slowly due to diminished ROM/strength, stiff/sore joints, and cardiopulmonary compromise.*

Home Care

- Assess home environment for barriers and a support system for emergency and contingency care (e.g., Lifeline). *Immobility and wheelchair use may pose a threat during health crises.* **EB:** *In two connected studies, 37% of respondents at home had fallen from wheelchairs, and 46% of fallers had injuries; 36% had not made home modifications (Berg, Hines, & Allen, 2002).*
- Recommend the following changes to the home to accommodate the use of a wheelchair:
  - Arrange traffic patterns so they are wide enough to maneuver a wheelchair.
  - Recognize a 5-foot turning space is necessary to maneuver wheelchairs; doorways need to be 32 to 36 inches wide; and entrance ramps/paths should slope 1 inch per foot.
  - Replace door hardware with fold-back hinges, remove doorway encasements (if too narrow), remove/replace thresholds (if too high), hang wall-mounted sinks/handrails, grade floors in showers for roll-in chairs, use non-skid/non-slip floor coverings (e.g., nonwaxed wood, linoleum, or Berber carpet).
  - Rearrange room functions, furniture, and storage so that toileting, sleeping, bathing, and preparing/eating meals can safely take place on one level of the home.
  The ability to perform these activities is critical for staying in one's own home. Modifications make homes more accessible/safe (Bogert, 2008).
- ▲ Request PT/OT referrals to evaluate wheelchair skills and safety, to suggest home modifications and ways to propel wheelchairs on irregular surfaces and get back into a chair after a fall (Berg, Hines, & Allen, 2002). **EB:** *A study concluded the Wheelchair Skills Test (WST) is a short, reliable test for professionals to assess clients' manual wheelchair skills (Kirby et al, 2004).*
- Suggest community resources for servicing and tuning up wheelchairs and/or locating parts so clients can service their own chairs; an annual tune-up is recommended.

 Client/Family Teaching and Discharge Planning

- ▲ Assess pain levels of long-term wheelchair users and make referrals to therapists or wheelchair clinics for modifications. **EB:** *Most subjects experienced pain relief with ergonomic, individualized seating interventions (Samuelsson et al, 2001). Seating prototype testing found seat adjustability and low-back support improved comfort (Crane & Hobson, 2003).*
- Instruct and have client return demonstrate re-inflation of pneumatic tires; encourage client to monitor tire pressure every 2 to 3 weeks. **EB:** *Tire pressure that is at or below 50% of what the manufacturer recommends increases wheeling/rolling resistance and energy expenditure (Sawatzky, Denison, & Kim, 2002).*
- Instruct clients to remove large wheelchair parts (leg rests, arm rests) when lifting wheelchair into car for transport; when reassembling it, check that all parts are fastened securely and temperature is tepid. *This reduces weight that needs to be lifted; locked parts and a safe temperature prevent injury/burns.*
- Teach the importance of using seatbelts or chair tie-downs when riding in motor vehicles; if unavailable, clients in wheelchairs should be transported in large heavy vehicles only. *Clients need restraint protection in case of abrupt vehicle maneuvers (Shaw, 2000).*
- For further information, refer care plans for **Impaired Transfer ability** and **Impaired bed Mobility.**

Ⓔvolve   See the EVOLVE website for Weblinks for client education resources.

REFERENCES

American Geriatric Society (AGS): Guidelines for the prevention of falls in older persons, *JAGS* 49: 664–672, 2001.

Baptiste A, McCleerey M, Matz M et al: Proper sling selection and application while using client lifts, *Rehabil Nurs* 33(1):22–32, 2008.

Berg K, Hines M, Allen S: Wheelchair users at home: few modifications and many injurious falls, *Am J Pub Health* 92(1):48, 2002.

Berry BE, Ignash S: Assistive technology: providing independence for individuals with disabilities, *Rehabil Nurs* 28(1):6–14, 2003.

Bogert S: Stay-at-home solutions for seniors: home modification for aged and disabled on the rise, *Rehabil Manag,* 21(2):22–25, 2008.

Brienza DM, Karg PE, Geyer MJ et al: The relationship between pressure ulcer incidence and buttock-seat cushion interface pressure in at-risk elderly wheelchair users, *Arch Phys Med Rehabil* 82(4):529–533, 2001.

Brienza D: A randomized clinical trial on preventing pressure ulcers with seat cushions. *25th International Seating Symposium,* Department of Rehabilitation Science and Technology Continuing Education, School of Health and Rehabilitation Sciences, University of Pittsburgh, Orlando FL, paper presented March 12, 2009.

Buning ME, Angelo JA, Schmeler MR: Occupational performance and the transition to powered mobility: a pilot study, *Am J Occup Ther* 55(3):339–344, 2001.

Coggrave MJ, Rose LS: A specialist seating assessment clinic: changing pressure relief practice, *Spinal Cord,* 41:692–695, 2003.

● = Independent   ▲ = Collaborative   **EBN** = Evidence-Based Nursing   **EB** = Evidence-Based

Consortium for Spinal Cord Medicine Clinical Practice Guidelines: Preservation of upper limb function following spinal cord injury: A clinical practice guideline for health-care professionals. *Clinical practice guideline,* 1–40, Washington DC, 2005.

Cooper RA, Cooper R, Boninger ML: Push for power, *Rehabil Manag* 17(2):32–36, 2004.

Cooper RA, Schmeler MR, Cooper R et al: Long-term rehab: advanced seating systems, parts I and II, *Rehabil Manag* 13(2–3):58, 2000.

Corfman TA, Cooper RA, Fitzgerald SG et al: Tips and falls during electric-powered wheelchair driving: effects of seatbelt use, legrests, and driving speed, *Arch Phys Med Rehabil* 84(12):1797–1802, 2003.

Cox DI: Not your parent's wheelchair, *Rehabil Manag* 17(7):26–27, 2004.

Crane B, Hobson D: No room for discomfort, *Rehabil Manag* 16(1):30, 2003.

Fauci A, Braunwald E, Kasper DL et al, editors: *Harrison's principles of internal medicine,* ed 17, New York, 2008, McGraw-Hill.

Gavin-Dreschnack D: Effects of wheelchair posture on patient safety, *Rehabil Nurs* 29(6):221–226, 2004.

Gavin-Dreschnack D, Schonfeld L, Nelson A et al: Development of a screening tool for safe wheelchair seating. In Agency for Healthcare Research and Quality (AHRQ), Department of Defense (DoD)—Health Affairs: *Advances in patient safety: from research to implementation,* www.ncbi.nlm.nih.gov/books/bv.fcgi?rid=aps.section.6773. Accessed September 15, 2009.

Kirby RL, Dupuis DJ, Macphee AH et al: The wheelchair skills test (version 2.4): measurement properties, *Arch Phys Med Rehabil* 85(5):794–804, 2004.

Koontz AM, Boninger M: Proper propulsion, *Rehabil Manag* 16(6):18–22, 2003.

Leipzig RM, Cumming RG, Tinetti ME: Drugs and falls in older people: a systematic review and meta-analysis: II. Cardiac and analgesic drugs, *J Am Geriatr Soc* 47(1):40–50, 1999.

Minkel JL: Seating and mobility considerations for people with spinal cord injury, *Phys Ther* 80(7):701–709, 2000.

Minkel JL: Sitting outside of the box, *Rehabil Manag* 14(8):50, 2001.

Mortenson WB, Miller WC, Boily J et al: Perceptions of power mobility use and safety within residential facilities, *Can J Occup Ther* 72(3):142–152, 2005.

Murray E, Burns, J, See TS et al: Interactive Health Communication Applications for people with chronic disease. *Cochrane Database Syst Rev,* 4:CD004274, 2005.

Nelson, A, Lloyd JD, Menzel N et al: Preventing nursing back injuries: redesigning patient handling tasks, *AAOHN J* 51(3):126-134, 2003.

Ouslander JG, Griffiths PC, McConnell E et al: Functional incidental training: a randomized, controlled, crossover trial in Veterans Affairs nursing homes, *J Am Geriatr Soc* 53(7):1091–1100, 2005.

Paleg G: The prevention struggle, *Rehabil Manag* 15(8):40–42, 2002.

Pellow TR: A comparison of interface pressure readings to wheelchair cushions and positioning: a pilot study, *Can J Occup Ther* 66(3):140, 1999.

Pierce LL: Barriers to access: frustrations of people who use a wheelchair for full-time mobility, *Rehabil Nurs* 23(3):120–125, 1998.

Pierce LL, Steiner V, Govoni AL: Internet-based support for rural caregivers of persons with stroke shows promise, *Rehabil Nurs* 29(3):95–99, 2004.

Purk JK: Support groups: why do people attend? *Rehabil Nurs* 29(2):62–67, 2004.

Rader J, Jones D, Miller LL: Individualized wheelchair seating: reducing restraints and improving comfort and function, *Top Geriatr Rehabil* 15(2):34, 1999.

Rader J, Jones D, Miller L: The importance of individualized wheelchair seating for frail older adults, *J Gerontol Nurs* 26(11):24–32, 2000.

Samuelsson K, Larsson H, Thyberg M et al: Wheelchair seating intervention: results from a client-centered approach, *Disabil Rehabil* 23(15):677–682, 2001.

Sawatzky BJ, Denison I, Kim W: Rolling, rolling, rolling, *Rehabil Manag* 15(6):36–39, 2002.

Shaw G: Wheelchair rider risk in motor vehicles: a technical note, *J Rehabil Res Dev* 37(1):89–100, 2000.

Smith R: Devising a system: new tools help therapists find seating solutions, *Rehabil Manag* 21(3):10, 12–15, 2008.

Stinson MD, Porter-Armstrong AP, Eakin PA: Pressure mapping systems: reliability of pressure map interpretation, *Clin Rehabil* 17(5):504–511, 2003.

Szabo RM, Kwak C: Natural history and conservative management of cubital tunnel syndrome, *Hand Clin* 23:311–318, 2007.

Taylor SJ: An overview of evaluation for wheelchair seating for people who have had strokes, *Top Stroke Rehabil* 10(1):95, 2003.

Trefler E, Fitzgerald SG, Hobson DA et al: Outcomes of wheelchair systems intervention with residents of long-term care facilities, *Assist Technol* 16(1):18–27, 2004.

Wound, Ostomy, and Continence Nurses Society (WOCN): *Guideline for prevention and management of pressure ulcers,* Glenview IL, 2003, The Society.

Dysfunctional gastrointestinal Motility

Nancy Albright Beyer, RN, CEN, MS, Betty J. Ackley, MSN, EdS, RN, and Joan Klehr, RNC, BS, MPH

NANDA-I

Definition

Increased, decreased, ineffective, or lack of peristaltic activity within the gastrointestinal system

Defining Characteristics

Absence of flatus; abdominal cramping; abdominal distension; abdominal pain; accelerated gastric emptying; bile-colored gastric residual; change in bowel sounds (e.g., absent, hypoactive, hyperactive); diarrhea; dry stool; difficulty passing stool; hard stool; increased gastric residual; nausea; regurgitation; vomiting

Related Factors (r/t)

Aging; anxiety; enteral feedings; food intolerance (e.g., gluten, lactose); immobility; ingestion of contaminates (e.g., food, water); malnutrition; pharmaceutical agents (e.g., narcotics/opiates, laxatives, antibiotics, anesthesia); prematurity; sedentary lifestyle; surgery

• = Independent ▲ = Collaborative **EBN** = Evidence-Based Nursing **EB** = Evidence-Based

(Nursing Outcomes Classification)

Suggested NOC Outcomes

Gastrointestinal Function, Electrolyte and Acid-Base Balance, Fluid Balance, Hydration, Nausea & Vomiting Control, Treatment Behavior: Illness or Injury

Example **NOC Outcome with Indicators**
Gastrointestinal Function as evidenced by the following indicators: Bowel sounds/Stool soft and formed/Appetite present without evidence of reflux, nausea, or vomiting/Reported normal abdominal comfort (Rate the outcome and indicators of **Gastrointestinal Function:** 1= severely compromised, 2=substantially compromised, 3=moderately compromised, 4= mildly compromised, 5= not compromised [see Section I].)

Client Outcomes

Client Will (Specify Time Frame):

- Have abdomen circumference normal for client's body, free of abdominal distention
- Be free of abdominal pain
- Have normal bowel sounds
- Pass gas rectally at intervals
- Defecate formed, soft stool every day to every third day
- State has an appetite
- Be able to eat food without nausea and vomiting
- Be free of gastric reflux

NIC **(Nursing Interventions Classification)**

Suggested NIC Intervention

Gastric Motility Management

Example **NIC Activities—Gastric Motility Management**
Evaluate use of prokinetics for delayed gastric motility; Suggest change in dietary habits to either increase gastric motility or decrease it, depending on the presenting complaint

Nursing Interventions and *Rationales*

- Assess for abdominal distention, and presence of abdominal pain. *Abdominal distention is often found with decreased gastric motility, and abdominal pain is found in both increased and decreased gastric motility (Bickley & Szilagyi, 2009).*
- Inspect the abdomen, auscultate for bowel sounds noting characteristics and frequency, palpate, and percuss the abdomen. *Physical assessment of the abdomen can be helpful to find abnormalities or changes associated with either increased or decreased gastric motility (Bickley & Szilagyi, 2009).*
- Review history noting any anorexia, dyspepsia, nausea/vomiting, abnormal characteristics of bowel movements, including frequency, consistency, and the presence of gas. *These are signs of abnormal gastric motility (King, 2006).*
- Have client keep a diary of time food and fluid was consumed as it compares to pattern of defecation, including, but not limited to, consistency, amount, and frequency of stool *(Holman, Roberts, & Nicol, 2008).*
- Monitor and record intake and output daily. *GI dysfunction can cause rapid fluid loss, making it important to monitor a client's input and output (Dillon, 2007).*
- Weigh the client daily and note decreased weight. **EB:** *Systematic reviews demonstrated that measurement of body weight is an effective technique to assess hydration status (Armstrong, 2005; Wakefield, 2008).*
- ▲ Assess for fluid and nutritional deficits by assessing skin turgor, texture of hair, and obtain and review laboratory studies that affirm difficulties, such as albumin, protein, liver profile, glucose, and an electrolyte panel (Dillon, 2007).

 = Independent   ▲ = Collaborative   **EBN** = Evidence-Based Nursing   **EB** = Evidence-Based

▲ Review diet history. Obtain nutritional consult, considering diets lower or higher in liquids or solids, especially fats, depending on gastric motility (Shakil, Church, & Rao, 2008). *For the person with diminished gastric emptying, s/he may be advised to avoid fatty meals while more liquid intake of nutrients may be advised (Barrett, 2005).*

▲ Evaluate medication profile for gastrointestinal side effects. *Many medications have GI effects (Dillon, 2007).*

▲ Review results of laboratory studies and other diagnostic tests that will determine delayed versus rapid gastric emptying. **EB:** *Rapid gastric emptying is more common than gastroparesis in clients with autonomic dysfunction, as noted in a case series that reviewed paradoxical similarity in symptom complex in case of both delayed and accelerated gastric function (Lawal et al, 2007).*

Slowed Gastric Motility

• Assess the client for signs and symptoms of decreased gastric motility, which may include delayed emptying, nausea after meals, vomiting, heartburn, diarrhea, feeling full quickly while eating, abdominal bloating and/or pain, anorexia, and reflux (NIDDK, 2007; Shakil, Church, & Rao, 2008).

▲ Monitor daily laboratory studies, assuring that daily glucose levels are done. *Elevated blood glucose levels can cause delayed gastric emptying; therefore, it is important to normalize blood glucose levels (Shakil, Church, & Rao, 2008).*

▲ Assess for dehydration if client has continued nausea and vomiting, and to correct, provide an antiemetic and intravenous fluids as ordered (Kee, Paulanka, & Purnell, 2004). Refer to the care plans for **Nausea** and **Deficient Fluid volume.**

▲ Evaluate medications the client is taking. *Recognize that opioids and anticholinergics can cause gastric slowing, along with aluminum hydroxide antacids, beta-adrenergic receptor agonists; calcium channel blockers, diphenhydramine , histamine H2 antagonists, interferon alfa, levodopa, proton pump inhibitors, sucralfate, and tricyclic antidepressants (Shakil, Church, & Rao, 2008).*

• Observe for complications of delayed gastric and or intestinal motility, such as an ileus. Symptoms include abdominal pain, nausea, cramping, anorexia, and sometimes bloating. Also abdominal distention, and tympany to percussion, with absence of flatus or bowel movements, and lack of bowel sounds (Woodard, Rastinehad, & Richstone, 2008). Be alert to possible gastrointestinal complaints in clients that have a documented history of migraines. **EB:** *Clients with migraines may suffer from gastric stasis both during and outside an acute migraine attack (Aurora et al, 2006).*

• Obtain a thorough gastrointestinal history if the client has diabetes, as they are at high risk for gastroparesis and gastric reflux. *Gastroparesis is a manifestation of diabetic autonomic neuropathy. Gastrointestinal autonomic neuropathy contributes to increased morbidity, mortality, reduced quality of life, and increased health care costs of a client with diabetes mellitus (Feigenbaum, 2006).*

▲ Review possible laboratory and other diagnostic tools, including complete blood count (CBC), amylase, thyroid-stimulating hormone level, glucose with other metabolic studies, upper endoscopy, and gastric-emptying scintigraphy. *The diagnosis of diabetic gastroparesis is made when other causes are excluded and postprandial gastric stasis is confirmed by gastric emptying scintigraphy, which is considered the gold standard for diagnosing gastroparesis (Feigenbaum, 2006; Shakil, Church, & Rao, 2008). Other gastric emptying tests include the Breath Test and the Smart Pill (NIDDK, 2007).*

▲ If client is unable to eat or retain food, consult with the registered dietician and physician, considering further nutritional support in form of enteral or parenteral for the client with gastroparesis. *Some clients require supplementation with either enteral or parenteral nutrition for survival (Abell, Malinowski, & Minocha, 2006; Feigenbaum, 2006).*

▲ If client is receiving gastric enteral nutrition (EN), evaluate gastric residual volumes (GRV) per hospital protocol. If residual volumes are consistently greater than 150 mL, discuss with physician the benefits of prokinetic therapy, specifically erythromycin and/or metoclopramide. **EB:** *Starting prokinetic therapy speeds gastric emptying (Landzinski, Fish, & MacLaren, 2008).* **EB:** *Of all options in managing elevated GRV, treatment with a prokinetic agent is considered first-line therapy (MacLaren et al, 2008).*

▲ Administer prokinetic medications as ordered. *Metoclopramide (Reglan) has central antiemetic effects, and thus is useful for improving symptoms of postprandial fullness and nausea. Erythromycin stimulates antral contractility and increases the rate of stomach emptying by stimulating motilin receptors, smooth muscles, and nerves (Shakil, Church, & Rao, 2008).*

▲ For the client with nausea and vomiting associated with gastroparesis, review use of tricyclics, in addition to the traditional antiemetics and other prokinetic drugs. *Though the mechanism of action*

• = Independent   ▲ = Collaborative   **EBN** = Evidence-Based Nursing   **EB** = Evidence-Based

of tricyclic antidepressants for nausea and vomiting is unknown, tricyclic antidepressants are used in the treatment of many functional gastrointestinal disorders (Stapleton & Wo, 2009).

Increased Gastric Motility

- Assess for nausea, vomiting, bloating, cramping, diarrhea, dizziness, and fatigue. *These are common signs and symptoms of **early** rapid gastric emptying (NIDDK, 2007).*
- Assess for low blood sugar, weakness, sweating, and dizziness 1 to 3 hours after eating as this is when **late** rapid gastric emptying may occur. *Experiencing both early and late forms of gastric emptying is not uncommon (NIDDK, 2007).*
- ▲ Order a nutritional consult to discuss diet changes. Encourage several small meals per day that are low in carbohydrates, and higher in fiber supplements and fat. Space fluids around meal times, not with them (Barrett, 2005; NIDDK, 2007).
- ▲ Give intravenous fluids as ordered for the client complaining of diarrhea with weakness and dizziness. *Severe diarrhea can cause deficient fluid volume with extreme weakness (Mentes, 2006).*
- ▲ Review the client's medication profile, including current medication list, noting those that may increase gastric motility. *Medications such as beta-adrenergic receptor antagonists and prokinetic agents can cause increased gastrointestinal motility (Shakil, Church, & Rao, 2008).*
- Review indications for the prescribed medications to slow their digestion such as opioids and anticholinergics (Schragg, 2006).
- Observe for complications of gastric surgeries such as dumping syndrome. *This syndrome is the effect of changes in the motor functions of the stomach, including disturbances in the gastric reservoir and transporting function. Gastrointestinal hormones play an important role in dumping by mediating responses to surgical resection. Treatment options of dumping syndrome include diet, medications, and surgical revision (Ukleja, 2005).*
- Offer bathroom, commode, or bedpan assistance; depending on frequency, amount of diarrhea, and condition of client.
- Refer to the care plans for the nursing diagnoses of **Deficient Fluid volume**, **Nausea, Diarrhea**, and **Constipation** as relevant.

Pediatric

- Assess infants with suspected delayed gastric emptying (DGE) for fullness and vomiting. *Babies with DGE take longer to get hungry again, and throw up undigested, or partially digested food several hours after feeding (MacLean, 2007).*
- Continue to encourage the mother of a baby diagnosed with delayed gastric emptying to breast-feed, reinforcing the benefits of breastfeeding. *Breast milk moves through the digestive system almost twice as fast as formula (MacLean, 2007).*
- If the infant is already on a bottle, encourage parents to discuss with the pediatrician a switch to a hypoallergenic formula. *Hypoallergenic formula is already partially digested, making the transit time out of the stomach potentially faster (Skillman & Wischmeyer, 2008).*
- Observe for nutritional and fluid deficits with assessment of skin turgor, mucous membranes, fontanels, furrows of the tongue, electrolyte panel, fluid status, and cardiopulmonary function (Skillman & Wischmeyer, 2008).
- ▲ For the pediatric client presenting with symptoms suggestive of delayed gastric emptying, review the importance of further diagnostic tests as ordered, to include measurement of solid-phase gastric emptying with a gastric scintigraphy, in order to make a definitive diagnosis. **EB:** *The symptoms in children that are suggestive of delayed gastric motility can be from other gastrointestinal disorders that have either normal or rapid gastric emptying (Aktay, Werlin, & Hellman, 2003).*

Geriatric

- Closely monitor diet and medication use/side effects as they affect the gastrointestinal system. Watch for constipation. *Gastrointestinal functions are slowed in the elderly (Kee, Paulanka, & Purnell, 2004).*
- Along with assessments as indicated above, in the elderly assess more specifically for dysphagia, dyspepsia, anorexia, and fecal incontinence. *These are the most frequent gastrointestinal motor problems encountered of the elderly when they seek medical care (Firth & Prather, 2002).*

● = Independent   ▲ = Collaborative   **EBN** = Evidence-Based Nursing   **EB** = Evidence-Based

▲ If client takes metoclopramide for gastroesophageal reflux disease or slowed gastric motility, assess indication and side effects. Recognize that metoclopramide can cause drug-induced Parkinson's disease in the elderly, in addition to other neurotoxic side effects (Esper & Factor, 2008). *This medication should be used with great caution in the elderly client because of their increased side effect profile (Firth & Prather, 2002).*

Home Care

- Review safety in the home, especially if client is discharged home in a weakened state.
- Encourage a diary of nutritional intake and subsequent bowel activity.

Client/Family Teaching and Discharge Planning

- Teach the client and caregivers about their medications, reinforcing the side effects as it relates to gastrointestinal function (Firth & Prather, 2002).
- With clients newly diagnosed with diabetes, teach risks, which may include gastroparesis and gastric reflux disease.
- Review possible exercise programs. *Exercise may increase gastric motility (Shakil, Church, & Rao, 2008).*
- Give literature and resources about smoking cessation programs. *Tobacco slows gastric emptying by decreasing esophageal sphincter tone (Shakil, Church, & Rao, 2008).*
- Teach client and caregivers to report signs and symptoms that may indicate further complications including increased abdominal girth, projectile vomiting, and unrelieved acute cramping pain (bowel obstruction).
- Review signs and symptoms of dehydration with client and caregivers.

⊖volve   See the EVOLVE website for Weblinks for client education resources.

REFERENCES

Abell TL, Malinowski S, Minocha A: Nutrition aspects of gastroparesis and therapies for drug-refractory patients, *Nutr Clin Pract* 21(1):23–33, 2006.

Aktay AN, Werlin SL, Hellman RS: The impact of solid-phase gastric emptying studies in the management of children with dyspepsia, *Clin Pediatr* 42(7):621–625, 2003.

Armstrong LE: Hydration assessment techniques, *Nutr Rev* 63(6 Part 2): S40–S54, 2005.

Aurora SK, Kori SH, Barrodale P et al: Gastric stasis in migraine: more than just a paroxysmal abnormality during a migraine attack, *Headache* 46(1):57–63, 2006.

Barrett K: *Gastrointestinal physiology*, New York, 2005, MacGraw-Hill.

Bickley LS, Szilagyi P: *Guide to physical examination*, ed 10, Philadelphia, 2009, Lippincott Williams & Wilkins.

Dillon P: *Nursing health assessment: a critical thinking, case studies approach*, Philadelphia, 2007, F.A. Davis.

Esper CD, Factor SA: Failure of recognition of drug-induced parkinsonism in the elderly, *Mov Disord* 23(3):401–404, 2008.

Feigenbaum K: Update on gastroparesis, *Gastroenterol Nurs* 29(3):239–246, 2006.

Firth M, Prather CM: Gastrointestinal motility problems in the elderly patient, *Gastroenterol* 122:1688–1700, 2002.

Holman C, Roberts S, Nicol M: Preventing and treating constipation in later life, *Nurs Older People* 20(5):22–24, 2008.

Kee JL, Paulanka BJ, Purnell L: *Fluids and electrolytes with clinical applications*, ed 7, Cincinnati, 2004, Delmar Publishers.

King, JE: What is gastroparesis? *Nursing 2006* 36(9):18, 2006.

Landzinski J, Fish DN, MacLaren R: Gastric motility function in critically ill patients tolerant vs intolerant to gastric nutrition. *JPEN J Parenter Enteral Nutr* 32(1):45–50, 2008.

Lawal A, Barboi A, Massey BT et al: Rapid gastric emptying is more common than gastroparesis in patients with autonomic dysfunction, *Am J Gastroenterol* 102:618–623, 2007.

MacLaren R, Kiser TH, Fish DN et al: Erythromycin vs metoclopromide for facilitating gastric emptying and tolerance to intragastric nutrition in critically ill patients, *J Parenter Enteral Nutr* 32(4):412–419, 2008.

MacLean R: Gastroparesis, modified 2007. http://infantrefluxdisease.com/gastroparesis.php/. Accessed July 23, 2009.

Mentes J: Oral hydration in older adults: greater awareness is needed in preventing, recognizing, and treating dehydration, *Am J Nurs* 106(6):40–49, 2006.

NIDDK: Rapid gastric emptying, 2007, http://digestive.niddk.nih.gov/ddiseases/pubs/rapidgastricemptying/index.htm. Accessed July 9, 2009.

NIDDK: Gastroparesis, 2007, http://digestive.niddk.nih.gov/ddiseases/pubs/gastroparesis/. Accessed July 9, 2009.

Schraag J: Rapid gastric emptying, 2006, www.endonurse.com/articles/6c1diagnosis.html#. Accessed July 9, 2009.

Shakil A, Church, R, Rao SS: Gastrointestinal complications of diabetes, *Am Fam Physician* 77(12):1697–1703, 2008.

Skillman HE, Wischmeyer PE: Nutrition therapy in critically ill infants and children, *J Parenter Enteral Nutr* 32(5):520–534, 2008.

Stapleton J, Wo JM: Current treatment of nausea and vomiting associated with gastroparesis: antiemetics, prokinetics, tricyclics, *J Alt Complement Med* 14(7):833–39, 2009.

Ukleja A: Dumping syndrome: pathophysiology and treatment, *Nutr Clin Pract* 20(5):517–525, 2005.

Wakefield B: Fluid management guideline. In Ackley BA, Ladwig GL, Swan BA et al: *Evidence-based nursing care guidelines: medical-surgical interventions,* Philadelphia, 2008, Mosby.

Woodard E, Rastinehad AR, Richstone L: Management of postoperative ileus, *Urol Times* 36(Suppl):S8–S14, 2008.

Risk for dysfunctional gastrointestinal Motility

Betty J. Ackley, MSN, EdS, RN, and Joan Klehr, RNC, BS, MPH

NANDA-I

Definition

Risk for increased, decreased, ineffective, or lack of peristaltic activity within the gastrointestinal system

Risk Factors

Abdominal surgery; aging; anxiety; change in food; change in water; decreased gastrointestinal circulation; diabetes mellitus; food intolerance (e.g., gluten, lactose); gastroesophageal reflux disease (GERD); immobility; infection (e.g., bacterial, parasitic, viral): pharmaceutical agents (e.g., antibiotics, laxatives, narcotics/opiates, proton pump inhibitors); prematurity; sedentary lifestyle; stress; unsanitary food preparation.

NOC, NIC, Client Outcomes, Nursing Interventions, Client/Family Teaching and Discharge Planning, *Rationales*, and References

Refer to care plan for **Dysfunctional gastrointestinal Motility.**

Nausea *Janelle M. Tipton, MSN, RN, AOCN®* ⊖volve

NANDA-I

Definition

A subjective, unpleasant, wavelike sensation in the back of the throat, epigastrium, or the abdomen that may lead to the urge or need to vomit

Defining Characteristics

Aversion to food; gagging sensation; increased salivation; increased swallowing; report of nausea; sour taste in mouth

Related Factors (r/t)

Biophysical

Biochemical disorders (e.g., uremia, diabetic ketoacidosis, pregnancy); esophageal disease; gastric distention; gastric irritation; increased intracranial pressure; intraabdominal tumors; labyrinthitis; liver capsule stretch; localized tumors (e.g., acoustic neuroma, primary or secondary brain tumors, bone metastases at base of skull); meningitis; Ménière's disease; motion sickness; pain; pancreatic disease; splenetic capsule stretch; toxins (e.g., tumor-produced peptides, abnormal metabolites due to cancer)

Situational

Anxiety; fear; noxious odors; noxious taste; pain; psychological factors; unpleasant visual stimulation

Treatment-Related

Gastric distention; gastric irritation: pharmaceuticals

NOC (Nursing Outcomes Classification)

Suggested NOC Outcomes

Comfort Level, Hydration, Nausea & Vomiting Severity, Nutritional Status: Food and Fluid Intake, Nutrient Intake

• = Independent ▲ = Collaborative **EBN** = Evidence-Based Nursing **EB** = Evidence-Based

Client Outcomes

Client Will (Specify Time Frame):

- State relief of nausea
- Explain methods they can use to decrease nausea and vomiting (N&V)

NIC   (Nursing Interventions Classification)

Suggested NIC Interventions

Distraction, Medication Administration, Progressive Muscle Relaxation, Simple Guided Imagery, Therapeutic Touch

Example NIC Activities—Distraction

Encourage the individual to choose the distraction technique(s) desired, such as music, engaging in conversation or telling a detailed account of event or story, guided imagery, or humor; Advise patient to practice the distraction technique before the time needed, if possible

Nursing Interventions and *Rationales*

- ▲ Determine cause or risk for nausea and vomiting (N&V) (e.g., medication effects, infectious causes, disorders of the gut and peritoneum, central nervous system causes [including anxiety], endocrine and metabolic causes [including pregnancy], postoperative-related status). *Since most episodes of N&V are now preventable, it is important for the cause to be determined and appropriate plan and interventions to be developed (Steele & Carlson, 2007).*
- ▲ Evaluate and document the client's history of N&V, with attention to onset, duration, timing, volume of emesis, frequency of pattern, setting, associated factors, aggravating factors, and past medical and social histories. *The onset and duration of nausea and vomiting may be distinctly associated with specific events, and may be treated differently (Steele & Carlson, 2007).*
- Document each episode of nausea and/or vomiting separately, as well as effectiveness of interventions. Consider an assessment tool for consistency of evaluation. *A systematic approach can provide consistency, accuracy, and measurement needed to direct care. It is important to recognize that nausea is a subjective experience (Steele & Carlson, 2007; Kearney et al, 2009).*
- Identify and eliminate contributing causative factors. This may include eliminating unpleasant odors or medications that may be contributing to nausea. *These interventions are theory-based; however, there is no research evidence to support outside of expert opinion (Steele & Carlson, 2007).*
- ▲ Implement appropriate dietary measures such as NPO status as appropriate, small, frequent meals, and low-fat meals. It may be helpful to avoid foods that are spicy, fatty, or highly salty. Reverting to previous practices when ill in the past, and consuming "comfort foods" may also be helpful at this time. *Expert opinion consensus recommends these interventions, with no research data available (Tipton et al, 2007).*
- ▲ Recognize, implement interventions, and monitor complications associated with N&V. This may include administration of intravenous fluids and electrolytes. *Recognition of complications of N&V is critical to prevent and manage untoward complications of dehydration and electrolyte imbalance (Steele & Carlson, 2007).*
- ▲ Administer appropriate antiemetics, according to emetic cause, by most effective route, considering the side effects of the medication. *Antiemetic medications are effective at different receptor sites and treat different causes of N&V. A combination of agents may be more effective than single agents (Steele & Carlson, 2007).*
- Consider nonpharmacologic interventions such as acupressure, acupuncture, music therapy, distraction, and slow, deliberate movements. *Nonpharmacologic interventions can augment pharmaco-*

● = Independent   ▲ = Collaborative   **EBN** = Evidence-Based Nursing   **EB** = Evidence-Based

logic interventions because they predominantly affect the higher cortical centers that trigger N&V. Nonpharmacologic interventions are often low cost, relatively easy to use, and have few adverse events (Steele & Carlson, 2007). **EBN:** *A review of acupressure studies suggest effectiveness in reducing chemotherapy-induced nausea and vomiting (CINV) when combined with antiemetics (Lee et al, 2008).*

- Provide oral care after the client vomits. *Oral care helps remove the taste and smell of vomitus, thus reducing the stimulus for further vomiting.*

Nausea in Pregnancy

- Recommend that the woman eat dry crackers or dry toast in bed before arising and then get up slowly. Also advise to eat small frequent meals, drink small amounts of fluids often, avoid foods with offensive odors, and avoid preparing food or shopping when nauseated. *These are traditional strategies for alleviating nausea during pregnancy (Sheehan, 2007).*
- ▲ Discuss with the primary care practitioner the possibility of using the P6 acupuncture point stimulation to help relieve nausea. **EB:** *The results of a systematic review of the studies showed that the results of using P6 acupressure during pregnancy are equivocal (Ezzo, Streitberger, & Schneider, 2006).*
- ▲ Recognize that ginger ingestion may help nausea. Ginger is available in a number of forms including tea, biscuits, and capsules. There are scant randomized controlled clinical trials for use of ginger in pregnancy. **EB:** *Ginger, when compared to placebo, showed benefit in reducing N&V with no adverse events (Vutyavanich, Kraisarin, & Ruangsri, 2001).*
- ▲ Recognize that there are currently no FDA-approved drugs for the treatment of morning sickness, N&V of pregnancy, or hyperemesis gravidarum. There are, however, several pharmacologic treatments outlined by the American College of Obstetrics and Gynecology (ACOG). These include pyridoxine (vitamin B_6), doxylamine, dimenhydrinate, diphenhydramine, phenothiazines such as promethazine, and serotonin antagonists such as ondansetron. *A step-wise, cost-effective strategy may be helpful in approaching nausea with pregnancy. Considerable N&V with associated dehydration may require intravenous antiemetics (Reichmann & Kirkbride, 2008).*

Nausea Following Surgery

- ▲ Evaluate for risk factors for postoperative nausea and vomiting (PONV). Strong evidence suggests that female gender, history of PONV, history of motion sickness, nonsmoking behavior, postoperative opioid use, and volatile anesthetics may increase the risk for PONV. *It is important to determine this risk in the preoperative period, to better plan interventions (ASPAN, 2006).*
- ▲ Medicate the client prophylactically for nausea as ordered. **EB:** *Antiemetic medications can reduce the incidence of PONV, and use of more than one medication may be needed (ASPAN, 2006).*
- ▲ Alleviate postoperative pain using ordered analgesic agents (refer to care plan for **Acute Pain**). *Pain is known to be a factor in the development of PONV.*
- ▲ Ensure that the client is well hydrated. *Intravenous fluids with lactated ringers solution have been shown to decrease PONV in high-risk clients (ASPAN, 2006).*
- Consider the use of nonpharmacological techniques, such as P6 acupoint stimulation, as an adjunct for controlling PONV. **EB:** *Acupuncture and acustimulation have been studied with the most consistent results, similarly effective across methods of stimulation (acupuncture or non-invasive with acupressure or wrist-like electrical stimulation) (Ezzo, Streitberger, & Schneider, 2006).*
- Use relaxation, imagery, and distraction techniques for nausea; encourage the client to take slow, deep breaths. *Deep breaths can serve as a distraction technique and can help rid the body of the anesthetic agent.*
- Include client education on the management of PONV for all outpatients, and discuss key assessment criteria (ASPAN, 2006).

Nausea Following Chemotherapy

- Perform risk assessment prior to chemotherapy administration. Risk factors include female gender, younger age, history of low alcohol consumption, history of morning sickness during pregnancy, anxiety, previous history of chemotherapy, and emetic potential of the regimen. *It is important to recognize the many risk factors individual clients may have, and tailor the antiemetic strategy accordingly. Far too often, the degree of N&V is underestimated by health care providers (Grunberg et al, 2004; Hawkins & Grunberg, 2009).*

● = Independent   ▲ = Collaborative   **EBN** = Evidence-Based Nursing   **EB** = Evidence-Based

▲ Consult with physician regarding antiemetic strategy, either prophylactic or when N&V occurs. *Preventing N&V is important; one failure in antiemetic therapy can result in anticipatory nausea for the remainder of the client's treatments (Hawkins & Grunberg, 2009).*

▲ Use antiemetics and a nursing intervention program of increased access to support and increase information. **EBN:** *A creative education strategy using the addition of a video to standard education resulted in a higher recall of information about predictable chemotherapy side effects and reporting of treatment-related symptoms (Kinnane et al, 2008).*

• Consider teaching your client to learn how to use acupressure for nausea, applying pressure bilaterally at P6 points using fingers or bands to decrease the amount and severity of nausea. **EBN and EB:** *Finger acupressure can be effective to relieve chemotherapy-induced nausea (Ezzo, Streitberger, & Schneider, 2006; Lee et al, 2008). Use of acupressure bands yielded negative results (Lee et al, 2008). Research supports the use of acupressure as an adjunct to pharmacologic interventions. Acupressure is a safe, inexpensive, non-invasive technique that has promise for CINV (Lee et al, 2008).*

▲ Consider the use of ginger root *(Zingiber officinale)* to relieve nausea. **EB:** *A small randomized study showed that protein meals in addition to ginger reduced the delayed CINV and use of antiemetics. This nutritionally based treatment requires further study, but shows promise (Levine et al, 2008). A large Phase II trial showed no additional benefit for reduction in the prevalence or severity of acute or delayed CINV when given with serotonin receptor antagonists and/or a precipitant (Zick et al, 2009).*

• Consider massage for symptom relief of nausea. **EB/EBN:** *Two systematic reviews of massage in cancer clients show suggestion of benefit in the reduction of nausea; however, the variability of areas massaged and the poor quality of studies make it difficult to draw definitive conclusions (Wilkinson, Barnes, & Storey, 2008; Ernst, 2009).*

• Consider the use of yoga for CINV. **EB:** *A small study in breast cancer clients showed a significant decrease in postchemotherapy nausea frequency, nausea intensity, and intensity of anticipatory N&V compared to a control group. This may be a possible stress-reduction technique in conjunction with antiemetics to decrease CINV (Raghavendra et al, 2007).*

Home Care

• Previously mentioned interventions may be adapted for home care use.

▲ In hospice care clients, assess for causes of nausea, such as constipation, bowel obstruction, adverse effects of medications, and onset of increased intracranial pressure. Refer the client to a primary care practitioner if needed. *There can be multiple causes of nausea in clients with advanced cancer (Pantilat & Issac, 2008).*

• Assist the client and family with identifying and avoiding irritants in the home that exacerbate nausea (e.g., strong odors from food, plants, perfume, and room deodorizers). All medications except antiemetics should be given after meals to minimize the risk of nausea.

Client/Family Teaching and Discharge Planning

• Teach the client techniques to use prior to and after chemotherapy, including relaxation techniques, guided imagery, hypnosis, and music therapy (Tipton, et al, 2007).

⊖volve   See the EVOLVE website for Weblinks for client education resources.

REFERENCES

American Society of PeriAnesthesia Nurses (ASPAN): ASPAN'S evidence-based clinical practice guideline for the prevention and/or management of PONV/PDNV, *J PeriAnesth Nurs* 21(4):230–250, 2006.

Ernst E: Massage therapy for cancer palliation and supportive care: a systematic review of randomised clinical trials, *Support Care Cancer* 17: 333–337, 2009.

Ezzo J, Streitberger K, Schneider A: Cochrane systematic reviews examine P6 acupuncture-point stimulation for nausea and vomiting, *J Altern Compl Med* 12(5):489–495, 2006.

Grunberg SM, Deuson RR, Mavros P et al: Incidence of chemotherapy-induced nausea and emesis after modern antiemetics, *Cancer* 100(10):2261–2268, 2004.

Hawkins R, Grunberg S: Chemotherapy-induced nausea and vomiting: challenges and opportunities for improved patient outcomes, *Clin J Oncol Nurs* 13(1):54–64, 2009.

Kearney N, McCann L, Norrie J et al: Evaluation of a mobile phone-based, advanced symptom management system (ASyMS(c)) in the management of chemotherapy-related toxicity, *Support Care Cancer* 17:437–444, 2009.

• = Independent   ▲ = Collaborative   **EBN** = Evidence-Based Nursing   **EB** = Evidence-Based

Kinnane N, Stuart E, Thompson L et al: Evaluation of the addition of video-based education for patients receiving standard pre-chemotherapy education, *Eur J Cancer Care* 17:328–339, 2008.

Lee J, Dodd M, Dibble S et al: Review of acupressure studies for chemotherapy-induced nausea and vomiting control, *J Pain Symp Manage,* 36(5):529–544, 2008.

Levine ME, Gillis MG, Koch SY et al: Protein and ginger for the treatment of chemotherapy-induced delayed nausea, *J Alt Complement Med* 14(5):545–551, 2008.

Raghavendra RM, Nagarathna R, Nagendra HR et al: Effects of an integrated yoga programme on chemotherapy-induced nausea and emesis in breast cancer patients, *Eur J Cancer Care* 16:462–474, 2007.

Reichmann, JP, Kirkbride, MS: Nausea and vomiting of pregnancy: cost-effective pharmacologic treatments, *Manag Care* 17(12):41–45, 2008.

Pantilat SZ, Issac M: End-of-life care for the hospitalized patient, *Med Clin North Am* 92:349–370, 2008.

Sheehan P: Hyperemesis gravidarum, *Aust Fam Phys* 36(9):698–701, 2007.

Steele A, Carlson KK: Nausea and vomiting: applying research to bedside practice, *AACN Adv Crit Care* 18(1):61–75, 2007.

Tipton JM, McDaniel RW, Barbour L et al: Putting evidence into practice: evidence-based interventions to prevent, manage, and treat chemotherapy-induced nausea and vomiting, *Clin J Oncol Nurs* 11(1):69–78, 2007.

Vutyavanich T, Kraisarin T, Ruangsri R: Ginger for nausea and vomiting in pregnancy: randomised, double-masked, placebo controlled trial, *Obstet Gynecol* 97:577–582, 2001.

Wilkinson S, Barnes K, Storey L: Massage for symptom relief in patients with cancer: systematic review, *J Adv Nurs* 63(5):430–439, 2008.

Zick SM, Ruffin MT, Lee J et al: Phase II trial of encapsulated ginger as a treatment for chemotherapy-induced nausea and vomiting, *Support Care Cancer* 17:563–572, 2009.

Self Neglect   *Susanne W. Gibbons, PhD, C-ANP, C-GNP*  ⓔvolve

NANDA-I

Definition

A constellation of culturally framed behaviors involving one or more self-care activities necessary to maintain a socially-accepted standard of health and well-being (Gibbons, Lauder & Ludwick, 2006)

Defining Characteristics

Inadequate personal hygiene; inadequate environmental hygiene; nonadherence to health activities

Related Factors (r/t)

Capgras syndrome; cognitive impairment (i.e., dementia); depression; learning disability; fear of institutionalization; frontal lobe dysfunction and executive processing ability; functional impairment; lifestyle/choice; maintaining control; malingering; obsessive compulsive disorder; schizotypal personality disorder; paranoid personality disorder; substance abuse; major life stressor (i.e., coping difficulty); mental retardation

NOC   (Nursing Outcomes Classification)

Suggested NOC Outcomes

Self-Care Status, Self-Care: Activities of Daily Living (ADL), Hygiene, Grooming, Cognition, Risk Control, Personal Safety Behavior, Nutritional Status

Examples of NOC Outcome with Indicator

Self-Care Status as evidenced by the following indicators: maintains personal cleanliness, recognizes safety needs in the home (Rate outcome and indicators of **Self-Care Status:** 1 = severely compromised, 2 = substantially compromised, 3 = moderately compromised, 4 = mildly compromised, 5 = not compromised [see Section I].)

Client Outcomes

Client Will (Specify Time Frame):

- Demonstrate improved personal hygiene
- Show improved environmental hygiene
- Demonstrate adherence to health activities

NOTE: Because self-neglect is a culturally framed and socially defined phenomenon, change in a client's status must occur in such a way that it respects individual rights while ensuring individual health and well-being, and this is accomplished through client-nurse partnership.

• = Independent   ▲ = Collaborative   **EBN** = Evidence-Based Nursing   **EB** = Evidence-Based

NIC   (Nursing Interventions Classification)

Suggested NIC Interventions

Self-Care Assistance: Dressing/Grooming, Abuse Protection Support

> **Example NIC Activities—Self-Care Assistance: Dressing/Grooming**
>
> Be available for assistance in dressing, as necessary; Reinforce efforts to dress self; Maintain privacy while the patient is dressing

Nursing Interventions and *Rationales*

- Monitor individuals with acute or chronic mental and complex physical illness for defining characteristics for self-neglect. **EBN and EB:** *In a sample of 538 impaired older adults referred by their local APS, cardiovascular disorders (84%) and hypertension (51.6%); mental disorders (53%), of which dementia and depression were the most common; and endocrine disorders (30.2%), of which diabetes was the most common (25.2%), were the most frequent medical diagnoses seen with self-neglect (Gibbons, Lauder, & Ludwick, 2006; Dyer et al, 2007).*
- Assist individuals with complex mental and physical health issues to adopt positive health behaviors so that they may maintain their health status. **EB:** *A variety of mental illnesses have been correlated with self-neglect in younger adults. However, in the older adult population, depression has been particularly associated with self-neglecting behavior, with inadequately treated medical disease identified more often in self-neglecters who are also depressed (Dyer et al, 2000; Lauder, Anderson, & Barclay, 2005; Burnett et al, 2006; Gibbons, 2007; Tomkins, 2008).*
- Assess persons with complex health issues for adequate coping abilities and assist those with coping problems to maintain their health and well-being in the community. **EB:** *Personal control and protecting self are coping strategies seen in community-dwelling self-neglecters and in those identified by adult protective services (APS). Individuals use these strategies to compensate, which sometimes causes them to appear uncooperative or resistant to care and change (Rathbone-McCuan & Fabian, 1992; Bozinovski, 2000; Gibbons, 2007).*
- Assist individuals whose self-care is failing with managing their medication regimen. **EBN:** *Individuals who exhibit self-neglect may have difficulty managing medication (Gibbons, 2007; Naik et al, 2008).*
- Assess individuals with failing self-care for noncompliance (i.e., diagnostic testing, medication regimen, therapeutic regimen, and safety precautions). **EBN:** *Individuals who exhibit self-neglect may demonstrate noncompliance (Gibbons, 2007; Naik et al, 2008).*
- Assist persons with self-care deficits due to ADL or IADL impairments. **EBN:** *Individuals with self-care deficits may have difficulty with ADLs (Gibbons, 2007; Naik et al, 2008).*
- Assess persons with failing self-care for changes in cognitive function (i.e., psychiatric illness or dementia). **EBN:** *Individuals with failing self-care may have changes in cognition (Abrams et al, 2002; Gibbons, 2007).*
- ▲ Refer persons with failing self-care to appropriate specialists (i.e., psychologist, psychiatrist, social work) and therapists (i.e., physical therapy, occupational therapy, etc.). **EBN:** *Individuals with self-care deficits may need assistance of medical professional service. (Gibbons, 2007; Naik et al, 2008).*
- Utilize behavioral modification as appropriate to bring about client changes that lead to improvement in personal hygiene, environmental hygiene, and adherence to medical regimen. **EB:** *Behavioral modification approaches have been effective in reversing self-neglect in older adults where triggers or events brought about the behavior (Fraser, 2006; Thibault, 2008).*
- ▲ Refer persons with failing self-care who are significantly impaired cognitively or functionally and who are suspected victims of abuse to APS. **EBN and EB:** *Self-neglect has been associated with mistreatment in older adults, especially those who live alone (NEAIS, 1998; Dyer et al, 2007).*
- Monitor clients with changes in cognitive function for adequate safety. **EB:** *Dementia is one of the leading causes for self-neglect (NEAIS, 1998; Abrams et al, 2002).*
- Monitor clients with functional impairments for adequate safety. **EBN and EB:** *Functional impairment, often associated with depression in the older adult, is correlated with self-neglect (NEAIS, 1998; Lachs et al, 2002; Gibbons, 2007).*

• = Independent   ▲ = Collaborative   **EBN** = Evidence-Based Nursing   **EB** = Evidence-Based

- Assist individuals with complex mental and physical health needs with maintaining their health and well-being in the community. **EB:** *Those self-neglecters institutionalized in nursing homes have a higher mortality rate than those never identified, and for this reason, maintaining a client's health and well-being in the community setting is essential to a positive outcome (Lachs et al, 1998; Lachs et al, 2002).*
- Monitor persons with substance abuse problems (i.e., drugs, alcohol, smoking) for adequate safety. **EB:** *As mental health and substance use disorders can go unrecognized and untreated in this population, identified self-neglecting clients should be screened as appropriate by nurses and other health professionals (Gibbons, 2007; Paveza, Vande Weerd, & Laumann, 2008).*

Geriatric

- ▲ Assess client's socioeconomic status and refer for appropriate support. **EB:** *The findings in this study show that elder self-neglect/neglect is, in large part, attributable to frail older adults' and their families' lack of resources to pay for essential goods and services, and the inadequate health care and other formal support programs for the older adults and their caregivers (Choi, Kim, & Asseff, 2009).*
- ▲ Refer persons demonstrating a significant decline in self-care abilities (i.e., posing a threat to themselves or to their community) for evaluation of competency and executive function. **EB:** *Current evidence indicates that executive dyscontrol contributes to self-neglect in the older adult population (Dyer et al, 2007).*

Multicultural

- Deliver health care that is sensitive to the culture and philosophy of individual's whose self-care appears inadequate. **EBN:** *Nurses must be careful not to prematurely judge client's health choices or living arrangements as personal choice or lifestyle do not necessarily indicate self-neglect, until client behavior poses a risk to themselves and/or others. For this reason, it is imperative that nurses assess values and beliefs of persons with inadequate self-care to better identify their individual health needs (Lauder, Anderson, & Barclay, 2005; Gibbons et al, 2006).*

⊖volve   See the EVOLVE website for Weblinks for client education resources.

REFERENCES

Abrams RC, Lachs M, McAvay G et al: Predictors of self-neglect in community dwelling elders, *Am J Psychiatry* 159:10, 1724–1730, 2002.

Bozinovski SD: Older self-neglecters: interpersonal problems and the maintenance of self-continuity, *J Elder Abuse Neglect* 12(1):37–56, 2000.

Burnett J, Coverdale J, Pickens S et al: What is the association between self-neglect, depressive symptoms and untreated medical conditions? *J Elder Abuse Neglect* 18(4):25–34, 2006.

Choi NG, Kim J, Asseff J: Self-neglect and neglect of vulnerable older adults: reexamination of etiology, *J Gerontol Soc Work* 52(2):171–187, 2009.

Dyer C, Goodwin JS, Pickens-Pace S et al: Self-neglect among the elderly: a model based on more than 500 patients seen by a geriatric medicine team, *Am J Public Health* 97(9):1671–1676, 2007.

Dyer C, Pavlik V, Murphy K et al: The high prevalence of depression and dementia in elder abuse or neglect, *J Am Geriatr Soc* 48(2):205–208, 2000.

Fraser A: Psychological therapies in the treatment of abused adults, *J Adult Protect* 8(2):31–38, 2006.

Gibbons S: Characteristics and behaviors of self-neglect among community-dwelling older adults, [dissertation: The Catholic University of America] (UMI No.AAI3246949), 2007.

Gibbons S, Lauder W, Ludwick R: Self-neglect: a proposed new NANDA diagnosis, *Int J Nurs Terminol Classif* 17(1):10–18, 2006.

Lachs MS, Williams CS, O'Brien S et al: The mortality of elder mistreatment, *JAMA* 280(5):428–432, 1998.

Lachs MS, Williams CS, O'Brien S et al: Adult protective services use and nursing home placement, *Gerontologist* 42(6):734–739, 2002.

Lauder W, Anderson I, Barclay A: A framework for good practice in interagency interventions with cases of self-neglect, *J Psychiatr Mental Health Nurs* 12:192–198, 2005.

Naik A, Lai J, Kunik M et al: Assessing capacity in suspected cases of self-neglect, *Geriatr* 63(2):24–31, 2008.

National Elder Abuse Incidence Study [NEAIS]: Administration for Children and Families and the Administration on Aging. The U.S. Department of Health and Human Services. Available from National Center on Elder Abuse website, http://www.aoa.gov/AoARoot/AoA_Programs/Elder_Rights/Elder_Abuse/docs/ABuseReport_Full.pdf, 1998. Accessed on October 30, 2009.

Paveza G, Vande Weerd C, Laumann E: Elder self-neglect: a discussion of typology, *J Am Geriatr Soc* 56(Suppl 2):S271–S275, 2008.

Rathbone-McCuan, E, Fabian, DR: *Self-neglecting elders: a clinical dilemma*, Westport CT, 1992, Auburn House.

Thibault JM: Analysis and treatment of self-neglectful behaviors in three elderly female patients, *J Elder Abuse Neglect* 19(3/4):151–166, 2008.

Tomkins J: Starting out: student experiences in the real world of nursing. I stopped blaming the patient for the problems in her life, *Nurs Stand* 22(51):27, 2008.

● = Independent   ▲ = Collaborative   **EBN** = Evidence-Based Nursing   **EB** = Evidence-Based

Unilateral Neglect   *Lori M. Rhudy, PhD, RN*

 NANDA-I

Definition

Impairment in sensory and motor response, mental representation, and spatial attention of the body and the corresponding environment characterized by inattention to one side and overattention to the opposite side; left-side neglect is more severe and persistent than right-side neglect

Defining Characteristics

Appears unaware of positioning of neglected limb; difficulty remembering details of internally represented familiar scenes that are on the neglected side; displacement of sounds to the nonneglected side; distortion of drawing on the half of the page on the neglected side; failure to cancel lines on the half of the page on the neglected side; failure to eat food from portion of the plate on the neglected side; failure to dress neglected side; failure to groom neglected side; failure to move eyes, head, limbs, trunk in the neglected hemispace, despite being aware of a stimulus in that space; failure to notice people approaching from the neglected side; lack of safety precautions with regard to the neglected side; marked deviation of the eyes to the nonneglected side to stimuli and activities on that side; marked deviation of the head to the nonneglected side to stimuli and activities on that side; marked deviation of the trunk to the nonneglected side to stimuli and activities on that side; omission of drawing on the half of the page on the neglected side; perseveration of visual motor tasks on nonneglected side; substitution of letters to form alternative words that are similar to the original in length when reading; transfer of pain sensation to the nonneglected side; use of only vertical half of page when writing

Related Factors (r/t)

Brain injury from cerebrovascular problems; brain injury from neurological illness; brain injury from trauma; brain injury from tumor, hemianopsia

NOTE: Because the right hemisphere plays a role in focusing attention while the left hemisphere specializes in global attention, unilateral neglect is more common if neurological pathology occurs in the right hemisphere of the brain, which results in left-sided neglect (Jepson, Despain & Keller, 2008).

NOC   **(Nursing Outcomes Classification)**

Suggested NOC Outcomes

Body Image, Body Positioning: Self-Initiated, Mobility, Self-Care: Activities of Daily Living (ADLs)

Example NOC Outcome with Indicators
Mobility as evidenced by the following indicators: Balance/Coordination/Gait/Muscle movement (Rate the outcome and indicators of **Mobility:** 1 = severely compromised, 2 = substantially compromised, 3 = moderately compromised, 4 = mildly compromised, 5 = not compromised [See Section I].)

Client Outcomes

Client Will (Specify Time Frame):

- Use techniques that can be used to minimize unilateral neglect
- Care for both sides of the body appropriately and keep affected side free from harm
- Return to the highest functioning level possible based on personal goals and abilities
- Remain free from injury

NIC   **(Nursing Interventions Classification)**

Suggested NIC Intervention

Unilateral Neglect Management

 = Independent   ▲ = Collaborative   **EBN** = Evidence-Based Nursing   **EB** = Evidence-Based

Example NIC Activities—Unilateral Neglect Management
Ensure that affected extremities are properly and safely and positioned; Rearrange the environment to use the right or left visual field; Position personal items, television, or reading materials within view on unaffected side

Nursing Interventions and *Rationales*

- Assess the client for signs of unilateral neglect (UN; e.g., not washing, shaving, or dressing one side of the body; sitting or lying inappropriately on affected arm or leg; failing to respond to environmental stimuli contralateral to the side of lesion; eating food on only one side of plate; or failing to look to one side of the body). *Looking, listening, touching, and searching deficits occur on the affected side of the body and may or may not be associated with a loss of vision, sensation, or motion on the affected side (Menon-Nair et al, 2006). Many tests for UN exist, but there is no consensus about which is the most valid. Joint assessments of UN that include both clinical observation and precise testing perform better than either used alone (Jepson, Despain, & Keller, 2008).*
- ▲ Collaborate with physician for referral to a rehabilitation team (including, but not limited to, rehabilitation clinical nurse specialist, physical medicine and rehabilitation physician, neuropsychologist, occupational therapist, physical therapist, and speech and language pathologist) for continued help in dealing with UN. **EB:** *There is some evidence that cognitive rehabilitation for unilateral spatial neglect improves performance, but its effect on disability is not clear. Further studies are needed (Bowen et al, 2009).*
- Use the principles of rehabilitation to progressively increase the client's ability to compensate for UN by using assistive devices, feedback, and support. **EB:** *Studies demonstrate rate that recovery from UN is most rapid in the first 10 days with significant neglect rare at 6 months (Jones & Shinton, 2006).*
- Set up environment so that most activity is on unaffected side:
  - Place the client's personal items within view and on unaffected side.
  - Position the bed so that client is approached from the unaffected side.
  - Monitor and assist the client to achieve adequate food and fluid intake.
  Helps in focusing attention and aids in maintenance of safety.
- Implement fall prevention interventions. **EB:** *Unilateral neglect has been strongly associated with increased risk of injury an higher incidence of falls (Wee & Hopman 2008).*
- Position affected extremity in a safe and functional manner. **EB:** *A study found that clients with UN had higher rates of shoulder-hand complications than those without UN (Wee & Hopman, 2008).*
- Teach the client to be aware of the problem, and modify behavior and environment. **EB:** *Awareness of the environment decreases risk of injury. There is some evidence that use of scanning techniques may decrease visual neglect (Jones & Shinton, 2006).*
- Use cues and anchors to promote attention to the neglected side and help the client develop compensatory mechanisms to deal with the neglect syndrome.
- Use reminders to keep the client scanning the entire environment.
- Use bright yellow or red stickers on outer margins in reading or writing exercises. Have the client look for the sticker while reading or writing. Similar markers can be applied to a meal tray or plate to encourage scanning of the entire meal.
- Encourage the client to bathe and groom the affected side first.
- Focus touch and talking on affected side; use a positive approach (e.g., "Mary, turn your head to the left and you'll see your daughter").
- Implement a discharge plan to ensure continuity of care. **EB:** *A study demonstrated that clients with UN have longer length of stay and less likelihood of discharge to home than subjects without UN (Wee & Hopman 2008).*

Home Care

- Many of the previously listed interventions may be adapted for use in the home care setting.
- Position bed at home so that client gets out of bed on unaffected side. *Positioning the bed so that the client gets out on the unaffected side can increase safety.*

● = Independent   ▲ = Collaborative   **EBN** = Evidence-Based Nursing   **EB** = Evidence-Based

Client/Family Teaching and Discharge Planning

- Explain pathology and symptoms of unilateral neglect to both the client and family.
- Teach the client how to scan regularly to check the position of body parts and to regularly turn head from side to side for safety when ambulating, using a wheelchair, or doing self-care tasks.
- Reinforce the client's use of adaptive devices such as prisms prescribed by rehabilitation professionals.
- Teach caregivers to cue the client to the environment.

evolve   See the EVOLVE website for Weblinks for client education resources.

REFERENCES

Bowen A, West C, Hesketh A et al: Rehabilitation for apraxia. Evidence for short-term improvements in activities of daily living, *Stroke*, April 2, 2009, Epub ahead of print.

Jepson R, Despain K, Keller DC: Unilateral neglect: assessment in nursing practice, *J Neurosci Nurs* 40:142, 2008.

Jones SA, Shinton RA: improving outcome in stroke patients with visual problems, *Age Ageing* 35:560, 2006.

Menon-Nair A, Korner-Bitensky N, Wood-Dauphinee S et al: Assessment of unilateral neglect post stroke in Canadian acute care hospitals: are we neglecting neglect? *Clin Rehabil* 20(7):623–634, 2006.

Wee JYM, Hopman WM: Comparing consequences of right and left unilateral neglect in a stroke rehabilitation population, *Am J Phys Med Rehabil* 87:910, 2008.

Noncompliance   *Betty J. Ackley, MSN, EdS, RN*

NANDA-I

Definition

Behavior of person and/or caregiver that fails to coincide with a health-promoting or therapeutic plan agreed on by the person (and/or family and/or community) and health care professional; in the presence of an agreed-on, health-promoting, or therapeutic plan, person's or caregiver's behavior is fully or partially nonadherent and may lead to clinically ineffective or partially ineffective outcomes

Defining Characteristics

Behavior indicative of failure to adhere; evidence of development of complications; evidence of exacerbation of symptoms; failure to keep appointments; failure to progress; objective tests (e.g., physiological measures, detection of physiological markers)

Related Factors (r/t)

Health System

Access to care; client/provider relationships; communication skills of the provider; convenience of care; credibility of provider; individual health coverage; provider continuity; provider regular follow-up; provider reimbursement; satisfaction with care; teaching skills of the provider

Health Care Plan

Complexity; cost; duration; financial flexibility of plan; intensity

Individual Factors

Cultural influences; developmental abilities; health beliefs; individual's value system; knowledge relevant to the regimen behavior; motivational forces; personal abilities; significant others; skill relevant to the regimen behavior; spiritual values

Network

Involvement of members in health plan; perceived beliefs of significant others; social value regarding plan

NOTE: The nursing diagnosis **Noncompliance** is judgmental and places blame on the client. The authors recommend use of the diagnosis **Ineffective self Health management** in place of the diagnosis

Noncompliance. The diagnosis **Ineffective self Health management** has interventions that are developed by both the health care providers and the client. It is a more respectful and efficacious nursing diagnosis than **Noncompliance.**

NOC, NIC, Client Outcomes, Nursing Interventions, Client/Family Teaching and Discharge Planning, *Rationales,* and References

Refer to care plans for **Ineffective self Health management.**

Imbalanced Nutrition: less than body requirements   ⊖volve
Betty J. Ackley, MSN, EdS, RN

NANDA-I

Definition

Intake of nutrients insufficient to meet metabolic needs

Defining Characteristics

Abdominal cramping; abdominal pain; aversion to eating; body weight 20% or more under ideal; capillary fragility; diarrhea; excessive loss of hair; hyperactive bowel sounds; lack of food; lack of information; lack of interest in food; loss of weight with adequate food intake; misconceptions; misinformation; pale mucous membranes; perceived inability to ingest food; poor muscle tone; reported altered taste sensation; reported food intake less than RDA (recommended daily allowance); satiety immediately after ingesting food; sore buccal cavity; steatorrhea; weakness of muscles required for swallowing or mastication

Related Factors (r/t)

Biological factors; economic factors; inability to absorb nutrients; inability to digest food; inability to ingest food; psychological factors

NOC   (Nursing Outcomes Classification)

Suggested NOC Outcomes

Nutritional Status, Nutritional Status: Food and Fluid Intake, Nutrient Intake, Weight Control

Example NOC Outcome with Indicators
Nutritional Status as evidenced by the following indicators: Food and fluid intake/Body mass index/Weight-height ratio/Hematocrit (Rate the outcome and indicators of **Nutritional Status:** 1 = severe deviation from normal range, 2 = substantial deviation from normal range, 3 = moderate deviation from normal range, 4 = mild deviation from normal range, 5 = no deviation from normal range [see Section I].)

Client Outcomes

Client Will (Specify Time Frame):

- Progressively gain weight toward desired goal
- Weigh within normal range for height and age
- Recognize factors contributing to underweight
- Identify nutritional requirements
- Consume adequate nourishment
- Be free of signs of malnutrition

NIC   (Nursing Interventions Classification)

Suggested NIC Interventions

Feeding, Nutrition Management, Nutrition Therapy, Weight Gain Assistance

• = Independent   ▲ = Collaborative   **EBN** = Evidence-Based Nursing   **EB** = Evidence-Based

Example NIC Activities—Nutrition Management
Ascertain the client's food preferences; provide the client with high-protein, high-calorie, nutritious finger foods and drinks that can be readily consumed, as appropriate

Nursing Interventions and *Rationales*

▲ Utilize a nutritional screening tool to determine possibility of malnutrition upon admission into any health care facility. Watch for recent weight loss of over 10 pounds, 10% under healthy weight, not eating for more than three days, ½ normal eating for greater than 5 days, and body mass index (BMI) of less than 20, or other reasons why the client may be malnourished and refer to a dietitian for a complete nutritional assessment (Thomas et al, 2005; Lutz & Przytulski, 2010). **EB:** *Research has shown that up to 50% of all clients are malnourished on admission, and the presence of malnutrition influences the length of stay (de Luis et al, 2006; Baldwin, Parsons, & Logan, 2007).*

• Recognize that clients with wounds, recent surgery, trauma, and a fever need increased calories to maintain nutrition.

• Monitor for signs of malnutrition including: brittle hair that is easily plucked, bruises, dry skin, pale skin and conjunctiva, muscle wasting, smooth red tongue, cheilosis, "flaky paint" rash over lower extremities, and disorientation (Fauci et al, 2008).

• Recognize that severe protein calorie malnutrition can result in septicemia from impairment of the immune system, and organ failure including heart failure, liver failure, and respiratory dysfunction, especially in the critically ill client. *Untreated malnutrition can result in death (Fauci et al, 2008).*

▲ Note laboratory test results as available: serum albumin, prealbumin, serum total protein, serum ferritin, transferrin, hemoglobin, hematocrit, and electrolytes. *A serum albumin level of less than 3.5 is considered an indicator of risk of poor nutritional status (DiMaria-Ghalili & Amella, 2005). Prealbumin was reliable in evaluating the existence of malnutrition (Devoto et al, 2006).*

• Weigh the client daily in acute care, weekly in extended care at the same time (usually before breakfast), with same amount of clothing.

▲ Monitor food intake; record percentages of served food that is eaten (25%, 50%). Keep a 3-day food diary to determine actual intake, consult with dietitian for actual calorie count if needed. *Use of a food diary is helpful for both the client and the nurse, to examine usual foods eaten, patterns of eating, and presence of deficiencies in the diet (Shay, Shobert, & Seibert, 2009).*

• Observe the client's relationship to food. Attempt to separate physical from psychological causes for eating difficulty. *Refusing to eat may be the only way the client can express some control, and it may also be a symptom of depression.*

• Compare usual food intake with the Food Guide Pyramid, noting slighted or omitted food groups. *Omission of entire food groups increases risk of deficiencies.*

• If the client is a vegetarian, evaluate vitamin B_{12} and iron intake. *Strict vegetarians (vegans) may be at particular risk for vitamin B_{12} and iron deficiencies. Special care should be taken when implementing vegetarian diets for pregnant women, infants, children, and the elderly. A dietitian can furnish a balanced vegetarian diet (with adequate substitutes for omitted foods) for inpatients and can provide instruction for outpatients (O'Regan, 2009).*

• Observe the client's ability to eat (time involved, motor skills, visual acuity, and ability to swallow various textures). If the client needs to be fed, allocate **at least 35 minutes** to feeding. *Clients in institutions are susceptible to protein-calorie malnutrition (PCM) when they are unable to feed themselves.* **EB:** *Research demonstrates it takes at least 35 minutes to feed the client who is willing to eat (Simmons, Osterweil, & Schnelle, 2001; Simmons & Schnelle, 2004; Simmons, 2008).*

NOTE: If the client is unable to feed self, refer to Nursing Interventions for **Feeding Self-Care deficit.** If the client has difficulty swallowing, refer to Nursing Interventions for **Impaired Swallowing.** If the client is receiving tube feedings, refer to the Nursing Interventions for **Risk for Aspiration.**

• If the client has a minimally functioning gastrointestinal tract and is on clear fluids, consult with dietitian regarding use of a clear liquid product that contains increased amounts of protein and calories such as Ensure Alive, Resource Breeze Fruit Beverage, or citrotein (Lutz & Przytulski, in press).

• For the client with anorexia, who will not eat foods, consider offering 30 mL of a nutritional supplement in a medication cup every hour, often during medication rounds (Capra et al, 2007). **EB:** *A*

• = Independent   ▲ = Collaborative   **EBN** = Evidence-Based Nursing   **EB** = Evidence-Based

Cochrane Review demonstrated that there was a small but consistent weight gain along with a positive effect on mortality in elderly clients who received a nutritional supplement (Milne et al, 2009).

- For the client who is malnourished and can eat, offer small quantities of energy-dense and protein-enriched food, served in an appetizing fashion, at frequent intervals. **EB:** *Fortified foods, such as those with increased protein, were acceptable to clients if they tasted the same as regular foods (Dunne & Dahl, 2007).*
- For the client who is able to eat, but has a decreased appetite, try the following activities:
  - Offer foods that are familiar to the client, and do not offend their beliefs. *All people like to eat foods to which they are accustomed, especially when ill (O'Regan, 2009).*
  - Avoid interruptions during mealtimes; meals should be eaten in a calm and peaceful environment. *Interruptions have a negative effect on client's nutrition. Some hospitals in Britain have started a "protected mealtime" effort to ensure that clients are not disturbed during mealtime (Hallpike, 2008; O'Regan, 2009).*
  - Make food available as desired between early evening and breakfast. *Have food available 24 hours as desired, including additional meals, snack boxes, and "light bites." There can be a 14-hour time span between the evening meal and breakfast; having foods available in the evening and before bedtime, as well as any time desired, can increase nutritional intake (O'Regan, 2009).*
- Use colored trays to identify clients who need help eating or who are at nutritional risk. *This system is a visible reminder of client's nutritional needs (O'Regan, 2009).*
- If the client lacks endurance, schedule rest periods before meals, and open packages and cut up food for the client. *Nursing assistance will conserve the client's energy for eating.*
- When the client is malnourished, watch carefully for signs of infection and maintain every action possible to protect the client from infection. *Protein-energy malnutrition is associated with a significant decrease in immunity (Ritz & Gardner, 2006).*
- Provide companionship at mealtime to encourage nutritional intake. *Mealtime usually is a time for social interaction; often clients will eat more food if other people are present at mealtimes.*
- Monitor state of oral cavity (gums, tongue, mucosa, teeth). Provide good oral hygiene before each meal. *Good oral hygiene enhances appetite; the condition of the oral mucosa is critical to the ability to eat. The oral mucosa must be moist, with adequate saliva production to facilitate and aid in the digestion of food.*
- If a client has anorexia and dry mouth from medication side effects, offer sips of fluids throughout the day, along with sugarless hard candy and chewing gum. *These actions help to stimulate saliva formation (DiMaria-Ghalili & Amella, 2005).*
- Determine relationship of eating and other events to onset of nausea, vomiting, diarrhea, or abdominal pain.
- Determine time of day when the client's appetite is the greatest. Offer highest calorie meal at that time. *Clients with liver disease often have their greatest appetite at breakfast time.*
- ▲ Administer antiemetics and pain medications as ordered and needed before meals. *The presence of nausea or pain decreases the appetite.*
- Prepare the client for meals. Clear unsightly supplies and excretions. Avoid invasive procedures before meals. *A pleasant environment helps promote intake.*
- If client is nauseated, remove cover of food tray before bringing it into the client's room. *The sudden, concentrated food odors that come when the cover is removed in front of the client can trigger nausea.*
- Work with the client to develop a plan for increased activity. *Immobility leads to negative nitrogen balance that fosters anorexia.*
- If the client is anemic, offer foods rich in iron and vitamins B_{12}, C, and folic acid. *Iron in meat, fish, and poultry is absorbed more readily than iron in plants. Vitamin C increases the solubility of iron. Vitamin B_{12} and folic acid are necessary for erythropoiesis (Lutz & Przytulski, 2010).*
- For the agitated pacing client, offer finger foods (sandwiches, fresh fruit) and fluids. *If a client cannot be still, food can be consumed while pacing.*
- ▲ If client has been malnourished for a significant length of time, consult with dietitian and refeed carefully after correcting electrolyte balance. Watch for heart and respiratory failure. *Refeeding syndrome, a potentially fatal condition, occurs in some malnourished clients when nutrients are given (orally, by tube feeding, or parenterally) in excess of the client's ability to metabolize them. Clients at*

risk of refeeding syndrome must be monitored carefully for electrolyte imbalances, congestive heart failure, and respiratory failure (Adkins, 2009).

Critical Care

- Recognize the need to begin enteral feedings within 24 to 48 hours of entrance into the critical care environment, once the client is free of hemodynamic compromise, if the client is unable to eat. *Providing nutrition early helps maintain muscle and immune system function, lower infection rate, decrease gut permeability, decrease incidence of multiple organ failure, help wounds heal, and reduce hospital length of stay (McClave et al, 2009; Racco, 2009).*
- Recognize that it is important to get the ordered feedings into the client, and that frequently checking for gastric residual, checking placement of the tube, can be a limiting factors to adequate nutrition in the tube-fed client. **EBN:** *A study found that critical care clients received only 50% of the ordered enteral formula because of frequent interruptions of tube feedings due to problems with small-bore feeding tubes, checking placement, and other care of the tube-fed client (O'Meara et al, 2008).*

Pediatric

- If the client is pregnant, ensure that she is receiving adequate amounts of folic acid by eating a balanced diet and taking prenatal vitamins as ordered. *All women of child-bearing potential are urged to consume 400 mcg of synthetic folic acid from fortified foods or supplements in addition to food folate from a varied diet (Lutz & Przytulski, 2010).*
- Watch for symptoms of malnutrition including short stature, thin arms and legs, poor condition of skin and hair, visible vertebrae and rib cage, wasted buttocks, wasted facial appearance, lethargy, and in extreme cases, edema (Paediatric Nursing, 2006).
- Weigh and measure the length (height) of the child and utilize a growth chart to help determine growth pattern, which reflects nutrition. *Age-related growth charts are available from this website: www.keepkidshealthy.com/welcome/welcome.html.*
- Determine the child's BMI after the child is 3 years old *(Fowler-Brown & Kahwati, 2004).*
- ▲ Refer to a physician and a dietician a child who is underweight for any reason. *Good nutrition is extremely important for children to ensure sufficient growth and development of all body systems.*
- Work with parents of the underweight child to improve the child's nutritional status as needed by:
  - Referring to a breastfeeding specialist if needed
  - Teaching how to select, prepare, and handle appropriate food for the age of the child
  - Teaching when to introduce solid foods and progress weaning
  - Advising on the appropriate range of food and portion sizes for children
  - Advising the parent to accept the child's natural size and shape; the child needs the parents' unconditional love
  - Making family meals a priority (Neumark-Sztainer et al, 2003)
  - Involving the child in helping plan menus, and doing cooking and preparation as appropriate for the child's age
  - Encouraging children to love their bodies

  Areas of concern that may be causing malnutrition should be discussed with the parents, and referrals made as necessary including to physician, dietitian, or specialist such as speech therapist to help with swallowing (Paediatric Nursing, 2006).
- Work with the child and parent to develop an appropriate weight gain plan. *The goal with a child is sometimes to maintain existing weight as the body grows taller (Fowler-Brown & Kahwati, 2004).*
- Recognize that a large percentage of girls and teenagers are dieting, which can result in nutritional problems.

Geriatric

- Assess for protein-energy malnutrition in elderly clients regardless of setting. Use a screening tool such as the Nutritional Risk Screening (NRS) if in acute care, or the Mini Nutritional Assessment (MNA) if in long-term care or living in the community (Sieber, 2006). *Malnutrition is common in the*

• = Independent   ▲ = Collaborative   **EBN** = Evidence-Based Nursing   **EB** = Evidence-Based

elderly population, and malnutrition increases the risk for illness and death in the elderly (DiMaria-Ghalili & Amella, 2005, 2008). **EB:** *Underweight elderly with a BMI less than 20 who had difficulty feeding themselves, or bathing, were found to be at greatest risk of dying in the hospital (Thomas et al, 2005). Malnutrition was found to be a predisposing cause to hip fracture (Stolee et al, 2009).*

- Assess for factors contributing to a current acute illness, such as dehydration and the presence of diarrhea. **EBN:** *Dehydration is the most common fluid and electrolyte imbalance in older adults. Offering fluids and maintaining intake of 1600 mL/day ensures adequate hydration (Hodgkinson, Evans, & Wood, 2003).*

▲ Interpret laboratory findings cautiously. Compromised kidney function makes reliance on blood and urine samples for nutrient analyses less reliable in the elderly than in younger persons. Watch the color of urine for an indication of fluid balance, darker urine demonstrating dehydration. **EBN:** *Because it is correlated to urine specific gravity and urine osmolality, observing urine color is a low-cost method of monitoring dehydration (Wakefield et al, 2002).*

- Recognize that constipation is a common problem with the elderly, therefore they avoid many types of food for fear of problems with their bowel regimen. **EBN:** *A fiber supplement in the form of raw bran is not always tolerated by the elderly. Studies indicate that daily consumption of fruit and fiber-rich porridge has a positive effect on stool frequency and consistency when compared to laxative use (Wisten, 2005). If constipation is present, please refer to the interventions and rationales in the* **Constipation** *care plan.*

- Give the client a choice of nutritional supplements to increase personal control, including a taste test. If the client is unwilling to drink a glass of liquid supplement, offer 30 mL/hr in a medication cup. *Often the elderly will take medications when they will not take food. The supplement is then served as a medicine (Capra et al, 2007).* **EB:** *A Cochrane Review demonstrated that there was a small but consistent weight gain along with a positive effect on mortality and a shorter length of hospital stay in elderly clients who received a nutritional supplement (Milne et al, 2009).*

- Encourage client to increase intake of protein, unless medically contraindicated by organ failure. Aim for 1.5 g of protein per kilogram of body weight. *Increased protein is thought to increase muscle protein anabolism, and help decrease the development of progressive muscle loss, sarcopenia, with aging. Combining increased protein with resistance exercises is even more effective in maintaining or increasing the muscle mass in the elderly (Shepherd, 2009).*

- Serve food in a restaurant-style manner if possible. **EB:** *Food served family style resulted in increased food ingestion and decreased number of elderly clients with malnutrition in a nursing home (Nijs et al, 2006).*

- Encourage physical activity throughout the day. **EB:** *Exercise is vital and may improve oral food and fluid consumption during meals in nursing home residents (Simmons, 2004; Shephard, 2009).*

- Assess intake of components of bone health: calcium intake, the elderly adult needs 1200 mg of calcium and adequate amount of vitamin D (Lutz & Przytulski, 2010).

- Recognize that older women may continue their younger preoccupation with weight and recurrent dieting, despite being at normal weight.

- Assess for psychological and mental factors that impact nutrition. Watch for signs of depression. *Malnutrition is commonly found with depression in the elderly (Stewart, 2004), but malnutrition may also cause depression in the elderly (Smith, 2008).*

- Provide a restful, homelike environment during meals where the clients are treated with respect and are encouraged to maintain autonomy as they are able. **EBN:** *A study of dementia clients conducted in extended care facilities found that when caregivers were given courses on and expected to follow these guidelines—maintaining client's integrity, interacting with client in an attentive manner, and providing a calmer, homelike atmosphere—the client gained weight (Mamhidir et al, 2007).*

- Recommend to families that enteral feedings may or may not be indicated for clients with dementia; instead use hand-feeding assistance, modified food consistency as needed, or environmental alterations (Easterling & Robbins, 2008). **EBN:** *Research has demonstrated that tube feedings in this population do not prevent malnutrition or aspiration, improve survival, or reduce infections. Instead there is an increased risk for aspiration pneumonia (Keithley & Swanson, 2004).*

NOTE: If the client is unable to feed self, refer to Nursing Interventions and Rationales for **Feeding Self-Care deficit.** If client has impaired physical function, malnutrition, depression, and cognitive impairment, please refer to care plan on **Adult Failure to thrive.**

● = Independent   ▲ = Collaborative   **EBN** = Evidence-Based Nursing   **EB** = Evidence-Based

Multicultural

- Assess for dietary intake of essential nutrients. *African American adolescents have some of the highest levels of vitamin D deficiency (Gordon et al, 2004).*
- Assess for the influence of cultural beliefs, norms, and values on the client's nutritional knowledge. *What the client considers normal dietary practices may be based on cultural perceptions (Leininger & McFarland, 2002). Among African Americans, there was a general perception that "eating healthy" meant giving up part of their cultural heritage, trying to conform to the dominant culture, and feeling that friends and relatives usually were not supportive of dietary changes (James, 2004).*
- Discuss with the client those aspects of their diet that will remain unchanged. Negotiate with the client regarding the aspects of his or her diet that will need to be modified. *Aspects of the client's life that are meaningful and valuable to them should be understood and preserved without change (Leininger & McFarland, 2002).*
- Encourage family meals. **EB:** *Frequency of family meals was positively associated with intake of fruits, vegetables, grains, and calcium-rich foods, and negatively associated with soft drink consumption (Neumark-Sztainer et al, 2003).*

 Home Care

- The above interventions may be adapted for home care use.
- Screen for malnutrition using the Malnutrition Universal Screen Tool (MUST), which is simple and can be done rapidly. *MUST is evidence-based, and the results are reproducible to identify malnourished clients in the home (Scott, 2008).*
- Monitor food intake. Instruct the client in intake of small frequent meals of foods with increased calories and protein.
- Assess clients' willingness to eat; fashion interventions accordingly. **EBN:** *Older adults reported that factors influencing appetite included mood, personal value, wholesomeness, food (preparation, consistency, and freshness), pleasantness of eating environment, and meal companionship (Wikby & Fagerskiold, 2004).*
- ▲ Assess the client for depression. Refer for mental health services as indicated. *Decreased appetite with weight loss is part of the syndrome of depression. Return of appetite is unlikely unless the underlying depression is treated.*
- Consider social factors that may interfere with nutrition (e.g., lack of transportation, inadequate income, lack of social support).
- ▲ Monitor the effect of total parenteral nutrition (TPN) as ordered by physician, and appropriate including weight, blood glucose levels, electrolytes, symptoms of fluid overload or deficit, and symptoms of infection at entry site of catheter (Gorski, 2008).

 Client/Family Teaching and Discharge Planning

- Help the client/family identify the area to change that will make the greatest contribution to improved nutrition.
- Build on the strengths in the client's/family's food habits. Adapt changes to their current practices.
- Select appropriate teaching aids for the client's/family's background.
- Implement instructional follow-up to answer the client's/family's questions.
- Suggest community resources as suitable (food sources, counseling, Meals on Wheels, senior centers).
- Teach the client and family how to manage tube feedings or parenteral therapy at home.

ⓔvolve   See the EVOLVE website for Weblinks for client education resources.

REFERENCES

Adkins SM: Recognizing and preventing refeeding syndrome, *Dimen Crit Care Nurs* 28(2):53–60, 2009.

Baldwin C, Parsons T, Logan S: Dietary advice for illness-related malnutrition in adults, *Cochrane Database Syst Rev* (1):CD002008, 2007.

Capra S, Collins C, Lamb M et al: Effectiveness of interventions for undernourished older inpatients in the hospital setting, *Best Pract Joanna Briggs Inst* 11(2):1–4, 2007.

de Luis DA, Izaola O, Cuellar L et al: Nutritional assessment: predictive variables at hospital admission related with length of stay, *Ann Nutr Metabol* 50(4):394–398, 2006.

Devoto G, Gallo F, Marchello C et al: Prealbumin serum concentrations as a useful tool in the assessment of malnutrition in hospitalized patients, *Clin Chem* 52(12):2281–2285, 2006.

DiMaria-Ghalili RA, Amella E: Nutrition in older adults, *Am J Nurs* 105(3):40, 2005.

DiMaria-Ghalili RA, Amella E: The Mini nutritional assessment: this tool can identify malnutrition in older adults before changes in biochemistry or weight are evidence, *Am J Nurs* 108(2):50–54, 57–60, 2008.

Dunne JL, Dahl WJ: A novel solution is needed to correct low nutrient intakes in elderly long-term care residents, *Nutr Rev* 65(3):135–139, 2007.

Easterling CS, Robbins E: Dementia and dysphagia, *Geriatr Nurs* 29(4):275–285, 2008.

Fauci A, Braunwald, Kasper et al: *Harrison's principles of internal medicine*, ed 17, New York, 2008, McGraw-Hill.

Fowler-Brown A, Kahwati LC: Prevention and treatment of overweight in children and adolescents, *Am Fam Physician* 69(11):2591–2598, 2004.

Gordon CM et al: Prevalence of vitamin D deficiency among healthy adolescents, *Arch Pediatr Adolesc Med* 158(6):531–537, 2004.

Gorski LA: Total parenteral nutrition administration. In Ackley BA, Ladwig GB, Swan BA et al: *Evidence-based nursing care guidelines: medical surgical interventions*, Philadelphia, 2008, Mosby.

Hallpike B: Promoting good nutrition in patients with dementia, *Nurs Stand* 22(29):37–43, 2008.

Hodgkinson B, Evans D, Wood J: Maintaining oral hydration in older adults: a systematic review, *Int J Nurs Pract* 9(3):S19–S28, 2003.

James DC: Factors influencing food choices, dietary intake, and nutrition-related attitudes among African Americans: application of a culturally sensitive model, *Ethn Health* 9(4):349–367, 2004.

Keithley JK, Swanson B: Enteral nutrition: an update on practice recommendations, *Medsurg Nurs* 13(2):131, 2004.

Leininger MM, McFarland MR: *Transcultural nursing: concepts, theories, research and practices*, ed 3, New York, 2002, McGraw-Hill.

Lutz CA, Przytulski KR: *Nutrition and diet therapy*, ed 5, Philadelphia, in press, F.A. Davis.

Mamhidir A, Karlsson I, Norbert A et al: Weight increase in patients with dementia, and alteration in meal routines and meal environment after integrity promoting care, *J Clin Nurs* 16:987–996, 2007.

McClave S, Martindale R, Vanek V et al: Guidelines for the provision and assessment of nutrition support therapy in the adult critically ill patient: Society of Critical Care Medicine (SCCM) and American Society for Parenteral and Enteral Nutrition (A.S.P.E.N.), *JPEN J Parenter Enteral Nutr* 33(3):277–316, 2009.

Milne AC, Potter J, Vivanti A et al: Protein and energy supplementation in elderly people at risk from malnutrition, *Cochrane Database Syst Rev* (2):CD003288, 2009.

Neumark-Sztainer D, Hannan PJ, Story M et al: Family meal patterns: associations with sociodemographic characteristics and improved dietary intake among adolescents, *J Am Diet Assoc* 103(3):317–322, 2003.

Nijs KA, de Graaf C, Siebelink E et al: Effect of family-style meals on energy intake and risk of malnutrition in Dutch nursing home residents: a randomized controlled trial, *J Gerontol A Biol Sci Med Sci* 61(9):935–942, 2006.

O'Meara D, Mireles-Cabodevila E, Frame F et al: Evaluation of delivery of enteral nutrition in critically ill patients receiving mechanical ventilation, *Am J Criti Care* 17(1):53–61, 2008.

O'Regan P: Nutrition for patients in hospital, *Nurs Stand* 23(23):35–41, 2009.

Racco M: Nutrition in the ICU, *RN* 72(1):26–30, 2009.

[No Author]: Recognizing malnutrition, *Paediatr Nurs* 18(5):30, 2006.

Ritz BS, Gardner EM: Recent advances in nutritional sciences, *J Nutr* 136(5):1141–1145, 2006.

Scott A: Screening for malnutrition in the community: the MUST tool, *Br J Community Nurs* 13(9):406–412, 2008.

Shay LE, Shobert JL, Seibert D et al: Adult weight management: translating research and guidelines into practice, *J Am Acad Nurse Pract* 21(4):197–206, 2009.

Shepherd A: Nutrition through the life span. Part 3: adults aged 65 years and over. *Br J Nurs* 18(5):301–307, 2009.

Sieber CC: Nutritional screening tools—how does the MNA compare? Proceedings of the session held in Chicago May 2–3, 2006, *J Nutr Health Aging* 10(6):488–492, 2006.

Simmons S: Effects of an exercise and scheduled toileting intervention on appetite and constipation in nursing home residents, *J Nutr Health Aging* 8(2):116–121, 2004.

Simmons SF: Feeding. Guideline. In Ackley B, Ladwig G, Swan BA et al, editors: *Evidence-Based Nursing Care Guidelines*, Philadelphia, 2008, Mosby.

Simmons SF, Osterweil D, Schnelle JF: Improving food intake in nursing home residents with feeding assistance: a staffing analysis, *J Gerontol A Biol Sci Med Sci* 56(12):M790–M794, 2001.

Simmons SF, Schnelle JF: Individualized feeding assistance care for nursing home residents: staffing requirements to implement two interventions, *J Gerontol A Biol Sci Med Sci* 59(9):M966–M973, 2004.

Smith A: Nutrition in care homes: going back to the basics, *Nurs Resident Care* 10(2):68–72, 2008.

Stewart JT: Why don't physicians consider depression in the elderly? *Postgrad Med* 115(6):57, 2004.

Stolee P, Poss J, Cook RJ et al: Risk factors for hip fracture in older home care clients, *J Gerontol Ser A Biol Sci Med Sci* 64(3):403–410, 2009.

Thomas DR, Kamel H, Azharrudin M et al: The relationship of functional status, nutritional assessment, and severity of illness to in-hospital mortality, *J Health Nutr Aging* 9(3):169–175, 2005.

Wakefield B, Mentes J, Diggelmann L et al: Monitoring hydration status in elderly veterans, *West J Nurs Res* 24:132, 2002.

Wikby K, Fagerskiold A: The willingness to eat: an investigation of appetite among elderly people, *Scand J Caring Sci* 18:120, 2004.

Wisten A: Fruit and fiber (Pajala porridge) in the prevention of constipation, *Scand J Caring Sci* 19(1):71–76, 2005.

Imbalanced Nutrition: more than body requirements

Betty J. Ackley, MSN, EdS, RN

NANDA-I

Definition

Intake of nutrients that exceeds metabolic needs

• = Independent ▲ = Collaborative **EBN** = Evidence-Based Nursing **EB** = Evidence-Based

Defining Characteristics

Concentrating food intake at the end of the day; dysfunctional eating pattern (e.g., pairing food with other activities); eating in response to external cues (e.g., time of day, social situation); eating in response to internal cues other than hunger (e.g., anxiety); sedentary activity level; triceps skin fold >25 mm in women, >15 mm in men, weight 20% over ideal for height and frame

Related Factors (r/t)

Excessive intake in relation to metabolic need

(Nursing Outcomes Classification)

Suggested NOC Outcomes

Nutritional Status: Food and Fluid Intake, Nutrient Intake, Weight Loss Behavior

Example NOC Outcome with Indicators
Weight Loss Behavior as evidenced by the following indicators: Uses diary to monitor food and fluid intake/ Selects a healthy target weight/Selects nutritious food and fluid/Controls food portions/Establishes an exercise routine/ Monitors body weight/Maintains progress toward target weight (Rate the outcome and indicators of **Weight Loss Behavior:** I = never demonstrated, 2 = rarely demonstrated, 3 = sometimes demonstrated, 4 = often demonstrated, 5 = consistently demonstrated [see Section I].)

Client Outcomes

Client Will (Specify Time Frame):

- State pertinent factors contributing to weight gain
- Identify behaviors that remain under client's control
- Design dietary modifications to meet individual long-term goal of weight control
- Lose weight in a reasonable period (1 to 2 lb per week)
- Incorporate appropriate activities requiring energy expenditure into daily life

NIC (Nursing Interventions Classification)

Suggested NIC Interventions

Eating Disorders Management, Nutrition Management, Nutritional Counseling, Weight Management, Weight Reduction Assistance

Example NIC Activities—Weight Management
Determine client's motivation for changing eating habits; develop with client a method to keep daily record of intake

Nursing Interventions and *Rationales*

- Ask the client to keep a 1- to 3-day food diary where everything eaten or drunk is recorded. **EB:** *Use of self-monitoring tools that meet the needs of clients increase dietary reporting and promote self-efficacy (Mossavar-Rahmani et al, 2004).*
- Advise the client to measure food periodically. Help the client learn usual portion sizes. *Measuring food alerts the client to normal portion sizes. Estimating amounts can be extremely inaccurate.* **EB:** *A study where women were served either larger portions, or more calorie-dense foods in the same portion size demonstrated that extra calories were eaten, and the women subjects did not realize it and decrease their calories for dinner (Kral, Roe, & Rolls, 2004). A study of young adults who self-selected portion sizes for breakfast and dinner demonstrated significantly increased portion sizes than recommended, which predisposed to weight gain (Schwartz & Byrd-Bredbenner, 2006). Another study found that group training was effective at teaching individuals to accurately estimate and measure food portion sizes (Ayala, 2006).*
- Help the client determine their body mass index (BMI). Use a chart or a website such as *www.bcm. edu/cnrc/caloriesneed.htm. A normal BMI is 20 to 25; 26 to 29 is overweight; and a BMI of greater than 30 is obese. Clients with increased muscle mass may be labeled overweight, when in reality they*

● = Independent   ▲ = Collaborative   **EBN** = Evidence-Based Nursing   **EB** = Evidence-Based

are very physically fit. Also, clients who have lost large amounts of muscle mass may be in the healthy range, when in reality they may be malnourished (Camden, 2009). **EB:** *An analysis of 57 studies demonstrated that mortality was lowest for people with a BMI of 22.5 to 25. Each 5–unit increase above a BMI of 25 resulted in an increased mortality rate by 30% (Whitlock et al, 2009).*

- Recommend the client follow the U.S. Dietary Guidelines to determine foods to eat, which can be found at www.healthierus.gov/dietaryguidelines. *Dietary guidelines are written by national experts and based on research in nutrition.*
- Recommend the client use the interactive Food Guide Pyramid site at www.MyPyramid.gov to determine the number of calories to eat, and gain more information on how to eat in a healthy fashion. To lose weight, the client must eat fewer calories. **EB:** *A systematic review found that safe choices for weight loss included low-calorie diets such as the DASH diet or a Weight Watchers–type of diet (Strychar, 2006). A study of the National Weight Control Registry members, with almost 5000 members of the registry who had maintained weight loss of at least 33 kg for more than 5 years, indicated that eating a low-calorie, low-fat diet was one of many factors associated with maintenance of the weight loss (Wing & Phelan, 2005).*
- Recommend that clients lose weight slowly, no more than 1 to 2 lb per week, based on a healthy eating pattern and increased exercise. The number of calories consumed should be at least 1600 for men, and 1300 for women. *Slower weight loss is generally more likely to be lasting weight loss. It is important that increased activity is included to help burn more calories (Ruser, Federman, & Kashaf, 2005).*
- Demonstrate the use of food labels to make healthful choices. Alert the client/family to focus on serving size, total fat, and simple carbohydrate. The standardized food label in bold type simplifies the search for information. *Fats and sugars contribute the least to a healthful diet and the most to excessive calorie intake. Generally clients should eat foods that are no more than 30% fat (Lutz & Przytulski, in press).*
- ▲ Watch the client for signs of depression: flat affect, poor sleeping habits, lack of interest in life. Refer for counseling/treatment as needed. *Depression is found in a large percentage of obese persons (Ruser, Federman, & Kashaf, 2005; Camden, 2009).*

Pattern of Dietary Intake

- Recommend the client eat a healthy breakfast every morning. **EB:** *A study demonstrated that people who skipped breakfast were 450 times more likely to be obese (Ma et al, 2003). A study of people who binge eat found that less than half of the people ate breakfast (43%), and those people who ate breakfast weighed less than subjects who did not eat breakfast (Masheb & Grillo, 2006). A descriptive study of the National Weight Control Registry members who had maintained weight loss of at least 33 kg for more than 5 years indicated that eating breakfast regularly was one of many factors associated with maintenance of the weight loss (Wing & Phelan, 2005). Another study found that men on a weight reduction diet who received more protein for breakfast had increased satiety that lasted during the day (Leidy et al, 2009).*
- Recommend the client avoid eating in fast food restaurants. **EB:** *A 15–year study demonstrated that people who often eat fast foods gain an average of 10 lb more than those who eat fast food less often, and were two times more likely to develop insulin resistance, which can lead to diabetes (Pereira, Kartashov, & Ebbeling, 2005).*

Nursing Care of Obese Client

- Treat the obese client with respect and concern. *The obese client needs a healing, caring environment where dignity is maintained (Kirkpatrick, 2008; Camden, 2009).*
- Recognize that obese clients have an increased incidence of venous thromboembolism (VTE), and ensure use of supportive stockings, movement, and other methods of prevention of VTE are utilized (Maiocco, 2008; Pettit, 2009).
- ▲ Recognize that it can be difficult to obtain and maintain intravenous access in the obese client. Request an order for a peripherally inserted central catheter or midline catheter if intravenous therapy is being utilized (Camden, 2009).
- Recognize that obese clients commonly have sleep-disordered breathing problems that can result in hypercapnia, and somnolence during the day. *The client with disordered sleep, loud snoring, periods of apnea during sleep should receive a sleep study for possible use of CPAP (Berger, 2008).*

● = Independent   ▲ = Collaborative   **EBN** = Evidence-Based Nursing   **EB** = Evidence-Based

- Utilize special equipment as needed: larger beds, commodes, wheelchairs, stretchers for the obese client (Pettit, 2009).
- Utilize assistive devices to lift obese clients. *Manual lifting of clients may be a cause of injuries to the nurse as well as the client (Drake et al, 2008; Pettit, 2009).*
▲ Obtain a thorough history. Refer to a dietitian if the client has a medical condition. *The most appropriate clients for the nursing intervention of weight management are adults with no other major health problems requiring medical nutritional therapy.*

Recommended Foods/Fluids

- Encourage the client to increase intake of vegetables and fruits to at least five servings per day, preferably nine servings per day. *Vegetables are low in calories: 10 to 50 calories per serving, yet packed with vitamins, minerals, and phytochemicals, which can protect from disease (Liebman & Hurley, 2009).* **EB:** *A study demonstrated that women who increased their fruit and vegetable intake to four servings per day had a 24% lower risk of obesity than those who ate only two servings per day (He et al, 2004).*
- Encourage the client to eat at least three whole grain servings per day, preferably more. **EB:** *A study demonstrated that men who ate more whole grains had decreased weight gain (Koh-Banerjee et al, 2004). A review of studies found strong evidence that eating whole grains is associated with a decreased BMI, and reduced the risk of being overweight (Williams, Grafenauer, & O'Shea, 2008).*
- Evaluate the client's usual intake of fiber. Recommended intake is 25 g per day for women and 38 g per day for men. Increase intake of whole grains, legumes, fruits, and vegetables to obtain needed fiber. *In general, high-fiber foods take longer to eat, increase satiety, and contain fewer calories than most other foods (Slavin, 2008).* **EB:** *Increased dietary fiber was associated with lower body weight and waist-to-hip ratios, as well as decreased fiber ingestion predicted weight gain more strongly than did fat consumption (Slavin, 2008).*
- Discuss the possibility of using a primarily plant-based or vegetarian diet to lose weight. **EB:** *A systematic review demonstrated that the weight and BMI of vegetarians was on average 3% to 20% lower than that of nonvegetarians (Berkow & Barnard, 2006). Another study demonstrated that people who voluntarily chose a lacto-ovo-vegetarian diet as part of a weight loss treatment were able to continue with the diet for 18 months (Burke et al, 2006).*
- Encourage the client to **decrease** intake of sugars including intake of soft drinks, desserts, and candy. *Sugar predisposes to dental caries, and also is a source of calories that is empty of other nutrients (ADA, 2009).*
- Recommend client increase intake of water to at least 2000 mL or 2 quarts per day. A guideline is 1 to 1.5 mL of fluid per each calorie needed, so an average intake would be between 2000 and 3000 mL/day, or at least 8 cups of fluid. *The adequate intake recommendation is 3 L for the 19- to 30-year-old male and 2.2 L for the 19- to 30-year-old female. Water balance studies suggest that adult men require 2.5 L per day (Institute of Medicine, 2004).*
- For more information on healthy eating, refer to Nursing Interventions for **Readiness for enhanced Nutrition.**

Behavioral Methods for Weight Loss

- Familiarize the client with the following behavior modification techniques:
  - Self-monitoring of food intake, including keeping a food and exercise diary
  - Graphing weight weekly
  - Controlling stimuli that causes overeating, such as watching television with frequent food-related commercials
  - Limiting food intake to one site in the home
  - Sitting down at the table to eat
  - Planning food intake for each day
  - Rearranging the schedule to avoid inappropriate eating
  - Avoiding boredom that results in eating; keeping a list of activities on the refrigerator
  - For a party, eating before arriving, sitting away from the snack foods, and substituting lower-calorie beverages for alcoholic ones
  - Deciding beforehand what to order in a restaurant
  - Bringing only healthy foods into the house to decrease temptation

• = Independent   ▲ = Collaborative   **EBN** = Evidence-Based Nursing   **EB** = Evidence-Based

- Slowing mealtime by swallowing food before putting more food on the utensil, pausing for a minute during the meal and attempting to increase the number of pauses, and trying to be the last one to finish eating
- Drinking a glass of water before each meal; taking sips of water between bites of food
- Charting one's progress
- Making an agreement with oneself or a significant other for a meaningful reward and not rewarding oneself with food
- Changing one's mindset, as in control of eating behavior
- Viewing exercise as a means of controlling hunger
- Practicing relaxation techniques
- Visualizing oneself enjoying a fresh apple in preference to apple pie

EB: *A Cochrane review found that cognitive-behavior therapy, when combined with a diet and exercise intervention, resulted in more weight loss than diet and exercise alone. Behavioral therapy used independently as a stand-alone therapy also resulted in significant weight loss (Shaw et al, 2006). Another Cochrane review found that weight loss methods including dietary, exercise, or behavioral interventions resulted in significant weight loss among people with prediabetes, and a decrease in diabetes development (Norris et al, 2005).*

Physical Activity

- Assess for reasons why the client would be unable to participate in an exercise program; refer for evaluation by a primary care practitioner as needed. Encourage activity to help with weight loss.
- Use the Outcome Expectation for Exercise Scale to determine client's self-efficacy expectations and outcomes expectations toward exercise. **EBN:** *The client's self-efficacy expectations and outcome expectations for exercise will greatly influence his or her willingness to exercise. If the individual has a low outcome, interventions can be implemented to strengthen the expectations and hopefully improve exercise behavior (Resnick, Zimmerman, & Orwig, 2001).*
- Recommend the client enter an exercise program with a friend. **EBN:** *Findings from a study of exercise behavior found that friends have the strongest influence to keep on an exercise program, more than family members or experts (Resnick, Orwig, & Magaziner, 2002).*
- Recommend the client begin a walking program using the following guidelines:
    - Buy a pedometer.
    - Determine times when walking can be incorporated into usual lifestyle.
    - Set a goal of walking 10,000 steps per day, or 5 miles per day.
    - If, when clients come home from work, they do not have the required number of steps, have them go for a walk until they reach designated goal of 10,000 steps per day.

EB: *A study demonstrated that in middle-age women, women who walked more had lower BMIs, and that women who walked 10,000 or more steps per day were in the normal range for BMI (Thompson et al, 2004). A systematic review found that the use of pedometers resulted in increased physical activity (Bravata et al, 2007).*

 ### Pediatric

- Work with parents of the overweight child by encouraging the following behaviors:
    - Emphasize providing good food, not depriving children of food. *Trying to get children to eat less or move more for weight control generally backfires and makes the child preoccupied with food and unwilling to move unless forced.*
    - Accept the child's natural size and shape, the child needs the parents' unconditional love.
    - Make family meals a priority.
    - Involve the child in helping plan menus, and doing cooking and preparation as appropriate for the child's age.
    - Educate parents to participate in activities with children.
    - Encourage children to love their bodies.

    These methods can help children who are overweight without causing harm to the child (Satter, 2005).
- Determine the child's BMI after the child is 3 years old (Fowler-Brown & Kahwati, 2004). *The Centers for Disease Control and Prevention's (CDC) BMI chart for children and teens is available at*

www.cdc.gov/nccdphp/dnpa/bmi/bmi-for-age.htm. **EB:** *Research has demonstrated that kids who are overweight or obese have a higher risk for being overweight or obese as adults (Field, Cook, & Gillman, 2005).*

- Work with the child and parent to develop an appropriate weight maintenance plan, including behavioral methods of weight loss, as well as increased activity. *The goal with a child is often to maintain existing weight as the body grows taller (Fowler-Brown & Kahwati, 2004).* **EB:** *A Cochrane review showed that combined behavioral lifestyle interventions are more effective than self-help or other standard programs, and can lead to a significant reduction in obesity (Oude Luttikhuis, Baur, & Jansen, 2009).*
- Work with the parent to change the food that is available in the home, eliminating sugary drinks, and foods with a high saturated fat or trans fat content. *Foods with increased sugar cause dental cavities, and are empty calories for the child; high-fat foods with saturated fat and trans fats cause high cholesterol levels and obesity (Kline, 2009).*
- Encourage child to increase the amount of walking done per day; if the child is willing, ask them to wear a pedometer to measure number of steps. **EB:** *A study demonstrated that the recommended number of steps per day to have a healthy body composition for the -6 to 12–year-old is 12,000 for the girl and 15,000 for the boy (Tudor-Locke et al, 2004).*
- Do not use food as a reward for good behavior, especially foods that are concentrated sources of sugar or fat. *Avoid using foods as a reward, especially high-calorie foods. Making them a reward may only make them more desirable.*
- Recommend the child decrease television viewing, watching movies, and playing video games. Ask parents to limit television to 1 to 2 hours per day maximum (Calamaro & Faith, 2004). **EB:** *A study demonstrated that girls who watched more TV had a higher BMI and percentage of body fat (Davison, Downs, & Birch, 2006).*

Geriatric

- Assess changes in lifestyle and eating patterns. *Energy needs decrease an estimated 5% per decade after the age of 40 years, but often eating patterns remain unchanged from youth.*
- Assess fluid intake. Recommend routine drinks of fluids regardless of thirst. *Thirst sensation becomes dulled in the elderly.*
- Observe for socioeconomic factors that influence food choices (e.g., inadequate funds or cooking facilities). *Even those on restricted budgets and with limited facilities can be helped to choose food sources for a balanced diet.*
- Recognize that it is generally not appropriate to have an elderly client on a calorie-restrictive diet. *Once elderly, clients deserve to eat and not be hungry.*
- Encourage the client to do strength training to increase muscle strength after checking with physician. *Loss of muscle (sarcopenia) occurs with normal aging; when paired with excessive fat, it leads to increased weakness and disability (Jarosz & Bellar, 2009).*

Multicultural

- Recognize that the BMI's accuracy is different for some ethnic groups. *Blacks have 2% to 5% less body fat than whites, so it is suggested that the BMI cutoff number should be higher in blacks. Asians and Hispanics have more fat, so BMI cutoff numbers should be lower (Jackson et al, 2009).*
- Assess for the influence of cultural beliefs, norms, acculturation, and values on the client's nutritional knowledge and practices. *What the client considers normal dietary practices may be based on cultural perceptions (Leininger & McFarland, 2002). Among African Americans, there was a general perception that "eating healthfully" meant giving up part of their cultural heritage (James, 2004). A higher risk for obesity among Latino immigrants was associated with length of residence in the United States and may be due to acculturation processes such as the adoption of a diet high in fat and low in fruits and vegetables and sedentary lifestyles of the host country (Kaplan et al, 2004). Another study suggests that acculturation to the United States is a risk factor for obesity-related behaviors among Asian American and Hispanic adolescents (Unger et al, 2004).*
- Encourage parental efforts at increasing physical activity and decreasing dietary fat and sugars for their children. **EB:** *Physical activity and dietary fat consumption were inversely related among African*

American girls (Thompson et al, 2004). Interventions to increase physical activity among preadolescent African American girls may benefit from a parental component to encourage support and self-efficacy for daughters' physical activity (Adkins et al, 2004).

- Assess for the influence of cultural beliefs, norms, and values on the client's ideal of acceptable body weight and body size. **EB:** *African American women report more satisfaction with body size than other women (Miller et al, 2000).*
- Discuss with the client those aspects of his or her diet that will remain unchanged, and work with the client to adapt cultural core foods. *Aspects of the client's life that are meaningful and valuable to the client should be understood and preserved without change (Leininger & McFarland, 2002).*
- Negotiate with the client regarding the aspects of his or her diet that will need to be modified. *Give and take with the client will lead to culturally congruent care (Leininger & McFarland, 2002).*
- Validate the client's feelings regarding the impact of current lifestyle, finances, and transportation on the ability to obtain and prepare nutritious food.

Client/Family Teaching and Discharge Planning

- Provide the client and family with information regarding the treatment plan options. *If the client and family select the treatment plan, they are more likely to comply with it, particularly if the client does not do the shopping and cooking.*
- Inform the client about the health risks associated with obesity, which include cancer, diabetes, heart disease, strokes, hypertension, gastroesophageal reflux, gallstones, osteoarthritis, and venous thrombosis (Camden, 2009).
- Recommend the client weigh self frequently, ideally every day. *A systematic review found that clients who weighed themselves frequently had moderate weight loss, and less weight regain (Vanwormer et al, 2008).*
- Inform the client and family of the disadvantages of trying to lose weight by dieting alone, and encourage the client to include exercise into weight loss plan. *Resting metabolic rate is decreased as much as 45% with extreme calorie restriction. The decrease persists after the diet period has ended, which leads to the "yo-yo effect." With a reduced-calorie diet alone, as much as 25% of the weight lost can be lean body mass rather than fat. Resting energy expenditure is positively related to lean body mass (Lutz & Przytulski, in press).* **EB:** *A metaanalysis found that diet plus exercise resulted in significantly greater weight loss than a diet-only intervention for weight loss (Wu, Gao, & Chen, 2009).*
- Recommend the client receive adequate amounts of sleep. **EB:** *Sleep deprivation, less than 7 hours per night, is associated with an increased risk of obesity (Tufts University, 2005). Sleep curtailment in young healthy men resulted in increased hunger and appetite (Spiegel et al, 2004). A review found that decreased sleep was associated with increased obesity in both children and adults (Van Cauter & Knutson, 2008).*
- Teach stress reduction techniques as alternatives to eating. *The client should have available a variety of healthy behaviors to substitute for unhealthy ones.*

evolve   See the EVOLVE website for Weblinks for client education resources.

REFERENCES

Adkins S, Sherwood NE, Story M et al: Physical activity among African-American girls: the role of parents and the home environment, *Obes Res* 12(Suppl):S38–S45, 2004.

American Dental Association (ADA): A to Z Topics. www.ada.org/prof/resources/topics/index.asp. Accessed July 1, 2009.

Ayala GX: An experimental evaluation of a group- versus computer-based intervention to improve food portion size estimation skills, *Health Educ Res* 21(1):133–145, 2006.

Berger KI: Obesity hypoventilation syndrome: diagnosing and treating an old problem, *RT J Respir Care Pract* 21(11):12–15, 2008.

Berkow SE, Barnard N: Vegetarian diets and weight status, *Nutr Rev* 64(4):175–188, 2006.

Bravata DM, Smith-Spangler C, Sundaram V et al: Using pedometers to increase physical activity and improve health: a systematic review, *JAMA* 298:2296–2304, 2007.

Burke LE, Choo J, Music E et al: PREFER study: A randomized clinical trial testing treatment preference and two dietary options in behavioral weight management–rationale, design and baseline characteristics, *Contemp Clin Trials* 27(1):34–48, 2006.

Calamaro CJ, Faith MS: Preventing childhood overweight, *Nutr Today* 39(5):194, 2004.

Camden S: Obesity: an emerging concern for patients and nurses, *Online J Issues Nurs* 14(1):5–17, 2009.

Davison KK, Downs DS, Birch LL: Pathways linking perceived athletic competence and parental support at age 9 years to girls' physical activity at age 11 years, *Res Q Exerc Sport* 77(1):23–31, 2006.

Drake DJ, Baker G, Keenher Engelke M et al: Challenges in caring for the morbidly obese: differences by practice settings. *South Online J Nurs Res* 8(3), 2008.

● = Independent   ▲ = Collaborative   **EBN** = Evidence-Based Nursing   **EB** = Evidence-Based

Field AE, Cook NR, Gillman MW: Weight status in childhood as a predictor of becoming overweight or hypertensive in early adulthood, *Obes Res J* 13(1):163, 2005.

Fowler-Brown A, Kahwati LC: Prevention and treatment of overweight in children and adolescents, *Am Family Physician* 69(11):2591, 2004.

He K, Hu FB, Colditz GA et al: Changes in intake of fruits and vegetables in relation to risk of obesity and weight gain among middle-aged women, *Int J Obes Relat Metab Disord* 28(12):1569, 2004.

Institute of Medicine: Applications of dietary reference intakes for electrolytes and water, *National Academy of Sciences*, 2004, National Academies Press.

Jackson AS, Ellis KJ, McFarlin BK et al: Body mass index bias in defining obesity of diverse young adults: the Training Intervention and Genetics of Exercise Response (TIGER) study, *Br J Nutr* 102(7):1084–1090, 2009.

James DC: Factors influencing food choices, dietary intake, and nutrition-related attitudes among African Americans: application of a culturally sensitive model, *Ethn Health* 9(4):349–367, 2004.

Jarosz, P, Bellar A: Sarcopenic obesity: an emerging cause of frailty in older adults, *Geriatr Nursi* 30(1):64–70, 2009.

Kaplan MS, Huguet N, Newsom JT et al: The association between length of residence and obesity among Hispanic immigrants, *Am J Prev Med* 27(4):323–326, 2004.

Kirkpatrick MK: A caring, healing environment for the overweight/obese client, *Int J Hum Caring* 12(3):93–94, 2008.

Kline A: Pediatric obesity in acute and critical care, *AACN Adv Crit Care* 19(1):38–46, 2009.

Koh-Banerjee P, Franz M, Sampson L et al: Changes in whole-grain, bran, and cereal fiber consumption in relation to 3 year weight gain among men, *Am J Clin Nutr* 80(5):1237, 2004.

Kral TV, Roe LS, Rolls BJ: Combined effects of energy density and portion size on energy intake in women, *Am J Clin Nutr* 79(6):962, 2004.

Leidy HJ, Bossingham MJ, Mattes RD et al: Increased dietary protein consumed at breakfast leads to an initial and sustained feeling of fullness during energy restriction compared to other meal times, *Br J Nutr* 101(6):798–803, 2009.

Leininger MM, McFarland MR: *Transcultural nursing: concepts, theories, research and practices,* ed 3, New York, 2002, McGraw-Hill.

Liebman B, Hurley J: Rating rutabagas: not all vegetables are created equal, *Nutr Action Healthletter* Jan/Feb:13–15, 2009.

Lutz CA, Przytulski KR: *Nutrition and diet therapy,* ed 5, Philadelphia, in press, F.A. Davis.

Ma Y, Bertone ER, Stanek EJ III et al: Association between eating patterns and obesity in a free-living U.S. adult population, *Am J Epidiomol* 158(1):85, 2003.

Maiocco G: DVT prevention for the obese patient: evidence-based nursing interventions, *Bariatr Nurs Surg Patient Care* 3(4):279–284, 2008.

Masheb RM, Grillo CM: Eating patterns and breakfast consumption in obese patients with binge eating disorder. *Behav Res Ther* 44(11):1545–1553, 2006.

Miller KJ, Gleaves DH, Hirsch TG et al: Comparisons of body image dimensions by race/ethnicity and gender in a university population, *Int J Eat Disord* 27(3):310–316, 2000.

Mossavar-Rahmani Y, Henry H, Rodabough R et al: Additional self-monitoring tools in the dietary modification component of the women's health initiative, *J Am Diet Assoc* 104(1):76, 2004.

Norris SL, Zhang X, Avenell A et al: Long-term non-pharmacological weight loss interventions for adults with prediabetes, *Cochrane Database Syst Rev* (2):CD005270, 2005.

Oude Luttikhuis H, Baur L, Jansen H: Interventions for treating obesity in children, *Cochrane Database Syst Rev* (1):CD001872, 2009.

Pereira MA, Kartashov AI, Ebbeling CB: Fast-food habits, weight gain, and insulin resistance (the CARDIA study): 15–year prospective analysis, *Lancet* 365(9453):36, 2005.

Pettit E: Treating morbid obesity, *RN* 72(2):30–34, 2009.

Resnick B, Orwig D, Magaziner J: The effect of social support on exercise behavior in older adults, *Clin Nurs Res* 11(1):52, 2002.

Resnick B, Zimmerman S, Orwig D: Model testing for reliability and validity of the outcome expectations for exercise scale, *Nurs Res* 50:5, 2001.

Ruser CB, Federman DG, Kashaf SS: Whittling away at obesity and overweight, *Postgrad Med* 117(1):31, 2005.

Satter E: *Your child's weight, helping without harming.* Madison, WI, 2005, Kelcy Press.

Schwartz J, Byrd-Bredbenner C: Portion distortion: typical portion sizes selected by young adults, *J Am Diet Assoc* 106(9):1412–1418, 2006.

Shaw K, Gennat H, O'Rourke P et al: Exercise for overweight or obesity, *Cochrane Database Syst Rev* (4):CD003817, 2006.

Slavin JL. Position of the American Dietetic Association: health implications of dietary fiber, *J Am Diet Assoc* 108(10):1716–1731, 2008.

Spiegel K, Tasali E, Penev P et al: Brief communication: sleep curtailment in healthy young men is associated with decreased leptin levels, elevated ghrelin levels, and increased hunger and appetite, *Ann Intern Med* 141(11):846, 2004.

Strychar I: Diet in the management of weight loss, *CMAJ*, 174(1):56–63, 2006.

Thompson DL, Jago R, Baranowski T et al: Covariability in diet and physical activity in African-American girls, *Obes Res* 12(Suppl):S46–S54, 2004.

Thompson DL, Rakow J, Perdue SM: Relationship between accumulated walking and body composition in middle-aged women, *Med Sci Sports Exerc* 36(5):911, 2004.

Tudor-Locke C, Pangrazi RP, Corbin CB et al: BMI-referenced standards for recommended pedometer-determined steps/day in children, *Prev Med* 38(6):857, 2004.

Tufts University: Getting enough sleep helps you stay slim, *Health Nutr Let* 22(11):2, 2005.

Unger JB, Reynolds K, Shakib S et al: Acculturation, physical activity, and fast-food consumption among Asian-American and Hispanic adolescents, *J Community Health* 29(6):467–481, 2004.

Van Cauter E, Knutson KL: Sleep and the epidemic of obesity in children and adults, *Eur J Endocrinol* 159(Suppl 1):S59–S66, 2008.

Vanwormer JJ, French SA, Pereira MA et al: The impact of regular self-weighing on weight management: a systematic literature review, *Int J Behav Nutr Phys Act* 5:54, 2008.

Whitlock G, Lewington S, Sherliker P et al: Body-mass index and cause-specific mortality in 900,000 adults: collaborative analyses of 57 prospective studies, *Lancet* 373(9669):1083–1096, 2009.

Williams PG, Grafenauer SJ, O'Shea JE: Cereal grains, legumes, and weight management: a comprehensive review of the scientific evidence, *Nutr Rev* 66(4):171–182, 2008.

Wing RR, Phelan S: Long-term weight loss maintenance, *Am J Clin Nutr* 82(1 Suppl):222S-225S, 2005.

Wu T, Gao X, Chen M: Long-term effectiveness of diet-plus-exercise interventions vs. diet-only interventions for weight loss: a meta-analysis. *Obes Rev*10(3):313–323, 2009.

Risk for imbalanced Nutrition: more than body requirements

Betty J. Ackley, MSN, EdS, RN

Definition

At risk for intake of nutrients that exceeds metabolic needs

Risk Factors

Concentrating food at the end of day; dysfunctional eating patterns; eating in response to external cues (e.g., time of day, social situation); eating in response to internal cues other than hunger (e.g., anxiety); higher baseline weight at beginning of each pregnancy; observed use of food as comfort measure; observed use of food as reward; pairing food with other activities; parental obesity; rapid transition across growth percentiles in children; reported use of solid food as major food source before 5 months of age

NOC, NIC, Client Outcomes, Nursing Interventions, Client/Family Teaching and Discharge Planning, *Rationales,* and References

See care plan for **Imbalanced Nutrition: more than body requirements.**

Readiness for enhanced Nutrition   *Betty J. Ackley, MSN, EdS, RN*

Definition

A pattern of nutrient intake that is sufficient for meeting metabolic needs and can be strengthened

Defining Characteristics

Attitude toward drinking is congruent with health goals; attitude toward eating is congruent with health goals; consumes adequate fluid; consumes adequate food; eats regularly; expresses knowledge of health fluid choices; expresses knowledge of health food choices; expresses willingness to enhance nutrition; follows an appropriate standard for intake (e.g., the food pyramid or American Diabetic Association guidelines); safe preparation for fluids; safe preparation for food; safe storage for food and fluids

NOC   (Nursing Outcomes Classification)

Suggested NOC Outcomes

Nutritional Status, Nutritional Status: Food and Fluid Intake, Nutrient Intake, Weight Control

Example **NOC** Outcome with Indicators
Nutritional Status as evidenced by the following indicators: Food and fluid intake/Hydration/Body mass index/ Weight-height ratio/Hematocrit (Rate the outcome and indicators of **Nutritional Status:** 1 = severe deviation from normal range, 2 = substantial deviation from normal range, 3 = moderate deviation from normal range, 4 = mild deviation from normal range, 5 = no deviation from normal range [see Section I].)

Client Outcomes

Client Will (Specify Time Frame):

- Explain how to eat according to the U.S. Dietary Guidelines
- Design dietary modifications to meet individual long-term goal of health, using principles of variety, balance, and moderation
- Weigh within normal range for height and age

• = Independent   ▲ = Collaborative   **EBN** = Evidence-Based Nursing   **EB** = Evidence-Based

| NIC | (Nursing Interventions Classification) |

Suggested NIC Interventions

Nutrition Management, Nutritional Counseling, Weight Reduction Assistance

Example NIC Activities—Nutrition Management

Determine the client's motivation for changing eating habits; Develop with the client a method to keep a daily record of intake

Nursing Interventions and *Rationales*

- Ask the client to keep a 1- to 3-day food diary where everything eaten or drunk is recorded. Analyze the quality, quantity, and pattern of food intake. *Use of a food diary is helpful for both the client and the nurse, to examine usual foods eaten and patterns of eating (Shay et al, 2009).* **EB:** *Development of self-monitoring tools that meet the needs of clients increases dietary reporting and promote self-efficacy (Mossavar-Rahmani et al, 2004).*
- Advise the client to measure food periodically. Help the client learn usual portion sizes. *Measuring food alerts the client to normal portion sizes. Estimating amounts can be extremely inaccurate.* **EB:** *A study where women were served either larger portions, or more calorie dense foods in the same portion size demonstrated that extra calories were eaten, and the women subjects did not realize it and decrease their calories for dinner (Kral, Roe, & Rolls, 2004). A study demonstrated that obese people had significantly larger portion sizes, plus ate later in the day (Berg et al, 2009).*
- Help the client determine their body mass index (BMI). Use a chart or a website such as *www.bcm .edu/cnrc/caloriesneed.htm. A normal BMI is 20 to 25; 26 to 29 is overweight; and a BMI of greater than 30 is obese (Nix, 2005). If BMI is greater than 25, refer to* **Imbalanced Nutrition: more than body requirements.**
- Recommend the client use the interactive Food Pyramid site at www.MyPyramid.gov to determine the number of calories to eat and gain more information on how to eat in a healthy fashion.
- Recommend the client follow the Dietary Guidelines for Americans: www.healthierus.gov/ dietaryguidelines. Use the Food Guide Pyramid to analyze the quality of the diet. *Dietary Guidelines are written by national experts and based on research in nutrition (Dietary Guidelines for Americans, 2005).*
- Recommend the client eat a healthy breakfast every morning. **EB:** *A study found that that people who skip breakfast are more likely to overeat in the evening (Masheb & Grillo, 2006). Another study demonstrated that people who skipped breakfast were 450 times more likely to be obese (Ma et al, 2003).*
- Recommend the client avoid eating in fast food restaurants. **EB:** *A 15–year study demonstrated that people who frequently eat fast foods gain an average of 10 lb more than those who eat fast food less often, and were two times more likely to develop insulin resistance, which can lead to diabetes (Peirera et al, 2005).*
- Review the client's current exercise level. With the client and primary health care provider, design a long-term exercise program. Encourage the client to adopt an exercise program that involves walking 3 to 5 hours per week at an average pace. *This is the amount of exercise recommended by the U.S. Dietary Guidelines for Americans and results in lowering the risk for cardiovascular disease, diabetes, osteoporosis, and other chronic illnesses (Wright, 2007).*
- Demonstrate the use of food labels to make healthful choices. Alert the client/family to focus on serving size, total fat, and simple carbohydrate. *The standardized food label in bold type simplifies the search for information. Fats and sugars contribute the least to a healthful diet and the most to excessive calorie intake. Generally clients should eat foods that are no more than 30% fat (Welland, 2007).*
- Determine the client's knowledge of the need for supplements. Discourage the client from taking excessive amounts of vitamins unless prescribed by a physician. If the client eats a healthy diet, there is generally no need for supplementation until the client is 50 years of age or older. *If the client is over age 50 years, one multivitamin per day is generally recommended.* **EB:** *A review of 14*

randomized trials demonstrated that intake of antioxidant supplementation did not prevent gastrointestinal (GI) cancers, and intake seemed to increase mortality (Bjelakovic et al, 2004).

Carbohydrates

- Encourage the client to **decrease** intake of sugars including intake of soft drinks, desserts, and candy. Limit sugar intake to 12 teaspoons of added sugar daily. *Sugar predisposes to dental caries, and also is a source of calories that is empty of other nutrients (ADA, 2009). A 20–ounce cola drink contains 17 teaspoons of sugar (Tufts University, 2004).*
- Recommend the client eat whole grains whenever possible, and explain how to find whole grains using the food label. **EB:** *A review of studies found strong evidence that eating whole grains is associated with a decreased BMI, and reduced the risk of being overweight (Williams, Grafenauer, & O'Shea, 2008). Intake of whole grains has been shown to decrease the incidence of heart failure (Nettleton et al, 2008), and when eaten with other healthier foods, resulted in lower incidence of diabetes in a multiethnic study (Nettleton et al, 2008). Intake of refined grains in women was associated with an increased risk of hemorrhagic strokes (Oh et al, 2005).*
- Evaluate the client's usual intake of fiber. Recommended intake is 25 g per day for women and 38 g per day for men. Increase intake of whole grains, legumes, fruits, and vegetables to obtain needed fiber. *In general, high-fiber foods take longer to eat, increase satiety, and contain fewer calories than most other foods (Slavin, 2008).* **EB:** *Increased dietary fiber was associated with lower body weight and waist-to-hip ratios, as well as predicted weight gain more strongly than did fat consumption (Slavin, 2005).*
- Recommend the client eat five to nine fruits and vegetables per day, with a minimum of two servings of fruit and three servings of vegetables. Encourage client to eat a rainbow of fruits and vegetables because bright colors are associated with increased nutrients. *Both fruits and vegetables are excellent sources of vitamins and also phytochemicals that help protect from disease, strokes, some kinds of cancer, and possibly macular degeneration (Liebman & Hurley, 2009).* **EB:** *A study done on women following breast cancer found that those who ate 5 to 9 fruits and vegetables per day, as well as exercising, had a reduced reoccurrence of cancer (Pierce et al, 2007). A study done on older men found that if they ingested increased foods high in vitamin C, it resulted in decreased thickening of the carotid arteries (Ellingsen et al, 2009). Another study found ingesting increased foods containing vitamin C resulted in increased bone strength in older men (Sahni, Hannan, & Gagnon, 2008).*

Fats

- Recommend the client limit intake of saturated fats and trans-fatty acids; instead increase intake of vegetable oils such as canola and olive oil. Limit fat intake to around 30% of total calories per day. *Intake of both saturated fat and trans-fatty acids raises the low-density lipoprotein (LDL) level, which predisposes to atherosclerosis (Welland, 2007). Eating even small amounts of trans fats increases the risk of heart disease, strokes, and diabetes (EN Comments, 2007).*
- Recommend client use low-fat choices when selecting and cooking meat; also when selecting dairy products.
- Recommend that the client eat cold-water fish such as salmon, tuna, or mackerel at least two times per week to ensure adequate intake of omega-3 fatty acids. If unwilling to eat fish, suggest sources such as flaxseed, soy, or walnuts. NOTE: Fish oil capsules should be taken cautiously; some brands can be contaminated with mercury or pesticides. Intake of excessive omega-3 fatty acids can result in bleeding. *Ingestion of omega-3 fats results in lower triglycerides and total cholesterol, also decrease the risk of heart disease and stroke (Neville, 2009).* **EB:** *The intake of omega-3 fatty acids by fish intake or fish oil capsules results in decreased incidence of sudden cardiac death (von Schacky, 2007). Consumption of fish was associated with a significantly reduced progression of coronary artery atherosclerosis in postmenopausal women with coronary artery disease (Erkkilä et al, 2004). Omega-3 fatty acids were found to be effective in helping psychiatric clients with both unipolar and bipolar depression (Freeman et al, 2006).*

Protein

- Recommend the client decrease intake of red meat and processed meats, instead eat more poultry, fish, soy, and dairy sources of protein. **EB:** *Red and processed meat intakes were associated with increases in mortality for cancer, and cardiovascular disease (Sinha et al, 2009). Women who eat more*

● = Independent   ▲ = Collaborative   **EBN** = Evidence-Based Nursing   **EB** = Evidence-Based

red and processed meats, along with processed grains and increased sweets consumption, have higher rates of cerebrovascular accidents (CVAs) (Fung et al, 2004).

- Recommend the client eat meatless meals at intervals and try alternative sources of protein, including nuts, especially almonds (one handful), and nut butters. **EB:** *Consumption of nuts and peanut butter was shown to decrease the incidence of cardiovascular disease in women with type 2 diabetes (Li et al, 2009). A study demonstrated that intake of almonds in a regular diet resulted in decreased risk factors for cardiovascular disease and other chronic diseases (Jaceldo-Siegl et al, 2004).*
- Recommend the client eat beans and especially soy as an alternative to animal proteins at intervals. Introduce the client to soy products such as flavored soy milk and tofu. *Eating soy as a substitute for animal products reduces the incidence of coronary artery disease by reducing blood lipids, oxidized LDL, homocysteine, and blood pressure (Jenkins et al, 2002). NOTE: Women with diagnosed estrogen-dependent cancer of the breast should generally avoid eating soy foods. New research has shown that intake of soy foods as a child may cut the incidence of breast cancer by half, and protect women from breast cancer in a Chinese study, but further research is needed (Welland, 2007).*

Fluid and Electrolytes

- Recommend the client choose and prepare foods with less salt, aiming for a maximum of 1500 mg per day, less than a teaspoon. *The CDC (2009) recommends that all salt-sensitive Americans, including everyone 40 years or older, should decrease daily sodium intake.* **EB:** *A study found that decreased sodium intake helped lower blood pressure, as well as increase flexibility in blood vessels, improving the health of the blood vessels (CDC, 2009).*
- If the client drinks alcohol, encourage him or her to drink in moderation—no more than one drink per day for women and two drinks per day for men. *Consuming more than a moderate amount of alcohol is one of the main causes of hypertension in both men and women (Krousel-Wood et al, 2004).* **EB:** *A study found an increased incidence of cancer of the upper gastrointestinal tract, liver cancer, and also renal cancer (Thygesen et al, 2009).*
- Recommend client increase intake of water, to at least 2000 mL or 2 quarts per day. A guideline is 1 to 1.5 mL of fluid per each calorie needed, so an average intake would be between 2000 and 3000 mL/day, or at least 8 cups of fluid. *The adequate intake recommendation is 3 L for the 19– to 30–year-old male and 2.2 L for the 19– to 30–year-old female. Water balance studies suggest that adult men require 2.5 L per day (Institute of Medicine, 2004).*

Pediatrics

- Mealtime is family time. Aim for at least one meal per day eating together. *Mealtime to together has been shown to improve children's eating habits: children eat more fruits and vegetables when the family eats together.*
- Involve the family in planning meals and food preparation. Children can learn about nutrition as they help plan and make meals. *Children are more likely to eat foods that they help select or prepare.*
- Parents need to be a good role model of healthy eating. *Setting a good example is key for children, children learn the value of healthy eating early, and it can continue for a lifetime.*
- Try new foods, try either a new food or recipe every week. *More variety can increase the intake of fruits and vegetables.*
- Keep healthy snacks on hand. Store the snacks in your purse, the car, a desk drawer. *Suggestions include crackers and peanut butter, small boxes of cereal, fresh fruit, plain popcorn.*
- Plan ahead before eating out. *Visit restaurant websites to see the nutritional value of foods on the menu; also call ahead to see what is offered for healthy foods. Most mothers want their families to eat healthier, but with busy schedules, this can be difficult. Some of the ideas above can help mothers in accomplishing their goal to improve nutrition of their families (ADA, 2009).*

Geriatric

- Utilize a nutritional screening tool designed for the elderly such as the Mini Nutrition Assessment (MNA), the Malnutrition Universal Screening Tool (MUST), or the Nutrition Risk Screening

(NRS). *The MNA is helpful for the elderly person living in the community or in an extended care facility; the NRS is more helpful for clients in the acute care setting (Sieber, 2006).*

- Assess changes in lifestyle and eating patterns. *Energy needs decrease an estimated 5% per decade after age 40 years, but often, eating patterns remain unchanged from youth (Lutz & Przytulski, in press).*
- ▲ Recommend the client discuss the need for a low-dose balanced multiple vitamin and mineral supplement with physician. *It is generally recommended that anyone over age 50 should take a multivitamin every day to ensure that adequate amounts of vitamins and minerals are obtained.*
- Assess fluid intake. Recommend routine drinks of water regardless of thirst. Monitor elderly clients for deficient fluid volume carefully, noting new onset of weakness, dizziness, and postural hypotension. *Older adults have a higher osmotic point for thirst sensation and a diminished sensitivity to thirst, relative to younger adults (Wotton, Crannitch, & Munt, 2008).*
- Observe for socioeconomic factors that influence food choices (e.g., funds, cooking facilities). *Even those on restricted budgets and with limited facilities can be assisted to choose healthy food sources for a balanced diet.*

Multicultural

- Assess for dietary intake of essential nutrients. **EBN:** *African American adolescents have some of the greatest vitamin D deficiencies (Gordon et al, 2004).*
- Assess for the influence of cultural beliefs, norms, and values on the client's nutritional knowledge. *What the client considers normal dietary practices may be based on cultural perceptions (Leininger & McFarland, 2002; Giger & Davidhizar, 2008). Among African Americans, there was a general perception that "eating healthfully" meant giving up part of their cultural heritage (James, 2004).*
- Discuss with the client those aspects of their diet that will remain unchanged. *Aspects of the client's life that are meaningful and valuable to them should be understood and preserved without change (Leininger & McFarland, 2002).*
- Negotiate with the client regarding the aspects of his or her diet that will need to be modified. *Give and take with the client will lead to culturally congruent care (Leininger & McFarland, 2002).*
- Explore strategies that appeal to the client. **EBN:** *A study using the Parents as Teachers site to deliver a dietary change program via personal visits, newsletters, and group meetings was successful in reducing the percentage of calories from fat and increasing fruit and vegetable consumption among participating parents (Haire-Joshu et al, 2003).*
- Validate the client's feelings regarding the impact of current lifestyle, finances, and transportation on ability to obtain nutritious food.
- Encourage family meals. **EB:** *Frequency of family meals was positively associated with intake of fruits, vegetables, grains, and calcium-rich foods and was negatively associated with soft drink consumption (Neumark-Sztainer et al, 2003).*

Client/Family Teaching and Discharge Planning

- The majority of interventions above involve teaching.
- Work with the family members regarding information on how to improve nutritional status
- Teach the importance of exercise in a weight control program.

ⓔvolve   See the EVOLVE website for Weblinks for client education resources.

REFERENCES

American Dental Association (ADA): Cleaning your teeth and gums, 2009, www.ada.org/public/topics/alpha.asp. Accessed July 1, 2009.

Berg C, Lappas G, Wolk A et al: Eating patterns and portion size associated with obesity in a Swedish population, *Appetite* 52(1):21–26, 2009.

Bjelakovic G, Nikolova D, Simonetti RG et al: Antioxidant supplements for prevention of gastrointestinal cancers: a systematic review and meta-analysis, *Lancet* 364(9441):1219–1228, 2004.

Centers for Disease Control and Prevention (CDC): Application of lower sodium intake recommendations to adults—United States, 1999–2006, *MMWR Morb Mortal Wkly Rep* 58(11):281–283, 2009.

Dietary Guidelines for Americans 2005, www.health.gov/Dietary Guidelines. Accessed July 14, 2009.

Ellingsen I, Seljeflot I, Arnesen H et al: Vitamin C consumption is associated with less progression in carotid intima media thickness in

● = Independent   ▲ = Collaborative   **EBN** = Evidence-Based Nursing   **EB** = Evidence-Based

elderly men: a 3–year intervention study, *Nutr Metab Cardiovasc Dis* 19(1):8–14, 2009.

EN Comments: Trans fats get the boot thanks to you; how to spur more change, *Environ Nutr* 30(3):3, 2007.

Erkkilä AT, Lichtenstein AH, Mozaffarian D et al: Fish intake is associated with a reduced progression of coronary artery atherosclerosis in postmenopausal women with coronary artery disease, *Am J Clin Nutr* 80(3):626, 2004.

Freeman MP, Hibbeln JR, Wisner KL et al: Omega-3 fatty acids: evidence bases for treatment and future research in psychiatry, *J Clin Psychiatry* 67(12):1954–1964, 2006.

Fung TT, Stampfer MJ, Manson JE et al: Prospective study of major dietary patterns and stroke risk in women, *Stroke* 35(9):2014, 2004.

Giger J, Davidhizar R: *Transcultural nursing: assessment and intervention*, ed 5, St Louis, 2008, Mosby.

Gordon CM, DePeter KC, Feldman HA et al: Prevalence of vitamin D deficiency among healthy adolescents, *Arch Ped Ad Med* 158(6):531–537, 2004.

Haire-Joshu D, Brownson RC, Nanney MS et al: Improving dietary behavior in African Americans: the Parents As Teachers High 5, Low Fat Program, *Prev Med* 36(6):684–691, 2003.

Institute of Medicine: Applications of dietary reference intakes for electrolytes and water, *National Academy of Sciences*, National Academies Press, 2004.

Jaceldo-Siegl K, Sabaté J, Rajaram S et al: Long-term almond supplementation without advice on food replacement induces favourable nutrient modifications to the habitual diets of free-living individuals, *Br J Nutr* 92(3):533–540, 2004.

James DC: Factors influencing food choices, dietary intake, and nutrition-related attitudes among African Americans: application of a culturally sensitive model, *Ethn Health* 9(4):349–367, 2004.

Jenkins DJ, Kendall CW, Jackson CJ et al: Effects of high-and low-isoflavone soyfoods on blood lipids, oxidized LDL, homocysteine, and blood pressure in hyperlipidemic men and women, *Am J Clin Nutr* 76(2):365, 2002.

Kral TV, Roe LS, Rolls BJ: Combined effects of energy density and portion size on energy intake in women, *Am J Clin Nutr* 79(6):962–968, 2004.

Krousel-Wood MA, Muntner P, He J et al: Primary prevention of essential hypertension, *Med Clin North Am* 88(1):223–238, 2004.

Leininger MM, McFarland MR: *Transcultural nursing: concepts, theories, research and practices*, ed 3, New York, 2002, McGraw-Hill.

Li TY, Brennan AM, Wedick NM et al: Regular consumption of nuts is associated with a lower risk of cardiovascular disease in women with type 2 diabetes, *J Nutr* 139(7):1333–1338, 2009.

Liebman B, Hurley J: Rating rutabagas: not all vegetables are created equal, *Nutr Action Healthletter* Jan:13–15, 2009.

Lutz CA, Przytulski KR: *Nutrition and diet therapy*, ed 5, Philadelphia, in press, F.A. Davis.

Ma Y, Bertone ER, Stanek EJ 3rd et al: Association between eating patterns and obesity in a free-living U.S. adult population, *Am J Epidiomol* 158(1):85–92, 2003.

Masheb RM, Grillo CM: Eating patterns and breakfast consumption in obese patients with binge eating disorder, *Behav Res Ther* 44(11): 1545–1553, 2006.

Mossavar-Rahmani Y et al: Additional self-monitoring tools in the dietary modification component of the women's health initiative, *J Am Diet Assoc* 104(1):76, 2004.

Nettleton JA, Steffen LM, Ni H et al: Dietary patterns and risk of incident type 2 diabetes in the Multi-Ethnic Study of Atherosclerosis (MESA), *Diabetes Care* 31(9):1777–1782, 2008.

Neumark-Sztainer D et al: Family meal patterns: associations with sociodemographic characteristics and improved dietary intake among adolescents, *J Am Diet Assoc*, 103(3):317–322, 2003.

Neville K: Focus on good fats: balancing Omega-3s with Omega-6s, *Environ Nutr* 32(3):1–4, 2009.

Nix S: *Williams' basic nutrition and diet therapy*, St Louis, 2005, Mosby.

Oh K, Hu FB, Cho E et al: Carbohydrate intake, glycemic index, glycemic load, and dietary fiber in relation to risk of stroke in women, *Am J Epidemiol* 161(2):161–169, 2005.

Pereira MA, Kartashov AI, Ebbeling CB et al: Fast-food habits, weight gain, and insulin resistance (the CARDIA study): 15–year prospective analysis, *Lancet* 365(9453):36, 2005.

Pierce JP, Stefanick ML, Flatt SW et al: Greater survival after breast cancer in physically active women with high vegetable-fruit intake regardless of obesity, *J Clin Oncol* 25(17):2345–2351, 2007.

Sahni S, Hannan MT, Gagnon D: High vitamin C intake is associated with lower 4–year bone loss in elderly men, *J Nutr* 138(10):1931–1938, 2008.

Shay LE, Shobert JL, Seibert D et al: Adult weight management: translating research and guidelines into practice, *J Am Acad Nurse Pract*; 21(4):197–206, 2009.

Sieber CC: Nutritional screening tools—how does the MNA compare? Proceedings of the session held in Chicago May 2–3, 2006 (15 Years of Mini Nutritional Assessment), *J Nutr Health Aging* 10(6):488–492, 2006.

Sinha R, Cross AJ, Graubard BI et al: Meat intake and mortality: a prospective study of over half a million people, *Arch Intern Med* 169(6): 562–5671, 2009.

Slavin JL: Dietary fiber and body weight, *Nutr* 21(3):411, 2005.

Slavin JL: Position of the American Dietetic Association: health implications of dietary fiber, *J Am Diet Assoc* 108(10):1716–1731, 2008.

Thygesen LC, Mikkelsen P, Andersen TV et al: Cancer incidence among patients with alcohol use disorders—long-term follow-up, *Alcohol Alcohol* 44(4):387–391, 2009.

Tufts University: How much sugar is right? *Health and Nutrition Letter* 22(4), 2004.

von Schacky C: Omega-3 fatty acids and cardiovascular disease, *Curr Opin Clin Nutr Metab Care* 10(2):129–135, 2007.

Welland D: Red-flagging food labels: 8 tips to sift fact from fiction, *Environ Nutr* 30(3):2, 2007.

Williams PG, Grafenauer SJ, O'Shea JE: Cereal grains, legumes, and weight management: a comprehensive review of the scientific evidence, *Nutr Rev* 66(4):171–182, 2008.

Wotton K, Crannitch K, Munt R: Prevalence, risk factors and strategies to prevent dehydration in older adults, *Contemp Nurse* 31(1):44–56, 2008.

Wright H: Get active to increase your chances of surviving cancer, *Environ Nutr* 30(3):1–4, 2007.

Impaired Oral mucous membrane   *Betty J. Ackley, MSN, EdS, RN*   ⊝volve

NANDA-I

Definition

Disruption of the lips and/or soft tissues of the oral cavity

Defining Characteristics

Bleeding; cheilitis; coated tongue; desquamation; difficult speech; difficulty eating; difficulty swallowing; diminished taste; edema; enlarged tonsils; fissures; geographic tongue; gingival hyperplasia; gingival pallor; gingival recession; halitosis; hyperemia; macroplasia; mucosal denudation; mucosal pallor; nodules; oral discomfort; oral lesions; oral pain; oral ulcers; papules; pocketing deeper than 4 mm; presence of pathogens; purulent drainage; purulent exudates; red or bluish masses (e.g., hemangiomas); reports bad taste in mouth; smooth atrophic tongue; spongy patches; stomatitis; vesicles; white; curd-like exudates; white patches/plaques; xerostomia

Related Factors (r/t)

Barriers to oral self-care; barriers to professional care; chemotherapy; chemical irritants (e.g., alcohol, tobacco, acidic foods, drugs, regular use of inhalers or other noxious agents); cleft lip; cleft palate; decreased platelets; decreased salivation; deficient knowledge of appropriate oral hygiene; dehydration; depression; diminished hormone levels (women); ineffective oral hygiene; infection; immunocompromised; immunosuppression; loss of supportive structures; malnutrition; mechanical factors (e.g., ill-fitting dentures, braces, tubes [endotracheal/nasogastric] surgery in oral cavity); medication side effects; mouth breathing; NPO for more than 24 hours; radiation therapy; stress; trauma

NOC   (Nursing Outcomes Classification)

Suggested NOC Outcomes

Oral Hygiene, Tissue Integrity: Skin and Mucous Membranes

Example NOC Outcome with Indicators
Oral Hygiene as evidenced by the following indicators: Cleanliness of mouth/Moisture of oral mucosa and tongue/Color of mucous membranes/Oral mucosa/tongue/gum integrity (Rate the outcome and indicators of **Oral Hygiene**: 1 = severely compromised, 2 = substantially compromised, 3 = moderately compromised, 4 = mildly compromised, 5 = not compromised [see Section I].)

Client Outcomes

Client Will (Specify Time Frame):

- Maintain intact, moist oral mucous membranes that are free of ulceration, inflammation, infection, and debris
- Demonstrate measures to maintain or regain intact oral mucous membranes

NIC   (Nursing Interventions Classification)

Suggested NIC Intervention

Oral Health Restoration

Example NIC Activities—Oral Health Restoration
Use a soft toothbrush for removal of dental debris; Instruct client to avoid commercial mouthwashes

Nursing Interventions and *Rationales*

▲ Inspect the oral cavity at least once daily and note any discoloration, lesions, edema, bleeding, exudate, or dryness. Refer to a physician or dental specialist as appropriate. *Oral inspection can reveal*

• = Independent   ▲ = Collaborative   **EBN** = Evidence-Based Nursing   **EB** = Evidence-Based

signs of oral disease, symptoms of systemic disease, drug side effects, or trauma of the oral cavity (Gonsalves, Chi, & Neville, 2007).

- If the client does not have a bleeding disorder and is able to swallow, encourage the client to brush the teeth with a soft toothbrush using fluoride-containing toothpaste at least twice per day. **EBN:** *A systematic review found that the toothbrush is the most important tool for oral care. Brushing the teeth is the most effective method for reducing plaque and controlling periodontal disease (McGuire et al, 2006).*
- Use foam sticks to moisten the oral mucous membranes, clean out debris, and swab out the mouth of the edentulous client. **Do not use foam sticks to clean the teeth** unless the platelet count is very low and the client is prone to bleeding gums. Foam sticks are useful for cleansing the oral cavity of a client who is edentulous (Curzio & McCowan, 2000). **EBN:** *Foam sticks are not effective for removing plaque; the toothbrush is much more effective (Pearson & Hutton, 2002).*
- If the client does not have a bleeding disorder, encourage the client to floss once per day or use an interdental cleaner. **EB:** *Floss is useful to remove plaque buildup between the teeth (ADA, 2009).*
- Encourage the client to brush the tongue with a toothbrush or use a tongue scraper twice a day. **EB:** *A Cochrane study found a small but statistically significant effect in reducing halitosis when a tongue scraper was utilized (Outhouse et al, 2006).* **EB:** *The tongue scraper was shown to be more effective than brushing in removing volatile sulfur compounds which are associated with halitosis (Pedrazzi, Sato, & de Mattos Mda, 2004). A review found that tongue scraping was effective in decreasing halitosis (Hughes & McNab, 2008).*
- ▲ Use an antimicrobial mouthwash as ordered or tap water or saline only for a mouth rinse. Do not use commercial mouthwashes containing alcohol or hydrogen peroxide. Also, do not use lemon-glycerin swabs. *Some antimicrobial mouthwashes have demonstrated effective action in decreasing bacterial counts in plaque and decreasing gingivitis (ADA, 2009). Alcohol dries the oral mucous membranes (Rogers, 2001).* **EBN:** *Hydrogen peroxide can cause mucosal damage and is extremely foul tasting to clients (Tombes & Gallucci, 1993). Use of lemon-glycerin swabs can result in decreased salivary amylase and oral moisture, as well as erosion of tooth enamel (Poland, 1987; Foss-Durant & McAffee, 1997).*
- If the client is unable to care for him- or herself, oral hygiene must be provided by nursing personnel. The nursing diagnosis **Bathing Self-Care deficit** is then applicable.
- If the client is unable to brush own teeth, follow this procedure:
  - Position the client sitting upright or on side.
  - Use a soft bristle baby toothbrush.
  - Use fluoride toothpaste and tap water or saline as a solution.
  - Brush teeth in an up-and-down manner.
  - Suction as needed.
  Each client must receive oral care including toothbrushing two times every day to maintain healthy teeth and mouth, and to prevent complications associated with periodontitis (the advanced form of gum disease that can cause tooth loss), which is associated with health problems such as cardiovascular disease, stroke, and bacterial pneumonia (ADA, 2009).
- Assess for mechanical agents such as ill-fitting dentures and chemical agents such as frequent exposure to tobacco that could cause or increase trauma to oral mucous membranes. **EB:** *Denture wearing and being edentulous can be related to a decreased quality of life and risk for undiagnosed oral disease (Weyant et al, 2004).*
- Monitor the client's nutritional and fluid status to determine if it is adequate. Refer to the care plan for **Deficient Fluid volume** or **Imbalanced Nutrition: less than body requirements** if applicable. *Dehydration and malnutrition predispose clients to impaired oral mucous membranes.*
- Encourage fluid intake of up to 3000 mL/day if not contraindicated by the client's medical condition. *Fluids help increase moisture in the mouth, which protects the mucous membranes from damage.*
- Determine the client's usual method of oral care and address any concerns regarding oral hygiene. *Whenever possible, build on the client's existing knowledge base and current practices to develop an individualized plan of care.*
- If the client has a dry mouth (xerostomia):
  - Provide saliva substitutes as ordered. *Saliva substitutes are helpful to decrease the discomfort of dry mouth and may help prevent stomatitis (ADA, 2009).*

• = Independent   ▲ = Collaborative   **EBN** = Evidence-Based Nursing   **EB** = Evidence-Based

- ■ Suggest the client chew sugarless gum or sugarless sour candy to promote salivary flow. *Both sugarless gum and candy stimulate the formation of saliva (ADA, 2009).*
- ■ Provide ice chips frequently to keep the mouth moist. **EB:** *There is some evidence that ice chips help prevent mucositis (Clarkson, Worthington, & Eden, 2003).*
- ■ Recommend the client decrease or preferably stop intake of soft drinks. *Sugar containing soft drinks can cause cavities and the low pH of the drink can cause erosion in teeth (ADA, 2009).* **EB:** *A study demonstrated a much higher incidence of caries in children who drank soft drinks, as well as increased processed foods (Llena & Forner, 2008).*
- • If client has halitosis, review good oral care with the client including brushing teeth, using floss, and brushing the tongue. *Halitosis can be a beginning sign of gingivitis, and can be eradicated by a good program of dental hygiene (Obesity, Fitness & Wellness Week, 2006; ADA, 2009).*
- • Instruct the client with halitosis to clean the tongue when performing oral hygiene. Brush tongue with tongue scraper and follow with a mouth rinse. **EB:** *A Cochrane review found that tongue cleaning was effective for short-term control of halitosis (Outhouse et al, 2006).*
- ▲ Assess the client for an underlying medical condition that may be causing halitosis. *Causes of halitosis can be subdivided into three categories: oral origin, where good mouth care can help prevention; halitosis from the upper respiratory tract including the sinuses and nose; and halitosis from systemic diseases that are blood-borne, volatilized in the lungs, and expelled from the lower respiratory tract. Potential sources of blood-borne halitosis are some systemic diseases, metabolic disorders, medication, and certain foods (Tangerman, 2002; ADA, 2009).*
- • Keep the lips well lubricated using a lip balm that is water or aloe-based. *This is a comfort measure.*

Client Receiving Chemotherapy/Radiation

- • Ensure that the client receives a comprehensive oral examination before initiation of chemotherapy or radiation, with aggressive preventative dental care given as needed (Keefe et al, 2007; Weikel, 2008).
- • Provide instructions both verbal and written about the need for and method of providing frequent oral care to the client before radiation therapy or chemotherapy (Keefe et al, 2007; Harris et al, 2008).
- • Assess the condition of the oral cavity daily in the client receiving radiation or chemotherapy (Harris et al, 2008).
- • For measurement of presence or severity of mucositis, use the Oral Mucositis Assessment Scale (OMAS). **EBN:** *This is an instrument that has two components; clinician's assessment of presence and severity of mucositis, and client report about pain, difficulty swallowing, and ability to eat (Harris et al, 2008).*
- • Utilize a protocol to prevent/treat mucositis that includes the following:
  - ■ Use of a soft toothbrush that is replaced on a regular basis
  - ■ Use of a validated tool to assess condition of the oral cavity
  - ■ Client teaching of the need for and method of performing oral care
  - ■ Use of a bland rinse to remove debris and moisten the oral cavity

  EBN and EB: *Use of an oral care protocol helps to decrease oral mucositis in clients receiving treatment for cancer (Rubenstein et al, 2004; Keefe et al, 2007; Harris et al, 2008).*
- • Use cryotherapy with ice chips dissolving in client's mouth before, during, and after bolus administration of fluorouracil (5–FU) to reduce the severity of mucositis (Worthington, Clarkson, & Eden, 2004; Keefe et al, 2007). Also use cryotherapy for clients receiving bolus edatrexate (Keefe et al, 2007) and melphalan (Aisa et al, 2005; Tartatone et al, 2005; Keefe et al, 2007).
- • Help the client use a mouth rinse of normal saline or salt and soda every 1 to 2 hours for prevention and treatment of stomatitis. A typical mixture is 1 teaspoon of salt or sodium bicarbonate per pint of water. Clients are directed to take a tablespoon of the rinse, swish it in the mouth for 30 seconds, and then expectorate. *Rinses are helpful to remove debris and hydrate the oral mucous membranes, and sodium bicarbonate can discourage yeast colonization (Harris et al, 2008).* **EBN:** *A study demonstrated that there was no difference in the rate of cessation of symptoms of stomatitis when three different mouthwashes were used: chlorhexidine, lidocaine, Benadryl and Maalox, and salt and soda (Dodd et al, 2000).*

▲ If the mouth is severely inflamed and it is painful to swallow, contact the physician for a topical anesthetic or analgesic order. Modification of oral intake (e.g., soft or liquid diet) may also be necessary to prevent friction trauma. The nursing diagnosis **Imbalanced Nutrition: less than body requirements** may apply.

• If the client's platelet count is lower than 50,000/mm³ or the client has a bleeding disorder, use a specially made toothbrush designed for sensitive or diseased tissue, or a toothette that is not soaked in glycerin or flavorings; if the client cannot tolerate a toothbrush or a toothette, a piece of gauze wrapped around a finger can be used to remove plaque and debris (Brown & Yoder, 2002).

Critical Care—Client on a Ventilator

• Use a pediatric-sized toothbrush to brush teeth; use suction to remove secretions. **EBN:** *Brushing the teeth is effective in removing dental plaque (Stiefel et al, 2000).*

• Recognize that good oral care can be effective to prevent ventilator-associated pneumonia. **EBN and EB:** *Increased plaque on the teeth is associated with increased contamination of the mouth and incidence of ventilator-associated pneumonia (Munro et al, 2006). Many studies have demonstrated the effectiveness of good oral care to decrease the incidence of ventilator-associated pneumonia (Coffin et al, 2008; Fields, 2008).*

▲ Apply chlorhexidine gluconate in the oral cavity by swab or spray early after intubation, and at intervals if ordered. **EBN:** *The use of chlorohexidine gluconate administered early after intubation and at intervals decreased positive cultures of bacteria and may decrease VAP (Grap et al, 2004; Koeman et al, 2006).*

 ### Geriatric

• Determine the functional ability of the client to provide his or her own oral care. *Interventions must be directed toward both treatment of the functional loss and care of oral health.*

• Provide appropriate oral care to the elderly client with a self-care deficit, brushing the teeth after every meal. **EBN:** *Oral care is often poor for clients with dementia in long-term facilities (Sigal, 2006; Jablonski et al, 2009).* **EB:** *Several studies have shown that the rate of pneumonia was decreased by providing oral care (Watando et al, 2004; Sarin et al, 2008).*

▲ Carefully observe the oral cavity and lips for abnormal lesions such as white or red patches, masses, ulcerations with an indurated margin, or a raised granular lesion. *Malignant lesions are more common in elderly persons than in younger persons, especially if there is a history of smoking or alcohol use, and many elderly persons rarely visit a dentist (Gonsalves, Chi, & Neville, 2007).*

• Ensure that dentures are removed and scrubbed at least once daily, removed and rinsed thoroughly after every meal, and removed and kept in an appropriate solution at night. *Denture plaque containing* Candida *organisms can cause denture-induced stomatitis, which is more common in clients with unhealthy lifestyles and poor oral hygiene than in others (Lyon et al, 2006).*

▲ If the client has xerostomia, evaluate medications to see if they could be the cause, provide synthetic saliva products to moisten the oral cavity as ordered, and offer frequent sips of water and sugarless gum or candy to provide lubrication. *Xerostomia is common in the elderly for many reasons, including medication use and aging. The goal is to keep the mouth moist to prevent stomatitis.*

 ### Home Care

• The interventions described previously may be adapted for home care use.

• If dryness is a side effect of the client's medication(s), instruct the client in the use of artificial saliva.

• Instruct the client to avoid alcohol-based or hydrogen peroxide–based commercial products for mouth care and to avoid other irritants to the oral cavity (e.g., tobacco, spicy foods). *Oral irritants can further damage the oral mucosa and increase the client's discomfort.*

• Instruct the client in ways to soothe the oral cavity (e.g., cool beverages, Popsicles, viscous lidocaine).

▲ If necessary, refer for home health aide services to support the family in oral care and observation of the oral cavity.

• = Independent ▲ = Collaborative **EBN** = Evidence-Based Nursing **EB** = Evidence-Based

Client/Family Teaching and Discharge Planning

- Teach the client how to inspect the oral cavity and monitor for signs and symptoms of infection or complications, and when to call the health care practitioner (Harris et al, 2008).
- Teach the client and family if necessary how to perform appropriate mouth care.
- Recommend the client use a powered toothbrush for removal of dental plaque and prevention of gingivitis. Please refer to the care plan **Impaired Dentition** for more interventions in caring for the teeth.

⊖volve   See the EVOLVE website for Weblinks for client education resources.

REFERENCES

Aisa Y, Mori T, Kudo M et al: Oral cryotherapy for the prevention of high-dose melphalan-induced stomatitis in allogeneic hematopoietic stem cell transplant recipients, *Support Care Cancer* 13(4):266–269, 2005.

American Dental Association (ADA): Cleaning your teeth and gums, 2009, www.ada.org/public/topics/alpha.asp. Accessed July 1, 2009.

Brown CG, Yoder LH: Stomatitis: an overview, *Am J Nurs* 102(Suppl 4): 20, 2002.

Clarkson JE, Worthington HV, Eden OB: Interventions for preventing oral mucositis or oral candidiasis for patients with cancer receiving chemotherapy, *Cochrane Database Syst Rev* (3):CD000978, 2003.

Coffin SE, Klompas M, Classen D et al: Strategies to prevent ventilator-associated pneumonia in acute care hospitals, *Infect Control Hosp Epidemiol* 29(1):S31–S37, 2008.

Curzio J, McCowan M: Getting research into practice: developing oral hygiene standards, *Br J Nurs* 9(7):434–438, 2000.

Dodd MJ, Dibble SL, Miaskowski C et al: Randomized clinical trial of the effectiveness of three commonly used mouthwashes to treat chemotherapy-induced mucositis, *Oral Surg Oral Med Oral Pathol Oral Radiol Endod* 90(1):39, 2000.

Fields LB: Oral care intervention to reduce incidence of ventilator-associated pneumonia in the neurologic intensive care unit, *J Neurosci Nurs* 40(5):291–298, 2008.

Foss-Durant AM, McAffee A: A comparison of three oral care products commonly used in practice, *Clin Nurs Res* 6:1, 1997.

Gonsalves WC, Chi AC, Neville BW: Common oral lesions: part I. Superficial mucosal lesions, *Am Fam Physician* 75(4):501–506, 2007.

Grap MJ, Munro CL, Elswick RK Jr et al: Duration of action of a single, early oral application of chlorhexidine on oral microbial flora in mechanically ventilated patients: a pilot study, *Heart Lung* 33(2):83, 2004.

Harris DJ, Eilers J, Harriman A et al: Putting evidence into practice: evidence-based interventions for the management of oral mucositis, *Clin J Oncol Nurs* 12(1):141–152, 2008.

Hughes FJ, McNab R: Oral malodour—a review, *Arch Oral Biol* 53(Suppl 1):S1–S7, 2008.

Jablonski RA, Munro CL, Grap MG et al: Mouth care in nursing homes: knowledge, beliefs, and practices of nursing assistants, *Geriatr Nurs* 30(2):99–107, 2009.

Keefe DM, Schubert M, Elting LS et al: Updated clinical practice guidelines for the prevention and treatment of mucositis, *Am Cancer Soc* 109(5):820–831, 2007.

Koeman M, van der Ven AJ, Hak E et al: Oral decontamination with chlorhexidine reduces the incidence of ventilator-associated pneumonia, *Am J Respir Crit Care Med* 173(12):1348–1356, 2006.

Llena C, Forner L: Dietary habits in a child population in relation to caries experience, *Caries Res* 42(5):387–393, 2008.

Lyon JP, da Costa SC, Totti VM et al: Predisposing conditions for *Candida spp.* carriage in the oral cavity of denture wearers and individuals with natural teeth, *Can J Microbiol* 52(5):462–468, 2006.

McGuire DB, Correa ME, Johnson J et al: The role of basic oral care and good clinical practice principles in the management of oral mucositis, *Support Care Cancer* 14(6):541–547, 2006.

Munro CL, Grap MJ, Elswick RK Jr et al: Oral health status and development of ventilator-associated pneumonia: a descriptive study, *Am J Crit Care* 15(5):453–461, 2006.

[No author]: Dental research: gingival bleeding and halitosis are greatly reduced after a two-week oral hygiene program, *Obesity, Fitness & Wellness Week,* Aug 26:843, 2006.

Outhouse, TL, Fedorowicz, A, Keenan JV et al: A Cochrane systematic review finds tongue scrapers have short-term efficacy in controlling halitosis, *Gen Dent* 54(5):352–359; 360, 367–358, 2006.

Pedrazzi V, Sato S, de Mattos Mda G: Tongue-cleaning methods: a comparative clinical trial employing a toothbrush and a tongue scraper, *J Periodontol* 75(7):1009–1012, 2004.

Pearson LS, Hutton JL: A controlled trial to compare the ability of foam swabs and toothbrushes to remove dental plaque, *J Adv Nurs* 39:5, 2002.

Poland JM: Comparing Moi-Stir to lemon-glycerin swabs, *Am J Nurs* 87(4):422, 1987.

Rogers BB: Mucositis in the oncology patient, *Nurs Clin North Am* 36:4, 2001.

Rubenstein EB, Peterson DE, Schubert M et al: Clinical practice guidelines for the prevention and treatment of cancer therapy-induced oral and gastrointestinal mucositis, *Cancer* 100(9 Suppl):2026–2046, 2004.

Sarin, J, Balasubramaniam R, Corcoran AM et al: Reducing the risk of aspiration pneumonia among elderly patients in long-term care facilities through oral health interventions, *J Am Med Dir Assoc* 9(2):128–135, 2008.

Sigal MJ: Dental considerations for persons with dementia, *Oral Health* 96(9):53–58, 2006.

Stiefel KA, Damron S, Sowers NJ et al: Improving oral hygiene for the seriously ill patient: implementing research-based practice, *Medsurg Nurs* 9(1):40, 2000.

Tangerman A: Halitosis in medicine: a review, *Int Dent J* 52(Suppl 3): 201–206, 2002.

Tartarone A, Matera R, Romano G et al: Prevention of high-dose melphalan-induced mucositis by cryotherapy, *Leuk Lymphoma* 46(4): 633–634, 2005.

Tombes MB, Gallucci B: The effects of hydrogen peroxide rinses on the normal oral mucosa, *Nurs Res* 42(6):332, 1993.

Watando A, Ebihara S, Ebihara T et al: Daily oral care and cough reflex sensitivity in elderly nursing home patients, *Chest* 126(4):1066, 2004.

Weikel DS: Oral health maintenance guideline. In Ackley B, Ladwig G, Swan T et al, editors: *Evidence-based nursing care guidelines,* Philadelphia, 2008, Mosby.

Weyant RJ, Pandav RS, Plowman JL et al: Medical and cognitive correlates of denture wearing in older community-dwelling adults, *J Am Geriatr Soc* 52(4):596, 2004.

Worthington HV, Clarkson JE, Eden OB: Interventions for treating oral mucositis for patients with cancer receiving treatment, *Cochrane Database Syst Rev* (2):CD001973, 2004.

Acute Pain Susan J. Dempsey, MN, CNS, RN-BC ⊘volve

NANDA-I

Definition

Unpleasant sensory and emotional experience arising from actual or potential tissue damage or described in terms of such damage (International Association for the Study of Pain, 1979); sudden or slow onset of any intensity from mild to severe with an anticipated or predictable end and a duration of less than 6 months.

Pain is whatever the experiencing person says it is, existing whenever the person says it does (McCaffery, 1968; APS, 2008)

Defining Characteristics

Subjective

Pain is a subjective experience, and its presence cannot be proved or disproved. Self-report is the most reliable method of evaluating pain presence and intensity (APS, 2008). A client with cognitive ability who is able to speak or provide information about pain in other ways, such as pointing to numbers or words, should use a self-report pain tool (e.g., Numerical Rating Scale [NRS]) to identify the current pain level and establish a comfort-function goal (Pasero, 2009a; Puntillo et al, 2009).

Objective

Pain is a subjective experience, and objective measurement is impossible (APS, 2008; Breivik et al, 2008). If a client cannot provide a self-report, there is no pain intensity level (Pasero & McCaffery, 2005). Behavioral or physiological responses should never serve as the basis for pain management decisions if self-report is possible (Pasero & McCaffery, 2005; Herr et al, 2006; Erstad et al, 2009). However, observation of these responses may be helpful in recognition of pain presence for clients who are unable to provide a self-report (Herr et al, 2006; Bjoro & Herr, 2008). Observable pain responses may include loss of appetite and inability to deep breathe, ambulate, sleep, and perform ADLs; demonstrate pain-related behaviors such as guarding, self-protective behavior, and self-focusing; and distraction behavior ranging from crying to laughing, as well as muscle tension or rigidity (Puntillo et al, 2009). Acute pain may be associated with neurohumoral responses that can lead to increases in heart rate, blood pressure, and respiratory rate (Dunwoody et al, 2008; Polomano, Rathmell et al, 2008). However, physiological responses are not sensitive indicators of pain presence and intensity as they do not discriminate pain from other sources of distress, pathologic conditions, hemostatic changes, or medications (Herr et al, 2006). Behavioral or physiologic indicators may be used to confirm other findings; however, the absence of these indicators does not indicate the absence of pain.

NOTE: The defining characteristics are modified from the work of NANDA-I.

Related Factors (r/t)

Injury agents (biological, chemical, physical, psychological)

NOC (Nursing Outcomes Classification)

Suggested NOC Outcomes

Comfort Level, Pain Control, Pain Level

Example NOC Outcome with Indicators

Pain Level as evidenced by the following indicators: Reported pain/Length of pain episodes/Moaning and crying/Facial expressions of pain (Rate the outcome and indicators of **Pain Level:** 1 = severe, 2 = substantial, 3 = moderate, 4 = mild, 5 = none ([see Section I].)

Client Outcomes

Client Will (Specify Time Frame):

For the client who is able to provide a self-report:
- Use a self-report pain tool to identify current pain level and establish a comfort-function goal
- Report that pain management regimen achieves comfort-function goal without adverse effects
- Describe nonpharmacological methods that can be used to help achieve comfort-function goal
- Perform activities of recovery or ADLs easily
- Describe how unrelieved pain will be managed
- State ability to obtain sufficient amounts of rest and sleep
- Notify member of the health care team promptly for pain level greater than the comfort-function goal, or occurrence of adverse effects

For the client who is unable to provide a self-report:
- Decrease in pain-related behaviors
- Use clinical judgment to evaluate intervention effectiveness if the client is unable to demonstrate behaviors
- Perform activities of recovery or ADLs easily as determined by client condition
- Demonstrate the absence of nonopioid analgesic or opioid-induced adverse effects

NIC   (Nursing Interventions Classification)

Suggested NIC Interventions

Analgesic Administration, Pain Management, Patient-Controlled Analgesia (PCA) Assistance

Example NIC Activities—Pain Management

Assure that the client receives attentive analgesic care; Perform a comprehensive assessment of pain to include location, characteristics, onset/duration, frequency, quality, intensity or severity of pain, and precipitating factors

Nursing Interventions and *Rationales*

▲ Determine if the client is experiencing pain at the time of the initial interview. If pain is present, conduct and document a comprehensive pain assessment and implement pain management interventions to achieve comfort. Components of this initial assessment include: location, quality, onset/duration, temporal profile, intensity, aggravating and alleviating factors, and effects of pain on function and quality of life. *Determining location, temporal aspects, pain intensity, characteristics, and the impact of pain on function and quality of life are critical to determine the underlying cause of pain and effectiveness of treatment (Breivik et al, 2008; Ming Wah, 2008). This initial assessment includes all pain information that the client can provide and provides data for the development of the individualized pain management plan. Self-report is considered the single most reliable indicator of pain presence and intensity (APS, 2008).*

- Assess pain level in a client using a valid and reliable self-report pain tool, such as the 0–10 numerical pain rating scale. *The first step in pain assessment is to determine if the client can provide a self-report. Ask the client to rate pain intensity or select descriptors of pain intensity using a valid and reliable self-report pain tool (Breivik et al, 2008; Pasero et al, 2009).* **EB:** *Single-dimension pain ratings are valid and reliable as measures of pain intensity level (Breivik et al, 2008).* **EBN:** *An investigation of nursing attitudes and beliefs about pain assessment revealed that effective use of pain rating scales is often determined by the nurse's personal attitude about its effectiveness (Layman-Young, Horton, & Davidhizar, 2006).*

- Assess the client for pain presence routinely at frequent intervals, often at the same time as vital signs are taken, and during activity and rest. Also assess for pain with interventions or procedures

● = Independent   ▲ = Collaborative   **EBN** = Evidence-Based Nursing   **EB** = Evidence-Based

likely to cause pain. *Pain assessment is as important as physiological vital signs and pain is considered as the "fifth vital sign" (APS, 2008). Acute pain should be reliably assessed both at rest (important for comfort) and during movement (important for function and decreased client risk of cardiopulmonary and thromboembolic events (Breivik et al, 2008).*

- Ask the client to describe prior experiences with pain, effectiveness of pain management interventions, responses to analgesic medications including occurrence of adverse effects, and concerns about pain and its treatment (e.g., fear about addiction, worries, or anxiety) and informational needs. **EBN:** *Obtaining an individualized pain history helps to identify potential factors that may influence the client's willingness to report pain, as well as, factors that may influence pain intensity, the client's response to pain, anxiety, and pharmacokinetics of analgesics (Kalkman et al, 2003; Deane & Smith, 2008; Dunwoody et al, 2008). Pain management regimes must be individualized to the client and consider medical, psychological, and physical condition; age; level of fear or anxiety; surgical procedure; client goals and preference; and previous response to analgesics (Bhavani-Shankar & Oberol, 2009).*

- Ask the client to identify a comfort-function goal, a pain level, on a self-report pain tool, that will allow the client to perform necessary or desired activities easily. This goal will provide the basis to determine effectiveness of pain management interventions. If the client is unable to provide a self-report, it will not be possible to establish a comfort-function goal. *The relationship between pain level and functional goals should be a major focus of the development of individualized pain management plans (Pasero & McCaffery, 2004b). Effective pain relief with function such as mobilization, coughing, and deep breathing is critical for decreasing risk factors for cardiopulmonary and thromboembolic complications after surgery (Breivik et al, 2008). Immobilization also is a major risk factor for chronic hyperalgesic pain after surgery (Stubhaug & Breivik, 2007).*

- Describe the adverse effects of unrelieved pain. **EBN:** *Unrelieved acute pain can have physiological and psychological consequences that facilitate negative client outcomes. Ineffectively managing acute pain has the potential for neurohumoral changes, neuronal remodeling, an impact on immune-function, and long-lasting physiological, psychological, and emotional distress, and may lead to chronic pain syndromes (Brennan, Carr, & Cousins, 2007; Dunwoody et al, 2008; Evans et al, 2009).*

- ▲ If the client is unable to provide a self-report, 1) consider the client's condition and search for possible causes of pain (e.g., presence of tissue injury, pathological conditions, or exposure to procedures/interventions that typically result in pain); 2) observe for behaviors that may indicate pain presence (e.g., facial expressions, crying, restlessness, and changes in activity); 3) evaluate physiological indicators, with the understanding that these are the least sensitive indicators of pain and may be related to conditions other than pain (e.g., shock, hypovolemia, anxiety); and 4) conduct an analgesic trial. *The absence of behaviors thought to be indicative of pain does not necessarily mean that pain is absent (Pasero & McCaffery, 2005).* **EBN:** *Certain behaviors have been shown to be indicative of pain and can be used to assess pain in clients who cannot use a self-report pain tool (e.g., the cognitively impaired client) (Puntillo et al, 2004; Puntillo et al, 2009). However, behaviors vary among individuals, and behavior that may indicate pain in one client may not indicate pain for another. A surrogate who knows the client well may be able to provide information about the underlying painful pathology and behaviors specific to the client that may signal pain (Pasero, 2009a). Pain assessment cannot not be standardized and must take into account cognitive ability, the underlying painful condition or procedure, level of fear or anxiety, and the client ability to provide a self-report (Herr et al, 2006; Pasero et al, 2009).*

- Assume that pain is present if the client is unable to provide a self-report and has tissue injury, a pathological condition, or has undergone a procedure that typically results in pain. *Pain is associated with actual or potential tissue damage such as pathological conditions (e.g., cancer) and procedures (e.g., surgery or trauma, fractures). In the absence of self-report (e.g., anesthetized, critically ill, or cognitively impaired client), the clinician should assume pain is present and implement pain management interventions accordingly (Pasero & McCaffery, 2005; Herr et al, 2006; Pasero, 2009b).*

- ▲ Conduct an analgesic trial for clients who are unable to provide a self-report and have an underlying pathology/condition that is thought to be painful, or who demonstrate behaviors that may indicate pain is present. Administer a nonopioid if pain is thought to be mild and an opioid if pain is thought to be moderate to severe. Reassess the client to evaluate intervention effectiveness within

---

• = Independent   ▲ = Collaborative   **EBN** = Evidence-Based Nursing   **EB** = Evidence-Based

a specific period of time based on pharmacokinetics (intravenous 6–10 minutes; oral 60 minutes; subcutaneous 30 minutes). *For clients who are able to demonstrate behaviors, use a valid and reliable behavioral pain tool (e.g. Critical Care Observation Tool or Checklist of Nonverbal Pain Indicators) to assess behaviors that may indicate pain. If client is unable to demonstrate behaviors (e.g. receiving goal-directed sedation, neuromuscular blocking agent, or is paralyzed) and clinical judgment must be used to evaluate pain presence, behavioral observation tools should not be used, pain should be assumed to be present, and recommended analgesic doses administered (Pasero, 2009b). The purpose of the trial is to help confirm the presence of pain and provide a basis for the development of an individualized pain management plan (Herr et al, 2006; Pasero, 2009a).*

▲ Prevent pain during procedures if possible (e.g. venipuncture, heel punctures, and peripherally inserted intravenous catheters). Use a topical or intravenous local anesthetic as determined by individualized client status and need. *Intravenous catheter placement is one of the most common painful procedures performed in all ages and health care settings, often without anesthetic, despite research demonstrating effectiveness (Valdovinos et al, 2009).* **EBN:** *Topical anesthetic creams can decrease venipuncture and IV insertion pain significantly (Fetzer, 2002; Brown, 2009; Valdovinos et al, 2009).*

• Determine the client's current medication use. Obtain an accurate and complete list of medications the client is taking or has taken. *Accurate medication reconciliation can prevent errors associated with incorrect medications, dosages, omission of components of the home medication regime, drug-drug interactions, and toxicity that can occur when incompatible drugs are combined or when allergies are present. This history will provide the clinician with an understanding of what medications have been tried and were or were not effective in treating the client's pain (APS, 2008; Krenzischek et al, 2008; The Joint Commission, 2009).*

▲ Manage acute pain using a multimodal approach. *Multimodal analgesia combines two or more medications, or methods, from different pharmacological classes that target different mechanisms along the pain pathway, including opioid, nonopioid, and adjuvant analgesics (Pasero, 2003a, 2009a). Specifically, an acute pain multimodal regime may include an opioid, acetaminophen, a nonsteroidal antiinflammatory drug (NSAID), an anticonvulsant, a local anesthetic, or combinations (Pasero, 2007, 2009a). The advantage of this approach is that the lowest effective dose of each drug can be administered, resulting in fewer or less severe adverse effects such as oversedation and respiratory depression (Pasero, 2003a; Parvizi et al, 2007; APS, 2008; Polomano, Rathmall et al, 2008).*

▲ Obtain a prescription to administer an opioid analgesic if indicated, especially for moderate to severe pain. *Opioids are indicated for the treatment of moderate to severe pain (Pasero, 2003a; Goodman et al, 2006; APS, 2008; Krenzischek et al, 2008; Ming Wah, 2008; DeSandre & Quest, 2009).*

▲ Administer opioids orally or intravenously (IV) as ordered. Provide PCA, perineural infusions, and intraspinal analgesia as ordered, when appropriate and available. *The least invasive route of administration capable of providing adequate pain control is recommended. The IV route is preferred for rapid control of severe pain. For constant pain (expected to be present approximately 50% of the day), administer the opioid every 4 hours (based on half-life) around-the-clock (ATC) (DeSandre & Quest, 2009). For intermittent or breakthrough pain, prn dosing is appropriate (Pasero, 2003a; Pasero & McCaffery, 2007; APS, 2008).* **EBN:** *Patient-controlled analgesia was more effective in controlling pain than on-demand IM injections (Chang, Ip, & Cheung, 2004; Bainbridge, Martin, & Cheng, 2006).*

• Avoid giving pain medication intramuscularly (IM). *IM injections are painful, result in unreliable absorption, and lead to variable blood levels of the administered medication (Pasero, 2003a; APS, 2008). Repeated IM injections can cause sterile abscesses and fibrosis of muscle and soft tissue. IM injection also may lead to nerve injury with subsequent chronic neuropathic pain (APS, 2008).* **EBN:** *Patient-controlled analgesia was more effective in controlling pain than on-demand IM injections (Chang, Ip, & Cheung, 2004).*

• Explain to the client the pain management approach, including pharmacological and nonpharmacological interventions, the assessment and reassessment process, potential adverse effects, and the importance of prompt reporting of unrelieved pain. *One of the most important steps toward improved control of pain is a better client understanding of the nature of pain, its treatment, and the role the client needs to play in pain control (APS, 2008).*

• Plan nursing care when the client is comfortable based on pharmacokinetics and the maximum serum concentration (C_{MAX}) of the opioid. *For opioids administered orally, C_{MAX} is approximately 60* *minutes, subcutaneously administered is approximately 30 minutes, and intravenously administered varies from 6 to 10 minutes most transdermal medications become effective in 12–16 hours, with steady state blood levels within 48 hours (APS, 2008; DeSandre & Quest, 2009). Pain diminishes the client's activity. Knowing when the medication becomes effective helps guide nursing practice of checking back on the client, ensuring that adequate pain relief has been obtained, and also planning nursing activities.*

- Discuss the client's fears of under treated pain, overdose, and addiction. *Because of the many misconceptions regarding pain and its treatment, education about the ability to control pain effectively and correction of myths about the use of opioids should be included as part of the treatment plan. Addiction is unlikely when clients use opioids for pain management (McCaffery, Pasero, & Portenoy, 2004; APS, 2008; DeSandre & Quest, 2009).* **EBN:** *Clients often harbor unrealistic anxieties and misconceptions about the use of opioids, risk of addiction, and management of adverse effects (Brennan, Carr, & Cousins, 2007).*

▲ Assess pain level, sedation level, and respiratory status at regular intervals during pain management with opioid administration. Assess sedation and respiratory status at least every 1 to 2 hours during the first 24 hours of opioid therapy, then every 4 hours if respiratory status has been stable without episodes of hypoventilation, and more frequently as determined by individualized client status. Awaken sleeping clients for assessment if the respiratory rate is inadequate, or if respirations are shallow, ineffective, irregular, or noisy (snoring), or periods of apnea occur. Discontinue continuous opioid infusions immediately, and decrease subsequent opioid doses by 25% to 50% if the client develops oversedation (Pasero & McCaffery, 2002; Pasero, 2009b; Pasero et al, 2009). *Life-threatening respiratory depression is the most serious of opioid adverse effects. All clients receiving opioids for pain management are at risk for sedation that may progress to oversedation and lead to clinically significant, opioid-induced respiratory depression. Clients are at the highest risk for opioid-induced respiratory depression during the first 24 hours of therapy, when the dose is increased, the opioid has been changed to a different opioid, or within the first 4 hours of arrival to the nursing care unit from PACU (Lucas, Vlahos, & Ledgerwood, 2007; ASA, 2009; Pasero, 2009b).* **Sedation always precedes opioid-induced respiratory depression (Pasero & McCaffery, 2002).** *Less opioid is required to produce sedation than to produce respiratory depression. Opioid-induced respiratory depression can be prevented by performing systematic sedation assessment and reducing the opioid dose when oversedation is identified (Pasero & McCaffery, 2002; Pasero, 2009b). Sedation scales that are used to assess purposeful, goal-directed sedation are not recommended when the desired client outcome is prevention of sedation (Pasero, 2009). Use a valid and reliable sedation tool that identifies distinct changes in the level of alertness and arousability to prevent oversedation (Nisbet & Mooney-Cotter, 2008; Dempsey et al, 2009; Jarzyna et al, 2009).*

▲ Review the client's pain flowsheet and medication administration record to evaluate effectiveness of pain relief, previous 24–hour opioid requirements, and occurrence of adverse effects. **EBN:** *Systematic tracking of pain was an important factor in improving pain management and making adjustments to the pain management regime (Faries et al, 1991). If pain is constant, a dose of an immediate-release opioid should be administered every 4 hours ATC. If pain remains uncontrolled after 24 hours, increase the routine dose by an amount equal to the total dose of opioid administered during the previous 24 hours, or by 25% to 50% of mild-moderate pain, and 50% to 100% for severe pain (NCI, 2007).*

▲ Administer supplemental opioid doses as ordered to keep the client's pain level at or below the comfort-function goal, or desired outcome if client is unable to provide a self-report based on clinical judgment or behaviors. *An order for prn supplementary opioid doses between regular doses is an essential backup (McCaffery & Pasero, 2003; Pasero & McCaffery, 2004b; APS, 2008).*

▲ Obtain prescriptions to increase or decrease opioid doses as needed; base prescriptions on the client's report of pain severity (clinical judgment of effectiveness if the client is unable to provide a self-report), response to the previous dose in terms of pain relief, occurrence of adverse effects, and ability to perform the activities of recovery or ADLs. *It is important that nurses knowledgeable in pain management have an "as needed" range of opioid doses available to provide appropriate pain relief (Pasero, Manworren, & McCaffery 2007; APS, 2008).*

▲ When the client is able to tolerate oral analgesics, obtain a prescription to change to the oral route; use an equianalgesic chart to determine the initial dose and adjust for incomplete cross tolerance. *The oral route is preferred because it is the most convenient and cost effective (APS, 2008).*

• = Independent ▲ = Collaborative **EBN** = Evidence-Based Nursing **EB** = Evidence-Based

Equianalgesic doses should be used when changing from one opioid or route of administration to help prevent loss of pain control from underdosing and adverse effects from overdosing (McCaffery, 2003).

- In addition to administering analgesics, support the client's use of nonpharmacological methods to help control pain, such as distraction, imagery, relaxation, and application of heat and cold. *Cognitive-behavioral strategies can restore the client's sense of self-control, personal efficacy, and active participation in his or her own care (Lassetter, 2006; APS, 2008).*
- Teach and implement nonpharmacological interventions when pain is relatively well-controlled with pharmacological interventions. *Nonpharmacological interventions should be used to supplement, not replace, pharmacological interventions (APS, 2009).*
- ▲ Ask the client to describe appetite, bowel elimination, and ability to rest and sleep. Administer medications and treatments to improve these functions. Obtain a prescription for a combination stool softener plus peristaltic stimulant to prevent opioid-induced constipation. *Opioid-induced constipation is a common and significant problem in pain management. Prevention and early detection are much easier than management of opioid-induced constipation. Opioids cause constipation by decreasing intestinal motility and reducing mucosal secretions (Friedman & Dello Buono, 2001; Panchal, Muller-Schwefe, & Wurzelmann, 2007). A peripherally acting mu-opioid receptor antagonist reverses opioid-induced constipation without affecting analgesia in clients with advanced-illness (Thomas et al, 2008).*

Pediatric

- As with adults, use nonpharmacological interventions to supplement, not replace, pharmacologic interventions. **EBN:** *Complementary therapies such as relaxation, distraction, hypnotics, art therapies, and imagery may play an important role in holistic pain management (Lassetter, 2006; Golianu et al, 2007; APS, 2008; Bouza, 2009; Lago et al, 2009). Nonpharmacological interventions reduce procedure-related distress (APS, 2008).*
- Use environmental, behavioral, and nonpharmacological interventions for procedures likely to result in pain. *Pharmacological pain management interventions used in combination with environment, behavioral, and nonpharmacological methods have a synergistic effect in reducing procedural pain for neonates (Johnston et al, 2008; Lago et al, 2009).*
- For the neonate, use oral sucrose and nonnutritional sucking (NNS) or human milk for pain of short duration such as heel stick or venipuncture. *Neonates, especially preterm neonates, are more sensitive to pain than older children. Oral sucrose briefly produces analgesia in neonates up to age 6 months of age (Pasero, 2004; Taddio et al, 2008). Oral sucrose and NNS are more effective than EMLA for venipuncture (Stevens, Yamada, & Ohlsson, 2004; Shah, Aliwalas, & Shah, 2006; Lago et al, 2009).*
- Recognize that breastfeeding has been shown to reduce behavioral indicators of pain. *Breastfeeding, however, is not as effective in reducing pain as oral sucrose (Paseroa, 2007a; Codipietro, Ceccarelli, & Ponzone, 2008; Lago et al, 2009).*
- ▲ Use a topical local anesthetic such as EMLA cream or LMX-4 before performing venipuncture in an infant or child. *Venipunctures are a painful and stressful procedure for children (Jimenez et al, 2006). Topical anesthetics are more effective in reducing pain during venipuncture, circumcisions, arterial puncture, and percutaneous venous catheter placement than with heel punctures (Taddio et al, 1998; Lago et al, 2009).*
- ▲ For the neonate experiencing moderate to severe pain, use opioid analgesics and anesthetics in appropriate dosages. *Neonates experiencing endotracheal intubation, chest tube placement, or other procedures causing pain should receive adequate pain medication (Pasero, 2004; Anand, 2007).*
- Assess for pain presence using a valid and reliable pain scale based on age, cognitive development, and the child's ability to provide a self-report. **EB:** *Behavioral observation tools are helpful for pain recognition in neonates, infants, and children less than 4 years of age. Examples of valid and reliable pain tools for neonates, infants, and children include CRIES, COMFORT, FLACC, Faces Pain Scale-Revised (FPS-R), and the Finger Span Scale (Pasero, 2002; Walker, 2008). The CRIES is a behavioral tool that has demonstrated validity and reliability in assessment of postoperative pain in neonates (Krechel & Bildner, 1995). Pain and sedation in infants may be evaluated using the COMFORT tool, which assesses behavioral and physiological indicators (van Dijk et al, 2005). The FLACC scale is an*

evidence-based behavioral tool for pain assessment in infants and children between 2 months and 7 years of age. Self-report tools for children include the FPS-R and Finger Span Scale. The FPS-R is a self-report tool that has demonstrated validity for use in postoperative children ages 4 to 12 (Hicks & Lavender, 2001). It also has demonstrated validity with children ages 4 to 5 years receiving immunizations (Wood et al, 2003). Children are able to quantify pain using self-report tools that correlate pain levels with numbers (e.g. Numerical Rating Scale) or the Visual Analog Scale at 8 years of age (Spragrud, Piira, & Von Baeyer, 2003).

Geriatric

- Please refer to the interventions and rationales in the care plan for **Chronic Pain**.

Multicultural

- Assess for the influence of cultural beliefs, norms, and values on the client's perception and experience of pain. **EB:** *Native American clients may think that asking for pain medication is disrespectful because it implies that health care providers do not know what they are doing (Brant, 2001; Green et al, 2003). A study of African American elders found the use of prayer or faith for pain management, care, and prevention was very common (Green et al, 2003; Ibrahim et al, 2004). The Representational Intervention to Decrease Cancer Pain (RID) offers a flexible framework for nurses to help cancer clients delve deeply into their own belief systems about health, disease, pain, and so on, and to add sound concepts that will work for their pain management (Ward et al, 2008).*
- Assess for the effect of fatalism on the client's beliefs regarding the current state of comfort. **EBN:** *Fatalistic perspectives, which involve the belief that one cannot control one's own fate, may influence health behaviors in some African American and Latino populations (Ward et al, 2008).*
- Assess for pain disparities among racial and ethnic minorities. **EB:** *Racial and ethnic minorities tend to be undertreated for pain when compared with non-Hispanic whites (Green et al, 2003).* **EBN:** *Persons from various ethnic and cultural groups vary in their affective response to pain, requests for pain medication, tolerance to pain, and physiological reaction to pain medication (Davidhizar & Giger, 2004; Giger & Davidhizar, 2008.)*
- Incorporate safe and effective folk health care practices and beliefs into care whenever possible. *It is the responsibility of the caregiver to ensure that safe and effective pain management is provided. Although support of an individual's health care beliefs is recommended, when research does not support the safety or effectiveness of a method or when research does not exist, this should be explained fully to the client (McCaffery, 2002).* **EBN:** *Incorporating folk health care beliefs and practices into pain management care increased compliance with the treatment plan (Juarez, Ferrell, & Borneman, 1998).*
- Use a family-centered approach to care. **EBN:** *Involving the family in pain management care increased compliance with the treatment regimen (Juarez, Ferrell, & Borneman, 1998).*
- Teach information about pain medications and their side effects and how to work with health care providers to manage pain, and encourage use of religious faith as desired to cope with pain. **EB:** *Socioeconomically disadvantaged African American and Hispanic clients benefit from educational interventions on pain that dispel myths about opioids and teach clients to communicate assertively about their pain with their physicians and nurses (Anderson et al, 2002).*
- Use culturally relevant pain scales to assess pain in the client. **EBN:** *Clients from minority cultures may express pain differently than clients from the majority culture. The Faces Pain Scale-Revised was shown to be preferred over other self-report pain rating tools in older minority adults (Jowers-Ware, 2006). The Oucher Scale is available in African American and Hispanic versions and is used to assess pain in children (Beyer et al, 2003). A variety of pain assessment instruments are available for use with varying cultural and ethnic groups but tools must be evaluated for reliability and validity for and across cultures (Davidhizar & Giger, 2004).*
- Ensure that directions for medication use are available in the client's language of choice and are understood by the client and caregiver. **EB:** *Use of bilingual instructions for medication administration increased compliance with the pain management plan (Juarez, Ferrell, & Borneman, 1998). Using*

• = Independent   ▲ = Collaborative   **EBN** = Evidence-Based Nursing   **EB** = Evidence-Based

specific phrases in Spanish to assess acute pain in non–English-speaking Hispanic clients helps provide timely pain assessment and management (Collins, Gullette, & Schnepf, 2004).

Home Care

- Develop the treatment plan with the client and caregivers. *Client input into the plan of care improves the likelihood of successful management.*
- ▲ Develop a full medication profile, including medications prescribed by all physicians and all over-the-counter medications. Assess for drug interactions. Instruct the client to refrain from mixing medications without physician approval. *Pain medications may significantly affect or be affected by other medications and may cause severe side effects. Some combinations of drugs are specifically contraindicated (Pasero, 2003a; APS, 2008).*
- Assess the client's and family's knowledge of side effects and safety precautions associated with pain medications (e.g., use caution in operating machinery when opioids are first taken or dosage has been increased significantly). *The cognitive effects of opioids usually subside within a week of initial dosing or dosage increases. The use of long-term opioid treatment does not appear to affect neuropsychological performance.* **EB:** *Pain itself may reduce performance on neuropsychological tests more than oral opioid treatment (Sjogren et al, 2000).*
- ▲ If medication is administered using highly technological methods, assess the home for the necessary resources (e.g., electricity) and ensure that there will be responsible caregivers available to assist the client with administration.
- Assess the knowledge base of the client and family with regard to highly technological medication administration. Teach as necessary. Be sure the client knows when, how, and whom to contact if analgesia is unsatisfactory.

Client/Family Teaching and Discharge Planning

NOTE: To avoid the negative connotations associated with the words *drugs* and *narcotics,* use the term *pain medicine* when teaching clients.

- Provide written materials on pain control such as *Understanding Your Pain: Using a Pain Rating Scale* (McCaffery, Pasero, & Portenoy, 2001) (see instructions on the use of pain rating scales) and *Taking Oral Opioid Analgesics* (McCaffery, Pasero, & Portenoy, 2004).
- Discuss the various discomforts encompassed by the word *pain* and ask the client to give examples of previously experienced pain. Explain the pain assessment process and the purpose of the pain rating scale. *It is often difficult for clients to understand the concept of pain and describe their pain experience. Using alternative words and providing a complete description of the assessment process, including the use of scales, will ensure that an accurate treatment plan is developed (McCaffery, Pasero, & Portenoy, 2001).*
- Teach the client to use the self-report pain tool to rate the intensity of past or current pain. Ask the client to set a comfort-function goal by selecting a pain level on the self-report tool that makes it easy to perform desired or necessary activities of recovery easily (e.g., turn, cough, deep breathe, ambulate). If the pain level is above the comfort-function goal, the client should take action that decreases pain or notify a member of the health care team so that effective pain management interventions may be implemented promptly. (See information on teaching clients to use the pain rating scale.) *The use of comfort-function goals provides direction for the treatment plan. Changes are made according to the client's response and achievement of the goals of recovery or rehabilitation (Pasero & McCaffery, 2004b).*
- ▲ Demonstrate medication administration and the use of supplies and equipment. If PCA is ordered, determine the client's ability to press the appropriate button. Remind the client and staff that the PCA button is for client use only.
- Reinforce the importance of taking pain medications to maintain the comfort-function goal. *Teaching clients to stay on top of their pain and prevent it from getting out of control will improve the ability to accomplish the goals of recovery (Pasero & McCaffery, 2004b).*
- Reinforce that taking opioids for pain relief is not addiction and that addiction is very unlikely to occur. *The development of addiction when opioids are taken for pain relief is rare (APS, 2008).*

● = Independent   ▲ = Collaborative   **EBN** = Evidence-Based Nursing   **EB** = Evidence-Based

- Demonstrate the use of appropriate nonpharmacological approaches in addition to pharmacological approaches for helping to control pain, such as application of heat and/or cold, distraction techniques, relaxation breathing, visualization, rocking, stroking, music listening, and television watching. *Nonpharmacological interventions are used to complement, not replace, pharmacological interventions (APS, 2008).*

Ⓔvolve   See the EVOLVE website for Weblinks for client education resources.

REFERENCES

The American Pain Society (APS): *Principles of analgesic use in acute and chronic pain,* ed 6, Glenview, IL, 2008, The Society.

The American Pain Society (APS): Pain: current understanding of assessment, management and treatments, 2009. www. ampainsoc.org/ce/enduring.htm. Accessed July 6, 2009.

American Society of Anesthesiologists (ASA): Practice guidelines for the prevention, detection, and management of respiratory depression associated with neuraxial opioid administration, *Anesthesiology* 110:218–230, 2009.

Anand KJ: Pharmacological approaches to the management of pain in the neonatal intensive care unit, *J Perinatol* 27:S4–S11, 2007.

Anderson KO, Richman SP, Hurley J et al: Cancer pain management among underserved minority outpatients: perceived needs and barriers to optimal control, *Cancer* 94(8):2295–2304, 2002.

Bainbridge D, Martin JE, Cheng DC: Patient-controlled versus nurse-controlled analgesia after cardiac surgery—a meta-analysis, *Can J Anaesth* 53(5):492–499, 2006.

Beyer J, Turner S, Jones L et al: The Alternate Forms Reliability of the Oucher Pain Scale, *Pain Manage Nurs* 6(1):10–17, 2003.

Bhavani-Shankar K, Oberol JS: Management of postoperative pain; "Uptodate" version June 19, 2009; accessed July 2009. www.uptodate.com/patients/content/topic.do?topicKey=~9TD93y2rpud9.

Bjoro K, Herr K: Assessment of pain in the nonverbal or cognitively impaired older adult, *Clin Geriatr Med* 24:237, 2008.

Bouza H: The impact of pain in the immature brain, *J Matern Fetal Neonatal Med* 11:1–11, 2009.

Brant JM: *Cultural implications of pain education, a Native American example.* Presented at Cancer Pain and Education for Patients and the Public conference, City of Hope National Medical Center, Duarte, CA, October 18, 2001.

Breivik H, Borchgrevink PC, Allen SM et al: Assessment of pain, *Br J Anaesth* 101(1):17–24, 2008.

Brennan F, Carr DB, Cousins M: Pain management: a fundamental human right, *Anesth Analg* 105(1):205–211, 2007.

Chang AM, Ip WY, Cheung TH: Patient-controlled analgesia versus conventional intramuscular injection: a cost effectiveness analysis, *J Adv Nurs* 46(5):531, 2004.

Collins AS, Gullette D, Schnepf M: Break through language barriers, *Nurs Manag* 35(8):34–36, 2004.

Codipietro L, Ceccarelli M, Ponzone A: Breastfeeding or oral sucrose solution in term neonates receiving heel lance: a randomized, controlled trial, *Pediatrics* 122(3):e716–721, 2008.

Davidhizar R, Giger J: A nursing review of the literature on pain and culture, *Int Nurs Rev* 51(1):42–54, 2004.

Deane G, Smith HS: Overview of pain management in older persons, *Clin Geriatr Med* 24:185–201, 2008.

Dempsey SJ, Davidson J, Cahill D et al: *Selection of a sedation assessment scale for clinical practice: Inter-rater reliability, ease of use, and applicability of the Richmond-Agitation-Sedation Scale and Pasero Opioid-Induced Sedation Scale,* Poster presentation, National Association of Orthopedic Nurses Congress, Tampa, FL, May 6–10, 2009.

DeSandre PL, Quest TE: Management of cancer-related pain, *Emerg Med Clin N Am* 27:179–194, 2009.

Dunwoody CF, Krenzischek DA, Pasero C et al: Assessment, physiological monitoring, and consequences of inadequately treated pain, *J Perianesth Nurs* 23(1A):S15–S27, 2008.

Erstad BL, Puntillo K, Gilbert HC et al: Pain management principles in the critically ill, *Chest* 135(4):1075–7086, 2009.

Evans C, Galustian C, Kumar D et al: Impact of surgery on immunologic function: comparison between minimally invasive techniques and conventional laparotomy for surgical resection of colorectal tumors, *Am J Surg* 197:238–245, 2009.

Faries JE, Mills DS, Goldsmith KW et al: Systematic pain records and their impact on pain control, *Cancer Nurs* 14(6):306, 1991.

Fein JA, Gorelick MH: The decision to use topical anesthetic for intravenous insertion in the pediatric emergency department, *Acad Emerg Med* 13:264–268, 2006.

Fetzer SJ: Reducing venipuncture and intravenous insertion pain with eutectic mixture of local anesthetic: a meta-analysis, *Nurs Res* 51(2):119–124, 2002.

Friedman JD, Dello Buono FA: Opioid antagonists in the treatment of opioid-induced constipation and pruritus, *Ann Pharmacother* 35(1):85–91, 2001.

Giger J, Davidhizar R: *Transcultural assessment: assessment and intervention,* St Louis, 2008, Mosby.

Golianu B, Krane E, Seyboid J et al: Non-pharmcological techniques for pain management in neonates, *Semin Perinatol* 31(5):318–322, 2007.

Goodman LS, Gilman A, Brunton LL et al: *Goodman and Gilman's the pharmacological basis of therapeutics,* ed 11, New York, 2006, McGraw-Hill.

Green CR, Anderson KO, Baker TA et al: The unequal burden of pain: confronting racial and ethnic disparities in pain, *Pain Med* 4(3):277–294, 2003.

Harbuz MS, Chover-Gonzalea AJ, Jessop DS: Hypothalamo-pituitary-adrenal axis and chronic immune activation, *Ann NY Acad Sci* 992:99–106, 2003.

Harmon MP, Castro FG, Coe K: Acculturation and cervical cancer: knowledge, beliefs, and behaviors of Hispanic women, *Women Health* 24(3):37, 1996.

Harris T, Cameron, PA, Ugoni A: The use of pre-cannulation local anesthetic and factors affecting pain perception in the emergency department setting, *Emerg Med J* 18:175–177, 2001.

Herr K, Coyne P, McCaffery M et al: Pain assessment in the nonverbal patient: position statement with clinical recommendations, *Pain Manage Nurs* 7(2):44–52, 2006.

Hicks MD, Lavender R: Psychosocial practice trends in pediatric oncology, *J Pediatr Oncol Nurs* 18(4):143–153, 2001.

Hughes E: Principles of post-operative patient care, *Nurs Stand* 19:22–29, 2004.

Hurley RW, Cohen SP, Williams KA: The analgesic effects of perioperative gabapentin on postoperative pain: a meta-analysis, *Reg Anesth Pain Med* 31(3):237–247, 2006.

● = Independent   ▲ = Collaborative   **EBN** = Evidence-Based Nursing   **EB** = Evidence-Based

Ibrahim SA, Zhang A, Mercer MB et al: Inner city African-American elderly patients' perceptions and preferences for the care of chronic knee and hip pain: findings from focus groups, *J Gerontol Series A Biol Sci Med Sci* 59(12):1318–1322, 2004.

International Association for the Study of Pain: Pain terms: a list with definitions and notes on usage, *Pain* 6(3):249–252, 1979.

Jarzyna D, Pasero C, Junquist C et al: *Expert consensus panel for monitoring of opioid-induced sedation and respiratory depression: summary report and findings*, Oral Presentation, ASPMN annual meeting, Tampa, FL, September 11–15, 2009.

Jessop DS, Richards LJ, Harbuz MS: Effects of stress on inflammatory autoimmune disease: destructive or protective, *Stress* 7:261–266, 2004.

Jimenez J, Bradford H, Seidel KD et al: A comparison of a needle-free injection system for local anesthesia versus EMLA for intravenous catheter insertion in the pediatric patient, *Anesth Analg* 102:411–414, 2006.

Johnston CC, Filion F, Campbell-Yeo M et al: Kangaroo mother care diminishes pain from heel lance in very preterm neonates: a crossover trial, *BMC Pediatr* 8:13, 2008.

Joint Commission: *Hospital accreditation standards,* Oakbrook Terrace, IL, 2009, The Joint Commission.

Jowers Ware et al: Evaluation of the revised faces pain scale, verbal descriptor scale, numeric rating scale, and Iowa pain thermometer in older minority adults, *Pain Manag Nurs* 7(3):117–125, 2006.

Juarez G, Ferrell BR, Borneman T: Influence of culture on cancer pain management in Hispanic clients, *Cancer Pract* 6(5):262, 1998.

Kalkman CJ, Visser K, Moen J et al: Preoperative predication of severe postoperative pain, *Pain* 57:415–423, 2003.

Kleiber C, Sorenson M, Whiteside K et al: Topical anesthetics for intravenous insertion in children: a randomized equivalency study, *Pediatrics* 110:758–761, 2002.

Krechel SW, Bildner J: CRIES: a new neonatal postoperative pain measurement score. Initial testing of validity and reliability, *Paediatr Anaesth* 5(1):53–61, 1995.

Krenzischek DA, Dunwoody CJ, Polomano RC et al: Pharmacotherapy for acute pain: implications for practice, *J Perianesth Nurs* 23(1A):528–542, 2008.

Lago P, Garetti E, Merazzi D et al: Guidelines for procedural pain in the newborn, *Acta Paediatrica* 98(6):932–939, 2009.

Lassetter JH: The effectiveness of complementary therapies on the pain experience of hospitalized children, *J Holist Nurs* 24(3):196–211, 2006.

Layman-Young J, Horton F, Davidhizar R: Nursing attitudes and beliefs in pain assessment and management, *J Adv Nurs* 53(4):412–421, 2006.

Lemyre B, Hogan DL, Gaboury I et al: How effective is tetracaine 4% gel, before a venipuncture, in reducing procedural pain in infants: a randomized double-blind placebo controlled trail, *BMC Pediatr* 7:7, 2007.

Lucas CE, Vlahos AL, Ledgerwood AM: Kindness kills: the negative impact of pain as the fifth vital sign, *J Am Coll Surg* 205:101–107, 2007.

McCaffery M: *Nursing practice theories related to cognition, bodily pain, and man-environment interactions,* Los Angeles, 1968, University of California at Los Angeles Students' Store.

McCaffery M: What is the role of nondrug methods in the nursing care of patients with acute pain? *Pain Manage Nurs* 3(3):77–80, 2002.

McCaffery M: Switching from IV to PO, *Am J Nurs* 103(5):62–63, 2003.

McCaffery M, Pasero C: Pain control: breakthrough pain, *Am J Nurs* 103(4):83, 2003.

McCaffery M, Pasero C, Portenoy RK: *Understanding your pain: using a pain rating scale,* Chadds Ford, PA, 2001, Endo Pharmaceuticals.

McCaffery M, Pasero C, Portenoy RK: *Understanding your pain: taking oral opioid analgesics,* Chadds Ford, PA, 2004, Endo Pharmaceuticals.

Ming Wah IJ: Pain management in the hospitalized patient, *Med Clin N Am* 92:371–385, 2008.

National Cancer Institute (NCI): Education in palliative and end-of-life care for oncology (EPEC-O), Bethesda, MD, 2007, U.S. Department of Health and Human Services.

Nisbet A, Mooney-Cotter M: *Post opioid sedation scales. Validity, reliability, accuracy, and performance in adult non-critical care settings.* Poster presentation, ASPMN National Meeting, Tucson, AZ, September 4–6, 2008.

Panchal SJ, Muller-Schwefe P, Wurzelmann I: Opioid-induced bowel dysfunction: prevalence, pathophysiology and burden, *Int J Clin Pract* 61:1181–1187, 2007.

Parvizi J, Reines D, Steege J et al: CSI: investigating acute postoperative pain: improving outcomes and clinical horizons, 2007. www.com/viewarticle/549349_1. Accessed July 6, 2009.

Pasero C: Pain control: pain assessment in infants and children: neonates, *Am J Nurs* 102(8):61–64, 2002.

Pasero C: Multimodal balanced analgesia in the PACU, *J Perianesth Nurs* 18(4):265–268, 2003a.

Pasero C: No self-report means no pain-intensity rating, *Am J Nurs* 105(10): 50–53, 2005.

Pasero C: Breastfeeding may reduce neonatal procedural pain, *Am J Nurs* 107(4):30, 2007.

Pasero C: Challenges in pain assessment, *J Perianesth Nurs* 24(1):50–54, 2009a.

Pasero C: Assessment of sedation during opioid administration for pain management, *J Perianesth Nurs,* 24(3):186–190, 2009b.

Pasero C, Manworren RCB, McCaffery M: IV Opioid range orders, *Am J Nurs* 107(2):52–59, 2007.

Pasero C, McCaffery M: Pain control: patient's report of pain, *Am J Nurs* 101(12):73, 2001.

Pasero C, McCaffery M: Using the 0–10 pain rating scale, *Am J Nurs* 101(12):81–82, 2001b.

Pasero C, McCaffery M: Monitoring opioid-induced sedation, *Am J Nurs* 102(2):67–68, 2002.

Pasero C, McCaffery M: Pain control: controlled-release oxycodone, *Am J Nurs* 104(1):30, 2004a.

Pasero C, McCaffery M: Comfort-function goals: a way to establish accountability for pain relief, *Am J Nurs* 104(9):77–78, 2004b.

Pasero C, McCaffery M: No self report means no pain intensity, *Am J Nurs* 105(10):50–53, 2005.

Pasero C, McCaffery M: Orthopedic postoperative pain management, *J Perianesth Nurs* 22(4):160–172, 2007.

Polomano RC, Dunwoody CJ, Krenzischek DA et al: Perspective on pain management in the 21st century, *Pain Manage Nurs* 9(1):S3–S10, 2008.

Polomano RC, Rathmell JP, Krenzischek DA et al: Emerging trends and new approaches to acute pain, *Pain Manage Nurs* 9(Suppl 1):33–41, 2008.

Puntillo K, Morris A, Thompson C et al: Pain behaviors observed ruing six common procedures: result from Thunder Project II, *Crit Care Med* 32:421–427, 2004.

Puntillo K, Pasero C, Li D et al: Evaluation of pain in ICU patients, *Chest* 135(4):1069–1074, 2009.

Shah PL, Aliwalas LI, Shah V: Breastfeeding or breast milk for procedural pain in neonates, *Cochrane Data Base Syst Rev* 326:13–19, 2006.

Sjogren P, Olsen AK, Thomsen AB et al: Neuropsychological performance in cancer clients: the role of opioids, pain and performance status, *Pain* 86(3):237, 2000.

Spagrud LJ, Piira T, Von Baeyer CL: Children's self-report of pain intensity, *Am J Nurs* 103(12):62–64, 2003.

● = Independent ▲ = Collaborative **EBN** = Evidence-Based Nursing **EB** = Evidence-Based

Stevens B, Yamada J, Ohlsson A: Sucrose for analgesia in newborn infants undergoing painful procedures, *Cochrane Database Syst Rev* (3):CD001069, 2004.

Stubhaug A, Breivik H: Prevention and treatment of hyperalgesia and persistent pain after surgery. In Brevik H, Shipley M, editors: *Pain, best practice and research compendium*, London, 2007, Elsevier.

Taddio A, Ohlsson A, Einarson TR et al: A systematic review of lidocaine-prilocaine cream (EMLA) in the treatment of acute pain in neonates, *Pediatrics* 101(2):E1–9, 1998.

Taddio A, Shah B, Hancock R et al: Effectiveness of sucrose analgesia in newborns undergoing painful medical procedures, *CMAJ* 179:37–43, 2008.

Thomas J, Karver S, Cooney GA et al: Methylnaltrexone for opioid-induced constipation in advanced illness, *N Engl J Med* 358(22):2332–2343, 2008.

Valdovinos NC, Reddin C, Bernard C et al: The use of topical anesthesia during intravenous catheter insertion in adults: a comparison of pain scores using LMX-4 versus placebo, *J Emerg Nurs* 35(4):299–304, 2009.

van Dijk M, Peters WB, van Deventer, P, Tibboel D: The COMFORT Behavior Scale: a tool for assessing pain and sedation in infants, *Am J Nurs* 105(1):33–36, 2005.

Walker SM: Pain in children: recent advances and ongoing challenges, *Br J Anaesth* 101(1):101–110, 2008.

Ward S, Donovan H, Gunnarsdottir S et al: Randomized trial of a Representational Intervention to Decrease Cancer Pain (RID) *Health Psychol* 27(1):59–67, 2008.

Wood C, von Baeyer CL, Bourrillon A et al: *Self-assessment by the Faces Pain Scale: revised of immediate post-vaccination pain following administration of Priorix versus MMRII as a second dose in 4 to 6 year old children*, Poster, Sixth International Symposium on Pediatric Pain, Sydney, 2003, Special Interest Group on Pain in Childhood, International Association for the Study of Pain.

Chronic Pain   Susan J. Dempsey, MN, CNS, RN-BC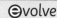

NANDA-I

Definition

Unpleasant sensory and emotional experience arising from actual or potential tissue damage or described in terms of such damage (International Association for the Study of Pain, 1979); sudden or slow onset of any intensity from mild to severe, constant or recurring without an anticipated or predictable end and a duration of >6 months

Pain is whatever the experiencing person says it is, existing whenever the person says it does (McCaffery, 1968; APS, 2008)

Defining Characteristics

Pain is a subjective experience and its presence cannot be proved or disproved. Self-report is the most reliable method of evaluating pain presence and intensity (APS, 2008). Please refer to the Defining Characteristics in the **Acute Pain** care plan for further characteristics of pain

Related Factors (r/t)

Actual or potential tissue damage; tumor progression and related pathology; diagnostic and therapeutic procedures; central or peripheral nerve injury (neuropathic pain)

NOTE: The cause of chronic nonmalignant pain may be unknown because pain study is a new science and an area encompassing diverse types of problems.

NOC   (Nursing Outcomes Classification)

Suggested NOC Outcomes

Comfort Level, Pain Control, Pain: Disruptive Effects, Pain Level

Example **NOC** Outcome with Indicators
Pain Level as evidenced by the following indicators: Reported pain/Length of pain episodes/Moaning and crying/Facial expressions of pain (Rate the outcome and indicators of **Pain Level:** 1 = severe, 2 = substantial, 3 = moderate, 4 = mild, 5 = none ([see Section I.]))

Client Outcomes

Client Will (Specify Time Frame):

For the client who is able to provide a self-report:

- Use a self-report pain tool to identify current pain level and establish a comfort-function goal

---

• = Independent   ▲ = Collaborative   **EBN** = Evidence-Based Nursing   **EB** = Evidence-Based

- Report that the pain management regimen achieves comfort-function goal without the occurrence of adverse effects
- Describe nonpharmacological methods that can be used to supplement, or enhance, pharmacological interventions and help achieve the comfort-function goal
- Perform necessary or desired activities at a pain level less than or equal to the Comfort-Function Goal
- Demonstrate the ability to pace activity, taking rest breaks before they are needed
- Describe how unrelieved pain will be managed
- State the ability to obtain sufficient amounts of rest and sleep
- Notify a member of the health care team promptly for pain level greater than the comfort-function goal or occurrence of adverse effect

For the client who is unable to provide a self-report:
- Demonstrate decrease or resolved pain-related behaviors
- Perform desired activities as determined by client condition
- Demonstrate the absence of adverse effects

(Nursing Interventions Classification)

Suggested NIC Interventions

Analgesic Administration, Pain Management

Example NIC Activities—Pain Management
Assure that the client receives attentive analgesic care; Perform comprehensive assessment of pain, including location, characteristics, onset and duration, frequency, quality, intensity or severity, and precipitating factors

Nursing Interventions and *Rationales*

▲ Determine if the client is experiencing pain at the time of the initial interview. If pain is present, conduct and document a comprehensive pain assessment and implement pain management interventions to achieve comfort. Components of this initial assessment include: location, quality/characteristics, onset/duration, temporal aspects, intensity, aggravating and alleviating factors, and impact of pain on function and quality of life. *Determining location, quality/characteristics, onset/ duration, temporal aspects, pain intensity, aggravating and alleviating factors, and the impact of pain on function and quality of life are critical to determine the underlying cause of pain and effectiveness of treatment (Breivik et al, 2008; Ming Wah, 2008). Additionally, a comprehensive initial assessment may reveal a new acute pain etiology rather than exacerbation of persistent pain (AGS, 2009). Self-report is considered the single most reliable indicator of pain presence and intensity (APS, 2008).*

- Assess the pain level in a client using a valid and reliable self-report pain tool. *The first step in pain assessment is to determine if the client can provide a self-report (Herr et al, 2006).* **EB:** *Single-dimension pain ratings are valid and reliable as measures of pain intensity level (Breivik et al, 2008).* **EBN:** *An investigation of nursing attitudes and beliefs about pain assessment revealed that effective use of pain rating scales is often determined by the nurse's personal attitude about its effectiveness (Layman-Young, Horton, & Davidhizar, 2006).*

- Assess the client for pain presence routinely at frequent intervals, often at the same time as vital signs are taken, and during activity and rest. *Pain assessment is as important as physiological vital signs and pain is considered as the "fifth vital sign" (APS, 2008). Routine monitoring of the effects of the pain management regime results in improved pain management and decreased risk of adverse effects.*

- Assess pain location, characteristics, intensity with every report of pain. *Pain should be assessed both at rest (important for comfort) and during movement (important for function) and decreased client risk of cardiopulmonary and thromboembolic events (Breivik et al, 2008). Regular assessment of clients is critical as changes in the underlying pain condition, presence of comorbidities, and changes in psychosocial circumstances can impact pain intensity and characteristics and require revision of the pain management plan (Chou et al, 2009).*

- Ask the client to identify the pain level, on a self-report pain tool, that will allow the client to perform desired activities and achieve an acceptable quality of life. This comfort-function goal will provide the basis to determine effectiveness of the individualized pain management plan. If the client is unable to provide a self-report, it will not be possible to establish a comfort-function goal. *Comfort-function goals should be established for managing pain to a level that allows improved function (e.g., performance of desired activities), decreased psychosocial suffering, and achievement of an acceptable quality of life (AGS, 2009).*
- Ask the client to describe prior experiences with pain, effectiveness of pain management interventions, responses to analgesic medications including occurrence of adverse effects, concerns about pain and its treatment (e.g., fear about addiction, worries, or anxiety) and informational needs. **EBN:** *The client's history provides important initial information. This information helps to identify possible causes of pain; concerns that may influence the willingness to report pain, factors that may influence pain intensity, response to pain, anxiety, pharmacokinetics of analgesics, and compliance with the pain management plan (Deane & Smith, 2008; Dunwoody et al, 2008). Pain management regimes must be individualized to the client and consider medical, psychological, and physical condition; age; level of fear or anxiety; client goals and preference; and previous response to analgesics (Bhavani-Shankar & Oberol, 2009).*
- Describe the adverse effects of persistent unrelieved pain. **EBN:** *Pain can have physiological and psychological consequences that facilitate negative client outcomes. Unrelieved pain can result in suppressed immune function, which can lead to infection, increased tumor growth, and other complications (Brennan, Carr, & Cousins, 2007; Dunwoody et al, 2008; Evans et al, 2009; Herr & Titler, 2009). Clients with persistent pain, or its inadequate treatment, often experience functional impairment, depression, anxiety, decreased socialization, sleep disturbances, disruption in relationships (work, family, social) and decreased quality of life (McDermott et al, 2006; Smith et al, 2007; Closs et al, 2008).*
- Ask the client to maintain a diary (if able) of pain ratings, timing, precipitating events, medications, and effectiveness of pain management interventions. **EBN:** *Systematic tracking of pain has been demonstrated to be an important factor in improving pain management (Schumacher et al, 2002; Hager & Brockopp, 2009).*
- ▲ If the client is unable to provide a self-report, use the Hierarchy of Importance of Pain Measures to determine the method to recognize or detect pain. 1) Attempt to obtain self-report; 2) consider the client's condition and search for possible causes of pain (e.g., presence of tissue injury, pathological conditions, or exposure to procedures/interventions that typically result in pain); 3) observe for behaviors that may indicate pain presence (e.g., facial expressions, crying, restlessness, and changes in activity); 4) evaluate physiological indicators, with the understanding that these are the least sensitive indicators of pain presence and may be related to conditions other than pain (e.g., shock, hypovolemia, anxiety); and 5) conduct an analgesic trial. *The absence of behaviors thought to be indicative of pain does not necessarily mean that pain is absent (Pasero & McCaffery, 2005).* **EBN:** *Certain behaviors have been shown to be indicative of pain and can be used to assess pain in clients who cannot use a self-report pain tool (e.g., the cognitively impaired client) (Puntillo et al, 2004, 2009). However, behaviors vary among individuals, and behavior that may indicate pain in one client may not indicate pain for another. A surrogate who knows the client well may be able to provide information about the underlying painful pathology and behaviors specific to the client that may signal pain (Pasero, 2009). Pain assessment cannot not be standardized and must take into account cognitive ability, the underlying painful condition or procedure, level of fear or anxiety, and the client's ability to provide a self-report (Herr et al, 2006; Pasero, 2009a).*
- Assume that pain is present if the client is unable to provide a self-report and has tissue injury, a pathological condition, or has undergone a procedure or intervention that typically results in pain. *Pain is associated with actual or potential tissue damage such as pathological conditions (e.g., cancer, fractures) and procedures (e.g., surgery or trauma). In the absence of self-report (e.g., anesthetized, critically ill, or cognitively impaired client), the clinician should assume pain is present and implement pain management interventions accordingly (Pasero & McCaffery, 2005; Herr et al, 2006; Pasero, 2009a).*
- Determine the client's current medication use. *Obtain an accurate and complete list of medications the client is taking or has taken. Accurate medication reconciliation can prevent withdrawal and errors associated with incorrect medications, dosages, omission of components of the home medication regime,*

drug-drug interactions, and toxicity that can occur when incompatible drugs are combined or when allergies are present. As history will provide the clinician with an understanding of what medications have been tried and were, or were not, effective in treating the client's pain (APS, 2008; Krenzischek, 2008; The Joint Commission (TJC), 2009).

▲ Manage persistent or chronic pain using a multimodal approach. *The most effective treatment for all pain is a multimodal and balanced approach that combines both pharmacologic and nonpharmacologic strategies (Gordon et al, 2004). Multimodal analgesia combines two or more medications, or methods, from different pharmacological classes that target different mechanisms along the pain pathway. This approach for chronic pain may include an opioid, nonopioid, and adjuvant (Pasero, 2003a; 2009a). Specifically, an acute pain multimodal regime may include an opioid, acetaminophen, a nonsteroidal antiinflammatory drug (NSAID), an anticonvulsant, a local anesthetic, or combinations (Pasero & McCaffery, 2007; Pasero, 2009a). The value of this physiological approach is that the lowest effective dose of each drug can be administered, resulting in fewer or fewer or less severe adverse effects such as oversedation and opioid-induced respiratory depression and more effective pain management (Pasero, 2003a; Pasero & McCaffery, 2007; APS, 2008; Fanelli, Berti, & Baciarello, 2008; Polomano et al, 2008).*

▲ Recognize that the oral route is preferred for pain management interventions. If the client is receiving parenteral analgesia, use an equianalgesic chart to convert to a controlled release, long-acting oral medication as soon as possible (McCaffery, 2003a; NCI, 2007). *The least invasive route of administration capable of providing adequate pain control is recommended. The oral route is always the preferred route because of its convenience and the relatively steady blood levels that can result (AGS, 2009). The intravenous route provides the most rapid time to peak serum concentration (6–10 minutes) and is preferred for rapid control of severe pain (NCI, 2007; AGS, 2009).*

▲ Avoid giving pain medication intramuscularly (IM). *Please refer to the care plan on **Acute Pain** for rationales on why not to utilize IM injections.*

▲ Recognize that opioid therapy may be indicated for clients experiencing chronic (persistent) pain which is unrelieved with nonopioids. *For clients who are opioid-naïve, initiate opioid therapy at a low dose and titrate slowly, to decrease the risk of opioid-induced adverse effects such as oversedation or opioid-induced respiratory depression. Some clients, such as frail older persons or those with comorbidities, require extreme cautious initiation and titration of opioid therapy. Immediate release opioids are safer for initial therapy related to a shorter half-life and may be associated with a lower risk of adverse effects related to overdose. Initiation of opioid therapy with immediate release opioids administered around-the-clock (ATC) followed by conversion to long-acting opioids may be beneficial for more consistent pain control and increased adherence to the pain management plan (Chou et al, 2009).*

▲ Administer supplemental opioid doses for breakthrough pain as needed to keep pain ratings at or below the comfort-function goal (Pasero & McCaffery, 2004b). *Please refer to the care plan on **Acute Pain** for rationales on use of opioids for breakthrough pain.*

▲ Ask the client to describe appetite, bowel elimination, and ability to rest and sleep. Administer medications and treatments to improve these functions. Obtain a prescription for a combination stool softener plus peristaltic stimulant to prevent opioid-induced constipation. *Opioid-induced constipation is a common and significant problem in pain management. Prevention and early detection are much easier than management of opioid-induced constipation. Opioids cause constipation by interrupting rhythmic contractions required for intestinal motility, reducing mucosal secretions, decreasing GI transit by inhibiting gastric emptying and slowing small and large bowel transit due to activation of mu opioid receptors located in the GI tract (Friedman & Dello Buono, 2001; Panchal, Muller-Schwefe, & Wurzelmann, 2007). Stool softeners alone are ineffective to prevent opioid-induced constipation. The client should be started on a combination of a stool softener plus stimulant laxative when the opioid is prescribed. Titrate doses to effect and add osmotic laxatives and enemas as needed (Furlan et al, 2006; NCI, 2007; Panchal, Muller-Schwefe, & Wurzelmann, 2007). A peripherally acting mu-opioid receptor antagonist reverses opioid-induced constipation without affecting analgesia in clients with advanced illness (Thomas et al, 2008).*

• Question the client about any disruption in sleep. **EB:** *Clients with low back pain had significant loss of sleep (Marin, Cyhan, & Miklos, 2006).*

• Watch for signs of depression in the clients with chronic pain, including sleeplessness, not eating, flat affect, statements of depression, or suicidal ideation. **EB:** *Chronic pain clients had twice the rate* *of suicide than the people without pain (Tang & Crane, 2006). Clients over 60 who committed suicide had physical illness, especially pain, breathlessness, and disability (Harwood et al, 2006).*

- Explain to the client the pain management approach that has been ordered, including therapies, medication administration, side effects, and complications. *One of the most important steps toward improved control of pain is a better client understanding of the nature of pain, its treatment, and the role the client needs to play in pain control (APS, 2004).*

- Discuss the client's fears of undertreated pain, addiction, and overdose. *Because of the many misconceptions regarding pain and its treatment, education about the ability to control pain effectively and correction of myths about the use of opioids should be included as part of the treatment plan (McCaffery, Pasero, & Portenoy, 2004). Opioid tolerance and physical dependence are expected with long-term opioid treatment and should not be confused with addiction (APS, 2004). Addiction is unlikely when clients use opioids for pain relief (McCaffery, Pasero, & Portenoy, 2004; Pasero & McCaffery, 2004b).*

- Review the client's pain diary, flow sheet, and medication records to determine the overall degree of pain relief, side effects, and analgesic requirements for an appropriate period (e.g., 1 week). **EBN:** *Pain diaries are valid and reliable methods of documenting pain severity, activity including aggravating and alleviating factors (Hoekstra, Bindels, & van Dujin, 2004; Hadjistavropoulous et al, 2007; Hager & Brockopp, 2009).*

- ▲ Obtain prescriptions to increase or decrease opioid doses as needed; base prescriptions on the client's report of pain severity (clinical judgment of effectiveness if the client is unable to provide a self-report), response to the previous dose in terms of pain relief, occurrence of adverse effects, and ability to perform the activities of recovery or ADLs. *It is important that nurses knowledgeable in pain management have an "as needed" range of opioid doses available to provide appropriate pain relief (APS, 2008; Gordon et al, 2004). Policies or protocols that require clinicians to begin at a certain opioid dose or administer a specific dose based on pain intensity levels are inappropriate and unsafe (Gordon et al, 2004). Safe and effective pain management requires opioid dose adjustment based on individualized, adequate pain and sedation assessment, opioid administration, and evaluation of the response to treatment. This ability to adjust the dose based on client assessment requires knowledge about opioid action, onset, time to peak serum concentration, duration of action, and potential adverse effects.*

- ▲ Assess pain level, sedation level, and respiratory status at regular intervals during pain management with opioid administration. Assess sedation and respiratory status at least every 1 to 2 hours during the first 24 hours of opioid therapy, then every 4 hours if no episodes of oversedation have occurred, respiratory status has been stable without episodes of hypoventilation, and more frequently as determined by individualized client status. Awaken sleeping clients for assessment if the respiratory rate is inadequate, or if respirations are shallow, ineffective, irregular, noisy (snoring), or periods of apnea occur. Discontinue continuous opioid infusions immediately, and decrease subsequent opioid doses by 25% to 50% if the client develops oversedation (Pasero & McCaffery, 2002; Pasero, 2009b). *Life-threatening respiratory depression is the most serious of opioid adverse effects. All clients receiving opioids for pain management are at risk for sedation, which may progress to oversedation and lead to clinically significant, opioid-induced respiratory depression. Clients are at the highest risk for opioid-induced respiratory depression during the first 24 hours of therapy, when the dose is increased, or the opioid has been changed to a different opioid (Lucas, Vlahos, & Ledgerwood, 2007; Benyamin et al, 2008; Pasero, 2009b; ASA, 2009). Sedation always precedes opioid-induced respiratory depression (Pasero & McCaffery, 2002). Less opioid is required to produce sedation than to produce respiratory depression. Opioid-induced respiratory depression can be prevented by performing systematic sedation assessment and reducing the opioid dose when oversedation is identified (Pasero & McCaffery, 2002; Dempsey & Davidson, 2009b; Pasero, 2009b). Use a valid and reliable sedation tool that identifies distinct changes in the level of alertness and arousability to prevent oversedation (Nisbet & Mooney-Cotter, 2008; Dempsey & Davidson, 2009b; Jarzyna et al, 2009).*

- ▲ In addition to the use of analgesics, support the client's use of nonpharmacological methods to help control pain, such as physical therapy, group therapy, distraction, imagery, relaxation, massage, and application of heat and cold. *Cognitive-behavioral strategies can restore the client's sense of self-control, personal efficacy, and active participation in his or her own care (Miaskowski et al, 2005; APS, 2008; Norelli & Harju, 2008). Teach and implement nonpharmacological interventions when pain is relatively well controlled with pharmacological means. Nonpharmacological interventions should be used to supplement, not replace, pharmacological interventions (APS, 2004; Miaskowski et al, 2005).*

- Encourage the client to plan activities around periods of greatest comfort whenever possible. Pain impairs function. *Clients will find it easier to perform their ADLs and enjoy social activities when they are rested and pain is under control (Pasero & McCaffery, 2004b).*
- Explore appropriate resources for management of pain on a long-term basis (e.g., hospice, pain care center). *Most clients with cancer or chronic nonmalignant pain are treated for pain in outpatient and home care settings. Plans should be made to ensure ongoing assessment of the pain and the effectiveness of treatments in these settings (NCI, 2007; APS, 2008).*
- If the client has progressive cancer pain, assist the client and family with handling issues related to death and dying. *Peer support groups and pastoral counseling may increase the client's and family's coping skills and provide needed support (NCI, 2007; APS, 2008).*

Pediatric

- Assess for pain presence using a valid and reliable pain scale based on age, cognitive development, and the child's ability to provide a self-report. *Please refer to the care plan on* **Acute Pain** *for rationales on pain assessment in children.*
- Help children and adolescents learn and utilize techniques such as relaxation and cognitive behavioral techniques to handle pain. **EBN:** *Studies have shown that the use of psychological interventions can reduce the frequency and severity of pain in children and adolescents (Eccleston et al, 2002).*

Geriatric

- Always take an older client's report of pain seriously and ensure that the pain is relieved. *Pain is not an expected part of normal aging (AGS, 2002, 2009; Herr, 2002). Pain in the elderly is often unrecognized, untreated, and undertreated. Consequences of persistent pain, or its inadequate treatment, is associated with adverse effects such as decreased cognition, delirium, mood changes (depression, anxiety), functional impairment, falls, decreased socialization, sleep disturbances, and decreased quality of life (Davis & Srivastava, 2003; Pasero & McCaffery, 2004b; Pasero et al, 2005). Additionally, a hospitalized older adult experiencing pain is at higher risk for physiological consequences such as atelectasis, nosocomical pneumonia, thromboembolism, and functional decline (Herr & Titler, 2009).*
- When assessing pain, speak clearly, slowly, and loudly enough for the client to hear, and if the client uses a hearing aid, be sure it is in place; repeat information as needed. Be sure the client can see well enough to read the pain scale (use an enlarged scale) and written materials. **EBN:** *Older clients often have difficulty hearing and seeing. Comprehension is improved when instructions are given slowly and clearly and when clients can see visual aids (Herr et al, 2004; Pasero et al, 2005).*
- Handle the client's body gently. Allow the client to move at his or her own speed. *Elders are particularly susceptible to injury during care activities. Caregivers must be patient and expect that older clients will move more slowly than younger clients; they may also perform better and experience less pain when they are allowed to move themselves (McCaffery & Pasero, 1999).*
- ▲ Use acetaminophen for pain relief and avoid the use of NSAIDs. *Acetaminophen should be used, unless contraindicated, for initial and ongoing treatment of pain in older persons (Zhang, Jones, & Doherty, 2004; AGS, 2009). Consider limiting the maximum single dose of acetaminophen to 650 mg, and the maximum daily dose to less than 4000 mg per 24 hours (FDA, 2009). Clients with chronic alcoholism and liver disease, or who are fasting, can develop severe hepatotoxicity even with therapeutic doses (Mehta & Rothstein, 2009). NSAIDs should be used rarely, and with extreme caution, as the elderly are at higher risk for adverse effects such as gastrointestinal, cardiovascular, and renal toxicity (AGS, 2002, 2009; Fine, 2004; Hutchinson, 2004). Clients taking NSAIDS for pain management should also use a proton pump inhibitor for gastrointestinal protection (NCI, 2007; AGS, 2009). Assess older clients taking NSAIDS for evidence of gastrointestinal and renal toxicity, hypertension, heart failure, and drug-drug and drug-disease interactions (AGS, 2009). Opioids may be safer than NSAIDs in some older clients with moderate to severe pain, or impaired function, and decreased quality of life related to pain (AGS, 2009).*

▲ Avoid or use with caution drugs with a long half-life, such as the NSAID piroxicam (Feldene), and the opioids methadone (Dolophine) and levorphanol (LevoDromoran). *The higher prevalence of renal insufficiency in elders compared with younger persons can result in toxicity from drug accumulation (AGS, 2002, 2009; Fick et al, 2003; APS, 2004).*

▲ Use opioids cautiously in the older client with moderate to severe pain. Initiate opioid therapy with a low dose, and carefully titrate the dose based on pain and sedation assessment. Titrate the dose using an immediate release opioid, and convert to an extended release opioid when the comfort-function goal has been achieved. **EBN:** *Consider opioid therapy for older clients with moderate to severe pain, pain-related functional impairment, or decreased quality of life related to pain (AGS, 2009). Opioid selection, initial dosing, and titration should be individualized and based on the client's health status, previous exposure to opioids, attainment of therapeutic goals, and predicted or observed adverse effects or harms. Conduct a therapeutic trial that includes individualization of the dose through incremental dose escalations, as long as no adverse events or serious harms occur (Chou et al, 2009). Consider administration of opioids every 4 hours "around-the-clock" (ATC) for clients with pain that is present approximately 50% of the day (constant pain) to achieve steady serum concentrations. Steady serum concentrations will be achieved with ATC dosing in approximately 4 to 5 half-lives (NCI, 2007). Older clients have demonstrated greater sensitivity to opioid-induced analgesic effects as well as higher risk for adverse effects (AGS, 2009). Initiate opioid therapy with a low dose (recommended adult starting opioid dosage by 25% to 50%) followed by careful titration (gradually increase the dosage by 25% to 50%) to facilitate safe and effective pain management without the occurrence of adverse effects (APS, 2003; Ardery et al, 2003).*

▲ Avoid the use of meperidine (Demerol) and propoxyphene (Darvon, Darvocet), in older clients. *Meperidine's metabolite, normeperidine, can produce central nervous system (CNS) irritability, seizures, and even death; propoxyphene's metabolite, norpropoxyphene, can produce CNS toxicity. Both of these metabolites are eliminated by the kidneys, which makes meperidine and propoxyphene particularly poor choices for older clients, many of whom have at least some degree of renal insufficiency (Ardery et al, 2003; Fick et al, 2003).*

▲ Monitor for signs of depression in older clients and refer to specialists with relevant expertise. **EB:** *Assessment of psychological factors and coping styles is critical in the development of an individualized plan for chronic pain (AGS, 2002; ASA, 2009). Depression is often associated with pain in the older client (AGS, 2009). Treatment of depression in the elderly with arthritis has been demonstrated to decrease pain and improve functional abilities (Lin et al, 2003). Older adults with good coping strategies have reported significantly lower pain and demonstrated less psychological disability. Treatment of depression has resulted in improved function in older clients (Callahan et al, 2005).*

Multicultural

- Please refer to the care plan on **Acute Pain** for multicultural interventions and rationales.

Home Care

- Please refer to the care plan on **Acute Pain** for interventions and rationales on home care.

Client/Family Teaching and Discharge Planning

NOTE: To avoid the negative connotations associated with the words *drugs* and *narcotics,* use the term *pain medicine* when teaching clients and *opioids* when speaking with colleagues.

- Provide written materials on pain control such as *Understanding Your Pain: Using a Pain Rating Scale* (McCaffery, Pasero, & Portenoy, 2001) (see instructions on the use of a pain rating scale) and *Taking Oral Opioid Analgesics* (McCaffery, Pasero, & Portenoy, 2004). *Written materials are provided in addition to verbal instructions so that the client will have a reference during treatment.*
- Discuss the various discomforts encompassed by the word "pain" and ask the client to give examples of previously experienced pain. Explain the pain assessment process and the purpose of the pain rating scale. *It is often difficult for clients to understand the concept of pain and describe their pain experience. Using alternative words and providing a complete description of the assessment pro-*

cess, including the use of scales, will ensure that an accurate treatment plan is developed (Pasero & McCaffery, 2004b). Teach clients to use the pain rating scale to rate the intensity of past or current pain.

▲ Ask the client to identify the pain level, on a self-report pain tool, that will allow the client to perform desired activities and achieve an acceptable quality of life. If pain is above this level, the client should take action that decreases pain or notify a member of the health care team so that pain assessment can be performed and effective interventions implemented promptly. *The use of comfort-function goals provides direction for the treatment plan. Changes are made according to the client's response and achievement of the goals of recovery or rehabilitation (Pasero & McCaffery, 2004b).*

▲ Discuss the total plan for pharmacological and nonpharmacological treatment, including the medication plan for ATC administration and supplemental doses, the maintenance of a pain diary, and the use of supplies and equipment. *Appropriate instruction increases the accuracy and safety of medication administration.*

• Reinforce the importance of taking pain medications to keep pain under control. *Teaching clients to stay on top of their pain and prevent it from getting out of control will improve their ability to perform ADLs and accomplish goals (Pasero & McCaffery, 2004b).*

• Reinforce that taking opioids for pain relief is not addiction and that addiction is very unlikely to occur. *The development of addiction when opioids are taken for pain relief is rare (APS, 2004; McCaffery, Pasero, & Portenoy, 2004).*

• Explain to a client with chronic neuropathic pain the process of taking adjuvant analgesics (e.g., tricyclic antidepressants). *A low dose of adjuvant analgesic is used initially and the dose is increased gradually. Pain relief is delayed, and the adjuvant analgesics must be taken daily. Teaching clients that, although the medicine is an antidepressant, it is used for analgesia and not depression will increase understanding of the drug. Comparable teaching should take place when an anticonvulsant is prescribed for analgesia.*

• Suggest the client with cancer try having a massage, with aromatherapy if desired. **EB:** *Both massage and aromatherapy massage have short-term benefits on psychological well-being for the client with cancer (Fellowes, Barnes, & Wilkinson, 2004).*

• Emphasize to the client the importance of pacing activity and taking rest breaks before they are needed. *Clients will find they are able to perform their ADLs and achieve goals better when they are rested (Pasero & McCaffery, 2004b).*

• Demonstrate the use of appropriate nonpharmacological approaches in addition to pharmacological approaches for helping to control pain (e.g., physical therapy, group therapy, distraction, imagery, and application of heat and cold) (Miaskowski et al, 2005).

• Teach and implement nonpharmacological interventions when pain is relatively well controlled with pharmacological means. *Nonpharmacological interventions are used to supplement, not replace, pharmacological interventions (APS, 2004; Miaskowski et al, 2005).*

ⓔvolve   See the EVOLVE website for Weblinks for client education resources.

REFERENCES

American Geriatric Society (AGS): Panel on Persistent Pain in Older Persons: The management of persistent pain in older persons, *J Am Geriatr Soc* 50:S205, 1–20, 2002.

American Geriatric Society (AGS) Panel on the Pharmacological Management of Persistent Pain in Older Persons: Pharmacological management of persistent pain in older persons, *J Am Geriatr Soc* 37(8):1331–1346, 2009.

The American Pain Society (APS): *Principles of analgesic use in acute and chronic pain,* ed 6, Glenview, IL: American Pain Society; 2008.

The American Pain Society (APS): Pain: current understanding of assessment, management and treatments, 2009. www.ampainsoc.org/ce/enduring.htm. Accessed December 21, 2009.

The American Pain Society (APS): *Principles of analgesic use for the treatment of acute pain and cancer pain,* Glenview, IL 2003, APS.

American Society of Anesthesiologists (ASA): Practice guidelines for the prevention, detection, and management of respiratory depression associated with neuraxial opioid administration, Anesthesiology 110:218–230, 2009.

Anderson KO et al: Cancer pain management among underserved minority outpatients: perceived needs and barriers to optimal control, *Cancer* 94(8):2295–2304, 2002.

Ardery G, Herr KA, Titler MG et al: Assessing and managing acute pain in older adults: a research base to guide practice, *Med-Surg Nurs* 12:1, 2003.

Benyamin R, Trescot AM, Datta S et al: Opioid complications and side effects, *Pain Physician* 11(2 Suppl):S105–120, 2008.

Bhavani-Shankar K, Oberol JS: Management of postoperative pain. "Uptodate" version June 19, 2009; accessed July 2009 from www.uptodate.com/patients/content/topic.do?topicKey=~9TD93y2rpud9.

• = Independent   ▲ = Collaborative   **EBN** = Evidence-Based Nursing   **EB** = Evidence-Based

Breivik H, Borchgrevink PC, Allen SM et al: Assessment of pain, *Br J Anaesth* 101(1):17–24, 2008.

Brennan F, Carr DB, Cousins M. Pain management: a fundamental human right, *Anesth Analg* 105(1):205–211, 2007.

Callahan CM, Kroenke K, Counsell SR et al: Treatment of depression improves physical functioning in older adults. *Am Geriatr Soc* 53(3):367–373, 2005.

Chou R, Fanciullo GJ, Fine PG et al: Clinical guidelines for the use of chronic opioid therapy in chronic noncancer pain, *The Journal of Pain* 10(2):113–130, 2009.

Closs Sj, Staples V, Reid I et al: The impact of neuropathic pain on relationships, *J Adv Nurs* 65(2):402–411, 2008.

Davis MP, Srivastava M: Demographics, assessment and management of pain in the elderly, *Drugs Aging* 20(1):23, 2003.

Deane G, Smith HS: Overview of pain management in older persons, *Clin Geriatr Med* 24:185–201, 2008.

Dempsey SJ, Davidson J: Improving pain assessment and management: application of the hierarchy of importance of pain measures in clinical practice, 2009a, submitted for publication.

Dempsey SJ, Davidson J: Reducing oversedation for patients receiving opioids for pain management: implementation of the Pasero Opioid-Induced Sedation Scale in clinical practice, 2009b, submitted for publication.

Dunwoody CF, Krenzischek DA, Pasero C et al: Assessment, physiological monitoring, and consequences of inadequately treated pain, *J PeriAnes Nursing* 23(1A):S15–S27, 2008.

Eccleston C, Morley S, Williams A et al: Systematic review of randomised controlled trials of psychological therapy for chronic pain in children and adolescents with a subset meta-analysis of pain relief, *Pain* 99(1–2):157–165, 2002.

Evans C, Galustian C, Kumar D et al: Impact of surgery on immunologic function: comparison between minimally invasive techniques and conventional laparotomy for surgical resection of colorectal tumors. *Am J Surg* 197(2):238–245, 2009.

Fanelli G, Berti M, Baciarello M: Updating postoperative pain management: from multimodal to context-sensitive treatment, *Minerva Anes* 74:489–500, 2008.

FDA: Joint Meeting of the Drug Safety and Risk Management Advisory Committee with the Anesthetic and Life Support Drugs Advisory Committee and the Nonprescription Drugs Advisory Committee Recommendations, June 30, 2009. Accessed November 19, 2009, from www.fda.gov/downloads/AdvisoryCommittees/CommitteesMeetingMaterials/Drugs/Drug.

Fellowes D, Barnes K, Wilkinson S: Aromatherapy and massage for symptom relief in patients with cancer, *Cochrane Database Syst Rev*. (2):CD002287, 2004.

Fick DM, Cooper JW, Wade WE et al: Updating the Beers criteria for potentially inappropriate mediation use in older adults, *Arch Int Med* 163:2716–2724, 2003.

Fine P: Pharmacological management of persistent pain in older patients, *Clin J Pain* 20(4):220–226, 2004.

Friedman JD, Dello Buono FA: Opioid antagonists in the treatment of opioid-induced constipation and pruritus, *Ann Pharmacother* 35(1):85–91, 2001.

Furlan AD, Sandoval JA, Mailis-Gagnon A et al: Opioids for chronic noncancer pain: a meta-analysis of effectiveness and side effects, *CMAJ* 174:1589–1594, 2006.

Gordon DB, Dahl J, Phillips P et al: The use of "as-needed" analgesics in the management of acute pain: a consensus statement of the American Society for Pain Management Nursing and the American Pain Society, *Pain Manag Nurs* 5(2):53–58, 2004.

Hadjistavropoulos T, Herr K, Turk DC et al: An interdisciplinary expert consensus statement on assessment of pain in older persons, *Clin J Pain* 23(1 Suppl):S1–43, 2007.

Hager K. Brockopp D: The use of a chronic pain diary in older people, *Br J Nurs* 18(8):490–494, 2009.

Harwood DM, Hawton K, Hope T et al: Life problems and physical illness as risk factors for suicide in older people: A descriptive and case-control study, *Psychol Med*, 36(9):1265–1274, 2006.

Herr K, Bjoro K: Assessment of pain in the nonverbal or cognitively impaired older adult, *Clin Geriatr Med* 24(2):237–262, 2008.

Herr K, Coyne P, McCaffery M et al: Pain assessment in the nonverbal patient: position statement with clinical recommendations, *Pain Manage Nurs* 7(2):44–52, 2006.

Herr K, Titler M: Acute pain assessment and pharmacological management practices for the older adult with a hip fracture: review of ED trends, *J Emer Nurs* 35(4):312–320, 2009.

Herr K, Titler MG, Schilling ML et al: Evidence-based assessment of acute pain in older adults: current nursing practices and perceived barriers, *Clin J Pain* 20(5):331–340, 2004.

Herr KJ: Chronic pain: challenges and assessment strategies, *Gerontol Nurs* 28(1):20–27, 2002.

Hoekstra J, Bindels P, van Dujin N et al: The symptom monitor. A diary for monitoring physical symptoms for cancer patients in palliative care: feasibility, reliability, and compliance, *J Pain Symptom Manag* 27(1):24–35, 2004.

Hutchison R: Cox-2–selective NSAIDS, *AJN* 104(3):52–55, 2004.

International Association for the Study of Pain, Subcommittee on Taxonomy: Classification of chronic pain: descriptions of chronic pain syndromes and definitions of pain terms, *Pain Suppl* 3:S1–S226, 1979.

Jarzyna D, Pasero C, Junquist C, et al: Expert consensus panel for monitoring of opioid-induced sedation and respiratory depression: summary report and findings, Oral Presentation, ASPMN annual meeting, Tampa, FL, September 11–15, 2009.

Krenzischek DA: Pharmacotherapy for acute pain: implications for practice *Pain Manag Nurs* 9(1 Suppl):S22–S32, 2008.

Layman-Young J, Horton F, Davidhizar R: Nursing attitudes and beliefs in pain assessment and management, *Journal of advanced nursing* 412–421, 2006.

Lin EHB, Katon W, Von Korff M et al: Effect of improving depression care on pain and functional outcomes among older adults with arthritis, *JAMA* 290(18):2428, 2003.

Lucas CE, Vlahos AL, Ledgerwood AM: Kindness kills: the negative impact of pain as the fifth vital sign, *J Am Coll Surg* 205:101–107, 2007.

Marin R, Cyhan T, Miklos W: Sleep disturbance in patients with chronic low back pain, *Am J Phys Med Rehabil* 85(5):430–435, 2006.

McDermott AM, Toelle TR, Rowbotham DJ et al: The burden of neuropathic pain: results from a cross-sectional survey, *Eur J Pain* 10:127–135, 2006.

McCaffery M: *Nursing practice theories related to cognition, bodily pain, and man-environment interactions*, Los Angeles, 1968, University of California at Los Angeles Students' Store.

McCaffery M, Pain control: switching from IV to PO, *Am J Nurs* 103(5):62–63, 2003.

McCaffery M, Pasero C: *Pain: clinical manual*, ed 2, St Louis, 1999, Mosby.

McCaffery M, Pasero C: Pain control: breakthrough pain, *Am J Nurs* 103(4):83, 84, 86, 2003.

McCaffery M, Pasero C, Portenoy RK: *Understanding your pain: using a pain rating scale*, Chadds Ford, PA, 2001, Endo Pharmaceuticals.

McCaffery M, Pasero C, Portenoy RK: *Understanding your pain: taking oral opioid analgesics*, Chadds Ford, PA, 2004, Endo Pharmaceuticals.

Mehta G, Rothstein KD: Health maintenance issues in cirrhosis. *Med Clin North Am*, 93(4):901–915, 2009.

● = Independent   ▲ = Collaborative   **EBN** = Evidence-Based Nursing   **EB** = Evidence-Based

Miaskowski C, Cleary J, Burney R et al: *Guideline for the management of cancer pain in adults and children,* Glenview, IL, 2005, American Pain Society.

Ming Wah IJ: Pain management in the hospitalized patient, *Med Clin N Am* 92:371–385, 2008.

National Cancer Institute (NCI): *Education in palliative and end-of-life care for oncology (EPEC-O),* Bethesda, MD, 2007, U.S. Department of Health and Human Services.

Nisbet A, Mooney-Cotter M: *Post opioid sedation scales. Validity, reliability, accuracy, and performance in adult non-critical care settings.* Poster presentation, ASPMN National Meeting, Tucson, AZ, September 4–6, 2008.

Norelli LJ, Harju SK: Behavioral approaches to pain management in the elderly, *Clin Geriatr Med* 24(2):335–344, 2008.

Panchal SJ, Muller-Schwefe P, Wurzelmann I: Opioid-induced bowel dysfunction: prevalence, pathophysiology and burden, *Int J Clin Pract* 61:1181–1187, 2007.

Pasero C: Multimodal analgesia in the PACU, *J PeriAnesthesia Nursing* 18(4):265–268, 2003a.

Pasero C: Pain in the critically ill, *J PeriAnesthesia Nursing* 18(6):422–425, 2003b.

Pasero C: Challenges in pain assessment, *J PeriAnesthesia Nurs* 24(1):50–54, 2009a.

Pasero C: Assessment of sedation during opioid administration for pain management, *J PeriAnes Nurs,* 24(3):186–190, 2009b.

Pasero C, McCaffery M: Pain control: patient's report of pain, *Am J Nurs* 101(12):73–74, 2001.

Pasero C, McCaffery M: Monitoring opioid-induced sedation, *Am J Nurs* 102(2):67–68, 2002.

Pasero C, McCaffery M: Pain control: controlled-release oxycodone, *Am J Nurs* 104(1):30–32, 2004a.

Pascro C, McCaffery M: Pain control: comfort-function goals, *Am J Nurs* 104(9):77–78, 81, 2004b.

Pasero C, McCaffery M: No self report means no pain intensity, *American Journal of Nursing* 105(10):50–53, 2005.

Pasero C, McCaffery M: Orthopedic postoperative pain management, *Journal of PeriAnesthesia Nursing* 22(3):160–174, 2007.

Pasero C, Rakel B, McCaffery M: *Pain in Older Persons,* Seattle, 2005, IASP.

Polomano RC, Dunwoody CJ, Krenzischek DA et al: Perspective on pain management in the 21st century, *Pain Manage Nurs* 9(1):S3–S10, 2008.

Puntillo K, Morris A, Thompson C et al: Pain behaviors observed during six common procedures: result from Thunder Project II, *Crit Care Med* 32:421–427, 2004.

Puntillo K, Pasero C, Li D et al: Evaluation of pain in ICU patients, *Chest* 135(4):1069–1074, 2009.

Schumacher KL, Koresawa S, West C et al: The usefulness of a daily pain management diary for outpatients with cancer-related pain, *Oncol Nurs Forum* 29(9):1304, 2002.

Smith BH, Torrance N, Bennett MI et al: Health and quality of life associated with chronic pain of predominantly neuropathic origin in the community, *Clin J Pain* 23(2):143–149, 2007.

Tang NK, Crane C: Suicidality in chronic pain: a review of the prevalence, risk factors and psychological links, *Psychol Med,* 36(5):575–586, 2006.

The Joint Commission: *2009 Hospital accreditation standards,* Oakbrook Terrace, IL, 2009, The Commission.

Thomas J, Karver S, Cooney GA et al: Methylnaltrexone for opioid-induced constipation in advanced illness, *N Engl J Med* 358(22):2332–2343, 2008.

Zhang W, Jones A, Doherty M: Does paracetamol (acetaminophen) reduce the pain of osteoarthritis? A meta-analysis of randomized controlled trains, *Ann Rheum Dis* 63:901–907, 2004.

Impaired Parenting   *Gail B. Ladwig, MSN, RN, CHTP*

Definition

Inability of the primary caretaker to create, maintain, or regain an environment that promotes the optimum growth and development of the child

Defining Characteristics

Infant/Child

Behavioral disorders; failure to thrive; frequent accidents; frequent illness; incidence of abuse; incidence of trauma (e.g., physical and psychological); lack of attachment; lack of separation anxiety; poor academic performance; poor cognitive development; poor social competence; runaway

Parental

Abandonment; child abuse; child neglect; frequently punitive; hostility to child; inadequate attachment; inadequate child health maintenance; inappropriate caretaking skills; inappropriate stimulation (e.g., visual, tactile, auditory); inappropriate child care arrangements; inconsistent behavior management; inconsistent care; inflexibility in meeting needs of child; little cuddling; maternal-child interaction deficit; negative statements about child; paternal-child interaction deficit; poor parent-child interaction; rejection of child; statements of inability to meet child's needs; unsafe home environment; verbalization of inability to control child; verbalization of frustration; verbalization of role inadequacy

● = Independent   ▲ = Collaborative   **EBN** = Evidence-Based Nursing   **EB** = Evidence-Based

Related Factors (r/t)

Infant/Child

Altered perceptual abilities; attention deficit–hyperactivity disorder; developmental delay; difficult temperament; handicapping condition; illness; multiple births; not desired gender; premature birth; separation from parent; temperamental conflicts with parental expectations

Knowledge

Deficient knowledge about child development; deficient knowledge about child health maintenance; deficient knowledge about parenting skills; inability to respond to infant cues; lack of cognitive readiness for parenthood; lack of education; limited cognitive functioning; poor communication skills; preference for physical punishment; unrealistic expectations

Physiological

Physical illness

Psychological

Closely spaced pregnancies; depression; difficult birthing process; disability; high number of pregnancies; history of mental illness; history of substance abuse; lack of prenatal care; sleep deprivation; sleep disruption; young parental age

Social

Change in family unit; chronic low self-esteem; father of child not involved; financial difficulties; history of being abused; history of being abusive; inability to put child's needs before own; inadequate child care arrangements; job problems; lack of family cohesiveness; lack of parental role model; lack of resources; lack of social support networks; lack of transportation; lack of valuing of parenthood; legal difficulties; low socioeconomic status; maladaptive coping strategies; marital conflict; mother of child not involved; single parent; social isolation; poor home environment; poor parental role model; poor problem-solving skills; poverty; presence of stress (e.g., financial, legal, recent crisis, cultural move); relocations; role strain; situational low self-esteem; unemployment; unplanned pregnancy; unwanted pregnancy

 (Nursing Outcomes Classification)

Suggested NOC Outcomes

Abuse Cessation, Abuse Protection, Abuse Recovery: Abusive Behavior Self-Restraint, Child Development (all), Coping, Family Functioning, Family Social Climate, Knowledge: Child Physical Safety, Neglect Recovery, Parent-Infant Attachment, Parenting Performance, Parenting: Psychosocial Safety, Role Performance, Social Support

Example **NOC Outcome with Indicators**
Parenting: Psychosocial Safety as evidenced by the following indicators: Fosters open communication/Recognizes risk(s) for abuse/Uses strategies to eliminate risk(s) of abuse/Selects appropriate supplemental caregiver(s)/Uses strategies to prevent high-risk social behaviors/Provides required level of supervision/Sets clear rules for behavior/Maintains structure and daily routine in child's life (Rate the outcome and indicators of **Parenting: Psychosocial Safety:** 1 = never demonstrated, 2 = rarely demonstrated, 3 = sometimes demonstrated, 4 = often demonstrated, 5 = consistently demonstrated [see Section I].)

Client Outcomes

Client Will (Specify Time Frame):

- Initiate appropriate measures to develop a safe, nurturing environment
- Acquire and display attentive, supportive parenting behaviors and child supervision
- Identify appropriate strategies to manage a child's inappropriate behaviors
- Identify strategies to protect child from harm and/or neglect and initiate action when indicated

(Nursing Interventions Classification)

Suggested NIC Interventions

Abuse Protection Support: Child, Attachment Promotion, Caregiver Support, Developmental Enhancement: Adolescent, Child, Environmental Management: Environmental Management: Family Integrity Promotion, Impulse Control Training, Infant Care, Parent Education: Adolescent, Childrearing Family, Infant, Parenting Promotion, Role Enhancement, Substance Use Prevention, Treatment, Teaching: Infant Stimulation, Toddler Nutrition, Toddler Safety

Example NIC Activities—Family Integrity Promotion

Identify typical family coping mechanisms; Determine typical family relationships for each family; Counsel family members on additional effective coping skills for their own use; Assist family with conflict resolution; Monitor current family relationships; Facilitate a tone of togetherness within and among the family; Encourage family to maintain positive relationships; Refer for family therapy, as indicated

Nursing Interventions and *Rationales*

- Use the Parenting Sense of Competence (PSOC) to measure parental self-efficacy. **EB:** *The PSOC contains three useful factors that reflect satisfaction with the parental role, parenting efficacy, and interest in parenting. In this study mothers reported higher efficacy than fathers, and fathers reported greater satisfaction with the parenting role than did mothers. The study provides normative data against which at-risk groups can be compared (Gilmore & Cuskelly, 2009).*
- Examine the characteristics of parenting style and behaviors. Consider dysfunctional child-centered and parent-centered cognitions as potentially critical correlates of abusive behavior. **EB:** *Child abuse is a major social concern around the world. Important to tackling the problem is an understanding of the mechanisms contributing to abusive parenting. This study brings together research on the cognitive variables associated with abusive or high-risk parenting. Interactions with additional factors, such as an ability to inhibit aggression, problem-solving capabilities, parenting skills, social isolation, and societal context are examined (Seng & Prinz, 2008).*
- ▲ Institute abuse/neglect protection measures if evidence exists of an inability to cope with family stressors or crisis, signs of parental substance abuse are observed, or a significant level of social isolation is apparent. **EBN:** *Maternal difficult life circumstances, psychiatric-mental health symptoms, educational level, maternal experience in the family of origin, and parenting stress explained 74% of the variance in maternal sensitivity and responsiveness of mothers with their toddlers in the laboratory setting (LeCuyer-Maus, 2003).*
- ▲ For a mother with a toddler, assess maternal depression. Make appropriate referral. **EB:** *Women who report symptoms of depression when their children are young are highly likely to continue to report such symptoms. These results support the need to screen for elevated depressive symptoms at varying intervals depending on prior screening results and for screening in locations where women most at risk routinely visit, such as well-child clinics. Further, these results point to the need for a system to identify and manage this common treatable condition (Horwitz et al, 2009).*
- Appraise the parent's resources and the availability of social support systems. Determine the single mother's particular sources of support, especially the availability of her own mother and partner. Encourage the use of healthy, strong support systems. **EB:** *To reduce chronic supervisory neglect, mothers may need assistance with both informal and formal child care support. The results of this study showed the mothers who provided inadequate supervision received less child care support from their partners and relatives, but not their friends (Coohey, 2007).*
- Provide education to at-risk parents on behavioral management techniques such as looking ahead, giving good instructions, providing positive reinforcement, redirecting, planned ignoring, and instituting time-outs. **EB:** *These behavioral management techniques are effective approaches for dealing with ineffective parent-child interactions and improving family relationships (Nicholson et al, 2002). Parents with low levels of knowledge and confidence in their parenting may be at greater risk of dysfunctional parenting and might benefit from interventions designed to enhance both knowledge and confidence (Morawska, Winter, & Sanders, 2009).*

● = Independent ▲ = Collaborative **EBN** = Evidence-Based Nursing **EB** = Evidence-Based

- Promotion of better-quality relationships between parents and children is an effective strategy that can lead to enhanced learning. Good-quality parenting leads to improved cognitive and social skills for the children. **EB:** *Research supports that effective early interventions lead to enhanced short-term gains in cognitive and social skills, particularly for children at risk of low educational achievement (National Literacy Trust, 2005).*
- Support parents' competence in appraising their infant's behavior and responses. **EBN:** *Parents must be supported and welcomed as active collaborators in their infant's care (Lawhon, 2002).*
- Aim supportive interventions at minimizing parents' experience of strain. *Research supports interventions that lead to parents becoming empowered in their parenthood (Nystrom & Ohrling, 2004).*
- Model age-appropriate and cognitively appropriate caregiver skills by doing the following: communicating with the child at an appropriate cognitive level of development, giving the child tasks and responsibilities appropriate to age or functional age/level, instituting safety considerations such as the use of assistive equipment, and encouraging the child to perform activities of daily living as appropriate. *These activities illustrate parenting and childrearing skills and behaviors for parents and family (McCloskey & Bulechek, 2008).*
- Encourage mothers to understand and capitalize on their infants' capacity to interact, particularly in the early months of life. **EBN:** *A study suggested that nurses should routinely assess parent-child interactions in all high-risk, disadvantaged families with very young children (Schiffman, Omar, & McKelvey, 2003).*
- ▲ Provide programs for homeless mothers with severe mental illness who have lost physical custody of their children. **EBN:** *Programs for homeless mothers with severe mental illness can effect changes that promote family reunification. Changes in housing, psychosis, substance use, and therapeutic relationships predicated reunification (Hoffman & Rosenheck, 2001).*
- ▲ Provide a recovery program that includes instruction in parenting skills and child development for mothers who are addicted to cocaine. **EBN:** *Women addicted to cocaine who are parenting children need strong encouragement from the health care system to begin a recovery program and also gain parenting skills. Lack of parenting knowledge may be a major barrier for them (Coyer, 2003).*
- Refer to **Readiness for enhanced Parenting** for additional interventions.

Multicultural

- Acknowledge that value conflicts from acculturation stresses may contribute to increased anxiety and significant conflict with children. **EBN:** *Immigrant mothers scored significantly lower on the evaluation of parenting knowledge than U.S.-born mothers (Bornstein & Cote, 2004). Chinese immigrant mothers identified that a larger perceived acculturation gap was associated with more parenting difficulties (Buki et al, 2003).*
- Approach individuals of color with respect, warmth, and professional courtesy. **EBN:** *Instances of disrespect have special significance for individuals of color (D'Avanzo & Naegle, 2001).*
- Clarify parents' feelings, expectations, perceptions, and availability regarding participation in the care of their sick child. **EBN:** *Cultural differences in regard to parent participation in the care of ill or hospitalized children should be considered (Pongjaturawit & Harrigan, 2003).*
- Carefully assess meaning of terms used to describe health status when working with Native Americans. **EB:** *This study of American Indians over 50 indicates that Native Americans engage in "positive talk" with regards to health status so their distress may be underestimated and their satisfaction over estimated (Garroutte et al, 2006).*
- Provide support for Chinese families caring for children with disabilities. **EBN:** *The care of children with handicaps strains and violates the Chinese culturally expected order of parental obligations. The following themes emerged: disruptions to natural order, public opinions on what constitutes personhood and ordered bodies, and the establishment of moral reputations linked to shame and blame and the gendered division of parenting (Holroyd, 2003).*
- Facilitate modeling and role playing to help the family improve parenting skills. **EBN:** *It is helpful for the family and the client to practice parenting skills in a safe environment before trying them in real-life situations (Rivera-Andino & Lopez, 2000).*

● = Independent   ▲ = Collaborative   **EBN** = Evidence-Based Nursing   **EB** = Evidence-Based

Home Care

- The interventions previously described may be adapted for home care use.
- Assess parenting stress at each home visit to provide appropriate support and anticipatory guidance to families of children with a chronic disease. **EB:** *Parents found it difficult to set limits or discipline children with heart disease; older age of the child was associated with higher parenting stress scores (Uzark & Jones, 2003). This study demonstrated the effectiveness of a home visitation program in enhancing the early parenting history of infants born at medical risk—a population that is at risk for mistreatment (Bugental & Schwartz, 2009).*
- ▲ Assess the single mother's history regarding childhood and partner abuse and current status regarding depressive symptoms, abusive parenting attitudes (lack of empathy, favorable opinion of corporal punishment, parent-child role-reversal, and inappropriate expectations). Refer for mental health services as indicated. **EBN:** *History of partner and child abuse predicted higher daily stress, leading to lower self-esteem. The presence of more depressive symptoms and daily stressors was associated with greater anger. Greater anger was associated with lower parental empathy. Partner abuse predicted higher levels of abusive parenting attitudes (Lutenbacher, 2002).*
- Provide a parenting program of Planned Activities Training (PAT). **EB:** *Planned Activities Training (PAT) is a five-session intervention aimed at improving parent-child interactions, increasing child engagement in daily activities, and reducing challenging child behaviors. Parents in this program demonstrated improvements in their parenting behaviors (Bigelow, Carta, & Lefever, 2008).*
- Provide follow up support for the PAT via cell phone and text messaging. **EB:** *Cellular phones afford the opportunity for home visitors to maintain regular communication with parents between intervention visits and thus retain high-risk families in parenting interventions. The use of cellular phones may also increase the dosage of intervention provided to families and the fidelity with which parents implement the intervention, thus resulting in improved outcomes for parents and children. Parents have rated text messaging and cellular phone call enhancements very positively (Bigelow, Carta, & Lefever, 2008).*

 Client/Family Teaching and Discharge Planning

- Consider individual and/or group-based parenting programs for teenage mothers. **EB:** *A systematic review indicated that results favored those engaged in individual and/or group parenting programs in the areas of mother-infant interaction, language development, parental attitudes, parental knowledge, maternal mealtime communication, maternal self-confidence, and maternal identity (Barlow & Coren, 2004).*
- Consider group-based parenting programs for parents of children younger than 3 years with emotional and behavioral problems. **EB:** *A metaanalysis indicated that results favored those engaged (Barlow & Parsons, 2003).*
- Consider group-based parenting programs for parents with anxiety, depression, and/or low self-esteem. **EB:** *Parenting programs can make a significant contribution to the short-term psychosocial health of mothers and have a potential role to play in the promotion of mental health (Barlow & Coren, 2004).*
- ▲ Refer adolescent parents for comprehensive psychoeducational parenting classes. **EBN:** *A study indicated that a comprehensive psychoeducational parenting group can be effective in changing parenting attitudes and beliefs (Thomas & Looney, 2004).*
- Parent training is one of the most effective interventions for behavior problems in young children. **EB:** *Parent training implementation and parental engagement may be improved by the introduction of a cognitive component. Parent training programs can be delivered to the parents alone, to the parents and children in separate group meetings, or to the parents and children together in sessions for at least part of the time. An overview of findings from research on these programs indicates that these programs have consistent and replicated effects on children's behavior, on parents' improved use of effective discipline strategies, and on improved family functioning (Cartwright-Hatton, McNally, & White, 2005; Omara, 2007).*
- Encourage positive parenting: respect for children, understanding of normal development, and creative and loving approaches to meet parenting challenges. **EBN:** *Understanding normal development is a first step for parents to distinguish common behaviors for a given stage of development from*

"problems." Central to positive parenting is developing approaches that can be used in place of anger, manipulation, punishment, and rewards (Ahmann, 2002).

▲ Initiate referrals to community agencies, parent education programs, stress management training, and social support groups. Consider the use of technology and the media. *The parent needs support to manage angry or inappropriate behaviors. Use of support systems and social services can provide an opportunity to decrease feelings of inadequacy (Baker, 1994). This study demonstrated that media interventions (a parenting television series with and without Web support) depicting evidence-based parenting programs may be a useful means of reaching hard-to-engage families in population-level child maltreatment prevention programs (Calam et al, 2008).*

• Provide information regarding available telephone counseling services and Internet support. *In this study both the telephone and the Web-based support improved the children's well-being and decreased their perceived burden of problem (Fukkink & Hermanns, 2009). The authors of this study report on the adaptation of a parenting program for delivery via the Internet, enhanced with participant-created videos of parent-infant interactions and weekly staff contact, which enable distal treatment providers to give feedback and make decisions informed by direct behavioral assessment. This Internet-based, parent-education intervention has the potential to promote healthy and protective parent-infant interactions in families who might not otherwise receive needed mental health services (Feil et al, 2008).*

• Refer to the care plans for **Delayed Growth and development**, **Risk for impaired Attachment**, and **Readiness for enhanced Parenting** for additional teaching interventions.

⊖volve   See the EVOLVE website for Weblinks for client education resources.

REFERENCES

Ahmann E: Promoting positive parenting: an annotated bibliography, *Pediatr Nurs* 28(4):382, 2002.

Baker NA: Avoid collisions with challenging families, *MCN Am J Matern Child Nurs* 19:97, 1994.

Barlow J, Coren E: Parent-training programmes for improving maternal psychosocial health, *Cochrane Database Syst Rev* (1):CD002020, 2004.

Barlow J, Parsons J: Group-based parent-training programmes for improving emotional and behavioral adjustment in 0–3 year old children, *Cochrane Database Syst Rev* (1):CD003680, 2003.

Bigelow KM, Carta JJ, Lefever JB: Txt u ltr: using cellular phone technology to enhance a parenting intervention for families at risk for neglect, *Child Maltreat* 13(4):362–367, 2008.

Bornstein MH, Cote LR: "Who is sitting across from me?" Immigrant mothers' knowledge of parenting and children's development, *Pediatrics* 114(5):e557–e564, 2004.

Bugental DB, Schwartz A: A cognitive approach to child mistreatment prevention among medically at-risk infants, *Dev Psychol* 45(1):284–288, 2009.

Buki LP, Ma TC, Strom RD et al: Chinese immigrant mothers of adolescents: self-perceptions of acculturation effects on parenting, *Cultur Divers Ethnic Minor Psychol* 9(2):127–140, 2003.

Calam R, Sanders MR, Miller C et al: Can technology and the media help reduce dysfunctional parenting and increase engagement with preventative parenting interventions? *Child Maltreat* 13(4):347–361, 2008.

Cartwright-Hatton S, McNally D, White C: A new cognitive behavioural parenting intervention for families of young anxious children: a pilot study, *Behav Cogni Psychother* 33:243–247, 2005.

Coohey C: Social networks, informal child care, and inadequate supervision by mothers, *Child Welfare* 86(6):53–66, 2007.

Coyer SM: Women in recovery discuss parenting while addicted to cocaine, *MCN Am J Matern Child Nurs* 28(1):45, 2003.

D'Avanzo CE, Naegle MA: Developing culturally informed strategies for substance-related interventions. In Naegle MA, D'Avanzo CE, editors: *Addictions and substance abuse: strategies for advanced practice nursing*, St Louis, 2001, Mosby.

Feil EG, Baggett KM, Davis B et al: Expanding the reach of preventive interventions: development of an Internet-based training for parents of infants, *Child Maltreat* 13(4):334–346, 2008.

Fukkink RG, Hermanns JM: Children's experiences with chat support and telephone support, *J Child Psychol Psychiatr* 50(6):759–766, 2009.

Garroutte EM, Kunovich RM, Buchwald D et al: Medical communication in older American Indians: variations by ethnic identity, *J Appl Gerontol* 25(Suppl 1):27S-43S, 2006.

Gilmore L, Cuskelly M: Factor structure of the Parenting Sense of Competence scale using a normative sample, *Child Care Health Dev* 35(1):48–55, 2009.

Hoffman D, Rosenheck R: Homeless mothers with severe mental illnesses and their children: predictors of family reunification, *Psychiatr Rehabil J* 25(2):163, 2001.

Holroyd EE: Chinese cultural influences on parental caregiving obligations toward children with disabilities, *Qual Health Res* 13(1):4, 2003.

Horwitz SM, Briggs-Gowan MJ, Storfer-Isser A et al: Persistence of maternal depressive symptoms throughout the early years of childhood, *J Womens Health* 18(5):637–645, 2009.

Lawhon G: Facilitation of parenting the premature infant within the newborn intensive care unit, *J Perinat Neonatal Nurs* 16(1):71, 2002.

LeCuyer-Maus E: Stress and coping in high-risk mothers: difficult life circumstances, psychiatric-mental health symptoms, education, and experiences in their families of origin, *Public Health Nurs* 20(2):132, 2003.

Lutenbacher M: Relationships between psychosocial factors and abusive parenting attitudes in low-income single mothers, *Nurs Res* 51:158, 2002.

McCloskey JC, Bulechek GM, editors: *Nursing interventions classification (NIC)*, St Louis, 2008, Mosby.

Morawska A, Winter L, Sanders MR: Parenting knowledge and its role in the prediction of dysfunctional parenting and disruptive child behaviour, *Child Care Health Dev* 35(2):217–226, 2009.

National Literacy Trust: *Birth to school study: a longitudinal evaluation of the Peers Early Education Partnership (PEEP) 1998–2005*, 2005.

www.literacytrust.org.uk/talktoyourbaby/PEEPstudy2005.html, accessed January 2007.

Nicholson B, Anderson M, Fox R et al: One family at a time: a prevention program for at-risk parents, *J Couns Dev* 80(3):362, 2002.

Nystrom K, Ohrling K: Parenthood experiences during the child's first year: literature review, *J Adv Nurs* 46(3):319–330, 2004.

Omara L: A cognitive behavioural parenting intervention reduced conduct problems in children and improved parenting skill and confidence, *Evid Based Nurs* 10(2):46, 2007.

Pongjaturawit Y, Harrigan R: Parent participation in the care of hospitalized child in Thai and Western cultures, *Issues Comp Pediatr Nurs* 26(3):183–199, 2003.

Rivera-Andino J, Lopez L: When culture complicates care, *RN* 63(7):47, 2000.

Schiffman RF, Omar MA, McKelvey LM: Mother-infant interaction in low-income families, *MCN Am J Matern Child Nurs* 28(4):246–251, 2003.

Seng AC, Prinz RJ: Parents who abuse: what are they thinking? *Clin Child Fam Psychol Rev* 11(4):163–175, 2008.

Thomas DV, Looney SW: Effectiveness of a comprehensive psychoeducational intervention with pregnant and parenting adolescents: a pilot study, *J Child Adolesc Psychiatr Nurs* 17(2):66–77, 2004.

Uzark K, Jones K: Parenting stress and children with heart disease, *J Pediatr Health Care* 17(4):163–168, 2003.

Risk for impaired Parenting   *Gail B. Ladwig, MSN, RN, CHTP*

Definition

Risk for inability of the primary caretaker to create, maintain, or regain an environment that promotes the optimum growth and development of the child

Risk Factors

Infant/Child

Altered perceptual abilities; attention deficit–hyperactivity disorder; developmental delay; difficult temperament; handicapping condition; illness; multiple births; not gender desired; premature birth; prolonged separation from parent; temperamental conflicts with parental expectation

Knowledge

Deficient knowledge about child development; deficient knowledge about child health maintenance; deficient knowledge about parenting skills; inability to respond to infant cues; lack of cognitive readiness for parenthood; low cognitive functioning; low educational level; poor communication skills; preference for physical punishment; unrealistic expectations of child

Physiological

Physical illness

Psychological

Closely spaced pregnancies; depression; difficult birthing process; disability; high number of pregnancies; history of mental illness; history of substance abuse; sleep deprivation; sleep disruption; young parental age

Social

Change in family unit; chronic low self-esteem; father of child not involved; financial difficulties; history of being abused; history of being abusive; inadequate child care arrangements; job problems; lack of access to resources; lack of family cohesiveness; lack of parental role model; lack of prenatal care; lack of resources; lack of social support network; lack of transportation; lack of valuing of parenthood; late prenatal care; legal difficulties; low socioeconomic class; maladaptive coping strategies; marital conflict; mother of child not involved; parent-child separation; poor home environment; poor parental role model; poor problem-solving skills; poverty; role strain; single parent; situational low self-esteem; social isolation; stress; relocation; unemployment; unplanned pregnancy; unwanted pregnancy

NOC, NIC, Client Outcomes, Nursing Interventions, Client/Family Teaching and Discharge Planning, *Rationales*, and References

Refer to care plans **Readiness for enhanced Parenting** and **Impaired Parenting**.

Readiness for enhanced Parenting   *Gail B. Ladwig, MSN, RN, CHTP*

Definition

A pattern of providing an environment for children or other dependent person(s) that is sufficient to nurture growth and development and can be strengthened

Defining Characteristics

Child satisfaction with home environment, emotional support of children; emotional support of other dependent persons; evidence of attachment; exhibits realistic expectations of children; exhibits realistic expectations of other dependent person(s); expresses willingness to enhance parenting; needs of children are met (e.g., physical and emotional); other dependent person(s) expresses(es) satisfaction with home environment

NOC   (Nursing Outcomes Classification)

Suggested NOC Outcomes

Child Development, Knowledge: Child Physical Safety, Parenting Performance, Parenting: Psychosocial Safety

---

Example NOC Outcome with Indicators

Parenting Performance as evidenced by the following indicators: Provides preventive and episodic health care/ Stimulates cognitive and social development/Stimulates emotional and spiritual growth/Empathizes with child/Expresses satisfaction with parental role/Expresses positive self-esteem (Rate the outcome and indicators of **Parenting Performance:** 1 = never demonstrated, 2 = rarely demonstrated, 3 = sometimes demonstrated, 4 = often demonstrated, 5 = consistently demonstrated [see Section I].)

Client Outcomes

Client/Family Will (Specify Time Frame):

- Affirm desire to improve parenting skills to further support growth and development of children
- Demonstrate loving relationship with children
- Provide a safe, nurturing environment
- Assess risks in home/environment and takes steps to prevent possibility of harm to children
- Meet physical, psychosocial, and spiritual needs or seek appropriate assistance

NIC   (Nursing Interventions Classification)

Suggested NIC Interventions

Anticipatory Guidance, Attachment Promotion, Developmental Enhancement: Adolescent, Child, Family Integrity Promotion: Childbearing Family, Infant Care, Newborn Care, Parent Education: Adolescent, Childrearing Family, Infant, Parenting Promotion, Teaching: Infant Stimulation

---

Example NIC Activities—Parenting Promotion

Assist parents to have realistic expectations appropriate to developmental and ability level of child; Assist parents with role transition and expectations of parenthood

---

Nursing Interventions and *Rationales*

- Use family-centered care and role modeling for holistic care of families. **EBN:** *Specific techniques of role modeling and reflective practice are suggested as effective approaches to teach the family sensitive care in clinical settings in which families are part of the care environment (Tomlinson et al, 2002).*

• = Independent   ▲ = Collaborative   **EBN** = Evidence-Based Nursing   **EB** = Evidence-Based

EBN: *This study demonstrated that family-centered care enhanced the overall quality of NICU care, resulting in less stressed, more informed, and more confident parents (Cooper et al, 2007).*

- Assess parents' feelings when dealing with a child who has a chronic illness. **EB:** *It is essential for health care professionals who provide support to children with disabilities to understand the process that parents as primary caregivers undergo to accept the conditions of their child's disability (Anan & Yamaguchi, 2007). EBN: Parents needs must be continuously reassessed (Nuutila & Salanterä, 2006).*

- Encourage positive parenting: respect for children, understanding of normal development, and use of creative and loving approaches to meet parenting challenges. **EBN:** *Understanding normal development is a first step so that parents can distinguish common behaviors for a given stage of development from "problems" (Ahmann, 2002).*

- Promote low-technology interventions, such as massage and multisensory interventions (maternal voice, eye-to-eye contact, and rocking) and music to reduce maternal and infant stress and improve mother-infant relationship. **EBN:** *These are strategies aimed at reducing maternal and infant stress and improving the mother-infant relationship (White-Traut, 2004). Incorporating infant massage into a planned parenting enhancement program may promote effective parenting through a special focus on infant stimulation through massage (Porter & Porter, 2004). **EB:** Musical activities were used in this study to promote positive parent-child relationships and children's behavioral, communicative, and social development (Nicholson et al, 2008).*

- Support kangaroo care for infants at risk at birth; keep infants in an upright position in skin-to-skin contact until they no longer tolerate it. **EB:** *Kangaroo Mother Care has a positive impact on family and home environment. The results of this study also suggest, first, that both parents should be involved as direct caregivers in the Kangaroo Mother Care procedure and secondly, that this intervention should be directed more specifically at infants who are more at risk at birth (Tessier et al, 2009).*

- Provide the parent with the opportunity to assist in the newborn's first bath, allowing a flexible bath time. **EBN:** *A flexible bathing time is recommended depending on the characteristics and stability of the newborn and family desires (Behring, Vezeau, & Fink, 2003).*

- When the person who is ill is the parent, use family-centered assessment skills to determine the impact of an adult's illness on the child and then guide the parent through those topics that are most likely to be of concern. **EBN:** *The pediatric nurse, by embracing core principles of openness and honesty and by providing concrete developmental information, can empower parents to support their own children (McCue & Bonn, 2003).*

- Provide practical and psychological assistance for parents of clients with psychiatric diagnoses, such as schizophrenia. **EBN:** *Parents may be overloaded with their long-term caring tasks, and provision of practical and psychological assistance can be of benefit (Jungbauer et al, 2003). Women who are mothers and who are also users of mental health services face particular challenges in managing the contradictory aspects of their dual identity. Professionals need to help the person both with parenting and with their mental health needs (Davies & Allen, 2007).*

- Refer to the care plan for **Impaired Parenting** for additional interventions.

 Multicultural

- Assess the influence of cultural beliefs, norms, and values on the client's perception of parenting. **EBN:** *What the client considers normal parenting may be based on cultural perceptions (Leininger & McFarland, 2002).*

- Acknowledge racial and ethnic differences at the onset of care and provide appropriate health information and social support. **EBN:** *Acknowledgment of racial and ethnicity issues enhances communication, establishes rapport, and promotes treatment outcomes (Gaston-Johansson et al, 2007; Campbell-Grossman et al, 2009).*

- Support programs for parents of young children in Jewish communities. *These programs combine Jewish themes with content about parenting and child development, both to provide information and support and to inspire families to become more involved with Jewish religion and tradition. Families benefit the most when Jewish organizations partner with local experts, combining religious/cultural knowledge with early childhood expertise (Wertlieb & Rosen, 2008).*

• = Independent ▲ = Collaborative **EBN** = Evidence-Based Nursing **EB** = Evidence-Based

- Clarify parents' feelings, expectations, perceptions, and availability regarding participation in the care of their sick child. **EBN:** *Cultural differences in regard to parent participation in the care of ill or hospitalized children should be considered (Pongjaturawit & Harrigan, 2003).*
- Acknowledge and praise parenting strengths noted. *Clinicians could explore and support the positive qualities of authoritative parenting in Mexican descent families (Varela et al, 2004).*

 ### Home Care

- The nursing interventions previously described should be used in the home environment with adaptations as necessary.
- ▲ Refer to a parenting program to facilitate learning of parenting skills. **EB:** *Results of this study indicate that parents who took part in the U.S. Navy New Parent program improved their perceptions of their parenting and coping skills, and the program enhanced the family's quality of life (Kelley et al, 2007).* **EB:** *This study demonstrated that a psychoeducational program with modest dosage (eight sessions), delivered in a universal framework through childbirth education programs and targeting the coparenting relationship, had a positive impact on observed family interaction and child behavior at 6–month follow-up (child age 1 year) (Feinberg, Kan, & Goslin, 2009).*

 ### Client/Family Teaching and Discharge Planning

- Refer to Client/Family Teaching and Discharge Planning for **Impaired Parenting** for suggestions that may be used with minor adaptations.
- Teach parents home safety: reduction of hot water temperature, proper poison storage, use of smoke alarms, and installation of safety gates for stairs. **EB:** *Counseling and convenient access to reduced-cost products appear to be an effective strategy for promoting children's home safety (Gielen, McDonald & Wilson, 2002).*
- Teach parents and young teens conflict resolution by using a hypothetical conflict solution with and without a structured conflict resolution guide. Support self direction of the families with minimal therapist intervention. **EBN:** *Parents and young teens do not use a systematic method of solving disagreements, but with structured guidance the parents and teens are able to resolve conflicts (Riesch et al, 2003).* **EB:** *This research suggests that a self-directed behavioral family intervention with minimal therapist contact may be an effective early intervention for adolescent problems (Stallman & Ralph, 2007).*
- Refer mothers of children with type 1 diabetes for community support in babysitting, child care, or respite. **EBN:** *Mothers raising young children older than 4 years with type 1 diabetes highlight the importance of identifying family and/or community resources that could reduce some of the tremendous stress and burden of responsibility experienced after a child is diagnosed with diabetes (Sullivan-Bolyai et al, 2003).*
- Teach families the importance of monitoring television viewing and limiting exposure to violence. **EBN:** *Media violence can be hazardous to children's health, and studies overwhelmingly point to a causal connection between media violence and aggressive attitudes, values, and behaviors in some children (Muscari, 2002).*
- Promotion of better-quality relationships between parents and children is an effective strategy that can lead to enhanced learning. Good-quality parenting leads to improved cognitive and social skills for the children. **EB:** *Research supports that effective early interventions lead to enhanced short-term gains in cognitive and social skills, particularly for children at risk of low educational achievement (National Literary Trust, 2005).*

⊖volve   See the EVOLVE website for Weblinks for client education resources.

REFERENCES

Ahmann E: Promoting positive parenting: an annotated bibliography, *Pediatr Nurs* 28(4):382, 2002.

Anan A, Yamaguchi M: Process of parental acceptance of a child's disability: literature review, *J UOEH* 29(1):73–85, 2007.

Behring A, Vezeau TM, Fink R: Timing of the newborn first bath: a replication, *Neonatal Netw* 22(1):39, 2003.

Campbell-Grossman C, Hudson DB, Keating-Lefler R et al: Community leaders' perceptions of Hispanic, single, low-income mothers' needs, concerns, social support, and interactions with health care services, *Compr Pediatr Nurs* 32(1):31–46, 2009.

Cooper LG, Gooding JS, Gallagher J et al: Impact of a family-centered care initiative on NICU care, staff and families, *J Perinatol* 27(Suppl 2):S32–S37, 2007.

Davies B, Allen D: Integrating 'mental illness' and 'motherhood': the positive use of surveillance by health professionals. A qualitative study, *Int J Nurs Stud* 44(3):365–376, 2007.

Feinberg ME, Kan ML, Goslin MC: Enhancing coparenting, parenting, and child self-regulation: effects of family foundations 1 year after birth, *Prev Sci* 10(3):276–285, 2009.

Gaston-Johansson F, Hill-Briggs F, Oguntomilade L et al: Patient perspectives on disparities in healthcare from African-American, Asian, Hispanic, and Native American samples including a secondary analysis of the Institute of Medicine focus group data, *J Nat Black Nurses Assoc* 18(2):43–52, 2007.

Gielen AC, McDonald EM, Wilson ME: Effects of improved access to safety counseling, products, and home visits on parents' safety practices: results of a randomized trial, *Arch Pediatr Adolesc Med* 156(1):33, 2002.

Jungbauer J, Wittmund B, Dietrich S et al: Subjective burden over 12 months in parents of patients with schizophrenia, *Arch Psychiatr Nurs* 17(3):126–134, 2003.

Kelley ML, Schwerin MJ, Farrar KL et al: A participant evaluation of the U.S. Navy Parent Support Program, *J Fam Violence* 22(3):131–139, 2007.

Leininger MM, McFarland MR: *Transcultural nursing: concepts, theories, research and practices,* ed 3, New York, 2002, McGraw-Hill.

McCue K, Bonn R: Helping children through an adult's serious illness, *Pediatr Nurs* 29(1):47, 2003.

Muscari M: Media violence: advice for parents, *Pediatr Nurs* 28(6):585, 2002.

National Literacy Trust: *Birth to school study: a longitudinal evaluation of the Peers Early Education Partnership (PEEP) 1998–2005,* 2005. www.literacytrust.org.uk/talktoyourbaby/PEEPstudy2005.html, accessed January 2007.

Nicholson JM, Berthelsen D, Abad V et al: Impact of music therapy to promote positive parenting and child development, *J Health Psychol* 13(2):226–238, 2008.

Nuutila L, Salanterä S: International pediatric column. Children with a long-term illness: parents' experiences of care, *J Pediatric Nurs* 21(2):153–160, 2006.

Pongjaturawit Y, Harrigan R: Parent participation in the care of hospitalized child in Thai and Western cultures, *Issues Compr Pediatr Nurs* 26(3):183–199, 2003.

Porter LS, Porter BO: A blended infant massage-parenting enhancement program for recovering substance-abusing mothers, *Pediatr Nur* 30(5):363–372, 389–390, 401, 2004.

Riesch SK, Gray J, Hoeffs M et al: Conflict and conflict resolution: parent and young teen perceptions, *J Pediatr Health Care* 17(1):22, 2003.

Stallman HM, Ralph A: Reducing risk factors for adolescent behavioural and emotional problems: a pilot randomised controlled trial of a self-administered parenting intervention, *Aus e-J Advance Ment Health* 6(2):1–4, 2007.

Sullivan-Bolyai S, Deatrick J, Gruppuso P et al: Constant vigilance: mothers' work parenting young children with type 1 diabetes, *J Pediatr Nurs* 18(1):21, 2003.

Tessier R, Charpak N, Giron M et al: Kangaroo Mother Care, home environment and father involvement in the first year of life: a randomized controlled study, *Acta Paediatr* 98(9):1444–1450, 2009.

Tomlinson PS, Thomlinson E, Peden-McAlpine C et al: Clinical innovation for promoting family care in paediatric intensive care: demonstration, role modeling and reflective practice, *J Adv Nurs* 38(2):161, 2002.

Varela RE, Vernberg EM, Sanchez-Sosa JJ et al: Parenting style of Mexican, Mexican American, and Caucasian non-Hispanic families: social context and cultural influences, *J Fam Psychol* 18(4):651–657, 2004.

Wertlieb D, Rosen MI: Inspiring Jewish connections: outreach to parents with infants and toddlers, *Zero Three* 28(3):11–17, 2008.

White-Traut R: Providing a nurturing environment for infants in adverse situations: multisensory strategies for newborn care, *J Midwifery Womens Health* 49(4 Suppl 1):36, 2004.

Risk for ineffective renal Perfusion *Jennifer Hafner, RN, BSN, TNCC, and Joan Klehr, RNC, BS, MPH*

NANDA-I

Definition

At risk for a decrease in blood circulation to the kidney that may compromise health

Risk Factors

Abdominal compartment syndrome; advanced age; bilateral cortical necrosis; burns; cardiac surgery; cardiopulmonary bypass; diabetes mellitus; exposure to toxins; female glomerulonephritis; hyperlipidemia; hypertension; hypovolemia; hypoxemia; hypoxia; infection (e.g., sepsis, localized infection); malignancy; malignant hypertension; metabolic acidosis; multitrauma; polynephritis; renal artery stenosis; renal disease (polycystic kidney); smoking; systemic inflammatory response syndrome; treatment-related side effects (medications); vascular embolism; vasculitis

NOC (Nursing Outcomes Classification)

Suggested NOC Outcomes

Tissue Perfusion: Renal, Kidney Function

• = Independent ▲ = Collaborative **EBN** = Evidence-Based Nursing **EB** = Evidence-Based

Example NOC Outcome with Indicators
Kidney Function as evidenced by: 24–hour intake and output balance/Blood urea nitrogen/Serum creatinine/Urine color/ Serum electrolytes (Rate the outcome and indicators of **Kidney Function:** 1 = severely compromised, 2 = substantially compromised, 3 = moderately compromised, 4 = mildly compromised, 5 = not compromised [see Section I].)

Client Outcomes

Client Will (Specify Time Frame):

- Maintain normal blood urea nitrogen and serum creatinine levels
- Maintain urine output of 0.5 mL/kg/hr
- Maintain urine output that is yellow and clear
- Maintain serum electrolytes within normal limits

NIC   (Nursing Interventions Classification)

Suggested NIC Interventions

Medication Management, Acid/Base Monitoring, Fluid/Electrolyte Management, Laboratory Data Interpretation, Electrolyte Management.

Example NIC Activities—Fluid/Electrolyte Management
Monitor for serum electrolytes levels, as available; Weigh daily and monitor trends; Monitor vital signs, as appropriate

Nursing Interventions and *Rationales*

- Assess client for history of or risk factors for renal insufficiency, renal artery stenosis, and acute renal failure. Risk factors include history of diabetes, hypertension, heart failure, obesity, smoking, advanced age, extrarenal atherosclerosis, cardiovascular surgery, and thoracoabdominal aortic surgery. *Clients who have undergone cardiac and thoracoabdominal surgeries are at risk for acute renal failure due to renal parenchymal damage possibly related to such factors as hypovolemia, inflammation, ischemia-reperfusion, and other factors (Nigwekar & Kandula, 2009).*
- Monitor vital signs. Compare blood pressure to client's normal range. *Long-term hypertension can cause decreased renal perfusion; it also can be a symptom of decreased renal function (Broscious & Castagnola, 2006).*
- ▲ Utilize continuous cardiac monitoring as needed. **EBN:** *Monitor for dysrhythmias due to possible increased serum potassium and phosphorus due to poor kidney function from ineffective renal perfusion (Broscious & Castagnola, 2006).*
- Measure intake and output on a regular basis. Calculate intake against the output to monitor fluid status. *Oliguria and/or anuria are signs of acute renal failure. Intake greater than output is a sign of fluid retention and renal insufficiency which may be caused by ineffective renal perfusion (Broscious & Castagnola, 2006).*
- Monitor for edema. *Edema may be present with increased fluid retention due to impaired renal function related to decreased renal perfusion (Broscious & Castagnola, 2006).*
- Listen to lung sounds, noting presence of adventitious lung sounds. *Crackles or rales are signs of fluid overload due to acute or chronic renal failure (Broscious & Castagnola, 2006).*
- Monitor for changes in mental status. *Changes in mental status from impaired renal function can range from seizures, confusion, difficulty in concentration, and coma as the result of uremic toxins and electrolyte imbalances that can cause encephalopathy (Broscious & Castagnola, 2006).*
- Weigh the client daily. *Increased fluid retention related to decreased renal perfusion will cause weight to increase (Broscious & Castagnola, 2006).*
- ▲ Monitor peak and trough blood levels carefully in clients receiving nephrotoxic antibiotics including Vancomycin, and aminoglycosides. *The antibiotics are excreted via the renal system and are nephrotoxic. Peak and trough testing reflects antibiotic levels in the serum. Elevated levels can cause renal impairment (Decker & Molitoris, 2009; Drew, 2009).*
- ▲ Ensure the clients having diagnostic testing with contrast are well hydrated with IV saline as ordered before and after the examination. *Hydration with crystalloids has been shown to prevent renal*

• = Independent   ▲ = Collaborative   **EBN** = Evidence-Based Nursing   **EB** = Evidence-Based

insufficiency by diluting the IV contrast. Fluids without salt have been shown to increase acute renal failure (Rudnick & Tumlin, 2009).

▲ Collect a 24–hour urine specimen for a creatinine clearance test as ordered. *Evaluate the rate and efficiency of the kidney filtration of the blood over a 24 period of time (Lab Tests Online, 2005a).*

▲ Note the results of diagnostic studies as available: renal ultrasound, radionuclide scanning, abdominal/pelvic CT, MRA, arteriography. *These tests are commonly done for diagnosing renal failure (Spinowitz & Rodriguez, 2006).*

▲ Perform a complete pain assessment. Assess and document the onset, intensity, character, location, duration, aggravating factors and relieving factors. Notify the provider of any increase in pain or discomfort or if comfort measures are not effective. **EBN:** *A buildup of uric acid due to decreased kidney function will deposit in the joints and soft tissue, causing joint pain and swelling (Broscious & Castagnola, 2006).*

▲ Monitor laboratory data as ordered or per protocol. Laboratory data could include BUN, serum creatinine, serum and urine electrolytes, calcium, phosphate, complete blood count, urine total protein, albumin, alkaline phosphatase, and urinalysis. Report abnormalities to attending provider. *The above laboratory studies are used in the diagnosis and monitoring of renal insufficiency and renal failure. Monitoring these labs will help direct therapy (Lab Tests Online, 2005b).*

Client/Family Teaching and Discharge Planning

● Provide client teaching related to risk factors for renal insufficiency or acute renal failure, including signs and symptoms of acute renal failure, and lifestyle changes that can improve renal function. *Client education is a vital part of nursing care for the client with possible renal disease. Start with the client's base level of understanding and use that as a foundation for further education (National Kidney Foundation, 2009).*

▲ Teach client about any medications prescribed. *Medication teaching includes the drug name, its purpose, administration instructions such as taking it with or without food, and any side effects to be aware of. Instruct the client to report any adverse side effects to his/her provider (Broscious & Castagnola, 2006).*

▲ Stress the importance of stopping smoking. Effects of nicotine include increasing pulse and blood pressure and constricting of blood vessels. *Smoking causes vasoconstriction and atherosclerosis which can exacerbate problems with tissue perfusion, including perfusion of the kidneys (Spinowitz & Rodriguez, 2006).*

 See the EVOLVE website for Weblinks for client education resources.

REFERENCES

Broscious SK, Castagnola J: Chronic kidney disease: acute manifestations and role of critical care nurses, *Crit Care Nurse* 26(4):17–27, 2006.

Decker BS, Molitoris BA: *Manifestations of and risk factors for aminoglycoside nephrotoxicity,* 2009. www.uptodate.com/online/content/topic.do?topicKey=renlfail/10385&selectedTitle=2~150&source=search_result#, accessed April 9, 2009.

Drew RH: *Vancomycin dosing and serum concentration monitoring in adults,* 2009. www.uptodate.com/online/content/topic.do?topicKey=antibiot/7122&selectedTitle=2~150&source=search_result, accessed April 9, 2009.

Lab Tests Online: *Creatinine clearance,* 2005a. http://labtestsonline.org/understanding/analytes/creatinine_clearance/test.html, accessed April 9, 2009.

Lab Tests Online: *Kidney and urinary tract function, disorders, and diseases,* 2005b. http://labtestsonline.org/understanding/conditions/kidney-4.html, accessed March 20, 2009.

Moorhead S, Johnson M, Maas M L et al: *Nursing outcomes classification,* ed 4, St Louis, MO, 2008, Mosby.

National Kidney Foundation: *Chronic kidney disease,* 2009. www.kidney.org/kidneyDisease/ckd/index.cfm, accessed March 20, 2009.

Nigwekar S, Kandula P: N-Acetylcysteine in cardiovascular surgery associated renal failure: a meta-analysis, *Ann Thorac Surg* 87:139–147, 2009.

Rudnick MR, Tumlin JA: *Prevention of radiocontrast media-induced acute kidney injury (acute renal failure),* 2009. www.uptodate.com/online/content/topic.do?topicKey=renlfail/14655&selectedTitle=1~150&source=search_result#. Accessed April 9, 2009.

Spinowitz BS, Rodriguez J: *Renal artery stenosis,* 2006. www.emedicine.com/med/topic2001.htm. Accessed October 23, 2006.

● = Independent   ▲ = Collaborative   **EBN** = Evidence-Based Nursing   **EB** = Evidence-Based

Risk for decreased cardiac tissue Perfusion

⊖volve

Jennifer Hafner, RN, BSN, TNCC, and Joan Klehr, RNC, BS, MPH

NANDA-I

Definition

Risk for a decrease in cardiac (coronary) circulation

Risk Factors

Cardiac surgery; hyperlipidemia; hypertension; hypovolemia; hypoxemia; hypoxia; coronary artery spasm; cardiac tamponade; birth control pills; diabetes mellitus; drug abuse; elevated C-reactive protein; family history of coronary artery disease; lack of knowledge of modifiable risk factors (e.g., smoking, sedentary lifestyle, obesity)

NOC   (Nursing Outcomes Classification)

Suggested NOC Outcomes

Cardiac Pump Effectiveness, Circulation Status, Tissue Perfusion: Cardiac, Tissue Perfusion: Cellular, Vital Signs

Example NOC Outcome with Indicators
Tissue Perfusion: Cardiac as evidenced by: Angina/Arrhythmia/Tachycardia/Bradycardia/Nausea/Vomiting/Profuse diaphoresis (Rate the outcome and indicators of **Tissue Perfusion: Cardiac:** 1 = severe, 2 = substantial, 3 = moderate, 4 = mild, 5 = none [see Section I].)

Client Outcomes

Client Will (Specify Time Frame):

- Be free from chest pain related to angina
- Have absence of arrhythmias, tachycardia, or bradycardia
- Deny nausea and be free from vomiting
- Have skin that is dry and of normal temperature

NIC   (Nursing Interventions Classification)

Suggested NIC Interventions

Cardiac Care, Cardiac Precautions, Embolus Precautions, Dysrhythmia Management, Vital Signs Monitoring, Shock Management: Cardiac

Example NIC Activity—Cardiac Precautions
Avoid causing intense emotional situations; Avoid overheating or chilling the patient; Provide small frequent meals; Substitute artificial salt and limit sodium intake if appropriate; Promote effective techniques for reducing stress; Restrict smoking

Nursing Interventions and *Rationales*

- Monitor for chest, neck and jaw pain, shortness of breath, diaphoresis, nausea, and vomiting. *These symptoms are signs of decreased cardiac perfusion and a heart attack (American Heart Association, 2009a).*
- ▲ If chest pain is present, administer oxygen per nasal cannula as ordered. *Maintaining a SaO_2 level of 90% or more will decrease the pain associated with myocardial ischemia by increasing the amount of oxygen delivered to the myocardium (Overbaugh, 2009).*
- ▲ Give client an aspirin tablet if ordered and not contraindicated. *Aspirin inhibits platelet aggregation to help stop clotting and also inhibits vasoconstriction by preventing the production of thromboxane A2. Contradictions are: active peptic ulcer disease, bleeding disorders, and aspirin allergy (Overbaugh, 2009).*

• = Independent   ▲ = Collaborative   **EBN** = Evidence-Based Nursing   **EB** = Evidence-Based

▲ Administer nitroglycerin tablets sublingually every 5 minutes until the chest pain is resolved, for a maximum of three doses as ordered. *Nitroglycerin causes arterial and venous dilation, thus reducing preload and afterload, which decreases myocardial oxygen demand (Overbaugh, 2009).*

▲ Administer morphine sulfate as ordered if the pain continues after the nitroglycerin is administered. *Morphine sulfate causes arterial and venous dilation, thus reducing afterload and preload which decreases the workload of the heart (Overbaugh, 2009).*

• Perform a full respiratory assessment and look for signs of tachypnea, rales, pleural friction rub, diminished breath sounds, and dullness on percussion. *All are signs of a pulmonary embolism. Rales may be heard at the site of the embolism. A pleural effusion may be present during an acute pulmonary infarction; the breath sounds will be diminished and dullness may be heard on percussion (Sharma, 2006).*

▲ Obtain a 12–lead electrocardiogram. *A 12–lead echocardiogram should be performed within 10 minutes of emergency department arrival for all clients who are having chest discomfort. Electrocardiograms are used to identify the area of ischemia or injury and guide treatment (Antman et al, 2004).*

• Review the client's medical, surgical, and social history. *Certain conditions place clients at higher risk for decreased cardiac tissue perfusion (e.g., hypertension, diabetes mellitus, hyperlipidemia, family history, tobacco use, obesity, low HDL-C, sedentary lifestyle). A medical history must be concise and detailed to determine the possibility of a myocardial infarction (Antman et al, 2004; Fung, 2008).*

• Perform a cardiovascular physical and neurological assessment. *A physical assessment will aid in the extent, location and presence of, and complications resulting from a myocardial infarction. It will promote rapid triage and treatment. It is also important to assess if the client had a prior stroke (Antman et al, 2004).*

Critical Care

▲ Monitor electrocardiography, heart rate and rhythm, blood pressure, central venous pressure, and SaO_2 (pulse oximetry), SvO_2, or $ScvO_2$. **EBN:** *Central venous pressure is a measurement of fluid status. Tachycardia and bradycardia may be present due to the decreased perfusion to the coronaries. A decrease in blood pressure will be observed as cardiac function is impaired and cardiac output decreases. Oxygenation of the cells will be lower due to hypoperfusion, hypotension, misdistribution of blood flow, increased capillary wall thickness, and inability of the cells to use oxygen; monitoring of SvO_2 and $ScvO_2$ will monitor the oxygen consumption. The duo of pulse oximetry and SvO_2 or $ScvO_2$ monitors oxygen demand and delivery (Bridges & Dukes, 2005; Goodrich, 2006; Sharma, 2006).*

▲ Monitor cardiac output, cardiac index, and systemic vascular resistance. **EBN:** *Cardiac output will increase and systemic vascular resistance will decrease when the client develops vasodilatation. Cardiac output and cardiac index will both decrease when there is injury to the cardiac muscle (Bridges & Dukes, 2005; Sharma, 2006).*

▲ Monitor and evaluate intake and output. **EBN:** *Elevated fluid levels is a sign of congestive heart failure which may be due to poor coronary perfusion (Varughese, 2007).*

▲ Monitor pulmonary artery occlusion pressure. *A decreased pulmonary artery occlusion pressure is an indicator of low intravascular volume. This value is used to determine the amount of fluid resuscitation needed and will help guide therapy (Bridges & Dukes, 2005).*

▲ Monitor cardiac enzymes, chemistries, hematology, and coagulation studies. *Elevated cardiac enzymes indicate cardiac tissue injury (Lab Tests Online, 2008).*

▲ Prepare the client for the following procedures as ordered: 2D echocardiogram, trans-esophageal echocardiogram, cardiac catheterization, stress test, and cardiac computed tomography (CT). *Evaluation of the left ventricular function is essential to determine treatment. It also helps determine long-term survival. Early reperfusion via cardiac catheterization improves morbidity and mortality by reperfusing the area of ischemia (Krumholz et al, 2008). A stress test is used to determine cardiac disease, evaluate treatment and predict myocardial infarction (American Heart Association, 2009b). A cardiac CT scan assesses coronary artery disease, atherosclerosis, and cardiac function (Budoff et al, 2006).*

▲ Prepare the client for central line placement. *Adequate IV and central line access is required for fluid resuscitation and medication delivery. Large amounts of fluid can be delivered more efficiently through central lines. Most vasopressive agents can only be delivered through central lines due to risk of tissue sloughing. Central venous pressure can only be monitored through a central line (Bridges & Dukes, 2005).*

● = Independent   ▲ = Collaborative   **EBN** = Evidence-Based Nursing   **EB** = Evidence-Based

▲ Monitor arterial blood gasses, coagulation, chemistries, point of care blood glucose, cardiac enzymes, blood cultures, and hematology. *Abnormalities can identify the cause of the decreased perfusion, and identify complications related to the decreased perfusion or shock. Elevated cardiac enzymes are indicative of a myocardial infarction and the low perfusion could be cardiogenic shock (Bridges & Dukes, 2005).*

• Complete a full physical examination. *A full nursing assessment is crucial in identifying multiple complications of shock such as: hypoperfusion of internal organs that manifest as decreased bowel sounds and shortness of breath (Bridges & Dukes, 2005).*

Client/Family Teaching and Discharge Planning

• Provide client teaching related to risk factors for decreased cardiac tissue perfusion, such as hypertension, hypercholesterolemia, diabetes mellitus, tobacco use, advanced age, and gender (female). *Client education is a vital part of nursing care for the client. Start with the client's base level of understanding and use that as a foundation for further education. It is important to factor in cultural and/or religious beliefs in the education provided (Alzamora et al, 2007; Mieres & Redberg, 2007; Fung, 2008).*

• Teach client about any medications prescribed. *Medication teaching includes the drug name, its purpose, administration instructions such as taking it with or without food, and any side effects to be aware of. Instruct the client to report any adverse side effects to his/her provider.*

• Stress the importance of ceasing tobacco use. *Tobacco use can cause or worsen decreased blood flow in the coronaries. Effects of nicotine include increasing pulse and blood pressure and constricting of blood vessels. Tobacco use is a primary factor in heart disease.* **EBN:** *Smoking causes vasoconstriction, which can lead to atherosclerotic disease (Alzamora et al, 2007; Fung, 2008).*

• Teach client the benefits of a heart healthy diet. *Clients with hypercholestemia are at an increased risk for decreased cardiac perfusion.* **EB:** *A diet high in cholesterol places the client at a higher risk of atherosclerosis and decreased tissue perfusion (Alzamora et al, 2007; Mieres & Redberg, 2007).*

• Teach the importance of exercise. *Exercise helps control blood pressure and weight which are the most important controlled risk factors for cardiovascular disease (Mieres & Redberg, 2007).*

ⓔvolve   See the EVOLVE website for Weblinks for client education resources.

REFERENCES

Alzamora MT, Baena-Diez JM, Sorribes M et al: Peripheral arterial disease study (perart): prevalence and predictive values of asymptomatic peripheral arterial occlusive disease related to cardiovascular morbidity and mortality, *BMC Public Health* 7:348, 2007.

American Heart Association: *Heart attack symptoms and warning signs,* 2009a. www.americanheart.org/presenter.jhtml?identifier=4595, accessed April 15, 2009.

American Heart Association: *Exercise stress test,* 2009b. www .americanheart.org/presenter.jhtml?identifier=4568, accessed April 15, 2009.

Antman EM, Anbe, DT, Armstrong PW et al: ACC/AHA guidelines for the management of patients with ST-elevation in myocardial infarction: a report of the American College of Cardiology/American Heart Association Task Force on Practice Guidelines, *Circulation* 110(9):e82–e292, 2004.

Bridges EJ, Dukes MS: Cardiovascular aspects of septic shock: pathophysiology, monitoring, and treatment, *Crit Care Nurse* 25(2):14–42, 2005.

Budoff MJ, Achenbach S, Blumenthal RS et al: Assessment of coronary artery disease by cardiac computed tomography, *Circulation* 114:1761–1791, 2006.

Fung G: *Cardiovascular risk factor reduction: where are we going?* May 21, 2008. www.ahalibrary.com/pt/re/aha/addcontent.82812555.htm, accessed March 10, 2009.

Goodrich C: Endpoints of resuscitation: what should we be monitoring? *AACN Adv Crit Care* 17(3):308–316, 2006.

Krumholz HM, Anderson JL, Bachelder BL et al: ACC/AHA 2008 performance measures for adults with ST-elevation and non-ST-elevation myocardial infarction, *Circulation* 118(24):2596–2648, 2008.

Lab Tests Online: *Cardiac biomarkers.* July 30, 2008. http://labtestsonline .org/understanding/analytes/cardiac_biomarkers/glance-3.html, accessed April 15, 2009.

Mieres JH, Redberg R: *Cardiovascular disease prevention in women: comments on the AHA Guideline: evidenced -based guidelines for cardiovascular disease prevention in women: 2007 update.* www .hahlibrary.com/pt/re/aha/addcontent.1062217, accessed March 10, 2009.

Overbaugh KJ: Acute coronary syndrome, *Am J Nurs* 109(5):42–52, 2009.

Sharma S: *Pulmonary embolism,* from EMedicine, 2006. www.emedicine .com/med/TOPIC1958.htm, accessed December 12, 2007.

Varughese S: Management of acute decompensated heart failure, *Crit Care Nurse* 30(2):94–103, 2007.

Risk for ineffective cerebral tissue Perfusion

⊖volve

Jennifer Hafner, RN, BSN, TNCC, and Joan Klehr, RNC, BS, MPH

NANDA-I

Definition

Risk for decrease in cerebral tissue circulation

Risk Factors

Abnormal partial thromboplastin time; abnormal prothrombin time; a kinetic left ventricular segment; aortic atherosclerosis; arterial dissection; atrial fibrillation; atrial myxoma; brain tumor; carotid stenosis; cerebral aneurysm; coagulopathy (e.g., sickle cell anemia); dilated cardiomyopathy; disseminated intravascular coagulation; embolism; head trauma; hypercholesterolemia; hypertension; infective endocarditis; left atrial appendage thrombosis; mechanical prosthetic valve; mitral stenosis; recent myocardial infarction; sick sinus syndrome; substance abuse; thrombolytic therapy; treatment-related side effects (cardiopulmonary bypass, medications)

NOC   (Nursing Outcomes Classification)

Suggested NOC Outcomes

Acute Confusion Level, Tissue Perfusion: Cerebral, Agitation Level, Neurological Status, Cognition, Seizure Control

Example NOC Outcome with Indicators
Tissue Perfusion: Cerebral as evidenced by: Headache/Restlessness/Listlessness/Agitation/Vomiting/Fever/Impaired Cognition/Decreased Level of Consciousness (Rate the outcome and indicators of **Tissue Perfusion: Cerebral:** 1 = severe, 2 = substantial, 3 = moderate, 4 = mild, 5 = none [see Section I].)

Client Outcomes

Client Will (Specify Time Frame):

- State absence of headache
- Demonstrate appropriate orientation to person, place, time, and situation
- Demonstrate ability to follow simple commands

NIC   (Nursing Interventions Classification)

Suggested NIC Interventions

Medication Management, Neurologic Monitoring, Positioning: Neurologic, Cerebral Perfusion Promotion, Fall Prevention, Cognitive Stimulation, Environmental Management: Safety

Example NIC Activities—Neurologic Monitoring
Monitor pupillary size, shape, symmetry, and reactivity; Monitor level of consciousness; Monitor level of orientation; Monitor trend of Glasgow Coma Scale; Monitor facial symmetry; Note complaint of headache

Nursing Interventions and *Rationales*

- Review the client's past medical and surgical history. *Certain conditions place clients at higher risk for ineffective tissue perfusion (e.g., hypertension, atrial fibrillation, diabetes mellitus, abdominal surgery, cardio/thoracic surgery, trauma, mechanical ventilation, hypovolemia, traumatic brain injury). In addition to medical or surgical conditions, lifestyle choices such as smoking affect tissue perfusion. Hypertension increases stroke risk four to six times. Diabetes triples a client's stroke risk (Palmieri, 2006).*
- ▲ If the client has a period of syncope or other signs of a possible transient ischemic attack, assist the client to a resting position, perform a neurological and cardiovascular assessment, and report findings to the physician. *Syncope may be caused by dysrhythmias, hypotension caused by decreased tone*

● = Independent   ▲ = Collaborative   **EBN** = Evidence-Based Nursing   **EB** = Evidence-Based

or volume, cerebrovascular disease, or anxiety. Clients with syncope associated with cerebrovascular disease often have additional symptoms such as leg or arm weakness, double vision, difficulty speaking, ataxia, or sensory problems (Fauci et al, 2008).

- If the client experiences dizziness because of postural hypotension when getting up, teach the client methods to decrease dizziness, such as rising slowly, remaining seated for several minutes before standing, flexing feet up and down several times while seated, rising slowly, sitting down immediately if feeling dizzy, and trying to have someone present when standing. *These are methods to decrease postural hypotension and possible falling causing injury (Fauci et al, 2008).*

▲ If symptoms of a new cerebrovascular accident occur (e.g., slurred speech, change in vision, hemiparesis, hemiplegia, or dysphasia), notify a physician immediately. **EB:** *New onset of these neurological symptoms can signify a stroke. If the stroke is caused by a thrombus and the client receives thrombolytic treatment within 3 hours, effects can often be reversed and function improved, although there is an increased risk of intracranial hemorrhage (Wardlaw et al, 2003).*

- If symptoms of a stroke are present, use the National Institute of Health Stroke Scale (NIHSS) to evaluate the condition of the client. *The scale includes evaluation of level of consciousness, field of vision testing, facial nerve function, checking for ataxia, and ability to speak. Information on the scale is available at http://stroke.nih.gov/resources/scale.htm.* **EB:** *The NIHSS score as an outcome measure in acute stroke is a useful analytic and communication tool (Bruno, Saha, & Williams, 2009).*

▲ Provide fluid resuscitation carefully as ordered, generally with an isotonic solution such as 0.9% normal saline. *Poor fluid resuscitation of clients is associated with an increased incidence of morbidity and mortality (Cottingham & Bridges, 2006).*

▲ Avoid periods of physiologic stress which can lead to hypoxemia. Minimize environmental stressors. Monitor oxygen saturation and provide oxygen therapy as ordered. Take steps to prevent hypovolemia and hypotensive episodes. **EBN:** *Physiologic stress that is often associated with critical illness can cause the body to initiate protective mechanisms to shunt blood to the vital organs to perfuse the brain and heart, and decrease perfusion to the gastrointestinal and other nonvital organs (Martin, 2007; Gregory, 2008; Singh et al, 2008).*

- Perform a neurological assessment every hour to every 4 hours as appropriate. **EB:** *Clinical symptoms of cerebral vasospasm include fluctuations in level of consciousness, motor weakness, and aphasia (Sakowitz & Unterberg, 2006).*

- Complete Glasgow Coma Scale assessment as ordered and indicated. The *Glasgow Coma Scale is a neurological assessment tool used to assess the extent and progression of neurological injury. A declining score over time can be an indicator of the need for acute management or neurosurgical intervention (Iacono & Lyons, 2005).*

- Monitor for changes in mental status or behavior. **EBN:** *Decreased mental status is suggestive of decreased cerebral perfusion (Goodrich & Bridges, 2006).*

▲ Monitor vital signs at least three times daily or hourly if needed. Notify provider of any deviations from baseline. *Clients with unstable vital signs should be monitored continuously using invasive or non-invasive methods.* **EBN:** *Systemic hypertension is common following neurologic injury/insult. Continuous monitoring may allow clinicians to observe trends and respond as appropriate (Blissitt, 2006).*

- Monitor pupil size and reactivity. **EBN:** *Changes in pupil size and reactivity can indicate cranial nerve involvement in the brain injured person, increased intracranial pressure, and herniation (Meeker et al, 2005).*

▲ Monitor laboratory data as ordered. **EBN:** *Trending serial laboratory measures including lactate, base deficit, and venous oxygen saturation is used for assessing systemic tissue perfusion (Cottingham & Bridges, 2006).*

- Provide safety measures to prevent falls. **EBN:** *Clients suffering neurological insults are at increased risk for falls. History of stroke, altered mental status, dementia, and disorientation are risk factors for falls (Chelly et al, 2008).*

▲ Administer medications as ordered. Discuss with provider ordering a AT1–R blocker such as candesartan if client is hypertensive. **EB:** *Candesartan is shown to protect against stroke in hypertensive clients and has been shown to have a beneficial effect on cerebrovascular and cardiovascular events during a 12–month follow-up (Liu et al, 2008). Common pharmaceutical agents used in managing increased intracranial pressure include mannitol, barbiturates, sedation, analgesic, and hypertonic saline (Blissitt, 2006).*

• = Independent ▲ = Collaborative **EBN** = Evidence-Based Nursing **EB** = Evidence-Based

▲ Maintain invasive intracranial monitoring, central venous pressure monitoring and continuous mixed venous oxygen saturation as ordered. *Systemic hemodynamic monitoring alone is of limited use in assessing and managing cerebral hypoxia. SvO₂ monitoring can provide insight into intracranial oxygen supply and demand (Blissitt, 2006).*

Client/Family Education and Discharge Planning

- Teach the client risk factors for stroke. *Risk factors include atherosclerosis, hypertension, smoking, diabetes mellitus, hyperlipidemia, and systemic inflammation (Palmieri, 2006).*
- Teach family/client warning signs of impending stroke. Warning signs include headache focused on one side of the head, changes in mentation, ability to speak. *Stress the importance of reporting any new symptoms to his/her provider (Palmieri, 2006).*
- Encourage the client to participate in smoking cessation. *Tobacco smoking almost doubles the risk of ischemic stroke (Palmieri, 2006).*
- Teach lifestyle changes that can help lower cholesterol levels. *Lifestyle changes include weight loss, low fat/low cholesterol diet, and exercise (Palmieri, 2006).*
- Teach client the importance of stress reduction. *Anger and other negative emotions may play a role in triggering ischemic stroke (Palmieri, 2006).*

ℰvolve   See the EVOLVE website for Weblinks for client education resources.

REFERENCES

Blissitt P: Hemodynamic monitoring in the care of the critically ill neuroscience patient, *AACN Adv Crit Care* 17(3):327–340, 2006.

Bruno A, Saha C, Williams LS: Percent change on the National Institutes of Health Stroke Scale: a useful acute stroke outcome measure, *J Stroke Cerebrovasc Dis* 18(1):56–59, 2009.

Chelly J, Conroy L, Miller G et al: Risk factors and injury associated with falls in elderly hospitalized patients in a community hospital, *J Patient Saf* 4(3):178–183, 2008.

Cottingham C, Bridges E: Resuscitation of traumatic shock: a hemodynamic review, *AACN Adv Crit Care* 17(3):317–326, 2006.

Fauci A, Braunwald E, Kasper DL et al: *Harrison's principles of internal medicine,* ed 17, New York, 2008, McGraw Hill.

Goodrich C, Bridges E: Endpoints of resuscitation: what should we be monitoring? *AACN Adv Crit Care* 17(3):306–316, 2006.

Gregory K: Clinical predictors of necrotizing enterocolitis in premature infants, *Nurs Res* 57(4):260–270, 2008.

Iacono L, Lyons K: Making GCS as easy as 1, 2, 3, 4, 5, 6, *J Trauma Nurs* 12(3):77–81, 2005.

Liu H, Kitazato K, Uno M et al: Protective mechanisms of the angiotensin II type 1 receptor blocker candesartan against cerebral ischemia: in-vivo and in-vitro studies, *J Hypertens* 26(7):1435–1445, 2008.

Martin B: Prevention of gastrointestinal complications in the critically ill patient, *AACN Adv Crit Care* 18(2):158–160, 2007.

Meeker M, Du R, Bacchetti P et al: Pupil examination: validity and clinical utility of an automated pupillometer, *J Neurosci Nurs* 37(1):34–40, 2005.

Palmieri R: Cerebral artery stenosis paves the way for a stroke, *Nursing* 36(6):36–41, 2006.

Sakowitz O, Unterberg A: Detecting and treating microvascular ischemia after subarachnoid hemorrhage, *Curr Opin Crit Care* 12(2):103–111, 2006.

Singh H, Houy T, Singh N et al: Gastrointestinal prophylaxis in critically ill patients, *Crit Care Nurs Q* 31(4):291–301, 2008.

Wardlaw JM, Zoppo G, Yamaguchi T et al: Thrombolysis for acute ischaemic stroke, *Cochrane Database Syst Rev* (3):CD000213, 2003.

Risk for ineffective gastrointestinal tissue Perfusion   *Joan Klehr, RNC, BS, MPH*

NANDA-I

Definition

At risk for decrease in gastrointestinal circulation

Risk Factors

Abdominal aortic aneurysm; abdominal compartment syndrome; abnormal partial thromboplastin time; abnormal prothrombin time; acute gastrointestinal bleed; acute gastrointestinal hemorrhage; age >60 years; anemia; coagulopathy (e.g., sickle cell anemia); diabetes mellitus; disseminated intravascular coagulation; female gender; gastric paresis (e.g., diabetes mellitus); gastroesophageal varicies; gastrointestinal disease (e.g., duodenal or gastric ulcer, ischemic colitis, ischemic pancreatitis); hemodynamic instability; liver dysfunction; myocardial infarction; poor left ventricular performance; renal failure; stroke; trauma; smoking; treatment-related side effects (e.g., cardiopulmonary bypass, medica-

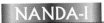
• = Independent   ▲ = Collaborative   **EBN** = Evidence-Based Nursing   **EB** = Evidence-Based

tion, anesthesia, gastric surgery); vascular disease (e.g., peripheral vascular disease, aortoiliac occlusive disease)

 (Nursing Outcomes Classification)

Suggested NOC Outcomes

Tissue Perfusion: Abdominal Organs, Gastrointestinal Function, Tissue Perfusion: Cellular, Circulation Status, Knowledge: Treatment Regimen

---

Example NOC Outcome with Indicators

Tissue Perfusion: Abdominal Organs as evidenced by the following indicators: Diastolic, systolic, and mean arterial blood pressure within normal limits/Bowel sounds active/Urine output within normal limits for age/Electrolyte and acid/base balance within normal limits (Rate the outcome and indicators of **Tissue Perfusion: Abdominal Organs:** 1 = severe deviation from normal range, 2 = substantial deviation from normal range, 3 = moderate deviation from normal range, 4 = mid deviation from normal range, 5 = no deviation from normal range [see Section I].)

Client Outcomes

Client Will (Specify Time Frame):

- Maintain blood pressure within normal limits
- Remain free from abdominal distention
- Tolerate feedings without nausea, vomiting, or abdominal discomfort
- Pass stools of normal color, consistency, frequency, and amount
- Describe prescribed diet regimen
- Describe prescribed medication regimen including medication actions and possible side effects
- Verbalize understanding of treatment regimen including monitoring for signs and symptoms that may indicate problems with gastrointestinal tissue perfusion, the importance of diet and exercise to gastrointestinal health

NIC **(Nursing Interventions Classification)**

Suggested NIC Interventions

Vital Signs Monitoring, Surveillance, Bowel Management, Electrolyte Monitoring, Laboratory Data Interpretation, Medication Management, Teaching: Prescribed Diet, Teaching: Disease Process, Teaching: Prescribed Medication, Nutrition Monitoring

---

Example NIC Activities—Surveillance

Monitor gastrointestinal function; Monitor vital signs

Nursing Interventions and *Rationales*

▲ Monitor vital signs at least three times a day. Notify physician if significant deviation from baseline. **EBN:** *Splanchnic hypoperfusion is a common pathophysiologic mechanism leading to mucosal ischemia and GI dysfunction. The gastrointestinal vasculature is not able to compensate for reduced systemic blood pressure. Any state of decreased cardiac output, vasopressor usage, or mechanical ventilation can lead to splanchnic hypoperfusion, which then leads to ischemia, decreased bicarbonate secretion, and decreased upper gastrointestinal motility (Martin, 2007; Gregory, 2008).*

▲ Avoid periods of physiologic stress which can lead to hypoxemia. Minimize environmental stressors. Monitor oxygen saturation and provide oxygen therapy as ordered. Take steps to prevent hypovolemia and hypotensive episodes. **EBN:** *Physiologic stress that is often associated with critical illness can cause the body to initiate protective mechanisms, to shunt blood to the vital organs, to perfuse the brain and heart, and decrease perfusion to the gastrointestinal and other nonvital organs (Martin, 2007; Gregory, 2008; Singh et al, 2008).* **EB:** *The use of vasopressive agents such as epinephrine or norepinephrine for treatment of hypotension decreases regional mesenteric blood flow in the intestine even though arterial blood pressure and systemic oxygen delivery increase (Krejci, Hiltebrand, & Gisli, 2006).*

• = Independent   ▲ = Collaborative   **EBN** = Evidence-Based Nursing   **EB** = Evidence-Based

- Encourage the client to eat small, frequent meals rather than three larger meals. Encourage the client to rest after eating to maximize blood flow to the stomach and improve digestion. *Smaller meals will reduce pressure on the lower esophageal sphincter (O'Malley, 2008).*

- Complete a physical abdominal examination including inspection, auscultation, percussion, and palpation. *Associated signs and symptoms of common gastrointestinal complications can be distinguished through physical assessment for example; increased peristaltic waves and high-pitched or "tinkling" bowel sounds can be an indicator of paralytic ileus (Martin, 2007). Marked visible peristaltic waves accompanied by abdominal distention is indicative of intestinal obstruction (Jarvis, 2008).*

- Monitor frequency, consistency, color, and amount of stools. *Loose watery stools without blood, pus, or mucous may indicate infection or a reaction to pharmaceutical agents; bloody diarrhea may indicate mesenteric ischemia (Martin, 2007). Clients presenting with sudden cramping, left lower abdominal pain, a strong urge to pass stool and bright red or maroon blood mixed with the stool should be evaluated for colon ischemia (Frishman et al, 2008).*

- Assess for abdominal distension. Measure abdominal girth and compare to client's accustomed waist or belt size. *Common causes of abdominal distension include fat, flatus, fluid, fetus, feces, and tumor (Jarvis, 2008). Abdominal distension from bowel obstruction occurs almost immediately after the obstruction develops and is due to accumulation of fluids and gases (Martin, 2007).*

▲ Monitor for gastrointestinal side effects from medication administrations, particularly NSAIDs. Discuss with the provider the possibility of prescribing a gastroprotective agent such as a proton pump inhibitor for clients requiring long-term administration of NSAIDs. *Nonsteroidal anti-inflammatory drugs (NSAIDs) have significant gastrointestinal toxicity. The mechanisms of damage include disruption of the mucus layer, inhibition of bicarbonate secretion, local tissue hypoxia caused by vasoconstriction, and others. Up to 60% of clients taking these types of medications have some injury and serious adverse events, including gastric and duodenal ulcers; perforation and hemorrhage can occur, and the damage may be asymptomatic especially in the elderly. The relative risk of injury increases with age (Jones et al, 2008).*

- Review the client's past medical and surgical history. Recognize that certain conditions place clients at higher risk for ineffective tissue perfusion (e.g., diabetes mellitus, abdominal surgery, cardio/thoracic surgery, trauma, mechanical ventilation). In addition to medical or surgical conditions, lifestyle choices such as smoking affect tissue perfusion. **EB:** *Gastrointestinal complications following cardiac surgery are rare, but substantially increase morbidity and mortality. Risk factors include age, intraoperative hypoperfusion, and need for high-dose vasopressors (Abboud et al, 2008).*

▲ Complete pain assessment. Assess and document the onset, intensity, character, location, duration, aggravating factors, and relieving factors. Determine whether the pain is exacerbated by eating. Notify the provider of any increase in pain or discomfort or if comfort measures are not effective. *Abdominal pain is a sensitive indicator of GI pathology (Martin, 2007). A significant symptom of mesenteric ischemia is pain that is disproportionate to the physical examination findings. Acute arterial mesenteric ischemia often has the most abrupt onset of pain. Clients presenting with acute mesenteric ischemia may have a history of abdominal angina, which is a syndrome of pain starting soon after eating and lasting for several hours (Stamatakos et al, 2008).*

- Encourage the client to ambulate or perform activity as tolerated, but vigorous activity or heavy lifting should be avoided for several hours after meals. *Decreasing activity reduces the risk of reflux during digestion of food (O'Malley, 2008).*

▲ Assess fluid and electrolyte balance by monitoring intake and output, and reviewing laboratory data as ordered. *Vomiting and diarrhea are common gastrointestinal symptoms and can cause depletion of fluids and electrolytes if not replaced. Gastrointestinal disease is the most common cause of fluid and electrolyte imbalance. Large amounts of fluid and electrolytes may be lost from the GI tract or pooled in the ileus (Macafee, Allison, & Lobo, 2005).*

▲ Prepare client for diagnostic or surgical procedures. Diagnostic studies may include abdominal x-ray to rapidly rule out intestinal obstruction, CT, angiography, and abdominal ultrasound. Surgical procedures include exploratory laparotomy, thrombectomy, surgical revascularization, and/or stent placement (Stamatakos et al, 2008). **EB:** *Elderly clients with serum ferritin concentration in the low normal range should be considered for GI investigation using endoscopy. Anemic clients without evidence of iron deficiency have a low incidence of bleeding GI lesions and should not undergo GI investigation (Powell & McNair, 2008).*

• = Independent   ▲ = Collaborative   **EBN** = Evidence-Based Nursing   **EB** = Evidence-Based

Client/Family Teaching and Discharge Planning

- Provide client teaching related to risk factors for ineffective gastrointestinal tissue perfusion, signs and symptoms, lifestyle changes that can improve gastrointestinal functioning. Start with the client's base level of understanding and use that as a foundation for further education. *Client education is most effective and efficient when the education involves the learner and is individualized to his/her needs including culture specific needs (London, 2008).*
- ▲ Teach client about any medications prescribed. Medication teaching includes the drug name, its purpose, administration instructions such as taking it with or without food, and any side effects to be aware of. Instruct the client to report any adverse side effects to his or her provider. *Assessing and instructing clients about medications on focusing on important details can help prevent client medication errors (Polzien, 2007).*

Ⓔvolve   See the EVOLVE website for Weblinks for client education resources.

REFERENCES

Abboud B, Daher R, Sleilaty G et al: Is prompt exploratory laparotomy the best attitude for mesenteric ischemia after cardiac surgery? *Interact Cardiovasc Thorac Surg* 7:1079–1083, 2008.

Frishman W, Novak S, Brandt L et al: Pharmacologic management of mesenteric occlusive disease, *Cardiol Rev* 16(2):59–68, 2008.

Gregory K: Clinical predictors of necrotizing enterocolitis in premature infants, *Nurs Res* 57(4):260–270, 2008.

Jarvis C: *Physical Examination & Health Assessment,* ed 5, Philadelphia, 2008, Saunders, Elsevier.

Jones R, Rubin G, Berenbaum F et al: Gastrointestinal and cardiovascular risks of nonsteroidal anti-inflammatory drugs, *Am J Med* 121(6):464–474, 2008.

Krejci V, Hiltebrand L, Gisli H: Effects of epinephrine, norepinephrine, and phenylephrine on microcirculatory blood flow in the gastrointestinal tract in sepsis, *Crit Care Med,* 34(5):1456–1463, 2006.

London, F: Meeting the challenge: patient education in a diverse America, *J Nurses Staff Dev* 24(6):283–285, 2008.

Macafee D, Allison S, Lobo D: Some interactions between gastrointestinal function and fluid and electrolyte homeostasis, *Currnt Opin Clini Nutr Metabol Care* 8(2):197–203, 2005.

Martin B: Prevention of gastrointestinal complications in the critically ill patient, *AACN Adv Crit Care* 18(2):158–166, 2007.

O'Malley P: *Screening for GERD in hospitalized patients, Clinical Updates,* 2008. www.nursingconsult.com/das/stat/view/124538266–4/cup?nid=191270&sid=813547978&SEQNO=2. Accessed May 12, 2009.

Polzien G: Prevent medication errors: a New Year's resolution: teaching patients about their medications, *Home Healthc Nurse* 25(1):59–62, 2007.

Powell N, McNair A: Gastrointestinal evaluation of anaemic patients without evidence of iron deficiency, *Eur J Gastroenterol Hepatol* 20(11), 2008.

Singh H, Houy T, Singh N et al: Gastrointestinal prophylaxis in critically ill patients, *Crit Care Nurs Q* 31(4):291–301, 2008.

Stamatakos M, Stefanaki C, Mastrokalos D et al: Mesenteric ischemia: still a deadly puzzle for the medical community, *Tohoku J Exp Med* 216(3):197–204, 2008.

Ineffective peripheral tissue Perfusion   Ⓔvolve

Lorraine A. Duggan, MSN, RN, APNC, Maryanne Crowther, MSN, APN, CCRN, and Jennifer Hafner, RN, BSN, TNCC

NANDA-I

Definition

Decrease in blood circulation to the periphery that may compromise health

Defining Characteristics

Absent pulses; altered motor function; altered skin characteristics (color, elasticity, hair, moisture, nails, sensation, temperature); blood pressure changes in extremities; claudication; color does not return to leg on lowering it; delayed peripheral wound healing; diminished pulses; edema; extremity pain; paraesthesia; skin color pale on elevation

Related Factors (r/t)

Deficient knowledge of aggravating factors (e.g., smoking, sedentary lifestyle, trauma, obesity, salt intake, immobility); deficient knowledge of disease process (e.g., diabetes, hyperlipidemia); diabetes mellitus; hypertension; sedentary lifestyle; smoking

NOC   (Nursing Outcomes Classification)

Suggested NOC Outcomes

Circulation Status, Fluid Balance, Hydration, Tissue Perfusion: Peripheral

Example NOC Outcome with Indicators

Demonstrates adequate **Circulation Status** as evidenced by the following indicators: Peripheral pulses strong/ Peripheral pulses symmetrical/Peripheral edema not present (Rate the outcome and indicators of **Circulation Status:** 1 = severely compromised, 2 = substantially compromised, 3 = moderately compromised, 4 = mildly compromised, 5 = not compromised [see Section I].)

Client Outcomes

Client Will (Specify Time Frame):

- Demonstrate adequate tissue perfusion as evidenced by palpable peripheral pulses, warm and dry skin, adequate urine output, and absence of respiratory distress
- Verbalize knowledge of treatment regimen, including appropriate exercise and medications and their actions and possible side effects
- Identify changes in lifestyle needed to increase tissue perfusion

NIC   (Nursing Interventions Classification)

Suggested NIC Intervention

Circulatory Care: Arterial Insufficiency

Example NIC Activities—Circulatory Care: Arterial Insufficiency

Evaluate peripheral edema and pulses; Inspect skin for arterial ulcers and tissue breakdown

Nursing Interventions and *Rationales*

- ▲ Check the brachial, radial, dorsalis pedis, posterior tibial, and popliteal pulses bilaterally. If unable to find them, use a Doppler stethoscope and notify the physician immediately if new onset of pulses is not present. *Diminished or absent peripheral pulses indicate arterial insufficiency with resultant ischemia (Fauci et al, 2008).*
- Note skin color and feel the temperature of the skin. *Skin pallor or mottling, cool or cold skin temperature, or an absent pulse can signal arterial obstruction, which is an emergency that requires immediate intervention (Dillon, 2003). Rubor (reddish-blue color accompanied by dependency) indicates dilated or damaged vessels. Brownish discoloration of the skin on the anterior tibia indicates chronic venous insufficiency (Simon, Dix, & McCollum, 2004; Bickley & Szilagyi, 2007).*
- Check capillary refill. *Nail beds usually return to a pinkish color within 2 to 3 seconds after compression (Dillon, 2003).*
- Note skin texture and the presence of hair, ulcers, or gangrenous areas on the legs or feet. *Thin, shiny, dry skin with hair loss; brittle nails; and gangrene or ulcerations on toes and anterior surfaces of the feet are seen in clients with arterial insufficiency. If ulcerations are on the side of the leg, they are usually associated with venous insufficiency (Bickley & Szilagyi, 2007).*
- Note the presence of edema in the extremities and rate severity on a four-point scale. Measure the circumference of the ankle and calf at the same time each day in the early morning.
- Assess for pain in the extremities, noting severity, quality, timing, and exacerbating and alleviating factors. Differentiate venous from arterial disease. *In clients with venous insufficiency the pain lessens with elevation of the legs and exercise. In clients with arterial insufficiency the pain increases with elevation of the legs and exercise (Fauci et al, 2008). Some clients have both arterial and venous insufficiency. Arterial insufficiency is associated with pain when walking (claudication) that is relieved by rest. Clients with severe arterial disease have foot pain while at rest, which keeps them awake at night. Venous insufficiency is associated with aching, cramping, and discomfort (Fauci et al, 2008).*

Arterial Insufficiency

▲ Monitor peripheral pulses. If there is new onset of loss of pulses with bluish, purple, or black areas and extreme pain, notify the physician immediately. *These are symptoms of arterial obstruction that can result in loss of a limb if not immediately reversed.*

▲ Measure Ankle Brachial Index (ABI) via Doppler. **EB:** *A study revealed that neither pulse palpation nor automatic oscillometric devices can be recommended as reliable methods for ABI measurement (Aboyans et al, 2008).*

• Do not elevate the legs above the level of the heart. *With arterial insufficiency, leg elevation decreases arterial blood supply to the legs.*

▲ For early arterial insufficiency, encourage exercise such as walking or riding an exercise bicycle from 30 to 60 minutes per day as ordered by the physician. *Exercise therapy should be the initial intervention in nondisabling claudication (Treat-Jacobson & Walsh, 2003; Fauci et al, 2008).* **EB:** *Participation in an exercise program was shown to increase walking times more effectively than angioplasty and antiplatelet therapy (Leng, Fowler & Ernst, 2004).* **EB:** *A study showed that brief exercise results in an improvement in cutaneous perfusion, particularly in individuals with diabetes (Williams, Harding, & Price, 2007). A study showed treadmill and resistance training both improve quality of life (Gupta, 2009).*

• Keep the client warm and have the client wear socks and shoes or sheepskin-lined slippers when mobile. Do not apply heat. *Clients with arterial insufficiency report being constantly cold; keep extremities warm to maintain vasodilation and blood supply. Heat application can easily damage ischemic tissues.*

• Use a variety of leg positions after surgical intervention for peripheral arterial disease (either supine with legs extended, sitting with legs extended, or supine with legs elevated 20 degrees) when getting this population out of bed. **EBN:** *There were no significant changes in transcutaneous oxygen measurements between positions used (Rich, 2004).* **EBN:** *Significant to the nursing care of clients with vascular disease is the finding that any of the leg/body positions in this study could be used postoperatively on the revascularized extremity without decreasing oxygenation (Rich, 2008).*

▲ Pay meticulous attention to foot care. Refer to a podiatrist if the client has a foot or nail abnormality. *Ischemic feet are vulnerable to injury; meticulous foot care can prevent further injury.*

• If the client has ischemic arterial ulcers, refer to the care plan for **Impaired Tissue integrity**.

▲ If client smokes, aggressively counsel the client to stop smoking and refer to the physician for medications to support nicotine withdrawal and a smoking withdrawal program. **EB:** *A combination of psychosocial and pharmacological interventions was more effective than either intervention alone to stop smoking behavior (van der Meer et al, 2003). A recent Cochrane review found that use of the medication varenicline (Chantix) increased the rate of smoking withdrawal two to three times more than smoking withdrawal without use of medications (Cahill, Stead, & Lancaster, 2008).*

Venous Insufficiency

▲ Elevate edematous legs as ordered and ensure no pressure under the knee and heels to prevent pressure ulcers. *Elevation increases venous return, helps decrease edema, and can help heal venous leg ulcers (Simon, Dix, & McCollum, 2004). Pressure under the knee decreases venous circulation.* **EBN:** *When the heels are elevated, tissue perfusion to the area is substantially increased, alleviating tissue hypoxia, evidenced by the heel capillary bed hyperemia (Huber et al, 2008).*

▲ Apply graduated compression stockings as ordered. Ensure proper fit by measuring accurately. Remove the stocking at least twice a day, in the morning with the bath and in the evening, to assess the condition of the extremity, then reapply. Knee-length is preferred rather than thigh length. **EBN and EB:** *The use of graduated compression stockings reduced the incidence of deep vein thrombosis in a high-risk orthopedic surgical population. Implementation of additional antithrombotic measures along with stocking use decreased the incidence even further (Joanna Briggs Institute, 2001). Graduated compression stockings, alone or used in conjunction with other prevention modalities, help prevent deep vein thrombosis in hospitalized clients (Amarigiri & Lees, 2005).* **EBN:** *A study that assessed use of knee-length graduated compression stockings found they are as effective as thigh-length graduated compression stockings. They are more comfortable for clients, are easier for staff and clients to use, pose less risk of injury to clients, and are less expensive as recommended in this study (Hilleren-Listerud, 2009).*

• = Independent ▲ = Collaborative **EBN** = Evidence-Based Nursing **EB** = Evidence-Based

- Encourage the client to walk with compression stockings on and perform toe-up and point-flex exercises. *Exercise helps increase venous return, builds up collateral circulation, and strengthens the calf muscle pumps (Simon, Dix, & McCollum, 2004).*
- If the client is overweight, encourage weight loss to decrease venous disease. *Obesity is a risk factor for development of chronic venous disease (Fauci et al, 2008).*
- If the client has venous leg ulcers, encourage the client to avoid prolonged sitting, standing, and elevation of the involved leg. **EBN:** *Wound perfusion was lower when the client with venous leg ulcers was sitting, standing, or elevating the involved leg than when the client was lying supine (Wipke-Tevis et al, 2001).*
- Discuss lifestyle with the client to determine if the client's occupation requires prolonged standing or sitting, which can result in chronic venous disease (Fauci et al, 2008).
- ▲ If the client is mostly immobile, consult with the physician regarding use of a calf-high pneumatic compression device for prevention of deep vein thrombosis. *Pneumatic compression devices can be effective in preventing deep vein thrombosis in the immobile client (Van Gerpen & Mast, 2004; Roman, 2005).*
- Observe for signs of deep vein thrombosis, including pain, tenderness, swelling in the calf and thigh, and redness in the involved extremity. Take serial leg measurements of the thigh and calf circumferences. In some clients a tender venous cord can be felt in the popliteal fossa. Do not rely on Homans' sign. *Thrombosis with clot formation is usually first detected as swelling of the involved leg and then as pain. Homans' sign is not reliable. Symptoms of existing deep vein thrombosis are nonspecific and cannot be used alone to determine the presence of DVT (Fauci et al, 2008).*
- ▲ Note the results of a D-dimer test and ultrasounds. *High levels of d-dimer, a fibrin degradation fragment, are found in deep vein thrombosis and pulmonary embolism (Sadovsky, 2005), but results should be confirmed with a duplex venous ultrasonogram (Fauci et al, 2008).*
- If deep vein thrombosis is present, observe for symptoms of a pulmonary embolism, including dyspnea, tachypnea, and tachycardia, especially with a history of trauma. **EB:** *Fatal pulmonary embolisms are reported in one third of trauma clients (Agency for Healthcare Research and Quality, 2009).*
- If client is receiving heparin subcutaneously, do not change the needle after drawing up the dose. **EBN:** *Changing the subcutaneous needle after withdrawing heparin from a vial did not reduce the size of ecchymoses at the injection site of study subjects (Klingman, 2000).*
- ▲ If client develops deep vein thrombosis, after treatment and hospital discharge recommend client wear below-the-knee elastic compression stockings during the day on the involved extremity. **EB:** *Clients who wore compression stockings had a 50% less likely incidence of developing postthrombotic syndrome than did clients who did not wear the stockings (Shaughnessy, 2005). There is substantial evidence that compression stockings reduce the occurrence of postthrombotic syndrome after deep vein thrombosis (Kolbach et al, 2004).*

Geriatric

- Change the client's position slowly when getting the client out of bed. *Postural hypotension can be detected in up to 30% of elderly clients (Tinetti, 2003).*
- Recognize that the elderly have an increased risk of developing pulmonary embolism; if it is present, the symptoms are nonspecific and often mimic those of heart failure or pneumonia (Berman, 2001).

Home Care

- The interventions previously described may be adapted for home care use.
- Differentiate between arterial and venous insufficiency. *Accurate diagnostic information directs nursing care.*
- If arterial disease is present and the client smokes, aggressively encourage smoking cessation.
- Examine the feet carefully at frequent intervals for changes and new ulcerations. *Lower Extremity Amputation Prevention Program (LEAP) documentation forms are available at www.hrsa.gov/leap (Health Resources and Service Administration, 2009).*
- ▲ Assess the client's nutritional status, paying special attention to obesity, hyperlipidemia, and malnutrition. Refer to a dietitian if appropriate. *Malnutrition contributes to anemia, which further*

• = Independent   ▲ = Collaborative   **EBN** = Evidence-Based Nursing   **EB** = Evidence-Based

compounds the lack of oxygenation to tissues. Obese clients have poor circulation in adipose tissue, which can create increased hypoxia in the tissues.

- Monitor for development of gangrene, venous ulceration, and symptoms of cellulitis (redness, pain, and increased swelling in an extremity). *Cellulitis often accompanies peripheral vascular disease.*
- Assess pain management strategies and their effectiveness. **EBN:** *Effective pain management is recommended to assist adherence to the medical regimen (Van Hecke, Grypdonck, & Defloor, 2009).*
- Assess support systems available at home and in the community. **EBN:** *Effective social support by family or significant others should be encouraged to assist adherence to the medical regimen (Van Hecke, Grypdonck, & Defloor, 2009).*

Client/Family Teaching and Discharge Planning

- Explain the importance of good foot care. Teach the client and family to wash and inspect the feet daily. Recommend that the diabetic client wear padded socks, special insoles, and jogging shoes. *Use of cushioned footwear can decrease pressure on the feet, decrease callus formation, and help save the feet.*
- ▲ Teach the diabetic client that he or she should have a comprehensive foot examination at least annually, including assessment of sensation using the Semmes-Weinstein monofilaments. If good sensation is not present, refer to a footwear professional for fitting of therapeutic shoes and inserts, the cost of which is covered by Medicare. **EB:** *A research study found that use of 6–gm monofilaments was helpful in detecting loss of sensation in clients with Type II diabetes (Thomson et al, 2008).*
- For arterial disease, stress the importance of not smoking, following a weight loss program (if the client is obese), carefully controlling a diabetic condition, controlling hyperlipidemia and hypertension, maintaining intake of antiplatelet therapy, and reducing stress. *All these risk factors for atherosclerosis can be modified (Treat-Jacobson, 2003).*
- Teach the client to avoid exposure to cold; limit exposure to brief periods if going out in cold weather and wear warm clothing.
- For venous disease, teach the importance of wearing compression stockings as ordered, elevating the legs at intervals, and watching for skin breakdown on the legs (Shaughnessy, 2005).
- Teach the client to recognize the signs and symptoms that should be reported to a physician (e.g., change in skin temperature, color, or sensation or the presence of a new lesion on the foot).
- Provide clear, simple instructions about plan of care. **EBN:** *Health care professionals should give clear, unambiguous and tailored information according to this study (Van Hecke, Grypdonck & Defloor, 2009).*

NOTE: If the client is receiving anticoagulant therapy, see the care plan for **Ineffective Protection**.

ⓔvolve   See the EVOLVE website for Weblinks for client education resources.

REFERENCES

Aboyans V, Lacroix P, Doucet S et al: Diagnosis of peripheral arterial disease in general practice: can the ankle-brachial index be measured either by pulse palpation or an automatic blood pressure device? *Int J Clin Pract* 62(7):1001–1007, 2008.

Agency for Healthcare Research and Quality: *Prevention of venous thromboembolism after injury.* www.ahrq.gov/clinic/epcsums/vtsumm.htm. Accessed May 1, 2009.

Amarigiri SV, Lees TA: Elastic compression stockings for prevention of deep vein thrombosis, *Cochrane Database Syst Rev* (3):CD001484, 2005.

Berman AR: Pulmonary embolism in the elderly, *Clin Geriatr Med* 17(1):107, 2001.

Bickley LS, Szilagyi PG: *Bates guide to physical examination and history taking,* ed 9, Philadelphia, 2007, Lippincott.

Cahill K, Stead LF, Lancaster T: Nicotine receptor partial agonists for smoking cessation, *Cochrane Database Syst Rev* (3):CD006103, 2008.

Dillon PM: *Nursing health assessment,* Philadelphia, 2003, F.A. Davis.

Fauci A Braunwald E, Kasper DL et al: *Harrison's principles of internal medicine,* ed 17, New York, 2008, McGraw-Hill.

Gupta S: Endurance and strength training have different benefits for people with peripheral arterial disease, but both improve quality of life *Aust J Physiother* 55(1):63, 2009.

Health Resources and Service Administration. *Lower extremity amputation prevention.* www.hrsa.gov/leap. Accessed on May 1, 2009.

Hilleren-Listerud AE: Graduated compression stocking and intermittent pneumatic compression device length selection *Clin Nurse Spec* 23(1):21–24, 2009.

Huber J, Reddy R, Pitham T et al: Increasing heel skin perfusion by elevation, *Adv Skin Wound Care* 21(1):37–41, 2008.

Joanna Briggs Institute: Best practice: graduated compression stockings for the prevention of post-operative venous thromboembolism, *Evidence based practice information sheets for health professions.* www.joannabriggs.edu.au/pubs/best_practice.php?pageNum_rsBestPractice_/&totalRows_ersBestPractice_47, *Australia* 5:2, 2001. Accessed April 27, 2007.

Klingman L: Effects of changing needles prior to administering heparin subcutaneously, *Heart Lung* 29(1):70, 2000.

Kolbach DN, Sandbrink MW, Hamulyak K et al: Non-pharmaceutical measures for prevention of post-thrombotic syndrome, *Cochrane Database Syst Rev* (1):CD004174, 2004.

Leng GC, Fowler B, Ernst E: Exercise for intermittent claudication, *Cochrane Database Syst Rev* (2):CD000990, 2004.

Rich KA: *The effects of leg/body position on transcutaneous oxygen measurements in age-matched healthy subjects and PAD subjects after lower extremity arterial revascularization* [thesis], Chicago, 2004, Rush University College of Nursing.

Rich KA: The effects of leg/body position on transcutaneous oxygen measurements after lower-extremity arterial revascularization *J Vasc Nur* 26(1):6–14, 2008.

Roman M: Deep vein thrombosis: an overview, *Med-Surg Matters* 14(1), 2005.

Sadovsky R: D-Dimer assays for prediction of venous thromboembolism, *Am Fam Physician* 71(4):775–806, 2005.

Shaughnessy AF: Compression stockings and post-thrombotic syndrome, *Am Fam Physician* 71(1):139–188, 2005.

Simon DA, Dix FP, McCollum CN: Management of venous leg ulcers, *BMJ* 328(7452):1358, 2004.

Thomson MP, Potter J, Finch PM et al: Threshold for detection of diabetic peripheral sensory neuropathy using a range of research grade monofilaments in persons with Type 2 diabetes mellitus, *J Foot Ankle Res* 1(1):9, 2008.

Tinetti ME: Preventing falls in elderly persons, *N Engl J Med* 348(1):421, 2003.

Treat-Jacobson D, Walsh ME: Treating patients with peripheral arterial disease and claudication, *J Vasc Nurs* 21(1):5, 2003.

van der Meer RM, Wagena EJ, Ostelo RW et al: Smoking cessation for chronic obstructive pulmonary disease, *Cochrane Database Syst Rev* (2):CD002999, 2003.

Van Gerpen RV, Mast ME: Thromboembolic disorders in cancer, *Clin J Oncol Nurs* 8(3):289, 2004.

Van Hecke A, Grypdonck M, Defloor T: A review of why patients with leg ulcers do not adhere to treatment, *J Clin Nurs* 18(3):337–344, 2009.

Williams DT, Harding KG, Price PE: The influence of exercise on foot perfusion in diabetes, *Diabet Med* 24(10):1105–1111, 2007.

Wipke-Tevis DD, Stotts NA, Williams DA et al: Tissue oxygenation, perfusion, and position in patients with venous leg ulcers, *Nurs Res* 50(1):24, 2001.

Risk for Peripheral neurovascular dysfunction

Noreen C. Miller, RN, MSN, ONC, and Betty J. Ackley, MSN, EdS, RN

NANDA-I

Definition

At risk for disruption in circulation, sensation, or motion of an extremity

Risk Factors

Burns; fractures; immobilization; mechanical compression (e.g., tourniquet, cane, cast, brace, dressing, restraint); orthopedic surgery; trauma; vascular obstruction

NOC   (Nursing Outcomes Classification)

Suggested NOC Outcomes

Circulation Status, Neurological Status: Spinal Sensory/Motor Function, Tissue Perfusion: Peripheral

Example **NOC** Outcome with Indicators
Tissue Perfusion: Peripheral as evidenced by the following indicators: Radial or pedal pulse strength/Capillary refill in fingers or toes/Extremity skin temperature/Localized extremity pain/Numbness/Tingling/Skin color/Muscle strength/Skin integrity/Peripheral edema (Rate the outcome and indicators of **Tissue Perfusion: Peripheral:** 1 = severe deviation from normal range, 2 = substantial deviation from normal range, 3 = moderate deviation from normal range, 4 5 = mild deviation from normal range, 5 = no deviation from normal range [see Section I].)

Client Outcomes

Client Will (Specify Time Frame):

- Maintain circulation, sensation, and movement of an extremity within client's own normal limits
- Explain signs of neurovascular compromise and ways to prevent venous stasis
- Explain and demonstrate low molecular weight heparin or fondaparinux injections which would be expected to be ordered in orthopedic cases and other high-risk conditions unless contraindicated. These injections may be ordered to continue at home after discharge.

 = Independent   ▲ = Collaborative   **EBN** = Evidence-Based Nursing   **EB** = Evidence-Based

| NIC | (Nursing Interventions Classification) |

Suggested NIC Interventions

Exercise Therapy: Joint Mobility, Peripheral Sensation Management

| **Example NIC Activities—Peripheral Sensation Management** |
| Monitor for paresthesia: numbness, tingling, hyperesthesia, and hypoesthesia; Monitor for thrombophlebitis and deep vein thrombosis |

Nursing Interventions and *Rationales*

▲ Perform neurovascular assessment every 15 minutes to every 4 hours as ordered or needed based on client's condition. Use the six Ps of assessment as outlined below. *The goal is to prevent ischemia (cell death). Delay in recognizing compartment syndrome can lead to paralysis, painful dysaesthesia, contracture and amputation of limb. Missing compartment syndrome can lead to ligation (Giannoudis, Tzioupis, & Pape, 2009).*

- **Pain:** Assess severity (on a scale of 1 to 10), quality, radiation, and relief by medications. *Excessive pain relative to injury incurred, pain on passive stretch and any numbness, tingling, or weakness (sensorimotor deficits) can indicate compartment syndrome (Gonzalez et al, 2009).*

- **Pulses:** Check the pulses distal to the injury. *Palpation of pulses in area of concern, such as tibia fracture, assess dorsalis pedis and posterior tibial pulses. Vascular assessment also includes checking color, temperature, and capillary refill. Compartment syndrome can occur in the face of an intact pulse (Miller & Askew, 2007). Always assess uninjured or unaffected side and compare with area of concern.*

- **Pallor/Poikilothermia:** Check color and temperature changes below the injury site. Check capillary refill. *If pallor is present, record the level of coldness carefully. A cold, pale, or bluish extremity indicates arterial insufficiency or arterial damage, and a physician should be notified (Bickley & Szilagyi, 2007). A reddened, warm extremity may indicate infection (Kasper et al, 2005). A capillary refilling time >3 seconds is abnormal (Lobos & Menon, 2008).*

- **Paresthesia** (change in sensation): Check by lightly touching the skin proximal and distal to the injury. Ask if the client has any unusual sensations such as hypersensitivity, tingling, prickling, decreased feeling, or numbness. Check nerve function (e.g., can the client feel a touch to the area of concern, such as the first web space of the foot [deep peroneal nerve] with tibia fracture). *Irreversible damage from compartment syndrome occurs when compression to tissue and nerves is left unchecked (Weinstein & Buckwalter, 2005).*

- **Paralysis:** Ask the client to perform appropriate range-of-motion exercises in the unaffected and then the affected extremity. *Loss of movement (paralysis) is a late symptom of compartment syndrome (Mamaril, Childs, & Sortman, 2007). Decreased range of motion and loss of movement can indicate impending muscle, nerve and vascular cellular death (ishcemia) (Mamaril, Childs, & Sortman, 2007).*

- **Pressure:** Check by feeling the extremity; note new onset of firmness of the extremity. *Internal pressure or external confinement or restriction can proceed to the point at which cellular exchange is diminished. Swelling and tightness of the involved compartment are indications of increased pressure (Rockwood, Green, & Bucholtz, 2006).*

▲ Monitor the client for symptoms of compartment syndrome evidenced by pain greater than expected, pain with passive movement, decreased sensation, weakness, loss of movement, absence of pulse, and tension in the skin that surrounds the muscle compartment. All of *the six P's may not be present, and they are not specific for compartment syndrome. Have a high index of suspicion for any of the six P's. Noting two or more of the six P's increases the probability of compartment syndrome (Giannoudis, Tziouspis, & Pape, 2009).*

- Monitor appropriate application and function of corrective device (e.g., cast, splint, traction) every 1 to 4 hours as needed. *Compartment syndrome can result from improper casting or splinting and is the most serious complication of casting or splinting. The condition results from increased pressure within a closed space that compromises blood flow. After immobilization (casting or splinting), if pain worsens, any tingling or numbness, swelling, delayed capillary refill or change in color of exposed digit, immediate evaluation is needed. Casting or splinting can cause thermal injuries or skin break down therefore proper padding is essential (Boyd, Benjamin, & Asplund, 2009).*

- Position the extremity in correct alignment with each position change; check every hour to ensure appropriate alignment.

Prevention of Deep Vein Thrombosis (DVT), Pulmonary Embolism (PE)

Prevention of fatal pulmonary embolism is top priority for prophylaxis programs as is the prevention of symptomatic DVT, PE, and postphlebitis syndrome (Geerts et al, 2008).

▲ Get the client out of bed as early possible and ambulate frequently after consultation with the physician. *Immobility is a risk factor for DVT; early ambulation can help prevent clot formation (Roman, 2005; Geerts et al, 2008).*

▲ Monitor for signs of DVT, especially in high-risk populations, including clients of increasing age; clients with immobility or obesity; clients taking estrogen or oral contraceptives, pregnancy and the postpartum period; inherited or acquired thrombophilia (e.g., Factor V Leiden) persons with a history of trauma, surgery, or previous DVT; and persons with a cerebrovascular accident, varicose veins, malignancy, or cardiovascular disease (Geerts et al, 2008).

- Recognize that mechanical methods for DVT prophylaxis such as graduated compression stocking (GCS), the use of intermittent pneumatic compression (IPC) devices, and the venous foot pump (VFP), increase venous outflow and/or reduce stasis within the leg veins.

▲ Apply graduated compression stockings if ordered; measure carefully to ensure proper fit, removing at least daily to assess circulation and skin condition. **EBN and EB:** *Graduated compression stockings reduced the incidence of DVT in a high-risk orthopedic surgical population and additional antithrombotic measures, along with stocking use, decreased the incidence even further (Joanna Briggs Institute, 2008). The use of graduated compression stockings, alone or in conjunction with other prevention modalities, prevents DVT in hospitalized clients (Amarigiri & Lees, 2005) by increasing venous outflow and/or reducing stasis within the leg veins (Geerts et al, 2008).*

▲ Apply intermittent pneumatic compression (IPC) device if ordered. *IPC is another mechanical prophylaxis used in addition to graduated compression stockings in the hospitalized or surgical client. Typically IPC device is used as much of the time as possible when client is in bed or sitting in a chair. Mechanical methods of prevention of VTE have advantage due to lack of bleeding potential that exists with LMWH (Geerts et al, 2008; Joanna Briggs Institute, 2008).*

▲ Watch for and report signs of DVT as evidenced by pain, deep tenderness, swelling in the calf and thigh, and redness in the involved extremity. Take serial leg measurements of the thigh and leg circumferences. In some clients, a tender venous cord can be felt in the popliteal fossa. Do not rely on Homans' sign. *Thrombosis with clot formation is usually first detected as edema of the involved leg and then as pain. Homans' sign is not reliable (Kasper et al, 2005).*

- Help the client perform prescribed exercises every 4 hours as ordered.
- Provide a nutritious diet and adequate fluid replacement. *Good nutrition and sufficient fluids are needed to promote healing and prevent complications.*

Geriatric

- Use heat and cold therapies cautiously. *Elderly clients often have decreased sensation and circulation.*
- Recognize that older clients have an increased risk of developing DVTs. *Being older than 60 (although DVT can occur at any age) increases risk for deep vein thrombosis (Link, 2008).*

Home Care

- Assess the knowledge base of the client and family after hospitalization.
- Teach about the disease process and care as necessary. *The shorter length of stay in hospital decreases time for teaching and may have been too short and insufficient for learning. Neurovascular status can deteriorate after discharge.*
- If risk is related to fractures and cast care, teach the family to complete a neurovascular assessment; it may be performed as often as every 4 hours but is more commonly done two to three times per

day. *A risk requiring monitoring more often than every 4 hours for longer than 24 hours indicates a need for evaluation.*

- If the fracture is peripheral, position the limb for comfort and change position frequently, avoiding dependent positions for extended periods. *Changes in position enhance circulation.*
- ▲ Refer to physical therapy services as necessary to establish an exercise program and safety in transfers or mobility within limitations of physical status.
- Establish an emergency plan.

Client/Family Teaching and Discharge Planning

- Teach the client and family to recognize signs of neurovascular dysfunction and report signs immediately to the appropriate person.
- Teach the client and family to recognize side effects of anticoagulant such as irritation, pain, tenderness, and redness that may occur at the site of injection.
- Teach the client and family to notify the doctor if the client experiences increased bruising, bleeding, or black stools.
- Emphasize proper nutrition to promote healing.
- ▲ If necessary, refer the client to a rehabilitation facility for instruction in proper use of assistive devices and measures to improve mobility without compromising neurovascular function.
- See **Ineffective peripheral tissue Perfusion** (venous insufficiency) for further interventions to prevent deep vein thrombosis.

eVolve   See the EVOLVE website for Weblinks for client education resources.

REFERENCES

Amarigiri SV, Lees TA: Elastic compression stockings for prevention of deep vein thrombosis, *Cochrane Database Syst Rev* (3):CD001484, 2005.

Bickley LS, Szilagyi PG: *Bates' guide to physical examination*, ed 9, Philadelphia, 2007, Lippincott Williams & Wilkins.

Boyd AS, Benjamin HJ, Asplund C: Principles of casting and splinting, *Am Fam Physician* 79(1):16–22, 2009.

Geerts WH, Bergqvist D, Pineo GF et al: Prevention of venous thromboembolism: American College of Chest Physicians Evidence-Based Clinical Practice Guidelines, ed 8, *Chest* 133(6 Suppl):381S-453S, 2008.

Giannoudis PV, Tzioupis C, Pape HC: Early diagnosis of tibial compartment syndrome: continuous pressure measurement or not? *Injury* 40(4):341–342, 2009.

Gonzalez RP, Scott W, Wright A et al: Anatomic location of penetrating lower-extremity trauma predicts and compartment syndrome development, *Am J Surg* 197(3):371–375, 2009.

Joanna Briggs Institute: Best practice: graduated compression stockings for the prevention of post-operative venous thromboembolism, *EB Pract Inform Sheets Health Profes* 12:4, 2008.

Kasper DL et al: *Harrison's principles of internal medicine,* ed 16, New York, 2005, McGraw-Hill.

Link R: National Heart, Lung and Blood Institute programs for deep vein thrombosis, *Arterioscler Thromb Vasc Biol* 28(30):392–393, 2008.

Lobos AT, Menon K: A multidisciplinary survey on capillary refill time: inconsistent performance and interpretation of a common clinical test, *Ped Crit Care Med* 9(4):386–391, 2008.

Mamaril ME, Childs SG, Sortman S: Care of the orthopedic trauma patient, *J PeriAnesth Nurs* 22(3):184–194, 2007.

Miller NC, Askew AE: Tibia fractures. An overview of evaluation and treatment, *Orthop Nurs* 26(4):215–223, 2007.

Rockwood CA, Green DP, Bucholz RW: *Rockwood and Green's fractures in adults,* ed 6, vol 2, Philadelphia, 2006, Lippincott Williams & Wilkins.

Roman M: Deep vein thrombosis: an overview, *Medsurg Matters* 14(1), 2005.

Weinstein SL, Buckwalter JA: *Turek's orthopaedics principles and their applications,* ed 6, Philadelphia, 2005, Lippincott, Williams & Wilkins.

Risk for Poisoning   *Mary E. B. Stahl, RN, MSN, CEN, and Betty J. Ackley, MSN, EdS, RN*

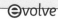

NANDA-I

Definition

Accentuated risk of accidental exposure to, or ingestion of, drugs or dangerous products in doses sufficient to cause poisoning

Risk Factors

External

Availability of illicit drugs potentially contaminated by poisonous additives; dangerous products placed within reach of children; dangerous products placed within reach of confused individuals or children; large supplies of drugs in house; medicines stored in unlocked cabinets; medicines stored in unlocked cabinets accessible to confused individuals or children; medications not maintained in original containers; breastfeeding mothers who are drug addicted; use of over-the-counter cold and cough medication for children

Internal

Cognitive difficulties; emotional difficulties; lack of drug education; lack of proper precaution; lack of safety education; reduced vision; verbalization that occupational setting is without adequate safeguards

 (Nursing Outcomes Classification)

Suggested NOC Outcomes

Knowledge: Child Physical Safety, Medication, Personal Safety, Parenting Performance, Risk Control, Risk Control: Alcohol Use, Drug Use, Risk Detection, Safe Home Environment

Example **NOC** Outcome with Indicators
Risk Control as evidenced by the following indicators: Monitors environmental risk factors/Develops effective risk control strategies (Rate the outcome and indicators of **Risk Control:** 1 = never demonstrated, 2 = rarely demonstrated, 3 = sometimes demonstrated, 4 = often demonstrated, 5 = consistently demonstrated [see Section I].)

Client Outcomes

Client Will (Specify Time Frame):

- Prevent inadvertent ingestion of or exposure to toxins or poisonous substances
- Explain and undertake appropriate safety measures to prevent ingestion of or exposure to toxins or poisonous substances
- Verbalize appropriate response to apparent or suspected toxic ingestion or poisoning

 (Nursing Interventions Classification)

Suggested NIC Interventions

Environmental Management: Safety, First Aid, Health Education, Medication Management, Surveillance, Surveillance: Safety

Example **NIC** Activities—Environmental Management: Safety
Identify safety hazards in the environment (i.e., physical, biological, and chemical); Remove hazards from the environment, when possible

Nursing Interventions and *Rationales*

- When a client comes to the hospital with possible poisoning, begin care following the ABCs and administer oxygen if needed. *Poisoning is an emergency and should be treated as such (Broderick, 2004). Nursing assessment should center on ventilation, perfusion, cognition, and elimination of the poison. Assess and reassess these areas because changes occur rapidly (Madden, 2008).*
- ▲ It is important for the triage nurse to call the poison control center. *The Poison Control hotline, 1–800–222–1222, serves as a key source of medical information (Madden, 2008).*
- Obtain a thorough history of what was ingested, how much, and when, and ask to look at the container. Note the client's age, weight, medications, any medical conditions, and any history of vomiting, choking, coughing, or change in mental status. Also take note of any interventions performed before seeking treatment. *A thorough history is critical to success of treatment (Broderick, 2004; Madden, 2008).*

• = Independent   ▲ = Collaborative   **EBN** = Evidence-Based Nursing   **EB** = Evidence-Based

- Carefully inspect for signs of ingestion of poisons, including an odor on the breath, a trace of the substance on the clothing, burns, or redness around the mouth and lips, as well as signs of confusion, vomiting, or dyspnea. **EB:** *It is important to look for signs of ingestion of poison before initiating treatment because up to 40% of children who present with poisoning have not actually been exposed to the suspected toxin (Hwang, Foot, & Eddie, 2003).*
- ▲ Note results of toxicology screens, arterial blood gasses, blood glucose levels, and any other ordered laboratory tests. *If information about what was ingested is incomplete or inaccurate, laboratory tests may be needed to determine treatment (Broderick, 2004).*
- ▲ Initiate any ordered treatment for poisoning quickly. *Activated charcoal is the first-line defense in GI decontamination and should be given to the client if a significant ingestion has occurred within preferably 1 hour since ingestion of poison (Krawczyk, Gharahbaghian, & Rutowski, 2006; Madden, 2008).*

Safety Guidelines for Medication Administration.

- Prevent iatrogenic harm to the hospitalized client by following these guidelines for administering medications:
  - Use at least two methods to identify the client before administering medications or blood products, such as the client's name and medical record number or birth date. Do not use the client's room number.
  - When taking verbal or telephone orders, the orders should be written down and then read back for verification to the individual giving the order. The person who gave the orders for the medication then needs to confirm the information that was read back.
  - Standardize use of abbreviations, acronyms, symbols, and dose designations and eliminate those that are prone to cause errors. (Please refer to The Joint Commission, Critical Access Hospital National Patient Safety goals for list of abbreviations, acronyms, symbols and dose designations that should not be used.)
  - Be aware of the medications that look/sound alike and ensure that the correct medication is ordered.
  - Take high-alert medications off the nursing unit, such as potassium chloride. Standardize concentrations of medications such as morphine in PCA pumps.
  - Label all medications, and medication containers or other solutions that are on or off a sterile field for a procedure. Label them when they are first taken out of the original packaging to another container. Label with medication name, strength, amount, and expiration date/time. Review the labels whenever there is a change of personnel.
  - Use only IV pumps that prevent free flow of IV solution when the tubing is taken out of the pump.
  - Identify all the client's current medications on admission to a health care facility, and compare the list with the current ordered medications. Reconcile any differences in medications. Reconcile the list of medications if the client is transferred from one unit to another, when there is a handoff to the next provider of care, and reconcile the list of medications when the client is discharged. *Accurate and complete medication reconciliation can prevent numerous prescribing and administration errors (The Joint Commission, 2006).*
- ▲ Detect possible interactions and cumulative or other adverse effects among prescribed medications, self-administered over-the-counter products, culturally based home treatments, herbal remedies, and foods. *Serious consequences may occur if interactions are not identified; herbal preparations can be toxic (The Joint Commission, 2009).*

Pediatric

- Recognize that some children may haves been exposed to methamphetamines or the components used to make methamphetamines. *From year 2000 through the first quarter of 2005, more than 15,000 children were reported as being affected in clandestine laboratory-related incidents (Grant, 2007).*
- Evaluate/educate breastfeeding mothers who may use methamphetamines. *Because methamphetamine is secreted in breast milk, breastfeeding is not recommended for mothers who use the drug after delivery (Bradford, Voorhees, & Pehl, 2007).*
- ▲ Evaluate lead exposure risk and consult the health care provider regarding lead screening measures as indicated (public/ambulatory health). *Lead poisoning is the most common preventable poisonings of childhood (American Academy of Child & Adolescent Psychiatry, 2004). Children can be exposed to*

• = Independent   ▲ = Collaborative   **EBN** = Evidence-Based Nursing   **EB** = Evidence-Based

lead from multiple sources: house paint, dust, soil, imported toys, imported and traditional medications, and housewares (Woolf, Goldman, & Bellinger, 2007).

- Supply "Mr. Yuk" labels for families with children. *Information on how to obtain "Mr. Yuk" labels is available at www.chp.edu/CHP/mryuk.php.*
- Provide guidance for parents and caregivers regarding age-related safety measures, including the following:
  - Store prescription and over-the-counter medications and alcohol in a locked cabinet far from children's reach.
  - Store cleaning products including things like dishwashing liquids in a high cabinet, out of children's reach.
  - Use safety latches on cabinets that contain poisonous substances.
  - Store potentially harmful substances in the original containers with safety closures intact.
  - Recognize that no container is completely childproof.
  - Do not store medications or toxic substances in food containers.
  - Do not leave alcoholic drinks, cosmetics, or toiletries where children can reach them.
  - Remove poisonous houseplants from the home. Teach children not to put leaves or berries in their mouths.
  - Do not suggest that medications are candy.
  - If interrupted when using a harmful product, take it with you; children can get into it within seconds.
  - Discard used button batteries safely and store unused batteries away from children's reach.
  - Store poisonous automotive or gardening supplies in a locked area.
  - Use extreme caution with pesticides and gardening materials close to children's play areas.

  Infants have a high level of hand-to-mouth behavior and ingest anything. Young children may inadvertently ingest poisonous materials, particularly if those materials are thought to be food or a beverage (Broderick, 2004; Madden, 2008). **EB:** *A study of poisoning incidences in children in which the child was brought to the emergency department demonstrated that 73% of the parents received no instructions on how to prevent another incidence of poisoning (Demorest et al, 2004).*
- Teach the family to keep the home safe for children by keeping harmful cleaning products and all liquids containing hydrocarbons away from children and using child-resistant packaging as available. *Liquid products that contain more than 10% hydrocarbons (e.g., cosmetics such as hair oils, automotive chemicals, cleaning solvents, or water repellents) are now required to be in child-resistant packaging. When these products enter the lungs inadvertently, they can cause chemical pneumonia and death in children (Barone, 2002).*
- ▲ Advise families that syrup of ipecac is no longer recommended to be kept and used in the home (Madden, 2008).
- ▲ Advise families that over-the-counter cough and cold suppressant medications are not recommended and are no longer considered safe. *Over-the-counter cold and cough medications are no longer recommended for children under the age of 2 unless recommended by a health care provider (U.S. Food and Drug Administration, 2010). Minimal data exist to support their effectiveness, and overuse can cause harm (Krawcdzyk, Gharahbaghian, & Rutkowski, 2006; Woo, 2008).*

Geriatric

- Caution the client and family to avoid storing medications with similar appearances close to one another (e.g., nitroglycerin ointment near toothpaste or denture creams). *Confusion and visual impairment can place the older person at risk of incorrectly identifying the contents. Place medications in a medication box that indicates when they are to be taken. Failing eyesight, the use of multiple drugs, and difficulty in remembering whether a medication was taken are among the causes of accidental poisoning in older persons.* **EB:** *A study that reviewed causes of calls to poison information centers by adults older than 50 years demonstrated that most of the calls related to errors in taking drugs, and then adverse drug reactions (Skarupski, Mrvos, & Krenzelok, 2004).*
- Remind the older client to store medications out of reach when young children come to visit. *Children are inquisitive and may ingest medicines in containers without safety caps.*

- Perform medication reconciliation on all elderly clients entering the health care system as well as on discharge. *Elderly clients do not compare drugs that they have at home with new prescriptions and often take multiple drugs with the same indications, leading to toxicity.*

Home Care

NOTE: The Home Safety Council (2009) lists poisoning as the second leading cause of accidental injury leading to death in the home.
- The interventions previously described may be adapted for home care use.
- Provide the client and/or family with a poison control poster to be kept on the refrigerator or a bulletin board. Ensure that the telephone number for local poison control information is readily available.
- Pre-pour medications for a client who is at risk of ingesting too much of a given medication because of mistakes in preparation. Delegate this task to the family or caregivers if possible. *Elderly clients who live alone are at greatest risk of poisoning.*
- Identify poisonous substances in the immediate surroundings of the home, such as a garage or barn, including paints and thinners, fertilizers, rodent and bug control substances, animal medications, gasoline, and oil. Label with the name, a poison warning sign, and a poison control center number. Lock out of the reach of children. *Dangerous poisonous substances can be found in areas other than the internal home setting. Curious children are at risk for ingestion when exploring.*
- Identify the risk of toxicity from environmental activities such as spraying trees or roadside shrubs. Contact local departments of agriculture or transportation to obtain material substance data sheets or to prevent the activity in desired areas. *Very young children, women who are of childbearing age or who are pregnant, and the elderly are at greatest risk of poisoning.*
- To prevent carbon monoxide poisoning, instruct the client and family in the importance of using a carbon monoxide detector in the home, having the chimney professionally cleaned each year, having the furnace professionally inspected each year, ensuring that all combustion equipment is properly vented, and installing a chimney screen and cap to prevent small animals from moving into the chimney. *Carbon monoxide poisoning can kill quickly (Home Safety Council, 2009).*

Multicultural

- Assess housing for pathways of lead poisoning. **EB:** *Minority individuals are more likely to reside in older and substandard housing. Approximately 74% of privately owned, occupied housing units in the United States built before 1980 contain lead-based paint (Centers for Disease Control and Prevention, 2005).*
- Prompt caregivers to take action to prevent lead poisoning. **EB:** *A lead poisoning–awareness campaign targeted at ethnic minority parents of preschool-age children respondents reported an increase in steps to prevent lead poisoning after exposure to the campaign (McLaughlin et al, 2004).*
- Inform minority parents of children who present for treatment of a poisoning episode of poisoning prevention education as part of the medical encounter. **EB:** *Research suggests that young children experiencing a first poisoning episode will have a second occurrence and that poisoning prevention education may prevent repeat poisoning occurrence (Demorest et al, 2004).*
- Poison control centers should offer information in bilingual and bicultural manner. **EB:** *Research suggests that poison control centers are underused by low-income minority and Spanish-speaking parents because of lack of knowledge and misconception. A videotape intervention was highly effective in changing knowledge, attitudes, behaviors, and behavioral intentions concerning the poison control center within this population (Shepherd et al, 2004).*

Client/Family Teaching and Discharge Planning

- Counsel the client and family members regarding the following points of medication safety:
  - Avoid sharing prescriptions.
  - Always use good light when preparing medication. Do not dispense medication during the night without a light on.

• = Independent ▲ = Collaborative **EBN** = Evidence-Based Nursing **EB** = Evidence-Based

- Read the label before you open the bottle, after you remove a dose, and again before you give it.
- Always use child-resistant caps and lock all medications away from your child or confused elder.
- Give the correct dose. NEVER guess.
- Do not increase or decrease the dose without calling the physician.
- Always follow the weight and age recommendations on the label.
- Avoid making conversions. If the label calls for 2 tsp and you have a dosing cup labeled only with ounces, do not use it.
- Be sure the physician knows if you are taking more than one medication at a time.
- Never let young children take medication by themselves.
- Read and follow labeling instructions on all products; adjust dosage for age.
- Avoid excessive amounts and/or frequency of doses. ("If a little does some good, a lot should do more.")

Each year, thousands of adverse drug-related events occur, including poisoning. Poisoning is a major cause of morbidity and mortality (American Academy of Pediatrics Committee on Injury, Violence, and Poison Prevention, 2003).

- Advise the family to post first-aid charts and poison control center instructions in an accessible location. Poison control center telephone numbers should be posted close to each telephone and the number programmed into cell phones. *A poison control center should always be called immediately before initiating any first-aid measures. The national toll-free number is (800) 222–1222; the agency will connect the caller to the closest poison control center (Broderick, 2004; Madden, 2008).*
- Advise family when calling the poison control center to do the following:
  - Give as much information as possible, including your name, location, and telephone number, so that the poison control operator can call back in case you are disconnected or to summon help if needed.
  - Give the name of the potential poison ingested and, if possible, the amount and time of ingestion. If the bottle or package is available, give the trade name and ingredients if they are listed.
  - Be prepared to tell the person the child's height, weight, and age.
  - Describe the state of the poisoning victim. Is the victim conscious? Does he or she have any symptoms? What is the person's general appearance, skin color, respiration, breathing difficulties, mental status (alert, sleepy, unusual behavior)? Is the person vomiting? Having convulsions?

Rapid initiation of proper treatment reduces mortality and morbidity rates and decreases emergency department visits and inpatient admissions. Consultation with a poison control center is necessary to assess and treat poisoned clients (Broderick, 2004; Ressel, 2004).

- Encourage the client and family to take first-aid and other types of safety-related programs. *These programs raise participants' level of emergency preparation.*
- ▲ Initiate referrals to peer group interventions, peer counseling, and other types of substance abuse prevention/rehabilitation programs when substance abuse is identified as a risk factor. Teach parents and other caregivers that cough and cold medication bought over-the-counter are not safe for a child under 2 unless specifically ordered by a health care provider. *"Educational campaigns to decrease the use of over-the-counter cough and cold medications in infants need to be increased" (Rimsza & Newberry, 2008).*

evolve   See the EVOLVE website for Weblinks for client education resources.

REFERENCES

American Academy of Child & Adolescent Psychiatry: *Lead exposure in children affects brain and behavior,* updated November, 2004. www.aacap.org/cs/root/facts_for_families/lead_exposure_in_children_affects_brain_and_behavior. Accessed May 24, 2009.

American Academy of Pediatrics Committee on Injury, Violence, and Poison Prevention: Poison treatment in the home. American Academy of Pediatrics Committee on Injury, Violence, and Poison Prevention, *Pediatrics* 112(5):1182–1185, 2003.

Barone S: Child-resistant packaging, *Consumer Product Safety Review* 6(3):3, 2002.

Bradford T, Voorhees K, Pehl K: Methamphetamine abuse, *Am Fam Physician* 76:1169–1176, 2007.

Broderick M: Pediatric poisoning! *RN* 67(9):37–38, 40–42, 2004.

Centers for Disease Control and Prevention: *Preventing lead poisoning in young children,* Atlanta, 2005, CDC.

Demorest RA, Posner JC, Osterhoudt KC et al: Poisoning prevention education during emergency department visits for childhood poisoning, *Pediatr Emerg Care* 20(5):281, 2004.

Grant P: Evaluation of children removed from a clandestine methamphetamine laboratory, *J Emerg Nurs* 33:31–41, 2007.

• = Independent   ▲ = Collaborative   **EBN** = Evidence-Based Nursing   **EB** = Evidence-Based

Home Safety Council, *How to prevent accidental poisoning in the home.* www.associatedcontent.com/pop_print.shtml?content_type=article&content_type_id=1. Accessed March 29, 2009.

Hwang CF, Foot CL, Eddie G: The utility of the history and clinical signs of poisoning in childhood: a prospective study, *Ther Drug Monit* 25(6):728, 2003.

Krawcdzyk J, Gharahbaghian L, Rutkowski A: *Toxicity, cough and cold preparation,* updated July 14, 2006. http://emedicine.medscape.com/article/1010513–print. Accessed March 28, 2009.

Madden M: Responding to pediatric poisoning, *Nursing* 38(8):52–55, 2008.

McLaughlin TJ, Humphries O Jr, Nguyen T et al: "Getting the lead out" in Hartford, Connecticut: a multifaceted lead-poisoning awareness campaign, *Environ Health Perspect* 112(1):1–5, 2004.

Ressel GW: AAP releases policy statement on poison treatment in the home, *Am Family Physician* 69(3):741, 2004.

Rimsza M, Newberry S: Unexpected infant deaths associated with use of cough and cold medications, *Pediatrics* 122(2):e318–e322, 2008.

Shepherd G, Larkin GL, Velez LI et al: Language preferences among callers to a regional Poison Center, *Vet Hum Toxicol* 46(2):100–101, 2004.

Skarupski KA, Mrvos R, Krenzelok EP: A profile of calls to a poison information center regarding older adults, *J Aging Health* 16(2):228, 2004.

The Joint Commission: *Accreditation Program: Critical Access Hospital National Patient Safety Goals. The Joint Commission on Accreditation of Health Care Organizations, 2009.* http://www.jointcommission.org/NR/rdonlyres/E6FF3F84–280A-48DB-AA67–B9CE7CA693FE/0/RevisedChapter_CAH_NPSG_20090924.pdf . accessed August 9, 2009.

The Joint Commission: *Sentinel event alert.* www.jointcommission.org/SentinelEvents/SentinelEventAlert/sea_35.htm, January 25, 2006, accessed May 24, 2009.

U.S. Food and Drug Administration, 2010: Public Health Advisory: FDA Recommends that over-the-counter (OTC) cough and cold products not be used for infants and children under 2 years of age, 2010. www.fda.gov/drugs/drugsafety/publichealthadvisories/ucm051137.html. Accessed January 10, 2010.

Woolf AD, Goldman R, & Bellinger DC: Update on the clinical management of childhood lead poisoning, *Pediatr Clin North Am* 54(2):271–294, 2007.

Woo T: Pharmacology of cough and cold medicines, *J Pediatr Health Care* 22(2):73–79, 2008.

Post-Trauma syndrome   *Gail B. Ladwig, MSN, RN, CHTP*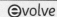

Definition

Sustained maladaptive response to a traumatic, overwhelming event

Defining Characteristics

Aggression; alienation; altered mood state; anger; anxiety; avoidance; compulsive behavior; denial; depression; detachment; difficulty concentrating; enuresis (in children); exaggerated startle response; fear; flashbacks; gastric irritability; grieving; guilt; headaches; hopelessness; horror; hypervigilance; intrusive dreams; intrusive thoughts; irritability; neurosensory irritability; nightmares; palpitations; panic attacks; psychogenic amnesia; rage; rape; reports feeling numb; repression; shame; substance abuse

Related Factors (r/t)

Abuse (physical and psychosocial); being held prisoner of war; criminal victimization; disasters; epidemics; events outside range of usual human experience; serious accidents (e.g., industrial, motor vehicle); serious injury/threat to self or loved ones; sudden destruction of one's home or community; torture; tragic occurrence involving multiple deaths; wars; witnessing of mutilation/violent death

   (Nursing Outcomes Classification)

Suggested NOC Outcomes

Abuse Cessation; Abuse Protection; Abuse Recovery: Aggression Self-Control, Anxiety Self-Control, Emotional, Sexual; Coping; Grief Resolution Impulse Self-Control; Self-Mutilation Restraint; Sleep

Example NOC Outcome with Indicators
Abuse Recovery: Emotional as evidenced by the following indicators: Trauma-induced psychoneurotic behaviors, conduct disorders, and learning difficulties (Rate outcome and indicators of **Abuse Recovery Emotional:** 1 = extensive, 2 = substantial, 3 = moderate, 4 = limited, 5 = none [see Section I].)

Client Outcomes

Client Will (Specify Time Frame):

• Return to pretrauma level of functioning as quickly as possible.

• = Independent   ▲ = Collaborative   **EBN** = Evidence-Based Nursing   **EB** = Evidence-Based

- Acknowledge traumatic event and begin to work with the trauma by talking about the experience and expressing feelings of fear, anger, anxiety, guilt, and helplessness.
- Identify support systems and available resources and be able to connect with them.
- Return to and strengthen coping mechanisms used in previous traumatic event.
- Acknowledge event and perceive it without distortions.
- Assimilate event and move forward to set and pursue life goals.

NIC (Nursing Interventions Classification)

Suggested NIC Interventions

Counseling, Support System Enhancement

Example **NIC Activities—Counseling**
Encourage expression of feelings; Assist patient to identify strengths and reinforce them

Nursing Interventions and *Rationales*

- Observe for a reaction to a traumatic event in all clients regardless of age or sex. **EB:** *Women are more likely to meet the criteria for posttraumatic stress disorder (PTSD), although they are less likely to experience posttraumatic events. Women are more likely than men to experience sexual assault and child sexual abuse but less likely to experience accidents, nonsexual assaults, witness of death injury, disaster, fire, or combat during war (Tolin & Foa, 2006).*
- After a traumatic event assess for intrusive memories, avoidance and numbing, and hyperarousal. **EB:** *Of three categories of symptoms associated with PTSD—intrusive memories, avoidance and numbing, and hyperarousal—avoidance and numbing appear to be the most specific for identification of PTSD (North et al, 2009).*
- Provide a safe and therapeutic environment. *This will assist the client in regaining control (Townsend, 2003).*
- Remain with the client and provide support during periods of overwhelming emotions. **EBN:** *The importance of trust was found to be a key element in a nurse-client relationship (Bell & Duffy, 2009).*
- Help the individual try to comprehend the trauma if possible. **EB:** *A stronger sense of coherence as the ability to perceive a stressor as comprehensible, manageable, and meaningful renders the client somewhat resilient to symptoms of PTSD (Engelhan, van den Hout, & Vheyen, 2003).*
- Use touch with the client's permission (e.g., a hand on the shoulder, holding a hand). **EB:** *TT has been found to reduce tension, confusion, anxiety, and pain and increases quality of life or general well-being (Collinge, Wentworth, & Sabo, 2005).*
- Explore and enhance available support systems. **EB:** *Support systems decrease isolation and encourage communication, which may reduce negative affect and enhance the understanding and assimilation of the event (Engelhan, van den Hout, & Vheyen, 2003).*
- Help the client regain previous sleeping and eating habits. **EBN:** *Associated behavioral symptoms after a traumatic event may include substance abuse, eating disorders, high-risk sexual behavior, suicidality, and revictimization (Seng et al, 2004).*
- ▲ Provide the client pain medication if he or she has physical pain. **EB:** *Pain may act as a proprioceptive trigger, stimulating posttraumatic reactions (Martz, 2004).*
- ▲ Assess the need for pharmacotherapy. **EB:** *Selective serotonin reuptake inhibitors are the medications most commonly prescribed for reexperiencing and avoidance/withdrawal symptoms of PTSD. Selective serotonin reuptake inhibitors and anticonvulsants are the medications most commonly prescribed for hyperarousal, irritability, or paranoia (Rosen et al, 2004).*
- ▲ Refer for appropriate psychotherapy: cognitive therapy, exposure therapy, eye movement desensitization and reprocessing (EMDR), cognitive behavior therapy. *All of these approaches can help the client gain control of the fear and distress that happen after a traumatic event (Mayo Clinic, 2009).*
- Help the client use positive cognitive restructuring to reestablish feelings of self-worth. **EB:** *Veterans with and without PTSD were found to have temporal fluctuations in self-esteem and negative effect, which are associated with diminished well-being (Kashdan et al, 2006). This study suggests that*

• = Independent   ▲ = Collaborative   **EBN** = Evidence-Based Nursing   **EB** = Evidence-Based

cognitive-behavioral approaches to the treatment of chronically traumatized populations have been successful (Cloitre, 2009).

- Provide the means for the client to express feelings through therapeutic drawing. **EBN:** *Expressive techniques such as therapeutic drawing can be used to facilitate the emotional work of coping with chronic trauma or life-threatening events, and facilitate a better understanding of the experience to health care professionals (Locsin et al, 2003).*
- Encourage the client to return to the normal routine as quickly as possible. *PTSD leads to disruption of normal daily and nighttime routines. Early treatment includes collaboration to develop a plan to establish normal daily routines (Carr, 2004).*
- Talk to and assess the client's social support after a traumatic event. **EB:** *Informal social networks play a critical role in buffering the negative effects of stressful life events. For women experiencing the stress of a violent relationship, family and friends are among the first sources of support sought (Trotter & Allen, 2009).*

Pediatric

- Refer to nursing care plan **Risk for Post-Trauma syndrome**.

Geriatric

- Carefully screen elderly for signs of PTSD, especially after a disaster. **EB:** *Clients with PTSD are often not recognized or incorrectly diagnosed. Increased knowledge on vulnerability factors for PTSD can facilitate diagnostic procedures and health management in the elderly. Because of age-related changes and associated disease processes, stress reaction in older adults may lead to a deterioration of function and a worsening of existing conditions (Marren & Christianson, 2005).*
- Consider using the Horwitz Impact of Event Scale, which is an appropriate instrument to measure the subjective response to stress in the senior population. *The Impact of Event Scale is recognized as one of the earliest self-report tools developed to assess posttraumatic stress (Marren & Christianson, 2005).*
- ▲ Monitor the client for clinical signs of depression and anxiety; refer to a physician for medication if appropriate. **EB:** *Depression is common in old age. Most late-life depression occurs in persons with a history of depression. The recurrence rate of depressive syndromes does not differ between men and women (Luijendijk et al, 2008).*
- Instill hope. **EBN:** *In this study of elderly palliative care clients, the participants described their main concern as wanting to "live with hope" and they achieved this through the basic social process of transforming hope. Transforming hope involved acknowledging "life the way it is," searching for meaning, and positive reappraisal (Duggleby & Wright, 2009).*

Multicultural

- Assess the influence of cultural beliefs, norms, and values on the client's ability to cope with a traumatic experience. **EBN:** *What the client views as healthy coping may be based on cultural perceptions (Leininger & McFarland, 2002).*
- Acknowledge racial and ethnic differences at the onset of care. **EBN:** *Acknowledgment of race and ethnicity issues enhances communication, establishes rapport, and promotes positive treatment outcomes (D'Avanzo & Naegle, 2001). Black veterans' rate of service connection for PTSD was 43% compared with 56% for other respondents (P = .003) even after adjusting for differences in PTSD severity and functional status (Murdoch et al, 2003). Race has been identified as a factor in who receives treatment for trauma (Koenen et al, 2003).*
- ▲ Carefully assess refugees for PTSD and refer for treatment as appropriate; encourage them to learn the language of their new residence. **EB:** *This study of Bosnian traumatized refugees suggests that traumatized refugees, especially women, are vulnerable to PTSD. English proficiency was correlated with lesser better adjustment (Vojvoda et al, 2008).*
- Use a family-centered approach when working with Latino, Asian, African American, and Native American clients. **EBN:** *Latinos may perceive the family as a source of support, solver of problems, and*

source of pride. Asian Americans may regard the family as the primary decision maker and influence on individual family members (D'Avanzo & Naegle, 2001). A school-based program using a family approach to treat traumatized immigrant children showed modest decline in trauma-related mental health problems (Kataoka et al, 2003).

- When working with Asian American clients, provide opportunities by which the family can save face. **EBN:** *Asian American families may avoid situations and discussion of issues that they perceive will bring shame on the family unit (D'Avanzo & Naegle, 2001).*
- Incorporate cultural traditions as appropriate. **EB:** *Activities such as tundra walks and time with elders were supported in treatment of trauma for the Yup'ik and Cup'ik Eskimo of Southwest Alaska (Mills, 2003).*

 ### Home Care

- ▲ Assess family support and the response to the client's coping mechanisms. Refer the family for medical social services or other counseling as necessary. **EB:** *It is recommended that treatment for PTSD include support of the family and interpersonal skills training for military personnel suffering while healing from trauma (Ray & Vanstone, 2009).*
- Assess the impact of the trauma on significant others (e.g., a father may have to take over his partner's parenting responsibility after she has been raped and injured). Provide empathy and caring to significant others. Refer for additional services as necessary. *Traumatic events can pose a crisis for both significant others and the involved client. Trying to help parents with PTSD implement a behavioral program for their children is likely to lead to a failed experience. Parents with PTSD should be offered an opportunity to undergo treatment for their own PTSD (Carr, 2004).*

 ### Client/Family Teaching and Discharge Planning

- Teach positive coping skills and avoidance of negative coping skills. *Cognitive coping skills teach the individual to challenge fearful or threatening cognitions and appraise anxiety-evoking situations in less-threatening ways (Carr, 2004).*
- Teach stress reduction methods such as deep breathing, visualization, meditation, and physical exercise. Encourage their use especially when intrusive thoughts or flashbacks occur. **EB:** *After a traumatic event, clients may be tempted to cope maladaptively with their overwhelming emotions, which can establish unhealthy patterns for the future (Lang et al, 2003).*
- Encourage other healthy living habits of proper diet, adequate sleep, regular exercise, family activities, and spiritual pursuits. *A wide range of preventive, educational, and supportive interventions for trauma survivors are used. Despite this, research is lacking to prove their effectiveness (Schnurr & Green, 2004).*
- Refer the client to peer support groups. **EB:** *Peer support decreases the sense of social isolation and enhances knowledge, which may reduce the negative effects and enhance the understanding and assimilation of the event (Engelhan, van den Hout, and Vheyen, 2003).*
- Consider the use of complementary and alternative therapies. **EB:** *Evidence suggests that Sudarshan kriya yoga is potentially beneficial as a low-risk adjunct treatment for stress, anxiety, PTSD, depression, and stress-related medical illnesses (Brown & Gerbarg, 2005). Preliminary observations from four cases and a review of the literature support the potential efficacy of incorporating qigong and tai chi into the treatment of survivors of torture and refugee trauma (Grodin et al, 2008).*

ⓔvolve   See the EVOLVE website for Weblinks for client education resources.

REFERENCES

Bell L, Duffy A: A concept analysis of nurse-patient trust, *Br J Nurs* 8(1):46–51, 2009.

Brown RP, Gerbarg PL: Sudarshan kriya yogic breathing in the treatment of stress, anxiety, and depression: Part II—clinical applications and guidelines, *J Altern Complement Med* 11(4):711–717, 2005.

Carr A: Interventions for post-traumatic stress disorder in children and adolescents, *Pediatr Rehab* 7(4):231–244, 2004.

Cloitre M: Effective psychotherapies for posttraumatic stress disorder: a review and critique, *CNS Spectr*14(1 Suppl 1):32–43, 2009.

Collinge W, Wentworth R, Sabo S: Integrating complementary therapies into community mental health practice: an exploration, *J Alt Complement Med* 11(3):569–574, 2005.

D'Avanzo CE, Naegle MA: Developing culturally informed strategies for substance-related interventions. In Naegle MA, D'Avanzo CE, editors: *Addictions and substance abuse: strategies for advanced practice nursing,* St Louis, 2001, Mosby.

Duggleby W, Wright K: Transforming hope: how elderly palliative patients live with hope. *Can J Nurs Res* 41(1):204–217, 2009.

Engelhan I, van den Hout M, Vheyen J: The sense of coherence in early pregnancy and crisis support and posttraumatic stress after pregnancy loss: a prospective study, *Behav Med* 29:80–84, 2003.

Grodin MA, Piwowarczyk L, Fulker D et al. Treating survivors of torture and refugee trauma: a preliminary case series using qigong and t'ai chi, *J Altern Complement Med*14(7):801–806, 2008.

Kashdan TB, Uswatte G, Steger MF et al: Fragile self-esteem and affective instability in posttraumatic stress disorders, *Behav Res Ther* 44(11):1609–1619, 2006.

Kataoka SH, Stein BD, Jaycox LH et al: A school-based mental health program for traumatized Latino immigrant children, *J Am Acad Child Adolesc Psychiatry* 42(3):311–318, 2003.

Koenen KC, Goodwin R, Struening E et al: Posttraumatic stress disorder and treatment seeking in a national screening sample, *J Trauma Stress* 16(1):5–16, 2003.

Lang A, Rodgers C, Laffaye C et al: Sexual trauma, posttraumatic stress disorder, and health behavior, *Behav Med* 28:150–158, 2003.

Leininger MM, McFarland MR: *Transcultural nursing: concepts, theories, research and practices,* ed 3, New York, 2002, McGraw-Hill.

Locsin R, Barnard A, Matua A et al: Surviving Ebola: understanding experience through artistic expression, *Int Nurs Rev* 50:156–166, 2003.

Luijendijk HJ, van den Berg JF, Dekker MJ et al: Incidence and recurrence of late-life depression, *Arch Gen Psychiatry* 65(12):1394–1401, 2008.

Marren J, Christianson S: Horowitz's Impact of Event Scale: an assessment of post traumatic stress in older adults, *Medsurg Nurs* 14(5):329–330, 2005.

Martz E: Death anxiety as a predictor of posttraumatic stress levels among individuals with spinal cord injuries, *Death Stud* 28:1–17, 2004.

Mayo Clinic: *PTSD, treatment and drugs.* www.mayoclinic.com/health/post-traumatic-stress-disorder/ds00246/dsection=treatments-and-drugs April 2009, accessed July 9, 2009.

Mills PA: Incorporating Yup'ik and Cup'ik Eskimo traditions into behavioral health treatment, *J Psychoactive Drugs* 35(1):85–88, 2003.

Murdoch M, Hodges J, Cowper D et al: Racial disparities in VA service connection for posttraumatic stress disorder disability, *Med Care* 41(4):536–549, 2003.

North CS, Suris AM, Davis M et al: Toward validation of the diagnosis of posttraumatic stress disorder, *Am J Psychiatry* 166(1):34–41, 2009.

Ray SL, Vanstone Mp; The impact of PTSD on veterans' family relationships: an interpretative phenomenological inquiry, *Int J Nurs Stud* 46(6):838–847, 2009.

Rosen CS, Chow HC, Finney JF et al: VA practices patterns and practice guidelines for treating posttraumatic stress disorder, *J Traum Stress* 17(3):213–222, 2004.

Schnurr PP, Green BL: Understanding relationships among trauma, post-traumatic stress disorder, and health outcomes, *Adv Mind Body Med* 20(1):18–29, 2004.

Seng J, Low L, Sparbel K et al: Abuse-related post-traumatic stress during the childbearing year, *J Adv Nurs* 46(6):604–613, 2004.

Tolin DF, Foa EB: Sex differences in trauma and posttraumatic stress disorder: a quantitative review of 25 years of research, *Psychol Bull* 132(6):959–992, 2006.

Townsend M: *Psychiatric mental health nursing: concepts of care,* ed 4, Philadelphia, 2003, F.A. Davis.

Trotter JL, Allen NE: The good, the bad, and the ugly: domestic violence survivors' experiences with their informal social networks, *Am J Community Psychol* 43(3–4):221–231, 2009.

Vojvoda D, Weine SM, McGlashan T et al: Posttraumatic stress disorder symptoms in Bosnian refugees 3 1/2 years after resettlement, *J Rehabil Res Devel* 45(3):421–426, 2008.

Risk for Post-Trauma syndrome   *Gail B. Ladwig, MSN, RN, CHTP*   ⊖volve

NANDA-I

Definition

At risk for sustained maladaptive response to a traumatic, overwhelming event

Risk Factors

Diminished ego strength; displacement from home; duration of event; exaggerated sense of responsibility; inadequate social support; occupation (e.g., police, fire, rescue, corrections, emergency department, mental health worker); perception of event; survivor's role in the event; unsupportive environment

NOC   (Nursing Outcomes Classification)

Refer to the care plan for **Post-Trauma syndrome**.

Example NOC Outcome with Indicators

Risk Detection as evidenced by the following indicators: Recognizes signs and symptoms that indicate risk/Uses health care services congruent with need (Rate the outcome and indicators of **Risk Detection:** 1 = never demonstrated, 2 = rarely demonstrated, 3 = sometimes demonstrated, 4 = often demonstrated, 5 = consistently demonstrated [see Section I].)

• = Independent   ▲ = Collaborative   **EBN** = Evidence-Based Nursing   **EB** = Evidence-Based

Client Outcomes

Client Will (Specify Time Frame):

- Identify symptoms associated with PTSD and seek help
- Identify the event in realistic, cognitive terms
- State that he or she is not to blame for the event

NIC (Nursing Interventions Classification)

Refer to the care plan for **Post-Trauma syndrome**.

Nursing Interventions and *Rationales*

- Assess for PTSD in a client who has chronic/critical illness, anxiety, or personality disorder; was a witness to serious injury or death; or experienced sexual molestation. **EB:** *Women are more likely than men to meet the criteria for PTSD, although they are less likely to have experienced posttraumatic events (Tolin & Foa, 2006). This review suggests a significantly increased risk for symptoms of PTSD among survivors of critical illness and the families of clients who survive or die after critical illness (Kross, Gries, & Curtis, 2008).*
- Consider the use of a self-reported screening questionnaire. **EB:** *Client self-reported screening questionnaires are efficient ways to assess for PTSD (National Center for PTSD, 2007). This research supports the use of the posttraumatic checklist as a brief self-report measure of* PTSD *symptomatology (Keen et al, 2008).*
- Assess for ongoing symptoms of dissociation, avoidant behavior, hypervigilance, and reexperiencing. **EB:** *A study of acute stress disorder as a predictor of PTSD identified these symptoms as being 79% predictable of subsequent PTSD cases (Brink, 2004).*
- Assess for past experiences with traumatic events. **EB:** *As individuals become accustomed to traumatic situations, they can develop stress inoculation and acquire coping skills. This is supported by previous research suggesting that prolonged exposure results in habituation (Ronen, Gahav, & Appel, 2004).*
- Consider screening for PTSD in a client who is a high user of medical care. **EB:** *Traumatic stress is associated with increased health complaints, health services utilization, morbidity, and mortality (National Center for PTSD, 2007).*
- ▲ Provide deployed combat veterans with previous history of low mental or physical health status before deployment with appropriate referral after deployment. **EB:** *Low mental or physical health status before combat exposure significantly increases the risk of symptoms or diagnosis of posttraumatic stress disorder after deployment. More vulnerable members of a population could be identified and benefit from interventions targeted to prevent new-onset posttraumatic stress disorder (Leardmann et al, 2009).*
- Provide peer support to contact co-workers experiencing trauma to remind them that others in the organization are concerned about their welfare. *Peer supporters are not counselors. Their tasks include contacting co-workers to remind them that others in the organization are concerned about their welfare, providing the opportunity to discuss the incident, and assessing for the need for further posttrauma services (Post Trauma Resources, 2001).*
- Provide posttrauma debriefings. Effective posttrauma coping skills are taught, and each participant creates a plan for his or her recovery. During the debriefing, the facilitators assess participants to determine their needs for further services in the form of posttrauma counseling. For maximal effectiveness, the debriefing should occur within 2 to 5 days of the incident. *Current treatment strategies for PTSD involve a combination of posttrauma debriefing, education, pharmacotherapy, and psychotherapy (Guess, 2006).*
- Provide posttrauma counseling. Counseling sessions are extensions of debriefings and include continued discussion of the traumatic event and posttrauma consequences and the further development of coping skills. *Immediate posttrauma responses cannot be prevented. Long-term problems can develop if posttrauma consequences are not managed. Current treatment strategies for PTSD involve a combination of posttrauma debriefing, education, pharmacotherapy, and psychotherapy (Guess, 2006).*
- Consider exposure therapy for civilian trauma survivors following a nonsexual assault or motor vehicle crash. **EB:** *In this study exposure-based therapy lead to greater reduction in subsequent PTSD symptoms in clients with acute stress disorder (ASD) when compared with cognitive restructuring.*

Exposure should be used in early intervention for people who are at high risk for developing PTSD (Bryant et al, 2008).

- Instruct the client to use the following critical incident stress management techniques:

Things to Try: Critical Incident Stress Debriefing

- Within the first 24 to 48 hours, engaging in periods of appropriate physical exercise alternated with relaxation to alleviate some of the physical reactions.
- Structure your time; keep busy.
- You are normal and are having normal reactions; do not label yourself as "crazy."
- Talk to people; talk is the most healing medicine.
- Be aware of numbing the pain with overuse of drugs or alcohol; you do not need to complicate the stress with a substance abuse problem.
- Reach out; people do care.
- Maintain as normal a schedule as possible.
- Spend time with others.
- Help your co-workers as much as possible by sharing feelings and checking out how they are doing.
- Give yourself permission to feel rotten and share your feelings with others.
- Keep a journal; write your way through those sleepless hours.
- Do things that feel good to you.
- Realize that those around you are under stress.
- Do not make any big life changes.
- Do make as many daily decisions as possible to give you a feeling of control over your life (e.g., if someone asks you what you want to eat, answer the person even if you are not sure).
- Get plenty of rest.
- Reoccurring thoughts, dreams, or flashbacks are normal; do not try to fight them because they will decrease over time and become less painful.
- Eat well-balanced and regular meals (even if you do not feel like it).
- The critical incident stress debriefing process is specifically designed to prevent or mitigate the development of PTSD among emergency services professions. Critical incident stress debriefing interventions are especially directed toward the mitigation of posttraumatic stress reactions (International Critical Incident Stress Foundation, 2009).

▲ Assess for a history of life-threatening illness such as cancer and provide appropriate counseling. *The physical and psychological impact of having a life-threatening disease, undergoing cancer treatment, and living with recurring threats to physical integrity and autonomy constitute traumatic experiences for many cancer clients (National Cancer Institute, 2007).*

 Pediatric

- Children with cancer should continue to be assessed for PTSD into adulthood. **EB:** *Childhood cancer survivors require lifelong monitoring, with prompt identification and treatment of adverse late effects (Haddy, Mosher, & Reaman, 2009).*
- Provide protection for a child who has witnessed violence or who has had traumatic injuries. Help the child acknowledge the event and express grief over the event. **EB:** *Violence-exposed adolescents reporting parental alcohol or drug use had the highest rates of psychiatric diagnoses (Hanson et al, 2006). There is an urgent need to address the needs of all children in Iraq by means of preventive programs such as life skills education and care programs within the school setting (Razokhi et al, 2006).*
- Assess for a medical history of anxiety disorders. **EB:** *The conditional risk for PTSD was increased for youth with anxiety disorders (Breslau, Lucia, & Alvarado, 2006).*
▲ Assess children of deployed parents for PTSD and provide appropriate referrals. **EB:** *In this study in child care centers on a large military base, children aged 3 years or older with a deployed parent exhibited increased behavioral symptoms compared with peers without a deployed parent after controlling for caregiver's stress and depressive symptoms (Chartrand et al, 2008).*

- Consider implementation of a school-based program for children to decrease PTSD after catastrophic events. **EB:** *A three-tiered, integrative mental health program composed of school-wide dissemination of psychoeducation and coping skills (tier 1), specialized trauma- and grief-focused intervention for severely traumatized and traumatically bereaved youths (tier 2), and referral of youths at acute risk for community-based mental health services (tier 3) constitutes an effective and efficient method for promoting adolescent recovery in postwar settings (Layne et al, 2008).* **EB:** *Following disaster, systematic screening for psychological problems in children is suggested in this review. An integrated approach using psycho-socio-educational and clinical interventions is expected to be effective (Kar, 2009).*

Geriatric/Multicultural

- Refer to the care plan for **Post-Trauma syndrome**.

Home Care

- ▲ Evaluate the client's response to a traumatic or critical event. If screening warrants, refer to a therapist for counseling/treatment. *A review of psychological debriefing has concluded that little evidence exists to support its use. Early intervention recommendations are to assess the need for sustained treatment, provide psychological first aid, and provide education about trauma and information about treatment resources. Recommendations for secondary prevention of PTSD include education, anxiety management, cognitive restructuring, exposure, and relapse prevention (Litz et al, 2002).*
- Refer to the care plan for **Post-Trauma syndrome**.

Client/Family Teaching and Discharge Planning

- Instruct family and friends to use the following critical incident stress management techniques (International Critical Incident Stress Foundation, 2009):
  - Listen carefully.
  - Spend time with the traumatized person.
  - Offer your assistance and a listening ear, even if the person has not asked for help.
  - Help the person with everyday tasks such as cleaning, cooking, caring for the family, and minding children.
  - Give the person some private time.
  - Do not take the individual's anger or other feelings personally, and do not tell the person that he or she is "lucky it wasn't worse"; such statements do not console traumatized people. Instead, tell the person that you are sorry such an event has occurred and you want to understand and assist him or her.
- Teach the client and family to recognize symptoms of PTSD and seek treatment when the client does the following (McDermott & Cvitanovich, 2000):
  - Relives the traumatic event by thinking or dreaming about it often.
  - Is unsettled or distressed in other areas of his or her life such as in school, at work, or in personal relationships.
  - Avoids any situation that might cause him or her to relive the trauma.
  - Demonstrates a certain amount of generalized emotional numbness.
  - Shows a heightened sense of being on guard.
- Provide education to explain that acute stress disorder symptoms are normal when preparing combatants for their role in deployment. Instruct clients to seek help if the symptoms persist. **EB:** *Interventions focused on systematic preparation of personnel for the extreme stress of combat may help to lessen the psychological impact of deployment (Iversen et al, 2008).*

ⓔvolve   See the EVOLVE website for Weblinks for client education resources.

REFERENCES

Breslau N, Lucia VC, Alvarado GF: Intelligence and other predisposing factors in exposure to trauma and posttraumatic stress disorder: a follow-up study at age 17 years, *Arch Gen Psychiatry* 63(11):1238–1242, 2006.

Brink E: Acute stress disorder as a predictor of post-traumatic stress disorder in physical assault victims, *J Interpers Violence* 19(6):709–726, 2004.

Bryant RA, Mastrodomenico J, Felmingham KL et al: Treatment of acute stress disorder: a randomized controlled trial, *Arch Gen Psychiatry* 65(6):659–667, 2008.

Chartrand MM, Frank DA, White LF et al: Effect of parents' wartime deployment on the behavior of young children in military families, *Arch Pediatr Adolesc Med* 162(11):1009–1014, 2008.

Guess KF: Posttraumatic stress disorder: early detection is key, *Nurse Pract* 31(3):26–35, 2006.

Haddy TB, Mosher RB, Reaman GH: Late effects in long-term survivors after treatment for childhood acute leukemia, *Clin Pediatr* 48(6):601–608, 2009.

Hanson RF, Self-Brown S, Fricker-Elhai A et al: Relations among parental substance use, violence exposure and mental health: the national survey of adolescents, *Addict Behav* 31(11):1988–2001, 2006.

International Critical Incident Stress Foundation: *Critical incident stress information, signs and symptoms.* www.icisf.org/ www.icisf.org/ articles/Acrobat%20Documents/TerrorismIncident/CISInfoSheet. pdf. Accessed July 9, 2009.

Iversen AC, Fear NT, Ehlers A et al: Risk factors for post-traumatic stress disorder among UK Armed Forces personnel, *Psychol Med* 38(4):511–522, 2008.

Kar N: Psychological impact of disasters on children: review of assessment and interventions, *World J Pediatr* 5(1):5–11, 2009.

Keen SM, Kutter CJ, Niles BL et al: Psychometric properties of PTSD checklist in sample of male veterans, *J Rehabil Res Devel*; 45(3):465–474, 2008.

Kross EK, Gries CJ, Curtis JR: Posttraumatic stress disorder following critical illness, *Crit Care Clin* 24(4):875–87, ix-x, 2008.

Layne CM, Saltzman WR, Poppleton L et al: Effectiveness of a school-based group psychotherapy program for war-exposed adolescents: a randomized controlled trial, *J Am Acad Child Adolesc Psychiatry* 47(9):1048–1062, 2008.

Leardmann CA, Smith TC, Smith B et al: Baseline self reported functional health and vulnerability to post-traumatic stress disorder after combat deployment: prospective U.S. military cohort study, *BMJ* 338:b1273, 2009.

Litz BT, Gray MJ, Bryant RA et al: Early intervention for trauma: current status and future direction, *Clin Psychol Sci Pract* 9:112, 2002.

McDermott BM, Cvitanovich A: Posttraumatic stress disorder and emotional problems in children following motor vehicle accidents: an extended case series, *Aust N Z J Psychiatry* 34:446, 2000.

National Cancer Institute: *Posttraumatic stress disorder.* www.cancer.gov/ cancerinfo/pdq/supportivecare/post-traumatic-stress/Health Professional. Accessed January 4, 2007.

National Center for PTSD: *Screening for PTSD in primary care settings.* www.ncptsd.va.gov/publications/assessment. Accessed January 4, 2007.

Post Trauma Resources: *Tools for an unsafe world,* 2001. www .posttrauma.com/tools.htm. Accessed January 4, 2007.

Razokhi A, Taha I, Taib N et al: Mental health of Iraqi children, *Lancet* 368(9538):838–839, 2006.

Ronen T, Gahav G, Appel N: Adolescent stress responses to a single acute stress and to continuous external stress: terrorist attacks, *J Loss Trauma* 8:261–282, 2004.

Tolin DF, Foa EF: Sex differences in trauma and posttraumatic stress disorder: a quantitative review of 25 years of research, *Psychol Bull* 132(6):959–992, 2006.

Readiness for enhanced Power   *Marie Giordano, RN, MS*   ⊖volve

NANDA-I

Definition

A pattern of participating knowingly in change that is sufficient for well-being and can be strengthened

Defining Characteristics

Expresses readiness to enhance awareness of possible changes to be made; expresses readiness to enhance freedom to perform actions for change; expresses readiness to enhance identification of choices that can be made for change; expresses readiness to enhance involvement in creating change; expresses readiness to enhance knowledge for participation in change; expresses readiness to enhance participation in choices for daily living; expresses readiness to enhance participation in choices for health; expresses readiness to enhance power

NOC   (Nursing Outcomes Classification)

Suggested NOC Outcomes

Health Beliefs: Perceived Control, Participation in Health Care Decisions, Personal Autonomy

● = Independent   ▲ = Collaborative   **EBN** = Evidence-Based Nursing   **EB** = Evidence-Based

Example NOC Outcome with Indicators
Health Beliefs: Perceived Control as evidenced by the following indicators: Belief that own actions and decisions control health outcomes/Perceived responsibility for health decisions/Efforts at gathering information (Rate the outcome and indicators of **Health Beliefs: Perceived Control** as 1 = very weak, 2 = weak, 3 = moderate, 4 = strong, 5 = very strong [see Section I].)

Client Outcomes

Client Will (Specify Time Frame):

- Describe power resources
- Identify realistic perceptions of control
- Develop a plan of action based on power resources
- Seek assistance as needed

NIC   (Nursing Interventions Classification)

Suggested NIC Interventions

Mutual Goal Setting, Self Esteem Enhancement, Self Responsibility Facilitation

Example NIC Activities—Mutual Goal Setting
Encourage the identification of specific life values; Identify with patient the goals of care; Assist patient in examining available resources to meet goals

Nursing Interventions and *Rationales*

- Develop partnerships for shared power. **EB:** *In a review of the history of shared power in medicine in the UK, this study concluded that shared power requires a partnership with clear expectations related to the roles of clients and health care professionals. In this partnership, clients are the experts on their symptoms and experiences. "It is only when power is shared, via good communication and mutual goals that trust will be established and choices truly explored within an agreed and analogous partnership that must be equally respected and valued by both medical [health care] professionals and patients" (McGregor, 2006).*
- Focus on the positive aspects of power, rather than prevention of powerlessness. **EBN:** *Numerous studies conducted during development of the health promotion model show that promotion differs from prevention and requires a positive rather than negative approach (Pender, Murdaugh, & Parsons, 2006).*
- Listen with intent. **EB:** *This study found that people are enacting a story as they deal with their illnesses. Physicians [and nurses] may be part the story. Listening to the person's story can reveal levels of complexity that affect perceptions of power and participation in illness management (Haidet, Kroll, & Sharf, 2006).* **EBN:** *A philosophical analysis of empowerment showed that listening to the client stories with intent to help is a dimension of helping older adults to achieve optimum self care (Hage & Lorensen, 2005).*
- Collaborate with the person to identify resources to put a plan into action. **EBN:** *In this conceptual analysis of client empowerment, it was concluded that client-centered collaboration is an essential aspect of client and provider empowerment (Anderson & Funnell, 2005).* **EB:** *A review of the health care literature identified eight dimensions of empowerment in prevention and health promotion as shared decision making, self-efficacy, social support and social capital, skills and competencies, health care utilization, goal setting and attainment, reflexive thought, and innovation (Kliche & Kroger, 2008).*
- Assess the meaning of the event to the person. **EBN:** *Understanding the meaning of side effects of chemotherapy through the use of a hand-held monitoring system was an important power resource for 12 clients undergoing this treatment for cancer (Forbat et al, 2009).* **EBN:** *In developing a methodology for creating partnerships with clients, it was found that talking about the meanings of events through focusing on the positive helped clients to visualize future goals to support and sustain self-care (Leenerts & Teal, 2006).* **EBN:** *In a study of parish nurses' experiences of client empowerment, the first step was to follow the client's agenda (Weis, Schank, & Matheus, 2006).*
- Identify the client's level of choice in decision making. **EB:** *Some clients want to be completely involved in all decisions; other clients prefer to have less involvement (Harkness, 2005).*

• = Independent   ▲ = Collaborative   **EBN** = Evidence-Based Nursing   **EB** = Evidence-Based

- Facilitate trust in self and others. **EBN:** *In a descriptive correlational study of men and women who were randomly selected from a national mailing list, there was a positive correlation of trust and power (Wright, 2004).* **EBN:** *In a study of parish nurses' experiences of client empowerment, trust was an important dimension of the process (Weis, Schank, & Matheus, 2006).*
- Help client to mobilize social supports, a power resource. **EBN:** *In a correlational study of women recruited from a community clinic, perceived social support explained a significant amount of variance in health empowerment (Shearer, 2004). Meaningful relationships were identified by women who had suffered a myocardial infarction as providing power and strength (Sundler, Dahlberg, & Ekenstam, 2009).*
- Support beliefs of power and perceptions of behavioral control. **EB:** *In an integration of eight studies the overall findings supported that power beliefs related to power intention and perceived behavioral control partially mediated power beliefs and intentions (Godin, Gagne, & Sheeran, 2004).*
- Promote the client's optimum level of physical functioning. **EBN:** *In a study of menopausal women, each woman perceived that her body and mind were empowered by regular exercise (Jeng et al, 2004).* **EB:** *In a study designed to test strength training programs, participants who received an empowerment intervention along with the strength-training program showed greater improvement than the group not receiving the intervention (Katula et al, 2006).*
- Reframe professional image, role and values to incorporate a vision of clients as the experts in their own care. **EBN:** *In a phenomenological study of the experiences of eight nurses who had been using an agency supported client-centered model of care for a year, it was found that the "nurses persistently described themselves as the experts who knew best"(Brown, William, & Ward-Griffin, 2006).* **EB:** *An intervention group of diabetics that received an empowerment-based intervention had significant changes in quality of life and metabolic control (n = 73) when measured 3 and 6 months afterwards, while there were no such changes in the control group (n = 35) (Pibernik-Okanovic et al, 2003).*

Home Care

- The above interventions may be adapted for home care use.

Client/Family Teaching and Discharge Planning

- Assess motivation to learn specific content. **EBN:** *Motivation is a basic element of a teaching model and of participation in health care decisions (Pender, Murdaugh & Parsons, 2006).*

⊖volve   See the EVOLVE website for Weblinks for client education resources.

REFERENCES

Anderson RM, Funnell MM: Patient empowerment: reflections on the challenge of fostering the adoption of a new paradigm, *Patient Educ Couns* 57:153–157, 2005.

Brown D, William C, Ward-Griffin C: Client-centred empowering partnering in nursing, *J Adv Nurs* 53(2):160–168, 2006.

Forbat L, Maguire R, McCann L et al: The use of technology in cancer care: applying Foucault's ideas to explore the changing dynamics of power in health care, *J Adv Nurs* 65(2):306–315, 2009.

Godin G, Gagne C, Sheeran P: Does perceived control mediate the relationship between power beliefs and intention? *Br J Health Psychol* 9:5557–5568, 2004.

Hage AM, Lorensen M: A philosophical analysis of the concept of empowerment: The fundament of an education programme to the frail elderly, *Nurs Philosophy* 6:235–246, 2005.

Haidet P, Kroll TL, Sharf BF: The complexity of patient participation: Lessons learned from patients' illness narratives, *Patient Educ Couns* 62(3): 323–329, 2006.

Harkness J: Patient involvement: a vital principle for patient-centered health care, *World Hosp Health Serv* 41(2):12–16, 40–43, 2005.

Jeng C, Yang S, Chang P et al: Menopausal women: perceiving continuous power through the experience of regular exercise, *J Clin Nurs* 13:447–454, 2004.

Katula JA, Sipe M, Rejeski WJ et al: Strength training in older adults: an empowering intervention, *Med Sci Sports Exerc* 38(1):106–111, 2006.

Kliche T, Kroger G: Empowerment in prevention and health prevention—a critical and conceptual evaluation of basic understanding, dimensions and assessment problems, *Gesundheitswesen* 70(12):715–720, 2008.

Leenerts MH, Teel CS: relational conversation as method for creating partnerships: A pilot study, *J Adv Nurs* 54(4):467–476, 2006.

McGregor S: Review: roles, power and subjective choice, *Patient Educ Couns* 60:5–9, 2006.

Pender NJ, Murdaugh CL, Parsons MA: *Health promotion in nursing practice*, ed 5, Stamford, CT, 2006, Appleton & Lange.

Pibernik-Okanovic M, Prasek M, Poljicanin-Filipovic T et al: Effects of an empowerment-based psychosocial intervention on quality of life and metabolic control in type 2 diabetic patients, *Patient Educ Couns* 52:193–199, 2003.

Shearer NB: Relationships of contextual and relational factors to health empowerment in women, *Res Theory Nurs Practice* 18(4):357–370, 2004.

Sundler AJ, Dahlberg K, Ekenstam C: The meaning of close relationships and sexuality: women's well being following a myocardial infarction, *Qual Health Res* 19(3):375–387, 2009.

Weis D, Schank MJ, Matheus R: The process of empowerment: a parish nurse perspective, *J Holist Nurs* 24(1):17–24, 2006.

Wright BW: Trust and power in adults: an investigation using Rogers' science of unitary human beings, *Nurs Sci Q* 17(2):139–146, 2004.

● = Independent   ▲ = Collaborative   **EBN** = Evidence-Based Nursing   **EB** = Evidence-Based

Powerlessness   *Kathleen L. Patusky, PhD, APRN-BC*

Definition

Perception that one's own actions will not significantly affect an outcome; a perceived lack of control over current situation or immediate happening

Defining Characteristics

Low

Expressions of uncertainty about fluctuating energy levels; passivity

Moderate

Anger; dependence on others that may result in irritability; does not defend self-care practices when challenged; does not monitor progress; expressions of dissatisfaction over inability to perform previous activities; expressions of dissatisfaction over inability to perform previous tasks; expressions of doubt regarding role performance; expressions of frustration over inability to perform previous activities; expressions of frustration over inability to perform previous tasks; fear of alienation from caregivers; guilt; inability to seek information regarding care; nonparticipation in care when opportunities are provided; nonparticipation in decision making when opportunities are provided; passivity; reluctance to express true feelings; resentment

Severe

Apathy; depression over physical deterioration; verbal expressions of having no control (e.g., over self-care, situation, outcome)

Related Factors (r/t)

Health care environment; illness-related regimen; interpersonal interactions; lifestyle of helplessness

NOC   (Nursing Outcomes Classification)

Suggested NOC Outcomes

Depression Self-Control, Health Beliefs, Health Beliefs: Perceived Ability to Perform, Perceived Control, Perceived Resources, Participation in Health Care Decisions

Example NOC Outcome with Indicators
Health Beliefs: Perceived Control as evidenced by the following indicators: Perceived responsibility for health decisions/Beliefs that own decisions and actions control health outcomes (Rate the outcome and indicators of **Health Beliefs: Perceived Control:** 1 = very weak belief, 2 = weak belief, 3 = moderately strong belief, 4 = strong belief, 5 = very strong belief [see Section I].)

Client Outcomes

Client Will (Specify Time Frame):

- State feelings of powerlessness and other feelings related to powerlessness (e.g., anger, sadness, hopelessness)
- Identify factors that are uncontrollable
- Participate in planning and implementing care; make decisions regarding care and treatment when possible
- Ask questions about care and treatment
- Verbalize hope for the future and sense of participation in planning and implementing care

 • = Independent   ▲ = Collaborative   **EBN** = Evidence-Based Nursing   **EB** = Evidence-Based

NIC (Nursing Interventions Classification)

Suggested NIC Interventions

Cognitive Restructuring, Complex Relationship Building, Mutual Goal Setting, Self-Esteem Enhancement, Self-Responsibility Facilitation

Example NIC Activities—Self-Responsibility Facilitation
Encourage independence but assist patient when unable to perform; Assist patient to identify areas in which they could readily assume more responsibility

Nursing Interventions and *Rationales*

NOTE: Before implementation of interventions in the face of client powerlessness, nurses should examine their own philosophies of care to ensure that control issues or lack of faith in client capabilities will not bias the ability to intervene sincerely and effectively. **EBN:** *Nurses and other health care professionals may feel that they, rather than clients, should make medical decisions, or profess a support of client empowerment that they find difficult to implement (Paliadelis et al, 2005; Ko & Muecke, 2006).*

- Observe for factors contributing to powerlessness (e.g., immobility, hospitalization, unfavorable prognosis, lack of support system, misinformation about situation, inflexible routine, chronic illness). **EBN:** *The essence of ill health is powerlessness, involving the sense of being imprisoned by circumstances (because of limited choices and abilities) and emotional suffering (Strandmark, 2004). Multiple client situations have been associated with powerlessness, including chronic disorders (Hagglund & Ahlstrom, 2007), cancer (Rydahl-Hansen, 2005), and domestic violence (Hyden, 2005), particularly when client perceptions are invalidated or ignored.*

- Assess for **Noncompliance**. Be alert to client behaviors that attempt to assert power, even if they seem confrontational. Help clients channel their behaviors in an effective manner. **EBN:** *Strategies women have used to regain control over uncertain illness trajectories included exiting (changing health care providers when dissatisfied), noncompliance (when medical advice did not seem to make sense), confrontation (especially when clients' perspectives were questioned or ignored), persuasion/insistence, making demands, and demonstrative distancing (refusing to participate in discussion) (Asbring & Narvanen, 2004).*

- Assess the client's locus of control related to his or her health. **EB:** *An external locus of control can negatively influence clients' perception of their power over a health situation, and religious faith may be a component of personal control beliefs (Sparks, Peterson, & Tangenberg, 2005).*

- Establish a therapeutic relationship with the client by spending one-on-one time with him or her, assigning the same caregiver, keeping commitments (e.g., saying, "I will be back to answer your questions in the next hour"), providing encouragement and support, and being empathetic. **EBN:** *Clients reported as empowering the support of family members, friends, and health care providers (Bolse et al, 2005) and believed they had to seek out nursing care as a means of alleviating powerlessness (Shattell, 2005).*

- Encourage the client to share his or her beliefs, thoughts, and expectations about his or her illness. *The Health Belief Model identifies perceived barriers and perceived susceptibility to disease, as powerful predictors of clients' motivation in taking action to prevent disease and participate in self-care management (Pender, Murdaugh, & Parsons, 2005).*

- Have the client assist in planning care whenever possible (e.g., determining what time to bathe, expressing food and fluid preferences). Document specifics in the care plan. *Self-regulation and self-care management promote feelings of self-efficacy, increasing confidence about managing chronic illness (Lorig et al, 2001).* **EBN:** *Cancer clients made use of the Internet to self-manage symptoms and empower decision making (Dickerson et al, 2006).*

- Help the client specify the health goals he or she would like to achieve, prioritizing those goals with regard to immediate concerns and identifying actions that will achieve the goals. Goals may need to be small to be attainable (e.g., dangle legs at bedside for 2 days, then sit in chair 10 minutes for 2 days, then walk to window). *People need goals that have value for them; the discrepancy between these goals and reality motivates action to reduce the discrepancy. Goals must be realistic and achiev-*

---

able; otherwise, the inability to perceive progress will increase hopelessness and powerlessness (Pender, Murdaugh, & Parsons, 2005).

- Encourage the client in goal-directed activities that promote a sense of accomplishment, especially regular exercise. *Goal direction enhances self-efficacy, an important antecedent of empowerment (Finfgeld, 2004).* **EBN:** *In a study of menopausal women, regular exercise promoted a sense of self-fulfillment and an increasing sense of power (Jeng, Yang, & Chang, 2004).*
- Recognize the client's need to experience a sense of reciprocity in dealing with others. Negotiate actions that the client can contribute to the caregiving partnership with both family and nurse (e.g., have the client prepare a cup of tea for the nurse during visits if the client is able). **EBN:** *Ill or injured individuals may make attempts to exchange what skills they can for physical care in attempts to gain a feeling of equity. For older adults, a lack of reciprocity (equitable exchange) was associated with depression (Patusky, 2007).*
- Allow time for questions (15 to 20 minutes each shift). Have the client write down questions, and encourage the client to record a summary of answers received, or provide written material that reinforces answers. *Encouraging the client to write down questions and answers emphasizes the importance of client input and nurses' willingness to attend to that input.* **EBN:** *For hospitalized clients, powerlessness was found to result from lack of staff support (in the form of not being listened to, especially during discharge planning) and lack of information about their illness or medical treatment (Blockley, 2003; Efraimsson et al, 2003).*
- Encourage the client to take control of as many ADLs as possible; keep the client informed of all care that will be given; and keep items the client uses and needs within reach (e.g., a urinal, tissues, telephone, and television controls). *Choice in ADLs such as eating, sleeping, and grooming contributes to a sense of control. Clients are more amenable to therapy if they know what to expect and can perform some tasks independently. Dependence can be alleviated by fostering an expectation of control over activities, which leads to the development of a sense of mastery (Pender, Murdaugh, & Parsons, 2005).*
- Give realistic and sincere praise for accomplishments. *Frequent positive reinforcement helps clients feel successful and competent, especially when it is immediate and is used to balance feedback about errors (Pender, Murdaugh, & Parsons, 2005).*
- In evaluating outcomes implemented to address powerlessness, look to changes in the client, changes in relationships with others, and changes in behavior. **EBN:** *In response to interventions, clients achieve increased self-confidence and self-esteem; improved relationships with families and friends as well as with health care providers; and the ability to make healthier choices for themselves (Falk-Rafael, 2001).*
- Consider using one of the measures of powerlessness that are available for general and specific client groups:
  - Measure of Powerlessness for Adult Patients (De Almeida & Braga, 2006)
  - Spreitzer's Psychological Empowerment Questionnaire (Boudrias, Gaudreau, & Laschinger, 2004)
  - Personal Progress Scale—Revised, tested with women (Johnson, Worell, & Chandler, 2005)
  - Life Situation Questionnaire—Powerlessness subscale, tested with stroke caregivers (Larson et al, 2005)
  - Making Decisions Scale, tested in clients with mental illness (Hansson & Bjorkman, 2005)
- Refer to the care plans for **Hopelessness** and **Spiritual distress**.

Pediatric

- Two key issues that lead to powerlessness for children and their families are hospitalization and peer victimization or bullying.
- Encourage emotional expression through processes that are appropriate to the child's level of development. **EBN:** *Qualitative analysis of play therapy using expressive arts allowing hospitalized children free self-expression revealed a theme of powerlessness as well as the ability of expressive arts to facilitate the child's communication (Wikstrom, 2005).*
- Recognize that a sense of powerlessness can prevent children and adolescents from reporting peer victimization. Be supportive, encourage disclosure without pressure, and help the child or adolescent problem solve options to deal with their stressors. **EBN:** *Pregnant teens reported family, partner, and gang violence that they had not mentioned to health care providers, with powerlessness as a theme*

(Renker, 2006). **EB:** *Disclosure of bullying was found to be inhibited by perceived powerlessness, with active listening and validation recommended as approaches (Mishna & Aleggia, 2005).*

- Provide instruction and visual aids to family members so they may better understand a child's illness and how the family members can help. **EBN:** *New mothers found instruction on child care to be empowering, helping them to be independent, increasing their confidence, and using their strengths (Aston et al, 2006).* **EB:** *Family members of a child with acquired brain injury who were new to medical and special education systems benefited from videos and informational booklets that addressed the child's needs (Forsyth et al, 2005).*

 Geriatric

- In addition to the above interventions as appropriate:
  - Initiate focused assessment questioning and education regarding syndromes common in the elderly. **EBN:** *Studies indicate that disease management programs led by nurses have a positive effect on the perception of powerlessness, loneliness, and disease management (Murchie et al, 2004).*
  - Assess for the presence of elder abuse. Initiate referral to Adult Protective Services and help client regain a sense of safety and control. *Older adults who need assistance are particularly vulnerable to feelings of powerlessness and dependence on caregivers.* **EB:** *Psychosocial assessment, relationship building, and empowerment were important in helping abused elders gain independence and control over their daily lives (Dayton, 2005).*
  - Explore feelings of powerlessness—the feeling that the client's behavior will not affect outcomes. **EBN:** *Older adults who engaged in effective strategies to control their health problems had fewer depressive symptoms, particularly in the presence of acute physical symptoms (Wrosch, Schulz, & Heckhausen, 2002).*
  - Explore personality resources and inner strengths that the client has used in the past. Incorporate these into the treatment plan. **EBN:** *Although resources and strengths cultivated by older adults over the years often go unrecognized, they contribute to the older adult's sense of coherence (perception that life is meaningful, comprehensible, and manageable) and have been shown to optimize quality of life in older women with chronic health problems (Nesbitt & Heidrich, 2000).*
  - Establish therapeutic relationships by listening; participate with the client in generating choices and incorporate his or her statement of limitations. **EBN:** *An individualized approach to health promotion, providing education that will support the individual client's needs, creates a partnership relationship that permits the nurse to enhance self-care practices of the older adult and thereby promote self-care ability and activity (Leenerts, Teel, & Pendleton, 2002).*
  - Instruct caregivers in effective means of managing the behavior of clients with dementia. **EBN:** *Dementia caregivers reported a dichotomy between feeling powerless, with their lives in chaos, versus feeling capable, gaining control and confidence over their abilities to respond to client behaviors (Graneheim et al, 2005).*

 Multicultural

- Assess the influence of cultural beliefs, norms, and values on the client's feelings of powerlessness. **EBN:** *Older Chinese adults who had fallen reported powerlessness, fear, and care seeking (Kong et al, 2002). Elderly Taiwanese men with heart trouble identified powerlessness as arising from lacking choice in living arrangements, having no control over discomfort, being unable to obtain care and companionship from families and friends, failing to get medical information about their disease and treatment options, or expecting deteriorating health and receiving no assistance (Shih et al, 2000).* **EBN:** *When 58 African American and Latino homeless women were given social support and taught to build skills, health outcomes improved (Hatton & Kaiser, 2004).* **EBN:** *African American women gained energy and decreased depression scores when a closed group using meditative exercise with culturally specific scenarios was used (Kohn et al, 2002).*
- Assess the effect of fatalism on the client's expression of powerlessness. *Fatalistic perspectives, which involve the belief that one cannot control one's own fate, may influence health behaviors in some African American, Latino, and Native American populations (Ramirez et al, 2002; Green et al, 2004).*

- Encourage spirituality as a source of support to decrease powerlessness. *African Americans and Latinos may identify spirituality, religiousness, prayer, and church-based approaches as coping resources (Samuel-Hodge et al, 2000).*
- Validate the client's feelings regarding the impact of health status on current lifestyle. **EBN:** *When 326 African American women gained knowledge of breast cancer risk and screening and breast self-examination proficiency, breast self-examination skills scores significantly increased (Wood et al, 2002).*
- For inner-city clients, help the client redefine behaviors as ways of coping with a hostile environment and reconnecting with community supports. **EBN:** *Powerlessness among inner-city African Americans can arise in reaction to inner-city environments, poverty, and racism. Strategies that involve redefining behavior and reconnecting to the community promote empowerment (Dancy et al, 2001).*
- Use an empowerment approach when working with African American women. **EB:** *Three strategies of empowerment for working with African American women caregivers were identified as (1) raising critical group consciousness through storytelling, (2) teaching concrete problem-solving skills, and (3) teaching advocacy skills and mobilizing resources (Chadiha et al, 2004).* **EBN:** *By providing woman-focused intervention of culturally enriched content founded in empowerment theory and feminism/ skills training relative to HIV risk, African American women gained independence and increased personal power and control over behavioral choices (Wechsberg et al, 2003).*

 Home Care

- Develop a therapeutic relationship in the home setting that respects the client's domain. **EBN:** *Effective home care empowers and makes vulnerable both nurse and client (Spiers, 2002).*
- Empower the client by encouraging the client to guide specifics of care such as wound care procedures and dressing and grooming details. Confirm the client's knowledge and document in the chart that the client is able to guide procedures. Document in the home and in the chart the preferred approach to procedures. Orient the family and caregivers to the client's role. **EBN:** *Negotiation, reciprocity, shared decision making, creation of opportunities, and effective information and support are key elements of empowerment in the home (Houston & Cowley, 2002).*
- Identify the client's concerns and implement interventions to address the consequences of disability in clients with medical illness. **EB:** *In clients with cancer being cared for at home, primary factors influencing vulnerability to depression and suicide were identified as real or feared loss of autonomy and independence, concerns about being a burden on others, hopelessness about their condition, and fear of suffering (Filiberti et al, 2001).*
- Respect the client's choices regarding desired assistance. Identify knowledge deficits and provide education to ensure that the client's choice is accurately informed. **EBN:** *The client may identify a problem but choose not to receive help at this time. Assessment is an opportunity to discuss health needs, not a condition for treatment (Houston & Cowley, 2002).*
- Assess the affective climate within the family and family support system, including other caregivers. Instruct the family in appropriate expectations of the client and in the specifics of the client's illness. Encourage the family and client in efforts toward educating friends and co-workers regarding appropriate expectations for the client. **EBN:** *Recognize that clients with an illness requiring extensive physical assistance may become caught in a dilemma; they may be dependent on others for assistance, but that very dependence may hamper their ability to respond naturally within the relationship or require that caregivers meet certain standards. Abuse is also a possibility (Curry et al, 2001).* Refer to care plan for **Risk for other-directed Violence.** *Clients experiencing a catastrophic illness or injury felt distressed by family members' or friends' comments that indicated a lack of understanding of the illness experience (Dewar, 2001).*
- Evaluate the powerlessness of caregivers to ensure they continue their ability to care for the client. Provide assistance using interventions from this care plan. **EB:** *In next of kin of clients with cancer receiving palliative home care, powerlessness and helplessness were reported regarding client's suffering, fading away, and next of kin's feeling of inadequacy (Milberg, Strang, & Jakobsson, 2004).*
- Be aware of and assist clients with potential needs for help in negotiating the health care system. **EB:** *Among individuals with disabilities, powerlessness may arise as a response to failures of the system to provide needed services (Helgoy, Ravneberg, & Solvang, 2003).*

• = Independent   ▲ = Collaborative   **EBN** = Evidence-Based Nursing   **EB** = Evidence-Based

- Explain all relevant symptoms, procedures, treatments, and expected outcomes. **EBN:** *In a study of clients' perceptions of their health care, clients who expressed powerlessness described a lack of knowledge and information about treatment strategies (Nordgren & Fridlund, 2001).*
- Provide written instructions for treatments and procedures for which the client will be responsible. **EBN:** *This review recommends the use of both verbal and written health information when communicating about care issues with clients and/or significant others on discharge from hospital to home. The combination of verbal and written health information enables the provision of standardized care information to clients and/or significant others, which appears to improve knowledge and satisfaction (Johnson, Sandford, & Tyndall, 2003).*
- Teach stress reduction, relaxation, and imagery. Many audio recordings are available on relaxation and meditation. **EBN:** *In this study of clients with breast cancer, participants reported the importance of engaging passive and active imagery. Imagery practice improved mood state (Freeman et al, 2008).*
- Teach cognitive-behavioral activities, such as active problem solving, reframing (reappraising the situation from a different perspective), or thought stopping (in response to a negative thought, such as picturing a large stop sign and replacing the image with a prearranged positive alternative). Teach the client to confront his or her own negative thought patterns (cognitive distortions). *Through cognitive-behavioral interventions, clients become more aware of their cognitive choices in adopting and maintaining their belief systems, thereby exercising greater control over their own reactions (Hagerty & Patusky, 2008).*
- Identify the strengths of the caregiver and efforts to gain control of unpredictable situations. Help the caregiver stay connected with a client who may be behaving differently than usual to make life as routine as possible, help the client set goals and sustain hope, and allow the client space to experience progress. **EBN:** *Identifying positive caregiver responses to the client's illness assists the caregiver in tolerating his or her own feelings of powerlessness. The most frequently identified burden was "worry about the future." The greatest concern was "dealing with sadness and grief" (Rose, Mallinson, & Gerson, 2006).*
- ▲ Refer the client to support groups, pastoral care, or social services. *These services help decrease levels of stress, increase levels of self-esteem, and reassure clients that they are not alone.* **EB:** *Hospitalized clients value visitation by chaplains and appreciate both religious and supportive interventions (Piderman et al, 2008).*

Client/Family Teaching and Discharge Planning

- Teach specifics about the illnesses and treatment regimen so that client may regain a sense of control. **EBN and EB:** *Acquiring knowledge about their illnesses or treatment regimens helped clients regain a sense of control, whether the condition was chronic fatigue syndrome or fibromyalgia (Asbring & Narvanen, 2004), ventilator-dependence (Johnson, 2004), or diabetes (Panja, Starr, & Colleran, 2005; Siminerio, Piatt, & Zgibor, 2005).*
- Teach family members how they can assist in client's care to enhance family support. **EBN and EB:** *Family members of clients with mental illness or traumatic brain injury have identified empowerment as an important factor in their ability to cope with client behavior and care needs (Sjoblom, Pejlert, & Asplund, 2005; Gavois, Paulsson, & Fridlund, 2006).*
- Facilitate client's participation in discharge planning by allowing the client time and space to express feeling/concerns about discharge plans. Assist client to prepare questions for discharge planning conferences. **EBN:** *In an analysis of a discharge planning conference, researchers found that professionals controlled topics by using medical language and talking about rather than with the client. The client felt she was viewed as an object, had no right to make demands, and was dependent on others; she resisted by withholding comments (Efraimsson et al, 2003).*

ⓔvolve   See the EVOLVE website for Weblinks for client education resources.

REFERENCES

Asbring P, Narvanen A: Patient power and control: a study of women with uncertain illness trajectories, *Qual Health Res* 14(2):226, 2004.

Aston M, Meagher-Stewart D, Sheppard-Lemoin D et al: Family health nursing and empowering relationships, *Ped Nurs* 32:61, 2006.

• = Independent   ▲ = Collaborative   **EBN** = Evidence-Based Nursing   **EB** = Evidence-Based

Blockley C: Experiences of first time hospitalisation for acute illness, *Nurs Prax N Z* 19(2):19, 2003.

Bolse K, Hamilton G, Flanagan J et al: Ways of experiencing the life situation among United States patients with an implantable cardioverter-defibrillator: a qualitative study, *Prog Cardiovasc Nurs* 20(1):4, 2005.

Boudrias J, Gaudreau P, Laschinger HKS: Testing the structure of psychological empowerment: does gender make a difference? *Educ Psychol Meas* 64:861, 2004.

Chadiha LA, Adams P, Biegel DE et al: Empowering African American women informal caregivers: a literature synthesis and practice strategies, *Soc Work* 49(1):97–108, 2004.

Curry MA, Hassouneh-Phillips D, Johnston-Silverberg A: Abuse of women with disabilities: an ecological model and review, *Violence Against Women* 7(1):60, 2001.

Dancy BL, McCreary L, Daye M et al: Empowerment: a view of two low-income African-American communities, *J Natl Black Nurses Assoc* 12(2):49, 2001.

Dayton C: Elder abuse: the social worker's perspective, *Clin Gerontol* 28:135, 2005.

De Almeida LM, Braga CG: Construction and validation of an instrument to assess powerlessness, *Int J Nurs Terminol Classif* 17:67, 2006.

Dewar A: Protecting strategies used by sufferers of catastrophic illness and injuries, *J Clin Nurs* 19:600, 2001.

Dickerson SS, Boehmke M, Ogle C et al: Seeking and managing hope: patients' experiences using the Internet for cancer care, *Oncology Nurs Forum* 33:E8, 2006.

Efraimsson E, Rasmussen BH, Gilje F et al: Expressions of power and powerlessness in discharge planning: a case study of an older woman on her way home, *J Clin Nurs* 12:707, 2003.

Falk-Rafael AR: Empowerment as a process of evolving consciousness: a model of empowered caring, *Adv Nurs Sci* 24(1):1, 2001.

Filiberti A, Ripamonti C, Totis A et al: Characteristics of terminal cancer patients who committed suicide during a home palliative care program, *J Pain Symptom Manage* 22:544, 2001.

Finfgeld DL: Empowerment of individuals with enduring mental health problems: results from concept analyses and qualitative investigations, *Adv Nurs Sci* 27(1):44, 2004.

Forsyth RJ, Kelly TP, Wicks B et al: "Must try harder?" A family empowerment intervention for acquired brain injury, *Ped Rehab* 8(2):140, 2005.

Freeman L, Cohen L, Stewart M et al: The experience of imagery as a post-treatment intervention in patients with breast cancer: program, process, and patient recommendations, *Oncol Nurs Forum* 35(6): E116–121, 2008.

Gavois H, Paulsson G, Fridlund B: Mental health professional support in families with a member suffering from severe mental illness: a grounded theory model, *Scand J Caring Sci* 20:102, 2006.

Graneheim UH, Isaksson U, Ljung IP et al: Balancing between contradictions: the meaning of interaction with people suffering from dementia and "behavioral disturbances," *Intl J Aging Hum Devel* 60(2):145, 2005.

Green BL, Lewis RK, Wang MQ et al: Powerlessness, destiny, and control: the influence on health behaviors of African Americans, *J Community Health* 29(1):15–27, 2004.

Hagerty B, Patusky K: Mood disorders: depression and mania. In Fortinash KM, Holoday-Worret PA, editors: *Psychiatric mental health nursing*, ed 4, St Louis, 2008, Mosby.

Hagglund D, Ahlstrom G: The meaning of women's experience of living with long-term urinary incontinence is powerlessness, *J Clin Nurs* 16:1946, 2007.

Hansson L, Bjorkman T: Empowerment in people with a mental illness: reliability and validity of the Swedish version of an empowerment scale, *Scand J Caring Sci* 19:32, 2005.

Hatton D, Kaiser L: Methodological and ethical issues emerging from pilot testing an intervention with women in a transitional shelter, *West J Nurs Res* 26(1):129–136, 2004.

Helgoy I, Ravneberg B, Solvang P: Service provision for an independent life, *Disability Soc* 18(4):471, 2003.

Houston AM, Cowley S: An empowerment approach to needs assessment in health visiting practice, *J Clin Nurs* 11:640, 2002.

Hyden M: "I must have been an idiot to let it go on": agency and positioning in battered women's narratives of leaving, *Fem Psychol* 15:169, 2005.

Jeng C, Yang S, Chang P: Menopausal women: perceiving continuous power through the experience of regular exercise, *J Clin Nurs* 13:447, 2004.

Johnson A, Sandford J, Tyndall J: Written and verbal information versus verbal information only for patients being discharged from acute hospital settings to home, *Cochrane Database Syst Rev* (4):CD003716, 2003.

Johnson DM, Worell J, Chandler RK: Assessing psychological health and empowerment in women: The Personal Progress Scale Revised, *Women Health* 41(1):109, 2005.

Johnson P: Reclaiming the everyday world: how long-term ventilated patients in critical care seek to gain aspects of power and control over their environment, *Intensive Crit Care Nurs* 20:190, 2004.

Ko NY, Muecke MA: Prevailing discourses among AIDS care professionals about childbearing by couples with HIV in Taiwan, *AIDS Care* 18(1):82, 2006.

Kohn L, Oden T, Munoz R et al: Adapted cognitive behavioral group therapy for depressed low-income African American women, *Community Ment Health J* 38(6):497–504, 2002.

Kong KS, Lee FK, Mackenzie AE et al: Psychosocial consequences of falling: the perspective of older Hong Kong Chinese who had experienced recent falls, *J Adv Nurs* 37:234, 2002.

Larson J, Franzen-Dahlen J, Billing E et al: Spouse's life situation after partner's stroke: psychometric testing of a questionnaire, *J Adv Nurs* 52:300, 2005.

Leenerts MH, Teel CS, Pendleton MK: Building a model of self-care for health promotion in aging, *J Nurs Scholarsh* 34:355, 2002.

Lorig KR, Ritter P, Stewart AL et al: Chronic disease self-management program: 2–year health status and health care utilization outcomes, *Med Care* 39:1217, 2001.

Milberg A, Strang P, Jakobsson M: Next of kin's experience of powerlessness and helplessness in palliative home care, *Support Care Cancer* 12:120, 2004.

Mishna F, Aleggia R: Weighing the risks: a child's decision to disclose peer victimization, *Child Schools* 27:218, 2005.

Murchie P, Campbell N, Ritchie LD et al: Effects of secondary prevention clinics on health status in patients with coronary heart disease: 4 year follow-up randomized trial in primary care, *Fam Pract* 21(5):567–574, 2004.

Nesbitt BJ, Heidrich SM: Sense of coherence and illness appraisal in older women's quality of life, *Res Nurs Health* 23:25, 2000.

Nordgren S, Fridlund B: Patients' perceptions of self-determination as expressed in the context of care, *J Adv Nurs* 35(1):117, 2001.

Paliadelis P, Cruickshank M, Wainohu D et al: Implementing family-centred care: an exploration of the beliefs and practices of paediatric nurses, *Austr J Adv Nurs* 23(1):31, 2005.

Panja S, Starr B, Colleran KM: Patient knowledge improves glycemic control: Is it time to go back to the classroom? *J Invest Med* 53:264, 2005.

Patusky KL: Event-generated dependence in older adults, *Int J Older People Nurs* 2:171–179, 2007.

Pender NJ, Murdaugh CL, Parsons MA: *Health promotion in nursing practice*, ed 5, Upper Saddle River, NJ, 2005, Prentice-Hall.

• = Independent ▲ = Collaborative **EBN** = Evidence-Based Nursing **EB** = Evidence-Based

Piderman KM, Marek DV, Jenkins SM et al: Patients' expectations of hospital chaplains, *Mayo Clin Proc* 83(1):58–65, 2008.

Ramirez JR, Crano WD, Quist R et al: Effects of fatalism and family communication on HIV/AIDS awareness variations in American and Anglo parents and children, *AIDS Educ Prev* 14(1):29, 2002.

Renker PR: Perinatal violence assessment: teenagers' rationale for denying violence when asked, *JOGNN* 35(1):56, 2006.

Rose LE, Mallinson RK, Gerson LD: Mastery, burden, and areas of concern among family caregivers of mentally ill persons, *Arch Psychiatr Nurs* 20(1):41–51, 2006.

Rydahl-Hansen S: Hospitalized patients experienced suffering in life with incurable cancer, *Scand J Caring Sci* 19:213, 2005.

Samuel-Hodge CD, Headen SW, Skelly AH et al: Influences on day-to-day self-management of type 2 diabetes among African American women: spirituality, the multi-caregiver role, and other social context factors, *Diabetes Care* 23(7):928, 2000.

Shattell M: Nurse bait: strategies hospitalized patients use to entice nurses within the context of the interpersonal relationship, *Issues Ment Health Nurs* 26:205, 2005.

Shih SN, Shih FJ, Chen CH et al: The forgotten faces: the lonely journey of powerlessness experienced by elderly single Chinese men with heart disease in Taiwan, *Geriatr Nurs* 21:254, 2000.

Siminerio LM, Piatt G, Zgibor JC: Implementing the chronic care model for improvements in diabetes care and education in a rural primary care practice, *Diabetes Educ* 31:225, 2005.

Sjoblom L, Pejlert A, Asplund K: Nurses' view of the family in psychiatric care, *J Clin Nurs* 14:562, 2005.

Sparks A, Peterson NA, Tangenberg K: Belief in personal control among low-income African American, Puerto Rican, and European American single mothers, *Affilia J Women Soc Work* 20:401, 2005.

Spiers JA: The interpersonal contexts of negotiating care in home care nurse-patient interactions, *Qual Health Res* 12:1033, 2002.

Strandmark M: Ill heath is powerlessness: a phenomenological study about worthlessness, limitations and suffering, *Scand J Caring Sci* 18:135, 2004.

Wechsberg WM, Lam WK, Zule WA et al: Violence, homelessness, and HIV risk among crack-using African-American women, *Subst Use Misuse* 38:671–701, 2003.

Wikstrom B: Communicating via expressive arts: the natural medium of self-expression for hospitalized children, *Ped Nurs* 31:480, 2005.

Wood R, Duffy M, Morris S et al: The effect of an education intervention on promoting breast self-examination in older African-American and Caucasian women, *Oncol Nurs Forum* 29(7):1081–1090, 2002.

Wrosch C, Schulz R, Heckhausen J: Health stresses and depressive symptomatology in the elderly: the importance of health engagement control strategies, *Health Psychol* 21:340, 2002.

Risk for Powerlessness   *Betty J. Ackley, MSN, EdS, RN*

Definition

At risk for perceived lack of control over a situation and/or one's ability to significantly affect an outcome

Risk Factors (r/t)

Physiological

Acute injury; aging; dying; illness; progressive debilitating disease process (e.g., spinal cord injury, multiple sclerosis)

Psychosocial

Absence of integrality (e.g., essence of power); chronic low self-esteem; deficient knowledge (e.g., of illness or health care system); disturbed body image; inadequate coping patterns; lifestyle of dependency; situational low self-esteem

NOC, NIC, Client Outcomes, Nursing Interventions, Client/Family Teaching and Discharge Planning, *Rationales*, and References

See the care plan for **Powerlessness.**

Ineffective Protection   *Ruth M. Curchoe, RN, MSN, CIC*

Definition

Decrease in ability to guard self from internal or external threats, such as illness or injury

Defining Characteristics

Altered clotting; anorexia; chilling; cough; deficient immunity; disorientation; dyspnea; fatigue; immobility; impaired healing; insomnia; itching; maladaptive stress response; neurosensory alteration; perspiring; pressure ulcers; restlessness; weakness

Related Factors (r/t)

Abnormal blood profiles (e.g., leukopenia, thrombocytopenia, anemia, coagulation); alcohol abuse; cancer; drug therapies (e.g., antineoplastic, corticosteroid, immune, anticoagulant, thrombolytic); extremes of age; immune disorders; inadequate nutrition; treatments (e.g., surgery, radiation)

NOC (Nursing Outcomes Classification)

Suggested NOC Outcomes

Health-Promoting Behavior, Blood Coagulation, Endurance, Immune Status

Example **NOC Outcome with Indicators**
Immune Status as evidenced by the following indicators: Recurrent infections/Tumors/ Weight loss (Rate the outcome and indicators of **Immune Status:** 1 = severe, 2 = substantial, 3 = moderate, 4 = mild, 5 = none [see Section I].)

Client Outcomes

Client Will (Specify Time Frame):

- Remain free of infection
- Remain free of any evidence of new bleeding
- Explain precautions to take to prevent infection
- Explain precautions to take to prevent bleeding

NIC (Nursing Interventions Classification)

Suggested NIC Interventions

Bleeding Precautions, Infection Prevention, Infection Protection

Example **NIC Activities—Infection Protection**
Monitor for systemic and localized signs and symptoms of infection; Inspect skin and mucous membranes for redness, extreme warmth, or drainage

Nursing Interventions and *Rationales*

- Take temperature, pulse, and blood pressure (e.g., every 1 to 4 hours). *Prospective surveillance study for health care acquired infection on hematology-oncology units should include fever of unknown origin as the single most common and clinically important entity (Engelhart et al, 2002). Changes in vital signs can indicate the onset of bleeding or infection.*
- ▲ Observe nutritional status (e.g., weight, serum protein and albumin levels, muscle mass, and usual food intake). Work with the dietitian to improve nutritional status if needed. All clients diagnosed with HIV should have a dietary consult. **EB:** *Nutrient status is an important factor contributing to immune competence; undernutrition impairs the immune system (Calder & Kew, 2002).* **EBN:** *Nutrition complications of HIV infection, including wasting syndrome, nutrient*

• = Independent   ▲ = Collaborative   **EBN** = Evidence-Based Nursing   **EB** = Evidence-Based

deficiencies, and metabolic complications, have been well-documented over the last 25 years (Coyne-Meyers & Trombley, 2004).

- Observe the client's sleep pattern; if altered, see Nursing Interventions and Rationales for **Disturbed Sleep pattern.**
- Identify stressors in the client's life. If stress is uncontrollable, see Nursing Interventions and Rationales for **Ineffective Coping.** *Data shows one of the consequences of sleep deprivation is increased susceptibility to infection (Palma, Tufik, & Suchecki, 2007).*

Prevention of Infection

▲ Monitor for and report any signs of infection (e.g., fever, chills, flushed skin, drainage, edema, redness, abnormal laboratory values, and pain) and notify the physician promptly. *The immunocompromised host may present with a very different clinical picture when compared to an immunecompetent host. The progress of the infection may be more rapid, and the infection may quickly become life-threatening (Risi, 2009).* **EBN:** *While the white blood cell count may be in the normal range, an increased number of immature bands may be present (Risi, 2009).*

▲ If the client's immune system is depressed, notify the physician of elevated temperature, even in the absence of other symptoms of infection. *Clients with depressed immune function are unable to mount the usual immune responses to the onset of infection; fever may be the only sign of infection. A neutropenic client with fever represents an absolute medical emergency (Burney, 2000; Quadri & Brown, 2000).*

- If white blood cell count is severely decreased (i.e., absolute neutrophil count of less than 1000/mm³), initiate the following precautions:
  - Take vital signs every 4 hours.
  - Complete a head-to-toe assessment twice daily, including inspection of oral mucosa, invasive sites, wounds, urine, and stool; monitor for onset of new reports of pain.
  - Avoid any invasive procedures, including catheterization, injections, or rectal or vaginal procedures unless absolutely necessary. *Infectious agents can invade when a treatment damages the skin or mucous membranes, which are natural barriers against infection (Risi, 2009).*
- Consider warming the client before elective surgery. **EBN:** *In clients undergoing elective hernia repair, varicose vein surgery, or breast surgery, preoperative warming with a local device or a warm air blanket reduces the incidence of wound infection after surgery (Borbasi & Brougham, 2002). Normothermia is associated with low postoperative infection rates (Leaper, 2006).*

▲ Administer granulocyte growth factor therapy as ordered. *Clients most likely to benefit from therapy would be those with profound neutropenia or neutropenia with infections not responding to antimicrobial therapy (Risi, 2009). Clinical trials suggest that granulocyte macrophage colony-stimulating factor shortens the duration of mucositis and diarrhea, stimulating dendritic cells, preventing infection, acting as an adjuvant vaccine agent, and facilitating antitumor activity (Buchsel et al, 2002).*

- Take meticulous care of all invasive sites; use chlorhexidine gluconate for cleansing. **EBN:** *Use of chlorhexidine gluconate for vascular catheter site care reduces catheter-related bloodstream infections and catheter colonization more than use of povidone iodine (Chaiyakunapruk et al, 2002; Young, Commiskey, & Wilson, 2006).*
- Provide frequent oral care. *The effects of chemotherapy or radiation leave the mouth inflamed; combined with immunosuppression, this can result in stomatitis. Good oral care can help prevent complications (Frydrych & Davies, 2002; Cawley & Benson, 2005).*

▲ Refer for prophylactic medication to prevent oral candidiasis. **EB:** *Drugs absorbed or partially absorbed from the gastrointestinal tract prevent oral candidiasis in the client receiving treatment for cancer (Worthington, Clarkson, & Eden, 2007).*

▲ Refer for appropriate prophylactic antifungal treatment and avoid pathogen exposure (through air filtration, regular hand hygiene, and avoidance of plants and flowers). *Practical measures can be taken to avoid exposing the client to fungi (Risi, 2009).* **EB:** *IV amphotericin B is the only antifungal agent for which there is evidence suggesting that its use might reduce mortality (Gotzsche & Johansen, 2002).*

- Have the client wear a mask when leaving the room. **EB:** *To prevent health care–acquired pulmonary aspergillosis during hospital construction, neutropenic clients with hematological malignancy were required to wear high-efficiency filtering masks when leaving their rooms (Raad et al, 2002).*
- Limit and screen visitors to minimize exposure to contagion.
- Help the client bathe daily.

● = Independent   ▲ = Collaborative   **EBN** = Evidence-Based Nursing   **EB** = Evidence-Based

- Practice food safety; a neutropenic diet may not be necessary (Foodsafety.gov, 2009). *No clear evidence exists that the neutropenic diet makes a difference in overall rates of infection (DeMille et al, 2006).*
- ▲ Ensure that the client is well nourished. Provide food with protein, and consider vitamin supplements. If appetite is suppressed, institute a dietary referral. Keep track of serum albumin levels, as well as transferrin and prealbumin levels. **EB:** *Levels of the visceral proteins (albumin, transferrin, and prealbumin) are an indirect measure of nutritional status (Calder & Kew, 2002).*
- Help the client to cough and practice deep breathing regularly. Maintain an appropriate activity level.
- Obtain a private room for the client. Use high-energy particulate air filters if available and appropriate. Protective isolation is not recommended. Recognize that cotton cover gowns may not be effective in decreasing infection. **EB:** *High-risk clients, especially those with prolonged granulocytopenia or organ transplants, should be cared for in hospital units with HEPA-filtered air (Safdar, Crnich, & Maki, 2005).* **EBN:** *The routine use of cotton cover gowns in the care of neutropenic clients found that the rates of infection were no different than when cover gowns were not used (Kenny & Lawson, 2000). Abandoning protective isolation combined with increased hygienic measures in nursing of clients with severe neutropenia does not increase the risk of infections (Mank & van der Lilie, 2003).*
- ▲ Watch for signs of sepsis, including change in mental status, fever, shaking, chills, and hypotension. If present, notify the physician promptly. *Change in mental status, fever, shaking, chills, and hypotension are indicators of sepsis (Risi, 2009).*
- Refer to care plan for **Risk for Infection.**
- Refer to care plan for **Readiness for enhanced Nutrition** for additional interventions.

Pediatric

- Suggest kangaroo care, frequent and exclusive or nearly exclusive breastfeeding, and early discharge from hospital for low-birth-weight infants. **EBN:** *Kangaroo care appears to reduce severe infant morbidity without any serious deleterious effect reported (Conde-Agudelo & Belizán, 2003).*
- Treat postoperative fever in pediatric oncology clients promptly. **EBN:** *A postoperative fever in immunocompromised pediatric clients indicates infection and may lead to complications if not treated promptly (Chang, Hendershot, & Colapinto, 2006).*
- For hand hygiene with low-birth-weight infants, use alcohol hand rub and gloves. **EBN:** *The introduction of the alcohol hand rub and glove protocol was associated with a 2.8-fold reduction in the incidence of late-onset systemic infection and a significant decrease in the incidence of methicillin-resistant* Staphylococcus aureus *septicemia and necrotizing enterocolitis in very-low-birth-weight infants (Ng et al, 2004).*

Geriatric

- If not contraindicated, promote exercise to strengthen the immune system in the elderly. **EB:** *A study of adults 62 years and older suggest that lifestyle factors, including exercise, may influence immune response to influenza immunization. The practice of regular, vigorous exercise was associated with enhanced immune response after influenza vaccination in older adults (Kohut et al, 2002; Phillips, Burns, & Lord, 2007).*
- Give elderly clients with imbalanced nutrition a nutritional supplement to enhance immune function. **EB:** *Consumption of this complete liquid nutritional supplement may have a beneficial effect on antibody response to influenza vaccination in the elderly population (Wouters-Wesseling et al, 2002).*
- Refer to the care plan for **Risk for Infection** for more interventions related to the prevention of infection.

Prevention of Bleeding

- Monitor the client's risk for bleeding; evaluate results of clotting studies and platelet counts. *Laboratory studies give a good indication of the seriousness of the bleeding disorder.*
- Watch for hematuria, melena, hematemesis, hemoptysis, epistaxis, bleeding from mucosa, petechiae, and ecchymoses. *These types of bleeding can be detected in a bleeding disorder (Paschall, 1993; Martini et al, 2007).*

• = Independent   ▲ = Collaborative   **EBN** = Evidence-Based Nursing   **EB** = Evidence-Based

▲ Give medications orally or IV only; avoid giving them IM, subcutaneously, or rectally (Shuey, 1996).

• Apply pressure for a longer time than usual to invasive sites, such as venipuncture or injection sites. *Additional pressure is needed to stop bleeding of invasive sites in clients with bleeding disorders.*

• Take vital signs often; watch for changes associated with fluid volume loss. *Excessive bleeding causes decreased blood pressure and increased pulse and respiratory rates.*

• Monitor menstrual flow if relevant; have the client use pads instead of tampons. *Menstruation can be excessive in clients with bleeding disorders. Use of tampons can increase trauma to the vagina.*

▲ Have the client use a moistened toothette or a very soft child's toothbrush instead of an adult toothbrush. Follow the dentist recommendation for flossing and appropriate rinses to use. Control gum bleeding by applying pressure to gums with gauze pad soaked in ice water *These actions help prevent trauma to the oral mucosa, which could result in bleeding (Medline Plus, 2009).*

• Ask the client either to not shave or to use only an electric razor. *This helps prevent any unnecessary trauma that could result in bleeding (Shuey, 1996).*

• To decrease risk of bleeding, avoid administering salicylates or nonsteroidal antiinflammatory drugs (NSAIDs) if possible. **EB:** *Gastrointestinal bleeding due to NSAID, acetylsalicylic acid, or warfarin was the most common adverse drug reaction that resulted in hospital admission and represented 40% of all ADRs (12/30), according to WHO causality criteria (Brvar et al, 2009).*

Home Care

• Some of the interventions previously described may be adapted for home care use.

▲ Consider institution of a nurse-administered mobile care unit for monitoring anticoagulant therapy. **EBN:** *Establishment of anticoagulation therapy management clinics leads to improvements in quality of care in terms of improved control of international normalized ratio and reduced complications (Gill & Landis, 2002).*

▲ For terminally ill clients, teach and institute all of the aforementioned noninvasive precautions that maintain quality of life. Discuss with the client, family, and physician the consequences of contracting infection. Determine which precautions do not maintain quality of life and should not be used (e.g., physical assessment twice daily or multiple vital sign assessments). *Multiple assessments and other invasive procedures are recovery-based and cure-focused activities. The client and physician must agree on an approach to care for the client's remaining life.*

Client/Family Teaching and Discharge Planning

Depressed Immune Function

• Teach the client and family how to take a temperature. Encourage the family to take the client's temperature between 3 PM and 7 PM at least once daily. *For most people, the difference between high and low values throughout the day is approximately 2.0° F (1.1° C) (97° to 99° F [36.1° to 37.2° C]), with the lowest value typically occurring in the early morning hours (2 AM to 5 AM) and the highest values commonly occurring in the evening (7 PM to 10 PM) (Round-the-Clock Systems, 2009).*

• Teach precautions to use to decrease the chance of infection (e.g., avoiding uncooked fruits and vegetables, using appropriate self-care including good hand hygiene, and ensuring a safe environment). Teach the client to avoid crowds and contact with persons who have infections. Teach the need for good nutrition, avoidance of stress, and adequate rest to maintain immune system function. *Approaches to avoiding infection at home for the client with neutropenia include good hand hygiene and careful management of food, drink, and the client's environment (Nirenberg et al, 2006; Hawkins, 2009).*

Bleeding Disorder

▲ Teach the client to wear a medical alert bracelet and notify all health care personnel of the bleeding disorder. *Emergency identification schemes such as medical alert bracelets use emblems that alert health care professionals to potential problems and can ensure appropriate and prompt treatment (Morton et al, 2002).*

▲ Teach the client and family the signs of bleeding, precautions to take to prevent bleeding, and action to take if bleeding begins. Caution the client to avoid taking over-the-counter medications without the permission of the physician. *Medications containing salicylates can increase bleeding.*

• Teach the client to wear loose-fitting clothes and avoid physical activity that might cause trauma.

⊝volve See the EVOLVE website for Weblinks for client education resources.

REFERENCES

Borbasi S, Brougham L: Warming clients before clean surgery reduced the incidence of postoperative wound infection, *Evid Based Nurs* 5(2):48, 2002.

Brvar M, Fokter N, Bunc M et al: The frequency of adverse drug reaction related admissions according to method of detection, admission urgency and medical department specialty, *BMC Clin Pharmacol* 4(9):8, 2009.

Buchsel PC, Forgey A, Grape FB et al: Granulocyte macrophage colony-stimulating factor: current practice and novel approaches, *Clin J Oncol Nurs* 6(4):198–205, 2002.

Burney KY: Tips for timely management of febrile neutropenia, *Oncol Nurs Forum* 27(4):617–618, 2000.

Calder PC, Kew S: The immune system: a target for functional foods? *Br J Nutr* 88(Suppl 2):S165–S177, 2002.

Cawley MM, Benson LM: Current trends in managing oral mucositis, *Clin J Oncol Nurs* 9(5):584–592, 2005.

Chaiyakunapruk N, Veenstra DL, Lipsky BA et al: Chlorhexidine compared with povidone-iodine solution for vascular catheter-site care: a meta-analysis, *Ann Intern Med* 136(11):792–801, 2002.

Chang A, Hendershot E, Colapinto K: Minimizing complications-related to fever in the postoperative pediatric oncology patient, *J Pediatr Oncol* 23(2):75–81, 2006.

Conde-Agudelo A, Belizán JM: Kangaroo mother care to reduce morbidity and mortality in low birthweight infants, *Cochrane Database Syst Rev* (2):CD002771, 2003.

Coyne-Meyers K, Trombley LE: A review of nutrition in human immunodeficiency virus infection in the era of highly active antiretroviral therapy, *Nutr Clin Pract* 19(4):340–355, 2004.

DeMille D, Deming P, Lupinacci P et al: The effect of the neutropenic diet in the outpatient setting: a pilot study, *Oncol Nurs Forum* 33(2):337–343, 2006.

Engelhart S, Glasmacher A, Exner M et al: Surveillance for health care acquired infections and fever of unknown origin among adult hematology/oncology patients, *Infect Control Hosp Epidemiol* 23(5):244, 2002.

Foodsafety.gov: www.foodsafety.gov. Accessed Nov. 23, 2009.

Frydrych AM, Davies CR: Treatment for dry mouth, stomatitis and mucositis, *Aust Dent J* 47(3):249–253, 2002.

Gill JM, Landis MK: Benefits of a mobile, point-of-care anticoagulation therapy management program, *Jt Comm J Qual Improv* 28(11):625–630, 2002.

Gotzsche PC, Johansen HK: Routine versus selective antifungal administration for control of fungal infections in patients with cancer, *Cochrane Database Syst Rev* (2):CD000026, 2002.

Hawkins J: Supportive care: managing febrile neutropenia, *Paediatr Nurs* 21(4):33–37, 2009.

Kenny H, Lawson E: The efficacy of cotton cover gowns in reducing infection in nursing neutropenic patients: an evidence-based study, *Int J Nurs Pract* 6(3):135–139, 2000.

Kohut ML, Cooper MM, Nickolaus MS et al: Exercise and psychosocial factors modulate immunity to influenza vaccine in elderly individuals, *J Gerontol A Biol Sci Med Sci* 57(9):M557–M562, 2002.

Leaper D: Effects of local and systemic warming on postoperative infections, *Surg Infect (Larchmt)* 7(Suppl 2):S101–S103, 2006.

Mank A, van der Lilie H: Is there still an indication for nursing patients with prolonged neutropenia in protective isolation? An evidence based nursing and medical study of 4 years experience for nursing patients with neutropenia without isolation, *Eur J Oncol Nurs* 7(1):17–23, 2003.

Martini MZ, Lopez JS Jr, Gendler JL et al: Idiopathic thrombocytopenic purpura presenting as post-extraction hemorrhage, *J Contemp Dent Pract* 8(6):43–49, 2007.

Medline Plus: Bleeding gums. www.nlm.nih.gov/medlineplus/ency/article/003062.htm. Accessed July 1, 2009.

Morton L, Murad S, Omar RZ et al: Importance of emergency identification schemes, *Emerg Med J* 19(6):584–586, 2002.

Ng PC, Wong HL, Lyon DJ et al: Combined use of alcohol hand rub and gloves reduces the incidence of late onset infection in very low birthweight infants, *Arch Dis Child Fetal Neonatal Ed* 89(4):F336–F340, 2004.

Nirenberg A, Parry Bush A, Davis A et al: Neutropenia: state of the knowledge part II, *Oncol Nurs Forum* 33(6):1202–1208, 2006.

Palma BD, Tufik S, Suchecki D: The stress of inadequate sleep and immune consequences. In Pandi-Perumal SR, Cardinali DP, Chrousos GP, editors: *Neuroimmunology of sleep,* New York, 2007, Springer.

Paschall FE: Thrombotic thrombocytopenic purpura: the challenges of a complex disease process, *AACN Clin Issues Crit Care Nurs* 4(4):655–663, 1993.

Phillips AC, Burns VE, Lord JM: Stress and exercise: getting the balance right for aging immunity, *Exerc Sport Sci Rev* 35(1):35–39, 2007.

Quadri TL, Brown AE: Infectious complications in the critically ill patient with cancer, *Semin Oncol* 27(3):335–346, 2000.

Raad I, Hanna H, Osting C et al: Masking of neutropenic patients on transport from hospital rooms is associated with a decrease in nosocomial aspergillosis during construction, *Infect Control Hosp Epidemiol* 23(1):41–43, 2002.

Risi GF: The immunocompromised host, In *APIC text of infection control and epidemiology,* ed 3, Washington, DC, 2009, Association for Professionals in Infection Control and Epidemiology, Inc (APIC).

Round-the-Clock Systems: *Circadian rhythms:* www.matrices.com/Workplace/Learning/sw.circadian.html. Accessed Nov. 23, 2009.

Safdar N, Crnich CJ, Maki DG: The pathogenesis of ventilator-associated pneumonia: its relevance to developing effective strategies for prevention, *Respir Care* 50(6):725–741, 2005.

Shuey KM: Platelet-associated bleeding disorders, *Semin Oncol Nurs* 12(1):15–27, 1996.

Worthington HV, Clarkson JE, Eden OB: Interventions for preventing oral candidiasis for patients with cancer receiving treatment, *Cochrane Database Syst Rev* (1):CD003807, 2007.

Wouters-Wesseling W, Rozendaal M, Snijder M et al: Effect of a complete nutritional supplement on antibody response to influenza vaccine in elderly people, *J Gerontol A Biol Sci Med Sci* 57(9):M563–M566, 2002.

Young EM, Commiskey ML, Wilson SJ: Translating evidence into practice to prevent central venous catheter-associated bloodstream infections: a systems-based intervention, *Am J Infect Control* 34(8):503–506, 2006.

• = Independent   ▲ = Collaborative   **EBN** = Evidence-Based Nursing   **EB** = Evidence-Based

Rape-Trauma syndrome   *Mary T. Shoemaker, RN, MSN, SANE*

 NANDA-I

Definition

Sustained maladaptive response to a forced, violent sexual penetration against the victim's will and consent

Defining Characteristics

Aggression; agitation; anger; anxiety; change in relationships; confusion; denial; dependence; depression; disorganization; dissociative disorders; embarrassment; fear; guilt; helplessness; humiliation; hyperalertness; impaired decision making; loss of self-esteem; mood swings; muscle spasms; muscle tension; nightmares; paranoia; phobias; physical trauma; powerlessness; revenge; self-blame; sexual dysfunction; shame; shock; sleep disturbances; substance abuse; suicide attempts; vulnerability

Related Factors (r/t)

Rape

NOC   (Nursing Outcomes Classification)

Suggested NOC Outcomes

Abuse Cessation, Abuse Protection, Abuse Recovery: Emotional, Sexual, Coping, Impulse Self-Control, Self-Mutilation Restraint

Example NOC Outcome with Indicators
Abuse Recovery: Sexual as evidenced by the following indicators: Acknowledgment of right to disclose abusive situation/Expression of right to have been protected from abuse (Rate the outcome and indicators of **Abuse Recovery: Sexual:** 1 = none, 2 = limited, 3 = moderate, 4 = substantial, 5 = extensive [see Section I].)

Client Outcomes

Client Will (Specify Time Frame):

- Share feelings, concerns, and fears
- Recognize that the rape or attempt was not client's own fault
- State that, no matter what the situation, no one has the right to assault another
- Describe medical/legal treatment procedures and reasons for treatment
- Report absence of physical complications or pain
- Identify support resources and attend psychotherapy/group assistance in coping with the trauma and effects of the traumatic experience
- Function at same level as before crisis, including sexual functioning
- Recognize that it is normal for full recovery to take a minimum of 1 year

NIC   (Nursing Interventions Classification)

Suggested NIC Interventions

Counseling, Rape-Trauma Treatment

Example NIC Activities—Rape-Trauma Treatment
Explain rape protocol and obtain consent to proceed through protocol; Implement crisis intervention counseling

Nursing Interventions and *Rationales*

- Stress the importance of awareness throughout the community of the scope and severity of the effects of sexual abuse as a means of additional healing empowerment. **EBN:** *A better appreciation of the biopsychosocial repercussions of sexual assault will aid in developing a more holistic and*

• = Independent   ▲ = Collaborative   **EBN** = Evidence-Based Nursing   **EB** = Evidence-Based

individualized therapy to help alleviate the physical and emotional pain following the trauma of rape (Chivers-Wilson, 2006).

▲ For those interested in a spiritual connection, make the appropriate referrals. **EBN:** *Having a strong spiritual connection creates for survivors the possibility of being supported and guided in their struggles, obtaining new insights that aid in their recovery, and acquiring strength as a result of passing spiritual challenges (Knapik, Martsolf, & Draucker 2008).*

• Observe the client's responses, including anger, fear, self-blame, sleep-pattern disturbances, and phobias. Monitor the client's verbal and nonverbal psychological state (e.g., crying, hand wringing, avoidance of interactions or eye contact with staff, silence, and denial). **EB:** *This study demonstrates that individuals can respond in a variety of ways to violence and trauma (Carlson, 2005).*

• Stay with (or have a trusted person stay with) the client initially. If a law enforcement interview is permitted, provide support by staying with the client, but only at the client's request. **EBN:** *Allow the client to make the decision about whom the client wishes to have present during any interviews or examinations to allow a return of control to the client (Ledray, 1998a).*

• Explain the entire medical/legal examination to the client before beginning any procedures. **EBN:** *Explain to the client that the injuries or symptoms may require hospitalization and that the care provider in the hospital will be aware of their special needs (Sommers & Buschur, 2004).* **EBN:** *This returns control to the client. Explain that a speculum examination will be performed for the purpose of identifying any injury and collecting evidence (Hutson, 2002).*

• Do not wait for the client to ask questions; explain everything you are doing; and clarify why it must be done, and describe when and where you will touch. The biological, psychological, and sociological impacts and treatments should not remain mutually exclusive. **EBN:** *A better appreciation of the biopsychosocial repercussions of sexual assault will aid in developing a more holistic and individualized therapy to help alleviate the physical and emotional pain following the trauma of rape (Chivers-Wilson, 2006).*

• Observe for signs of physical injury as you are asking the client to undress and collecting the client's clothing for evidence. Ask the client where it hurts without asking leading questions. Do not ask specific questions but allow the client to give you a history of the sexual assault in the client's own words. If the examiner needs further clarification, ask the client to point to areas that were injured or touched. Inform the client that photographs of any injuries are necessary for forensic evidence. Obtain specific written permission for photographs to be taken and released to law enforcement personnel. **EBN:** *The aforementioned non-leading questions are recommended. Do not ask questions that could indicate to the defense attorney and the jury that the examiner was leading the client and may have influenced the client's report of the assault (Ledray, 1998b).*

• Documentation of a sexual assault examination is critical to evidentiary reports. It is important to document the client's exact description of the assault and then to collect evidence and photographs that validate the history the client reports. **EBN:** *Evidence collection kits prepared by sexual assault nurse examiners (SANEs) are more accurate and complete when compared with evidence collection kits prepared by non-SANE nurses and physicians (Sievers, Murphy, & Miller, 2003).*

• It is also very important for the examiner not to offer any opinions in the documentation about whether or not the assault occurred according to the physical findings. **EBN:** *These opinions should be offered to the legal system only when they are requested for prosecution (Ledray, 1998b).*

• Document a one- or two-sentence summary of what happened. The chief complaint of the client reporting sexual assault should always be listed as "reported sexual assault"; obtaining the details of the sequence of events is the police officer's job. **EBN:** *The chief complaint of the client reporting sexual assault should always be listed as "reported sexual assault" (Hutson, 2002).*

• Encourage the client to verbalize feelings. *Individuals at risk for developing long-term problems after an assault should be identified during the initial assessment (Campbell, 2008).*

• Escort the client to the treatment room immediately to remove the client from the general population; do not question the client in the triage area. Close curtains and door, and avoid other interruptions during contact with the client (e.g., telephone calls, absence from the room, outside stimuli such as radios). **EB and EBN:** *This not only serves the client but also allows for the accurate collection and preservation of evidence (Ledray, 1999; McGregor, Du Mont, & Myhr, 2002).*

▲ Provide a sexual assault response team (SART) that includes a sexual assault nurse examiner (SANE), rape counseling advocate, and representative of law enforcement for best possible outcomes. **EBN:** *The quality of care the client receives from "first responders" may determine the client's*

• = Independent   ▲ = Collaborative   **EBN** = Evidence-Based Nursing   **EB** = Evidence-Based

willingness to continue with long-term treatment (Ledray, 1998a). The importance of SANE examination for sexual assault victims is stressed for well-being for victims (Patterson, Campbell, & Townsend, 2006; Bechtel, Ryan, & Gallagher, 2008).

▲ A rape crisis center advocate should be part of the SART and respond when the SANE responds. *Because advocates are better trained and prepared to talk to clients of acute sexual assault, they are usually more successful in encouraging further follow-up than are the medical/nursing staff.* **EB:** *Trained professionals working together within the care setting ensures that survivors and their families' needs are met (Preston, 2003; Bechtel, Ryan, & Gallagher, 2008).*

- Provide items for self-care after examination (e.g., for cleansing the vaginal and rectal area). **EBN:** *Many facilities provide items for personal hygiene (i.e., shampoo, soap, toothbrush, toothpaste, new underwear, and outer clothing to replace those secured for evidential purposes) (Hutson, 2002).*

- Most states provide sexual assault evidence collection kits that have been reviewed by the SART members to provide adequate evidence for analysis by the forensic laboratory. Explain to the client that all or some of the client's clothing may be kept for evidential purposes. **EBN:** *If the client arrives at the medical facility with the evidentiary clothing already in a bag, explain to the client that you will notify law enforcement personnel to pick it up directly from the client (Hutson, 2002).*

- Discuss the possibility of pregnancy and sexually transmitted diseases (STDs) and the treatments available. **EBN:** *Most clients prefer to prevent pregnancy rather than face the possibility of terminating it in the future. The risk of human immunodeficiency virus (HIV) exposure is a special concern to rape victims; the nurse should bring up this issue and inform the client of locations and schedules for HIV testing (Stermac, Dunlap, & Bainbridge, 2005).*

- Encourage the client to report the rape to a law enforcement agency. **EBN:** *Reporting of forced sex is necessary so that individuals have access to resources and support (Amar, 2008).*

- Discuss the client's support system. Involve the support system if appropriate and if the client grants permission. **EB:** *Significant others are coping with their own responses to the trauma and may be incapable of supporting the victim (Mackey et al, 1992).*

- Stress the importance of follow-up care with a mental health professional to help with the problems associated with the effects of the traumatic experience. **EBN:** *Given the complex etiology of lifetime trauma, risk for future trauma, and the health needs of women who have experienced trauma, a broader range of intervention strategies that include attention to tangible support need to be developed and evaluated (Glass et al, 2007).*

 ### Geriatric

- Build a trusting relationship with the client. **EBN:** *Raising the awareness with older adults that elder abuse is a complex phenomenon that should be reported (McGarry, 2008).*

- Explain reporting and encourage the client to report. **EB and EBN:** *Older rape victims have reported having a greater fear that people will find out about their rape than have younger women (Tyra, 1993).* **EB:** *Timely reporting, although important, should not determine whether a client receives appropriate medical care. Clients requesting medical treatment, prophylactic antibiotics, and contraception should be treated the same whether they report the incident to the police or not (Schei et al, 2003).*

- Observe for psychosocial distress (e.g., memory impairment, sleep disturbances, regression, changes in bodily functions). *Exacerbation of a chronic illness may be a major consequence of sexual assault.* **EBN:** *Rape trauma in an elder increases the challenge for recovery; it can lead to further physical, cognitive, and psychological deterioration of a victim (Burgess & Clements, 2006).*

- All examinations should be done on the elderly as they would be done on any adult client after sexual assault. Evidence should be collected, and consent for collection, photography, and law enforcement contact should be obtained as in all cases. Special attention should be given to the explanation of the genital examination, especially as it relates to the use of a speculum. **EBN:** *Because of the altered levels of awareness in the elderly, it is important for members of the SART to evaluate the client's ability to give informed consent (Hutson, 2002).*

- Modify the rape protocol to promote comfort for the geriatric client. Consider positioning female clients with pillows rather than stirrups and consider using a smaller speculum. *Aging results in decreased muscle tone and thinning of the vaginal wall.*

- Assess for mobility limitations and cognitive impairment. *Elicit information from family or caregivers to verify the client's level of functioning before sexual assault.*

• = Independent   ▲ = Collaborative   **EBN** = Evidence-Based Nursing   **EB** = Evidence-Based

- Respect the client's need for privacy. *Older clients may be reluctant to have their children or younger family members present during the examination and treatment; give clients a choice.*
- Consider arrangements for temporary housing. *Most sexual assaults of older clients occur in the home (or nursing home).* **EBN:** *Older age increases the powerlessness of a person, especially if the individual is isolated as a result of living alone. Physical injury can have a much greater effect on older victims, and they may experience a compound reaction because they are older. Sexual violence against an older woman is a reflection of antiage and antiwoman attitudes (Delorey & Wolf, 1993).*

Male Rape

- Encourage men who are raped to report the assault. **EB:** *There are several misconceptions surrounding male rape which can result in the underreporting and secondary or sanctuary victimization of the survivor. Men who have been raped may believe that it attacks the very essence of what it is to be masculine and male. Many may not seek help unless they perceive a need for immediate attention, such as physical trauma requiring medical assistance (Ellis, 2002).*

Multicultural

- Assess for the influence of cultural beliefs, norms, and values on the client's ability to cope with the trauma of the rape experience. **EBN:** *What the client views as healthy coping may be based on cultural perceptions (Leininger & McFarland, 2002).*
- Assess to determine if physically abused women are also victims of sexual assault. **EB:** *Sexual assault is experienced by most physically abused women and associated with significantly higher levels of post-traumatic stress disorder (PTSD) compared with women physically abused only. The risk of reassault is decreased if contact is made with health or justice agencies (McFarlane et al, 2005; Moreland et al, 2007).* **EBN:** *The nurse's awareness of the impact of trauma and abuse on psychological health can facilitate more appropriate assessment and support during maternity care (Mezey et al, 2005). Rape is more likely to occur in certain ethnic minority and socially disadvantaged groups than in other groups. The incidence of rape varies with race and ethnicity. Women who are raped are likely to be African American women who have been raped by African American men. Of the number of rapes, 65% occur at night (between the hours of 8 PM and 4 AM, 43% occur near the victim's home, and 15% occur at a friend's house. Although a greater number of women report "stranger rape," the incidence of acquaintance rape (date rape) and domestic violence rape is greatly underreported (Giger & Davidhizar, 2008).*
- Provide opportunities by which the family and individual can save face when working with Asian American clients. **EBN:** *Asian American families may avoid situations and discussion of issues that they perceive will bring shame on the family unit (D'Avanzo & Naegle, 2001).*
- Assure the client of confidentiality. **EBN:** *Many Indo-Chinese women will not discuss rape if they think that other staff members, their families, their husbands, or their community may find out (Mollica & Lavelle, 1988).*
- Validate the client's feelings regarding the rape and allow the client to tell his or her rape story. **EBN:** *Interventions should reaffirm therapeutic strategies that emphasize effective listening, based on speech styles appropriate to the cultural experiences of the women in question (Bletzer & Koss, 2004).*
- A culturally sensitive approach should be part of the training of all SARTs and members of SARTs. *Compassion and familiarity in a care plan will allow all care providers to provide a comfortable environment for the client (Giger & Davidhizar, 2008).*

Home Care

- Some of the interventions described previously may be adapted for home care use.
- Interact with the client supportively and nonjudgmentally; this supports the client's self-worth. *Rape victims usually experience a loss of self-worth.*
- Assist the client with realistically assessing the home setting for safety and/or selecting a safe environment in which to live. *Rape clients may be unable to make a realistic assessment of home safety both immediately after the rape and during long-term recovery.*
- ▲ Ensure that the client has a support system in place for long-term support. Instruct the family that recovery may take a long time. Refer for medical social work services to assist in setting up a sup-

● = Independent   ▲ = Collaborative   **EBN** = Evidence-Based Nursing   **EB** = Evidence-Based

port system if necessary. Refer for counseling if necessary. *The long-term response to rape (up to 4 years) requires ongoing support for the client to reorganize and reintegrate.*

▲ Make sure that physical symptoms from the rape or other physical conditions are followed up. Follow-up should include a visit to the primary care physician or the local health department in 3 to 4 weeks for repeat pregnancy testing and STD testing. Explain to the client that additional medication may be necessary for the treatment of STDs or pregnancy (Ohio Chapter of IAFN, 2002). *Stress response to rape can precipitate reemergence of other physical conditions that may be ignored because of the rape.*

▲ If the client is homebound, refer for psychiatric home health care services for client reassurance and implementation of a therapeutic regimen. *Psychiatric home care nurses can address issues relating to the client's rape-trauma syndrome. Behavioral interventions in the home can help the client to participate more effectively in the treatment plan (Patusky, Rodning, & Martinez-Kratz, 1996).*

Client/Family Teaching and Discharge Planning

▲ Provide information on prophylactic antibiotic therapy, hepatitis B vaccination, and tetanus prophylaxis for nonimmunized clients with trauma. *Prophylactic treatment for STDs should be provided as part of the initial examination (Ohio Chapter of IAFN, 2002).*

• Discharge instructions should be written out for the client. *Anxiety can hamper comprehension and retention of information; repeat instructions and provide them in a written form.*

• Give instructions to significant others. *Significant others need many of the same supportive and caring interventions as the client; suggest that they too might benefit from counseling.*

• Explain the purpose of the "morning-after pill." *The morning-after pill (norgestrel [Ovral]) often prevents pregnancy and is used only in emergencies. It must be taken within 72 hours (3 days) of sexual contact to be effective. It will not cause a miscarriage if the client is already pregnant, but it could harm the fetus.*

• Explain the potential for common side effects related to treatment with norgestrel, such as breast swelling or nausea and vomiting. Call the emergency department if the client vomits within 1 hour of taking the pill because the pill may need to be taken again. Discuss any issues about prophylactic medications at the follow-up visit in 3 to 4 weeks. It may take 3 to 30 days for the menstrual period to start; if menstruation has not begun in 30 days, contact a physician.

• Explain the potential for severe side effects related to treatment with norgestrel, such as severe leg or chest pain, trouble breathing, coughing up of blood, severe headache or dizziness, and trouble seeing or talking.

• Advise the client to call or return if new problems develop. *Physical injuries may not be recognized because of the client's emotional numbness during the initial examination or because the client may have forgotten or not understood some of the instructions.*

• Discuss practical lifestyle changes within the client's control to reduce the risk of future attacks. *A client's financial situation may limit some options, such as moving to another home. Provide other alternatives such as keeping doors locked, checking the car before getting in, not walking alone at night, keeping someone informed of whereabouts, asking someone to check if the client has not arrived at a destination within a reasonable amount of time, keeping lights on in an entryway, having keys in hand when approaching the car or house, and having a remote key entry car or garage.*

• Teach the client to use self-defense techniques to surprise an attacker and create an opportunity to run for help. Refer the client to a self-defense school.

• Teach the client appropriate outlets for anger. Encourage the significant other to direct anger at the event and the attacker, not at the client.

• Emphasize the vulnerability of the client and ensure that reactions are appropriate for the victim of sexual assault. *Females are at higher risk for depression than males, and the risk is significantly higher between the ages of 18 and 44 (Mackey et al, 1992).*

NOTE: Posttraumatic stress disorder has a high probability of being a psychological sequelae to rape. Research demonstrated two effective treatments for improvement of PTSD in rape victims—prolonged exposure and stress inoculation training (Foa et al, 1991). Prolonged exposure involves reliving the rape experience by imagining it as vividly as possible, describing it aloud in the present tense, taping this description, and listening to the tape at least once daily. Stress inoculation training uses breathing exercises to diminish anxiety and instruction in coping skills, thought stopping, cognitive

• = Independent   ▲ = Collaborative   **EBN** = Evidence-Based Nursing   **EB** = Evidence-Based

restructuring, self-dialogue, and role playing. Research suggests that a combination of both treatments may provide the optimal effect.

ⓔvolve   See the EVOLVE website for Weblinks for client education resources.

REFERENCES

Amar AF: African-American college women's perceptions of resources and barriers when reporting forced sex, *J Natl Black Nurses Assoc* 19(2):35–41, 2008.

Bechtel K, Ryan E, Gallagher D: Impact of sexual assault nurse examiners on the evaluation of sexual assault in a pediatric emergency department, *Pediatr Emerg Care* 24(7):442–447, 2008.

Bletzer KV, Koss MP: Narrative constructions of sexual violence as told by female rape survivors in three populations of the southwestern United States: scripts of coercion, scripts of consent, *Med Anthropol* 23(2):113–156, 2004.

Burgess A, Clements P: Information processing of sexual abuse in elders, *J Forens Nurs* 2(3):113–120, 2006.

Campbell R: The psychological impact of rape victims, *Am Psychol* 63(8):702–717, 2008.

Carlson BE: The most important things learned about violence and trauma in the past 20 years, *J Interpers Violence* 20(1):119–126, 2005.

Chivers-Wilson K: Sexual assault and posttraumatic stress disorders: review of the biological, psychological and sociological factors and treatments, *Mcgill J Med* 9(2):111–118, 2006.

D'Avanzo CE, Naegle MA: Developing culturally informed strategies for substance related interventions. In Naegle MA, D'Avanzo CE, editors: *Addictions and substance abuse: strategies for advanced practice nursing,* St Louis, 2001, Mosby.

Delorey C, Wolf KA: Sexual violence and older women, *AWHONNS Clin Issues Perinat Womens Health Nurs* 4:173, 1993.

Ellis CD: Male rape—the silent victims, *Collegian,* 9(4):34–39, 2002.

Foa EB, Rothbaum BO, Riggs DS et al: Treatment of posttraumatic stress disorder in rape victims: a comparison between cognitive-behavioral procedures and counseling, *J Consult Clin Psychol* 59(5):715, 1991.

Giger J, Davidhizar R: *Transcultural nursing: assessment and intervention,* ed 5, St Louis, 2008, Mosby.

Glass N, Perrin N, Campbell J et al: The protective role of tangible support on post-traumatic stress disorder symptoms in urban women survivors of violence, *Res Nurs Health* 30(5):558–568, 2007.

Hutson L: Development of sexual assault nurse examiner programs, *Nurs Clin North Am* 37(1):79–88, 2002.

Knapik G, Martsolf D, Draucker C: Being delivered: spirituality in survivors of sexual violence, *Issues Ment Health Nurs* 29(4):335–350, 2008.

Ledray L: Sexual assault: clinical issues. SANE development and operation guide, *J Emerg Nurs* 24(2):197, 1998a.

Ledray L: Sexual assault: clinical issues. SANE expert and factual testimony, *J Emerg Nurs* 24(3):284, 1998b.

Ledray LE: Sexual assault: clinical issues. IAFN Sixth Annual Scientific Assembly highlights, *J Emerg Nurs* 25(1):63, 1999.

Leininger MM, McFarland MR: *Transcultural nursing: concepts, theories, research and practices,* ed 3, New York, 2002, McGraw-Hill.

Mackey T, Sereika SM, Weissfeld LA et al: Factors associated with long-term depressive symptoms of sexual assault victims, *Arch Psychiatr Nurs* 6(1):10–25, 1992.

McFarlane J, Malecha A, Watson K et al: Intimate partner sexual assault against women: frequency, health consequences, and treatment outcomes, *Obstet Gynecol* 105(1):99–108, 2005.

McGarry J: Identifying, reporting and preventing elder abuse in the practice setting, *Nurs Stand* 22(46):49–56, 2008.

McGregor MJ, Du Mont J, Myhr TL: Sexual assault forensic medical examination: is evidence related to successful prosecution? *Ann Emerg Med* 39(6):639–647, 2002.

Mezey G, Bacchus L, Bewley S et al: Domestic violence, lifetime trauma and psychological health of childbearing women, *BJOG* 112(2):197–204, 2005.

Mollica RF, Lavelle J: Southeast Asian refugees. In Comas-Diaz L, Griffith EEH, editors: *Clinical guidelines in cross-cultural mental health,* New York, 1988, John Wiley and Sons.

Moreland L, Goebert D, Onoye J et al: Posttraumatic stress disorder and pregnancy health: preliminary update and implications, *Psychosom* 48:304–308, 2007.

Ohio Chapter of the International Association of Forensic Nurses [IAFN]: *The Ohio adolescent and adult sexual assault nurse examiner training manual,* Cleveland, 2002, Ohio Office of the Attorney General.

Patterson D, Campbell R, Townsend SM: Sexual Assault Nurse Examiner (SANE) program goals and patient care practices, *J Nurs Scholarsh* 38(2):180–186, 2006.

Patusky KL, Rodning C, Martinez-Kratz M: Clinical lessons in psychiatric home care: a case study approach, *J Home Health Case Manag* 9:18, 1996.

Preston L: The sexual assault nurse examiner and the rape crisis center advocate: a necessary partnership, *Top Emerg Med* 3:244–246, 2003.

Schei B, Sidenius K, Lundvall L et al: Adult victims of sexual assault: acute medical response and police reporting among women consulting a center for victims of sexual assault, *Acta Obstet Gynecol Scand* 82(8):750–752, 2003.

Sievers V, Murphy S, Miller JJ: Sexual assault evidence collection more accurate when completed by sexual assault nurse examiners: Colorado's experience, *J Emerg Nurs* 29(6):511–514, 2003.

Sommers M, Buschur C: Injury in women who are raped: what every critical care nurse needs to know, *Dimens Crit Care Nurs* 23(2):62–68, 2004.

Stermac L, Dunlap H, Bainbridge D: Sexual assault services delivered by SANEs, *J Forens Nurs* 1(3):124–128, 2005.

Tyra PA: Older women: victims of rape, *J Gerontol Nurs* 19(5):7–12, 1993.

Readiness for enhanced Relationship   *Gail B. Ladwig, MSN, RN, CHTP*   ⓔvolve

NANDA-I

Definition

A pattern of mutual partnership that is sufficient to provide each other's needs and can be strengthened

● = Independent   ▲ = Collaborative   **EBN** = Evidence-Based Nursing   **EB** = Evidence-Based

Defining Characteristics

Express desire to enhance communication between partners; express satisfaction with sharing of information and ideas between partners; express satisfaction with fulfilling physical and emotional needs by one's partner; demonstrates mutual respect between partners; meets developmental goals appropriate for family life-cycle stage; demonstrates well-balanced autonomy and collaboration between partners; demonstrates mutual support in daily activities between partners; identifies each other as a key person; demonstrates understanding of partner's insufficient (physical, social, psychological) function; express satisfaction with complementary relation between partners

 (Nursing Outcomes Classification)

Suggested NOC Outcomes

Coping, Family Functioning/Integrity, Role Performance, Social Support

Example NOC Outcome with Indicators
Family Integrity: Members share thoughts, feelings, interests, concerns/Members communicate openly and honestly with one another/Members encourage individual autonomy and independence/Members assist one another in performing roles and daily tasks (Rate the outcome and indicators of **Family Integrity**: 1 = never demonstrated, 2 = rarely demonstrated, 3 = sometimes demonstrated, 4 = often demonstrated, 5 = consistently demonstrated [see Section I].)

Client Outcomes

Family/Client Will (Specify Time Frame):

- Share thoughts and feelings with each other
- Communicate openly with each other
- Assist in performing family roles and tasks
- Provide support for each other
- Obtain appropriate assistance

 (Nursing Interventions Classification)

Suggested NIC Interventions

Coping Enhancement, Family Integrity Promotion, Role Enhancement

Example NIC Activities—Family Integrity Promotion
Facilitate a tone of togetherness within/among the family; Encourage family to maintain positive relationships; Facilitate open communication among family members

Nursing Interventions and *Rationales*

- ▲ Assess for signs of depression in the family when one partner is depressed, and make appropriate referrals. **EB:** *Depressive symptoms affect functioning of the whole family (Hinton et al, 2009).*
- Support "relationship talk" between couples (talking with a partner about the relationship, what one needs from one's partner, and/or the relationship implications of a shared stressor). *Such discussions in couples with lung cancer have been shown to help partners better define their relationships and repair relationships that are functioning poorly (Badr, Acitelli, & Taylor, 2008).*
- Encourage couples to participate and share in exciting and satisfying leisure activities. **EB:** *This study demonstrated that couples feel connected with their partners and more satisfied with their relationships when they engage in these types of activities (Graham, 2008).*
- Assist couples in establishing boundaries between work and home. *This study demonstrates that for both men and women, job demands foster their own work-family conflict (WFC), which in turn contributes to their partners' home demands, family-work conflict (FWC), and exhaustion. In addition, social undermining mediates the relationship between individuals' WFC and their partners' home demands (Bakker, Demerouti, & Dollard, 2008).*
- Assist couples in regulating negative emotions. **EB:** *The results of this study of newlyweds support theories suggesting that the ability to regulate negative emotions may help intimates avoid perpetrating*

• = Independent   ▲ = Collaborative   **EBN** = Evidence-Based Nursing   **EB** = Evidence-Based

intimate partner violence (IPV), particularly when faced with a partner's IPV perpetration (McNulty & Hellmuth, 2008).

- Assist couples in dealing with anger when the diagnosis is cancer. **EB:** *The anger-expression styles of both clients and their partners seem to modify the family atmosphere, and together, they are important determinants of the long-term quality of life of the cancer clients. Interventions for couples facing cancer should include a focus on ways of dealing with anger and thereby support dyadic coping with cancer (Julkunen, Gustavsson-Lilius, & Hietanen, 2009).*
- Refer to care plans **Readiness for enhanced Family processes** and **Readiness for enhanced family Coping.**

Pediatric

- Provide guidance and information on communication techniques for teenagers especially those involved in intimate relationships. **EBN:** *The findings of this study suggest that many adolescents desired the love of a male partner and were willing to concede to his request of practicing unprotected sex. Findings support the urgent need for interventions that will promote skill-building techniques to negotiate safer sex behaviors among youth who are most likely to be exposed to STIs through risky behaviors (Bralock & Koniak-Griffin, 2009).*

Geriatric

- ▲ Assess for spousal depression when one partner has cardiovascular disease and make appropriate referrals. **EB:** *Exposure to spousal suffering is an independent and unique source of distress in married couples that contributes to psychiatric and physical morbidity (Schulz et al, 2009).*
- ▲ Assess for depression and anxiety and make appropriate referrals for "prewidows" caring for spouses with chronic life-limiting conditions. **EB***: In this study health deficits associated with spousal bereavement may be evident earlier in the marital transition than previously thought, warranting attention to the health of elderly persons whose spouses have chronic/life-limiting conditions (Williams et al, 2008).*
- Support older couples positive collaborative communication. **EB:** *In this study of older couples they displayed a unique blend of warmth and control, during collaboration, suggesting a greater focus on emotional and social concerns during problem solving (Smith et al, 2009).*
- Encourage collaborative coping (i.e., spouses pooling resources and problem solving jointly) among older adults. **EB:** *This study of older adults whose husband's had prostrate cancer suggested that collaborative coping may be associated with better daily mood and greater marital satisfaction because of heightened perceptions of efficacy in coping with stressful events and problems surrounding illness (Berg et al, 2008).*

Multicultural

- Provide culturally tailored community-level interventions to raise awareness about HIV and bisexuality, and decrease HIV and sexual orientation stigma. **EB:** *Culturally tailored interventions may increase African American and Latino MSMW's (men who have sex with men and women) comfort in communicating with their female partners about sexuality, HIV, and condoms (Mutchler et al, 2008). Sociocultural factors and HIV-related misinformation contribute to the increasing number of Chilean women living with HIV. Future HIV prevention should stress partner communication, empowerment, and improving the education of women vulnerable to HIV (Cianelli, Ferrer, & McElmurry, 2008).*

Home Care

- Provide home-based psychoeducation to assist new parent couples with parenting and their couple relationship. **EB:** *The best outcomes for psychoeducational interventions for effective parenting of infants and sustaining a mutually satisfying couple relationship seem to be achieved when programs are accessible by couples at home, when skill-training is provided, and possibly when programs target couples at high-risk of maladjustment to parenthood (Petch & Halford, 2008).*

● = Independent   ▲ = Collaborative   **EBN** = Evidence-Based Nursing   **EB** = Evidence-Based

Client/Family Teaching and Discharge Planning

- Encourage clients and spouses to participate together in interventions to lower low-density lipoprotein cholesterol. Teach spouses how to provide emotional and instrumental support, allow clients to decide which component of the intervention they would like to receive, and have clients determine their own goals and action plans. Provide telephone calls to clients and spouses separately. During each client telephone call, clients' progress is reviewed, and clients create goals and action plans for the upcoming month. During spouse telephone calls, which occur within one week of client calls, spouses are informed of clients' goals and action plans and devise strategies to increase emotional and instrumental support. **EB:** *Almost 50% of Americans have elevated low-density lipoprotein cholesterol (LDL-C). The behaviors required to lower LDL-C levels may be difficult to adhere to if they are inconsistent with spouses' health practices, and, alternatively, may be enhanced by enlisting support from the spouse. Given the social context in which self-management occurs, interventions that teach spouses to provide instrumental and emotional support may help clients initiate and adhere to behaviors that lower their LDL-C levels. Moreover, allowing clients to retain autonomy by deciding which behaviors they would like to change and how may improve adherence and clinical outcomes (Voils et al, 2009). Interventions to reduce cardiovascular risk factors should be addressed jointly to both members of a marital couple (Di Castelnuovo et al, 2009).*

ⓔvolve   See the EVOLVE website for Weblinks for client education resources.

REFERENCES

Badr H, Acitelli LK, Taylor CL: Does talking about their relationship affect couples' marital and psychological adjustment to lung cancer? *J Cancer Surviv* 2(1):53–64, 2008.

Bakker AB, Demerouti E, Dollard MF: How job demands affect partners' experience of exhaustion: integrating work-family conflict and crossover theory, *J Appl Psychol* 93(4):901–911, 2008.

Berg CA, Wiebe DJ, Butner J et al: Collaborative coping and daily mood in couples dealing with prostate cancer, *Psychol Aging* 23(3):505–516, 2008.

Bralock A, Koniak-Griffin D: What do sexually active adolescent females say about relationship issues? *J Pediatr Nurs* 24(2):131–140, 2009.

Cianelli R, Ferrer L, McElmurry BJ: HIV prevention and low-income Chilean women: machismo, marianismo and HIV misconceptions, *Cult Health Sex* 10(3):297–306, 2008.

Di Castelnuovo A, Quacquaruccio G, Donati MB et al: Spousal concordance for major coronary risk factors: a systematic review and meta-analysis, *Am J Epidemiol* 169(1):1–8, 2009.

Graham JM: Self-expansion and flow in couples' momentary experiences: an experience sampling study, *J Pers Soc Psychol* 95(3):679–694, 2008.

Hinton L, Hagar Y, West N et al: Longitudinal influences of partner depression on cognitive functioning in Latino spousal pairs, *Dement Geriatr Cogn Disord* 27(6):491–500, 2009.

Julkunen J, Gustavsson-Lilius M, Hietanen P: Anger expression, partner support, and quality of life in cancer patients, *J Psychosom Res* 66(3):235–244, 2009.

McNulty JK, Hellmuth JC: Emotion regulation and intimate partner violence in newlyweds, *J Fam Psychol* 22(5):794–797, 2008.

Mutchler MG, Bogart LM, Elliott MN et al: Psychosocial correlates of unprotected sex without disclosure of HIV-positivity among African-American, Latino, and white men who have sex with men and women, Arch Sex Behav 37(5):736–747, 2008.

Petch J, Halford WK: Psycho-education to enhance couples' transition to parenthood, *Clin Psychol Rev* 28(7):1125–1137, 2008.

Schulz R, Beach SR, Hebert RS et al: Spousal suffering and partner's depression and cardiovascular disease: the Cardiovascular Health Study, *Am J Geriatr Psychiatry* 17(3):246–254, 2009.

Smith TW, Berg CA, Florsheim P et al: Conflict and collaboration in middle-aged and older couples: I. Age differences in agency and communion during marital interaction, *Psychol Aging* 24(2):259–273, 2009.

Voils CI, Yancy WS Jr, Kovac S et al: Study protocol: couples partnering for lipid enhancing strategies (CouPLES)—a randomized, controlled trial, *Trials* 6(10):10, 2009.

Williams BR, Sawyer P, Roseman JM et al: Marital status and health: exploring pre-widowhood, *J Palliat Med* 11(6):848–856, 2008.

Impaired Religiosity   Lisa Burkhart, PhD, RN   ⓔvolve

NANDA-I

Definition

Impaired ability to exercise reliance on beliefs and/or participate in rituals of a particular faith tradition

Defining Characteristics

Difficulty adhering to prescribed religious beliefs; difficulty adhering to prescribed religious rituals (e.g., religious ceremonies, dietary regulations, clothing, prayer, worship/religious services, private

 • = Independent   ▲ = Collaborative   **EBN** = Evidence-Based Nursing   **EB** = Evidence-Based

religious behaviors/reading religious materials/media, holiday observances, meetings with religious leaders); expresses emotional distress because of separation from faith community; expresses a need to reconnect with previous belief patterns; expresses an need to reconnect with previous customs; questions religious belief patterns; questions religious customs

Related Factors (r/t)

Developmental and Situational
Aging; end-stage life crises; life transitions

Physical
Illness; pain

Psychological
Anxiety; fear of death; ineffective coping; ineffective support; lack of security; personal crisis; use of religion to manipulate

Sociocultural
Cultural barriers to practicing religion; environmental barriers to practicing religion; lack of social integration; lack of sociocultural interaction

Spiritual
Spiritual crises; suffering

 (Nursing Outcomes Classification)

Suggested NOC Outcomes
Client Satisfaction: Cultural Needs Fulfillment

Example NOC Outcome with Indicators
Client Satisfaction: Cultural Needs Fulfillment as evidenced by the following indicators: Respect for religious beliefs/Respect for cultural health behaviors/Incorporation of cultural beliefs in health teaching/Respect for personal values (Rate each indicator of **Client Satisfaction: Cultural Needs Fulfillment**: 1 = not at all satisfied, 2 = somewhat satisfied, 3 = moderately satisfied, 4 = very satisfied, 5 = completely satisfied [see Section I].)

Client Outcomes

Client Will (Specify Time Frame):
- Express satisfaction with the ability to express religious practices
- Express satisfaction with access to religious materials and rituals
- Demonstrate balance between religious practices and healthy lifestyles
- Avoid high-risk, controlling religious relationships that inflict physical, sexual, or emotional harm and/or exploitation

NIC **(Nursing Interventions Classification)**

Suggested NIC Interventions
Religious Ritual Enhancement, Cultural Brokerage, Religious Addiction Prevention

Example NIC Activities—Religious Ritual Enhancement
Encourage the use of and participation in usual religious rituals that are not detrimental to health

Nursing Interventions and *Rationales*
- Identify client's concerns regarding religious expression. **EB:** *Religious salience is associated with being satisfied by one's health care (Benjamin, 2006). In a cross-sectional descriptive study of 85*

• = Independent ▲ = Collaborative **EBN** = Evidence-Based Nursing **EB** = Evidence-Based

individuals with visual impairment, religious well-being predicted 7% of coping behaviors (Yampolsky et al, 2008).

- Encourage and/or coordinate the use of and participation in usual religious rituals or practices that support coping. **EB:** *In a cross-sectional descriptive study of 85 individuals with visual impairment, religious well-being predicted 7% of coping behaviors (Yampolsky et al, 2008). In a prospective study of antepartal women, participating in organized religious activities was associated with less postpartum depression (Mann et al, 2008).*

- Encourage the use of prayer or meditation as appropriate. **EB:** *Controlled study of 84 college students revealed that those who participated in a religious spiritual mediation exercise experienced significantly less anxiety and more positive mood, spiritual health, and spiritual experiences and higher pain tolerance (Wachholtz & Pargament, 2005).*

- Determine family's religious practices and encourage use of religious practices (if used) to help cope with loss. **EB:** *In a cross-sectional, retrospective survey of parents of children who have died, participants identified spirituality and religion as shaping their perspective of the grief process (Arnold & Gemma, 2008).*

- ▲ Refer to religious leader, professional counseling, or support group as needed. **EBN:** *In a grounded theory study, it was found that chaplains promoted spirituality (Burkhart & Hogan, 2008).*

Geriatric

- Promote established religious practices in the elderly. **EB:** *Qualitative study of 26 older women who had not experienced a recent loss or terminal illness identified a need to feel connected, spiritual questioning, existential angst, thoughts about death and dying, and reliance on organized religion as important. Those who relied on religion don't experience the other themes (Moremen, 2005).*

Multicultural

- Promote religious practices that are culturally appropriate. **EBN:** *In a study of 274 older Caucasian and African American women, religious coping strategies were associated with health care utilization, with African American women using more religious coping strategies than Caucasian women (Ark et al, 2006). In a sample of 203 African American professional women, 69% rated attending church as a coping mechanism to deal with stress (Bacchus, 2008). In a semistructured interview with Hawaiian women in churches, integrating religious and spiritual practices in health promotion were viewed as important in promoting breast cancer screening (Ka'opua, 2008).*

ⓔvolve   See the EVOLVE website for Weblinks for client education resources.

REFERENCES

Ark PD, Hull PC, Husaini BA et al: Religiosity, religious coping styles, and health service use, *J Gerontol Nurs* 32(8):20–29, 2006.

Arnold J, Gemma PB: The continuing process of parental grief, *Death Stud* 32:658–673, 2008.

Bacchus DN: Coping with work-related stress: a study of the use of coping resources among professional black women, *J Ethnic Cultur Divers Soc Work* 17(1):60–81, 2008.

Benjamin MR: Does religion influence patient satisfaction? *Am J Health Behav* 30(1):85–91, 2006.

Burkhart L, Hogan N: An experiential theory of spiritual care in nursing practice, *Qual Health Res* 18(7):928–938, 2008.

Ka'opua LS: Developing a culturally responsive breast cancer screening promotion with native Hawaiian women in churches, *Health Soc Work* 33(3):169–177, 2008.

Mann JR, McKeown RE, Bacon J et al: Do antenatal religious and spiritual factors impact the risk of postpartum depressive symptoms? *J Womens Health* 17(5):745–755, 2008.

Moremen RD: What is the meaning of life? Women's spirituality at the end of life span, *Omega* 50(4):309–330, 2005.

Wachholtz AB, Pargament KI: Is spirituality a critical ingredient of meditation? Comparing the effects of spiritual meditation, secular meditation, and relaxation on spiritual, psychological, cardiac, and pain outcomes, *J Behav Med* 28(4):367–384, 2005.

Yampolsky MA, Wittich W, Webb G et al: The role of spirituality in coping with visual impairment, *J Vis Impair Blind* 102(1):28–39, 2008.

Risk for impaired Religiosity   *Betty J. Ackley, MSN, EdS, RN*

NANDA-I

At risk for an impaired ability to exercise reliance on religious beliefs and/or participate in rituals of a particular faith tradition

Related Factors (r/t)

Developmental

Life transitions

Environmental

Barriers to practicing religion; lack of transportation

Physical

Hospitalization; illness; pain

Psychological

Depression; ineffective caregiving; ineffective coping; ineffective support; lack of security

Sociocultural

Cultural barrier to practicing religion; lack of social interaction; social isolation

Spiritual

Suffering

NOC, NIC, Client Outcomes, Nursing Interventions, *Rationales,* and References

Refer to care plan for **Impaired Religiosity**.

Readiness for enhanced Religiosity   *Lisa Burkhart, PhD, RN*

NANDA-I

Definition

Ability to increase reliance on religious beliefs and/or participate in rituals of a particular faith tradition

Defining Characteristics

Expresses desire to strengthen religious belief patterns that have provided comfort in the past; expresses desire to strengthen religious belief patterns that have provided religion in the past; expresses desire to strengthen religious customs that have provided comfort in the past; questions belief patterns that are harmful; questions customs that are harmful; rejects belief patterns that are harmful; rejects customs that are harmful; requests assistance expanding religious options; request for assistance to increase participation in prescribed religious beliefs (e.g., religious ceremonies, dietary regulations/rituals, clothing, prayer, worship/religious services, private religious behaviors, reading religious materials/media, holiday observances); requests forgiveness; requests meeting with religious leader/facilitators; requests reconciliation; requests religious experiences; requests religious materials

NOC, NIC, Client Outcomes, Nursing Interventions, *Rationales,* and References

See care plan for **Impaired Religiosity**.

• = Independent   ▲ = Collaborative   **EBN** = Evidence-Based Nursing   **EB** = Evidence-Based

Pediatric

- Provide spiritual care for children based on developmental level. *When nurses are comfortable providing spiritual care, they can implement numerous spiritual care activities and interventions to meet the spiritual needs of the child and family. After determining the child's spiritual beliefs and spiritual needs, a plan of care is developed based on the child's developmental age (Elkins & Cavendish, 2004).*
  - **Infants:** Have the same nurse care for the child on a daily basis. Encourage holding, cuddling, rocking, playing with, and singing to the infant. *Continuity of care will promote the establishment of trust because nurses provide much of the needed ongoing support. The infant who is ill or dying still needs to be sung to, talked to, played with, held, cuddled, and rocked (Elkins & Cavendish, 2004).*
  - **Toddlers:** Provide consistency in care and familiar toys, music, stories, clothing blankets, pillows, and any other individual object of contentment. Schedule home religious routines into the plan of care and support home routines regarding good and bad behavior. *The importance of consistency in care and routine with this age group cannot be overemphasized. The nurse should support parents' home routines during hospitalization as much as possible and encourage them to continue to have the same expectations regarding good and bad behavior. If particular religious routines are carried out at certain times of the day, the nurse should schedule them in the care plan (Elkins & Cavendish, 2004).*
  - **School-age children and adolescents:** Encourage both groups to express their feelings regarding spirituality. Ask them, "Do you wish to pray and what do want to pray about?" Offer age-appropriate complementary therapies such as music, art, videos, and connectedness with peers through cards, letters, and visits. *School-age children and adolescents should be encouraged to express their feelings, concerns, and needs regarding spirituality. For adolescents, nurses need to accept their beliefs and wishes even if they are different from their caregiver's. The nurse needs to facilitate the child's participation in religious rituals and spiritual practices. Referrals to clergy and other spiritual support may be necessary (Elkins & Cavendish, 2004).*

** evolve**   See the EVOLVE website for Weblinks for client education resources.

REFERENCE

Elkins M, Cavendish R: Developing a plan for pediatric spiritual care, *Holist Nurs Pract* 18(4):179–184, 2004.

Relocation stress syndrome   *Rebecca A. Johnson, PhD, RN*

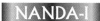

Definition

Physiological and/or psychosocial disturbances that result from transfer from one environment to another

Defining Characteristics

Alienation; aloneness; anger; anxiety (e.g., separation); concern over relocation; dependency; depression; fear; frustration; increased illness; increased physical symptoms; increased verbalization of needs; insecurity; loneliness; loss of identity; loss of self-esteem; loss of self-worth; pessimism; sleep disturbance; verbalizes unwillingness to move; withdrawal; worry

Related Factors (r/t)

Decreased health status; feelings of powerlessness; unpredictability of experience; impaired psychosocial health; isolation; lack of adequate support system; lack of predeparture counseling; language barrier; losses; move from one environment to another; passive coping

---

● = Independent   ▲ = Collaborative   **EBN** = Evidence-Based Nursing   **EB** = Evidence-Based

(Nursing Outcomes Classification)

Suggested NOC Outcomes

Anxiety Self-Control, Child Adaptation to Hospitalization, Coping, Depression Level, Depression Self-Control, Loneliness Severity, Psychosocial Adjustment: Life Change, Quality of Life

> **Example NOC Outcome with Indicators**
>
> **Anxiety Self-Control** as evidenced by the following indicators: Seeks information to reduce anxiety/Plans coping strategies for stressful situations/Uses effective coping strategies/Uses relaxation techniques to reduce anxiety/Maintains social relationships/Maintains adequate sleep/Controls anxiety response (Rate the outcome and indicators of **Anxiety Self-Control:** 1 = never demonstrated, 2 = rarely demonstrated, 3 = sometimes demonstrated, 4 = often demonstrated, 5 = consistently demonstrated [see Section I].)

Client Outcomes

Client Will (Specify Time Frame):

- Recognize and know the name of at least one staff member
- Express concern about move when encouraged to do so during individual contacts
- Carry out activities of daily living (ADLs) in usual manner
- Maintain previous mental and physical health status (e.g., nutrition, elimination, sleep, social interaction, physical activity)

 (Nursing Interventions Classification)

Suggested NIC Interventions

Anxiety Reduction, Coping Enhancement, Discharge Planning, Hope Instillation, Self-Responsibility Facilitation, Animal Assisted Therapy, Art Therapy, Music Therapy, Massage, Mood Management

> **Example NIC Activities—Anxiety Reduction**
>
> Stay with patient to promote safety and reduce fear; Provide objects that symbolize safeness

Nursing Interventions and *Rationales*

- Be aware that relocation to supportive housing may be a positive change. **EBN:** *Relocation stress syndrome is not a universally occurring phenomenon. Relocation was found to be no more stressful than other life changes (Walker, Curry, & Hogstel, 2007).*
- Begin relocation planning as early in the decision process as possible. **EB:** *Having a well-organized plan for the move with support and advocacy through the process may reduce anxiety (Talerico, 2004; Davis, 2005; Johnson, 2008).*
- Obtain a history, including the reason for the move, the client's usual coping mechanisms, history of losses, and family support for the client. *A history helps the nurse determine the amount of support needed and appropriate interventions to decrease relocation stress.*
- Identify to what extent the client can participate in the relocation decisions and advocate for this participation. **EBN:** *Older adults with poor mental functioning may be less able to be involved in the decisions and more vulnerable to disempowerment by others (Dwyer, 2005; Popejoy, 2005).*
- Assess client's readiness to relocate and relocation self-efficacy. **EBN:** *A validated relocation readiness instrument was used successfully with older adults (Rossen, 2007; Rossen & Gruber, 2007).*
- Consult an evidence-based practice guide for relocation. **EBN:** *Researchers compiled latest findings to develop a protocol to assist relocating elders (Hertz et al, 2007).*
- Assess family members' perceptions of clients' ability to participate in relocation decisions. **EB:** *Family members' and health care providers' perceptions of older adults' physical functioning may block elders' decision-making participation (Nolan & Dellesega, 2000).*
- Consider the clients' and families' cultural and ethnic values as much as possible when choosing roommates, foods, and other aspects of care. **EBN:** *Nurses need to be aware of the differences in*

• = Independent   ▲ = Collaborative   **EBN** = Evidence-Based Nursing   **EB** = Evidence-Based

values and practices of different cultures and ensure they give culturally appropriate care that is respectful of elders and family caregivers' beliefs about elder care (Johnson & Tripp-Reimer, 2001a, 2001b; Caron & Bowers, 2003; Johnson, 2008).

- Promote clear communication between all participants in the relocation process. **EBN:** *Case studies revealed the importance of using integrated approach to planning with clear communication among practitioners (LeClerc & Wells, 2001).*
- Observe the following procedures if the client is being transferred to an extended care facility or assisted living facility:
  - Facilitate the client's participation in decisions and choice of placement and arrange a preadmission visit if possible. *Clients who are more involved in the decision-making process appear to have less problems adjusting to the new environment (Newson, 2008b).* **EB and EBN:** *Research has shown a link between the loss of independence with transfer to a nursing home and depression (Loeher et al, 2004; Johnson, 2008). Decreased relocation control was significantly related to poorer adjustment (Bekhet, Zauszniewski, & Wykle, 2008).*
  - If the client cannot visit the new facility, arrange for a visit or telephone call by a member of the staff to welcome the client and show a videotape or at least provide pictures of the new care facility.
  - Have a familiar person accompany the client to the new facility. *This lessens client and family anxiety, confusion, and dissatisfaction.*
  - Recommend that the caregiver write a journal of thoughts and feelings regarding the relocation of their loved one. *Writing has been found to improve physical and emotional health among caregivers of older adults (Dellasega & Haagen, 2004).*
- Validate the caregiver's feelings of difficulty with deciding to relocate a loved one to a different environment. *This is a distressing experience, and caregivers feel responsible.*
- Identify previous routines for ADLs. Try to maintain as much continuity with the previous schedule as possible. *Continuity of routines has been shown to be a crucial factor in positively influencing adjustment to a new environment (Kao, Travis, & Acton, 2004).*
- Bring in familiar items from home (e.g., pictures, clocks, afghans).
- Establish the way the client would like to be addressed (Mr., Mrs., Miss, first name, nickname). *Calling clients by their desired name shows respect.*
- Thoroughly orient the client and the family to the new environment and routines; repeat directions as needed. *The stress of the move may interfere with the client's ability to remember directions. A progressive introduction and orientation for both the client and the family should be done (Kao, Travis, & Acton, 2004).*
- Spend one-to-one time with the client. Allow the client to express feelings and convey acceptance of them; emphasize that the client's feelings are real and individual and that it is acceptable to be sad or angry about moving. *Expressing feelings can help the client deal with the change and facilitate grief work that accompanies loss of independence (Tracy & DeYoung, 2004).*
- Allocate a caring staff member to help the client adjust to the move. Assign the same staff members to the client for care if compatible with client; maintain consistency in the personnel the client interacts with. *Consistency hastens adjustment and increases quality of care (Iwasiw et al, 2003). A caring practitioner can support the client through the journey of adapting to a new environment (Newson, 2008b).*
- Ask the client to state one positive aspect of the new living situation each day. *Helping the client focus on the positive aspects of the move can help change attitude and reframe the situation in a positive fashion.* **EBN:** *Learned resourcefulness through positive thinking significantly affected relocation adjustment (Bekhet, Zauszniewski, & Wykle, 2008).*
- Monitor the client's health status and provide appropriate interventions for problems with social interaction, nutrition, sleep, new onset of infection, or elimination problems. **EB and EBN:** *Health problems may appear first as declines in ADLs (e.g., bathing, eating, dressing) (Chen & Wilmoth, 2004). Morbidity and mortality outcomes for elders are similar between assisted living and nursing home (Pruchno & Rose, 2000). Clients who moved showed lower natural killer cell immunity 1 month after moving than was shown by a control group of elderly who did not move (Lutgendorf et al, 1999). Older adults who were relocated had lower natural killer cell cytotoxicity than those who did not move,*

but the clients generally recovered normal immune function by 3 months (Lutgendorf et al, 2001). Older adults who moved in the previous year reported increased comorbidity, disability, functional limitation, and worse self-rated health (Hong & Chen, 2009).

- If the client is being transferred within a facility, have staff members from the new unit visit the client before transfer.
- Work with the caregivers and family members helping them deal with stages of "making the best of it," "making the move," and "making it better." **EBN:** *A study demonstrated that relatives of clients entering a nursing home can work in partnership with health care staff to ease the transition for their loved one more effectively (Davies & Nolan, 2004; Newson, 2008b).*
- If a client is being transferred from the intensive care unit (ICU), have previous staff make occasional visits until the client is comfortable in the new surroundings. Ensure that the family is told relevant information. **EBN:** *Leaving the ICU staff may be the most negative component of transfer (McKinney & Deeny, 2002). A review of the literature in this area demonstrated that information needs were most important to families of clients transferred out of ICU (Mitchell, Courtney, & Coyer, 2003).*
- Watch for coping problems (e.g., withdrawal, regression, angry behavior, impaired sleeping, refusal to eat, flat affect) and intervene immediately. **EB:** *Research has shown a link between the loss of independence with transfer to a nursing home and depression (Loeher et al, 2004; Johnson, 2008).*
- Encourage the client to express grief for the loss of the old situation; explain that it is normal to feel sadness over change and loss. **EB:** *Older adults in long-term care grieve loss of home, possessions, and independence (Pilkington, 2005; Newson, 2008a).*
- Encourage the client to participate in care as much as possible and make own decisions when possible (e.g., placement of the bed, choice of roommate, bathing routines).
- Make an effort to accommodate the client. *Having choices helps prevent feelings of powerlessness that may lead to depression.* **EB:** *Research showed that residents who viewed the nursing home move negatively after 3 months felt powerless, vulnerable, and isolated (Iwasiw et al, 2003).*

Pediatric

- Assess family history and contact information from children relocated to rescue shelters. **EB:** *No unified system exists in the United States to reunite children with their families after natural disaster or terrorist attack, so nursing has a major role to play in locating children's families and facilitation reunification (Chung & Shannon, 2007).*
- Be aware that community relocation may be beneficial for children, and assess community resources of new location. **EB:** *African American children who relocated from an inner city to a suburb benefitted especially from available institutional resources (Keels, 2008).*
- Provide support for a child and family who must relocate to be near a transplant center. **EBN:** *Recognizing the unique needs of parents who must relocate for a child's transplantation procedure supports the delivery of individualized nursing care and the effective allocation of program resources (Stubblefield & Murray, 2002).*
- Encourage child to verbalize concerns in divorce situations when they and/or a parent relocate. **EB:** *Relocation of a parent in divorce has been linked with children's financial concerns, hostility toward parents, views of parents as not socially supportive, and poorer self-perceived health (Braver, Ellman, & Fabricius, 2003).*
- Assess presence of allergies before and after relocation. **EB:** *Six-year-old children who relocated were found to have significant allergy sensitization over those who did not relocate (Herberth et al, 2007).*
- If the client is an adolescent, try to avoid a move in the middle of the school year, find a newcomers' club for the adolescent to join, and refer for counseling if needed. *Most adolescents who relocate suffer a brief period of loss of companionship and intimacy with close friends (Vernberg, Greenhoot, & Biggs, 2006).*
- Assess adolescents' perceptions of their acceptance by peers. **EB:** *Poor perceptions of peer acceptance have been related to less initiation of social interactions in new settings (Aikins, Bierman, & Parker, 2005).*

Geriatric

- Monitor the need for transfer and transfer only when necessary. **EB:** *Older adults often experience loss of function after relocation (Chen & Wilmoth, 2004).* **EBN:** *Relocation has been associated with death (Laughlin et al, 2007).*
- Implement discharge planning early so that it is not rushed. **EBN:** *Early discharge planning enhanced elders' information levels and decreased their concerns (Kleinpell, 2004).*
- Protect the client from injuries such as falls. *Older adults who fell were more likely to be admitted to a nursing home (Seematter-Bagnoud et al, 2006). Having one fall increases the likelihood of additional falls (Quadri et al, 2005).*
- After the transfer, determine the client's mental status. *Document and observe for any new onset of confusion. Confusion can follow relocation because of the overwhelming stress and sensory overload.*
- Facilitate visits from companion animals. **EB:** *A randomized trial of 6 weeks of animal-assisted therapy (dog visits) decreased loneliness among nursing home residents (Banks & Banks, 2002).*
- Encourage reminiscence of happy times. **EB:** *Nine weeks of group reminiscence therapy enhanced self-esteem among 24 nursing home residents in a two-group, nonrandomized study (Chao et al, 2006).*
- ▲ Refer for music therapy. **EBN:** *One case study indicated that music therapy may facilitate a resident's adjustment to life in a long term–care facility (Kydd, 2001).*
- ▲ Monitor for neuroleptic prescriptions. **EB:** *A cohort study showed that 60% of older adults admitted to nursing homes were prescribed these drugs (most commonly Haloperidol) and 10% in doses over recommended levels within 100 days of admission (Bronskill et al, 2004).*

Client/Family Teaching and Discharge Planning

- Teach family members and remind direct care staff about relocation stress syndrome. Encourage them to monitor for signs of the syndrome. **EBN:** *Relocation Stress Syndrome begins to ease at approximately 4 weeks after the move (Hodgson et al, 2004).*
- Help significant others learn how to support the client in the move by setting up a schedule of visits, arranging for holidays, bringing familiar items from home, and establishing a system for contact when the client needs support. **EBN:** *Social support of family and friends was significantly related to relocation adjustment (Bekhet, Zauszniewski, & Wykle, 2008).*

 See the EVOLVE website for Weblinks for client education resources.

REFERENCES

Aikins JW, Bierman KL, Parker JG: Navigating the transition to junior high school: the influence of pre-transition friendship and self-system characteristics, *Soc Dev* 14:42–60, 2005.

Banks M, Banks W: The effects of animal-assisted therapy on loneliness in an elderly population in long-term care facilities, *J Gerontol A Biol Sci Med Sci* 57A(7):M428–M432, 2002.

Bekhet AK, Zauszniewski JA, Wykle ML: Milieu change and relocation adjustment in elders, *West J Nurs Res* 30:113–129, 2008.

Braver SL, Ellman IM, Fabricius WV: Relocation of children after divorce and children's best interests: new evidence and legal considerations, *J Fam Psychol* 17(2):206–219, 2003.

Bronskill SE, Anderson GM, Sykora K et al: Neuroleptic drug therapy in older adults newly admitted to nursing homes: incidence, dose, and specialist contact, *J Am Geriatr Soc* 52(5):749–755, 2004.

Caron CD, Bowers BJ: Deciding whether to continue, share, or relinquish caregiving: caregiver views, *Qual Health Res* 13(9):1252–1271, 2003.

Chao S, Lui H, Wu C et al: Effects of group reminiscence therapy on depression, self-esteem and life satisfaction of elderly nursing home residents, *J Nurs Res* 14(1):36–45, 2006.

Chen PC, Wilmoth J: The effects of residential mobility on ADL and IADL limitations among the very old living in the community, *J Gerontol B Soc Sci* 59B(3):S164–S172, 2004.

Chung S, Shannon M: Reuniting children with their families during disasters: a proposed plan for greater success, *Am J Disaster Med* 2(3):113–117, 2007.

Davies S, Nolan M: Making the move: relatives' experiences of the transition to a care home, *Health Soc Care Comm* 12(6):517, 2004.

Davis S: Melies' theory of nursing transitions and relatives' experiences of nursing home entry, *J Adv Nurs* 52:658–671, 2005.

Dellasega C, Haagen B: A different kind of caregiving support group, *J Psychosoc Nurs Ment Health Serv* 42(8):46–55, 2004.

Dwyer S: Older people and permanent care: whose decision? *Br J Soc Work* 35:1081–1092, 2005.

Herberth G, Weber A, Lehmann I et al: The stress of relocation and neuropeptides: an epidemiological study in children, *J Psychosomatic Res* 63:451–452, 2007.

Hertz JE, Rossetti J, Koren, ML et al: Management of relocation in cognitively intact older adults, *J Gerontol Nurs* 33(11):12–18, 2007.

Hodgson N, Freedman V, Granger D et al: Biobehavioral correlates of relocation in the frail elderly: salivary cortisol, affect, and cognitive function, *J Am Geriatr Soc* 52(11):1856–1862, 2004.

Hong SI, Chen LM: Contribution of residential relocation and lifestyle to the structure of health trajectories, *J Aging Health* 21:244–265, 2009.

● = Independent ▲ = Collaborative **EBN** = Evidence-Based Nursing **EB** = Evidence-Based

Iwasiw C, Goldenberg D, Bol N et al: Resident and family perspectives: the first year in a long-term care facility, *J Gerontol Nurs* 29(1):45, 2003.

Johnson RA, Tripp-Reimer T: Aging, ethnicity & social support: a review—part 1, *J Gerontol Nurs*, 27(6):15–21, 2001a.

Johnson RA, Tripp-Reimer T: Relocation among ethnic elders: a review—part 2, *J Gerontol Nurs*, 27(6):22–27, 2001b.

Johnson RA: Relocation stress syndrome guideline. In Ackley B, Ladwig G, Swan BA et al: *Evidence-based nursing care guidelines: medical-surgical interventions*, Philadelphia, 2008, Mosby.

Kao HF, Travis SS, Acton GJ: Relocation to a long-term care facility: working with patients and families before, during, and after, *J Psychos Nurs Ment Health Serv* 42(3):10, 2004.

Keels M: Neighborhood effects examined through the lens of residential mobility programs. *Am J Comm Psychol* 42(3–4):235–250, 2008.

Kleinpell R: Randomized trial of an intensive care-based early discharge planning intervention for critically ill elderly patients, *Am J Crit Care* 13:335–345, 2004.

Kydd P: Using music therapy to help a client with Alzheimer's disease adapt to long-term care, *Am J Alzheimers Dis Other Demen* 16(2):103, 2001.

Laughlin A, Parsons M, Kosloski KD et al: Predictors of mortality following involuntary interinstitutional relocation, *J Gerontol Nurs* 33(9):20–26, 2007.

LeClerc M, Wells DL: Process evaluation of an integrated model of discharge planning, *Can J Nurs Leadersh* 14(2):19–26, 2001.

Loeher KE, Bank AL, MacNeill SE et al: Nursing home transition and depressive symptoms in older medical rehabilitation patients, *Clin Gerontol* 27(1/2):59–70, 2004.

Lutgendorf SK, Reimer TT, Harvey JH et al: Effects of housing relocation on immunocompetence and psychosocial functioning in older adults, *J Gerontol A Biol Sci Med Sci* 56(2):M97, 2001.

Lutgendorf SK, Vitaliano PP, Tripp-Reimer T et al: Sense of coherence moderates the relationship between life stress and natural killer cell activity in healthy older adults, *Psychol Aging* 14(4):552, 1999.

McKinney AA, Deeny P: Leaving the intensive care unit: a phenomenological study of the patients' experience, *Intens Crit Care Nurs* 18(6):320, 2002.

Mitchell ML, Courtney M, Coyer F: Understanding uncertainty and minimizing families' anxiety at the time of transfer from intensive care, *Nurs Health Sci* 5(3):207, 2003.

Newson P: Relocation to a care home, part one: exploring reactions, *Nurs Resident Care* 10(7):321–324, 2008a.

Newson P: Relocation to a care home, part two: exploring helping strategies, *Nurs Resident Care* 10(8):373–377, 2008b.

Nolan M, Dellesega C: "I feel I've let him down": supporting family carers during long-term care placement for elders, *J Adv Nurs* 31(4):759–767, 2000.

Pilkington FB: Grieving a loss: the lived experience for elders residing in an institution, *Nurs Sci Q* 18(3):233–242, 2005.

Popejoy L: Health related decision making by older adults and their families: how clinicians can help, *J Gerontol Nurs* 13(9):12–18, 2005.

Pruchno R, Rose M: The effect of long-term care environments of health outcomes, *Gerontologist* 40(4):422–428, 2000.

Quadri P, Tettamanti M, Bernasconi S et al: Lower limb function as predictor of falls and loss of mobility with social repercussions one year after discharge among elderly inpatients, *Aging Clin Exper Res* 17(2):82–89, 2005.

Rossen EJ: Assessing older persons' readiness to move to independent congregate living, *Clin Nurs Spec* 21:292–296, 2007.

Rossen EJ, Gruber KJ: Development and psychometric testing of the Relocation Self-Efficacy Scale, *Nurs Res* 56:244–251, 2007.

Seematter-Bagnoud L, Wietlisbach V, Yersin B et al: Healthcare utilization of elderly persons hospitalized after a noninjurious fall in a Swiss academic medical center, *J Am Geriatr Soc* 54(6):891–897, 2006.

Stubblefield C, Murray RL: Waiting for lung transplantation: family experiences of relocation, *Pediatr Nurs* 28(5):501, 2002.

Talerico KA: Relocation to a long-term care facility: working with patients and families before, during, and after, *J Psychosoc Nurs* 42(3):10–16, 2004.

Tracy JP, DeYoung S: Moving to an assisted living facility: exploring the transitional experience of elderly individuals, *J Gerontol Nurs* 30(10):26, 2004.

Vernberg E, Greenhoot A, Biggs B: Intercommunity relocation and adolescent friendships: who struggles and why? *J Consult Clin Psychol* 74(3):511–523, 2006.

Walker CA, Curry LC, Hogstel MO: Relocation stress syndrome in older adults transitioning from home to a long-term care facility: Myth or reality? *J Psychosoc Nurs* 45:35–45, 2007.

Risk for Relocation stress syndrome   *Betty J. Ackley, MSN, EdS, RN*

NANDA-I

Definition

At risk for physiological and/or psychosocial disturbances that result from transfer from one environment to another

Risk Factors

Decreased health status; lack of adequate support system; lack of predeparture counseling; losses; moderate to high degree of environmental change; moderate mental competence; move from one environment to another; passive coping; unpredictability of experiences; verbal expression of powerlessness

NOC, NIC, Client Outcomes, Nursing Interventions, Client/Family Teaching and Discharge Planning, *Rationales*, and References

Refer to care plan for **Relocation stress syndrome.**

Risk for compromised Resilience
Shelly Eisbach, PhD, RN, and Angela Kueny, PhD(c), MSN, BA

NANDA-I

Definition

At risk for decreased ability to sustain a pattern of positive responses to an adverse situation or crisis

Risk Factors

Chronicity of existing crises; multiple coexisting adverse situations; presence of an additional new crisis (e.g., unplanned pregnancy, death of a spouse, loss of job, illness, loss of housing, death of family member)

NOC   (Nursing Outcomes Classification)

Suggested NOC Outcomes

Personal Resiliency, Family Resiliency, Knowledge: Health Resources

Example NOC Outcome with Indicators
Personal Resiliency as evidenced by the following indicator: Takes responsibility for own actions (Rate the outcome and indicators of **Personal Resiliency**: 1 = never demonstrated, 2 = rarely demonstrated, 3 = sometimes demonstrated, 4 = often demonstrated, 5 = consistently demonstrated [See Section I].)

Client Outcomes

Client Will (Specify Time Frame):

- Identify available community resources
- Propose practical, constructive solutions for disputes
- Identify and access community resources for assistance
- Accept assistance with activities of daily living from family and friends
- Verbalize an enhanced sense of control

NIC   (Nursing Interventions Classification)

Suggested NIC Interventions

Resiliency Promotion, Assertiveness Training, Values Clarification, Parenting Promotion

Example NIC Activities—Resiliency Promotion
Encourage family involvement with child's schoolwork and activities; Assist family in providing atmosphere conducive to learning

Nursing Interventions and *Rationales*

- Determine how family behavior affects client. **EB:** *The model of resilience is based on the presupposition that individuals and families are connected to each other and their community and have collective strengths, which will help them to compensate for their adversity (Landau, 2007).*
- Help to identify personal rights, responsibilities, and conflicting norms. **EBN:** *Maintaining a sense of control and positive perspective about one's environment helps individuals to positively cope with adversity (Jackson, Firtko, & Edenborough, 2007).*
- Encourage consideration of values underlying choices and consequences of the choice. **EBN:** *Improving social skills, enhancing problem solving abilities, and considering values behind choices will identify the positive and/or negative impact of individuals' life choices (Tuttle, Campbell-Heider, & David, 2006).*
- Help client to practice conversational and social skills. **EB:** *Social competence and social support have been shown to improve academic achievement for minority, low-income school children; cognitive skills are protective factors to assist individuals with resilience (Elias & Haynes, 2008).*

• = Independent   ▲ = Collaborative   **EBN** = Evidence-Based Nursing   **EB** = Evidence-Based

- Assist client to prioritize values. **EB:** *Nurses can help individuals to prioritize positive values, in order to resist engagement in risky behaviors such as smoking, drinking, or violence (Veselska et al, 2009).*
- Create an accepting, nonjudgmental atmosphere. **EB:** *Assisting families and individuals create stable and positive communication skills help to minimize unreasonable expectations and concentrate on positive outcomes (Anthony, Alter, & Jenson, 2009).*
- Help identify self-defeating thoughts. **EB:** *Self-esteem increases the potential for optimism; women with high self-esteem are more likely to adjust to changing life situations and transitions (Lee et al, 2008).*
- ▲ Refer to community resources as appropriate. **EBN:** *Attending community resources, such as support groups, helps to disseminate and develop health promotion activities that improve well-being and quality of life (Donze & Tercyak, 2006).*
- Help clarify problem areas in interpersonal relationships. **EBN:** *Individuals who were socially connected to their environment, family, and to their sense of self are able to maintain a supportive mindset and experience a good quality of life despite compromising health conditions, serious diagnosis, and poor prognosis (Denz-Penhey & Murdoch, 2008).*
- Identify and enroll high-risk families in follow-up programs. **EBN:** *Families with adequate resources and positive relationships have a better chance of managing stress and restoring balance in the presence of adversity and limited resources (Van Riper, 2007).*

ⓔvolve   See the EVOLVE website for Weblinks for client education resources.

REFERENCES

Anthony EK, Alter CF, Jenson JM: Development of a risk and resilience-based out-of-school time program for children and youths, *Soc Work* 54(1):45–55, 2009.

Denz-Penhey H, Murdoch JC: Personal resiliency: serious diagnosis and prognosis with unexpected quality outcomes, *Q Health Res* 18(3):391–404, 2008.

Donze JR, Tercyak KP: The survivor health and resilience education (SHARE) program: development and evaluation of a health behavior intervention for adolescent survivors of childhood cancer, *J Clin Psychol Med Sett* 13(2):169–176, 2006.

Elias J, Haynes NM: Social competence, social support, and academic achievement, in minority low income urban elementary school children, *School Psychol Q* 32(4):474–495, 2008.

Jackson D, Firtko A, Edenborough M: Personal resilience as a strategy for surviving and thriving in the face of workplace adversity: a literature review, *J Adv Nurs* 60(1):1–9, 2007.

Landau J: Enhancing resilience: families and communities as agents for change, *Fam Proc* 46(3):351–365, 2007.

Lee H, Brown SL, Mitchell MM et al: Correlates of resilience in the face of adversity for Korean women immigrants to the US, *J Immigr Minor Health* 10:415–422, 2008.

Tuttle J, Campbell-Heider N, David TM: Positive adolescent life skills training for high-risk teens: results of a group intervention study, *J Pediatr Health Care* 20(3):184–191, 2006.

Van Riper M: Families of children with Down syndrome: responding to a change in plans with resilience, *J Pediatr Nurs* 22(2):116–127, 2007.

Veselska Z, Geckova AM, Orosova O et al: Self-esteem and resilience: the connection with risky behavior among adolescents, *Addict Behav* 34:287–291, 2009.

Impaired individual Resilience   *Shelly Eisbach, PhD, RN, and Angela Kueny, PhD(c), MSN, BA*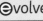

NANDA-I

Definition

Decreased ability to sustain a pattern of positive responses to an adverse situation or crisis

Defining Characteristics

Decreased interest in academic activities; decreased interest in vocational activities; depression; guilt; isolation low self-esteem; lower perceived health status; renewed elevation of distress; shame; social isolation; using maladaptive coping skills (i.e., drug use, violence, etc.)

Related Factors (r/t)

Demographics that increase chance of maladjustment; drug use; gender; inconsistent parenting; low intelligence; low maternal education; large family size; minority status; parental mental illness; poor

● = Independent   ▲ = Collaborative   **EBN** = Evidence-Based Nursing   **EB** = Evidence-Based

impulse control; poverty; psychological disorders; vulnerability factors which encompass indices that exacerbate the negative effects of the risk condition; violence; violence in neighborhood

 (Nursing Outcomes Classification)

Suggested NOC Outcomes

Personal Resiliency, Decision Making, Self-Esteem

Example **NOC Outcome with Indicators**
Personal Resiliency as evidenced by the following indicators: Adapts to unexpected crises or challenges (Rate the outcome and indicators of **Personal Resiliency**: 1 = never demonstrated, 2 = rarely demonstrated, 3 = sometimes demonstrated, 4 = often demonstrated, 5 = consistently demonstrated [See Section I].)

Client Outcomes

Client Will (Specify Time Frame):

- Demonstrate reduced or cessation of drug and alcohol usage
- State effective life events on feelings about self
- Will seek help when necessary
- Verbalize or demonstrate cessation of abuse
- Adapt to unexpected crises or challenges
- Verbalize positive outlook on illness, family, situation, and life
- Use available resources to meet coping needs
- Identify role models
- Identify available assets and resources

 (Nursing Interventions Classification)

Suggested NIC Interventions

Resiliency Promotion, Self-Esteem Enhancement

Example **NIC Activities—Resiliency Promotion**
Encourage positive health-seeking behaviors; Facilitate family communication

Nursing Interventions and *Rationales*

- Encourage positive, health-seeking behaviors. **EBN:** *Promoting health will provide a foundation for enhancing the abilities of individuals to cope, find resources, use resources, and evaluate resources for appropriate decision making (Landau, 2007).*
- Foster communication skills through basic communication skill training. **EBN:** *Individuals who are skilled communicators have fewer problems with family relationships and are able to articulate their own viewpoint (Tuttle, Campbell-Heider, & David, 2006).*
- Foster cognitive skills in decision making. **EBN:** *Assist in the identification of problems and situational factors that contribute to problems, offering options for resolution (Pierce & Hicks, 2001).*
- Facilitate supportive family environments and communication. **EBN:** *Individuals found to be resilient if raised in families with greater levels of parental supervision and consistent expectations, rules, and consequences for problem behaviors, and effective systems for monitoring children and adolescents (Scudder, Sullivan, & Copeland-Linder, 2008).*
- Promote engagement in positive social activities. **EB:** *Facilitating involvement with positive peers decreases the potential for involvement in risky behavior (Veselska et al, 2009).*
- Assist client to identify strengths, and reinforce these. **EBN:** *Positive self-esteem can be seen as an essential feature of mental health, and also a facilitator of social engagement (Veselska et al, 2009).*
- Help the client to identify positive emotions in the midst of adverse situations. **EBN:** *Those individuals who are able to recover from negative emotions in the midst of adverse situations and focusing on positive emotions helps to buffer against life adversity (Jackson, Firtko, & Edenborough, 2007).*

• = Independent   ▲ = Collaborative   **EBN** = Evidence-Based Nursing   **EB** = Evidence-Based

- Build on supportive counseling and therapy. **EB:** *Facilitating and mobilizing supportive systems external to individuals and families promote social connectedness, problem-solving, and resource-accessing, and cognitive restructuring (Landau, 2007).*
- Identify protective factors such as assets and resources to enhance coping. **EB:** *According to the protective factor model of resilience, a protective factor interacts with a stressor reduces the likelihood of negative outcomes (Steinhardt & Dolbier, 2008).*
- Provide positive reinforcement and emotional support during the learning process. **EBN:** *Positive outcomes and adherence to interventions are attained when clients are supported and reinforced for positive behavior or steps in the learning process (Tetlie, Heimsnes, & Almvik, 2009).* **EB:** *Clients with positive, supportive educational environments show self-efficacy to attaining goals in the midst of adverse situations (Rigby, Thornton, & Young, 2008).*

Pediatric

- The above interventions may be adapted for the pediatric client.
- Support the seeking of opportunities to improve cognitive abilities, such as tutoring and other resources; the development of positive and supportive relations such as family, community members or mentors; and the improvement of general health. **EBN:** *These activities help to encourage the promotion of protective factors of adolescent resilience such as positive coping and positive self-esteem (Ahern, 2006).*
- Promote the development of positive mentor relationships. **EBN:** *Avoidance of risk-taking behavior is linked to attachment with caring adults (Tuttle, Campbell-Heider, & David, 2006).* **EB:** *Children exposed early to caring adults experienced support, encouragement, guidance, and admonishment (Anthony, Alter, & Jenson, 2009).*

ⓔvolve   See the EVOLVE website for Weblinks for client education resources.

REFERENCES

Ahern NR: Adolescent resilience: an evolutionary concept analysis, *J Pediatr Nurs* 21(3):175–185, 2006.

Anthony EK, Alter CF, Jenson JM: Development of a risk and resilience-based out-of-school time program for children and youths, *Soc Work* 54(1):45–55, 2009.

Jackson D, Firtko A, Edenborough M: Personal resilience as a strategy for surviving and thriving in the face of workplace adversity: a literature review, *J Adv Nurs* 60(1):1–9, 2007.

Landau J: Enhancing resilience: families and communities as agents for change, *Fam Process* 46(3):351–365, 2007.

Pierce P, Hicks F: Patient decision-making behavior: an emerging paradigm for nursing science, *Nurs Res* 50(5):267–274, 2001.

Rigby SA, Thornton EW, Young CA: A randomized group intervention trial to enhance mood and self-efficacy in people with multiple sclerosis, *Br J Health Psychol* 13(Pt 4):619–631, 2008.

Scudder L, Sullivan K, Copeland-Linder N: Adolescent resilience: lessons for primary care, *J Nurse Pract* 4(7):535–543, 2008.

Steinhardt M, Dolbier C: Evaluation of a resilience intervention to enhance coping strategies and to decrease symptomatology, *J Am Coll Health* 56(4):445–453, 2008.

Tetlie T, Heimsnes MC, Almvik R: Using exercise to treat patients with severe mental illness: how and why? *J Psychosoc Nurs Mental Health Serv* 47(2):32–40, 2009.

Tuttle J, Campbell-Heider N, David TM: Positive adolescent life skills training for high-risk teens: results of a group intervention study, *J Pediatr Health Care* 20(3):184–191, 2006.

Veselska Z, Geckova AM, Orosova O et al: Self-esteem and resilience: the connection with risky behavior among adolescents, *Addict Behav* 34:287–291, 2009.

Readiness for enhanced Resilience

Shelly Eisbach, PhD, RN, and Angela Kueny, PhD(c), MSN, BA

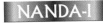

Definition

A pattern of positive responses to an adverse situation or crisis that can be strengthened to optimize human potential

Defining Characteristics

Access to resources; demonstrates positive outlook; effective use of conflict management strategies; enhances personal coping skills; expressed desire to enhance resilience; identifies available resources; identifies support systems; increases positive relationships with others; involvement in activities;

• = Independent   ▲ = Collaborative   **EBN** = Evidence-Based Nursing   **EB** = Evidence-Based

makes progress toward goals; presence of a crisis; safe environment is maintained; sets goals; takes responsibilities for actions; use of effective communication skills; verbalizes an enhanced sense of control; verbalizes self-esteem

Related Factors (r/t)

Demographics that increase chance of maladjustment; drug use; gender; inconsistent parenting; low intelligence; low maternal education; large family size; minority status; parental mental illness; poor impulse control; poverty; psychological disorders; vulnerability factors which encompass indices that exacerbate the negative effects of the risk condition; violence

 (Nursing Outcomes Classification)

Suggested NOC Outcomes

Personal Resiliency, Family Resiliency, Quality of Life

Example **NOC** Outcome with Indicators
Personal Resiliency as evidenced by the following indicator: Adapts to adversities and challenges (Rate the outcome and indicators of **Personal Resiliency:** 1 = never demonstrated, 2 = rarely demonstrated, 3 = sometimes demonstrated, 4 = often demonstrated, 5 = consistently demonstrated [See Section I].)

Client Outcomes

Client Will (Specify Time Frame):

- Adapt to adversities and challenges
- Communicate clearly and appropriately for age
- Take responsibility for own actions
- Make progress towards goals
- Use effective coping strategies
- Express emotions

 (Nursing Interventions Classification)

Suggested NIC Interventions

Resiliency Promotion, Self-Efficacy Enhancement, Counseling, Emotional Support

Example **NIC** Activities—Self-Efficacy Enhancement
Explore individual's perception of his/her capability to perform the desired behavior

Nursing Interventions and *Rationales*

- Listen to and encourage expressions of feelings and beliefs. **EBN:** *Communication assists individuals and families to resolve conflicts and to facilitate potential for growth, to identify inherent strengths, and problem solve effectively (Black & Lobo, 2008).*
- Establish a therapeutic relationship based on trust and respect. **EBN:** *Therapeutic relationships between therapists, nurses, and clients are essential to help individuals establish goals to communicate concerns, and to empower the client (Halldorsdottir, 2008).*
- Assist client to identify strengths and reinforce these. **EB:** *Fostering the use of protective factors will promote the ability of an individual to overcome adverse situations (Fergus & Zimmerman, 2005).*
- Provide positive reinforcement and emotional support during implementation of care. **EB:** *Providing positive reinforcement and emotional support will enhance a client's self-esteem, which is a key component of physical and mental health; individuals with higher self-esteem are more likely to be resilient then peers with less self-esteem (Veselska et al, 2008).*
- ▲ Facilitate the development of mentorship opportunities. **EB:** *Mentoring programs have been shown to prevent negative outcomes and to improve adolescent's transition to young adulthood (Osterling & Hines, 2006).*

● = Independent   ▲ = Collaborative   **EBN** = Evidence-Based Nursing   **EB** = Evidence-Based

- Determine how family behavior affects the client. **EB:** *The model of resilience is based on the presupposition that individuals and families are connected to each other and their community and have collective strengths, which will help them to compensate for their adversity (Landau, 2007).*
- Provide assistance in decision making. **EB:** *Decision making helps individuals to feel more in control of their situation, and nurses can create an atmosphere which helps clients participate in activities that develop life skills (Karapetian-Alvord & Grados, 2005).*
- Establish individual/family/community goals. **EB:** *Individuals, families, and communities who set goals will focus on attaining or achieving positive outcomes despite adversity (Armstrong, Birnie-Lefcovitch, & Ungar, 2005).*

Pediatric

- The above interventions may be adapted for the pediatric client.
- Encourage the promotion of protective factors by fostering the seeking of opportunities to improve cognitive abilities such as tutoring and other resources; the development of positive and supportive relations such as family, community members or mentors; and the improvement of general health. **EBN:** *These factors are associated with adolescent resilience and promote positive coping and positive self-esteem (Ahern, 2008).*

Multicultural

- Use teaching strategies that are culturally and age-appropriate. **EB:** *Nurses who use currently existing family and community resources will promote a context that allows solutions to emerge in a culturally appropriate and sustainable way (Landau, 2007).*

⊖volve   See the EVOLVE website for Weblinks for client education resources.

REFERENCES

Ahern NR, Ark P, Byers J: Resilience and coping strategies in adolescents, *Paediatr Nurs* 20(10):32–36, 2008.

Armstrong M, Birnie-Lefcovitch S, Ungar M: Pathways between social support, family well being, quality of parenting, and child resilience: what we know, *J Child Fam Stud* 14(2):269–281, 2005.

Black K, Lobo M: A conceptual review of family resilience, *J Family Nurs* 14(1):33–55, 2008.

Fergus S, Zimmerman MA: Adolescent resilience: a framework for understanding healthy development in the face of risk, *Ann Rev Public Health* 26(1):399–419, 2005.

Halldorsdottir S: The dynamics of the nurse-patient relationship: introduction of a synthesized theory from the patient's perspective, *Scand J Caring Sci* 22(4):643–652, 2008.

Karapetian-Alvord M, Grados JJ: Enhancing resilience in children: a proactive approach, *Prof Psychol Res and Pr* 36(3):238–245, 2005.

Landau J: Enhancing resilience: families and communities as agents of change, *Fam Proc* 46(3):351–365, 2007.

Osterling KL, Hines AM: Mentoring adolescent foster youth: promoting resilience during developmental transitions, *Child Fam Soc Work* 11(3):242–253, 2006.

Veseska Z, Geckova AM, Gajdosva B et al: Self-esteem and resilience: the connection with risky behaviors among adolescents, *Addicti Behav* 34:287–291, 2008.

Ineffective Role performance   *Gail B. Ladwig, MSN, RN, CHTP*

NANDA-I

Definition

Patterns of behavior and self-expression that do not match the environmental context, norms, and expectations

Defining Characteristics

Altered role perceptions; anxiety; change in capacity to resume role; change in other's perception of role; change in self-perception of role; change in usual patterns of responsibility; deficient knowledge; depression; discrimination; domestic violence; harassment; inadequate adaptation to change; inadequate confidence; inadequate coping; inadequate external support for role enactment; inadequate motivation; inadequate opportunities for role enactment; inadequate role competency; inadequate self-management; inadequate skills; inappropriate developmental expectations; pessimism;

• = Independent   ▲ = Collaborative   **EBN** = Evidence-Based Nursing   **EB** = Evidence-Based

powerlessness; role ambivalence; role confusion; role conflict; role denial; role dissatisfaction; role overload; role strain; system conflict; uncertainty

Related Factors (r/t)

Knowledge

Inadequate role model; inadequate role preparation (e.g., role transition, skill rehearsal, validation); lack of education; lack of role model; unrealistic role expectations

Physiological

Body image alteration; cognitive deficits; depression; fatigue; low self-esteem; mental illness; neurological defects; pain; physical illness; substance abuse

Social

Conflict; developmental level; domestic violence; inadequate role socialization; inadequate support system; inappropriate linkage with the health care system; job schedule demands; lack of resources; lack of rewards; low socioeconomic status; stress; young age

 (Nursing Outcomes Classification)

Suggested NOC Outcomes

Coping, Psychosocial Adjustment: Life Change, Role Performance

Example NOC Outcome with Indicators
Role Performance as evidenced by the following indicators: Knowledge of role transition periods/Reported strategies for role change(s)/Reported comfort with role changes (Rate the outcome and indicators of **Role Performance:** 1 = not adequate, 2 = slightly adequate, 3 = moderately adequate, 4 = substantially adequate, 5 = totally adequate [see Section I].)

Client Outcomes

Client Will (Specify Time Frame):

- Identify realistic perception of role
- State personal strengths
- Acknowledge problems contributing to inability to carry out usual role
- Accept physical limitations regarding role responsibility and consider ways to change lifestyle to accomplish goals associated with role performance
- Demonstrate knowledge of appropriate behaviors associated with new or changed role
- State knowledge of change in responsibility and new behaviors associated with new responsibility
- Verbalize acceptance of new responsibility

 (Nursing Interventions Classification)

Suggested NIC Intervention

Role Enhancement

Example NIC Activities—Role Enhancement
Assist patient to identify behaviors needed for role development; Assist patient to identify positive strategies for managing role changes

Nursing Interventions and *Rationales*

Social

- Ask the client direct questions regarding new roles and how the health care system can help him or her continue in roles. **EBN:** *All participants in this study of client's who had had a stroke described the loss of valued roles which they had previously enjoyed. Health care professionals need to recognize and*

• = Independent   ▲ = Collaborative   **EBN** = Evidence-Based Nursing   **EB** = Evidence-Based

provide psychological support for client's and significant others who are adjusting to these changes (Thompson, 2008).

- Allow the client to express feelings regarding the role change. **EBN:** *Cancer affects men's role as fathers, and changes self-image as a man and as a parent. This consists of gaining control, balancing emotions, subjective well-being, being open or not toward the family, and challenges in family life and to family well-being (Elmberger & Bolund, 2002).*
- Reinforce the client's strengths and internalized values. **EB:** *Participants in this study whose intentions were more aligned with their moral norm were more likely to perform healthy behaviors (driving within speed limit, applying universal precautions, exercising, not smoking) (Godin, Conner, & Sheeran, 2005).*
- Have the client make a list of strengths that are needed for the new role. Acknowledge which strengths the client has and which strengths need to be developed. Work with the client to set goals for desired role. **EBN:** *Adversity can be an opportunity to focus on strengths and nurture resiliency. Clients should not subscribe to "victim" labels. Resilience should be celebrated (Engel, 2007).*
- Support the client's religious practices. **EB:** *The majority of well-conducted studies found that higher levels of religious involvement are positively associated with indicators of psychological well-being (life satisfaction, happiness, positive effect, and higher morale) and with less depression, suicidal thoughts and behavior, drug/alcohol use/abuse (Moreira-Almeida, Neto, & Koenig, 2006).* **EBN:** *Clients dealing with role change associated with health crisis may be at risk for spiritual crisis and need an interdisciplinary approach to assist them through this time (Agrimson & Taft, 2009).*

Physiological

- Identify ways to compensate for physical disabilities (e.g., have a ramp built to provide access to house, put household objects within the client's reach from wheelchair) and provide technological assistance when available. **EB:** *Among people with disability, use of assistive technology was associated with use of fewer hours of personal assistance (Hoenig, Taylor, & Sloan, 2003).*
- Refer to the care plans for **Readiness for enhanced family Coping, Readiness for enhanced Decision-Making, Impaired Home maintenance, Impaired Parenting, Risk for Loneliness, Readiness for enhanced community Coping, Readiness for enhanced Self-Care,** and **Ineffective Sexuality pattern.**

 ### Pediatric

- Assist new parents to adjust to changes in workload associated with childbirth. **EB:** *Expectant parents in this study anticipated increase in workload after childbirth. Work increases were greater for women than for men (Gjerdingen, 2000; Gjerdingen & Center, 2003).*
- ▲ Refer teen parents and families to a community-based, multifamily group (MFG) intervention strategy (e.g., Families and Schools Together [FAST] babies). **EB:** *This program showed statistically significant increases in parental self-efficacy for the teenage mothers, improved parent-child bonds, reduced stress and family conflict, and increased social support (McDonald et al, 2009).*
- Assist parents in coping with infants with colic, a condition common in infants. **EBN:** *Even though nursing interventions do not cure infant colic, the amount of crying may be reduced and life made easier for the families if the parents are offered help in coping with the situation (Helseth, 2002).*
- ▲ Refer to home health agency for home visits when there is an infant who has excessive crying. **EBN:** *Almost every aspect of family life was disrupted when there was an infant who cried excessively, resulting in strained relationships, feelings of guilt, and concerns about losing control. A health visitor needs to visit frequently, stay for a prolonged period, demonstrate engagement with the family and its difficulties, and impart specific messages with conviction and sincerity (Long & Johnson, 2001). Mother infant relationships can be improved through early home visiting interventions by trained nursing staff (Geçkil, Sahin, & Ege, 2009).*
- Provide parents with coping skills when the role change is associated with a critically and chronically ill child. **EBN:** *Results from mothers who received the Creating Opportunities for Parent Empowerment (COPE) program indicate the need to educate parents regarding their children's responses as they recover from critical illness and how they can assist their children in coping with the stressful experience (Melnyk, Feinstein, & Fairbanks, 2006). Involving parents of chronically ill children in*

• = Independent   ▲ = Collaborative   **EBN** = Evidence-Based Nursing   **EB** = Evidence-Based

ongoing discussions about their positions in management may help promote their active and informed participation (Swallow, 2008).

- Assist families how to manage day-to-day needs of a child with cerebral palsy (CP). Teach family members to value the small things children do, connect with other families, locate community resources, and understand the short- and long-term needs of the child. **EB:** *In families of children with CP, strategies for optimizing caregiver physical and psychological health include supports for behavioral management and daily functional activities as well as stress management and self-efficacy techniques. These data support clinical pathways that require biopsychosocial frameworks that are family centered (Raina et al, 2005).*
- Consider the use of media-based behavioral treatments for children with behavioral disorders. **EBN:** *Behaviors problems in children are quite common. For straightforward cases, media-based interventions may be enough to make clinically significant changes in a child's behavior. Media-based therapies appear to have both clinical and economic implications for the treatment of children with behavioral problems (Montgomery, 2005).*

Geriatric

- Provide support for grandparents raising grandchildren. **EBN:** *Grandparent caregivers are at risk for multiple physical, mental, and emotional problems due to the stresses and strains of care provision (Kolomer, 2008; Lo & Liu, 2009).*
- Provide support for spouses and families of clients with strokes. **EB:** *In this study three roles of spouses are described: (1) the role of caregiver, (2) the role of client, and (3) the role of family member. A family-centered approach is indicated in which the strengths and needs of all family members are addressed, including the client with the stroke (Visser-Meily et al, 2006).*
- Support the client's religious beliefs and activities and provide appropriate spiritual support persons. **EB:** *Usually the positive impact of religious involvement on mental health is more robust among people under stressful circumstances (the elderly and those with disability and medical illness) (Moreira-Almeida, Neto, & Koenig, 2006).*
- Explore community needs after assessing the client's strengths. Encourage elders to participate in volunteer programs. **EB:** *Engagement in social and generative activities has benefits for the well-being of older adults; programs such as Experience Corps Baltimore provide a social model for health promotion for older adult volunteers in public schools (Martinez et al, 2006).*
- ▲ Refer to appropriate support groups for adjustment to role changes. **EBN:** *Health care professionals should provide information on Parkinson's disease symptom management, identify appropriate resources to reduce caregiver burden, and use of support groups (Edwards & Scheetz, 2002).* **EBN:** *Significant differences were found for distress levels and quality of life, with the mutual support group having greater improvements than the control group for dementia family caregivers (Fung & Chien, 2002).*
- ▲ Refer clients to therapeutic recreation programs that use humor. **EB:** *Older adults' life satisfaction showed significant improvement when participating in "the happiness and humor group" (Mathieu, 2008).*
- ▲ Refer to therapy to improve memory for clients with Alzheimer's disease. **EB:** *The available evidence shows that alternative and innovative ways of memory rehabilitation for Alzheimer's clients can indeed be clinically effective or pragmatically useful with a great potential for use within the new culture of a more graded and proactive type of Alzheimer's disease care (De Vreese et al, 2001).* **EB:** *Facing an inevitable decline, persons with early-stage dementia and their care partners found it helpful to talk with one another and with peers in the same circumstances about the disease and its effects in this memory club (Zarit et al, 2004).*

Multicultural

- Assess for the influence of cultural beliefs, norms, values, and expectations on the individual's role. **EBN:** *The individual's role may be based on cultural perceptions (Leininger & McFarland, 2002). It is important to gain an understanding of cultural beliefs and traditional practices relating to the postpartum care of women and their babies (Geçkil, Sabin, & Ege, 2009).*
- Assess for conflicts between the caregiver's cultural role obligations and competing factors like employment or school. **EBN:** *Mexican immigrant children provide essential help to their families,*

• = Independent ▲ = Collaborative **EBN** = Evidence-Based Nursing **EB** = Evidence-Based

including translating, interpreting, and caring for siblings (Orellana, 2003). A recent study found that African American caregivers experienced a wide range of caregiver role strain (Wallace Williams, Dilworth-Anderson, & Goodwin, 2003).

- Negotiate with the client regarding the aspects of their role that can be modified and still honor cultural beliefs. **EBN:** *Give and take with the client will lead to culturally congruent care (Leininger & McFarland, 2002).*
- Encourage family to use support groups or other service programs to assist with role changes. **EBN:** *Studies indicate that minority families of clients with dementia use few support programs even though these programs could have a positive impact on caregiver well-being (Cox, 1999).*
- Refer new moms to a new-mothers, Internet-based, social support network. **EBN:** *Many single, low-income, African American mothers lack social support, experience psychological distress, and encounter difficulties caring for their infants during the transition to parenthood. The New Mothers Network may be an effective social support nursing intervention for improving single, low-income, African American mothers' psychological health outcome, parenting outcome, and health care utilization outcomes (Hudson et al, 2008).*

Home Care

- The above interventions may be adapted for home care use.
- ▲ Offer a referral to medical social services to assist with assessing the short- and long-term impacts of role change. **EB:** *The discharge planner's role especially with the elderly is important (Preyde, Macaulay, & Dingwall, 2009).*

Client/Family Teaching and Discharge Planning

- Provide educational materials to family members on client behavior management plus caregiver stress-coping management. **EB:** *Brief primary care interventions as described above may be effective in reducing caregiver distress and burden in the long-term management of the dementia client (Burns et al, 2003).*
- Help the client identify resources for assistance in caring for a disabled or aging parent (e.g., adult day care, nursing home placement). **EBN:** *There is a need for support when a family member is placed in a nursing home (Wilkes, Jackson & Vallido, 2008). In this study daycare was effective in reducing behavioral and psychological symptoms of dementia clients and in alleviating caregivers' burden (Mossello et al, 2008).*
- ▲ Refer to appropriate community agencies to learn skills for functioning in the new or changed role (e.g., vocational rehabilitation, parenting classes, hospice, respite care). **EB:** *Program Without Walls (PWW) is a person-centered, community-based approach for state rehabilitation counselors to provide vocational rehabilitation (VR) services to people with traumatic brain injury (TBI). This study demonstrated that the PWW showed promise as a systems change effort to improve VR services for people with TBI (O'Neill et al, 2004).*
- Consider pet therapy for college students in a new role, their first semester away from home. **EBN:** *In this study students away from home for the first time felt that a pet therapy program could temporarily fill the absence of previous support systems and be a catalyst for establishing new social relationships (Adamle, Riley, & Carlson, 2009).*

Ⓔvolve   See the EVOLVE website for Weblinks for client education resources.

REFERENCES

Adamle KN, Riley TA, Carlson T: Evaluating college student interest in pet therapy, *J Am Coll Health* 57(5):545–548, 2009.

Agrimson LB, Taft LB: Spiritual crisis: a concept analysis, *J Adv Nurs* 65(2):454–461, 2009.

Burns R, Nichols LO, Martindale-Adams J et al: Primary care interventions for dementia caregivers: 2–year outcomes from the REACH study, *Gerontologist* 43(4):547–555, 2003.

Cox C: Race and caregiving: patterns of service use by African American and white caregivers of persons with Alzheimer's, *J Gerontol Soc Work* 32(2):5, 1999.

De Vreese LP, Neri M, Fioravanti M et al: Memory rehabilitation in Alzheimer's disease: a review of progress, *Int J Geriatr Psychiatry* 16(8):794, 2001.

Edwards NE, Scheetz PS: Predictors of burden for caregivers of patients with Parkinson's disease, *J Neurosci Nurs* 34(4):184, 2002.

Elmberger E, Bolund C: Men with cancer. Changes in attempts to master the self-image as a man and as a parent, *Cancer Nurs* 25(6):477, 2002.

Engel B: Eagle soaring: the power of the resilient self, *J Psychosoc Nurs Ment Health Serv* 45(2):44–49, 2007.

Fung WY, Chien WT: The effectiveness of a mutual support group for family caregivers of a relative with dementia, *Arch Psychiatr Nurs* 16(3):134, 2002.

Geçkil E, Sahin T, Ege E: Traditional postpartum practices of women and infants and the factors influencing such practices in South Eastern Turkey, *Midwifery* 25(1):62–71, 2009.

Gjerdingen D: Expectant parents' anticipated changes in workload after the birth of their first child, *J Fam Pract* 49(11):993, 2000.

Gjerdingen DK, Center BA: First-time parents' prenatal to postpartum changes in health, and the relation of postpartum health to work and partner characteristics, *J Am Board Fam Pract* 16(4):304–311, 2003.

Godin G, Conner M, Sheeran P: Bridging the intention-behavior "gap": the role of moral norm, *Br J Soc Psychol* 44(Pt 4):497–512, 2005.

Helseth S: Help in times of crying: nurses' approach to parents with colicky infants, *J Adv Nurs* 40(3):267–274, 2002.

Hoenig H, Taylor DH Jr, Sloan FA: Does assistive technology substitute for personal assistance among the disabled elderly? *Am J Public Health* 93(2):330–337, 2003.

Hudson DB, Campbell-Grossman C, Keating-Lefler R et al: New Mothers Network: the development of an Internet-based social support intervention for African American mothers, *Iss Comprehen Pediatr Nurs* 31(1):23–35, 2008.

Kolomer S: Grandparent caregivers, *J Gerontol Soc Work* 50(S1):321–44, 2008.

Leininger MM, McFarland MR: *Transcultural nursing: concepts, theories, research and practices,* ed 3, New York, 2002, McGraw-Hill.

Lo M, Liu YH: Quality of life among older grandparent caregivers: a pilot study, *J Adv Nurs* 65(7):1475–1484, 2009.

Long T, Johnson M: Living and coping with excessive infantile crying, *J Adv Nurs* 34(2):155, 2001.

Martinez IL, Frick K, Glass TA et al: Engaging older adults in high impact volunteering that enhances health: recruitment and retention in The Experience Corps Baltimore, *J Urban Health* 83(5):941–953, 2006.

Mathieu SI: Happiness and Humor Group promotes life satisfaction for the senior center participants, *Activities Adapt Aging* 32(2):134–148, 2008.

McDonald L, Conrad T, Fairtlough A et al: An evaluation of a group-work intervention for teenage mothers and their families, *Child Fam Soc Work* 14(1):45–57, 2009.

Melnyk BM, Feinstein N, Fairbanks E: Two decades of evidence to support implementation of the COPE program as standard practice with parents of young unexpectedly hospitalized/critically ill children and premature infants, *Pediatr Nurs* 32(5):475–481, 2006.

Montgomery M: Media-based behavioral treatments for behavioral disorders in children, *Cochrane Database Syst Rev* (1):CD002206, 2005.

Moreira-Almeida A, Neto FL, Koenig HG: Religiousness and mental health: a review, *Rev Bras Psiquiatr* 28(3):242–250, 2006.

Mossello E, Caleri V, Razzi E et al: Day care for older dementia patients: favorable effects on behavioral and psychological symptoms and caregiver stress, *Int J Geriatr Psychiatry* 23(10):1066–1072, 2008.

O'Neill JH, Zuger RR, Fields A et al: The Program Without Walls: innovative approach to state agency vocational rehabilitation of persons with traumatic brain injury, *Arch Phys Med Rehabil* 85(4 Suppl 2):S68–S72, 2004.

Orellana MF: Responsibilities of children in Latino immigrant homes, *New Dir Youth Dev* (100):25–39, 2003.

Preyde M, Macaulay C, Dingwall T: Discharge planning from hospital to home for elderly patients: a meta-analysis, *J Evid Based Soc Work* 6(2):198–216, 2009.

Raina P, O'Donnell M, Rosenbaum P et al: The health and well-being of caregivers of children with cerebral palsy, *Pediatrics* 115(6):e626–e636, 2005.

Swallow V: An exploration of mothers' and fathers' views of their identities in chronic-kidney-disease management: parents as students? *J Clin Nurs* (23):3177–3186, 2008.

Thompson HS: A review of the psychosocial consequences of stroke and their impact on spousal relationships, *Br J Neurosci Nurs* 4(4):177–184, 2008.

Visser-Meily A, Post M, Gorter JW et al: Rehabilitation of stroke patients needs a family-centered approach, *Disabil Rehabil* 28(24):1557–1561, 2006.

Wallace Williams S, Dilworth-Anderson P, Goodwin PY: Caregiver role strain: the contribution of multiple roles and available resources in African-American women, *Aging Ment Health* 7(2):103–112, 2003.

Wilkes L, Jackson D, Vallido T: Placing a relative into a nursing home: family members' experiences after the move. A review of the literature, *Geriaction* 26(1):24–29, 2008.

Zarit SH, Femia EE, Watson J et al: Memory Club: a group intervention for people with early-stage dementia and their care partners, *Gerontologist* 44(2):262–269, 2004.

S

Readiness for enhanced Self-Care   *Susan Mee, RN, PhD, CPNP*   ⊖volve

NANDA-I

Definition

A pattern of performing activities for oneself that helps to meet health-related goals and can be strengthened

Defining Characteristics

Expresses desire to enhance independence in maintaining life; expresses desire to enhance independence in maintaining health; expresses desire to enhance independence in maintaining personal development; expresses desire to enhance independence in maintaining well-being; expresses desire to enhance knowledge of strategies for self-care; expresses desire to enhance responsibility for self-care; expresses desire to enhance self-care

• = Independent   ▲ = Collaborative   **EBN** = Evidence-Based Nursing   **EB** = Evidence-Based

(Nursing Outcomes Classification)

Suggested NOC Outcomes

Adherence Behavior, Health-Seeking Behavior, Self-Care Status

Example NOC Outcome with Indicators
Health-Seeking Behavior as evidenced by the following indicators: Completes health-related tasks/Performs self-screening when indicated/Seeks assistance from health professionals when indicated (Rate the outcome and indicators of **Health-Seeking Behavior:** 1 = never demonstrated, 2 = rarely demonstrated, 3 = sometimes demonstrated, 4 = often demonstrated, 5 = consistently demonstrated [see Section I].)

Client Outcomes

Client Will (Specify Time Frame):

- Evaluate current levels of self-care as optimum for abilities
- Express the need or desire to continue to enhance levels of self-care
- Seek health-related information as needed
- Identify strategies to enhance self-care
- Perform appropriate interventions as needed
- Monitor level of self-care
- Evaluate the effectiveness of self-care interventions at regular intervals

NIC   **(Nursing Interventions Classification)**

Suggested NIC Interventions

Coping Enhancement, Energy Management, Learning Facilitation, Multidisciplinary Care Conference, Mutual Goal Setting, Self-Care Assistance, Teaching: Decision Process, Individual

Example NIC Activity—Self-Care Assistance
Encourage person to perform normal activities of daily living to level of ability

Nursing Interventions and *Rationales*

- For assessment of self-care, use a valid and reliable screening tool if available for specific characteristics of the person, e.g., arthritis, diabetes, stroke, heart failure, dementia. **EBN and EB:** *Assessment using a valid and reliable tool enables clinicians to identify factors that are known from research to be important for people with the specific problem (Czaja et al, 2009; Lewin et al, 2009; Pallant et al, 2009; Sousa et al, 2009).*
- Conduct mutual goal setting with the person. **EBN:** *In a study of a mutual goal-setting intervention with 27 heart failure clients, the intervention helped to promote receptivity to health-promotion behaviors (Meyerson & Kline, 2009).*
- Support the person's awareness that enhanced self-care is an achievable, desirable, and positive life goal. **EBN:** *In a review of 24 scholarly papers about psychological aspects of rehabilitation, setting self-care goals was identified as an important part of achieving optimum self-care (Scobbie, Wyke, & Dixon, 2009). In a study to examine the relation of self-care to heart failure status, self-care of heart failure explained a significant amount of variance in heart failure status (Lee, Suwanno & Riegel, 2009).*
- Show respect for the person, regardless of characteristics and/or background. **EBN:** *Respect for an individual is a necessary condition for the experience of participation in health care decisions (Eldh, Ekman, & Ehnfors, 2006).*
- Promote trust and enhanced communication between the person and health care providers. **EBN:** *In a qualitative study using semistructured interviews with 42 heart failure clients, factors such as faith in health professionals and belief in the local health system affected self-care practices (Clark et al, 2009). In an integrative review of 18 studies of people's experiences with heart failure, it was confirmed*

● = Independent   ▲ = Collaborative   **EBN** = Evidence-Based Nursing   **EB** = Evidence-Based

that experiences vary, and nurses should ask clients about their experiences (Welstand, Carson, & Rutherford, 2009).

- Promote opportunities for spiritual care and growth. **EBN:** *People may use their spirituality to make decisions, guide actions, and to accept, reorder, and transcend life events (Callaghan, 2005; Cavendish et al, 2006).*
- Promote social support through facilitation of family involvement. **EBN:** *In a review of 10 studies of discharge interventions and client characteristics, it was identified that clients with adequate social support experienced fewer hospital readmissions (Jacob & Poletick, 2008).*
- Provide opportunities for ongoing group support through establishment of self-help groups on the Internet. **EB:** *In a study to examine the feasibility and benefits of a videoconferencing health care support program with 18 older adults divided into three groups, the findings were that the participants appreciated the information shared by others about self-care and responded positively to the professional and peer support (Marziali, 2009).*
- Help the person identify and reduce the barriers to self-care. **EBN:** *In a secondary analyses of data from 61 older women with breast cancer, three barriers were studied and found to be amenable to interventions: negative beliefs about managing symptoms, perceived negative attitudes of health care providers, and difficulties in communicating about symptoms (Yeom & Heidrich, 2009).*
- Provide literacy-appropriate education for self-care activities. **EBN:** *Low health literacy is more prevalent than previously thought, so education materials should be designed at the fifth-grade reading level (Harvard School of Public Health: Health Literacy Studies, 2009). Client comprehension of discharge instructions should be determined before discharge (Chugh et al, 2009). Literacy-appropriate educational materials and brief counseling improved diabetes self-management (Wallace et al, 2009).*
- Facilitate self-efficacy by ensuring the adequacy of self-care education. **EBN and EB:** *In nursing and other studies, self-efficacy was shown to improve with education and also was an essential correlate to optimum self-care (Schmutte et al, 2009; Sousa et al, 2009; Wallace et al, 2009).*
- Conduct demonstrations and evaluate return demonstrations of self-care procedures such as use of an inhaler for asthma. **EB:** *In a 24–week prospective randomized control trial of 95 adults with moderate to severe asthma, individualized instruction such as how to use the peak flow meter improved clinical markers for asthma control (Janson et al, 2009).*
- Provide alternative mind-body therapies such as reiki, guided imagery, yoga, and self-hypnosis. **EBN:** *A study with 11 nurses who use Reiki to optimize self-care showed that this method helped them to achieve their goals (Vitale, 2009).* **EB:** *The National Health Survey data from 2002 indicated that 16.6% of people in the United States use mind-body therapies that they perceive as helpful in managing medical conditions (Bertisch et al, 2009).*
- Promote the person's hope to maintain self-care. **EBN:** *A study with 207 clients with acute coronary syndrome showed that it was important to assess for and address hopelessness in order to improve recovery (Dunn et al, 2009).*

 Pediatric

- Assess and evaluate a child's level of self-care and adjust strategies as needed. *Caring for or doing for are appropriate interventions for nursing young infants or children. Guiding and supporting older children in their self-care actions is appropriate. Nurses should help adolescents to develop beneficial self-care practices (Orem, 2001).* **EBN:** *Parents of children with asthma needed to be able to detect, interpret, and monitor meaningful symptoms to adequately control them. When barriers exist for enhanced self-care activities, treatment in an emergency room is the consequence even if the parents are well intended (Cox & Taylor, 2005).*
- Assist families to engage in and maintain social support networks. **EBN:** *Children with cancer are competent agents, performing many practices in the area of universal and developmental self-care requisites (Moore & Beckwitt, 2004).* **EBN:** *Improved caregiver-child relationship suggests participation in an Internet support group as soon as possible for primary caregivers of a child with special health care needs (Baum, 2004).* **EBN:** *Both social support and self-esteem have been linked to positive health practices. Social support is a powerful variable in positive health practices in adolescents; self-esteem is not as powerful a variable in positive health practices in this group of early adolescents (Yarcheski, Mahon, & Yarcheski, 2003).*

- Encourage activities that support or enhance spiritual care. **EBN:** *Spiritual growth is significantly related to an adolescent's initiation and responsibility for self-care. With spiritual growth comes the adolescent's assumption of responsibilities for self-care (Callaghan, 2005).* **EBN:** *When opportunities that enhance spiritual growth are explicated by research, nurses can assess and intervene to promote positive health outcomes. A spectrum of life events can promote a spiritual response leading to spiritual enhancement (Cavendish et al, 2006). Every child is born with an intrinsic spiritual essence that can be enhanced. Nurses must realize that a child's spirituality can affect his or her health and illness states. For an infant, the needs for love and trust, intrinsically related to spiritual care, must be addressed. School-aged children can play, attend religious services, and receive visits from clergy (Elkins & Cavendish, 2004).*

Multicultural

- Identify cultural beliefs, values, lifestyle practices, and problem-solving strategies when assessing the client's level of self-care. *Self-care needs are not inborn. Activities of self-care are learned according to one's cultural way of life. Hence, there are many variations in self-care practice (Orem, 2001). For common minor illnesses, many people use self-care with medicines, vitamins, herbs, exercise, or foods that they believe have healing powers. Many self-care practices are handed down from generation to generation. When self-care measures do not work, only then will people turn to professional or folk healing systems (Andrews & Boyle, 2003). As nurses we need to be aware of our client's health beliefs, practice-related folklore, and ethnocultural knowledge. Health promotion and protection practices can range from seeing a physician to wearing a clove of garlic around one's neck (Spector, 2004).*
- Enhance cultural knowledge by seeking out information regarding different cultural or ethnic groups. *To provide culturally competent and appropriate care, nurses need to skillfully and artfully use transcultural knowledge. The transcultural nurse must be guided by acquired knowledge in the assessment, diagnosis, planning, implementation, and evaluation of the client's needs, based on culturally relevant information (Giger & Davidhizar, 2004). Cultural self-assessment is the first step in providing culturally competent care. Through self-assessment one can overcome ethnocentric tendencies and cultural stereotypes that often lead to prejudice and discrimination against members of certain groups (Andrews & Boyle, 2003).*
- Recognize the impact of culture on self-care behaviors. **EB:** *Self-care practices play a critical role in the management of chronic illness, yet little is known about the self-care practices of chronically ill African Americans or how lack of access to health care affects health. Self-care practices are culturally based; the cultural component of self-care has been underemphasized, and self-care strategies to maximize chronic illness management have not been realized for people who lack access to health care (Becker, Gates, & Newsom, 2004).* **EB:** *In noting the factors that influence self-efficacy in HIV risk reduction among Asian and Pacific Islanders, variations in reported self-efficacy for female respondents are explained by acculturation, comfort in asking medical practitioners about HIV/AIDS, and to a lesser degree such variables as age, education, and HIV knowledge (Takahashi et al, 2006).*
- Provide culturally competent care. *Culturally competent care implies that within the delivered care the provider understands and attends to the total context of the client's situation. It is a complex combination of knowledge, attitude, and skills (Spector, 2004). Cultural competence is a continuous process of awareness, knowledge, skill, interaction, and sensitivity that is demonstrated among those who render care and the services they provide (Giger & Davidhizar, 2004).*
- Support independent self-care activities. **EB:** *In a study of self care practices of migrant and seasonal farm workers, a majority of self-care practices were judged as appropriate for the health problem (Anthony et al, 2009).*

Home Care

- The nursing interventions described above may also be used in home care settings.
- Implement standardized nursing languages such as NANDA-I nursing diagnoses, NIC, and NOC in home care documentation. **EBN:** *In a home care study that examined the effects of using the NOC and the Outcomes and Information Data Set (OASIS) for measuring client outcomes, the NOC was more sensitive to variations in client outcomes than OASIS and more effectively illustrated the need for nursing services (Schneider, Barkauskas, & Keenan, 2008).*
- Support the new sense of self that may occur with complex health problems. **EBN:** *In an integrative review of studies with heart failure clients, it was shown that a new sense of self permeated clients'*

● = Independent   ▲ = Collaborative   **EBN** = Evidence-Based Nursing   **EB** = Evidence-Based

attempts to deal with the day-to-day management (self-care) of the health problem (Welstand, Carson, & Rutherford, 2009).

- Assist individuals and families to prevent exacerbations of chronic illness symptoms so rehospitalization is not necessary. **EBN:** *Rehospitalization is expensive and demoralizing for clients and providers. In a database analyses of OASIS, of 145,191 people with heart failure in home care, 15% experienced rehospitalization (Madigan, 2008).*
- In complex chronic illnesses such as heart failure, help individuals and families to accept continued functional disabilities and work toward maintenance of optimum functional status, considering the reality of illness status. **EBN:** *In the database analysis of 145,191 cases in OASIS of people with heart failure at home, there was only a small improvement in functional status over an average of 44 home care visits (Madigan, 2008).*
- Use educational guidelines for stroke survivors. **EBN:** *Evidence-based educational guidelines were developed and tested in 1150 home visits (Ostwald et al, 2008).*
- Ensure appropriate interdisciplinary communication to support client safety. **EBN:** *In a study of an interdisciplinary Community of Practice across seven clinical sites in Canada, the focus on improved interprofessional communication was associated with improved quality of care and client safety (White et al, 2008).*
- Enhance individual and family coping with chronic illnesses. **EBN:** *In a study of 113 adults three weeks after hospital discharge, many difficulties with coping were identified (Fitzgerald Miller, Placentine, & Weiss, 2008).*
- Implement a community care management program. **EBN:** *For 12 years, a community care management program in Colorado with a focus on improving the quality of life and facilitating the self-efficacy of elderly chronically ill individuals and families has successively achieved its goals and demonstrated an 81% reduction in financial losses during 2006 for emergency and inpatient services (Luzinski et al, 2008).*

Client/Family Teaching and Discharge Planning

- Teach clients how to regularly assess their level of self-care.
- Instruct clients that a variety of interventions may be needed to enhance self-care.
- Help clients to understand that enhanced self-care is an achievable goal.
- Empower clients.
- Teach clients about the decision-making process and self-care activities needed to manage their illness state and promote well-being.
- Continuously stress that all self-care activities must be regularly evaluated to ensure that enhanced levels of self-care can be maintained.

evolve   See the EVOLVE website for Weblinks for client education resources.

REFERENCES

Andrews M, Boyle J: *Transcultural concepts in nursing care,* ed 4, Philadelphia, 2003, Lippincott Williams & Wilkins.

Anthony MJ, Martin EG, Avery AM et al: Self care and health-seeking behavior of migrant farmworkers, *J Immigr Minor Health* [Epub ahead of print], Apr 24, 2009.

Baum L: Internet parent support groups for primary caregivers of a child with special health care needs, *Pediatr Nurs* 30(5):381–401, 2004.

Becker G, Gates R, Newsom E: Self-care among chronically ill African Americans: culture, health disparities, and health insurance status, *Am J Public Health* 94(12):2066–2073, 2004.

Bertisch SM, Wee CC, Phillips RS et al: Alternative mind-body therapies used by adults with medical conditions, *J Psychosom Res* 66:511–519, 2009.

Callaghan D: The influence of spiritual growth on adolescents' initiative and responsibility for self-care, *Pediatr Nurs* 31(2):91–97, 2005.

Cavendish R, Konecny L, Naradovy L et al: Patients' perceptions of spirituality and the nurse as a spiritual care provider, *Holist Nurs Pract* 20(1):41–47, 2006.

Chugh A, Williams MV, Grigsby J et al: Better transitions: improving comprehension of discharge instructions, *Front Health Serv Manage* 25(3):11–32, 2009.

Clark AM, Freydberg C, McAlister FA et al: Patient and informal caregiver's knowledge of heart failure: Necessary but insufficient for effective self care, *Eur J Heart Fail* 11(6):617–621, 2009.

Cox K, Taylor S: Orem's self-care deficit nursing theory: pediatric asthma as exemplar, *Nurs Sci Q* 18(3):249–257, 2005.

Czaja SJ, Gitlin LN, Schulz R et al: Development of the Risk Appraisal Measure: a brief screen to identify risk areas and guide interventions for dementia caregivers, *J Am Geriatric Soc* 57(6):1064–1072 , 2009.

Dunn SL, Stommel M, Corser WD et al: Hopelessness and its effect on cardiac rehabilitation exercise participation following hospitalization for acute coronary syndrome, *J Cardiopulm Rehabil Prev* 29(1):32–39, 2009.

Eldh A, Ekman I, Ehnfors M: Conditions for patient participation and non-participation in health care, *Nurs Ethics* 13(5):503–514, 2006.

Elkins M, Cavendish R: Developing a plan for pediatric spiritual care, *Holist Nurs Pract* 14(4):179–184, 2004.

Fitzgerald Miller J, Placentine LB, Weiss M: Coping difficulties after hospitalization, *Clin Nurs Res* 17:278–296, 2008.

Giger J, Davidhizar R: *Transcultural nursing*, ed 4, St Louis, 2004, Mosby.

Harvard School of Public Health: Health Literacy Studies. www.hsph.harvard.edu/healthliteracy. Accessed May 26, 2009.

Jacob L, Poletick EB: Systematic review: predictors of successful transition to community-based care for adults with chronic care needs, *Care Manag J* 9:154–165, 2008.

Janson SL, McGrath KW, Covington JK et al: Individualized asthma self-management improves medication adherence and markers of asthma control, *J Allergy Clin Immunol* 123:840–846, 2009.

Lee CS, Suwanno J, Riegel B: The relationship between self-care and health status domains in Thai patients with heart failure, *Eur J Cardiovasc Nurs* [Epub ahead of print], May 1, 2009.

Lewin AB, Lagreca AM, Geffken GR et al: Validity and reliability of an adolescent and parent rating scale of type 1 diabetes adherence behaviors: the self care inventory, *J Pediatr Psychol* 34(9):999–1007, 2009.

Luzinski CH, Stockbridge E, Craighead J et al: The community care management program: for 12 years, caring at its best, *Geriatr Nurs* 29:207–215, 2008.

Madigan EA: People with heart failure and home care resource use and outcomes, *J Clin Nurs* 17(7B):253–259, 2008.

Marziali E: E-health program for patients with chronic disease, *Telemed J E Health* 15:176–181, 2009.

Moore J, Beckwitt A: Children with cancer and their parents: self-care and dependent-care practices, *Issues Compr Pediatr Nurs* 27:1–17, 2004.

Meyerson KL, Kline KS: Qualitative analysis of a mutual goal-setting intervention in participants with heart failure, *Heart Lung* 38(1):1–9, 2009.

Orem D: *Nursing concepts of practice*, ed 6, St Louis, 2001, Mosby.

Ostwald SK, Davis S, Hersch G et al: Evidence-based educational guidelines for stroke survivors after discharge home, *J Neurosci Nurs* 40:173–179, 2008.

Pallant JF, Keenan AM, Misajon R et al: Measuring the impact and distress of osteoarthritis from the patients' perspective, *Health Qual Life Outcomes* 7:37, 2009.

Schmutte T, Flanagan E, Bedregal L et al: Self efficacy and self care: missing ingredients in health and healthcare among adults with serious mental illnesses, *Psychiatr Q* 80(1):1–8, 2009.

Schneider JS, Barkauskas V, Keenan G: Evaluating home health care nursing outcomes with OASIS and NOC, *J Nurs Scholarsh* 40:76–82, 2008.

Scobbie L, Wyke S, Dixon D: Identifying and applying psychological theory to setting and achieving rehabilitation goals, *Clin Rehabil* 23:321–333, 2009.

Sousa VD, Hartman SW, Miller EH et al: New measures of diabetes self care agency, diabetes self efficacy, and diabetes self management for insulin-treated individuals with type 2 diabetes, *J Clin Nurs* 18:1305–1312, 2009.

Spector R: *Cultural diversity in health and illness*, ed 6, Upper Saddle River, NJ, 2004, Prentice Hall.

Takahashi LM, Magalong MG, Debell P et al: HIV and AIDS in suburban Asian and Pacific Islander communities: factors influencing self-efficacy in HIV risk reduction, *AIDS Educ Prev* 18(6):529–545, 2006.

Vitale A: Nurses' lived experience of Reiki for self care, *Holist Nurs Pract* 23:129–141, 2009.

Wallace AS, Seligman HK, Davis TC et al: Literacy appropriate educational materials and brief counseling improve diabetes self management, *Patient Educ Couns* 75(3):328–33, 2009.

Welstand J, Carson A, Rutherford P: Living with heart failure: An integrative review, *Int J Nurs Stud* 46(10):1374–1385, 2009.

White D, Suter E, Parboosingh IJ et al: Communities of practice: creating opportunities to enhance quality of care and safe practices, *Health Q* 11(3):80–84, 2008.

Yarcheski T, Mahon N, Yarcheski A: Social support, self-esteem, and positive health practices of early adolescents, *Psychol Rep* 92:99–103, 2003.

Yeom HE, Heidrich SM: Effect of perceived barriers to symptom management on quality of life in older breast cancer survivors, *Cancer Nurs* 32(4):309–316, 2009.

Bathing Self-Care deficit   *Linda S. Williams, MSN, RN*

NANDA-I

Definition

Impaired ability to perform or complete bathing/hygiene activities for self

Defining Characteristics

Inability to access bathroom; inability to dry body; inability to get bath supplies; inability to obtain water source; inability to regulate bath water; inability to wash body

Related Factors (r/t)

Cognitive impairment; decreased motivation; environmental barriers; inability to perceive body part; inability to perceive spatial relationship; musculoskeletal impairment; neuromuscular impairment; pain; perceptual impairment; severe anxiety; weakness

NOTE: Specify level of independence using a standardized functional scale.

NOC   (Nursing Outcomes Classification)

Suggested NOC Outcomes

Self-Care: Activities of Daily Living (ADL), Self-Care: Bathing, Self-Care: Hygiene

• = Independent   ▲ = Collaborative   **EBN** = Evidence-Based Nursing   **EB** = Evidence-Based

Example NOC Outcome with Indicators
Self-Care: Activities of Daily Living (ADL) as evidenced by the following indicators: Bathing/Hygiene (Rate outcome and indicators of **Self-Care: Activities of Daily Living (ADL):** 1 = severely compromised, 2 = substantially compromised, 3 = moderately compromised, 4 = mildly compromised, 5 = not compromised [see Section I].)

Client Outcomes

Client Will (Specify Time Frame):

- Remain free of body odor and maintain intact skin
- State satisfaction with ability to use adaptive devices to bathe
- Use methods to bathe safely with minimal difficulty
- Bathe with assistance of caregiver as needed and report satisfaction, and dignity maintained during bathing experience
- Bathe with assistance of caregiver as needed without exhibiting defensive (aggressive) behaviors

NIC (Nursing Interventions Classification)

Suggested NIC Intervention

Self-Care Assistance: Bathing/Hygiene

Example NIC Activities—Self-Care Assistance: Bathing/Hygiene
Determine amount and type of assistance needed; Consider the culture of the patient when promoting self-care activities; Provide assistance until patient is fully able to assume self-care

Nursing Interventions and *Rationales*

- Consider using a prepackaged bath, especially for high-risk clients (elderly, immunocompromised, invasive procedures, wounds, catheters, drains), to avoid client exposure to pathogens from contaminated bath basin, water source, and release of skin flora into bath water. **EBN:** *Use of cleansing cloths avoids exposure to bath basins (which are bacterial reservoirs), contaminated tap water, cross-contamination from use of one cloth to bathe the entire body and contamination of sink and surrounding area from bath water disposal (Johnson, Lineweave, & Maze, 2009).*
- Establish the goal of client's bathing as being a pleasant experience, especially for cognitively impaired clients, without the symptoms of unmet needs—hitting, biting, kicking, screaming, resisting—and plan for client preferences in timing, type and length of bathing, water temperature, and with silence or music. **EBN:** *Sensations that make bathing pleasant should be used for everyone to avoid behaviors that are symptoms of unpleasant bathing, which are often due to pain (Rader et al, 2006).*
- Role model and teach the sequence of behaviors for client-centered care: greet client, orient client to task, offer client choices and input, converse with client, and exhibit interest in client and convey approval of client as a person. **EBN:** *Nurses can role model person-centered caregiving during care and in communications with caregivers to allow caregivers to experience personalized interactions (Grosch, Medvene, & Wolcott, 2008).*
- Use client-centered bathing interventions: plan for client's comfort and bathing preferences, show respect in communications, critically think to solve issues that arise, and use a gentle approach. **EBN:** *Focusing on the client rather than the task of bathing results in greater comfort and fewer aggressive (defensive) behaviors (Hoeffer et al, 2006).*
- Develop a bathing care plan based on the client's own history of bathing practices that addresses skin needs, self-care needs, client response to bathing, and equipment needs. *Bathing is a healing rite and should be a comforting experience that concentrates on the client's needs, rather than being a routinely scheduled task (Rasin & Barrick, 2004).*
- Individualize bathing by identifying the function of bathing frequency required to achieve function (e.g., odor, urine removal), and best bathing form (e.g., towel bathing, tub, shower) to meet client preferences, preserve client dignity, make bathing a soothing experience, and reduce client aggression. **EB:** *Client behaviors labeled as aggressive are likely defensive behavior that results from feeling threatened or anxious and increases with shower (especially) and tub bathing. Towel bathing increases*

• = Independent ▲ = Collaborative **EBN** = Evidence-Based Nursing **EB** = Evidence-Based

privacy and eliminates need to move the client to central bathing area; therefore it is a more soothing experience than either showering or tub bathing (Perlmutter & Camberg, 2004).

- Provide a 41° C footbath for 40 minutes prior to bedtime. **EBN:** *Wakefulness decreased after footbath prior to bedtime (Liao, Chiu, & Landis, 2008).*

▲ Provide pain relief measures, such as ice packs, heat, and analgesics for sore joints 45 minutes before bathing; move extremities slowly and carefully; and inform the client before movements associated with pain occur (walking; transferring to a new location; moving joints; and washing genitals, face, and between toes and under arms). Have the client wash painful areas, recognize indicators of pain, and apologize for any pain caused. **EBN:** *Pain relief and client participation reduces discomfort, preserves dignity, and gives a sense of control (Rader et al, 2006).*

- Consider environmental and human factors that may limit bathing ability, such as bending to get into the tub, reaching for bathing items, grasping faucets, and lifting oneself. Adapt environment by placing items within easy reach, installing grab bars, lowering faucets, and using a handheld shower. **EB:** Adapting *environmental factors for bathing may help prevent bathing disability and promote bathing independence (Naik & Gill, 2005).*

- Use a comfortable padded shower chair with foot support, or adapt a chair: pad it with towels/washcloths, cover the cold back with dry towels, and cover the arms with foam pipe insulation. **EBN:** *Unpadded shower chairs with large openings and no foot support contribute to pain by allowing clients to sink into the opening with their feet unsupported (Rader et al, 2006).*

- Provide privacy, encourage a traffic-free bathing area, and post privacy signs. *The client perceives less privacy if more than one caregiver participates or if bathing takes place in a central bathing area in a high-traffic location that allows staff to enter freely during care (Calkins, 2005).*

- Have consistent caregiver assist with bathing. **EBN:** *Consistent caregiver allows development of a relationship and understanding of client's bathing wishes and needs (Rader et al, 2006).*

- Ensure bathing assistance preserves client dignity through conveyance of honor and recognition of the deservedness of respect and esteem of all persons, regardless of their dependency and infirmity. **EB:** *Needing assistance with bathing, being hospitalized, and having pain, were among the most significant issues fracturing a sense of the terminally ill client's dignity, which resulted in a higher desire for death and loss of will to live (Chochinov et al, 2002).*

- If the client is bathing alone, place the assistance call light within reach. *A readily available signaling device promotes safety and provides reassurance for the client.*

- For cognitively impaired clients, avoid upsetting factors associated with bathing: instead of using the terms *bath*, *shower*, or *wash*, use comforting words, such as *warm*, *relaxing*, or *massage*. Start at the client's feet and bathe upward; bathe the face last after washing hands and using a clean cloth. Use a beautician/barber or wash hair at another time to avoid water dripping in the face. **EBN:** *Some words are associated with unpleasant bathing experiences, whereas others convey a pleasant bathing experience. Starting with the face or hair is distressing, because water drips on the face and the head becomes cold and wet (Rader et al, 2006).*

- Use towel bathing to bathe client in bed using no-rinse soap, a bath blanket, and warm towels to keep the client covered the entire time. Warm and moisten towels/washcloths with no-rinse soap and place in plastic bags to keep them warm. Use the towels to massage large areas (front, back) and one washcloth for facial areas and another one for genital areas. No rinsing or drying is needed as is commonly thought for bathing. **EBN:** *Towel bathing is a gentle experience with less discomfort that significantly reduces aggression, as well as bathing time and soap residue over showering without accumulation of pathogenic bacteria (Sloane et al, 2004; Hoeffer et al, 2006).*

- For shower bathing: use client-centered techniques, keep client covered with towels and cleanse under the towels, use no-rinse products, use favorite bathing items, and use a handheld shower with adjustable spray. **EBN:** *Covering the client is an easy means to maintain dignity, reduce embarrassment, and keep the client warm and unexposed without increasing bathing time (Rader et al, 2006).*

- Allow the client to participate as able in bathing. Smile and provide praise for accomplishments in a relaxed manner. **EB:** *Improved client-centered communication decreases aggression during bathing and individualizes care (Perlmutter & Camberg, 2004).*

- Inspect skin condition during bathing. *Towel bathing facilitates inspection of skin to detect skin problems.*

Geriatric

- Design the bathing environment for comfort: **Visual.** Reduce clutter and use partitions to hide equipment storage. Laminate and put artwork or decorative objects in bather's view, or place cue cards to bathing process (wall, ceiling, shower). Stand or sit in bather's position to experience what he/she sees. Decrease glare from tiles, white walls, and artificial lights. Use contrasting colors and soft but adequate lighting on a dimming switch for adjustment. *Bathing rooms are sterile, institutional, and frightening spaces filled with unfamiliar equipment—tubs with sides that open up and look like they might swallow you, or gurneys with arms that look like construction cranes. Overhead lights can be bright and shine into the bather's eyes. Glare can cause visual discomfort, especially in clients with visual changes or cataracts (Calkins, 2005).*
- Arrange the bathing environment to promote sensory comfort: **Auditory.** Reduce noise of voices and water. Do not allow traffic into bathing room. Add fabric to absorb sound (three to four times the width of the opening for sound absorbing folds). Play soft music. *Noise discomfort can result from high-echo tiled walls, loud voices, and running water. Traffic can compromise privacy. Absorb negative sounds, and add positive sounds through music (Calkins, 2005).*
- Design the bathing environment for comfort: **Tactile.** Use heat lamps or radiant heat panels to keep the room warm. Use powder-coated grab bars in decorative colors with nonslip grip. Provide a soft rug to stand on. Ensure that flooring is not slippery (a high coefficient of friction, ideally above 80, is desired and obtained through flooring coatings). *If the caregiver is warm to the point of sweating, room temperature is about right for an older person being bathed. Appealing, stable grab bars are needed for balance. Preventing the floor from becoming slippery from water is essential (Calkins, 2005).*
- When bathing a cognitively impaired client, have all bathing items ready for the client's needs before bathing begins. *Injury often occurs when a cognitively impaired client is left alone while forgotten items are obtained.*
- Teach caregivers to use behaviors that validate the client's feelings, reassure the client, and segment tasks, and to explain the care process while bathing clients with Alzheimer's disease. **EBN:** *Caregivers should work to make bathing more therapeutic for individuals with Alzheimer's disease (Somboontanont et al, 2004).*
- Train caregivers bathing clients with dementia to avoid behaviors that can trigger assault: confrontational communication, invalidation of the resident's feelings, failure to prepare a resident for a task, initiating shower spray or touch during bathing without verbal prompts beforehand, washing the hair/face, speaking disrespectfully to the client, and hurrying the pace of the bath. **EBN:** *During bathing, assaults (defensive behavior) by nursing home residents with dementia are frequently triggered by caregiver actions that startle, frighten, hurt, or upset the resident. This might happen when caregivers spray water on a resident without warning or when they touch a resident's feet, axilla, or perineum, possibly due to the startle reflex (Somboontanont et al, 2004).*
- Limit total body bathing using tepid water to once a week; provide a towel bath at other times. **EBN:** *Frequent bathing and using hot water promotes skin dryness (Rader et al, 2006).*
- Use a prepackaged bath for older adults to prevent skin dryness. **EBN:** *A prepackaged bath regimen proved much more effective than the traditional soap and water method in preventing flaking and scaling and improving overall skin condition (Joanna Briggs Institute, 2007).*
- Test water temperature before use with a thermometer to prevent scalding. *With assistive bathing, temperature changes are not felt by the person controlling them (Fathers, 2004).*
- Teach caregiver to use gentle touch and massage for frail, older adult clients during bathing. *Gentle massage is desired by clients to reduce pain or agitation (Perimutter & Camberg, 2004).*

 Multicultural

- Ask the client for input on bathing habits and cultural bathing preferences. **EB:** *Creating opportunities for guiding personal care honors long-standing routines, increases control, and makes bath time more pleasant for client and caregiver (Perimutter & Camberg, 2004).*

Home Care

- If in a typical bathing setting for the client, assess the client's ability to bathe self via direct observation using physical performance tests for ADLs. *Observation of bathing performed in an atypical bathing setting may result in false data.*
- ▲ Request referrals for occupational and physical therapy if client has difficulty showering or getting into a tub. **EBN:** *Interdisciplinary team member's assessment of a client's functional abilities increases the client's mastery of self-care tasks by identifying aids, such as grab bars or bath seats, that allow the client to participate in the task more easily (Rader et al, 2006).*
- ▲ Based on functional assessment and rehabilitation capacity, refer for home health aide services to assist with bathing and hygiene. *Support by home health aides preserves the energy of the client and provides respite for caregivers.*
- Turn down temperature of hot water heater and recommend use of a water temperature–sensing shower valve to prevent scalding. *Older or disabled people have slower reflexes to respond to hot water and may be unable to regulate water temperature, yet they may be left unattended. Water at 130° F produces a first-degree burn in 20 seconds; at 135° to 140° F, exposure for 5 to 6 seconds causes third-degree burns (Fathers, 2004).*
- Cue cognitively impaired clients in the steps of hygiene. *Cognitively impaired clients can successfully participate in many activities with cueing, and participation in self-care can enhance their self-esteem.*
- If a terminally ill client requests hygiene care, make an extra effort to meet the request and provide care when the client and family will most benefit (e.g., before visitors arrive, at bedtime, in the early morning). *When desired, improved hygiene greatly boosts the morale of terminally ill clients.*

Client/Family Teaching and Discharge Planning

- Teach the client and family how to use adaptive devices for bathing (e.g., long-handled brushes, soap-on-a-rope, washcloth mitt, wall bars, tub bench, padded shower chair, commode chair without pan), and teach bathing techniques that promote safety and prevent burns (e.g., getting into tub before filling it with water if a temperature sensor valve is used; testing water with a thermometer; emptying water before getting out; using an antislip mat, wall-grab bars, and tub bench). **EB:** *Follow-up teaching in the home increases device use and safety of bathing (Chiu & Man, 2004).*
- Teach the client and family a client-centered bathing routine that includes a frequency schedule, privacy, skin inspection, no-rinse products, skin lubricants, chill prevention, and bathing options, such as sponge or towel. **EBN:** *Families and caregivers who are taught methods to meet the client's bathing needs can increase the client's satisfaction with the bathing experience in a quicker, easier, and less anxious manner (Rader et al, 2006).*

ⓔvolve See the EVOLVE website for Weblinks for client education resources.

REFERENCES

Calkins M: Designing bathing rooms that comfort, *Nurs Homes* 54(1):54–55, 2005.

Chiu C, Man D: The effect of training older adults with stroke to use home-based assistive devices, *OTJR* 24(3):113–120, 2004.

Chochinov H, Hack T, Hassard T et al: Dignity in the terminally ill: a cross-sectional, cohort study, *Lancet* 360(9350):2026–2030, 2002.

Fathers B: Bathing safety for the elderly and disabled, *Nurs Homes* 53(9):50–52, 2004.

Grosch K, Medvene L, Wolcott H: Person-centered caregiving instruction for geriatric nursing assistant students: development and evaluation, *J Gerontol Nurs* 34(8):23–31, 2008.

Hoeffer B, Amann Talerico K, Rasin J et al: Assisting cognitively impaired nursing home residents with bathing: effects of two bathing interventions on caregiving, *Gerontologist* 46(4):524–532, 2006.

Joanna Briggs Institute: Topical skin care in aged care facilities, *Best Practice* 11(3), 2007.

Johnson D, Lineweaver L, Maze L: Patient's bath basins as potential sources of infection: a multicenter sampling study, *Am J Crit Care* 18(1):31–38, 2009.

Liao W, Chiu M, Landis C: A warm footbath before bedtime and sleep in older Taiwanese with sleep disturbance, *Res Nurs Health* 31(5):514–528, 2008.

Naik A, Gill T: Underutilization of environmental adaptations for bathing in community-living older persons, *J Am Geriatr Soc* 53(9):1497–1503, 2005.

Perimutter J, Camberg L: Better bathing for residents with Alzheimer's, *Nurs Homes* 53(4):40–42, 2004.

Rader J, Barrick AL, Hoeffer B et al: The bathing of older adults with dementia: easing the unnecessarily unpleasant aspects of assisted bathing, *Am J Nurs* 106(4):4–49, 2006.

Rasin J, Barrick AL: Bathing patients with dementia, *Am J Nurs* 104(3):30–34, 2004.

• = Independent ▲ = Collaborative **EBN** = Evidence-Based Nursing **EB** = Evidence-Based

Sloane P, Hoeffer B, Mitchell C et al: Effect of person-centered showering and the towel bath on bathing-associated aggression, agitation,
   and discomfort in nursing home residents with dementia: a randomized, controlled trial, *J Am Geriatr Soc* 52(11):1795–1804, 2004.

Somboontanont W, Sloane P, Floyd F et al: Assaultive behavior in
   Alzheimer's disease: identifying immediate antecedents during bathing, *J Gerontol Nurs* 30(9):22–29, 2004.

Dressing Self-Care deficit   *Linda S. Williams, MSN, RN*

NANDA-I

Definition

Impaired ability to perform or complete dressing and grooming activities for self

Defining Characteristics

Inability to choose clothing; inability to put clothing on lower body; inability to maintain appearance at a satisfactory level; inability to pick up clothing; inability to put clothing on upper body; inability to put on shoes; inability to put on socks; inability to remove clothes; inability to remove shoes; inability to remove socks; inability to use assistive devices; inability to use zippers; impaired ability to fasten clothing; impaired ability to obtain clothing; impaired ability to put on necessary items of clothing; impaired ability to put on shoes; impaired ability to put on socks; impaired ability to take off necessary items of clothing; impaired ability to take off shoes; impaired ability to take off socks

Related Factors (r/t)

Cognitive impairment; decreased motivation; discomfort; environmental barriers; fatigue; musculoskeletal impairment; neuromuscular impairment; pain; perceptual impairment; severe anxiety; weakness

NOTE: Specify level of independence using a standardized functional scale.

NOC   (Nursing Outcomes Classification)

Suggested NOC Outcomes

Self-Care: Activities of Daily Living (ADL), Dressing, Hygiene, Grooming

Example NOC Outcome with Indicators
Self-Care: Dressing as evidenced by the following indicators: Gets clothing from drawer and closet/Puts clothing on upper body and lower body (Rate outcome and indicators of **Self-Care: Dressing:** 1 = severely compromised, 2 = substantially compromised, 3 = moderately compromised, 4 = mildly compromised, 5 = not compromised [see Section I].)

Client Outcomes

Client Will (Specify Time Frame):

- Dress and groom self to optimal potential
- Use adaptive devices to dress and groom
- Explain and use methods to enhance strengths during dressing and grooming
- Dress and groom with assistance of caregiver as needed

NIC   (Nursing Interventions Classification)

Suggested NIC Intervention

Self-Care Assistance: Dressing/Grooming

Example NIC Activities—Self-Care Assistance: Dressing/Grooming
Be available for assistance in dressing, as necessary; Reinforce efforts to dress self; Maintain privacy while the patient is dressing

• = Independent   ▲ = Collaborative   **EBN** = Evidence-Based Nursing   **EB** = Evidence-Based

Nursing Interventions and *Rationales*

- Assess a client's range of movement, upper limb strength, balance, coordination, functional grip, dexterity, sensation, and ability to detect limb position. *Dressing requires complex functions, and any impairment in these areas causes problems with dressing (Swann, 2008).*
- ▲ Provide pain medication 45 minutes before dressing and grooming as needed. *Time medication administration to make dressing or grooming easier (Swann, 2006).*
- Select adaptive clothing: loose clothing; elastic waistbands and cuffs; square, large arm holes; no seam lines; dresses that open down the back and short coats (for wheelchair users); Velcro fasteners; larger or magnetic buttons; zipper pulls for grasping; and for drooling, absorbent scarves that can be easily changed. *Adapting clothing can make dressing easier for those with impaired mobility or fine motor skills and help prevent pressure sores (Swann, 2008).*
- For clients with limited arm and shoulder movement use clothing that fastens at the front, such as for blouses, bras, and shirts. *Clients with stiff arms and shoulders, as with arthritis, may have difficulty with raising the arms to put on clothing over the head, such as with T-shirts (Nazarko, 2008).*
- Allow client with poor balance or postural hypotension to sit rather than stand when dressing, for safety. *Dressing and undressing may be carried out from a seated position (Swann, 2008).*
- Dress the affected side first, then the unaffected side; for undressing the affected side is done last. *Dressing the affected side first allows for easier manipulation of clothing (Swann, 2008).*
- Use adaptive dressing and grooming equipment as needed (e.g., long-handled brushes, long grasping devices, button hooks, elastic shoelaces, Velcro shoes, soap-on-a-rope, suction holders). *Adaptive devices increase self-care ability, and can decrease exertion (Swann, 2006).*
- For clients with a fine hand tremor, use weighted handles on grooming items or stabilize the client's arm on a table; for a weak or painful grip use lightweight, large-grip handles. *Adaptive handles or arm support can be helpful and may help control fine tremors (Swann, 2006).*
- ▲ Request referral for occupational therapy. **EB:** *Following a stroke, people were more independent in ADLs if they received treatment from an occupational therapist (Legg, Drummond, & Langhorne, 2006).*
- Maintain individuality with hairstyle, jewelry, and clothing. *Maintaining individuality helps to define a person's identity and promote self-esteem (Swann, 2008).*

Geriatric

- Determine the client's personal preferences for dressing and grooming by using the Self-maintenance Habits and Preferences in Elderly (SHAPE) questionnaire and focus on items most preferred by the client. **EB:** *The SHAPE questionnaire measures a client's customary daily routines to plan for personal preferences in dressing and grooming during self-care (Cohen-Mansfield & Jensen, 2007a).*
- Assist residents with goal setting and their highest ADL performance level rather than providing the care for them. *Participation in self-care improves functioning, self-esteem, and family and caregiver satisfaction while reducing functional decline and disability (Resnik et al, 2008).*
- Ensure clients can see clothing to select what to wear by administering annual vision testing and having client wear clean glasses. *Older adults' visual problems or dirty glasses impair clothing and color choices (Nazarko, 2008).*
- Encourage older clients to dress and groom rather than completing the tasks for them. *Performing self-care helps maintain independence and prevents functional decline, which is a common complication of institutionalization for older adults (Graf, 2006).*
- Use clocks, routines, and explanations for the client with dementia to convey that it is morning and time to get ready for the day's activities by dressing. *Clients with dementia often do not know the reason for needing to dress (Nazarko, 2008).*
- Lay clothing out (with label in back facing up) in the order that it will be put on by the client either one item at a time or in piles with first item on top of pile (dress bottom half first: underwear, then slacks, socks; then dress top half: bra, shirt, sweater). *Clients with dementia may have difficulty recognizing what a clothing item is and in what order and how to put it on (Nazarko, 2008).*
- ▲ Request referral for physical therapy. **EB:** *Physical rehabilitation for long-term care residents reduces disability to promote independence in ADLs (Forster et al, 2009).*

• = Independent ▲ = Collaborative **EBN** = Evidence-Based Nursing **EB** = Evidence-Based

Home Care

▲ Involve the client in planning of informal care and provide access to health professionals and financial support for the care. **EBN:** *To maintain self-care in dressing/grooming it is important to have continuity between past and present practices, so staff needs to be aware of and be sensitive to an individual's preferences and prior routines (Cohen-Mansfield & Jensen, 2007b).*

Client/Family Teaching and Discharge Planning

- Teach caregivers to see dressing as an opportunity to promote independence and a better quality of life for clients who are able, and as a time to increase social talk for others. **EB:** *The dressing process should not be viewed as a race for efficiency but rather a time to retain independence in dressing skills, and for social interaction that reduces isolation and loneliness by allowing residents to experience social contact and exercise (Cohen-Mansfield et al, 2006).*
- ▲ Consider referral for use of assistive technology to prompt independent learning of self-care skills such as dressing. **EB:** *Those with disabilities may be taught to dress independently with use of preferred stimuli–prompting assistive technology (visual—lights, auditory—music/verbal, vibratory) delivered upon failure to respond to a dressing task (Lancioni et al, 2007).*

Ѳvolve See the EVOLVE website for Weblinks for client education resources.

REFERENCES

Cohen-Mansfield J, Creedon MA, Malone T et al: Dressing of cognitively impaired nursing home residents: description and analysis, *Gerontologist* 46(1):89–96, 2006.

Cohen-Mansfield J, Jensen B: Self-maintenance Habits and Preferences in Elderly (SHAPE): reliability of reports of self-care preferences in older persons, *Aging Clin Exp Res* 19(1):61–68, 2007a.

Cohen-Mansfield J, Jensen B: Dressing and grooming: preferences of community-dwelling older adults, *J Gerontol Nurs* 33(2):31–39, 2007b.

Forster A, Lambley R, Hardy J et al: Rehabilitation for older people in long-term care, *Cochrane Database Syst Rev* (1):CD004294, 2009.

Graf C: Functional decline in hospitalized older adults, *Am J Nurs* 106(1):58–67, 2006.

Lancioni G, O'Reilly M, Singh N et al: Helping three persons with multiple disabilities acquire independent dressing through assistive technology, *J Vis Impair Blind* 12:768–773, 2007.

Legg L, Drummond A, Langhorne P: Occupational therapy for patients with problems in activities of daily living after stroke, *Cochrane Database Syst Rev*(4): CD003585, 2006.

Nazarko L: Dressed to impress: dressing in dementia, *Nurs Resident Care* 10(8):401–403, 2008.

Resnick B, Petzer-Aboff I, Galik, E et al: Barriers and benefits to implementing a restorative care intervention in nursing homes, *J Am Med Dir Assoc* 9:102–108, 2008.

Swann J: Keeping up appearances, *Nurs Resident Care* 8(11):517–520, 2006.

Swann J: Managing dressing problems in older adults in long-term care, *Nurs Resident Care* 10(11):564–567, 2008.

Feeding Self-Care deficit   *Linda S. Williams, MSN, RN*

Definition

Impaired ability to perform or complete self-feeding activities

Defining Characteristics

Inability to bring food from a receptacle to the mouth; inability to chew food; inability to complete a meal; inability to get food onto utensil; inability to handle utensils; inability to ingest food in a socially acceptable manner; inability to ingest food safely; inability to ingest sufficient food; inability to manipulate food in mouth; inability to open containers; inability to pick up cup or glass; inability to prepare food for ingestion; inability to swallow food; inability to use assistive device

Related Factors (r/t)

Cognitive impairment; decreased motivation; discomfort; environmental barriers; fatigue; musculoskeletal impairment; neuromuscular impairment; pain; perceptual impairment; severe anxiety; weakness

NOTE: Specify level of independence using a standardized functional scale.

● = Independent   ▲ = Collaborative   **EBN** = Evidence-Based Nursing   **EB** = Evidence-Based

(Nursing Outcomes Classification)

Suggested NOC Outcomes

Self-Care: Activities of Daily Living (ADL), Eating

Example NOC Outcome with Indicators
Self-Care: Eating as evidenced by the following indicators: Opens containers/Uses utensils/Completes a meal (Rate the outcome and indicators of **Self-Care: Eating:** 1 = severely compromised, 2 = substantially compromised, 3 = moderately compromised, 4 = mildly compromised, 5 = not compromised [see Section I].)

Client Outcomes

Client Will (Specify Time Frame):

- Feed self safely
- State satisfaction with ability to use adaptive devices for feeding
- Use assistance with feeding when necessary (caregiver)

 (Nursing Interventions Classification)

Suggested NIC Intervention

Self-Care Assistance: Feeding

Example NIC Activities—Self-Care Assistance: Feeding
Provide adaptive devices to facilitate the client's feeding self (e.g., long handles, handle with large circumference, or small strap-on utensils), as needed; Provide frequent cueing and close supervision as appropriate

Nursing Interventions and *Rationales*

- Assess for choking and swallowing risk for clients with learning disability and note condition of teeth, medication side effects, and abnormal eating behaviors. **EB:** *Choking is a serious hazard for many adults with learning disabilities, especially with these characteristics (Thacker et al, 2008).*
- ▲ Consult a speech-language pathologist for individualized feeding care plans. **EB:** *Speech-language pathologists design feeding plans to feed clients adequate nutrition in a safe, dignified manner, which nurses report using (McCullough et al, 2007).*
- ▲ Request referral for occupational therapy. **EB:** *Following a stroke, people were more independent in ADLs if they received treatment from an occupational therapist (Boczko & Feightner, 2007).*
- Consider use of protected mealtimes so that all non-urgent clinical activity stops and clients can eat without interruptions, and staff is available to assist. **EBN:** *Clients are more relaxed and eat more, without interruptions and availability of staff assistance, leading to better nutrition and better recovery (Murray, 2006).*
- To increase oral intake, use a feeding assistance intervention protocol: individual assistance, proper positioning, dining location preferences, and meal tray substitutions; use graduated prompting to enhance self-feeding ability as needed: (1) social stimulation and encouragement, (2) nonverbal cueing, (3) verbal cueing, (4) physical guidance, and (5) full physical assistance. **EB:** *Individualized nutritional care increased client daily oral intake for 90% of participants when one or both of the feeding assistance intervention protocols was used, or a between-meal snack was included (Simmons & Schnelle, 2004).*
- To increase oral intake, include between-meal snacks three times a day alone, or if intake is not increased 15% with the feeding assistance intervention protocol (discussed previously) delivered to the client on a movable cart with a variety of food/fluid choices. **EB:** *Individualized nutritional care increased client daily oral intake for 90% of participants when one or both of the feeding assistance intervention protocols was used or the between-meal snack was included (Simmons & Schnelle, 2004).*
- Presentation of feeding: provide 1 teaspoon of solid food or 10 to 15 mL of liquid at a time; wait until client has swallowed prior food/liquid. **EB:** *Feeding large volumes and feeding quickly occurred commonly because caregivers lacked knowledge that this could exacerbate dysphagia and increase the risk of health problems (Pelletier, 2004).*

• = Independent   ▲ = Collaborative   **EBN** = Evidence-Based Nursing   **EB** = Evidence-Based

- Individualize nutritional plan to promote a positive mealtime experience for clients after surgical and radiotherapy treatment for tongue cancer. **EB:** *After surgical and radiotherapy treatment for tongue cancer, clients experienced a negative impact related to time for meal consumption, pleasure in eating, chewing problems, food sticking in throat and mouth, and choking (Costa Bandeira et al, 2008).*
- Assist clients with cancer to plan self-care strategies to promote control (choosing foods), self-worth (food value for survival), and positive relationships (family meal interactions), and use distraction (humor) to manage eating problems. *Clients with cancer used self-care strategies to manage altered eating habits: taking control, promoting self-worth, relationship work, and distraction (Howard, 2008).*

 Geriatric

- Residents require an average of 35 to 40 minutes of staff time per meal to improve oral intake. *Adequate time must be provided for caregivers to assist with meals to promote improved oral intake (Simmons & Schnelle, 2006).*
- Use consistent volunteers or staff to assist residents with meals. **EB:** *Mealtime assistants who have time to develop social relationships with residents, which require consistency, can enhance the mealtime experience for residents in long-term care institutions (Steele, Rivera, & Bernick, 2007).*
- Consider use of slow music during meals. **EB:** *Slower music may improve feeding in older adults with dementia and facilitate caregivers offering more food and time for feeding (Watson & Green, 2006).*
- Use aromatherapy to increase appetite and pleasure in eating. *Making food pleasant and home-like helps prevent weight loss and maintains client independence (Pfeiffer et al, 2005).*
- ▲ Ensure CNAs know the signs/symptoms of dysphagia, such as choking, coughing, oral/chewing problems, throat clearing, wet voice, gurgling voice, or pneumonia; if any of these are exhibited during feeding, report them promptly. **EB:** *CNAs who were knowledgeable of symptoms and who indicated they would report them did not acknowledge or report symptoms during feeding other than to generally feed clients more slowly or with smaller volumes (Pelletier, 2004).*
- ▲ Provide CNAs with information on techniques to feed clients with dementia. **EB:** *This study indicated that nursing assistants stated they needed more training to address feeding difficulty in residents with dementia (Chang & Roberts, 2008).*
- Obtain and incorporate the client's view of the agency's food selection and presentation into agency food service. **EBN:** *The FoodEx-LTC, a 44–item questionnaire that measures food and food service satisfaction, can be used to promote the resident's enjoyment and increase nutritional intake of food (Evans & Crogan, 2005).*
- Provide a dignified assisted dining experience: create a home-like dining room; provide leisurely pace that will allow the client with dentures adequate time to chew; and support choices and independence. **EB:** *Assisted dining can be a dignified experience based on the environment and individualization of feeding (Ruigrok & Sheridan, 2006).*

 Multicultural

- Ask the client for input on methods to facilitate eating and feeding (e.g., cultural foods, other food and fluid preferences developed during a lifetime), and provide four entrée choices, including ethnic choices. **EBN:** *Using client input on preferences individualizes client care (Evans, Crogan, & Schultz, 2005).*
- For those who use chopsticks, suggest adapted chopsticks for those with impaired hand function. **EB:** *Adapted chopsticks can be inexpensive and easily constructed, for those with lower cervical spinal cord injury and residual gross grasp (Chang et al, 2006).*

 Home Care

- ▲ Based on functional assessment and rehabilitation capacity, refer for home health aide services to assist with feeding. *Support by home health aides preserves the energy of the client and provides respite for caregivers.*

Client/Family Teaching and Discharge Planning

- Educate family members about the benefits of hand feeding as long as possible and the benefits and risks of tube feeding for clients with dementia. **EB:** *Studies show that PEG tube feeding does not decrease aspiration or prolong survival for those with dementia (DiBartolo, 2006).*

 See the EVOLVE website for Weblinks for client education resources.

REFERENCES

Boczko F, Feightner K: Dysphagia in the older adult: the roles of speech-language pathologists and occupational therapists, *Top Geriatr Rehabil* 23(3):220–227, 2007.

Chang B, Huang B, Chou C et al: A new type of chopsticks for patients with impaired hand function, *Arch Phys Med Rehabil* 87(7):1013–1015, 2006.

Chang CC, Roberts BL: Cultural perspectives in feeding difficulty in Taiwanese elderly with dementia, *J Nurs Scholarsh* 40(3):235–240, 2008.

Costa Bandeira A, Azevedo E, Vartanian J et al: Quality of life related to swallowing after tongue cancer treatment, *Dysphagia* 23(2):183–192, 2008.

DiBartolo M: Careful hand feeding: a reasonable alternative to PEG tube placement in individuals with dementia, *J Gerontol Nurs* 32(5):25–35, 2006.

Evans BC, Crogan NL: Using the FoodEx-LTC to assess institutional food service practices through nursing home residents' perspectives on nutrition care, *J Gerontol A Biol Sci Med Sci*, 60(1):125–128, 2005.

Evans BC, Crogan NL, Schultz JA: The meaning of mealtimes: connection to the social world of the nursing home, *J Gerontol Nurs* 31(2):11–17, 2005.

Howard A: Patients with advanced cancer used 4 self-action strategies to manage eating-related problems, *Evid Based Nurs* 11(2):61, 2008.

McCullough K, Estes J, McCullough G et al: RN compliance with SLP dysphagia recommendations in acute care, *Top Geriatr Rehabil* 23(4):330–340, 2007.

Murray C: Improving nutrition for older people, *Nurs Older People* 18(6):18–22, 2006.

Pelletier C: What do certified nurse assistants actually know about dysphagia and feeding nursing home residents? *Am J Speech Lang Pathol* 13(2):99–113, 2004.

Pfeiffer NA, Rogers DA, Roseman MR et al: What's new in long-term care dining? *N C Med J* 66(4):287–291, 2005.

Ruigrok J, Sheridan L: Life enrichment programme; enhanced dining experience, a pilot project, *Int J Health Care Qual Assur Inc Leadersh Health Serv* 19(4–5):420–429, 2006.

Simmons S, Schnelle J: Individualized feeding assistance care for nursing home residents: staffing requirements to implement two interventions, *J Gerontol A Biol Sci Med Sci* 59(9):M966–M973, 2004.

Simmons S, Schnelle J: Feeding assistance needs of long-stay nursing home residents and staff time to provide care, *J Am Geriatr Soc* 54(6):919–924, 2006.

Steele C, Rivera T, Bernick L: Insights regarding mealtime assistance for individuals in long-term care: lessons from a time of crisis, *Top Geriatr Rehabil* 23(4):319–329, 2007.

Thacker A, Abdelnoor A, Anderson C et al: Indicators of choking risk in adults with learning disabilities: a questionnaire survey and interview study, *Disabil Rehabil* 30(15):1131–1138, 2008.

Watson R, Green S: Feeding and dementia: a systematic literature review, *J Adv Nurs* 54(1):86–93, 2006.

Toileting Self-Care deficit   *Linda S. Williams, MSN, RN*

NANDA-I

Definition

Impaired ability to perform or complete toileting activities for self

Defining Characteristics

Inability to carry out proper toilet hygiene; inability to flush toilet or commode; inability to get to toilet or commode; inability to manipulate clothing for toileting; inability to rise from toilet or commode; inability to sit on toilet or commode

Related Factors (r/t)

Cognitive impairment; decreased motivation; environmental barriers; fatigue; impaired mobility status; impaired transfer ability; musculoskeletal impairment; neuromuscular impairment; pain; perceptual impairment; severe anxiety; weakness

NOC   (Nursing Outcomes Classification)

Suggested NOC Outcomes

Self-Care: Activities of Daily Living (ADLs), Toileting

• = Independent   ▲ = Collaborative   **EBN** = Evidence-Based Nursing   **EB** = Evidence-Based

Client Outcomes

Client Will (Specify Time Frame):
- Remain free of incontinence and impaction with no urine or stool on skin
- State satisfaction with ability to use adaptive devices for toileting
- Explain and use methods to be safe and independent in toileting

NIC (Nursing Interventions Classification)

Suggested NIC Interventions

Environmental Management, Self-Care Assistance: Toileting

Example NIC Activities—Self-Care Assistance: Toileting
Assist patient to toilet/commode/bedpan/fracture pan/urinal at specified intervals; Institute a toileting schedule, as appropriate

Nursing Interventions and *Rationales*

- Assess ability to toilet, client's usual bowel and bladder toileting patterns, and personal toileting terminology; note specific deficits. *Functional assessment provides analysis data for ADL tasks for use in goal and intervention planning (Lekan-Rutledge, 2004).*
- ▲ Refer clients to occupational therapy. **EB:** *Clients who receive occupational therapy are more likely to be independent in their ability to perform ADLs (Legg, Drummond, & Langhorne, 2006).*
- Use any necessary assistive toileting equipment (e.g., raised toilet seat, bedside commode, suction mats, spill-proof urinals, support rails next to toilet, toilet safety frames, female urinal, fracture bedpans, long-handled toilet paper holders). *Adaptive devices promote independence and safety (Cohen, 2008).*
- Provide privacy. *Lack of privacy may contribute to incontinence or constipation (MacDonald & Butler, 2007).*
- Schedule toileting assistance to occur when the defecation urge is strongest or voiding is likely (e.g., in the morning, every 2 hours, after meals, at bedtime). **EBN:** *Medications (e.g., laxatives), briefs, linens, and enema use can be reduced with a scheduled toileting program (Engst et al, 2004).*
- Make assistance call button readily available to the client and answer call light promptly. **EBN:** *To decrease incontinence and promote safety, the client needs rapid access to toileting facilities (Joanna Briggs Institute, 1999).*

 ### Geriatric

- For residents who show occasional/frequent bowel/bladder incontinence on the Minimum Data Set, plan an individualized toileting schedule. **EBN:** *Assessment makes individualized planning possible and accurate and reduces incontinence (Morgan et al, 2008).*
- Assess the client's functional ability to manipulate clothing for toileting, and if necessary modify clothing with Velcro fasteners, elastic waists, drop-front underwear, or slacks. *For clients with impaired dexterity or weakness, wearing dresses, athletic bottoms, or skirts with a stretch waistband makes it easier to use the toilet than wearing clothing with buttons and zippers (Cohen, 2008).*
- Include regular exercise and a walking program in plan of care. **EB:** *Regular exercise improves functional abilities in clients in long-term care (de Carvalho & Filho, 2004).*
- Provide a small footstool in front of the toilet or commode. **EBN:** *Elevating the knees above the hips increases intraabdominal pressure, which facilitates elimination in elderly persons with weak abdominal muscles (Joanna Briggs Institute, 1999).*

● = Independent   ▲ = Collaborative   **EBN** = Evidence-Based Nursing   **EB** = Evidence-Based

- Avoid the use of indwelling catheters if possible, and use condom catheters in men without dementia. **EB:** *Using a condom catheter rather than an indwelling urinary catheter can reduce infection or death, especially in men without dementia (Saint, Kaufman, & Rodgers, 2006).*

Multicultural

- Remove barriers to toileting, support client's cultural beliefs, and preserve dignity. **EB:** *The physical and sociocultural environments in long-term care require older clients to overcome greater physical and cognitive challenges to maintain their participation, autonomy, and dignity in toileting than if they were at home (Sacco-Peterson & Borell, 2004).*

Home Care

- ▲ Request referral for occupational and physical therapy to identify barriers and suggest strategies for safe toileting. **EB:** *A multicomponent intervention targeting modifiable environmental and behavioral factors results in life quality improvements in community-dwelling older people, especially for toileting (Gitlin et al, 2006).*
- Assess home environmental factors leading to toileting disability. **EB:** *ADL dysfunction was greater in people who perceived an unmet need for accessibility in their home (Stineman et al, 2007).*

Client/Family Teaching and Discharge Planning

- Teach client and family to wash hands after toileting. **EB:** *Interventions that promote hand washing can reduce diarrhea episodes by about one third in children and adults (Ejemot et al, 2008).*
- Teach the client and family about bladder control and how to toilet the client with adaptive and safety devices. **EBN:** *Older clients want to learn about bladder control (Palmer & Newman, 2006).*
- Have the family install a toilet seat of a contrasting color. **EBN:** *Visualization of the toilet is aided by installing a toilet seat of a contrasting color (Gerdner, Buckwalter & Reed, 2002).*

⊖volve   See the EVOLVE website for Weblinks for client education resources.

REFERENCES

Cohen D: Providing an assist, *Rehab Manag* 21(8):16–19, 2008.

de Carvalho B, Filho W: Effect of an exercise program on functional performance of institutionalized elderly, *J Rehabil Res Dev* 41(5):659–668, 2004.

Ejemot RI, Ehiri JE, Meremikwu MM et al: Hand washing for preventing diarrhea, *Cochrane Database Syst Rev*(1): CD004265, 2008.

Engst C, Chhokar R, Robinson D et al: Implementation of a scheduled toileting program in a long term care facility, *AAOHN J* 52(10):427–435, 2004.

Gerdner LA, Buckwalter KC, Reed D: Impact of a psychoeducational intervention on caregiver response to behavioral problems, *Nurs Res* 51(6):363, 2002.

Gitlin LN, Winter K, Dennis MP et al: A randomized trial of a multicomponent home intervention to reduce functional difficulties in older adults, *J Am Geriatr Soc* 54(5):809–816, 2006.

Joanna Briggs Institute: Management of constipation in older adults, *Best Practice* 3(1), 1999.

Legg LA, Drummond AE, Langhorne P: Occupational therapy for patients with problems in activities of daily living after stroke, *Cochrane Database Syst Rev* (4): CD003585, 2006.

Lekan-Rutledge D: Urinary incontinence strategies for frail elderly women, *Urol Nurs* 24(4):281–283, 287–302, 2004.

MacDonald CD, Butler L: Silent no more: elderly women's stories of living with urinary incontinence in long-term care, *J Gerontol Nurs* 33(1):14, 2007.

Morgan C, Endozoa N, Paradiso C et al: Enhanced toileting program decreases incontinence in long term care, *Jt Comm J Qual Patient Saf* 34(4):206–208, 2008.

Palmer M, Newman D: Bladder control: educational needs of older adults, *J Gerontol Nurs* 32(1):28–32, 2006.

Sacco-Peterson M, Borell L: Struggles for autonomy in self-care: the impact of the physical and socio-cultural environment in a long-term care setting, *Scand J Caring Sci* 18(4):376–386, 2004.

Saint S, Kaufman S, Rodgers M: Condom versus indwelling urinary catheters: a randomized trial, *J Am Geriatr Soc* 54(7):1055–1061, 2006.

Stineman M, Ross R, Maislin G et al: Population-based study of home accessibility features and the activities of daily living: clinical and policy implications, *Disabil Rehabil* 29(15):1165–1175, 2007.

● = Independent   ▲ = Collaborative   **EBN** = Evidence-Based Nursing   **EB** = Evidence-Based

Readiness for enhanced Self-Concept   *Gail B. Ladwig, MSN, RN, CHTP*

NANDA-I

Definition

A pattern of perceptions or ideas about the self that is sufficient for well-being and can be strengthened

Defining Characteristics

Accepts limitations; accepts strengths; actions are congruent with verbal expression; expresses confidence in abilities; expresses satisfaction with body image; expresses satisfaction with personal identity; expresses satisfaction with role performance; expresses satisfaction with sense of worthiness; expresses satisfaction with thoughts about self; expresses willingness to enhance self-concept

NOC   (Nursing Outcomes Classification)

Suggested NOC Outcomes

Self-Esteem, Personal Well-Being, Psychosocial Adjustment Life Change

Example NOC Outcome with Indicators
Self-Esteem as evidenced by the following indicators: Verbalizations of self-acceptance/Open communication/Confidence level/Description of pride in self (Rate the outcome and indicators of **Self-Esteem:** 1 = never positive, 2 = rarely positive, 3 = sometimes positive, 4 = often positive, 5 = consistently positive [see Section I].)

Client Outcomes

Client Will (Specify Time Frame):

- State willingness to enhance self-concept
- State satisfaction with thoughts about self, sense of worthiness, role performance, body image, and personal identity
- Demonstrate actions that are congruent with expressed feelings and thoughts
- State confidence in abilities
- Accept strengths and limitations

NIC   (Nursing Interventions Classification)

Suggested NIC Intervention

Self-Esteem Enhancement

Example NIC Activities—Self-Esteem Enhancement
Encourage patient to identify strengths; Assist patient in setting realistic goals to achieve higher self-esteem

Nursing Interventions and *Rationales*

- Assess and support activities that promote self-concept developmentally. **EB:** *High self-esteem is associated with high academic achievement, involvement in sport and physical activity, and development of effective coping and peer pressure resistance skills (King, Vidourek, & Davis, 2002).* **EBN:** *Social support, self-esteem, and optimism were all positively related to positive health practices (McNicholas, 2002).*
- Refer to nutritional and exercise programs to support weight loss. **EB:** *Changes in weight using a community wellness center with exercise and nutrition information resulted in body satisfaction and an increase in the physical self-concept scale (Annesi, 2007).*
- Clients with cancer often use massage therapy as an adjunct treatment. **EB:** *Clients with advanced cancer who received six 30–minute massages over 2 weeks reported less pain and improved mood after each session (Kutner et al, 2008).*

● = Independent   ▲ = Collaborative   **EBN** = Evidence-Based Nursing   **EB** = Evidence-Based

- Support establishing a church-based community health promotion programs (CBHPPs) with the following key elements: partnerships, positive health values, availability of services, access to church facilities, community-focused interventions, health behavior change, and supportive social relationships. *CBHPPs, health promotion professionals, and churches can be dynamic partners (Peterson, Atwood, & Yates, 2002).* **EB:** *Clients in a faith-based weight loss program lost 3.6 lbs compared to 0.59 lbs in the control group (Kim et al, 2008).*
- ▲ For clients who have had breast surgery and need a prosthesis, provide the appropriate prosthesis before the client leaves the health care facility. *A diagnosis of breast cancer carries enormous implications for the client in terms of physical and psychological health. For this reason, it is vital that nurses respond sensitively to these needs and assist women to cope with the changes in body image and have the appropriate knowledge to fit the soft breast prosthesis (Keeton & McAloon, 2002).*
- Offer client choices in clothing when client is hospitalized. *Client clothes were experienced as being comfortable and practical, but also as being stigmatizing symbols of illness, confinement, and depersonalization (Edvardsson, 2009).*

Pediatric

- Consider the development of a Healthy Kids mentoring program that has four components: (1) relationship building, (2) self-esteem enhancement, (3) goal setting, and (4) academic assistance (tutoring). Mentors met with students twice each week for 1 hour each session on school grounds. During each meeting, mentors devoted time to each program component. **EB:** *The Healthy Kids Mentoring Program results indicated students' overall self-esteem, school connectedness, peer connectedness, and family connectedness were significantly higher at posttest than at pretest (King, Vidourek, & Davis, 2002). Results of this study suggest that healthy adolescent development includes positive resources from important others (e.g., parents, schools, and communities) (Youngblade et al, 2007).*
- ▲ Assess and provide referrals to mental health professionals for clients with unresolved worries associated with terrorism. **EBN:** *The National Association of Pediatric Nurse Practitioners (NAPNAP) initiated a new national campaign entitled Keep Your Children/Yourself Safe and Secure (KySS). Interventions are urgently needed to assist children and teens in coping with the multitude of stressors related to growing up in today's society (Melnyk et al, 2002).*
- Provide an alternative school-based program for pregnant and parenting teenagers. **EBN:** *The girls who attended this program developed close relationships with their peers and teachers. Many of them experienced academic success for the first time and reported that pregnancy and impending motherhood motivated them to do better in school (Spear, 2002).*

Geriatric

- Encourage clients to consider a Web-based support program when they are in a caregiving situation. **EBN:** *In this study of caregivers of clients with stroke, the caregivers came together and provided support for each other via a Web-based support program (Pierce, Steiner, & Govoni, 2004).*
- Encourage activity and a strength, mobility, balance, and endurance training program. **EB:** *This pilot study indicates that a physical training program may improve functional capacity for institutionalized elderly persons with multiple diagnoses (Rydwik, Frandin, & Akner, 2005). Participants in this physical activity program demonstrated increased self-worth (Huberty et al, 2008).*
- Provide opportunities for clients to engage in life skills (themed collections of everyday items based upon general activities that residents may have previously carried out). *Life-skill centers offer residents a means of purposeful occupation in tasks that they have undertaken for decades using skills that are inherent, and not forgotten (Swann, 2009).*
- Provide information on advance directives. **EBN:** *In this study elders stated that the optimal time for advance care planning was during periods of wellness. They are ready and eager to discuss advance planning (Malcomson & Bisbee, 2009).*

Multicultural

- Carefully assess each client and allow families to participate in providing care that is acceptable based on the client's cultural beliefs. **EBN:** *The results of this study contribute to the essential*

• = Independent ▲ = Collaborative **EBN** = Evidence-Based Nursing **EB** = Evidence-Based

knowledge about culturally sensitive nursing practices. An understanding of client suffering that is shaped by traditional cultural values helps nurses communicate empathy in a culturally sensitive manner to facilitate the therapeutic relationship and clinical outcomes (Hsiao et al, 2006).

- Provide support for health-promoting behaviors and self-concept for clients from diverse cultures. **EBN:** *In this convenience sample, regression analyses demonstrated that the internalization racial identity stage and self-esteem contributed to the variance in health-promoting lifestyles (Johnson, 2002).*

- Refer to the care plans **Disturbed Body image**, **Readiness for enhanced Coping**, **Chronic low Self-Esteem**, and **Readiness for enhanced Spiritual well-being**.

Home Care

- Previously discussed interventions may be used in the home care setting.

⊖volve See the EVOLVE website for Weblinks for client education resources.

REFERENCES

Annesi JJ: Relations of changes in exercise self-efficacy, physical self-concept, and body satisfaction with weight changes in obese white and African American women initiating a physical activity program, *Ethn Dis* 17(1):19–22, 2007.

Edvardsson D: Balancing between being a person and being a patient—a qualitative study of wearing patient clothing, *Int J Nurs Stud* 46(1):4–11, 2009.

Hsiao FH, Klimidis S, Minas H et al: Cultural attribution of mental health suffering in Chinese societies: the views of Chinese patients with mental illness and their caregivers, *J Clin Nurs* 15(8):998–1006, 2006.

Huberty JL, Vener J, Sidman C et al: Women Bound to Be Active: a pilot study to explore the feasibility of an intervention to increase physical activity and self-worth in women, *Women Health* 48(1):83–101, 2008.

Johnson RL: The relationships among racial identity, self-esteem, sociodemographics, and health-promoting lifestyles, *Res Theory Nurs Pract* 16(3):193–207, 2002.

Keeton S, McAloon L: The supply and fitting of a temporary breast prosthesis, *Nurs Stand* 16(41):43, 2002.

Kim KH, Linnan L, Campbell MK et al: The WORD (Wholeness, Oneness, Righteousness, Deliverance): a faith-based weight-loss program utilizing a community-based participatory research approach, *Health Educ Behav* 35(5):634–650, 2008.

King K, Vidourek R, Davis B: Increasing self-esteem and school connectedness through a multidimensional mentoring program, *J Sch Health* 72(7):294, 2002.

Kutner JS, Smith MC, Corbin L et al: Massage therapy versus simple touch to improve pain and mood in patients with advanced cancer: a randomized trial, *Ann Intern Med* 149(6):369–379, 2008.

Malcomson H, Bisbee S: Perspectives of healthy elders on advance care planning, *J Am Acad Nurse Pract* 21(1):18–23, 2009.

McNicholas SL: Social support and positive health practices, *West J Nurs Res* 24(7):772, 2002.

Melnyk BM, Feinstein NF, Tuttle J et al: Mental health worries, communication, and needs in the year of the U.S. terrorist attack: national KySS survey findings, *J Pediatr Health Care* 16(5):222, 2002.

Peterson J, Atwood JR, Yates B: Key elements for church-based health promotion programs: outcome-based literature review, *Public Health Nurs* 19(6):401, 2002.

Pierce LL, Steiner V, Govoni AL: Caregivers dealing with stroke pull together and feel connected, *J Neurosci Nurs* 36(1):32–39, 2004.

Rydwik E, Frandin K, Akner G: Physical training in institutionalized elderly people with multiple diagnoses—a controlled pilot study, *Arch Gerontol Geriatr* 40(1):29–44, 2005.

Spear HJ: Reading, writing, and having babies: a nurturing alternative school program, *J Sch Nurs* 18(5):293, 2002.

Swann J: Life-skill stations: tools for reminiscence and activity, *Nurs Resident Care* 11(2):96–98, 2009.

Youngblade LM, Theokas C, Schulenberg J et al: Risk and promotive factors in families, schools, and communities: a contextual model of positive youth development in adolescence, *Pediatrics* 119(suppl 1):S47–S53, 2007.

Chronic low Self-Esteem   *Mary Jane Roth, RN, BSN, MA*   ⊖volve

NANDA-I

Definition

Long-standing negative self-evaluating/feelings about self or self-capabilities

Defining Characteristics

Dependent on others' opinions; evaluates self as unable to deal with events; exaggerates negative feedback about self; excessively seeks reassurance; expressions of guilt; expressions of shame; frequent lack of success in life events; hesitant to try new things; indecisive behavior; lack of eye contact; nonassertive behavior; overly conforming; passive; rejects positive feedback about self

• = Independent   ▲ = Collaborative   **EBN** = Evidence-Based Nursing   **EB** = Evidence-Based

Related Factors (r/t)

Ineffective adaptation to loss; lack of affection; lack of approval; lack of membership in group; perceived discrepancy between self and cultural norms; perceived discrepancy between self and spiritual norms; perceived lack of belonging; perceived lack of respect from others; psychiatric disorder; repeated failures; repeated negative reinforcement; traumatic event; traumatic situation

NOC (Nursing Outcomes Classification)

Suggested NOC Outcome

Self-Esteem

Example NOC Outcome with Indicators
Demonstrates improved **Self-Esteem** as evidenced by the following indicators: Verbalizations of acceptance of self and limitations/Open communication (Rate the outcome and indicators of **Self-Esteem:** 1 = never positive, 2 = rarely positive, 3 = sometimes positive, 4 = often positive, 5 = consistently positive [see Section I].)

Client Outcomes

Client Will (Specify Time Frame):

- Demonstrate improved ability to interact with others (e.g., maintains eye contact, engages in conversation, expresses thoughts/feelings)
- Verbalize increased self-acceptance through positive self-statements about self
- Identify personal strengths, accomplishments, and values
- Identify and work on small, achievable goals
- Improve independent decision-making and problem-solving skills

NIC (Nursing Interventions Classification)

Suggested NIC Intervention

Self-Esteem Enhancement

Example NIC Activities—Self-Esteem Enhancement
Encourage patient to identify strengths; Assist in setting realistic goals to achieve higher self-esteem

Nursing Interventions and *Rationales*

- Actively listen to and respect the client. **EBN:** *Listening and nurturing are important aspects of care (Parrish, Penden, & Staten, 2008).*
- Assess the client's environmental and everyday stressors, including physical health concerns and the potential for abusive relationships. **EBN:** *It is difficult to determine whether a woman's depressive symptoms are related to physical abuse or to other risk factors (Al-Modallal, Peden & Anderson, 2008).*
- Assess existing strengths and coping abilities, and provide opportunities for their expression and recognition. **EBN:** *Supporting a client's beliefs and self-reflection and helping them cope can affect self-esteem (Räty & Gustaffson, 2006).*
- Reinforce the personal strengths and positive self-perceptions that a client identifies. **EBN:** *Clients with low self-esteem need to have their existence and value confirmed (Räty & Gustaffson, 2006).*
- Identify client's negative self-assessments. **EBN:** *Body-esteem and self-esteem are significantly related to one another (Jones et al, 2008).*
- Encourage realistic and achievable goal setting and resources and identify impediments to achievement. **EBN:** *This promotes self-acceptance, which is associated with psychological well-being (Macinnes, 2006).*
- Demonstrate and promote effective communication techniques; spend time with the client. **EBN:** *Presence and caring during communication is important (Mantha et al, 2008).*

● = Independent   ▲ = Collaborative   **EBN** = Evidence-Based Nursing   **EB** = Evidence-Based

- Encourage independent decision making by reviewing options and their possible consequences with client. **EBN:** *Decision-making capacity is vital to a sense of autonomy (Burke et al, 2008).*
- Assist client to challenge negative perceptions of self and performance. **EBN:** *Reduction in negative thinking will increase self-esteem (Day & Deutsch, 2004).*
- Use failure as an opportunity to provide valuable feedback. **EBN:** *This allows clients to change expectations of what would happen given the reality of what did happen (Pierce & Hicks, 2001).*
- Promote maintaining a level of functioning in the community. **EB:** *Driving cessation is one factor associated with increased depressive symptoms and decreased social integration among older adults (Mezuk & Rebok, 2008).*
- Assist client with evaluating the effect of family and peer group on feelings of self-worth. **EBN:** *Nurses are encouraged to assess actively the condition of social contacts among the elderly in their care and to assist their strengthening relationships with family members and others (Yao, Yu, & Chen, 2008).*
- Support socialization and communication skills. **EBN:** *Social support increases the client's ability to cope with problems (Johnson, 2008).*
- Encourage journal/diary writing as a safe way of expressing emotions. **EB:** *Daily diary writing has relevance as highlighted with reference to behavioral activation interventions for depression (Hopko & Mullane, 2008).*

Geriatric

- Support client in identifying and adapting to functional changes. **EBN:** *Changes in physical well-being decrease emotional resources to cope with stress/grief (Talerico, 2003).*
- Use reminiscence therapy to identify patterns of strength and accomplishment. *Identifying strengths and accomplishments counteracts pervasive negativity.*
- Encourage participation in peer group activities. **EBN:** *Withdrawal and social isolation are detrimental to feelings of self-worth (Stuart-Shor et al, 2003).*
- Encourage activities in which a client can support/help others. **EB:** *The findings of this study reveal that late-life productive engagement is widespread, with the majority of older individuals involved in multiple forms of activity concurrently. Non-market-based activities such as caregiving, informal assistance, and volunteering are most prevalent (Hinterlong, 2008).*

Multicultural

- Assess for the influence of cultural beliefs, norms, and values on the client's sense of self-esteem. **EBN:** *How the client values self may be based on cultural perceptions (Giger & Davidhizar, 2008). Asian American youths demonstrate lower levels of self-esteem than their non-Asian peers (Rhee, Chang, & Rhee, 2003).*
- Assess for evidence of client financial strain. **EB:** *A recent study of Mexican-origin individuals showed that financial strain was associated with cognitive self-esteem (Angel et al, 2003).*
- Assess for drug and alcohol use in individuals with low self-esteem. **EB:** *Among Mexican American female adolescents, poor self-confidence predicts higher levels of alcohol use (Swaim & Wayman, 2004).*
- Validate the client's feelings regarding ethnic or racial identity. **EBN:** *Individuals with strong ethnic affiliation have higher levels of self-esteem than others (Greig, 2003).*

Home Care

- Assess a client's immediate support system/family for relationship patterns and content of communication. **EBN:** *Family strength assessments help the nurse to incorporate family strengths into nursing care, especially in times of crisis (Sittner, Hudson, & DeFrain, 2007).*
- Encourage the client's family to provide support and feedback regarding client value or worth. **EBN:** *There are significant relationships between adolescents' practice of healthy behaviors, self-efficacy of those behaviors, self-care abilities and their support systems among other factors (Callaghan, 2006).*

• = Independent   ▲ = Collaborative   **EBN** = Evidence-Based Nursing   **EB** = Evidence-Based

▲ Refer to medical social services to assist the family in pattern changes that could benefit the client. *The best nursing plan may be to access specialty services for the client and family.*

▲ If a client is involved in counseling or self-help groups, monitor and encourage attendance. Help the client identify the value of group participation after each group encounter. *Discussion about group participation clarifies and reinforces group feedback and support.*

▲ If a client is taking prescribed psychotropic medications, assess for knowledge of medication side effects and reasons for taking medication. Teach as necessary. **EBN:** *Education that helps clients understand their illness, particular symptoms and how medications help them may be beneficial in promoting adherence (Wu et al, 2008).*

▲ Assess medications for effectiveness and side effects and monitor client for compliance. **EBN:** *A positive working relationship with the health care provider may result in improved adherence (Wu et al, 2008).*

Client/Family Teaching and Discharge Planning

▲ Refer to community agencies for psychotherapeutic counseling. **EB:** *Family-led programs are an effective resource for families with mental illness (Pickett-Schenk et al, 2008).*

▲ Refer to psychoeducational groups on stress reduction and coping skills **EB:** *CBT psychoeducation for anxiety disorders appears to be helpful for a number of clients and largely acceptable for most clients that attend (Houghton & Saxon, 2007).*

▲ Refer to self-help support groups specific to needs. **EB:** *Participation in mutual mental health groups leads to improved psychological and social functioning (Pistrang, Barker, & Humphreys, 2008).*

⊝volve   See the EVOLVE website for Weblinks for client education resources.

REFERENCES

Al-Modallal H, Peden A, Anderson D: Impact of physical abuse on adult depressive symptoms among women, *Issues Ment Health Nurs* 29:299–314, 2008.

Angel RJ, Frisco M, Angel JL et al: Financial strain and health among elderly Mexican-origin individuals, *J Health Soc Behav* 44(4):536–551, 2003.

Burke L, Steenkiste A, Music E et al: A descriptive study of past experiences with weight-loss treatment, *J Am Diet Assoc* 108:640–647, 2008.

Callaghan D: Basic conditioning factors' influences on adolescents' health, self efficacy, and self-care, *Issues Comp Pediatr Nurs* 29(4):191–204, 2006.

Day P, Deutsch S: Using mindfulness-based therapeutic interventions in psychiatric nursing practice—part 1: description and empirical support for mindfulness-based interventions and part 2: mindfulness-based approaches for all phases of psychotherapy-clinical case study, *Arch Psychiatr Nurs* 18(5):164–177, 2004.

Giger J, Davidhizar R: *Transcultural nursing: assessment and intervention,* ed 4, St Louis, 2008, Mosby.

Greig R: Ethnic identity development: implications for mental health in African-American and Hispanic adolescents, *Issues Ment Health Nurs* 24(3):317–331, 2003.

Hinterlong JE: Productive engagement among older Americans: prevalence, patterns, and implications for public policy, *J Aging Soc Policy* 20(2):141–164, 2008.

Hopko D, Mullane C: Exploring the relation of depression and overt behavior with daily diaries, *Behav Res Ther* 46:1085–1089, 2008.

Houghton S, Saxon D: An evaluation of large group CBT psychoeducation for anxiety disorders delivered in routine practice, *Patient Ed Couns* 68:107–110, 2007.

Johnson J: Informal social support networks and the maintenance of voluntary driving cessation by older rural women, *J Community Health Nurs* 25(2):65–72, 2008.

Jones JE, Robinson J, Barr W et al: Impact of exudate and odour from chronic venous leg ulceration, *Nurs Stand* 22(45):53–61, 2008.

Macinnes DL: Self-esteem and self-acceptance: an examination into their relationship and their effect on psychological health, *J Psychiatr Ment Health Nurs* 13(5):483, 2006.

Mantha S, Davies B, Moyer A et al: Providing responsive nursing care, *MCN Am J Matern Child Nurs* 33(5):307–314, 2008.

Mezuk B, Rebok G: Social integration and social support among older adults following driving cessation, *J Gerontol B Psychol Sci Soc Sci* 63(5):298–303, 2008.

Parrish E, Penden A, Staten R: Strategies used by advanced practice psychiatric nurses in treating adults with depression, *Perspect Psychiatr Care* 44(6):232–240, 2008.

Pickett-Schenk S, Lippincott R, Bennett C et al: improving knowledge about mental illness through family-led education: the journey of hope, *Psychiatr Serv* 59:49–56, 2008.

Pierce P, Hicks F: Patient decision-making behavior: an emerging paradigm for nursing science, *Nurs Res* 50(5):267, 2001.

Pistrang N, Barker C, Humphreys K: Mutual help groups for mental health problems: a review of effectiveness studies: *Am J Comm Psychol* 42(1–2):110–122, 2008.

Räty L, Gustaffson B: Emotions in relation to healthcare encounters affecting self-esteem, *J Neurosci Nurs* 38(1):42, 2006.

Rhee S, Chang J, Rhee J: Acculturation, communication patterns, and self-esteem among Asian and Caucasian American adolescents, *Adolescence* 38(152):749–768, 2003.

Sittner B, Hudson DB, DeFrain J: Using the concept of family strengths to enhance nursing care, *MCN Am J Matern Child Nurs* 32(6):353–357, 2007.

Stuart-Shor EM, Buselli EF, Carroll DL et al: Are psychosocial factors associated with the pathogenesis and consequences of cardiovascular disease in the elderly? *J Cardiovasc Nurs* 18(3):169, 2003.

Swaim RC, Wayman JC: Multidimensional self-esteem and alcohol use among Mexican American and white non-Latino adolescents: concurrent and prospective effects, *Am J Orthopsychiatry* 74(4):559–570, 2004.

• = Independent   ▲ = Collaborative   **EBN** = Evidence-Based Nursing   **EB** = Evidence-Based

Talerico K: Grief and older adults: differences, issues, and clinical approaches, *J Psychosoc Nurs Ment Health Serv* 41(7):12, 2003.

Wu J, Moser, D Lennie TA et al: Factors influencing medication adherence in patients with heart failure, *Heart Lung* 37(1):8–16, 2008.

Yao K, Yu S, Chen I: Relationships between personal, depression and social network factors and sleep quality in community-dwelling older adults, *J Nurs Res* 16(2):131–139, 2008.

Situational low Self-Esteem   *Mary Jane Roth, RN, BSN, MA*

Definition

Development of a negative perception of self-worth in response to a current situation (specify)

Defining Characteristics

Evaluation of self as unable to deal with events; evaluation of self as unable to deal with situations; expressions of helplessness; expressions of uselessness; indecisive behavior; nonassertive behavior; self-negating verbalizations; verbally reports current situational challenge to self-worth

Related Factors (r/t)

Behavior inconsistent with values; developmental changes; disturbed body image; failures; functional impairment; lack of recognition; loss; rejections; social role changes

NOC   (Nursing Outcomes Classification)

Refer to **Chronic low Self-Esteem.**

Client Outcomes

Client Will (Specify Time Frame):

- State effect of life events on feelings about self
- State personal strengths
- Acknowledge presence of guilt and not blame self if an action was related to another person's appraisal
- Seek help when necessary
- Demonstrate self-perceptions are accurate given physical capabilities
- Demonstrate separation of self-perceptions from societal stigmas

NIC   (Nursing Interventions Classification)

Refer to **Chronic low Self-Esteem.**

Nursing Interventions and *Rationales*

- ▲ Assess the client for signs and symptoms of depression and potential for suicide and/or violence. If present, immediately notify the appropriate personnel of symptoms. See care plans for **Risk for other-directed Violence** and **Risk for Suicide. EB:** *Well-documented suicide risk assessments are a core measure of quality of care (Simon, 2009).*
- Assess the client's environmental and everyday stressors, including evidence of abusive relationships. **EBN:** *High everyday stressors and a history of abuse in relationships are associated with low self-esteem and depression (Al-Modallal, Peden, & Anderson, 2008).*
- ▲ Assess for unhealthy coping mechanisms, such as substance abuse, and make appropriate referrals. **EB:** *Numerous factors influence the onset and continuation of alcohol use including the complex ways that genes interact with one another and with the environment (NIAAA, 2009).*
- Assist in the identification of problems and situational factors that contribute to problems, offering options for resolution. **EBN:** *Recognize the client's own personal resources strengthen client's self-determination (Meijers & Gustafsson, 2008).*
- Mutually identify strengths, resources, and previously effective coping strategies. **EBN:** *A common action for supporting self-determination is supplying the client with information and engaging the client in making a plan (Meijers & Gustafsson, 2008).*

• = Independent   ▲ = Collaborative   **EBN** = Evidence-Based Nursing   **EB** = Evidence-Based

- Have client list strengths. **EBN:** *Clients were found to use a variety of self-care strategies, medication management techniques, and emotional supports to alleviate symptoms of chronic heart failure (CHF) (Bennett et al, 2000).*
- Accept client's own pace in working through grief or crisis situations. **EBN:** *Recommended therapeutic communication skills such as eye contact, use of therapeutic touch, and active listening can be enhanced by an understanding of the grief process (Wright & Hogan, 2008).*
- Accept the client's own defenses in dealing with the crisis. **EBN:** *The SAUC modes (Sympathy-Acceptance-Understanding-Competence) helps strengthen and preserve the individual's positive self-relation (Meijers & Gustafsson, 2008).*
- Provide information about support groups of people who have common experiences or interests. **EBN:** *Cognitive-behavioral group therapy decreases depression levels and increases self-esteem in depressed clients (Chen et al, 2006).*
- Teach the client mindfulness techniques to cope more effectively with strong emotional responses. **EBN:** *Development of mindfulness strategies increased resolution of internal conflicts (Day & Deutsch, 2004).*
- Support problem-solving strategies but discourage decision making when in crisis. **EBN:** *Uncertainty is a significant negative predictor of resourcefulness (Dirsken, 2000).*
- Encourage objective appraisal of self and life events and challenge negative or perfectionist expectations of self. **EB:** *Positive life events improve self-esteem and positive affect (Drew & Mabry, 2004).*
- Provide psychoeducation to client and family. **EBN:** *Knowledge provides empowerment; however, written educational materials should be prepared by health professionals and by taking the target group into consideration (Demir, Ozsaker, & Ilce, 2008).*
- Validate confusion when feeling ill but looking well. **EBN:** *Validation of emotions is related to a client's experience of caring (Räty & Gustafsson, 2006).*
- Acknowledge the presence of societal stigma. Teach management tools. **EBN:** *Stigma towards mental illness is poorly understood, often unrecognized by nurses, and impacts both treatment seeking behavior and treatment adherence (Pinto-Foltz & Lodgson, 2008).*
- Validate the effect of negative past experiences on self-esteem and work on corrective measures. *People with low self-esteem have a need to be affirmed regarding their value (Räty & Gustaffson, 2006).*
- See care plan for **Chronic low Self-Esteem.**

Geriatric and Multicultural

- See care plan for **Chronic low Self-Esteem.**

Home Care

- Establish an emergency plan and contract with the client for its use. *Having an emergency plan is reassuring to the client. Establishing a contract validates the worth of the client and provides a caring link between the client and society.*
- Access supplies that support a client's success at independent living.
- See care plan for **Chronic low Self-Esteem.**

Client/Family Teaching and Discharge Planning

- Assess the person's support system (family, friends, and community) and involve them if desired. **EBN:** *Family strength assessments help the nurse to incorporate family strengths into nursing care, especially in times of crisis (Sittner, Hudson, & DeFrain, 2007).*
- Educate client and family regarding the grief process. *Understanding this process normalizes responses of sadness, anger, guilt, and helplessness. Recommended therapeutic communication skills such as eye contact, use of therapeutic touch, and active listening can be enhanced by an understanding of the grief process (Wright & Hogan, 2008).*
- Teach client and family that the crisis is temporary. *Knowing that the crisis is temporary provides a sense of hope for the future.*
- ▲ Refer to appropriate community resources or crisis intervention centers.

● = Independent   ▲ = Collaborative   **EBN** = Evidence-Based Nursing   **EB** = Evidence-Based

▲ Refer to resources for handicap and/or disability services.

● Refer to illness-specific consumer support groups. *Mutual help support groups aid the client with chronic illness to cope with their illness (Chen, Pai, & Li, 2008).*

● See care plan for **Chronic low Self-Esteem**.

ⓔvolve   See the EVOLVE website for Weblinks for client education resources.

REFERENCES

Al-Modallal H, Peden A, Anderson D: Impact of physical abuse on adult depressive symptoms among women, *Issues Men Health Nurs* 29:299–314, 2008.

Bennett SJ, Cordes DK, Westmoreland G et al: Self-care strategies for symptom management in patients with chronic heart failure, *Nurs Res* 49(3):139–145, 2000.

Chen, T, Lu RB, Chang AJ et al: The evaluation of cognitive-behavioral group therapy on patient depression and self-esteem, *Arch Psychiatr Nurs* 20(1):3–11, 2006.

Chen Y, Pai J, Li C: Haemodialysis: the effects of using the empowerment concept during the development of a mutual support group in Taiwan: *J Clin Nurs* 17(5):133–142, 2008.

Day P, Deutsch S: Using mindfulness-based therapeutic interventions in psychiatric nursing practice—part 1: description and empirical support for mindfulness-based interventions & part 2: mindfulness-based approaches for all phases of psychotherapy-clinical case study, *Arch Psychiatr Nurs* 18(5):164–177, 2004.

Demir F, Ozsaker E, Ilce A: The quality and suitability of written educational materials for patients, *J Clin Nurs* 17(2):259–265, 2008.

Dirsken SR: Predicting well-being among breast cancer survivors, *J Adv Nurs* 32(4):937, 2000.

Drew L, Mabry J: Predictors of positive life events: self-esteem and positive effect, *Gerontologist* 44(1):230, 2004.

Meijers KE, Gustafsson B: Patient's self-determination in intensive care: from an action- and confirmation theoretical perspective, *Intensive Crit Care Nurs* 24(4):222–232, 2008.

NIAAA Five Year Strategic Play FY09–14. www.niaaa.nih.gov/publications/Health Disparities/Strategic.html. Accessed March 21, 2009.

Pinto-Foltz M, Logsdon M: Stigma towards mental illness: a concept analysis using postpartum depression as an exemplar, *Issues Ment Health Nurs* 29:21–36, 2008.

Räty L, Gustafsson B: Emotions in relation to healthcare encounters affecting self-esteem, *J Neurosci Nurs* 38(1):42, 2006.

Simon R: Enhancing suicide risk assessment through evidence-based psychiatry, *Psychiatr Times*, January 1, 2009.

Sittner BJ, Hudson DB, DeFrain J: Using the concept of family strengths to enhance nursing care, *MCN Am J Maternal Child Nursing* (32)6:353–357, 2007.

Wright P, Hogan S: Grief theories and models applications to hospice nursing practice, *J Hospice Palliat Nurs* 10(6):350–356, 2008.

Risk for situational low Self-Esteem   Mary Jane Roth, RN, BSN, MA

NANDA-I

Definition

At risk for developing negative perception of self-worth in response to a current situation (specify)

Risk Factors

Behavior inconsistent with values; decreased control over environment; developmental changes; disturbed body image; failures; functional impairment; history of abandonment; history of abuse; history of learned helplessness; history of neglect; lack of recognition; loss; physical illness; rejections; social role changes; unrealistic self-expectations

NOC   (Nursing Outcomes Classification)

See **Chronic low Self-Esteem**.

Client Outcomes

Client Will (Specify Time Frame):

● State accurate self-appraisal

● Demonstrate the ability to self-validate

● Demonstrate the ability to make decisions independent of primary peer group

● Express effects of media on self-appraisal

● Express influence of substances on self-esteem

● Identify strengths and healthy coping skills

● State life events and change as influencing self-esteem

NIC   (Nursing Interventions Classification)

See **Chronic low Self-Esteem**.

● = Independent   ▲ = Collaborative   **EBN** = Evidence-Based Nursing   **EB** = Evidence-Based

Nursing Interventions and *Rationales*

- Identify environmental and/or developmental factors that increase risk for low self-esteem, especially in children/adolescents, to make needed referrals. **EBN:** *Self-esteem enhancement programs can improve self-esteem in school-age children (Dalgas-Pelish, 2006).*
- Assess the client's previous experiences with health care and coping with illness to determine the level of education and support needed. **EBN:** *Accessing illness self-concept in developing a treatment plan may prove useful (Morea, Friend, & Bennett, 2008).*
- Assess for low and negative affect (expression of feelings). **EBN:** *Self-esteem is more closely associated with affect than self-acceptance (Macinnes, 2006).*
- Encourage client to maintain highest level of community functioning. **EBN:** *Community volunteerism supports improved self-esteem (Messias, DeJong, & McLoughlin, 2005).*
- Treat the client with respect and as an equal to maintain positive self-esteem. **EBN:** *Clients with higher self-esteem need to be confirmed as being equal with care providers (Räty & Gustaffson, 2006).*
- Help the client to identify the resources and social support network available at this time. **EBN:** *Cognitive developmental transitions might be significantly enhanced by the presence of intimate ties, positive perceptions of one's health limitations, and residence in a healthy, safe, and resource-rich physical environment (Low, Molzahn, & Kalfoss, 2008).*
- Encourage the client to find a self-help or therapy group that focuses on self-esteem enhancement. **EBN:** *Cognitive-behavioral group therapy decreases depression levels and increases self-esteem in depressed clients (Chen et al, 2006).*
- Encourage the client to create a sense of competence through short-term goal setting and goal achievement. **EBN:** *Sense of competence is related to global self-esteem (Lauder et al, 2008).*
- ▲ Assess the client for symptoms of depression and anxiety. Refer to specialist as needed. *Prompt and effective treatment can prevent exacerbation of symptoms or safety risks.* **EB:** *Well-documented suicide risk assessments are a core measure of quality of care (Simon, 2009).*
- See care plans for **Disturbed personal Identity** and **Situational low Self-Esteem**.

Geriatric

- Support humor as a coping mechanism. **EB:** *This study identified a sense of humor as a mechanism for managing the inevitable stresses of aging (Marziali, McDonald, & Donahue, 2008).*
- Assist the client in life review and identifying positive accomplishments. *Life review is a developmental task that increases a person's sense of peace and serenity.*
- Help client to establish a peer group and structured daily activities. *Social isolation and lack of structure increase a client's sense of feeling lost and worthless.*
- See care plans for **Situational low Self-Esteem** and **Chronic low Self-Esteem**.

Home Care

- Assess current environmental stresses and identify community resources. *Accessing resources to help decrease environmental stress will increase the client's ability to cope.* **EBN:** *Nurses who identify older women with low self-esteem, high depressive symptoms, and low quality of life before relocation can make interventions to ease the transition process (Rossen & Knafl, 2007).*
- Encourage family members to acknowledge and validate the client's strengths. *Validation allows the client to increase self-reliance and to trust personal decisions.*
- Assess the need for establishing an emergency plan. *Openly assessing safety risks increases the client's sense of limits, boundaries, and safety.*
- See care plans for **Situational low Self-Esteem** and **Chronic low Self-Esteem**.

Client/Family Teaching and Discharge Planning

- ▲ Refer the client/family to community-based self-help and support groups. **EB:** *Participation in mutual mental health groups leads to improved psychological and social functioning (Pistrang, Barker, & Humphreys, 2008).*

● = Independent   ▲ = Collaborative   **EBN** = Evidence-Based Nursing   **EB** = Evidence-Based

▲ Refer the client to educational classes on stress management, relaxation training, and so on. **EB:** *CBT psychoeducation for anxiety disorders appears to be helpful for a number of clients and largely acceptable for most clients that attend (Houghton & Saxon, 2007).*

▲ Refer the client to community agencies that offer support and environmental resources.

• See care plans for **Situational low Self-Esteem** and **Chronic low Self-Esteem.**

⊖volve   See the EVOLVE website for Weblinks for client education resources.

REFERENCES

Chen, T, Lu RB, Chang AJ et al: The evaluation of cognitive-behavioral group therapy on patient depression and self-esteem, *Arch Psychiatr Nurs* 20(1):3–11, 2006.

Dalgas-Pelish P: Effects of a self-esteem intervention program on school-aged children, *Pediatr Nurs* 32(4):241, 2006.

Houghton S, Saxon D: An evaluation of large group CBT psycho-education for anxiety disorders delivered in routine practice, *Patient Educ Couns* 68:107–110, 2007.

Lauder W, Holland K, Roxburgh M et al: Measuring competence, self-reported competence and self-efficacy in pre-registration students, *Nurs Stand* 22(20):35–43, 2008.

Low G, Molzahn A, Kalfoss M: Quality of life in older adults in Canada and Norway: examining the Iowa model, *West J Nurs Res* 30(4):458–476, 2008.

Macinnes DL: Self-esteem and self-acceptance: an examination into their relationship and their effect on psychological health, *J Psychiatr Ment Health Nurs* 13(5):483, 2006.

Marziali E, McDonald L, Donahue P: The role of coping humor in the physical and mental health of older adults, *Aging Ment Health* 12(6):713–718, 2008.

Messias D, DeJong M, McLoughlin K: Being involved and making a difference: empowerment and well-being among women living in poverty, *J Holist Nurs* 23(1):66, 2005.

Morea J, Friend R, Bennett R: Conceptualizing and measuring illness self concept: a comparison with self-esteem and optimism in predicting fibromyalgia adjustment, *Res Nurs Health* 31:563–575, 2008.

Pistrang N, Barker C, Humphreys K: Mutual help groups for mental health problems: a review of effectiveness studies, *Am J Commun Psychol* 42(1–2):110–122, 2008.

Räty L, Gustaffson B: Emotions in relation to healthcare encounters affecting self-esteem, *J Neurosci Nurs* 38(1):42, 2006.

Simon R: Enhancing suicide risk assessment through evidenced-based psychiatry, *Psychiatr Times,* January 1, 2009.

Rossen E, Knafl K: Women's well-being after relocation to independent living communities, *West J Nurs Res* 29(2):183–199, 2007.

Readiness for enhanced Self Health management   ⊖volve

Dawn Fairlie, ANP, FNP, GNP, DNS(c)

 NANDA-I

Definition

A pattern of regulating and integrating into daily living a therapeutic regime for treatment of illness and its sequelae that is sufficient for meeting health-related goals and can be strengthened

Defining Characteristics

Choices of daily living are appropriate for meeting goals (e.g., treatment, prevention); describes reduction of risk factors; expresses desire to manage the illness (e.g., treatment, prevention of sequelae); expresses little difficulty with prescribed regimens; no unexpected acceleration of illness symptoms

NOC   **(Nursing Outcomes Classification)**

Suggested NOC Outcomes

Health-Promoting Behavior, Health-Seeking Behavior, Knowledge: Health Behavior, Health Promotion, Health Resources, Illness Care, Medication, Prescribed Activity, Treatment Regimen

Example **NOC** Outcome with Indicators
Health-Promoting Behavior as evidenced by the following indicators: Monitors personal behavior for risks/Seeks balance among exercise, work, leisure, rest, and nutrition/Performs healthy behaviors routinely/Uses financial and physical resources to promote health (Rate each indicator of **Health-Promoting Behavior:** 1 = never demonstrated, 2 = rarely demonstrated, 3 = sometimes demonstrated, 4 = often demonstrated, 5 = consistently demonstrated [see Section I].)

Client Outcomes

Client Will (Specify Time Frame):

- Describe integration of therapeutic regimen into daily living
- Demonstrate continued commitment to integration of therapeutic regimen into daily living routines

NIC   (Nursing Interventions Classification)

Suggested NIC Interventions

Anticipatory Guidance, Mutual Goal Setting, Patient Contracting, Self-Modification Assistance, Self-Responsibility Facilitation, Support System Enhancement, Teaching: Disease Process

Example NIC Activities—Mutual Goal Setting
Assist the patient in prioritizing (weighing) identified goals; Clarify with the patient roles of the health care provider and the patient, respectively

Nursing Interventions and *Rationales*

- Acknowledge the expertise that the client and family bring to self-management. **EBN:** *Older people diagnosed with asthma used three different models of self-management: a medical model, collaborative model, and self-agency model. To achieve optimal self-agency, it was recommended that health care professionals respect the expertise of clients (Koch, Jenkin, & Kralik, 2004). The Patient Education Department of Stanford University, Department of Medicine, directed by Dr. Kate Lorig, developed a client education program for self-management that is widely disseminated (Stanford University, 2007). Through 5 years of systematic research with more than 1000 clients, they established that client education in self-management is effective to improve health outcomes.*
- Review factors that contribute to the likelihood of health promotion and health protection. Use Pender's Health Promotion Model and Becker's Health Belief Model to identify contributing factors (Pender, Murdaugh, & Parsons, 2006). **EBN:** *Many studies using both the Health Promotion Model and the Health Belief Model support the view that individual perceptions and a variety of modifying factors affect the likelihood of improving health behaviors (Pender, Murdaugh, & Parsons, 2006). In post–myocardial infarction clients in the United Kingdom, adhering to physical activity was associated with health motivation, and adhering to smoking cessation was associated with self-efficacy (Leong, Molassiotis, & Marsh, 2004). Adherence to healthy diet was accounted for by the extent that family members encouraged the client to follow the therapeutic regimen.*
- Further develop and reinforce contributing factors that might change with ongoing management of the therapeutic regimen (e.g., knowledge, self-efficacy, self-esteem, and perceived benefits). **EBN:** *Illness care is associated with ongoing changes and, over time, management of therapeutic regimens can become increasingly tedious and difficult (Lubkin & Larsen, 2006).*
- Support all efforts to self-manage therapeutic regimens. **EBN:** *Ongoing support and assistance from health care providers is needed to identify and enhance factors that contribute to the likelihood of taking action for health promotion and health protection (Pender, Murdaugh, & Parsons, 2006).*
- Review the client's strengths in the management of the therapeutic regimen. **EBN:** *People who are doing the work of managing a therapeutic regimen may not even realize they are doing it well (Lubkin & Larsen, 2006).*
- Collaborate with the client to identify strategies to maintain strengths and develop additional strengths as indicated. **EBN:** *The client and provider working in partnership can facilitate, support, and reinforce the client's strengths (Bidmead & Cowley, 2005; Kettunen et al, 2006).*
- Identify contributing factors that may need to be improved now or in the future. **EBN:** *Health promotion and protection are complex behaviors that are difficult to implement on a daily basis. Based on the complexity of achieving these behaviors and the perceived barriers to implementation (e.g., time, energy, money), usually one or more contributing factors would benefit from increased focus and attention (Pender, Murdaugh, & Parsons, 2006).*
- Provide knowledge as needed related to the pathophysiology of the disease or illness, prescribed activities, prescribed medications, and nutrition. **EBN:** *Knowledge is a factor that contributes significantly to the client's taking action for health promotion and protection (Pender, Murdaugh, &*

● = Independent   ▲ = Collaborative   **EBN** = Evidence-Based Nursing   **EB** = Evidence-Based

Parsons, 2006). Remember, however, that knowledge is necessary but not sufficient to explain why people perform or do not perform actions for health promotion and protection (Pender, Murdaugh, & Parsons, 2006).

- Support positive health-promotion and health-protection behaviors. **EBN:** *Ongoing support may be needed to maintain these behaviors (Pender, Murdaugh, & Parsons, 2006).*
- Help the client maintain existing support and seek additional supports as needed. **EBN:** *In numerous research studies, social support was shown to be a factor contributing to ongoing maintenance of positive health behaviors (Lubkin & Larsen, 2006; Pender, Murdaugh, & Parsons, 2006). This study demonstrates that peer support programmes are a promising approach to enhance social and emotional support, assist clients in daily management and living with diabetes, and promote linkages to clinical care (Funnell, 2009; Heisler, 2009).* **EB:** *Clients using Internet discussion boards reported that knowledge and expertise accumulated over many years of self-management was instrumental to participants' self-reported ability to evaluate information posted and make decisions on its possible use (Armstrong & Powell, 2009).*

Geriatric

- Facilitate the client and family to obtain health insurance and drug payment plans whenever needed and possible. **EB:** *For older Americans, underuse of prescription medications because of cost was found to lead to adverse health effects (Heisler, 2004).*

Multicultural

- Assess client's perspectives on self-management. **EB:** *With the worldwide increase in migration, an understanding of the cultural factors that influence clients' perspectives on self-management behaviors is necessary. Participants are experts on their lives and, as such, they adopt appropriate disease control behaviors, based on their experience and knowledge, as well as integrate the illness and its symptoms into their lives (Chen et al, 2008).*
- Assess health literacy in clients of diverse backgrounds. **EB:** *Individuals with marginal or inadequate functional health literacy have difficulty reading, understanding, and interpreting most written health texts and instructions. In addition, clients with marginal or inadequate health literacy scores are more likely to misunderstand directions for health care (Redman, 2007).*
- Assess for depression. **EB:** *In diabetic clients in a Korean clinic, depression was an explanatory factor for those reporting low adherence with self-care (Park et al, 2004). In post–myocardial infarction clients in the United Kingdom, more than 19% had symptoms of depression, which were thought to contribute to low adherence (Leong, Molassiotis, & Marsh 2004).*
- Validate the client's feelings regarding the ability to manage his or her own care and the impact on current lifestyle. **EB:** *A recent study elicited the expectations of treatment in 93 hypertensive African-American clients. Client expectations of treatment could serve as the basis for client education and counseling about hypertension and its management in this client population (Ogedegbe, Mancuso, & Allegrante, 2004).*
- Facilitate the client and family to obtain health insurance and drug payment plans whenever needed and possible. **EB:** *In older Americans, underuse of prescription medications because of cost was found to lead to adverse health effects (Heisler, 2004).*
- Use electronic monitoring to improve medication adherence. **EB:** *A recent study showed that the use of electronic monitors had a positive effect on adherence for minority women (Robbins et al, 2004).*
- Discuss with clients their beliefs about medication and treatment to enhance medication and treatment adherence. **EB and EBN:** *Various cultures have different beliefs regarding medication and treatments (Leininger & McFarland, 2006). Fowles (2007) proposes that collaboration with underserved women is important to achieve health. In another study, the use of electronic monitors had a positive effect on adherence for minority women (Robbins et al, 2004).*

Community Teaching

- Review therapeutic regimens and their optimal integration with daily living routines.
- Teach disease processes and therapeutic regimens for management of these disease processes. Suggest peer support groups for clients with schizophrenia. **EB:** *In this study research supporting a more*

selective role for medication is reviewed along with the role of peer supporters in helping individuals to maximize their own unique medication needs with self-advocacy and negotiation skills (West, 2009).

ⓔvolve   See the EVOLVE website for Weblinks for client education resources.

REFERENCES

Armstrong N, Powell J: Patient perspectives on health advice posted on Internet discussion boards: a qualitative study, *Health Expect* 12(3):313–320, 2009.

Bidmead C, Cowley S: A concept analysis of partnership with clients, *Community Pract* 78:203–208, 2005.

Chen KH, Chen ML, Lee S et al: Self-management behaviours for patients with chronic obstructive pulmonary disease: a qualitative study, *J Adv Nurs* 64(6):595–604, 2008.

Fowles ER: Collaborative methodologies for advancing the health of underserved women, *Fam Community Health* 30:S53–S63, 2007.

Funnell MM: Peer-based behavioural strategies to improve chronic disease self-management and clinical outcomes: evidence, logistics, evaluation considerations and needs for future research, *Fam Pract* [Epub ahead of print], Jun 9, 2009.

Heisler M: The health effects of restricting prescription medication use because of cost, *Med Care* 42(7):626–634, 2004.

Heisler M: Different models to mobilize peer support to improve diabetes self-management and clinical outcomes: evidence, logistics, evaluation considerations and needs for future research, *Fam Pract* [Epub ahead of print] Mar 17, 2009.

Kettunen T, Liimatainen L, Villberg J et al: Developing empowering health counseling measurement. Preliminary results, *Patient Educ Couns* 64(1–3):159–166, 2006.

Koch T, Jenkin P, Kralik D: Chronic illness self management: locating the self, *J Adv Nurs* 48(5):484–492, 2004.

Leininger MM, McFarland MR: *Cultural care diversity and universality: a worldwide nursing theory*, ed 2, Boston, 2006, Jones and Bartlett.

Leong J, Molassiotis A, Marsh H: Adherence to health recommendations after a cardiac rehabilitation programme in post-myocardial infarction patients: the role of health beliefs, locus of control and psychological status, *Clin Effectiveness Nurs* 8(1):26–38, 2004.

Lubkin IM, Larsen PD: *Chronic illness: impact and interventions*, ed 6, Boston, 2006, Jones and Bartlett.

Ogedegbe G, Mancuso CA, Allegrante JP: Expectations of blood pressure management in hypertensive African-American patients: a qualitative study, *J Natl Med Assoc* 96(4):442–449, 2004.

Park H, Hong Y, Lee H et al: Individuals with type 2 diabetes and depressive symptoms exhibited low adherence with self care, *J Clin Epidemiol* 57:978–984, 2004.

Pender NJ, Murdaugh CL, Parsons MA: *Health promotion in nursing practice*, ed 5, Upper Saddle River, NJ, 2006, Prentice Hall.

Redman BK: *The practice of patient education: a case study approach*, ed 10, St Louis, 2007, Mosby.

Robbins B, Rausch KJ, Garcia RI et al: Multicultural medication adherence: a comparative study, *J Gerontol Nurs* 30(7):25–32, 2004.

Stanford University: *Patient education*. http://patient-education.stanford.edu/internet. Accessed April 25, 2007.

West C: Powerful choices: peer support and individualized medication self-determination. *Schizophr Bull* [Epub ahead of print] Jun 10, 2009.

Self-Mutilation   *Kathleen L. Patusky, PhD, APRN-BC*

NANDA-I

Definition

Deliberate self-injurious behavior causing tissue damage with the intent of causing nonfatal injury to attain relief of tension

Defining Characteristics

Abrading; biting; constricting a body part; cuts on body; hitting; ingestion of harmful substances; inhalation of harmful substances; insertion of object into body orifice; picking at wounds; scratches on body; self-inflicted burns; severing

Related Factors (r/t)

Adolescence; autistic individual; battered child; borderline personality disorder; character disorder; childhood illness; childhood sexual abuse; childhood surgery; depersonalization; developmentally delayed individual; dissociation; disturbed body image; disturbed interpersonal relationships; eating disorders; emotionally disturbed; family alcoholism; family divorce; family history of self-destructive behaviors; feels threatened with loss of significant relationship; history of inability to plan solutions; history of inability to see long-term consequences; history of self-injurious behavior; impulsivity; inability to express tension verbally; incarceration; ineffective coping; irresistible urge to cut self; irresistible urge to damage self; isolation from peers; labile behavior; lack of family confidant; living in nontraditional setting (e.g., foster, group institutional care); low self-esteem; mounting tension that is intolerable; needs quick reduction of stress; negative feelings (e.g., depression, rejection, self-hatred, separation anxiety, guilt, depersonalization); peers who self-mutilate; perfectionism; poor communication between parent

● = Independent   ▲ = Collaborative   **EBN** = Evidence-Based Nursing   **EB** = Evidence-Based

and adolescent; psychotic state (e.g., command hallucinations); sexual identity crisis; substance abuse; unstable body image; unstable self-esteem; use of manipulation to obtain nurturing relationship with others; violence between parental figures

NOC (Nursing Outcomes Classification)

Suggested NOC Outcomes

Self-Control, Distorted Thought Self-Control, Impulse Self-Control, Mood Equilibrium, Risk Detection, Self-Mutilation Restraint

Example NOC Outcome with Indicators

Self-Mutilation Restraint as evidenced by the following indicators: Refrains from gathering means for self-injury/ Obtains assistance as needed/Upholds contract not to harm self/Maintains self-control without supervision/Refrains from injuring self (Rate the outcome and indicators of **Self-Mutilation Restraint:** 1 = never demonstrated, 2 = rarely demonstrated, 3 = sometimes demonstrated, 4 = often demonstrated, 5 = consistently demonstrated [see Section I].)

Consider using a measure of self-harm risk that is available for clients: Self-Injury Questionnaire addresses intention for self-harm (Santa Mina et al, 2006).

Client Outcomes

Client Will (Specify Time Frame):

- Have injuries treated
- Refrain from further self-injury
- State appropriate ways to cope with increased psychological or physiological tension
- Express feelings
- Seek help when having urges to self-mutilate
- Maintain self-control without supervision
- Use appropriate community agencies when caregivers are unable to attend to emotional needs

NIC (Nursing Interventions Classification)

Suggested NIC Interventions

Active Listening, Anger Control Assistance, Behavior Management: Self-Harm, Calming Technique, Environmental Management: Safety, Limit Setting, Mood Management, Mutual Goal Setting, Risk Identification, Self-Responsibility Facilitation

Example NIC Activities—Behavior Management: Self-Harm

Anticipate trigger situations that may prompt self-harm and intervene to prevent it; Teach and reinforce patient for effective coping behaviors and appropriate expression of feelings

Nursing Interventions and *Rationales*

NOTE: Before implementing interventions in the face of self-mutilation, nurses should examine their own emotional responses to incidents of self-harm to ensure that interventions will not be based on countertransference reactions. **EBN and EB:** *Nurses have shown negative responses toward clients who self-mutilate (Anderson & Standen, 2007; Wilstrand et al, 2007; Fish & Duperouzel, 2008).*

▲ Provide medical treatment for injuries. Use careful aseptic technique when caring for wounds. Care for the wounds in a matter-of-fact manner. *A significant impediment to wound healing is infection. A matter-of-fact approach avoids promoting inappropriate attention-getting behavior and may decrease repetition of behavior.*

- Assess for risk of suicide or other self-damaging behaviors. **EB:** *Although self-mutilation should not be viewed simply as failed suicide, it is a significant indicator of suicide risk. Clients may also engage in other self-damaging behaviors, including substance abuse or eating disorders (Favaro, Ferrara, & Santonastaso, 2007).* Refer to the care plan for **Risk for Suicide**.

- Assess for signs of depression, anxiety, and impulsivity. Assess for an eating disorder, particularly bulimia nervosa. **EB:** *Self-mutilation has been associated with eating disorders, especially bulimia*

● = Independent   ▲ = Collaborative   **EBN** = Evidence-Based Nursing   **EB** = Evidence-Based

nervosa if the client experienced physical or sexual abuse before age 15 (Claes & Vandereycken, 2007; Ahren-Moonga et al, 2008; Murray, MacDonald, & Fox, 2008).

- Assess for presence of hallucinations. Ask specific questions such as, "Do you hear voices that other people do not hear? Are they telling you to hurt yourself?" *Command hallucinations occurring with schizophrenia or brief psychotic episodes may direct the client to hurt himself or herself, or others (Kress, 2003).*

- ▲ Assure the client that he or she will not be alone and will be safe during hallucinations. Provide referrals for medication. *Hallucinations can be very frightening; therefore clients need reassurance that they will not be left alone.*

- ▲ Assess for the presence of medical disorders, mental retardation, medication effects, or psychiatric disorders such as autism and dissociative disorders (DD) that may include self-mutilation. Initiate referral for evaluation and treatment as appropriate. **EB:** *Self-mutilation has been reported as a presenting symptom with medical disorders, such as the genetic Lesch-Nyhan syndrome (multiple types of behaviors) (Robey et al, 2003). (Additional relevant research: Izutsu et al, 2006; Singh et al, 2006; Ebrinc et al, 2008).*

- ▲ Case finding and referral by school nurses for psychological or psychiatric treatment is critical. *Treatment includes starting therapy and medications, increasing coping skills, facilitating decision making, encouraging positive relationships, and fostering self-esteem (McDonald, 2006).*

- Monitor the client's behavior, using 15–minute checks at irregular times so that the client does not notice a pattern. *When lack of control exists, client safety is an important issue and close observation is essential. Avoiding a pattern prevents clients from being self-abusive when they know a caregiver will not be present.*

- Establish trust, listen to client, convey safety, and assist in developing positive goals for the future. **EBN and EB:** *Clients reported that nurses were helpful when they took charge of unsafe situations, performed bodily interventions (e.g., holding hand), conveyed safety, and respected the autonomy of the client (Schoppmann et al, 2007). Clients expressed the need to be listened to; emphasized that staff relationships were important to help cope with strong emotions and daily stresses, cope with urges to self-injure. And provide a view of a positive future (Fish & Duperouzel, 2008).*

- Recognize that self-mutilation may serve a variety of functions for the person. *Self-mutilation may help with the regulation of dysphoric affect, the expression of emotions, or coping with dissociative states (Paris, 2005).*

- Be extremely cautious about touching the client when he or she is experiencing an abreaction (re-enactment of precipitating trauma). Sometimes physically holding a client is necessary to prevent self-injury. *Even well-intentioned or consoling touching may further upset the client. A therapist who is attempting to be consoling should always ask abreacting clients whether they may be touched. Clients may initially refuse, but they generally appreciate the offer (Weber, 2002).*

- Assess the client's ability to enter into a no-suicide or no-self-harm contract. Secure a written or verbal contract from the client to notify staff when experiencing suicidal ideation or the desire to self-mutilate. *Discussing feelings of self-harm with a trusted person provides relief for the client. A contract places some of the responsibility for safety with the client. Some clients are not appropriate for a contract: those under the influence of drugs or alcohol or unwilling to abstain from substance use, and those who are isolated or alone without assistance to keep the environment safe (Hauenstein, 2002).* **EB:** *The lack of willingness to self-disclose has been shown to discriminate the serious suicide attempter from the client with suicidal ideation or the mild attempter (Apter et al, 2001).* **EBN:** NOTE: *Although contracting is a common practice in psychiatric care settings, research has suggested that self-harm is not prevented by contracts. Thorough, ongoing assessment of suicide risk is necessary, whether or not the client has entered into a no-self-harm contract. Contracts may not be appropriate in community settings (Farrow, 2003; McMyler & Pryjmachuk, 2008).*

- ▲ Use a collaborative approach for care. *A collaborative approach to care is more helpful to the client.*

- Refer to the care plan for **Risk for Self-Mutilation** for additional information.

Home Care and Client/Family Teaching and Discharge Planning

- See the care plan for **Risk for Self-Mutilation.**

evolve   See the EVOLVE website for Weblinks for client education resources.

• = Independent   ▲ = Collaborative   **EBN** = Evidence-Based Nursing   **EB** = Evidence-Based

REFERENCES

Ahren-Moonga J, Holmgren S, van Knorring L et al: Personality traits and self-injurious behaviour in patients with eating disorders, *Eur Eating Dis Rev* 16:268, 2008.

Anderson M, Standen PJ: Attitudes towards suicide among nurses and doctors working with children and young people who self-harm, *J Psychiatr Ment Health Nurs* 14:470, 2007.

Apter A, Horesh N, Gothelf D et al: Relationship between self-disclosure and serious suicidal behavior, *Compr Psychiatry* 42(1):70, 2001.

Claes L, Vandereycken W: Is there a link between traumatic experiences and self-injurious behaviors in eating-disordered patients? *Eating Disord* 15:305, 2007.

Ebrinc S, Semiz UB, Basoglu C et al: Self-mutilating behavior in patients with dissociative disorders: the role of innate hypnotic capacity, *Isr J Psychiatry Relat Sci* 45(1):39–48, 2008.

Farrow TL: "No suicide contracts" in community crisis situations: a conceptual analysis, *J Psychiatr Ment Health Nurs* 10:199, 2003.

Favaro A, Ferrara S, Santonastaso P: Self-injurious behavior in a community sample of young women: relationship with childhood abuse and other types of self-damaging behaviors, *J Clin Psychiatry* 68:122, 2007.

Fish R, Duperouzel H: "Just another day dealing with wounds": self-injury and staff-client relationships, *Learning Disability Pract* 11: 12, 2008.

Hauenstein EJ: Case finding and care in suicide: children, adolescents, and adults. In Boyd MA, editor: *Psychiatric nursing: contemporary practice*, ed 2, Philadelphia, 2002, Lippincott Williams & Wilkins.

Izutsu T, Shimotsu S, Matsumoto T et al: Deliberate self-harm and childhood hyperactivity in junior high school students, *Eur Child Adolesc Psychiatry* 15:172, 2006.

Kress VEW: Self-injurious behaviors: assessment and diagnosis, *J Counsel Develop* 81(4):490, 2003.

McDonald C: Self-mutilation in adolescents, *J Sch Nurs* 22:193, 2006.

McMyler C, Pryjmachuk S: Do "no-suicide" contracts work? *J Psychiatr Ment Health Nurs* 15:512, 2008.

Murray CD, MacDonald S, Fox J: Body satisfaction, eating disorders and suicide ideation in an Internet sample of self-harmers reporting and not reporting childhood sexual abuse, *Psychol Health Med* 13:29, 2008.

Paris J: Understanding self-mutilation in borderline personality disorder, *Harv Rev Psychiatry* 13:179, 2005.

Robey KL, Reck JF, Giacomini KD et al: Modes and patterns of self-mutilation in persons with Lesch-Nyhan disease, *Dev Med Child Neurol* 45:167, 2003.

Santa Mina EE, Gallop R, Links P et al: The Self-Injury Questionnaire: evaluation of the psychometric properties in a clinical population, *J Psychiatr Ment Health Nurs* 13:221, 2006.

Schoppmann S, Schrock R, Schnepp et al: "Then I just showed her my arms..." Bodily sensations in moments of alienation related to self-injurious behaviour. A hermeneutic phenomenological study, *J Psychiatr Ment Health Nurs* 14:587, 2007.

Singh NN, Lancioni GE, Winton ASW et al: Mindful parenting decreases aggression, noncompliance, and self-injury in children with autism, *J Emot Behav Disord* 14:169, 2006.

Weber MT: Triggers for self-abuse: a qualitative study, *Arch Psychiatr Nurs* 16:118, 2002.

Wilstrand C, Lindgren BM, Gilje F et al: Being burdened and balancing boundaries: a qualitative study of nurses' experiences caring for patients who self-harm, *J Psychiatr Ment Health Nurs* 14:72, 2007.

Risk for Self-Mutilation   Kathleen L. Patusky, PhD, APRN-BC

NANDA-I

Definition

At risk for deliberate self-injurious behavior causing tissue damage with the intent of causing nonfatal injury to attain relief of tension

Risk Factors

Adolescence; autistic individuals; battered child; borderline personality disorders; character disorders; childhood illness; childhood sexual abuse; childhood surgery; depersonalization; developmentally delayed individuals; dissociation; disturbed body image; disturbed interpersonal relationships; eating disorders; emotionally disturbed child; family alcoholism; family divorce; family history of self-destructive behaviors; feels threatened with loss of significant relationship; history of inability to plan solutions; history of inability to see long-term consequences; history of self-injurious behavior; impulsivity; inability to express tension verbally; inadequate coping; incarceration; irresistible urge to damage self; isolation from peers; living in nontraditional setting (e.g., foster group, or institutional care); loss of control over problem-solving situations; loss of significant relationship(s); low self-esteem; mounting tension that is intolerable; needs quick reduction of stress; negative feelings (e.g., depression, rejection, self-hatred, separation anxiety, guilt); peers who self-mutilate; perfectionism; psychotic state (e.g., command hallucinations); sexual identity crisis; substance abuse; unstable self-esteem; use of manipulation to obtain nurturing relationship with others; violence between parental figures

NOC   (Nursing Outcomes Classification)

See care plan for **Self-Mutilation.**

• = Independent   ▲ = Collaborative   **EBN** = Evidence-Based Nursing   **EB** = Evidence-Based

Client Outcomes

Client Will (Specify Time Frame):

- Refrain from self-injury
- Identify triggers to self-mutilation
- State appropriate ways to cope with increased psychological or physiological tension
- Express feelings
- Seek help when having urges to self-mutilate
- Maintain self-control without supervision
- Use appropriate community agencies when caregivers are unable to attend to emotional needs

NIC   (Nursing Interventions Classification)

See care plan for **Self-Mutilation.**

Nursing Interventions and *Rationales*

- Assessment data from the client and family members may have to be gathered at different times; allowing a family member or trusted friend with whom the client is comfortable to be present during the assessment may be helpful. **EB:** *Self-mutilation sometimes occurs if clients have been victims of abuse (Claes & Vandereycken, 2007; Murray, MacDonald, & Fox, 2008). Clients or family members may be more willing to disclose the presence of abuse if greater privacy is afforded them. Presence of a trusted family member or friend may help clients to respond more comfortably to the interview situation.*
- Assess for risk factors of self-mutilation, including categories of psychiatric disorders (particularly borderline personality disorder, psychosis, eating disorders, autism); psychological precursors (e.g., low tolerance for stress, impulsivity, perfectionism); psychosocial dysfunction (e.g., presence of sexual abuse, divorce or alcoholism in the family, manipulative behavior to gain nurturing, chaotic interpersonal relationships); coping difficulties (e.g., inability to plan solutions or see long-term consequences of behavior); personal history (e.g., childhood illness or surgery, past self-injurious behavior); and peer influences (e.g., friends who mutilate, isolation from peers). *These risk factors have been associated with self-mutilation.* **EB:** *Self-mutilation has been associated with eating disorders, especially bulimia nervosa if the client experienced physical or sexual abuse before age 15 (Claes & Vandereycken, 2007; Ahren-Moonga et al, 2008; Murray, MacDonald, & Fox, 2008). Persons with borderline personality disorder who initiate self-harm as children will have the most serious course (Zanarini et al, 2005).*
- Assess for co-occurring disorders that require response, specifically childhood abuse, substance abuse, and suicide attempts. **EB:** *A relationship has been found between self-mutilating behavior, substance abuse, childhood abuse, alexithymia, and suicide attempts (Evren & Evren, 2005). Long-term glue sniffing has been associated with violent behavior and/or self mutilation (Shu & Tsai, 2003). Self-mutilation was found more often in drug-dependent persons than alcohol-dependent persons (Evren, Kural, & Cakmak, 2006).*
- Assess family dynamics and the need for family therapy and community supports. *Treatment generally focuses on increasing support for the client, improving family communication, and enhancing the client's sense of control over the environment (Derouin & Bravender, 2004).*
- Assess for a possible genetic disorder that results in severe and involuntary self-mutilation. *Lesch-Nyhan syndrome is a rare genetic disorder, which is characterized by compulsive self-mutilation (Zilli & Hasselmo, 2008).*
- Be alert to other risk factors of self-mutilation in clients with psychosis, including acute intoxication, dramatic changes in body appearance, preoccupation with religion and sexuality, and anticipated or perceived object loss. Monitor clients with obsessive-compulsive disorder or clients who have issues with gender identity. *Many psychiatric disorders have shown a connection with self-mutilation. Command hallucinations occurring with schizophrenia or brief psychotic episodes may direct the client to hurt himself or herself, or others (Kress, 2003).*
- Maintain ongoing surveillance of the client and environment. Monitor the client's behavior, using 15–minute checks at irregular times so that the client does not notice a pattern. *When lack of control exists, client safety is an important issue and close observation is essential. Not following a pattern prevents clients from being self-abusive when they know a caregiver will not be present.*

- When the client is experiencing extreme anxiety, use one-to-one staffing. Offer activities that will serve as a distraction. **EBN:** *The presence of a trusted individual may calm fears about personal safety. Distraction can be one way of preventing a self-injury episode (O'Donovan, 2007; Schoppmann et al, 2007).*
- Assess the client's ability to enter into a no-suicide or no-self-harm contract. Secure a written or verbal contract from the client to notify staff when experiencing suicidal ideation or the desire to self-mutilate. *Discussing feelings of self-harm with a trusted person provides relief for the client. A contract places some of the responsibility for safety with the client. Some clients are not appropriate for a contract: those under the influence of drugs or alcohol or unwilling to abstain from substance use, and those who are isolated or alone without assistance to keep the environment safe (Hauenstein, 2002).* **EB:** *The lack of willingness to self-disclose has been shown to discriminate the serious suicide attempter from the client with suicidal ideation or the mild attempter (Apter et al, 2001).* **EBN:** NOTE: *Although contracting is a common practice in psychiatric care settings, research has suggested that self-harm is not prevented by contracts. Thorough, ongoing assessment of suicide risk is necessary, whether or not the client has entered into a no-self-harm contract. Contracts may not be appropriate in community settings (McMyler & Pryjmachuk, 2008).*
- Establish trust, listen to client, convey safety, and assist in developing positive goals for the future. **EBN and EB:** *Clients reported that nurses were helpful when they took charge of unsafe situations, performed bodily interventions (e.g., holding hand), conveyed safety, and respected the autonomy of the client (Schoppmann et al, 2007). Clients expressed the need to be listened to; emphasized that staff relationships were important to help cope with strong emotions and daily stresses, cope with urges to self-injure, and to provide a view of a positive future (Fish & Duperouzel, 2008).*
- ▲ Refer to mental health counseling. Multiple therapeutic modalities are available for treatment. **EBN:** *Solution-focused brief therapy has been shown to be an effective treatment option for reducing repetitive self-harm (Wiseman, 2003).*
- When working with self-mutilative clients who have borderline personality disorder, develop an effective therapeutic relationship by avoiding labeling, seeking to understand the meaning of the self-mutilation, and advocating for adequate opportunities for care. **EBN and EB:** *Clients expressed a need to be respected and treated as an individual, with 1:1 time and awareness of moods. Mutual confidence and trust should be developed before working on issues in depth (O'Donovan, 2007; Schoppmann et al, 2007; Fish & Duperouzel, 2008).*
- Maintain a consistent relational distance from the client with borderline personality disorder who self-mutilates: neither too close nor too distant, neither rewarding unacceptable behavior nor trying to control or avoid the client. *Clients with borderline personality disorder recreate the chaos of their previous relationships in dealing with health care providers. Clients fear that they will be overwhelmed by or abandoned in relationships, and their reactions can change rapidly. The most effective posture is one that is consistent, allowing clients to react as they need to, while assuring clients that they will not be abandoned.*
- Inform the client of expectations for appropriate behavior and consequences within the unit. Emphasize that the client must comply with the rules. Give positive reinforcement for compliance and minimize attention paid to disruptive behavior while setting limits. *Clients benefit from clear guidance regarding behavioral expectations and consequences, providing much-needed structure. It is important to reinforce appropriate behavior to encourage repetition.* **EB:** *Treatment should involve assisting the client to learn healthier affective regulation skills (Claes & Vandereycken, 2007).*
- Clients need to learn to recognize distress as it occurs and express it verbally rather than as a physical action against the self. *Self-mutilation serves to act out feeling states that the client cannot express or process. Such acts may attempt to relieve pain or punish the self. Therapy helps the client to articulate emotions and needs (Derouin et al, 2004).* **EB:** *Treatment should involve assisting the client to learn healthier affective regulation skills (Claes & Vandereycken, 2007).*
- Assist the client to identify the motives/reasons for self-mutilation that have been perceived as positive. *Self-mutilation serves the following functions: releasing tension, returning to reality, regaining control of some aspect of self, expressing forbidden anger, escaping self-hatred associated with incest, aiming to decrease alienation from or influence others, relieving pressure from multiple personalities, and achieving sexual gratification. The sight of blood provides emotional release, and the pain and the blood stop feelings of emptiness. The client must learn alternative ways of securing these gains if they are to give up self-mutilation (McAllister, 2001).*

• = Independent   ▲ = Collaborative   **EBN** = Evidence-Based Nursing   **EB** = Evidence-Based

- Help the client identify cues that precede impulsive behavior. **EB:** *Dialectical behavior therapy (DBT) was found to be superior to non-DBT treatment in reducing self-mutilation among individuals with borderline personality disorder (Verheul et al, 2003).* **EBN:** *The DBT technique of behavioral chain analysis was found to reduce self-harm behaviors by processing events that precipitate self-mutilation (Alper & Peterson, 2001).*
- Assist clients to identify ways to soothe themselves and generate hopefulness when faced with painful emotions. **EBN:** *Women with a history of childhood abuse may not have developed the internal ability to comfort themselves, or self-soothe, resulting in neurobiological disruptions that lead to self-harm as a means of relieving pain (Gallop, 2002). Generating hopefulness is an important self-comforting intervention (Weber, 2002).*
- Reinforce alternative ways of dealing with depression and anxiety, such as exercise, engaging in unit activities, or talking about feelings. *Goal direction enhances self-efficacy, an important antecedent of empowerment (Fitzsimons & Fuller, 2002; Finfgeld, 2004).*
- Keep the environment safe; remove all harmful objects from the area. Use of unbreakable glass is recommended for the client at risk for self-injury. *Client safety is a nursing priority. Unbreakable glass would eliminate this type of injury.*
- Anticipate trigger situations and intervene to assist the client in applying alternatives to self-mutilation. **EB:** *When triggers occur, client stress level may obstruct ability to apply recent learning. Cognitive strategies can be useful to correct irrational beliefs that are part of the trigger (Claes & Vandereycken, 2007).*
- Reduce or eliminate use of caffeine, alcohol, and street drugs. *Caffeine can increase anxiety, which may trigger self-mutilation. Alcohol and street drugs alter mood and increase impulsivity while decreasing inhibitions (Derouin & Bravender, 2004).*
- If self-mutilation does occur, use a calm, nonpunitive approach. Whenever possible, assist the client to assume responsibility for consequences (e.g., dress self-inflicted wound). Refer to the care plan for **Self-Mutilation**. *This approach does not promote inappropriate attention-getting behavior, may decrease repetition of behavior, and reinforces self-responsibility and self-care management.*
- If the client is unable to control self-mutilation behavior, provide interactive supervision, not isolation. *Isolation and deprivation take away individuals' coping abilities and place them at risk for self-harm. Implementing seclusion for clients who have injured themselves in the past may actually facilitate self-injury. Clients are extraordinarily resourceful at identifying environmental objects with which to self-mutilate.*
- Involve the client in planning their care and problem solving, and emphasize that the client makes choices. **EB:** *Individuals who self-mutilate were found to use more problem avoidance behaviors and to perceive that they had less control over problem-solving options (Haines & Williams, 2003). Clients reported negative responses to having no input into their treatment plan (Fish & Duperouzel, 2008).*
- ▲ Use group therapy to exchange information about methods of coping with loneliness, self-destructive impulses, and interpersonal relationships as well as housing, employment, and health care system issues directly and noninterpretively. *The group's focus should be here and now, supportive and psychoeducative, while providing a comforting level of structure.*
- Internet groups may provide additional support. **EB:** *In a study of one Web support group (n=102), many participants reported a decrease in frequency and severity of self-mutilation (Murray & Fox, 2006).*
- ▲ Refer to protective services if evidence of abuse exists. *It is the nurse's legal responsibility to report abuse.*
- Refer to the care plan for **Self-Mutilation**.

 Pediatric

- Be aware of increasing incidence of self-mutilation, especially among teens and young adults. *The developmental stressors of adolescence, along with depression, may increase the incidence of self-mutilation (Derouin & Bravender, 2004).* **EBN:** *Teens who self-mutilate may be academically and socially successful, high-achieving, and outgoing, managing to hide evidence of problems or ineffective coping skills (Machoian, 2001).*
- Conduct a thorough physical examination, being alert for superficial scars that may be patterned, although in most cases scabbing or infection is not evident. *Apart from obvious sites, evidence of*

cutting or burning may be hidden in such areas as the axilla, abdomen, inner thighs, feet, and under breasts (Derouin & Bravender, 2004).

- Maintaining a therapeutic relationship with teens requires explicit assurances of confidentiality, consistency of clinical routines, and a nonjudgmental communication style. *Even adolescents younger than age 18 years need assurances that confidentiality will be maintained unless there is a serious risk of harm to themselves or others (Bravender, 2002). However, teens of all ages should be advised that parental notification will be made to ensure the teen's safety and to implement a treatment plan (Derouin & Bravender, 2004).*
- Attend to behavioral clues of self-mutilation; a brief self-report assessment can be useful. *Self-mutilators can exhibit mood swings, low self-esteem, poor impulse control, anxiety, self-disappointment, or an inability to identify positive elements in their lives (Machoian, 2001). The American Medical Association's Guidelines for Adolescent Preventive Services (GAPS) can be helpful and is available at www.ama-assn.org/ama/pub/physician-resources/public-health/promoting-healthy-lifestyles/adolescent-health/guidelines-adolescent-preventive-services.shtml (Derouin & Bravender, 2004).*
- Assess for the presence of an eating disorder or substance abuse. Attend to the themes that preoccupy teens with eating disorders who self-mutilate. **EB:** *Self-mutilation was shown to be more common among adolescents with dependence issues (drug abuse and eating disorders) (Bolognini et al, 2003). The thought processes of adolescents with eating disorders were found to center on feeling undeserving of receiving help, feeling helpless and hopeless in dealing with the eating disorder itself, having difficulty with recognizing and expressing feelings, feeling ambivalent about treatment, and mistrusting health care providers (Manley & Leichner, 2003).*
- Evaluate for suicidal ideation/suicide risk. Refer to the care plan for **Risk for Suicide** for additional information. **EB:** *Adolescents who attempted suicide by overdose admitted to some method of self-mutilation. The self-mutilators were significantly more likely than non–self-mutilators to be diagnosed with oppositional defiant disorder, major depression, and dysthymia, and had higher scores on measures of hopelessness, loneliness, anger, risk taking, and alcohol use (Guertin et al, 2001).*
- Be aware that there is not complete overlap between self-mutilation and suicidal behavior. The motivation may be different (coping with difficult feelings rather than ending life), and the method is usually different. **EB:** *In one study, about half of the participants reported both attempted suicide and self-mutilation; the other half reported no overlap in types of acts (Bolognini et al, 2003).*
- Use treatment approaches detailed previously, with modifications as appropriate for this age group.

Geriatric

- Provide hand or back rubs and calming music when elderly clients experience anxiety. **EBN:** *In a study of older adults in nursing homes, calming music and hand massage were found to soothe agitation for up to 1 hour. No additional benefit was found from combining the two interventions (Remington, 2002).*
- Provide soft objects for elderly clients to hold and manipulate when self-mutilation occurs as a function of delirium or dementia. Apply mitts, splints, helmets, or restraints as appropriate. *Delirious or demented clients may unconsciously scratch or pick at themselves. Soft objects may provide a substitute object to pick at; mitts or restraints may be necessary if the client is unable to exercise self-restraint.*
- Older adults who show self-destructive behaviors should be evaluated for dementia. **EB:** *In a study of nursing home residents, self-destructive behaviors were common and more likely related to dementia than to depression (Draper et al, 2002).*

Home Care

- Communicate degree of risk to family/caregivers; assess the family and caregiving situation for ability to protect the client and to understand the client's self-mutilative behavior. Provide family and caregivers with guidelines on how to manage self-harm behaviors in the home environment. *Client safety between home visits is a nursing priority. Appropriate family/caregiver support is important to the client. Appropriate support will only be forthcoming if all parties understand the basis of the behavior and how to respond to it.*
- Establish an emergency plan, including when to use hotlines and 911. Develop a contract with the client and family for use of the emergency plan. Role play access to the emergency resources with

the client and caregivers. *Having an emergency plan reassures the client and caregivers and promotes client safety. Contracting gives guided control to the client and enhances self-esteem.*

- Assess the home environment for harmful objects. Have family remove or lock objects as able. *Client safety is a nursing priority.*
- ▲ If client behaviors intensify, institute an emergency plan for mental health intervention. *The degree of disturbance and the ability to manage care safely at home determines the level of services needed to protect the client.*
- ▲ Refer for homemaker or psychiatric home health care services for respite, client reassurance, and implementation of therapeutic regimen. *Responsibility for a person at high risk for self-mutilation provides high caregiver stress. Respite decreases caregiver stress. The presence of caring individuals is reassuring to both the client and caregivers, especially during periods of client anxiety. A client with self-mutilative behavior, especially if accompanied by depression, can benefit from the interventions described previously, modified for the home setting.*
- ▲ If the client is on psychotropic medications, assess client and family knowledge of medication administration and side effects. Teach as necessary. *Knowledge of the medical regimen promotes compliance and promotes safe use of medications.*
- ▲ Evaluate the effectiveness and side effects of medications. *Accurate clinical feedback improves physician ability to prescribe an effective medical regimen specific to client needs.*

Client/Family Teaching and Discharge Planning

- Explain all relevant symptoms, procedures, treatments, and expected outcomes for self-mutilation that is illness based (e.g., borderline personality disorder, autism). **EB:** *Clients prefer to participate in their treatment planning to gain a sense of control (Fish & Duperouzel, 2008).*
- Assist family members to understand the complex issues of self-mutilation. Provide instruction on relevant developmental issues and on actions parents can take to avoid media that glorify self-harm behaviors. *Family members need to understand the behaviors they are dealing with, receive positive reinforcement that will promote their patience and perseverance, and know that they can take positive action to remove media triggers for self-mutilation (Derouin & Bravender, 2004).*
- Provide written instructions for treatments and procedures for which the client will be responsible. *A written record provides a concrete reference so that the client and family can clarify any verbal information that was given.*
- Instruct the client in coping strategies (assertiveness training, impulse control training, deep breathing, progressive muscle relaxation). *Clients who self-mutilate have difficulty dealing with stress and painful emotions, which serve as triggers to self-harm. Once clients are able to identify these triggers, they need to learn how to respond to them more effectively through assertiveness, impulse control, or relaxation, as appropriate.*
- Role play (e.g., say, "Tell me how you will respond if someone ignores you"). *Role playing is the most commonly used technique in assertiveness training. It deconditions the anxiety that arises from interpersonal encounters by allowing the client to practice how they might respond in a given situation. Anxiety levels tend to be higher in situations that are unfamiliar.*
- Teach cognitive-behavioral activities, such as active problem solving, reframing (reappraising the situation from a different perspective), or thought-stopping (in response to a negative thought, picture a large stop sign and replace the image with a prearranged positive alternative). Teach the client to confront his or her own negative thought patterns (or cognitive distortions), such as catastrophizing (expecting the very worst), dichotomous thinking (perceiving events in only one of two opposite categories), or magnification (placing distorted emphasis on a single event). *Cognitive-behavioral activities address clients' assumptions, beliefs, and attitudes about their situations, fostering modification of these elements to be as realistic and optimistic as possible. Through cognitive-behavioral interventions, clients become more aware of their cognitive choices in adopting and maintaining their belief systems, thereby exercising greater control over their own reactions (Claes & Vandereycken, 2007; Hagerty & Patusky, 2007).*
- ▲ Provide the client and family with phone numbers of appropriate community agencies for therapy and counseling. *Continuous follow-up care should be implemented; therefore, the method to access this care must be given to the client.*

▲ Give the client positive things on which to focus by referring to appropriate agencies for job-training skills or education. **EB:** *Clients expressed the desire for goals they could aim for as a means of regaining a positive view of the future (Fish & Duperouzel, 2008).*

ⓔvolve   See the EVOLVE website for Weblinks for client education resources.

REFERENCES

Ahren-Moonga J, Holmgren S, van Knorring L et al: Personality traits and self-injurious behaviour in patients with eating disorders, *Eur Eating Dis Rev* 16:268, 2008.

Alper G, Peterson SJ: Dialectical behavior therapy for patients with borderline personality disorder, *J Psychosoc Nurs Ment Health Serv* 39(10):38, 52, 2001.

Apter A, Horesh N, Gothelf D et al: Relationship between self-disclosure and serious suicidal behavior, *Compr Psychiatry* 42(1):70, 2001.

Bolognini M, Plancherel B, Laget J et al: Adolescents' self-mutilation: relationship with dependent behaviour, *Swiss J Psychol* 62(4):241, 2003.

Bravender T: *Adolescent medicine*, monograph ed. No. 279, Laewood, KS, 2002, American Academy of Family Physicians.

Claes L, Vandereycken W: Is there a link between traumatic experiences and self-injurious behaviors in eating-disordered patients? *Eating Disord* 15:305, 2007.

Derouin A, Bravender T: Living on the edge: the current phenomenon of self-mutilation in adolescents, *MCN Am J Matern Child Nurs* 29(1):12, 2004.

Draper B, Brodaty H, Lee-Fay L et al: Self-destructive behaviors in nursing home residents, *J Am Geriatr Soc* 50(2):354, 2002.

Evren C, Evren B: Self-mutilation in substance-dependent patients and relationship with childhood abuse and neglect, alexithymia and temperament and character dimensions of personality, *Drug Alcohol Depend* 80(1):15–22, 2005.

Evren C, Kural S, Cakmak D: Clinical correlates of self-mutilation in Turkish male substance-dependent inpatients, *Psychopathology* 39:248, 2006.

Finfgeld DL: Empowerment of individuals with enduring mental health problems: results from concept analyses and qualitative investigations, *Adv Nurs Sci* 27(1):44, 2004.

Fish R, Duperouzel H: "Just another day dealing with wounds": self-injury and staff-client relationships, *Learning Disability Pract* 11:12, 2008.

Fitzsimons S, Fuller R: Empowerment and its implications for clinical practice in mental health: a review, *J Ment Health* 11(5):481, 2002.

Gallop R: Failure of the capacity for self-soothing in women who have a history of abuse and self-harm, *J Am Psychiatr Nurses Assoc* 8:20, 2002.

Guertin T, Lloyd-Richardson E, Spirito A et al: Self-mutilative behavior in adolescents who attempt suicide by overdose, *J Am Acad Child Adolesc Psychiatry* 40(9):1062, 2001.

Hagerty B, Patusky K: Mood disorders: depression and mania. In Fortinash KM, Holoday-Worret PA, editors: *Psychiatric mental health nursing*, ed 4, St Louis, 2007, Mosby.

Haines J, Williams CL: Coping and problem solving of self-mutilators, *J Clin Psychol* 59(10):1097, 2003.

Hauenstein EJ: Case finding and care in suicide: children, adolescents, and adults. In Boyd MA, editor: *Psychiatric nursing: contemporary practice,* ed 2, Philadelphia, 2002, Lippincott Williams & Wilkins.

Kress VEW: Self-injurious behaviors: assessment and diagnosis, *J Counsel Develop* 81(4):490, 2003.

Machoian L: Cutting voices: self-injury in three adolescent girls, *J Psychosoc Nurs Ment Health Serv* 39(11):22, 2001.

Manley RS, Leichner P: Anguish and despair in adolescents with eating disorders: helping to manage suicidal ideation and impulses, *Crisis* 24(1):32, 2003.

McAllister MM: In harm's way: a postmodern narrative inquiry, *J Psychiatr Ment Health Nurs* 8:391, 2001.

McMyler C, Pryjmachuk S: Do "no-suicide" contracts work? *J Psychiatr Ment Health Nurs* 15:512, 2008.

Murray CD, Fox J: Do Internet self-harm discussion groups alleviate or exacerbate self-harming behavior? *Aust E J Adv Ment Health* 5:1, 2006.

Murray CD, MacDonald S, Fox J: Body satisfaction, eating disorders and suicide ideation in an Internet sample of self-harmers reporting and not reporting childhood sexual abuse, *Psychol Health Med* 13:29, 2008.

O'Donovan A: Pragmatism rules: the intervention and prevention strategies used by psychiatric nurses working with non-suicidal self-harming individuals, *J Psychiatr Ment Health Nurs* 14:64, 2007.

Remington R: Calming music and hand massage with agitated elderly, *Nurs Res* 51:317, 2002.

Schoppmann S, Schrock R, Schnepp et al: "Then I just showed her my arms..." Bodily sensations in moments of alienation related to self-injurious behaviour. A hermeneutic phenomenological study, *J Psychiatr Ment Health Nurs* 14:587, 2007.

Shu L, Tsai S: Long-term glue sniffing: report of six cases, *Intl J Psychiatry Med* 33:163, 2003.

Verheul R, Van den Bosch LMC, Koeter MWJ et al: Dialectical behaviour therapy for women with borderline personality disorder, *Br J Psychiatry* 182:135, 2003.

Weber MT: Triggers for self-abuse: a qualitative study, *Arch Psychiatr Nurs* 16:118, 2002.

Wiseman S: Brief intervention: reducing the repetition of deliberate self-harm, *Nurs Times* 99:35, 2003.

Zanarini MC, Frankenburg FR, Hennen J et al: The McLean Study of Adult Development (MSAD): overview and implications of the first six years of prospective follow-up, *J Personal Disord* 19:524, 2005.

Zilli EA, Hasselmo ME: A model of behavioral treatments for self-mutilation behavior in Lesch-Nyhan syndrome, *Neuroreport* 19(4):459–462, 2008.

Disturbed Sensory perception (Specify: Visual, Auditory, Kinesthetic, Gustatory, Tactile, Olfactory)   ⓔvolve

Major General (Ret) Gale S. Pollock, CRNA, MHA, FACHE, FAAN, and Betty J. Ackley, MSN, EdS, RN

NANDA-I

Definition

Change in the amount or patterning of incoming stimuli accompanied by a diminished, exaggerated, distorted, or impaired response to such stimuli

● = Independent   ▲ = Collaborative   **EBN** = Evidence-Based Nursing   **EB** = Evidence-Based

Defining Characteristics

Change in behavior pattern; change in problem-solving abilities; change in sensory acuity; change in usual response to stimuli; disorientation; hallucinations; impaired communication; irritability; poor concentration; restlessness; sensory distortions

Related Factors (r/t)

Altered sensory integration; altered sensory reception; altered sensory transmission; biochemical imbalance; electrolyte imbalance; excessive environmental stimuli; insufficient environmental stimuli; psychological stress

 (Nursing Outcomes Classification)

Suggested NOC Outcomes (Visual)

Body Image, Cognitive Orientation, Sensory Function: Vision, Vision Compensation Behavior

Example **NOC Outcome with Indicators**
Vision Compensation Behavior as evidenced by the following indicators: Uses adequate light for activity being performed/Wears eyeglasses correctly/Uses vision assistive devices/Uses computer assistive devices/Uses support services for low vision (Rate each indicator of **Vision Compensation Behavior:** 1 = never demonstrated, 2 = rarely demonstrated, 3 = sometimes demonstrated, 4 = often demonstrated, 5 = consistently demonstrated [see Section I].)

 (Nursing Outcomes Classification)

Suggested NOC Outcomes (Auditory)

Cognitive Orientation, Communication: Receptive, Distorted Thought Self-Control, Hearing Compensation Behavior

Example **NOC Outcome with Indicators**
Hearing Compensation Behavior as evidenced by the following indicators: Monitors symptoms of hearing deterioration/Positions self to advantage hearing/Reminds others to use techniques that advantage hearing/Eliminates background noise/Uses sign language/Uses lip reading/Uses closed captioning for television viewing/Uses hearing assistive devices/Uses hearing aid(s) correctly/Cares for internal hearing assistive devices correctly/Cares for external hearing assistive devices correctly/Uses support services for hearing impaired (Rate the outcome and indicators of **Hearing Compensation Behavior:** 1 = never demonstrated, 2 = rarely demonstrated, 3 = sometimes demonstrated, 4 = often demonstrated, 5 = consistently demonstrated [see Section I].)

Client Outcomes

Client Will (Specify Time Frame):

- Demonstrate understanding by a verbal, written, or signed response
- Demonstrate relaxed body movements and facial expressions
- Explain plan to modify lifestyle to accommodate visual or hearing impairment
- Incorporate use of lighting to maximize visual abilities
- Identify vision assistive devices that are appropriate in various settings
- Demonstrate familiarity with assistive devices
- Contact local vision or hearing support group
- Remain free of physical harm resulting from decreased balance or a loss of vision, hearing, or tactile sensation

 (Nursing Interventions Classification)

Suggested NIC Interventions

Cognitive Stimulation, Communication Enhancement: Hearing Deficit, Visual Deficit, Environmental Management

• = Independent   ▲ = Collaborative   **EBN** = Evidence-Based Nursing   **EB** = Evidence-Based

Example NIC Activities—Communication Enhancement: Visual Deficit

Identify yourself when you enter the patient's space; Build on patient's remaining vision, as appropriate

Nursing Interventions and *Rationales*

Visual—Loss of Vision

- Identify yourself whenever you enter the client's area, do not play guessing games about identity. *Good communication assists in the development of trust and decreases fear.*
- Provide environmental predictability. Consistently remind staff, family members, and visitors to tell the client when something is added or removed from the environment. *Consistency in placement of furniture and doors aids in location and decreases chances of injury (Houde & Huff, 2003).*
- Assist with feeding at mealtimes if blindness is temporary.
- Keep side rails up using half rails, maintain bed in a low position, keep call light readily available.
- Converse with and touch the client frequently during care if frequent touch is within the client's cultural norm. *Appropriate touch can decrease social isolation.*
- Walk the client by having the client grasp nurse's elbow or shoulder and walk partly behind nurse.
- Walk a frightened or confused client by having the client put both hands on nurse's shoulders; or nurse backs up in desired direction while holding the client around the waist. *These methods help the client feel secure and ensures safety.*
- Keep call light button within client's reach, and check location of call light button before leaving the room. **EB:** *A study demonstrated that a large percentage of hospitalized clients are unable to utilize the call light button and are very vulnerable as a result (Duffy et al, 2005).*
- Provide good lighting in rooms, task lights and night lights. *Good overall lighting is essential for safety, and task lighting makes everyday activities easier. Night lights allow safer navigation in the dark (Lighthouse International, 2009).*
- Make doorframes and light switches a contrasting color to the walls. *Contrast increases the likelihood of identifying them during navigation (Lighthouse International, 2009).*
- Ensure access to eyeglasses or magnifying devices as needed.
- Pay attention to the client's emotional needs. Encourage expression of feelings and expect grieving behavior. *Blind people grieve the loss of vision and experience a loss of identity and control over their lives.* **EB:** *A study of age-related macular degeneration clients found that a problem focused group was effective in helping client (Wahl et al, 2006).*
- Explore with the client the potential advantages of a vision loss self-management program. *Clients often do not recognize the value of learning problem solving for their disabilities (Rees et al, 2007).*
- Recommend client have vision evaluated by optometrist or ophthalmologist as appropriate to determine if an improvement in visual acuity is possible. *Clients may not have the correct prescription for their visual acuity (Park et al, 2005).*
- Provide a CD player, radio, or books on tape as desired. *Provides sensory stimulation, and can help deal with the boredom of hospitalization.*
- Explore and enhance available support systems to ensure a safe discharge. *Care givers and/or family may not have the ability to assist the client after discharge (Lighthouse International, 2009).*

Auditory—Hearing Loss

- Keep background noise to a minimum. Turn off television and radio when communicating with the client. If in a noisy environment, take the client to a private room and shut the door. *Background noise significantly interferes with hearing in the hearing-impaired client (Swann, 2008). Communication failure between health professionals and hearing-impaired clients is common (King, 2004).*
- Stand or sit directly in front of the client when communicating. Make sure adequate light is on nurse's face, avoid chewing gum or covering mouth or face with hands while speaking, establish eye contact, and use nonverbal gestures. *Clients with hearing impairment read lips and also interpret nonverbal communication, which is a significant part of communication. To increase communication, it is important that the client is able to see the face clearly of the person speaking (Swann, 2007).*
- Speak clearly in lower voice tones if possible. Do not over enunciate or shout at the client. *In many kinds of hearing loss, clients lose the ability to hear higher-pitched tones but can still hear lower-pitched*

● = Independent ▲ = Collaborative **EBN** = Evidence-Based Nursing **EB** = Evidence-Based

tones. Over-enunciating makes it difficult to read lips. Shouting makes the words less clear and may be painful (Swann, 2007).

- State the topic of conversation before beginning the conversation; make it clear when you change conversation topics. *This helps give the client a clear context for interpreting what you are saying.*
- Verify the client understands critical information by asking the client to repeat the information. *Hearing-impaired clients will often smile or nod when asked if they understand to avoid embarrassment; asking them to repeat the information is the best way to verify they understand what is being said.*
- If necessary, provide a communication board or personnel who know sign language. *Health care institutions are required to provide and pay for qualified interpreters under the Americans with Disabilities Act; an interpreter can be found through the Registry of Interpreters for the Deaf.*
- Prepare pictures or diagrams depicting tests or procedures; have books with relevant pictures available for more detailed discussions. *The use of visual aids can improve communication (Iezzoni et al, 2004).*
- ▲ Refer to appropriate resources such as a speech and hearing clinic; audiologist; or ear, nose, and throat physician. Refer children early for help. *Hearing loss can be treated with medical or surgical interventions or use of a hearing aid.*
- Encourage the client to wear hearing aid if available. **EB:** *A study demonstrated that nursing home clients with hearing loss who utilized a hearing aide had decreased level of depression (Goorabi, Hosseinabadi, & Share, 2008).*
- Observe emotional needs and encourage expression of feelings. *Hearing impairments may cause frustration, anger, fear, and self-imposed isolation.*
- For **Disturbed Sensory perception: kinesthetic, tactile**, see care plan for **Risk for Injury** or **Risk for Falls**. For **Disturbed Sensory perception: olfactory, gustatory**, see care plan for **Imbalanced Nutrition: less than body requirements**.

Pediatric

- ▲ Test hearing of infants and begin treatment/therapy early as needed. *Early treatment of a hearing loss can decrease the effects of a hearing loss on social, emotional, and academic development of a child (Smith, Bale, & White, 2005).*
- For classroom learning, ensure that ambient noise is minimized and devices are used to decrease reverberation in the environment. *For the hearing-impaired child, it is important that background noise is minimized and reverberation is controlled to increase the child's ability to hear and learn (Boothroyd, 2004; Crandell et al, 2004).*
- Recommend the child use a frequency-modulated system along with a hearing aid in school. **EB:** *For classroom learning, use of a frequency-modulated system in combination with a personal hearing aid substantially improved speech recognition (Anderson & Goldstein, 2004).*
- Refer the child to the use of a language wizard player with Baldi, a computer-animated tutor for teaching vocabulary. **EB:** *A study demonstrated that use of the computer system resulted in excellent retention of learned words 4 weeks after the end of the experiment (Massaro & Light, 2004).*

Geriatric

- Keep environment quiet, soothing, and familiar. Use consistent caregivers. *These measures are comforting to the elderly with a sensory loss and help decrease confusion.*
- If the client has a sensory deprivation, encourage family to provide appropriate sensory stimulation with music, voices, photographs, touch, and familiar smells.
- Increase the amount of light in the environment for elderly eyes; ensure it is nonglare lighting. *Increased lighting can help compensate for some of the visual changes of aging including reduced visual acuity, reduced contrast sensitivity, and reduced color discrimination (Boyce, 2003).*
- ▲ Determine origin of vision loss. If vision loss is from a stroke, watch for hemianopia, an ability to see to one side only. Encourage clients to scan environment by turning head from side to side. Also assess for visual spatial misconception. *Clients may underestimate distances and bump into doors and become confused.* **EB:** *Research demonstrated that mobility function improved after blind rehabilitation training for a group of older veterans (Kuyk & Elliot, 2004).*

● = Independent   ▲ = Collaborative   **EBN** = Evidence-Based Nursing   **EB** = Evidence-Based

▲ Refer to low-vision clinics or Independent Living Programs, which are designed for individuals who are vision impaired or blind to help maintain independence. *Clients with vision loss should be referred to clinics early, preferably before vision is gone, for help dealing with the loss (Kalinowski, 2008).* **EB:** *A research study demonstrated that mobility function improved after blind rehabilitation training for a group of older veterans (Kuyk & Elliot, 2004). Another study found that clients utilizing the Independent Living Program were highly satisfied with the quality, timeliness of services, and help in accomplishing independent living goals (Moore et al, 2006).*

- For a hearing impairment in the elderly, use the Hearing Handicap Inventory for the Elderly (HHIE-S) to determine how individuals perceive the emotional and social problems associated with a hearing loss. **EB:** *The HHIE-S is a valid and reliable instrument for screening of hearing loss (Yueh et al, 2003).*

- If the client has a hearing or vision loss, work with the client to ensure contact with others and to strengthen the social network. *Severe loneliness can accompany vision loss in the elderly as a result of self-imposed isolation (Swann, 2007).* **EBN and EB:** *Loss of hearing has a negative effect on psychosocial function with loneliness and increased rate of depression (Wallhagen, 2002; Mullins, 2004; Goorabi, Hosseinabadi, & Share, 2008). Loss of hearing has been associated with decreased cognitive function (Wallhagen, Strawbridge, & Shema, 2008).*

Home Care

- The listed interventions are applicable in the home care setting.

Client/Family Teaching and Discharge Planning

Low Vision

- Teach the client how to use a lighted magnification device to increase the ability to read text or see details.

- Teach the client to put a sheet of yellow acetate over text to make the text more visible. An alternative method is to highlight the text with a green or yellow highlighter.

- Put red, yellow, or orange identifiers on important items that need to be seen, such as a red strip at the edge of steps, red behind a light switch, or a red dot on a stove or washing machine to indicate how far to turn knob. *Color cues can improve the legibility of the environment and increase the ability to target objects quickly.*

- Use a watch or clock that verbally tells time, and a phone with large numbers and emergency numbers programmed into it.

- Teach blind client how to feed self; associate food on plate with hours on a clock so that the client can identify location of food.

- Use low-vision aids including magnifying devices for near vision and telescopes for seeing objects at a distance, a closed-circuit television that magnifies print, and guides for writing checks and envelopes. *Low vision aids can improve vision in clients with limited sight (Derrington, 2002).*

- Teach the client with vision loss to do the following:
  - Use a magnifying mirror to shave, apply makeup. Use electric razor only.
  - Put personal care products in brightly colored pump containers (red, yellow, or orange) for identification.
  - Use tactile clues such as safety pins or buttons placed in hems to help client match clothing.
  - Use prefilled medication organizer with large lettering or three-dimensional (3D) markers.
  These methods can help maintain the independence of the client (McGrory, Remington, & Secrest, 2004).

- Increase lighting in the home to help vision in the following ways:
  - Ensure adequate illumination of entire home, adding light fixtures and increasing wattage of existing bulbs as needed.
  - Decrease glare where light reflects on shiny surfaces; move or cover object.
  - Use nonglare wax on the floor.
  - Use motion lights that come on automatically when a person enters the room for nighttime use.
  - Add indoor strip or "runway"-type lighting to baseboards.

● = Independent   ▲ = Collaborative   **EBN** = Evidence-Based Nursing   **EB** = Evidence-Based

Visual acuity can be improved by taking steps to overcome age-related changes to vision.

- Work with the client to find rewarding recreational pursuits. *Recognize that advancing vision loss can often discourage people from the recreational pursuits they always enjoyed. When an activity becomes too much of a struggle, it simply isn't "fun" anymore. However, vision loss doesn't erase the basic need for the physical and mental rewards of play and relaxation.*

Hearing Loss

- Suggest installation of devices such as ring signalers for the telephone and doorbell, sensors that detect an infant's cry, alarm clocks that vibrate the bed, and closed caption decoders for television sets. Other helpful devices include telephone amplifiers, speakerphones, pocket talker personal listening system, and FM and infrared amplification systems that connect directly to a TV or audio output jack. Also available is a telecommunication device—a typewriter keyboard with an alphanumeric display that allows the hearing-impaired person to send typed messages over the telephone line; software and modems are available that allow a home computer to be used in this fashion. Use of hearing ear dogs—dogs specially trained to alert their owners to specific sounds—may also be helpful. *These devices can be helpful to increase communication and safety for the hearing-impaired client (Swann, 2007).*
- Teach client to avoid excessive noise at work or at home, wearing hearing protection when necessary. Any noise that hurts the ears or is above 90 decibels is excessive. *Hearing loss from excessive noise is common and preventable (Smith, Bale, & White, 2005).*

REFERENCES

Anderson KL, Goldstein H: Speech perception benefits of FM and infrared devices to children with hearing aids in a typical classroom, *Lang Speech Hear Serv Sch* 35(2):169, 2004.

Boothroyd A: Room acoustics and speech perception, *Semin Hear* 25(2):155, 2004.

Boyce PR: Lighting for the elderly, *Technol Disabil* 15(3):165, 2003.

Crandell CC, Kreisman BM, Smaldino JJ et al: Room acoustics intervention efficacy measures, *Semin Hear* 25(2):201, 2004.

Derrington D: Aids to low vision, *Nurs Res Care* 4:5, 2002.

Duffy S, Mallery L, Gordon J et al: Ability of hospitalized older adults to use their call bell: a pilot study in a tertiary care teaching hospital, *Aging Clin Exp Res* 17(5):390–393, 2005.

Goorabi K, Hosseinabadi R, Share H: Hearing aid effect on elderly depression in nursing home patients, *Asia Pac J Speech Lang Hear* 11(2):119–123, 2008.

Houde SC, Huff MA: Age-related vision loss in older adults: a challenge for gerontological nurses, *J Gerontol Nurs* 29(4):25, 2003.

Iezzoni L, O'Day B, Killeen M et al: Communicating about health care: observations from persons who are deaf or hard of hearing, *Ann Intern Med* 140(5):356–363, 2004.

Kalinowski MA: "Eye" dentifying vision impairment in the geriatric patient, *Geriatr Nurs* 29(2):125–132, 2008.

King A: Hearing and the elderly: a simple cure, *Geriatr Med* 34(6):9, 2004.

Kuyk T, Elliot JL: Mobility function in older veterans improves after blind rehabilitation, *J Rehabil Res Dev* 41(3):337, 2004.

Lighthouse International: "Tips for Confident Living." www.lighthouse.org/medical/tips-for-confident-living, accessed May 19, 2009.

Massaro DW, Light J: Improving the vocabulary of children with hearing loss, *Volta Rev* 104(3):141, 2004.

McGrory A, Remington R, Secrest JA: Optimizing the functionality of clients with age-related macular degeneration, *Rehabil Nurs* 29(3):90, 2004.

Moore JE, Steinman BA, Giesen JM et al: Functional outcomes and consumer satisfaction in the Independent Living Program for Older Individuals who are blind, *J Vis Impair Blind* 100(5):285–294, 2006.

Mullins T: Depression in older adults with hearing loss, *ASHA Leader* 9(1):12, 2004.

Park W, Mayer RS, Moghimi C et al: Rehabilitation of hospital inpatients with visual impairments and disabilities from systemic illness, *Arch Phys Med Rehabil* 86(1):79–81, 2005.

Rees G, Saw CL, Lamoureux EL et al: Self-management programs for adults with low vision: needs and challenges, *Patiet Educ Couns* 69(1–3):39–46, 2007.

Smith RJ, Bale JF, White KR: Sensorineural hearing loss in children, *Lancet* 365(9462):879, 2005.

Swann J: Helpful vibrations: assistive devices in hearing loss, *Nurs Residential Care*, 9(11):531–534, 2007.

Swann J: Understanding visual and auditory loss, *Nurs Residential Care* 10(4):195–197, 2008.

Wahl H, Kammerer A, Holz F et al: Psychosocial intervention for age-related macular degeneration: a pilot project, *J Vis Impair Blind* 100(9):533–545, 2006.

Wallhagen MI: Hearing impairment, *Annu Rev Nurs Res* 20:341, 2002.

Wallhagen MI, Strawbridge WJ, Shema SJ: The relationship between hearing impairment and cognitive function: a 5–year longitudinal study, *Res Gerontol Nurs* 1(2):80–86, 2008.

Yueh B, Shapiro N, MacLean CH et al: Scientific review and clinical applications. Screening and management of adult hearing loss in primary care: scientific review, *JAMA* 289(15):1976–1985, 2003.

Sexual dysfunction   *Elaine E. Steinke, PhD, RN, FAHA*

NANDA-I

Definition

The state in which an individual experiences a change in sexual function during the sexual response phases of desire, excitation, and/or orgasm, which is viewed as unsatisfying, unrewarding, or inadequate

Defining Characteristics

Alterations in achieving sexual satisfaction; alterations in achieving perceived sex role; actual limitations imposed by disease; actual limitations imposed by therapy; change of interest in others; change of interest in self; inability to achieve desired satisfaction; perceived alteration in sexual excitation; perceived deficiency of sexual desire; perceived limitations imposed by disease; perceived limitations imposed by therapy; seeking confirmation of desirability; verbalization of problem

Related Factors (r/t)

Absent role models; altered body function (e.g., pregnancy, recent childbirth, drugs, surgery, anomalies, disease process, trauma, radiation); altered body structure (e.g., pregnancy, recent childbirth, surgery, anomalies, disease process, trauma, radiation); biopsychosocial alteration of sexuality; deficient knowledge; ineffectual role models; lack of privacy; lack of significant other; misinformation; values conflict; psychosocial abuse (e.g., harmful relationships); physical abuse; vulnerability

NOC   (Nursing Outcomes Classification)

Suggested NOC Outcomes

Abuse Recovery: Sexual, Knowledge: Sexual Function, Physical Aging, Psychosocial Adjustment: Life Change, Risk Control: Sexually Transmitted Diseases (STDs), Sexual Functioning, Sexual Identity

Example NOC Outcome with Indicators
Sexual Functioning as evidenced by the following indicators: Expresses comfort with sexual expression/Expresses comfort with body/Expresses sexual interest (Rate the outcome and indicators of **Sexual Functioning:** 1 = never demonstrated, 2 = rarely demonstrated, 3 = sometimes demonstrated, 4 = often demonstrated, 5 = consistently demonstrated [see Section I].)

Client Outcomes

Client Will (Specify Time Frame):

- Identify individual cause of sexual dysfunction
- Identify stressors that contribute to dysfunction
- Discuss alternative, satisfying, and acceptable sexual practices for self and partner
- Identify the degree of sexual interest by the client and partner
- Adapt sexual technique as needed to cope with sexual problems
- Discuss with partner concerns about body image and sex role

NIC   (Nursing Interventions Classification)

Suggested NIC Interventions

Sexual Counseling, Teaching: Sexuality

Example NIC Activities—Sexual Counseling
Provide privacy and ensure confidentiality; Discuss necessary modifications in sexual activity, as appropriate; Provide referral/consultation with other members of the health care team, as appropriate

---

• = Independent   ▲ = Collaborative   **EBN** = Evidence-Based Nursing   **EB** = Evidence-Based

Nursing Interventions and *Rationales*

- Gather the client's sexual history, noting normal patterns of functioning and the client's vocabulary. **EB:** *A comprehensive sexual assessment includes a psychological, sexual, and social history that evaluates the client's life situation and relationships, including ruling out depression as a contributor to sexual problems (Archer et al, 2005).* **EBN:** *Health care professionals in urologic, gynecologic, and family practice offices and clinics are in key roles to identify females experiencing sexual dysfunction (Brassil & Keller, 2002).* **EB:** *Women who reported greater sexual satisfaction and who rated sex as important were less likely to experience low sexual desire; low genital arousal was less likely in those who were taking hormone therapy (Hayes et al, 2008).*

- Assess duration of sexual dysfunction and explore potential causes such as medications, medical problems, or psychosocial issues. Evaluate if sexual dysfunction may be related to either psychological or medical causes. **EB:** *New onset sexual dysfunction may be related to prescription and nonprescription medications as one cause, while sexual dysfunction of longer duration may be related to a disease process and can be a symptom of cardiovascular disease (Billups, 2005).* **EB:** *The most common sexual problems reported in a general practice were erectile failure and loss of desire for men, and loss of desire and failure in orgasmic response for women (Nazareth, Boynton, & King, 2003).* **EBN:** *Treatments for cancer often contribute to sexual dysfunction, and women identified chemotherapy and surgery as contributors to poor sexual functioning (Barton-Burke & Gustason, 2007). Additional relevant research: (Bruner & Calvano, 2007).*

- Assess for history of sexual abuse. **EB:** *In Australian women, 23% recalled past abuse and 12% recalled multiple episodes of abuse. Women who had been abused had lower scores on sexual satisfaction and frequency (Howard, O'Neill, & Travers, 2006).*

- Determine the client's and partner's current knowledge and understanding. **EB:** *This survey indicated that for those who have a partner, sexual disabilities and distress caused by them should be regarded from the partner relationship perspective (Fugl-Meyer & Fugl-Meyer, 2002).* **EB:** *Including couples in counseling improved overall male distress and male and female global sexual function at 3 months after treatment for prostate carcinoma (Canada et al, 2005).* **EB:** *In clients with chronic heart failure, 36% believed that sexual intercourse could harm their cardiac condition, and 75% of women and 60% of men reported that no physician had asked about potential sexual problems (Schwarz et al, 2008).*

- ▲ Assess and provide treatment for sexual dysfunction. Involve the person's partner in the process. Consider pharmacologic and nonpharmacological interventions. **EB:** *Of equal value—and necessity—is the involvement of the man's partner in both the assessment and treatment processes of erectile dysfunction (ED). Nonpharmacologic interventions should be considered as means to support and augment the effects of phosphodiesterase type 5 (PDE-5) inhibitors (Dunn, 2004).* **EB:** *Improved exercise tolerance and coronary dilatation occurred for those taking PDE-5 inhibitors. The safety profile of the drugs is excellent (Carson, 2005).* **EB:** *Postmenopausal women taking valsartan for hypertension reported positive improvements in sexual desire, changes in sexual behavior, and sexual fantasies (Fogari et al, 2004).*

- Observe for stress and anxiety as possible causes of dysfunction. **EBN:** *Sexual dysfunction can be attributed to many psychological factors. Anxiety is often high with cardiac illness, and decreased sexual satisfaction has been shown to heighten anxiety among myocardial infarction clients (Steinke & Wright, 2006).* **EBN:** *Clients with implantable cardioverter defibrillators (ICD) report fear of ICD discharge with sexual activity, and 44% avoided sexual encounters (Steinke, 2003; Steinke et al, 2005).* **EB:** *General anxiety and sexual anxiety were related in a sample of heart failure clients and healthy elders, and sexual self-concept, sexual anxiety, sexual self-efficacy, younger age, and marital status predicted sexual activity (Steinke et al, 2008).*

- Assess for depression as a possible cause of sexual dysfunction. Sexual problems and depression are common in chronic disease and those with chronic pain. **EBN:** *Global depression and sexual depression have been linked in heart failure and healthy elders (Steinke et al, 2008).* **EB:** *For women with advanced breast cancer, one third had a diagnosis of depression, affecting quality of life and with the potential of affecting sexual function (Grabsch et al, 2006).* **EBN:** *In those with diabetes it is often difficult to determine whether depression or diabetes cause the sexual dysfunction (Grandjean & Moran, 2007).*

- Observe for grief related to loss (e.g., amputation, mastectomy, ostomy). *A change in body image often precedes sexual dysfunction (see care plan for* **Disturbed Body image***).* **EB:** *An integrative* *review of 13 studies revealed that up to one half of women with prophylactic mastectomy suffered a negative effect on body image and changes in sexuality (McGaughey, 2006).* **EB:** *Among sexually active women, body image problems were associated with mastectomy and possible reconstruction, hair loss from chemotherapy, concern with weight gain/loss, poorer mental health, and decreased self-esteem (Fobair et al, 2006). Survivors of breast cancer report that issues of body image, sexuality, and partner communication are rarely addressed by traditional health care providers (Burwell et al, 2006).*

• Explore physical causes such as diabetes, arteriosclerotic heart disease, arthritis, benign prostatic hypertrophy, drug or medication side effects, or smoking (males). **EB:** *Erectile dysfunction is an early manifestation of arteriosclerosis and precedes systemic vascular disease as a result of endothelial dysfunction, a paradigm shift from the belief that ED occurred only as a result of cardiovascular disease or treatment (Billups, 2005).* **EBN:** *Research has demonstrated that the symptoms of rheumatoid arthritis can negatively impact a client's sexuality (Ryan & Wylie, 2005).* **EB:** *Studies reveal the detrimental effect of smoking on erectile function in males and sexual dysfunction in females, both in U.S. and international samples, and particularly when combined with other risk factors (Addis et al, 2005; Barqawi et al, 2005; Lam et al, 2006; Moreira et al, 2006; Oksuz & Malhan, 2006).*

• Provide privacy and be verbally and nonverbally nonjudgmental. *Privacy is important to ensure confidentiality. To facilitate communication, it is also vital that the nurse clarify personal values and remain nonjudgmental (Steinke, 2005).*

• Provide privacy to allow sexual expression between the client and partner (e.g., private room, "Do Not Disturb" sign for a specified length of time). *The hospital setting has little opportunity for privacy, so the nurse must ensure that it is available.*

• Explain the need for the client to share concerns with partner. **EBN:** *The partner should be involved in the assessment, diagnosis, client education, counseling, and choice of treatment for long-term treatment to be successful, unless the informed client is unwilling (Dorey, 2001).* **EB:** *Addressing client sexual concerns early in neurological disease processes is important in facilitating discussion with sexual partners and in prevention of future problems (Clayton & Ramamurthy, 2008).*

• Validate the client's feelings, let the client know that he or she is normal, and correct misinformation. **EB:** *Because men see the primary care physician's office as a natural and expected place in which to address issues of sexual health, those health care professionals who are prepared to initiate discussion of ED can offer clients and their partners the possibility of effective and enduring treatment success and the restoration of a satisfying relationship (Dunn, 2004).* **EBN:** *Women with spinal cord injury often believe that this disease process makes them infertile; however, it is believed that fertility is largely unaffected and approximately 90% of women report a return to their normal menstrual cycle at 1 year after their injury (Ricciardi, Szabo, & Poullos, 2007).*

▲ Refer to appropriate medical providers for consideration of medication for premature ejaculation, erectile dysfunction, or orgasmic problems. **EB:** *Phosphodiesterase-5 (PDE5) inhibitors are safe and effective in those with chronic stable coronary disease, although these drugs are contraindicated if the client is taking nitrates (Jackson, 2005).* **EBN:** *PDE5 inhibitors are well tolerated in the male spinal cord–injured population and may increase not only the quality and duration of erection, but also the frequency of reflex and psychogenic erections (Ricciardi, Szabo, & Poullos, 2007).*

▲ Refer women for possible pharmacologic intervention when sexual dysfunction is present. **EB:** *Common contributors to sexual dysfunction in women are decreased libido, vaginal dryness, dyspareunia, altered genital sensation, and difficulty with orgasm. Organic and psychological causes of dysfunction must be thoroughly evaluated (Archer et al, 2005).* **EB:** *For women with sexual dysfunction, pharmacotherapy may augment desire, arousability, and genital congestion, and lessen the pain of chronic dyspareunia (Basson, 2004).* **EB:** *Potential therapies for female sexual dysfunction include PDE5 inhibitors, androgen therapy, tibilone, and prostaglandins (Archer et al, 2005; Davis & Nijland, 2008).*

 Geriatric

▲ Carefully assess the sexuality needs of the elderly client and refer for counseling if needed. **EB:** *Older adults face several barriers to sexual expression. Because sexual issues are seldom volunteered, questions regarding sexuality and intimacy may have to be raised by the clinician, who can help his or her clients with sexual expression by providing appropriate assessment and counseling (Messinger-Rapport, Sandhu, & Hujer, 2003).*

• = Independent   ▲ = Collaborative   **EBN** = Evidence-Based Nursing   **EB** = Evidence-Based

- Carefully assess sexual functioning needs of clients with dementia and provide privacy for them and their spouse. *Assessment of decision-making potential is critical, with an emphasis on comprehension of the interests and intensions of both individuals, the understanding of physical intimacy and sexual activity, and expectations about the relationship (Rheaume & Mitty, 2008).* **EBN:** *Although women with dementia are particularly vulnerable to abuse, for some, if not most, sexual activity between loving spouses may be morally permissible even when one partner has dementia and cannot consent (Lingler, 2003).*
- Teach about normal changes that occur with aging: Female—reduction in vaginal lubrication, decrease in the degree and speed of vaginal expansion, reduction in duration and resolution of orgasm. Male—increase in time required for erection, increase in erection time without ejaculation, less firm erection, decrease in volume of seminal fluid, increase in time before another erection can occur (12–24 hours). **EBN:** *The older adult experiences a number of physiologic changes; however, these changes are gradual and vary from person to person (Salzman, 2006).* **EB:** *Erectile dysfunction may affect men as they age; however, there is high efficacy, reliability, and safety of the phosphodiesterase inhibitors in the treatment of ED in the elderly (Salonia et al, 2005).*
- Suggest the following to enhance sexual functioning: Female—use water-based vaginal lubricant, increase foreplay time, avoid direct stimulation of the clitoris if painful (clitoris may be exposed because of atrophy of the labia), practice Kegel exercises (alternately contracting and relaxing the muscles in the pelvic area), urinate immediately after coitus to prevent irritation of the urethra and bladder, and consult with a physician about use of systemic estrogen therapy or topical estrogen cream. Male—have female partner try a new coital position by bending her knees and placing a pillow under her hips to elevate pelvis (will more easily accommodate a partially erect penis); massage penis down using pressure at base, which puts pressure on major blood vessel and keeps blood in the penis; ask the female partner to push the penis into the vagina herself and flex her vaginal muscles that have been strengthened by Kegel exercises. If one of the partners has a protruding abdomen, experiment to find a position that allows the penis to reach the vagina (e.g., have woman lie on her back with legs apart and knees sharply bent while the man places himself over her with his hips under the angle formed by the raised knees). **EBN:** *The management of sexual problems in older adults should be guided by the same principles irrespective of age. Both partners should take part in therapy. A preliminary medical and social history may suggest contributing factors (Tallis, 2003).*
- Explore various sexual gratification alternatives (e.g., caressing, sharing feelings) with the client and partner. *Many satisfying alternatives are available for expressing sexual feelings. The many losses associated with aging leave the elderly with special needs for love and affection.*
- Discuss the difference between sexual function and sexuality. *All individuals possess sexuality from birth to death, regardless of the changes that occur over the life span.*
- ▲ If prescribed, instruct clients with chronic pain to take the pain medication prior to sexual activity. Nitroglycerine can be used for anginal pain, if prescribed. *Pain inhibits satisfying sexual activity.*
- See care plan for **Ineffective Sexuality pattern**.

 ### Multicultural

- Assess for the influence of cultural beliefs, norms, and values on the client's perceptions of normal sexual functioning. **EBN:** *Hasidic (ultraorthodox) Jews believe that male ejaculation must be vaginally contained. This belief will influence choice of interventions for certain sexual dysfunctions (Ribner, 2004). Most research on the sexual health of ethnic minority populations is typically focused on preventive sexual health without examination of the racial or ethnic aspects of sexual health (Lewis, 2004).* **EB:** *Cultural influences can impact on the sexual health of young people from culturally diverse backgrounds and in Australia's multicultural society, provision of sexual health services must acknowledge the specific needs of ethnically diverse young people (Rawson & Liamputtong, 2009).*
- Discuss with the client those aspects of sexual health/lifestyle that remain unchanged by his or her health status. **EBN:** *Aspects of the client's life that are valuable to him or her should be understood and preserved without change (Leininger & McFarland, 2002).* **EB:** *The most important contributors to sexual satisfaction for females were sexual self-confidence, frequency of orgasm, and relationship satisfaction, while for males contributors to sexual satisfaction were relationship satisfaction, sexual self-confidence, frequency of orgasm, health status, and social roles (Penhollow, Young, & Denny, 2009).*

● = Independent   ▲ = Collaborative   **EBN** = Evidence-Based Nursing   **EB** = Evidence-Based

- Validate the client's feelings and emotions regarding the changes in sexual behavior. *Validation lets the client know the nurse has heard and understands what was said, and it promotes the nurse-client relationship.* **EB:** *Sexual self-confidence was found to be the strongest predictor for participating in sexual intercourse among men and women, thus discussing sexual issues may enhance self-confidence and quality of life (Penhollow, Young, & Denny, 2009).* **EBN:** *A study of African American men treated for prostate cancer with prostatectomy or radiation found more positive attitudes than did Caucasian men toward seeking help for sexual problems, and were more likely to report seeking past help and intending to seek future help (Jenkins et al, 2004).*

 Home Care

- Previously discussed interventions may be adapted for home care use.
- Identify specific sources of concern about sexual activity. Provide reassurance and instruction on appropriate expectations as indicated. **EBN:** *Clients post-MI often have considerable anxiety about return to sexual activity, for some up to 5 months post-MI (Steinke & Swan, 2004; Steinke & Wright, 2006).* **EBN:** *An intervention with female myocardial infarction clients revealed that women had fewer symptoms and less concern about sexual activity after participating in the intervention (Varvaro, 2000).*
- Help the client and significant other to identify a place and time in the home and daily living for privacy to share sexual or relationship activity. If necessary, help the client to communicate the need for privacy to other family members. Consider periodic escapes to desirable surroundings. *The home setting can be one that affords little, if any, privacy without conscious effort on the part of members of the home.*
- Confirm that physical reasons for dysfunction have been addressed. Encourage participation in support groups or therapy if appropriate. **EBN:** *Sexual changes in clients after traumatic brain injury included a decreased importance and frequency of sexual activity, changes in sex drive and enjoyment of sexual activity, decline in ability to satisfy the partner and engage in sexual intercourse, and problems with arousal; these changes were exacerbated by fatigue, deceased mobility, low confidence levels, feelings of unattractiveness, pain, and difficulties with communication (Ponsford, 2003).* **EB:** *A survey of the Interstitial Cystitis Support Group revealed that most respondents reported frequency, urgency, and nocturia, with 49% that their condition presented considerable difficulties with sexual intercourse (Tincello & Walker, 2005).* **EB:** *Male renal transplant clients reported a better sexual relationship, sexual function, and sexual frequency than did those on hemodialysis, thus highlighting the importance of education and support for all renal clients (Tavallaii et al, 2009).*
- Reinforce or teach the client about sexual functioning, alternative sexual practices, and necessary sexual precautions. Update teaching as client status changes. **EBN:** *The PLISSIT model (giving permission to discuss sexual concerns, providing limited information, providing specific information, referral for intensive therapy) is a practical way for nurses to assess sexual concerns and provide information to clients (Katz, 2003).* **EBN:** *A link between sexual self-esteem and sexual function was noted in a study of women post pancreas and kidney transplant, although the majority had some difficulty with sexual function (Muehrer, Keller, & Powwattana, 2006).*

 Client/Family Teaching and Discharge Planning

- Provide accurate information for clients concerning sexual activity after a myocardial infarction (MI); consider use of a videotape. **EBN:** *Significant improvements in knowledge were found in clients who had a videotape to view at home on return to sexual activity. This intervention provides an alternative method for education to facilitate recovery post-MI (Steinke & Swan, 2004).*
- Teach the client and partner about condom use, for those at risk. **EB:** *A study of HIV-seropositive and -seronegative women revealed condom use by 68% of sexually active women, and those with HIV were more likely to use a condom (Wilson et al, 2003).*
- Teach the client that sexual activity can be resumed 1 to 2 weeks after an uncomplicated MI (Antman et al, 2004). Also discuss being well rested, reporting any cardiac warning signs, using foreplay to determine tolerance for sexual activity, not using alcohol or eating heavy meals prior to sex, and having sex with a familiar partner and in the usual setting to decrease any stress the couple might feel. **EB:** *Sexual activity can be discussed in the context of other usual activities, comparing the energy*

• = Independent ▲ = Collaborative **EBN** = Evidence-Based Nursing **EB** = Evidence-Based

expenditure for each as compared to sexual activity. The average energy expenditure for sex with a long-standing partner is 2.5 metabolic equivalent levels (METs) with the partner on top and 3.3 METs with the man on top, similar to walking at a moderate pace or doing a household chore like washing floors (Cheitlin, 2005).

- Provide written educational materials that address sexual issues for clients and families of clients with implantable cardiac defibrillators (ICDs). **EBN:** *Addressing the fears and concerns related to sexual function of ICD clients and partners is an essential aspect of rehabilitation and recovery. Study results suggest a need for written client education tools specific to sexual issues for clients and partners, as well as educational resources for health professionals (Steinke, 2003).*

▲ Refer to appropriate community resources, such as a clinical specialist, family counselor, or cardiac rehabilitation, including the partner if appropriate. For clients with complex issues, a referral to a sex counselor, urologist, gynecologist, or other specialist may be needed. **EB:** *Clients attending cardiac rehabilitation were nearly four times more likely to resume sexual activity compared to those who did not attend, thus highlighting the importance of providing education and support as part of education and counseling (Eyada & Atwa, 2007).* **EB:** *An expert in sexual counseling is recommended as part of the cardiac rehabilitation team (Klein et al, 2007).*

- Teach vaginal dilation to prevent stenosis. Inform the client to expect a bit of spotting after first session of intercourse. **EB:** *For women who had pelvic radio therapy, the use of vaginal dilators to prevent the development of vaginal stenosis is supported (Denton & Maher, 2003).*

- Teach how drug therapy affects sexual response (e.g., the possible side effects and the need to report them). **EB:** *Sexual dysfunction induced by selective serotonin reuptake inhibitors (SSRIs) affects 30% to 50% or more of individuals who take these drugs for depression (Keltner, McAfee, & Taylor, 2002).* **EBN:** *Medications that dry mucous membranes (e.g., antihistamines), those that affect blood flow (e.g., antihypertensive agents), and oral contraceptives, antipsychotics, and narcotics can affect sexual function (Grandjean & Moran, 2007).*

- Teach the importance of diabetic control and its effect on sexuality to clients with diabetes. **EBN:** *Sexual functioning may be changed by alterations in glucose levels, infections that affect comfort during sexual intercourse, changes in vaginal lubrication and penile erection, and changes in sexual desire and arousal. The cornerstone of therapy is tight glucose control and exercise, and PDE5 inhibitors can be considered if the client is not taking incompatible medications (Clayton & Ramamurthy, 2008).*

▲ Refer for medical advice for ED that lasts longer than 2 months or is recurring. *ED can be treated, and underlying causes need to be investigated (Mayo Foundation for Medical Education and Research, 2008). Cardiovascular disease and ED share common risk factors, therefore a common prevention strategy should be implemented using a client-centered approach (Hatzichristou & Tsimtsiou, 2005).*

- Teach the following interventions to decrease the likelihood of ED: limit or avoid the use of alcohol, stop smoking, exercise regularly, reduce stress, get enough sleep, deal with anxiety or depression, and see doctor for regular checkups and medical screening tests. **EB:** *These interventions may prevent or improve symptoms of ED (Guay, 2005; Mayo Foundation for Medical Education and Research, 2008).*

▲ Refer for medication to treat ED if necessary. **EB:** *The PDE-5 inhibitors are now widely used in selected clients (Jackson, 2005).* **EB:** *In this prospective, parallel-group, randomized, double-blind, placebo-controlled trial, sildenafil effectively improved erectile function and other aspects of sexual function in men with sexual dysfunction associated with the use of SSRI antidepressants (Nurnberg et al, 2003).*

- Discuss sexual problems and adaptations needed for sexual activity with spinal cord injury. **EBN:** *For erectile difficulties the PDE5 inhibitors can be safely used or other devices such as a vacuum pump and intracavernousal injections of vasoactive substances. The benefits of tactile stimulation to enhance sexual arousal should be addressed, as well as creativity in sexual positions. Discuss problems that can interfere with sexual arousal and sexual function, such as autonomic dysreflexia, urinary and bowel incontinence, altered thermoregulation, spasticity, and pain (Ricciardi, Szabo, & Poullos, 2007).*

- See Geriatric Interventions if a problem with erection is associated with stoma surgery.

evolve   See the EVOLVE website for Weblinks for client education resources.

• = Independent   ▲ = Collaborative   **EBN** = Evidence-Based Nursing   **EB** = Evidence-Based

REFERENCES

Addis IB, Ireland CC, Vittinghoff E et al: Sexual activity and function in postmenopausal women with heart disease, *Obstet Gynecol* 106:121–127, 2005.

Antman EM, Anbe DT, Armstrong PW et al: ACC/AHA guidelines for the management of patients with ST-elevation in myocardial infarction: a report of the American College of Cardiology/American Heart Association Task Force on Practice Guidelines, *Circulation* 110(9):e82–e292, 2004.

Archer SL, Gragasin FS, Webster L et al: Aetiology and management of male erectile dysfunction and female sexual dysfunction in patients with cardiovascular disease, *Drugs Aging* 22(10):823–844, 2005.

Barqawi A, O'Donnell C, Kumar R et al: Correlation between LUTS (AUA-SS) and erectile function (SHIM) in an age-matched racially diverse mail population: data from the Prostate Cancer Awareness Week (PCAW), *Int J Impot Res* 17:370–374, 2005.

Barton-Burke M, Gustason CJ: Sexuality in women with cancer, *Nurs Clin North Am* 42:531–554, 2007.

Basson R: Pharmacotherapy for sexual dysfunction in women, *Expert Opin Pharmacother* 5(5):1045–1059, 2004.

Billups K: Sexual dysfunction and cardiovascular disease: integrative concepts and strategies, *Am J Cardiol* 96(suppl 2):57M–61M, 2005.

Brassil DF, Keller M: Female sexual dysfunction: definitions, causes, and treatment, *Urol Nurs* 22(4):237, 284; quiz 245, 248, 2002.

Bruner DW, Calvano T: The sexual impact of cancer and cancer treatments in men, *Nurs Clin North Am* 42:555–580, 2007.

Burwell SR, Case LD, Kaelin C et al: Sexual problems in younger women after breast cancer surgery, *J Clin Oncol* 24:2815–2821, 2006.

Canada A, Neese L, Sui D et al: Pilot intervention to enhance sexual rehabilitation for couples after treatment for localized prostate carcinoma, *Cancer* 104:2689–2700, 2005.

Carson C III: Cardiac safety in clinical trials of phosphodiesterase 5 inhibitors, *Am J Cardiol* 96(12B):37M–41M, 2005.

Cheitlin MD: Sexual activity and cardiac risk, *Am J Cardiol* 96(suppl):24M–28M; 2005.

Clayton A, Ramamurthy S: The impact of physical illness on sexual dysfunction, *Adv Psychosom Med* 29:70–88, 2008.

Davis SR, Nijland EA: Pharmacologic therapy for female sexual dysfunction, *Drugs 2008* 68(3):259–264, 2008.

Denton AS, Maher EJ: Interventions for the physical aspects of sexual dysfunction in women following pelvic radiotherapy, *Cochrane Database Sys Rev* (1):CD003750, 2003.

Dorey G: Partners' perspective of erectile dysfunction: literature review, *Br J Nurs* 10(3):187, 2001.

Dunn ME: Restoration of couple's intimacy and relationship vital to reestablishing erectile function, *J Am Osteopath Assoc* 104(3):S6–S10, S16, 2004.

Eyada M, Atwa M: Sexual function in female patients with unstable angina or non-ST elevation myocardial infarction, *J Sex Med* 4:1373–1380, 2007.

Fobair P, Stewart SL, Chang S et al: Body image and sexual problems in young women with breast cancer, *Psychooncology* 15:579–594, 2006.

Fogari R, Preti P, Zoppi A et al: Effect of valsartan and atenolol on sexual behavior in hypertensive postmenopausal women, *Am J Hypertens* 17:77–81, 2004.

Fugl-Meyer K, Fugl-Meyer AR: Sexual disabilities are not singularities, *Int J Impot Res* 14(6):487, 2002.

Grabsch B, Clarke DM, Love A et al: Psychological morbidity and quality of life in women with advanced breast cancer: a cross-sectional study, *Palliat Support Care* 4(1):47–56, 2006.

Grandjean C, Moran B: The impact of diabetes on female sexual well-being, *Nurs Clin North Am* 42:581–592, 2007.

Guay AT: Relation of endothelial cell function to erectile dysfunction: implications for treatment, *Am J Cardiol* 96(12B):52M-56M, 2005.

Hatzichristou D, Tsimtsiou Z: Prevention and management of cardiovascular disease and erectile dysfunction: toward a common patient-centered care model, *Am J Cardiol* 96(12B):80M-84M, 2005.

Hayes RD, Dennerstein L, Bennett CM et al: Risk factors for female sexual dysfunction in the general population: exploring factors associated with low sexual function and sexual distress, *J Sex Med* 5,1681–1693, 2008.

Howard JR, O'Neill S, Travers C: Factors affecting sexuality in older Australian women: sexual interest, sexual arousal, relationships and sexual distress in older Australian women, *Climacteric* 9:355–367, 2006.

Jackson G: Hemodynamic and exercise effects of phosphodiesterase 5 inhibitors, *Am J Cardiol* 96(12B):32M-36M, 2005.

Jenkins R, Schover LR, Fouladi RT et al: Sexuality and health-related quality of life after prostate cancer in African-American and white men treated for localized disease, *J Sex Marital Ther* 30(2):79–93, 2004.

Katz A: Sexuality after hysterectomy: a review of the literature and discussion of nurses' role, *J Adv Nurs* 42(3):297–303, 2003.

Keltner NL, McAfee KM, Taylor CL: Mechanisms and treatments of SSRI-induced sexual dysfunction, *Perspect Psychiatr Care* 38(3):111, 2002.

Klein R, Bar-on E, Klein J et al: The impact of sexual therapy on patients after cardiac events participating in a cardiac rehabilitation program, *Eur J Cardiovasc Prev Rehabil* 14:672–678, 2007.

Lam TH, Abdullah AS, Ho LM et al: Smoking and sexual dysfunction in Chinese males: findings from men's health survey, *Int J Impot Res* 18:364–369, 2006.

Leininger MM, McFarland MR: *Transcultural nursing: concepts, theories, research and practices,* ed 3, New York, 2002, McGraw-Hill.

Lewis LJ: Examining sexual health discourses in a racial/ethnic context, *Arch Sex Behav* 33(3):223–234, 2004.

Lingler JH: Ethical issues in distinguishing sexual activity from sexual maltreatment among women with dementia, *J Elder Abuse Neglect* 15(2):85–102, 2003.

Mayo Foundation for Medical Education and Research: *Erectile dysfunction.* www.mayoclinic.com/health/erectile-dysfunction/DS00162, 2008. Accessed March 18, 2009.

McGaughey A: Body image after bilateral prophylactic mastectomy: an integrative literature review, *J Midwifery Womens Health* 51(6):e45–e49, 2006.

Messinger-Rapport BJ, Sandhu SK, Hujer ME: Sex and sexuality: is it over after 60? *Clin Geriatr* 11(10):45–55, 2003.

Moreira ED Jr, Kim SC, Glasser D et al: Sexual activity, prevalence of sexual problems, and associated help-seeking patterns in men and women aged 40–80 years in Korea: data from the Global Study of Sexual Attitudes and Behaviors (GSSAB), *J Sex Med* 3(2):201–211, 2006.

Muehrer RJ, Keller ML, Powwattana A: Sexuality among women recipients of a pancreas kidney transplant, *West J Nurs Res* 28:137–150, 2006.

Nazareth I, Boynton P, King M: Problems with sexual function in people attending London general practitioners: cross sectional study, *Brit Med J* 327:423–428, 2003.

Nurnberg HG, Hensley PL, Gelenberg AJ et al: Treatment of antidepressant-associated sexual dysfunction with sildenafil: a randomized controlled trial, *J Am Med Assoc* 289(1):56, 2003.

Oksuz E, Malhan S: Prevalence and risk factors for female sexual dysfunction in Turkish women, *J Urol* 175:654–658, 2006.

• = Independent   ▲ = Collaborative   **EBN** = Evidence-Based Nursing   **EB** = Evidence-Based

Penhollow TM, Young M, Denny G: Predictors of quality of life, sexual intercourse, and sexual satisfaction among sexually active older adults, *Am J Health Educ* 10(1):14–22, 2009.

Ponsford J: Sexual changes associated with traumatic brain injury *Neuropsychol Rehabil* 13(1/2): 275–289, 2003.

Rawson H, Liamputtong P: Influence of traditional Vietnamese culture on the utilisation of mainstream health services for sexual health issues by second-generation Vietnamese Australian young women, *Sex Health* 6(1):75–81, 2009.

Rheaume C, Mitty E: Sexuality and intimacy in older adults, *Geriatr Nurs* 29(5):342–349, 2008.

Ribner D: Ejaculatory restrictions as a factor in the treatment of Haredi (Ultraorthodox) Jewish couples, *Arch Sex Behav* 33(3):303–308, 2004.

Ricciardi R, Szabo CM, Poullos AY: Sexuality and spinal cord injury *Nurs Clin North Am* 42:675–684, 2007.

Ryan S, Wylie E: An exploratory survey of the practice of rheumatology nurses addressing the sexuality of patients with rheumatoid arthritis, *Musculoskeletal Care*, 3(1):44–53, 2005.

Salzman B: Myths and realities of aging, *Care Manage J* 7(3):141–150, 2006.

Salonia A, Briganti A, Montsori P et al: Safety and tolerability of oral erectile dysfunction treatments in the elderly, *Drugs Aging* 22(4):323–338, 2005.

Schwarz ER, Kapur V, Bionat S et al: The prevalence and clinical relevance of sexual dysfunction in women and men with chronic heart failure, *Int J Impot Res* 20:85–91, 2008.

Steinke EE: Sexual concerns of patients and partners after an implantable cardioverter defibrillator, *Dimens Crit Care Nurs* 22(2):89–96, 2003.

Steinke EE: Intimacy needs and chronic illness: strategies for sexual counseling and self-management, *J Gerontol Nurs* 31(5):40–50, 2005.

Steinke EE, Gill-Hopple K, Valdez D et al: Sexual concerns and educational needs after an implantable cardioverter defibrillator, *Heart Lung* 34(5):299–308, 2005.

Steinke EE, Swan JH: Effectiveness of a videotape for sexual counseling after myocardial infarction, *Res Nurs Health* 27(4):269–280, 2004.

Steinke EE, Wright DW: The role of sexual satisfaction, age, and cardiac risk factors in the reduction of post-MI anxiety, *Eur J Cardiovasc Nurs* 5:190–196, 2006.

Steinke EE, Wright DW, Chung ML et al: Sexual self-concept, anxiety, and self-efficacy predict sexual activity in heart failure and healthy elders, *Heart Lung* 37(5):323–333, 2008.

Tallis R: *Geriatric medicine and gerontology*, ed 6, Oxford, UK, 2003, Churchill Livingstone, 1140–1142.

Tavallaii SA, Mirzamani M, Heshmatzade Behzadi A et al: Sexual function: a comparison between male renal transplant recipients and hemodialysis patients, *J Sex Med* 6(1):142–148, 2009.

Tincello DG, Walker ACH: Interstitial cystitis in the UK: results of a questionnaire survey of members of the Interstitial Cystitis Support Group, *Eur J Obstet Gynecol Reprod Biol* 118(1):91–95, 2005.

Varvaro F: Family role and work adaptation in MI women, *Clin Nurs Res* 9:339–351, 2000.

Wilson T, Koenig L, Ickovics J et al: Contraception use, family planning, and unprotected sex: few differences among HIV-infected and uninfected postpartum women in four US states, *J Acquir Immune Defic Syndr* 33:608–613, 2003.

Ineffective Sexuality pattern   *Elaine E. Steinke, PhD, RN, FAHA*   ⊖volve

NANDA-I

Definition

Expressions of concern regarding own sexuality

Defining Characteristics

Alterations in achieving perceived sex role; alteration in relationship with significant other; conflicts involving values; reported changes in sexual activities; reported changes in sexual behaviors; reported difficulties in sexual activities; reported difficulties in sexual behaviors; reported limitations in sexual activities; reported limitations in sexual behaviors

Related Factors (r/t)

Absent role model; conflicts with sexual orientation preferences; conflicts with variant preferences; fear of acquiring a sexually transmitted infection; fear of pregnancy; impaired relationship with a significant other; ineffective role model; knowledge about alternative responses to health related transitions, altered body function or structure, illness, or medical treatment; lack of privacy; lack of significant other; skill deficit about alternative responses to health-related transitions, altered body function or structure, illness, or medical treatment

NOC   (Nursing Outcomes Classification)

Suggested NOC Outcomes

Abuse Recovery: Sexual, Body Image, Child Development: Middle Childhood/Adolescence, Client Satisfaction: Teaching, Knowledge: Sexual Function, Psychosocial Adjustment: Life Change, Risk Control: Sexually Transmitted Diseases (STDs), Risk Control: Unintended Pregnancy, Role Performance, Self-Esteem, Sexual Function, Sexual Identity

● = Independent   ▲ = Collaborative   **EBN** = Evidence-Based Nursing   **EB** = Evidence-Based

---

Example NOC Outcome with Indicators

Risk Control: Sexually Transmitted Diseases (STD) as evidenced by the following indicators: Acknowledges individual risk for STD/Uses methods to control STD transmission (Rate the outcome and indicators of **Risk Control: Sexually Transmitted Diseases (STD):** 1 = never demonstrated, 2 = rarely demonstrated, 3 = sometimes demonstrated, 4 = often demonstrated, 5 = consistently demonstrated [see Section I].)

Client Outcomes

Client Will (Specify Time Frame):

- State knowledge of difficulties, limitations, or changes in sexual behaviors or activities
- State knowledge of sexual anatomy and functioning
- State acceptance of altered body structure or functioning
- Describe acceptable alternative sexual practices
- Identify importance of discussing sexual issues with significant other
- Describe practice of safe sex with regard to pregnancy and avoidance of STDs

NIC (Nursing Interventions Classification)

Suggested NIC Interventions

Sexual Counseling, Teaching: Sexuality

Example NIC Activities—Sexual Counseling

Provide privacy and ensure confidentiality; Provide information about sexual functioning, as appropriate

Nursing Interventions and *Rationales*

- After establishing rapport or therapeutic relationship, give the client permission to discuss issues dealing with sexuality. Ask the client specifically, "Have you been or are you concerned about functioning sexually because of your health status?" *Start with more general questions and then ask those that are more personal. Discuss exercise recommendations and then discuss sex as another form of exercise. Recognize that some older adults may not be sexually active at the present time, but may want information for future reference (Steinke, 2005; Steinke & Jaarsma, 2008). The PLISSIT model (giving permission to discuss sexual concerns, providing limited information, providing specific information, referral for intensive therapy) as an assessment approach can uncover concerns that might not ordinarily be raised by the client (Hardin, 2007).*
- Use assessment questions and standardized instruments to assess sexual problems, where possible. **EB:** *The Prostate Cancer Index, The International Index of Erectile Function, and the Female Sexual Function Index have been used widely, including in cancer (Jeffrey et al, 2009).* **EBN:** *Specific assessment questions can be used to assess sexuality, such as: How important is intimacy in your relationship? Are you satisfied with the amount of intimacy you receive? Are you currently sexually active? Have you noticed any changes in your sexual performance, such as difficulty with decreased libido, vaginal dryness, orgasmic problems, or erectile problems? An assessment of current medication and supplements to determine if these are affecting sexual function is also important (Steinke & Jaarsma, 2008).*
- Encourage the client to discuss concerns with his or her partner. *Carefully assess a client's sexuality. A sexual relationship may be heterosexual or homosexual, and nurses must not lose sight of this (Silenzio, 2003). A daily walk together is an ideal time to discuss sexual concerns, while increasing the client's strength and stamina and promoting health (Steinke, 2005). Effective communication with one's partner includes listening and learning to express one's feelings, and is an important component of self-management for the client (Newman, 2007).*
- Assess psychosocial function such as anxiety, depression, and low self-esteem. **EBN:** *Psychosocial function was a powerful predictor of information needs at 6 months and at 1 year, including the need for sexual information among those who had coronary bypass or coronary angioplasty (Kattainen, Merilainen, & Jokela, 2004).* **EB:** *Sexual anxiety and sexual self-efficacy had a significant (p. 1) independent effect on sexual activity in a sample of those with heart failure and healthy elders, illustrating the importance of assessing psychosocial and sexual concerns (Steinke et al, 2008).*

● = Independent   ▲ = Collaborative   **EBN** = Evidence-Based Nursing   **EB** = Evidence-Based

- Discuss alternative sexual expressions for altered body functioning or structure. Closeness and touching are other forms of expression. *Recognize that the meaning of sex and sexuality is individually defined, with some engaging in sexual intercourse, while others may prefer touching, holding one another, or kissing (Steinke, 2005).* **EBN:** *For some clients with severe heart failure, activities such as mutual masturbation, oral sex, or sexual intercourse may not be possible if exercise capacity is compromised, making other expressions of intimacy of greater importance (Steinke & Jaarsma, 2008).*
- Some clients choose masturbation for sexual release. **EB:** *Parents of adults with intellectual disability had more conservative attitudes towards sexual behavior than did staff, and the older the adult child, the more conservative the parental attitudes. A difference in values regarding sexual expression may provide confusion to the adult with intellectual disability (Cuskelly & Bryde, 2004).* **EB:** *Community attitudes towards those with an intellectual disability are overall positive (Cuskelly & Gilmore, 2007).*
- Assess the client's sexual orientation and discuss prevention of illnesses for which the client may be at increased risk (e.g., anorectal cancer). *Ask about sexual orientation directly, for example, "Do you have sexual relationships with men, women, or both?" Assess use of safer sex practices (e.g., condom use); the frequency of anal intercourse; number of sexual partners during the last year; last HIV screening and results; and use of medications, alcohol, and illicit drugs (Ortiz, 2007; Blackwell, 2008).*
- The following are guidelines for sexual activity for clients who have had total hip replacement (THR) surgery:
  - When considering sexual positions, do not bend the affected leg more than 90 degrees at the hip. When lying on your back, do not turn or roll your affected leg toward the other leg. Do not turn the toes of the affected leg inward. When lying on your side, keep both legs separated with pillows between them. Do not let your knees touch and do not let the toes of your affected leg turn downward. When the client is in the bottom sexual position, place pillows under the affected thigh for support or comfort and keep toes of the affected leg pointed upward and slightly outward. Women should avoid the top position as it requires bending the hip more than 90 degrees; men should keep the affected leg out to the side with toes pointed outward. For men using a side-lying position, lie on your unaffected side with both you and your partner facing the same direction; you will be behind your partner in a "spooning" position. Your partner should place at least two pillows between her legs and your affected leg should rest on top of hers during intercourse. Do not bend your affected leg more than 90 degrees, and do not let the toes of your affected leg dangle or turn downward. For women in a side-lying position, lie on your unaffected side and place enough pillows between your legs to support the affected leg. Make sure the affected leg does not drop off the pillows during intercourse. Your partner should assume the "spooning" position behind you. Do not bend your affected hip more than 90 degrees, and do not let the toes of your affected leg turn downward. *Caution:* If you dislocate your hip during sexual intercourse, you will experience pain, your affected leg will appear shorter, and your foot will turn inward. Lie down, do not move, and tell your partner to call an ambulance. *The goal of rehabilitation after THR is to sustain and, if possible, increase clients' ability to function, including sexual function. Addressing issues about sexual activity should therefore be made a part of the standard instructions given to THR clients on how to protect the new hip (Rogers, 2003).*
- The following are suggestions to be used for those who have had a myocardial infarction (MI):
  - Sexual activity can be resumed in about 1 week to 10 days for those who had an uncomplicated MI. Sex should occur in familiar surroundings, in a comfortable room temperature, with the usual partner, and when well rested to minimize any cardiac stress. Heavy meals or alcohol should be avoided for 2 to 3 hours before sexual activity. Clients should choose the most comfortable position, one that minimizes any stress they may feel. *Anal sex stimulates the vagus nerve and is accompanied by slowed heart rate and rhythm and coronary blood flow; therefore, further evaluation by the physician may be needed before anal sex can be resumed (Steinke, 2005; Steinke & Jaarsma, 2008).*
- The following are suggestions for those who have had coronary artery bypass grafting (CABG):
  - Instructions are similar to those for MI, with the following additions. Clients may have incisional pain with sexual activity, generally a dull ache in the mid-sternal area, and pain that does not radiate (unlike prior experiences with chest pain). Reassure the client and partner that sexual activity will not harm the sternum. Sexual activity can be generally resumed in 3 to 6 weeks following CABG. **EBN:** *Women, particularly those with large breasts, may report more issues*

● = Independent   ▲ = Collaborative   **EBN** = Evidence-Based Nursing   **EB** = Evidence-Based

related to pain in the breast, chest numbness, and difficulty healing. Encouraging the woman to choose a position of comfort, support with pillows, and taking a pain reliever such as acetominophen prior to sexual activity may be helpful (Steinke & Jaarsma, 2008).

- The following are suggestions for those with an implantable cardioverter defibrillator (ICD):
  - Assure the client and partner that fears about being shocked during sexual activity are normal. Sex can be resumed after the ICD is placed as long as strain on the implant site is avoided. If the ICD does discharge with sexual activity, the client should stop and rest and later notify the physician that the device fired so that it can be evaluated whether changes in the device settings are needed. The client should be instructed to report any dyspnea, chest pain, or dizziness with sexual activity. *Partners are often fearful and overprotective of the client, and some have noted sensations when the client's ICD fired, though not harmful to the partner (Steinke, 2003; Steinke et al, 2005).*
- The following are suggestions for those with chronic lung disease:
  - Sexual activity should be planned when energy level is highest and using positions that minimize shortness of breath, such as a semireclining position. *Planning sexual activity when the medications may be at their peak effectiveness may also be helpful. An oxygen cannula can be used, if prescribed, to provide oxygen before, during, or after sex (Steinke, 2005). Pulmonary rehabilitation, including exercise and respiratory muscle training may improve physical and sexual function (Goodell, 2007).*
- The following are suggestions for those with multiple sclerosis:
  - Treatment of symptoms with prescribed medications and supportive therapies may assist with a more satisfying sexual experience. **EBN:** *Neuropathic pain may be treated with antiseizure medications, massage therapy, and acupuncture, as well as changing positions for sexual activity and discussing changes in sensation and stimulation with the partner. Exercise, stretching, taking antispasmodic medications 20 minutes prior to sexual activity, and trying alternative positions (e.g., side lying) may be beneficial. Routine bowel elimination and avoiding a distended bowel, as well as emptying the bladder can alleviate discomfort with sexual intercourse (Moore, 2007).*
- The following are suggestions for those with arthritis:
  - Those with either osteoarthritis or rheumatoid arthritis (RA) fear being in pain or causing pain to their partner. *The act of intercourse is often the most difficult, so encouraging the couple to have open communication between them and to allow plenty of time for sexual foreplay and intercourse is important. With open communication, the couple can discuss the type of stimulation preferred and trying new positions that may provide comfort during sexual activity. The use of touch through sexual stimulation can be enhanced with scented lotions, feathers, or vibrators, for example. It may take practice for the couple to determine which sexual position causes the least discomfort. Teaching the client and the partner relaxation techniques can be helpful in breaking the cycle of pain (Newman, 2007).* **EBN:** *Inflammation and fatigue are prominent symptoms in rheumatoid arthritis, and 50% of those with RA have loss of interest in sex, 60% are dissatisfied with their sexual quality of life, and 69% of men and 85% of women report that joint swelling affects the decision on whether to initiate sexual activity (Newman, 2007).* **EB:** *In one study, 41% of men and 51% of women had difficulty with joint pain during sexual activity (van Berso et al, 2007).* **EB:** *In female clients with RA, 62% reported problems with sexual performance, 17% were unable to engage in sexual activity due to RA, and sexual satisfaction was either diminished or lost by 92% (Abdel-Nasser & Ei, 2006).*
- Refer to the care plan **Sexual dysfunction** for additional interventions.

 Pediatric

- Provide age-appropriate information for adolescents regarding human immunodeficiency virus (HIV) or the acquired immunodeficiency syndrome (AIDS) and sexual behavior. **EB:** *Attempts should be made to make HIV education more relevant for teens so that they use the information they have when making decisions about safer sexual behavior (Hoppe, Graham, & Wilsdon, 2004).* **EBN:** *Pregnant adolescents and young mothers are vulnerable to acquiring HIV/AIDS through sexual transmission because they lack the resources, social status, and power to protect themselves (Lesser, Oakes, & Koniak-Griffin, 2003).*
- Provide support for the client's chosen ways to cope with HIV or AIDS. **EBN:** *Female adolescents infected with HIV/AIDS revealed that the most often used coping strategies identified by the adoles-*

cents were listening to music, thinking about good things, making your own decisions, being close to someone you care about, sleeping, trying on your own to deal with problems, eating, watching television, daydreaming, and praying (Lewis & Brown, 2002).

Geriatric

▲ Carefully assess the sexuality needs of the elderly client and refer for counseling if needed. *Being a sexual being and having sexual feelings are part of what it is to be a human being—there are no age limits to enjoying a healthy sex life and having the ability to love and be loved (Peate, 2004). The ability to form satisfying social relationships and to be intimate with others, including building strong emotional intimate connections, contributes to adaptation and successful aging (Steinke, 2005).* **EB:** *Many men and women in the United States report continued sexual interest and activity into middle age and beyond (Laumann et al, 2009).*

▲ Explore possible changes in sexuality related to health status, menopause, and medications, and make appropriate referrals. **EB:** *In a study of older Australian women, few reported low relationship satisfaction and sexual distress, although higher levels of distress were noted among younger women and those with partners (Howard, O'Neill, & Travers, 2006). To study sexual activity, the prevalence of sexual dysfunction and related help-seeking behaviors among mature adults in the United States of America, a telephone survey was conducted. Early ejaculation (26.2%) and erectile difficulties (22.5%) were the most common male sexual problems. A lack of sexual interest (33.2%) and lubrication difficulties (21.5%) were the most common female sexual problems. Less than 25% of men and women with a sexual problem had sought help for their sexual problem(s) from a health professional (Laumann et al, 2009).*

• Allow the client to verbalize feelings regarding loss of sexual partner or significant other. Acknowledge problems such as disapproval of children, lack of available partner for women, and environmental variables that make forming new relationships difficult. **EB:** *Similar to younger adults, older adults are often distressed about changes in their relationship, sexual satisfaction, and sexual intimacy (Svetlik et al, 2005).* **EB:** *Lack of an available partner is one of the most frequently reported barriers to maintaining sexual function as one ages (Ginsberg et al, 2005; Rheaume & Mitty, 2008).*

• Provide a milieu that allows for discussion of sexual issues and a higher level of sexual satisfaction. Allow couples to room together and bring in double beds from home. Place signs on the door to ensure privacy. *Sexuality among adults in long-term care facilities is a difficult issue for staff to address (Lantz, 2004). Lack of privacy may inhibit engaging in sexual behavior in the assisted living setting as few facilities are designed to accommodate those wishing to be sexually active, including potential interruptions by caregivers at any time of the day or night (Rheaume & Mitty, 2008).* **EBN:** *Sexual sensations can be a source of comfort and pleasure for older adults even as other biological systems are failing. Nursing home staff should foster an atmosphere that gives older adults permission to discuss sexual issues (Roach, 2004).*

• Provide clients with the following information:
  ▪ Exercise, such as walking, swimming, cycling, and riding a stationary bike will help control flabby thighs and weak musculature and make people feel more sexually attractive.
  ▪ Overindulgence in food or alcohol can affect sexual activity (see care plan for **Imbalanced Nutrition: more than body requirements**).
  ▪ Resting and sleeping on a firm mattress may augment sexual desire.
  ▪ Femininity and masculinity are still important.
  ▪ Pay attention to cleanliness, skin care, and clothing.
  ▪ Change the environment, and experiment with position changes.
  Because the majority of the elderly population maintains sexual interest, desire, and functioning, these interventions may be helpful during the rehabilitation process.

• See care plan for **Sexual dysfunction**.

Multicultural

• Assess for the influence of cultural beliefs, norms, and values on client's perceptions of normal sexual behavior. **EBN:** *What the client considers normal sexual behavior may be based on cultural perceptions (Leininger & McFarland, 2002). Religion may also influence one's perception of sexual* *behavior (Lazoritz & McDermott, 2002). Common cultural beliefs and behaviors of South Asian Indian clients around sexuality include the role of the individual client's duty to society, the client's sense of place in society, lack of formal sexual education, prearranged marriages, little premarital contraceptive education, and the dominance of the husband in contraceptive decisions (Fisher, Bowman, & Thomas, 2003).*

Home Care

- Previously discussed interventions may be adapted for home care use. Also see care plan for **Sexual dysfunction**.
- Help the client and significant other to identify a place and time in the home and daily living for privacy in sharing sexual or relationship activity. If necessary, help the client to communicate the need for privacy to other family members. Consider periodic escapes to desirable surroundings. *The home setting can be one that affords little, if any, privacy without a conscious effort made by members of the home.*
- Confirm that physical reasons for dysfunction have been addressed. Provide support for coping behaviors, including participation in support groups or therapy if appropriate. **EB:** *A study of clients with HIV/AIDS who were randomized to either a support group intervention or a coping group intervention revealed that the coping group intervention decreased episodes of unprotected sexual intercourse (Sikkema et al, 2008).* **EB:** *Women with cervical cancer with good quality of life were more likely to report greater social support and greater sexual pleasure; 69% reported that attendance at a support group after their initial treatment would have been helpful (Wenzel et al, 2005).* **EB:** *Women with metastatic breast cancer need ongoing support from others, including sexual concerns, although social support has been shown to decrease as women may find it difficult to discuss the challenges they face and responses from others may not be supportive (Vilhauer, 2008).*
- Reinforce or teach about sexual functioning, alternative sexual practices, and necessary sexual precautions. Update teaching as client status changes. *If the client or significant other has received information during an institutional stay, other stressors may have made the information a temporarily low priority or may have impaired learning. Depending on the cause for dysfunction, the client may experience changing status or feelings about the problem.*

Client/Family Teaching and Discharge Planning

- ▲ Refer to appropriate community agencies (e.g., certified sex counselor, Reach to Recovery, Ostomy Association). *Sexuality concerns should be addressed with all clients for which sexual function might be affected due to a acute or chronic condition.*
- Provide information regarding self-care and sexuality for the woman who has cancer and her partner. **EB:** *Women with breast cancer experience distress regarding body image, their sexual life, and the effect of stress on their illness (Vilhauer, 2008).*
- ▲ Sexuality education is important to all populations, whether hearing or deaf, sighted or blind, disabled or not disabled. Discuss contraceptive choices. Refer to appropriate health professional (e.g., gynecologist, nurse practitioner [NP]). *Physical and psychosocial health, including sexual counseling, should be included as part of preventive care for adolescents (Delisi & Gold, 2008). Sexuality education is vitally important for normal growth and development, including adolescents with developmental disabilities (Greydanus & Omar, 2008).*
- Teach safe sex to all clients including the elderly, including using latex condoms, washing with soap immediately after sexual contact, not ingesting semen, avoiding oral-genital contact, not exchanging saliva, avoiding multiple partners, abstaining from sexual activity when ill, and avoiding recreational drugs and alcohol when engaging in sexual activity. Adherence to antiretroviral therapy is important. **EB:** *Predictors of nonadherence to antiretroviral therapy include lack of trust between the health professional and the client, active drug and alcohol use, psychosocial issues such as depression or low social support, lack of client education about medications, and complex medication and management regimens. To increase adherence to medications and to support viral suppression, assess emotional and practical life supports; assist in determining ways to fit medications into daily routines and stress the importance of taking all doses; discuss that less than optimal adherence leads to resistance; and urge client to keep clinic appointments (U.S. Department Health & Human Services, 2008).* **EB:** *Older*

• = Independent ▲ = Collaborative **EBN** = Evidence-Based Nursing **EB** = Evidence-Based

adults can and will acquire new information regarding AIDS-related information when it is presented to them (Falvo & Norman, 2004). (Additional resource: CDC, 2008.)

ⓔvolve   See the EVOLVE website for Weblinks for client education resources.

REFERENCES

Abdel-Nasser AM, Ei A: Determinants of sexual disability and dissatisfaction in female patients with rheumatoid arthritis, *Clin Rheumatol* 25(6):822–830, 2006.

Blackwell CW: Anorectal carcinoma screening in gay men: Implications for nurse practitioners, *Am J Nurs Pract* 12(1):60–63, 2008.

Centers for Disease Control and Prevention (CDC): 2008 Compendium of Evidence-Based HIV Prevention Interventions, 2008, www.cdc.gov/hiv/topics/research/prs/evidence-based-interventions.htm. Accessed March 17, 2009.

Cuskelly M, Bryde R: Attitudes towards the sexuality of adults with an intellectual disability: parents, support staff, and a community sample, *J Intellect Dev Disabil* 29(3):255–264, 2004.

Cuskelly M, Gilmore L: Attitudes to sexuality questionnaire (Individuals with an Intellectual Disability): scale development and community norms, *J Intellect Dev Disabil* 32(3):214–221, 2007.

Delisi K, Gold MA: The initial adolescent preventative care visit, *Clin Obstet Gynecol* 51(2):190–204, 2008.

Falvo N, Norman S: Never too old to learn: the impact of an HIV/AIDS education program on older adults' knowledge, *Clin Gerontol* 27(1/2):103–117, 2004.

Fisher JA, Bowman M, Thomas T: Issues for South Asian Indian patients surrounding sexuality, fertility, and childbirth in the U.S. health care system, *J Am Board Fam Pract* 16(2):151–155, 2003.

Ginsberg TB, Pomerantz SC, Kramer-Feeley V: Sexuality in older adults: behaviours and preferences, *Age Aging* 34(5):475–480, 2005.

Goodell TT: Sexuality in chronic lung disease, *Nurs Clin North Am* 42:631–638, 2007.

Greydanus DE, Omar HA: Sexuality issues and gynecologic care of adolescents with developmental disabilities, *Pediatr Clin North Am* 55(6):1315–1335, 2008.

Hardin SR: Cardiac disease and sexuality: implications for research and practice, *Nurs Clin North Am* 42:593–603, 2007.

Hoppe MJ, Graham L, Wilsdon A: Teens speak out about HIV/AIDS: focus group discussions about risk and decision-making, *J Adolesc Health* 35(4):345–346, 2004.

Howard JR, O'Neill S, Travers C: Factors affecting sexuality in older Australian women: sexual interest, sexual arousal, relationships and sexual distress in older Australian women, *Climacteric* 9:355–367, 2006.

Jeffrey DD, Tzeng JP, Francis J et al: Initial report of the cancer Patient-Reported Outcomes Measurement Information System (PROMIS) sexual function committee: review of sexual function measures and domains used in oncology, *Cancer* 115(6):1142–1153, 2009.

Kattainen E, Merilainen P, Jokela V: CABG and PTCA patients' expectations of informational support in health-related quality of life themes and adequacy of information at 1–year follow-up, *Eur J Cardiovasc Nurs* 3:149–163, 2004.

Lantz MS: Consenting adults: sexuality in the nursing home, *Clin Geriatr* 12(6):33–36, 2004.

Laumann EO, Glasser DB, Neves RC et al: A population-based survey of sexual activity, sexual problems and associated help-seeking behavior patterns in mature adults in the United States of America, *Int J Impot Res* 21(3):171–178, 2009.

Lazoritz S, McDermott RT: Adolescent sexuality, cultural sensitivity and the teachings of the Catholic Church, *J Reprod Med* 47(8):603, 2002.

Leininger MM, McFarland MR: *Transcultural nursing: concepts, theories, research and practices,* ed 3, New York, 2002, McGraw-Hill.

Lesser J, Oakes R, Koniak-Griffin D: Vulnerable adolescent mothers' perceptions of maternal role and HIV risk, *Health Care Women Int* 24(6):513–528, 2003.

Lewis CL, Brown SC: Coping strategies of female adolescents with HIV/AIDS, *ABNF J* 13(4):72, 2002.

Moore LA: Intimacy and multiple sclerosis, *Nurs Clin North Am* 42:605–619, 2007.

Newman AM: Arthritis and sexuality, *Nurs Clin North Am* 42:605–619, 2007.

Ortiz MR: HIV, AIDS, and sexuality, *Nurs Clin North Am* 42:621–630, 2007.

Peate I: Sexuality and sexual health promotion for the older person, *Br J Nurs* 13(4):188–193, 2004.

Rheaume C, Mitty E: Sexuality and intimacy in older adults, *Geriatric Nursing* 29(5):342–349, 2008.

Roach SM: Sexual behavior of nursing home residents: staff perceptions and responses, *J Adv Nurs* 48(4):371–379, 2004.

Rogers D: New meaning for safe sex, *RN* 66(1):38–42, 2003.

Sikkema KJ, Wilson PA, Hansen NB et al: Effects of a coping intervention on transmission risk behavior among people living with HIV/AIDS and a history of childhood sexual abuse, *J Acquir Immune Defic Syndr* 47(4):506–513, 2008.

Silenzio VMB: Anthropological assessment for culturally appropriate interventions targeting men who have sex with men, *Am J Pub Health* 93(6):867–871, 2003.

Steinke EE: Sexual concerns of patients and partners after an implantable cardioverter defibrillator, *Dimens Crit Care Nurs* 22(2):89–96, 2003.

Steinke EE: Intimacy needs and chronic illness, *J Gerontol Nurs* 31(5):40–50, 2005.

Steinke EE, Gill-Hopple K, Valdez D et al: Sexual concerns and educational needs after an implantable cardioverter defibrillator, *Heart Lung* 34(5):299–308, 2005.

Steinke EE, Jaarsma T: Impact of cardiovascular disease on sexuality. In Moser D, Riegel B, editors: *Cardiac nursing: a companion to Braunwald's heart disease,* pp. 241–253, St Louis, Saunders, 2008.

Steinke EE, Wright DW, Chung ML et al: Sexual self-concept, anxiety and self-efficacy predict sexual activity in heart failure and healthy elders, *Heart Lung* 37:323–333, 2008.

Svetlik RN, Dooley WK, Weiner MF, Williamson GM, Walters AS: Declines in satisfaction with physical intimacy predict caregiver perceptions of overall relationship loss: a study of elderly caregiving spousal dyads, *Sexuality Disabil* 23(2):65–79, 2005.

U.S. Department of Health and Human Services: *Guidelines for the use of antiretroviral agents in HIV-1–infected adults and adolescents,* 2008, p. 25, http://aidsinfo.nih.gov/contentfiles/AdultandAdolescentGL.pdf. Accessed March 17, 2009.

van Berso WT, van de Weil HB, Taal E et al: Sexual functioning of people with rheumatoid arthritis: a multicenter study, *Clin Rheumatol* 26(1):30–38, 2007.

Vilhauer RP: A qualitative study of the experiences of women with metastatic breast cancer, *Palliat Support Care* 6(3):249–257, 2008.

Wenzel L, DeAlba I, Habbal R et al: Quality of life in long-term cancer survivors, *Gynecol Oncol* 97(2):310–317, 2005.

• = Independent   ▲ = Collaborative   **EBN** = Evidence-Based Nursing   **EB** = Evidence-Based

Risk for Shock   *Jennifer Hafner, RN, BSN, TNCC, and Joan Klehr, RNC, BS, MPH*   ⊝volve

NANDA-I

Definition

At risk for an inadequate blood flow to the body's tissues, which may lead to life-threatening cellular dysfunction

Risk Factors

Hypotension; hypovolemia; hypoxemia; hypoxia; infection; sepsis; systemic inflammatory response syndrome

NOC   (Nursing Outcomes Classification)

Suggested NOC Outcomes

Tissue Perfusion: Cellular, Fluid Balance, Circulation Status, Vital Signs

Example NOC Outcome with Indicators
Tissue Perfusion: Cellular as evidenced by the following indicators: Systolic blood pressure/Mean arterial blood pressure/Fluid balance/Urine output/Heart rate/Heart rhythm (Rate the outcome and indicators of **Tissue Perfusion: Cellular:** 1 = severe deviation from normal range, 2 = substantial deviation from normal range, 3 = moderate deviation from normal range, 4 = mild deviation from normal range, 5 = no deviation from normal range [see Section I].)

Client/Family Outcomes

Client Will (Specify Time Frame):

- Maintain a systolic blood pressure above 90 mm Hg
- Maintain a mean arterial blood pressure above 65 mm Hg
- Maintain a heart rate between 60-100 with a normal sinus rhythm
- Maintain urine output greater than 0.5 mL/kg/hr
- Have warm, dry skin

NIC   (Nursing Interventions Classification)

Suggested NIC Interventions

Shock Prevention, IV Therapy, Medication Administration, Fluid Resuscitation

Example NIC Activities—Shock Prevention
Monitor for early signs of systemic inflammatory response syndrome (e.g., increased temperature, tachycardia, tachypnea, hypocarbia, leukocytosis, or leukopenia); Monitor pulse oximetry; Monitor ECG

Nursing Interventions and *Rationales*

▲ Administer oxygen immediately and medications as prescribed. *Administration of oxygen, antibiotics, insulin, and vasoactive medications improve the survival of shock, and septic shock clients (Dellinger et al, 2009).*

● Monitor vital signs, blood pressure, pulse, respirations, and pulse oximetry. *Elevated heart rate, decreased blood pressure (below 90 mm Hg systolic), increased respiratory rate (greater than 20), and decreased SpO_2 (below 90%) are indicators of shock (Bridges & Dukes, 2005; Fauci et al, 2008; Dellinger et al, 2009). Temperature greater than 38° C or less than 36° C, along with a higher white blood cell count (12 x 103/mm³) or lower count (4 x 103/mm³) plus the symptoms above are indicators of septic shock (Dellinger et al, 2009; Nelson et al, 2009).*

▲ If sepsis or septic shock is suspected, obtain stat cultures as ordered. **EB and EBN:** *Systematic literature reviews identified that appropriate cultures should be obtained before the administration of antibiotics for evolving septic shock. At least two blood cultures are recommended, with at least one*

● = Independent   ▲ = Collaborative   **EBN** = Evidence-Based Nursing   **EB** = Evidence-Based

drawn percutaneously and one drawn through each vascular access line. Additional cultures of other sites such as urine, wounds, or other body fluids as indicated are also recommended (Dellinger et al, 2004; Kleinpell & Ahrens, 2008).

▲ Administer appropriate antibiotics as prescribed within 1 hour of diagnosis of severe sepsis or septic shock. Continue care with goal-directed therapy to treat condition. *Early goal directed therapy for sepsis results in a better rate of survival (Dellinger et al, 2008).*

• Review the client's medical and surgical history. *Certain conditions place clients at higher risk for shock such as: trauma, chest pain related to a myocardial infarction, head injury, dehydration, and infection. Certain co-morbidities require treatment to improve morbidity and mortality outcomes (Bridges & Dukes, 2005; Dellinger et al, 2009).*

• Monitor intake and output, and daily weights. *With the systemic inflammatory response associated with sepsis, the vascular membrane becomes permeable and third spacing occurs. This will increase the I/O ratio and weight due to edema (Dellinger et al, 2009). Blood is also shunted to the vital organs in shock, and urine output will decrease as a result (Goodrich, 2006).*

▲ Maintain IV access. Recognize that isotonic IV fluids such as 0.9% normal saline or ringers lactate rapidly may be administered for the client in shock. *Adequate IV access is required for fluid resuscitation and medication delivery (Bridges & Dukes, 2005; Dellinger et al, 2009). Crystalloids and isotonic IV solutions are commonly used for resuscitation of hypovolemic or septic shock clients. If the cause of shock is cardiac dysfunction, IV fluid administration of isotonic fluids may be harmful. Colloids are used for treatment of blood loss.* **EB:** *A study found that there was no difference in outcomes when the client needing fluid resuscitation was given crystalloids or colloids such as albumin (Younker, 2007).*

Critical Care

▲ Monitor: electrocardiography, invasive blood pressure monitoring, central venous pressure, and SvO_2 or $ScvO_2$ (mixed venous oxygen saturation). *Vasodilatation will decrease central venous pressure because the client will not have enough volume to properly fill the enlarged veins and arteries. Tachycardia may be present due to the decreased fluid volume, which will be seen prior to a decrease in blood pressure as a compensatory mechanism. A decrease in blood pressure will be observed as a later sign of distributive shock. Pulse oximetry may be lower as a result of increased oxygen demand. Oxygenation of the cells will be lower due to hypoperfusion, hypotension, misdistribution of blood flow, increased capillary wall thickness, and inability of the cells to use oxygen. Monitoring of SvO_2 and $ScvO_2$ will monitor the oxygen consumption. The duo of pulse oximetry and SvO_2 or $ScvO_2$ monitors oxygen demand and delivery (Bridges & Dukes, 2005; Goodrich, 2006; Dellinger et al, 2009).*

▲ Monitor mean arterial blood pressure. *Maintaining a mean arterial blood pressure at desired levels will maintain adequate perfusion to the organs (Bridges & Dukes, 2005; Dellinger et al, 2009). Mean arterial blood pressure is a more reliable indicator of tissue perfusion because it more closely reflects the autoregulatory limits of organ blood flow (Goodrich, 2006).*

▲ Monitor cardiac output and systemic vascular resistance. *Both cardiac output and systemic vascular resistance may temporarily increase with the onset of shock because of compensatory mechanisms. As shock progresses, cardiac output will decrease, along with systematic vascular resistance as the compensatory mechanisms fail (Bridges & Dukes, 2005; Dellinger et al, 2009).*

▲ Monitor intake and output carefully every hour. Insert a Foley catheter as ordered and measure hourly urine output, especially if the client has some renal insufficiency. *As shock progresses blood is shunted to the vital organs, and urine output will decrease as a result (Goodrich, 2006).*

▲ Maintain IV access. Recognize that isotonic IV fluids such as 0.9% normal saline or ringers lactate may be administered rapidly for the client in shock. **EBN:** *Adequate IV access is required for fluid resuscitation and medication delivery (Bridges & Dukes, 2005).*

▲ Prepare the client for central line placement. *Adequate IV and central line access is required for fluid resuscitation and medication delivery. Large amounts of fluid can be delivered more efficiently through central lines. Most vasopressive agents can only be delivered through central lines due to risk of tissue sloughing. Central venous pressure can only be monitored through a central line (Bridges & Dukes, 2005).*

▲ Monitor pulmonary artery occlusion pressure. *A decreased pulmonary artery occlusion pressure is an indicator of low intravascular volume. This value is used to determine the amount of fluid resuscitation needed and will help guide therapy (Bridges & Dukes, 2005).*

• = Independent ▲ = Collaborative **EBN** = Evidence-Based Nursing **EB** = Evidence-Based

▲ Monitor serum lactate level. *An elevated serum lactate level is an indicator of tissue hypoxia and anaerobic metabolism (Bridges & Dukes, 2005; Goodrich, 2006; Morton & Fontaine, 2008).*

▲ Monitor arterial blood gasses, coagulation, chemistries, point-of-care blood glucose, cardiac enzymes, blood cultures, and hematology. *Abnormalities can identify the cause of the decreased perfusion and identify complications related to the decreased perfusion or shock. Elevated cardiac enzymes are indicative of a myocardial infarction and the low perfusion could be cardiogenic shock (Bridges & Dukes, 2005). An elevated WBC count, or very low WBC count, and low blood pressure would be indicators of septic shock. Positive blood cultures are associated with septic shock.*

• Complete a full nursing physical examination including examination of the skin. *A full nursing assessment is crucial in identifying multiple complications of shock such as: hypoperfusion of internal organs that manifest as decreased bowel sounds and shortness of breath (Bridges & Dukes, 2005). Monitor for signs of a localized infection which may be present in septic shock. Cool, clammy skin and mottling are symptoms of tissue hypoperfusion (Dellinger et al, 2009). Pale, clammy skin will be present in shock states (Goodrich, 2006).* **EBN:** *Recognize that decreased capillary return may not be helpful in determining hypovolemia (Dufault et al, 2008).*

▲ Prepare the client for the following imaging studies: CT scan, x-ray (chest, abdominal, pelvic, and extremity) to assess for osteomyelitis, and lumbar puncture to rule out meningitis. *CT scan will assess for areas of injury, infection, and causality of hypoperfusion; and a head CT will assess causation for increased intracranial pressure, which may dilate the vessels in neurogenic shock (Dellinger et al, 2009).*

Client/Family Teaching and Discharge Planning

• Teach client about any medications prescribed. Instruct the client to report any adverse side effects to his/her provider. *Medication teaching includes the drug name, its purpose, administration instructions such as taking it with or without food, and any side effects to be aware of. Diuretic use remains a primary cause of low serum potassium levels (Muller & Bell, 2008). Assessing and instructing clients about medications and focusing on important details can help prevent medication errors (Polzien, 2007).*

• Explain the ordered imaging studies and laboratory tests. *The client will need to participate and cooperate with each procedure to prevent adverse effects or injury to the client. Continue to give the client verbal instruction during all procedures (Dellinger et al, 2009; Bridges & Dukes, 2005).*

• Instruct the client and family on disease process and rationale for care. **EBN:** *Helping clients and families understand the disease process and nursing procedures that best supports their conditions are an integral part of care. Knowledge empowers client and family members and allows them to be active participants in their care (Sanford, 2000).*

⊝volve   See the EVOLVE website for Weblinks for client education resources.

REFERENCES

Bridges EJ, Dukes MS: Cardiovascular aspects of septic shock: pathophysiology, monitoring, and treatment, *Crit Care Nurse* 25(2):14–42, 2005.

Dellinger RP, Carlet JM, Masur H et al : Surviving Sepsis Campaign guidelines for management of severe sepsis and septic shock, *Crit Care Med,* 32(3):858–873, 2004.

Dellinger RP, Cinel I, Sharma S et al: *Septic shock,* 12, 2009, Septic shock, www.emedicine.com/med/topic2101.htm. Accessed September 29, 2009.

Dellinger RP, Levy MM, Carlet JM et al: Surviving Sepsis Campaign: international guidelines for management of severe sepsis and septic shock: 2008, *Intens Crit Care Med* 34(1):17–60, 2008.

Dufault M, Davis B, Garman D et al: translating best practices in assessing capillary refill, *Worldviews Evid Based Nurs* 5(1):36–44, 2008.

Fauci A, Braunwald E, Kasper D et al: *Harrison's principles of internal medicine,* ed 17, New York, 2008, McGraw-Hill.

Goodrich C: Endpoints of resuscitation: what should we be monitoring? *AACN Adv Crit Care* 17(3):308–316, 2006.

Kleinpell R, Ahrens T: Shock prevention guideline. In Ackley B, Ladwig G, Swan BA et al, editors: *Evidence-based nursing care,* Philadelphia, 2008, Mosby.

Morton PG, Fontaine DK: *Critical care nursing: a holistic approach,* ed 9, Philadelphia, 2008, Lippincott Williams & Wilkins.

Muller A, Bell A: Electrolyte update: potassium, chloride, and magnesium, *Nurs Crit Care* 3(1):5–7, 2008.

Nelson D, LeMaster T, Plost G et al: Recognizing sepsis in the adult patient, *AJN* 109(3):40–45, 2009.

Polzien G: Prevent medication errors: a new year's resolution: teaching patients about their medications, *Home Healthc Nurse* 25(1):59–62, 2007.

Sanford RC: Caring through relation and dialogue: a nursing perspective for patient education, *Adv Nurs Sci* 22(3):1–15, 2000.

Younker J: Saline versus albumin fluid evaluation (SAFE). Effect of baseline serum albumin concentration on outcome of resuscitation with albumin or saline in patients in intensive care units: analysis of data from the saline versus albumin fluid evaluation (SAFE) study, *BM J* 333:1044–1046, 2007.

• = Independent   ▲ = Collaborative   **EBN** = Evidence-Based Nursing   **EB** = Evidence-Based

Impaired Skin integrity   *Sharon Baranoski, MSN, RN, CWCN, APN, FAAN*   ⊝volve

NANDA-I

Definition

Altered epidermis and/or dermis

Defining Characteristics

Destruction of skin layers; disruption of skin surface; invasion of body structures

Related Factors (r/t)

External

Chemical substance; extremes in age; humidity; hyperthermia; hypothermia; mechanical factors (e.g., friction, shearing forces, pressure, restraint); medications; moisture; physical immobilization; radiation

Internal

Changes in fluid status; changes in pigmentation; changes in turgor; developmental factors; imbalanced nutritional state (e.g., obesity, emaciation, chronic disease, vascular disease); immunological deficit; impaired circulation; impaired metabolic state; impaired sensation; skeletal prominence

NOC   (Nursing Outcomes Classification)

Suggested NOC Outcomes

Tissue Integrity: Skin and Mucous Membranes, Wound Healing: Primary Intention, Secondary Intention

Example NOC Outcome with Indicators
Tissue Integrity: Skin and Mucous Membranes will be intact as evidenced by the following indicators: Skin integrity/Skin lesions not present/Tissue perfusion/Skin temperature/Skin thickness (Rate the outcome and indicators of **Tissue Integrity: Skin and Mucous Membranes:** 1 = severely compromised, 2 = substantially compromised, 3 = moderately compromised, 4 = mildly compromised, 5 = not compromised [see Section I].)

Client Outcomes

Client Will (Specify Time Frame):

- Regain integrity of skin surface
- Report any altered sensation or pain at site of skin impairment
- Demonstrate understanding of plan to heal skin and prevent reinjury
- Describe measures to protect and heal the skin and to care for any skin lesion

NIC   (Nursing Interventions Classification)

Suggested NIC Interventions

Incision Site Care, Pain Management, Pressure Ulcer Care, Pressure Ulcer Prevention, Risk Identification, Skin Care: Topical Treatments, Skin Surveillance, Wound Care, Wound Irrigation

Example NIC Activities—Pressure Ulcer Care
Monitor color of wound bed, temperature, edema, errythema, moisture, and appearance of surrounding skin; Note characteristics of any drainage

Nursing Interventions and *Rationales*

- Assess site of skin impairment and determine cause (e.g., acute or chronic wound, burn, dermatological lesion, pressure ulcer, skin tear). **EB:** *The cause of the wound must be determined before*

• = Independent   ▲ = Collaborative   **EBN** = Evidence-Based Nursing   **EB** = Evidence-Based

appropriate interventions can be implemented. This will provide the basis for additional testing and evaluation to start the assessment process (Baranoski & Ayello, 2008; Krasner, Rodeheaver & Sibbald, 2007).

- Determine that skin impairment involves skin damage only (e.g., partial-thickness wound, stage I or stage II pressure ulcer). The following classification system is for pressure ulcers:
  - **Category/Stage I:** Intact skin with non-blanchable erythema of a localized area usually over a bony prominence. Discoloration of the skin, warmth, edema, hardness, or pain may also be present. Darkly pigmented skin may not have visible blanching. The area may be painful, firm, soft, warmer, or cooler as compared to adjacent tissue. *Category/Stage I may be difficult to detect in individuals with dark skin tones. May indicate "at -risk" persons (NPUAP, 2009).*
  - **Category/ Stage II:** Partial-thickness skin loss of dermis presenting as a shallow open ulcer with a red pink wound bed, without slough. May also present as an intact or open/ruptured serum-filled or serosanguineous-filled blister. Further description: presents as a shiny or dry shallow ulcer without slough or bruising. *This category should not be used to describe skin tears, tape burns, incontinence-associated dermatitis, maceration, or excoriation (NPUAP, 2009).*
  - NOTE: For wounds deeper into subcutaneous tissue, muscle, or bone (category/stage III or stage IV pressure ulcers), see the care plan for **Impaired Tissue integrity**.
- Monitor site of skin impairment at least once a day for color changes, redness, swelling, warmth, pain, or other signs of infection. Determine whether the client is experiencing changes in sensation or pain. Pay special attention to high-risk areas such as bony prominences, skinfolds, the sacrum, and heels. *Systematic inspection can identify impending problems early (Ayello & Braden, 2002; Ayello, Baranoski, & Salati, 2006).*
- Monitor the client's skin care practices, noting type of soap or other cleansing agents used, temperature of water, and frequency of skin cleansing. *Cleansing should not compromise the skin (Fore, 2006).*
- Individualize plan according to the client's skin condition, needs, and preferences. **EBN:** *Avoid harsh cleansing agents, hot water, extreme friction or force, or cleansing too frequently (WOCN, 2003, 2009; Fore, 2006).*
- Monitor the client's continence status, and minimize exposure of skin impairment and other areas of moisture from incontinence, perspiration, or wound drainage. **EBN:** *Moisture from incontinence contributes to pressure ulcer development by macerating the skin (WOCN, 2003, 2009).*
- ▲ If the client is incontinent, implement an incontinence management plan to prevent exposure to chemicals in urine and stool that can strip or erode the skin. Refer to a continence care specialist, urologist, or gastroenterologist for incontinence assessment (WOCN, 2003). **EB:** *Implementing an incontinence prevention plan with the use of a skin protectant or a cleanser protectant can significantly decrease skin breakdown and pressure ulcer formation (Fantl et al, 1996).*
- For clients with limited mobility, use a risk assessment tool to systematically assess immobility-related risk factors (Ayello & Braden, 2002). *A validated risk assessment tool such as the Norton or Braden scale should be used to identify clients at risk for immobility-related skin breakdown (Ayello & Braden, 2002; Braden & Maklebust, 2005).* **EB:** *Targeting variables (such as age and Braden Scale Risk Category) can focus assessment on particular risk factors (e.g., pressure) and help guide the plan of prevention and care (WOCN, 2003, 2009; Sussman & Bates-Jensen, 2006; Krasner, Rodeheaver, & Sibbald, 2007; Magnan, & Maklebust, 2009; NPUAP, 2009).*
- Do not position the client on site of skin impairment. If consistent with overall client management goals, turn and position the client at least every 2 hours. Transfer the client with care to protect against the adverse effects of external mechanical forces such as pressure, friction, and shear. **EB:** *Do not position an individual directly on a pressure ulcer. Continue to turn/reposition the individual regardless of the support surface in use. Establish turning frequency based on the characteristics of the support surface and the individual's response (NPUAP, 2009). If the goal of care is to keep the client (e.g., a terminally ill client) comfortable, turning and repositioning may not be appropriate (NPUAP, 2009).*
- Evaluate for use of specialty mattresses, beds, or devices as appropriate. Maintain the head of the bed at the lowest possible degree of elevation to reduce shear and friction, and use lift devices, pillows, foam wedges, and pressure-reducing devices in the bed *(NPUAP, 2009; WOCN, 2009).*
- Implement a written treatment plan for topical treatment of the site of skin impairment. *A written plan ensures consistency in care and documentation (Baranoski & Ayello, 2008).*

• = Independent ▲ = Collaborative **EBN** = Evidence-Based Nursing **EB** = Evidence-Based

- Select a topical treatment that will maintain a moist wound-healing environment and that is balanced with the need to absorb exudate. **EBN:** *Choose dressings that provide a moist environment, keep periwound skin dry, and control exudate and eliminate dead space (WOCN, 2003, 2009; NPUAP, 2009).*
- Avoid massaging around the site of skin impairment and over bony prominences. *Research suggests that massage may lead to deep-tissue trauma (Panel for the Prediction and Prevention of Pressure Ulcers in Adults, 1992).*
- ▲ Assess the client's nutritional status. Refer for a nutritional consult and/or institute dietary supplements as necessary. *Optimizing nutritional intake, including calories, fatty acids, protein, and vitamins, is needed to promote wound healing (NPUAP, 2009).* **EB:** *The benefit of nutritional evaluation and intensive nutritional support in clients at risk for and with pressure ulcers is not supported by rigorous clinical trials. Despite this lack of evidence, NPUAP (2006, 2009) endorses the application of reasonable nutritional assessment and treatment for clients at risk for and with pressure ulcers.*
- Identify the client's phase of wound healing (inflammation, proliferation, maturation) and stage of injury. **EBN:** *The selection of the dressing is based on the tissue in the ulcer bed, the condition of the skin around the ulcer bed and the goals of the person with the ulcer. Generally maintaining a moist ulcer bed is the ideal when the ulcer bed is clean and granulating to promote healing and closure (NPUAP, 2009). No single wound dressing is appropriate for all phases of wound healing.*

Home Care

- The interventions described previously may be adapted for home care use.
- Instruct and assist the client and caregivers in how to change dressings and maintain a clean environment. Provide written instructions and observe them completing the dressing change.
- Educate client and caregivers on proper nutrition, signs and symptoms of infection, and when to call the agency and/or physician with concerns.
- ▲ It may be beneficial to initiate a consultation in a case assignment with a wound, ostomy, continence (WOC) nurse (or wounds specialist) to establish a comprehensive plan for complex wounds.

Client/Family Teaching and Discharge Planning

- ▲ Teach skin and wound assessment and ways to monitor for signs and symptoms of infection, complications, and healing. *Early assessment and intervention help prevent serious problems from developing.*
- ▲ Teach the client why a topical treatment has been selected. **EBN:** *The type of dressing needed may change over time as the wound heals and/or deteriorates (WOCN, 2003, 2009; NPUAP, 2009).*
- ▲ If consistent with overall client management goals, teach how to turn and reposition at least every 2 hours. **EB:** *If the goal of care is to keep a client (e.g., terminally ill client) comfortable, turning and repositioning may not be appropriate (Krasner, Rodeheaver, & Sibbald, 2007; NPUAP, 2009).*
- ▲ Teach the client to use pillows, foam wedges, and pressure-reducing devices to prevent pressure injury. **EB:** *The use of effective pressure-reducing seat cushions for elderly wheelchair users significantly prevented sitting-acquired pressure ulcers (Brienza et al, 2008).*

ⓔvolve   See the EVOLVE website for Weblinks for client education resources.

REFERENCES

Ayello EA, Baranoski S, Salati D: Best practice in wound care prevention and treatment, Nursing Management, 37(9):42–48, 2006.

Ayello EA, Braden B: How and why to do pressure ulcer risk assessment, *Adv Skin Wound Care* 15(3):125, 2002.

Baranoski S, Ayello EA, editors: *Wound care essentials: practice principles,* ed 2, Ambler, PA, 2008, Lippincott Williams & Wilkins.

Braden B, Maklebust J: Wound wise: preventing pressure ulcers with the Braden scale, *Am J Nurs* 105(6):70–72, 2005.

Brienza DM, Geyer MJ, Springle S et al: Pressure redistribution: seating, positioning, and support surfaces. In Baranoski S, Ayello EA, editors:

Wound care essentials: practice principles, ed 2, Ambler, PA, 2008, Lippincott, Williams & Wilkins.

Fantl JA et al: *Urinary incontinence in adults: acute and chronic management,* Clinical Practice Guideline No 2, 1996 Update, Agency for Health Care Policy and Research, Pub No 96, Rockville, MD, 1996, Public Health Service, U.S. Department of Health and Human Services.

Fore J: A review of skin and the effects of aging on skin structure and function, *Ostomy Wound Manage* 52(9):24–35, 2006.

• = Independent   ▲ = Collaborative   **EBN** = Evidence-Based Nursing   **EB** = Evidence-Based

Krasner D, Rodeheaver G, Sibbald RG: *Chronic wound care: a clinical source book for healthcare professionals,* ed 4, Malvern, PA, 2007, HMP Communications.

Magnan MA, Maklebust J: The nursing process and pressure ulcer prevention: making the connection, *Adv Skin Wound Care* 22(2):83–91, 2009.

National Pressure Ulcer Advisory Panel (NPUAP): What is the role of nutritional support for patients in the prevention and treatment of pressure ulcers? Frequently asked questions, 2006, www.npuap.org/faq.htm. Accessed April 9, 2009.

National Pressure Ulcer Advisory Panel (NPUAP): *The new international guideline consensus on implementation, 11th Annual Biennial Conference,* Washington, DC, February 2009, NPUAP.

Panel for the Prediction and Prevention of Pressure Ulcers in Adults: *Pressure ulcers in adults: prediction and prevention,* Clinical Practice Guideline No. 3, Agency for Health Care Policy and Research, Pub No 92, Rockville, MD, 1992, Public Health Services, U.S. Department of Health and Human Services.

Sussman C, Bates-Jensen BM: *Wound care: a collaborative practice manual for healthcare professionals,* ed 3, Ambler, PA, 2006, Lippincott Williams & Wilkins.

Wound, Ostomy, and Continence Nurses Society (WOCN): *Guideline for prevention and management of pressure ulcers. WOCN clinical practice guideline series no 2,* Glenview, IL, 2003, The Society.

Wound, Ostomy, and Continence Nurses Society (WOCN): *Pressure ulcer assessment: best practice for clinicians,* Mt Laurel, NJ, 2009, The Society.

Risk for impaired Skin integrity   *Sharon Baranoski, MSN, RN, CWCN, APN, FAAN*

NANDA-I

Definition

At risk for skin being adversely altered

Risk Factors

External

Chemical substance; excretions and/or secretions; extremes of age; humidity; hyperthermia; hypothermia; mechanical factors (e.g., friction, shearing forces, pressure, restraint); moisture; physical immobilization; radiation

Internal

Alterations in skin turgor (change in elasticity); altered circulation; altered metabolic state; altered nutritional state (e.g., obesity, emaciation); altered pigmentation; altered sensation; chronic disease; developmental factors; history of pressure ulcers, immunological deficit; medication; psychogenetic, immunological factors; skeletal prominence, vascular disease

NOTE: Risk should be determined by the use of a risk assessment tool (e.g., Norton scale, Braden scale).

NOC   (Nursing Outcomes Classification)

Suggested NOC Outcomes

Immobility Consequences: Physiological, Tissue Integrity: Skin and Mucous Membranes

Example **NOC** Outcome with Indicators
Tissue Integrity: Skin and Mucous Membranes will be intact as evidenced by the following indicators: Skin intactness/Skin lesions not present/Tissue perfusion/Skin temperature (Rate the outcome and indicators of **Tissue Integrity: Skin and Mucous Membranes:** 1 = severely compromised, 2 = substantially compromised, 3 = moderately compromised, 4 = mildly compromised, 5 = not compromised [see Section I].)

Client Outcomes

Client Will (Specify Time Frame):

- Report altered sensation or pain at risk areas as soon as noted
- Demonstrate understanding of personal risk factors for impaired skin integrity
- Verbalize a personal plan for preventing impaired skin integrity

● = Independent   ▲ = Collaborative   **EBN** = Evidence-Based Nursing   **EB** = Evidence-Based

NIC   (Nursing Interventions Classification)

Suggested NIC Interventions

Positioning: Pressure Management, Pressure Ulcer Care, Pressure Ulcer Prevention, Skin Surveillance

Example NIC Activities—Pressure Ulcer Care

Monitor color of wound bed, temperature, edema, errythema, moisture, and appearance of surrounding skin; Note characteristics of any drainage

Nursing Interventions and *Rationales*

- Monitor skin condition at least once a day for color or texture changes, dermatological conditions, or lesions. Determine whether the client is experiencing loss of sensation or pain. *Systematic inspection can identify impending problems early (Krasner, Rodeheaver, & Sibbald, 2007; Baranoski & Ayello, 2008).*
- Identify clients at risk for impaired skin integrity as a result of immobility, chronological age, malnutrition, incontinence, compromised perfusion, immunocompromised status, or chronic medical condition, such as diabetes mellitus, spinal cord injury, or renal failure. **EB and EBN:** *These client populations are known to be at high risk for impaired skin integrity (McGuire, 2006; Stotts & Wipke-Tevis, 2007). Targeting variables (such as age and Braden Scale Risk Category) can focus assessment on particular risk factors (e.g., pressure) and help guide the plan of prevention and care (Magnan & Maklebust, 2009).*
- Monitor the client's skin care practices, noting type of soap or other cleansing agents used, temperature of water, and frequency of skin cleansing. *Individualize plan according to the client's skin condition, needs, and preferences (Baranoski & Ayello, 2008).*
- Avoid harsh cleansing agents, hot water, extreme friction or force, or too-frequent cleansing (Panel for the Prediction and Prevention of Pressure Ulcers in Adults, 1992).
- ▲ Monitor the client's continence status and minimize exposure of the site of skin impairment and other areas to moisture from incontinence, perspiration, or wound drainage. If the client is incontinent, implement an incontinence management plan to prevent exposure to chemicals in urine and stool that can strip or erode the skin; refer to a physician (e.g., continence care specialist, urologist, gastroenterologist) for an incontinence assessment (WOCN, 2003, 2009). **EB:** *Implementing an incontinence prevention plan with the use of a skin protectant or a cleanser protectant can significantly decrease skin breakdown and pressure ulcer formation (Fantl et al, 1996; Krasner, Rodeheaver, & Sibbald, 2007; Baranoski & Ayello, 2008).*
- For clients with limited mobility, monitor condition of skin covering bony prominences. *Pressure ulcers usually occur over bony prominences, such as the sacrum, coccyx, trochanter, and heels, as a result of unrelieved pressure between the prominence and support surface (WOCN, 2003, 2009; Sussman & Bates-Jensen, 2006; Krasner, Rodeheaver, & Sibbald, 2007; Baranoski & Ayello, 2008; Magnan & Maklebust, 2009).*
- Use a risk assessment tool to systematically assess immobility-related risk factors. *A validated risk assessment tool such as the Norton or Braden scale should be used to identify clients at risk for immobility-related skin breakdown (Ayello & Braden, 2002; Sussman & Bates-Jensen, 2006; Krasner, Rodeheaver, & Sibbald, 2007; Magnan & Maklebust, 2009; NPUAP, 2009; WOCN, 2003, 2009).*
- Implement a written prevention plan. **EB:** *A written plan ensures consistency in care and documentation (Baranoski & Ayello, 2008).* **EBN:** *Implementing a prevention protocol can significantly reduce costs and incidence of skin breakdown and pressure ulcers in the long-term care setting (CMS Manual System, 2006).*
- If consistent with overall client management goals, turn and position the client at least every 2 hours. Transfer the client with care to protect against the adverse effects of external mechanical forces (e.g., pressure, friction, shear) (WOCN, 2003, 2009).
- Evaluate for use of specialty mattresses, beds, or devices as appropriate (Fleck, 2007; Brienza et al, 2008). *If the goal of care is to keep the client (e.g., a terminally ill client) comfortable, turning and repositioning may not be appropriate. Maintain the head of the bed at the lowest possible degree of elevation to reduce shear and friction and use lift devices, pillows, foam wedges, and pressure-reducing devices in the bed (Krasner, Rodeheaver, & Sibbald, 2007; WOCN, 2003, 2009).*

● = Independent   ▲ = Collaborative   **EBN** = Evidence-Based Nursing   **EB** = Evidence-Based

- Avoid massaging over bony prominences. *Research suggests that massage may lead to deep-tissue trauma (WOCN, 2003).*
- ▲ Assess the client's nutritional status; refer for a nutritional consult, and/or institute dietary supplements. **EB:** *The benefit of nutritional evaluation and intensive nutritional support in clients at risk for or with pressure ulcers is not supported by rigorous clinical trials. Despite this lack of evidence, the National Pressure Ulcer Advisory Panel (NPUAP, 2006, 2009) endorses the application of reasonable nutritional assessment and treatment for clients at risk for and with pressure ulcers.*

 ### Geriatric

- Limit number of complete baths to two or three per week, and alternate them with partial baths. Use a tepid water temperature (between 90° and 105° F) for bathing. **EB:** *Excessive bathing, especially in hot water, depletes aging skin of moisture and increases dryness. The ability to retain moisture is decreased in aging skin due to diminished amounts of dermal proteins. One of the most common age-related changes to the skin is damage to the stratum corneum (Baranoski & Ayello, 2008).*
- Use lotions and moisturizers to prevent skin from drying out, especially in the winter (Sibbald & Cameron, 2007). *Avoid skin care products that contain allergens such as lanolin, latex, and dyes (Sibbald & Cameron, 2007).*
- Increase fluid intake within cardiac and renal limits to a minimum of 1500 mL per day. *Dry skin is caused by loss of fluid; increasing fluid intake hydrates the skin (Baranoski & Ayello, 2008).*
- Increase humidity in the environment, especially during the winter, by using a humidifier or placing a container of water on a warm object. *Increasing the moisture in the air helps keep moisture in the skin (Sibbald & Cameron, 2007).*

 ### Home Care

- Assess caregiver vigilance and ability. *In a limited study of the Braden Scale, caregiver vigilance and ability were recognized as potentially significant variables for determining the risk of developing pressure sores (Braden & Maklebust, 2005).*
- ▲ Initiate a consultation in a case assignment with a wound care specialist or wound, ostomy, and continence (WOC) nurse to establish a comprehensive plan as soon as possible.
- See the care plan for **Impaired Skin integrity**.

 ### Client/Family Teaching and Discharge Planning

- Teach the client skin assessment and ways to monitor for impending skin breakdown. *Early assessment and intervention help prevent the development of serious problems.* **EB:** *Basic elements of a skin assessment are assessment of temperature, color, moisture, turgor, and intact skin (Baranoski & Ayello, 2008).*
- If consistent with overall client management goals, teach how to turn and reposition the client at least every 2 hours. **EB:** *If the goal of care is to keep the client (e.g., a terminally ill client) comfortable, turning and repositioning may not be appropriate (Panel for the Prediction and Prevention of Pressure Ulcers in Adults, 1992). Do not position an individual directly on a pressure ulcer. Continue to turn/ reposition the individual regardless of the support surface in use. Establish turning frequency based on the characteristics of the support surface and the individual's response (NPUAP, 2009).*
- Teach the client to use pillows, foam wedges, and pressure-reducing devices to prevent pressure injury (WOCN, 2003, 2009; Krasner & Sibbald, 2007). **EB:** *The use of effective pressure-reducing seat cushions for elderly wheelchair users may significantly prevent sitting-acquired pressure ulcers (Brienza & Geyer, 2008).*

ⓔvolve See the EVOLVE website for Weblinks for client education resources.

• = Independent   ▲ = Collaborative   **EBN** = Evidence-Based Nursing   **EB** = Evidence-Based

REFERENCES

Ayello EA, Braden B: How and why to do pressure ulcer risk assessment, *Adv Skin Wound Care* 15(3):125, 2002.

Baranoski S, Ayello EA: Skin an essential organ. In Baranoski S, Ayello EA, editors: *Wound care essentials: practice principles,* ed 2, Ambler, PA, 2008, Lippincott, Williams & Wilkins.

Braden B, Maklebust J: Wound wise: preventing pressure ulcers with the Braden scale, *Am J Nurs* 105(6):70–72, 2005.

Brienza DM, Geyer MJ, Springle S et al: Pressure redistribution: seating, positioning, and support surfaces. In Baranoski S, Ayello EA, editors: *Wound care essentials: practice principles,* ed 2, Ambler, PA, 2008, Lippincott, Williams & Wilkins.

CMS Manual System: *Appendix PP, Tag F314. Guidance to surveyors for long term care facilities,* Baltimore, 2004, Department of Health and Human Services.

Fantl JA et al: *Urinary incontinence in adults: acute and chronic management,* Clinical Practice Guideline No. 2, 1996 Update, Agency for Health Care Policy and Research, Pub No 96, Rockville, MD, 1996, Public Health Service, U.S. Department of Health and Human Services.

Fleck C: Support surfaces: criteria and selection. In Krasner D, Rodeheaver G, Sibbald RG, editors: *Chronic wound care: a clinical source book for healthcare professionals,* ed 4, Malvern, PA, 2007, HMP Communications.

Krasner D, Rodeheaver G, Sibbald RG: Advanced wound caring for a new millennium. In Krasner D, Rodeheaver G, Sibbald RG, editors: *Chronic wound care: a clinical source book for healthcare professionals,* ed 4, Malvern, PA, 2007, HMP Communications.

Magnan MA, Maklebust J: The nursing process and pressure ulcer prevention: making the connection, *Adv Skin Wound Care* 22(2):83–91, 2009.

McGuire JB: Pressure redistribution strategies for the diabetic or at-risk foot part 1, *Adv Skin Wound Care* 19(5):270–277, 2006.

National Pressure Ulcer Advisory Panel (NPUAP): What is the role of nutritional support for patients in the prevention and treatment of pressure ulcers? Frequently asked questions, 2006, www.npuap.org/faq.htm. Accessed April 8, 2009.

National Pressure Ulcer Advisory Panel (NPUAP): *The new international guideline consensus on implementation, 11th Annual Biennial Conference,* Washington, DC, 2009, NPUAP.

Panel for the Prediction and Prevention of Pressure Ulcers in Adults: *Pressure ulcers in adults: prediction and prevention,* Clinical Practice Guideline No. 3, Agency for Health Care Policy and Research, Pub No 92, Rockville, MD, 1992, Public Health Service, U.S. Department of Health and Human Services.

Sibbald RG, Cameron J: Dermatological aspects of wound care. In Krasner D, Rodeheaver G, Sibbald RG, editors: *Chronic wound care: a clinical source book for healthcare professionals,* ed 4, Malvern, PA, 2007, HMP Communications.

Stotts NA, Wipke-Tevis D: Co-factors in impaired wound healing. In Krasner D, Rodeheaver G, Sibbald RG, editors: *Chronic wound care: a clinical source book for healthcare professionals,* ed 4, Malvern, PA, 2007, HMP Communications.

Sussman C, Bates-Jensen BM: *Wound care: a collaborative practice manual for healthcare professionals,* ed 3, Ambler, PA, 2006, Lippincott Williams and Wilkins.

Wound, Ostomy, and Continence Nurses Society (WOCN): *Guideline for prevention and management of pressure ulcers. WOCN clinical practice guideline series no 2,* Glenview, IL, 2003, The Society.

Wound, Ostomy, and Continence Nurses Society (WOCN): Pressure ulcer assessment: best practice for clinicians, Mt Laurel, NJ, 2009, The Society.

Sleep deprivation

 evolve

Judith A. Floyd, PhD, RN, FAAN, Jean D. Humphries, PhD(c), RN, and Elizabeth S. Jenuwine, PhD, MLIS

NANDA-I

Definition

Prolonged periods without sleep (sustained natural, periodic suspension of relative consciousness)

Defining Characteristics

Acute confusion; agitation; anxiety; apathy; combativeness; daytime drowsiness; decreased ability to function; fatigue; fleeting nystagmus; hallucinations; hand tremors; heightened sensitivity to pain; inability to concentrate; irritability; lethargy; listlessness; malaise; perceptual disorders (i.e., disturbed body sensation, delusions, feeling afloat); restlessness; slowed reaction; transient paranoia

Related Factors (r/t)

Aging-related sleep stage shifts; dementia; familial sleep paralysis; inadequate daytime activity; idiopathic central nervous system hypersomnolence; narcolepsy; nightmares; non–sleep-inducing parenting practices; periodic limb movement (e.g., restless leg syndrome, nocturnal myoclonus); prolonged discomfort (e.g., physical, psychological); sustained inadequate sleep hygiene; prolonged use of pharmacologic or dietary antisoporifics; sleep apnea; sleep terror; sleep walking; sleep-related enuresis; sleep-related painful erections; sundowner's syndrome; sustained circadian asynchrony; sustained environmental stimulation; sustained uncomfortable sleep environment

---

• = Independent   ▲ = Collaborative   **EBN** = Evidence-Based Nursing   **EB** = Evidence-Based

(Nursing Outcomes Classification)

Suggested NOC Outcomes

Rest, Sleep, Symptom Severity

Example NOC Outcome with Indicators
Sleep as evidenced by the following indicators: Hours of sleep/Sleep pattern/Sleep quality/Sleep efficiency/Feels rejuvenated after sleep/Sleeps through the night consistently (Rate the outcome and indicators of **Sleep:** 1 = severely compromised, 2 = substantially compromised, 3 = moderately compromised, 4 = mildly compromised, 5 = not compromised [see Section I].)

Client Outcomes

Client Will (Specify Time Frame):

- Wake up less frequently during night
- Awaken refreshed and be less fatigued during day
- Fall asleep without difficulty
- Verbalize plan that provides adequate time for sleep
- Identify actions that can be taken to improve quality of sleep

 (Nursing Interventions Classification)

Suggested NIC Intervention

Sleep Enhancement

Example NIC Activities—Sleep Enhancement
Monitor/record patient's sleep pattern and number of sleep hours; Encourage patient to establish a bedtime routine to facilitate transition from wakefulness to sleep

Nursing Interventions and *Rationales*

- Obtain a sleep history including bedtime routines, sleep patterns, use of medications and stimulants, use of complementary/alternative medical practices, responsibilities that limit sleep time, and daytime sequelae suggestive of sleep deprivation (e.g., drowsiness, inability to concentrate, slowed reactions). *Assessment of sleep–wake behavior and patterns is an important part of any health status examination (Lee & Ward, 2005; Mastin, Bryson, & Corwyn, 2006; Humphries, 2008).*
- From the history, assess factors leading to sleep deprivation. *Factors that most frequently limit sleep time for outpatients are work demands (including extended work hours and shift work), social activities, and domestic responsibilities (including child care and other family caregiving); for inpatients the most frequent causes of sleep loss are medical condition, their treatment, and environmental stimuli in the treatment setting (Baynard, Dinges, & Rogers, 2005; Fang & Wang, 2007; Humphries, 2008).*
- ▲ Assess for underlying physiological illnesses causing sleep loss (e.g., cardiovascular, pulmonary, gastrointestinal, hyperthyroidism, nocturia occurring with benign hypertrophic prostatitis or pain). *Symptomatology of disease states can cause insomnia (Sateia, 2009).*
- ▲ Assess for underlying psychiatric illnesses causing sleep loss (e.g., bipolar depression, anxiety disorders, schizophrenia). *Symptomatology of disease states can cause insomnia (Sateia, 2009).*
- ▲ Monitor for presence of nocturnal symptoms of restless leg syndrome with uncomfortable restless sensations in legs that occur before sleep onset or during the night. In addition, monitor for nocturnal panic attacks, and sleep-disordered breathing. Refer for treatment as appropriate. *Numerous nocturnal events and symptoms can contribute to sleep loss (Sateia, 2009).*
- Assess for chronic insomnia. *Chronic insomnia leads to sleep deprivation (Dement et al, 2005).* See the care plan for **Insomnia.**
- Minimize factors that disturb the client's sleep. Consolidate care. See **Disturbed Sleep pattern.**
- Keep the sleep environment quiet (e.g., avoid use of intercoms, lower the volume on radio and television, keep beepers on nonaudio mode, anticipate alarms on intravenous (IV) pumps, talk

• = Independent   ▲ = Collaborative   **EBN** = Evidence-Based Nursing   **EB** = Evidence-Based

quietly on unit). *Attention to environmental sources of noise can eliminate or markedly reduce noise (Floyd, 2002; Humphries, 2008).* **EBN:** *Effective sleep promotion protocols have been developed for minimizing sleep deprivation in intensive care settings (Patel et al, 2008).*

- Mask noise in sleep area if noise cannot be eliminated. See **Readiness for enhanced Sleep**.
- Encourage napping as a way to compensate for sleep deprivation when severely restricted sleep cannot be avoided. Set a regular schedule for napping. *Regular sleep schedules that include strategically placed nap periods can supplement total amounts of sleep obtained per circadian period (Dement, Dinges, & Walsh, 2005).*
- Monitor caffeine intake. *Sleep-deprived persons often use stimulants to overcome negative effects of sleep deprivation; caffeine may be helpful in the temporary management of sleepiness, but over-use and late-day use can contribute to subsequent sleep disruption (Roehrs & Roth, 2008).*

Geriatric

- Interventions identified above may be adapted for use with geriatric clients.
- See the Geriatric section of **Disturbed Sleep pattern**.

Home Care

- Interventions identified above may be adapted for home care use.
- See the Home Care section of **Disturbed Sleep pattern**.

Client/Family Teaching and Discharge Planning

- Teach family about the short-term and long-term consequences of inadequate amounts of sleep. *Insufficient sleep is associated with poor attention, decreased performance, increases in mortality and morbidity, and with cardiovascular risk factors including hypertension, insulin resistance, hormonal deregulation, and inflammation (Mullington et al, 2009).*
- Promote adoption of behaviors that assure adequate amounts of sleep for all family members. See **Readiness for enhanced Sleep**.
- Teach family about signs of sleep deprivation and how to avoid chronic sleep loss. See **Disturbed Sleep pattern**.
- Advise against the sleep deprived person's chronic use of stimulants (e.g., caffeine) to overcome daytime sequelae of sleep deprivation; focus on elimination of factors that lead to chronic sleep loss. *Caffeine may be helpful in the temporary management of sleepiness, but over-use and late-day use can contribute to subsequent sleep disruption and caffeine habituation (Roehrs & Roth, 2008).*

℮volve   See the EVOLVE website for Weblinks for client education resources.

REFERENCES

Baynard MD, Dinges DF, Rogers NL: Chronic sleep deprivation. In Kryger MH, Roth T, & Dement WC, editors: *Principles and practice of sleep medicine,* ed 4, Philadelphia, 2005, Elsevier.

Dement WC, Dinges DF, Walsh JK: Sleep medicine, public policy, and public health. In Kryger MH, Roth T, & Dement WC, editors: *Principles and practice of sleep medicine,* ed 4, Philadelphia, 2005, Elsevier.

Fang C, Wang R: Sleep quality and its associated factors among surgical intensive care unit patients, *J Evid Based Nurs* 3(1):63, 2007.

Floyd JA: Sleep and aging, *Nurs Clin North Am* 37:719, 2002.

Humphries JD: Sleep disruption in hospitalized adults, *Medsurg Nurs* 17(6):391, 2008.

Lee KA, Ward TM: Critical components of a sleep assessment for clinical practice, *Issues Ment Health Nurs* 26:739, 2005.

Mastin DF, Bryson J, Corwyn R: Assessment of sleep hygiene using the Sleep Hygiene Index, *J Behav Med* 29(3):223–227, 2006.

Mullington JM, Haack M, Toth M et al: Cardiovascular, inflammatory, and metabolic consequences of sleep deprivation, *Prog Cardiovasc Dis* 51(4):294–302, 2009.

Patel M, Chipman J, Carlin BW et al: Sleep in the intensive care unit setting, *Crit Care Nurs Q* 31(4):309–318, 2008.

Roehrs T, Roth T: Caffeine: sleep and daytime sleepiness, *Sleep Med Rev* 12(2):153, 2008.

Sateia MJ: Update on sleep and psychiatric disorders, *Chest* 135(5):1370, 2009.

Readiness for enhanced Sleep

Judith A. Floyd, PhD, RN, FAAN, Jean D. Humphries, PhD(c), RN, and Elizabeth S. Jenuwine, PhD, MLIS

Definition

A pattern of natural, periodic suspension of consciousness that provides adequate rest, sustains a desired lifestyle, and can be strengthened

Defining Characteristics

Expresses willingness to enhance sleep and interest in obtaining amount of sleep congruent with developmental needs; expresses a feeling of being rested after sleep; follows sleep routines that promote sleep habits; use of medications to induce sleep is infrequent (i.e., only occasional)

Related Factors (r/t)

Desire to improve sleep

 NOC   (Nursing Outcomes Classification)

Suggested NOC Outcomes

Personal Well-Being, Rest, Sleep

Example NOC Outcome with Indicators
Sleep as evidenced by the following indicators: Hours of sleep/Sleep pattern/Sleep quality/Sleep efficiency/Feels rejuvenated after sleep/Napping appropriate for age (Rate each indicator of **Sleep:** 1 = severely compromised, 2 = substantially compromised, 3 = moderately compromised, 4 = mildly compromised, 5 = not compromised [see Section I].)

Client Outcomes

Client Will (Specify Time Frame):

- Awaken naturally, feeling refreshed and is not fatigued during day
- Fall asleep without difficulty
- Verbalize plan to implement sleep promotion routines

NIC   (Nursing Interventions Classification)

Suggested NIC Intervention

Sleep Enhancement

Example NIC Activities—Sleep Enhancement
Assess patient's sleep/activity pattern; Assist/encourage patient to create an environment that facilitates sleep; Assist/encourage patient to adopt personal practices that enhance sleep

Nursing Interventions and *Rationales*

- Obtain a sleep history including bedtime routines, sleep patterns, use of medications and stimulants, and use of complementary/alternative medical practices. *Assessment of sleep behavior and patterns is an important part of any health status examination (Lee & Ward, 2005; Mastin, Bryson, & Corwyn, 2006; Humphries, 2008).*
- From the history assess the client's ability to initiate and maintain sleep, obtain adequate amounts of sleep, and manage daytime responsibilities free from fatigue and sleepiness. *Most adults who are satisfied with nighttime sleep average 7.5 hours of sleep per night (range of 6 to 9 hours), fall asleep within 20 minutes initially and more quickly if awakened during the night; daytime is characterized by no naps or regularly scheduled brief naps, and little fatigue or sleepiness (Floyd, 2002).* **EBN:** *Sleep patterns over the life span differ for men and women (Floyd, 2002). Cultural beliefs can influence sleep*

• = Independent   ▲ = Collaborative   **EBN** = Evidence-Based Nursing   **EB** = Evidence-Based

patterns and sleep preferences (Sok, 2008). **EB:** *Cigarette smokers take longer to fall asleep and have shorter and lighter nighttime sleep than nonsmokers; however, acute nicotine withdrawal causes even more sleep disruption (Zhang et al, 2006).* **EB:** *Difficulty sleeping can be a side effect of medications such as bronchodilators (Benca, 2005).*

- Based on assessment teach one or more of the listed sleep promotion practices as appropriate. **EBN:** *In adult acute-care settings, improved sleep quality and less use of sleeping medication has been reported when multicomponent sleep promotion protocols were tested (Robinson, Weitzel, & Henderson, 2005; Lareau et al, 2008).* **EBN:** *Breast cancer survivors reported improved sleep following teaching of a multicomponent sleep promotion program (Epstein & Dirksen, 2007).* **EBN:** *General medical practice clients with longstanding sleep complaints improved with short-term cognitive and behavioral counseling provided by sleep nurses (Espie et al, 2007).* **EB:** *Multicomponent psychoeducational programs that incorporated elements of sleep promotion listed below have been shown to effectively improve sleep in both men and women with sleep complaints (Benca, 2005).*

  - Establish a regular schedule for sleep, exercise, napping, and mealtimes. *Regular schedules are believed to promote sleep initiation and sleep maintenance by maintaining a circadian rhythm of alertness/drowsiness (Stepanski & Wyatt, 2003).*
  - Avoid long periods of daytime sleep. **EB:** *While regular, short napping in the morning or early afternoon improved mood and performance in older adults, long periods of sleep during the day appeared to replace nighttime sleep (Campbell, Murphy, & Stauble, 2005).*
  - Arise at the same time each day even if sleep was poor during the previous night. *Although many factors can interfere with falling and staying asleep, forcing a regular arise-time helps establish a circadian rhythm and assure better sleep the following night (Stepanski & Wyatt, 2003).*
  - If not contraindicated, have a high-glycemic-index carbohydrate dinner and/or bedtime snack. **EB:** *High-glycemic-index carbohydrate meals shortened sleep onset in adults (Afaghi, O'Connor, & Chow, 2007).*
  - Limit caffeine. *Caffeine is one of the most widely consumed psychoactive substances and it has profound effects on sleep-wake function; there are several hidden sources of caffeine such as over-the-counter medications, soft drinks, and chocolate (Roehrs & Roth, 2008).* **EBN:** *Caffeine abstinence improves sleep quality (Sin, Ho, & Chung, 2009).*
  - Limit alcohol use. **EB:** *Limited alcohol use (1 to 2 drinks) shortened time needed to fall asleep and increased depth of sleep the first 2 hours, but also suppressed REM sleep, which sometimes lead to REM-rebound, i.e., lighter more fragmented sleep later in the night (Feige et al, 2006; Van Reen et al, 2006).*
  - Avoid long-term use of sleeping pills. *Long-term use of sleeping pills is habit forming, and typically dependence and withdrawal symptoms occur while the therapeutic effect diminishes over time (Lemmer, 2007).*
  - Engage in relaxing activities before bed. *Several systematic reviews show that all forms of relaxation improve quantity and quality of sleep (Floyd, 2002).*

- Provide backrub or other forms of massage. **EBN:** *Use of a back massage has been shown effective for promoting relaxation, which likely leads to improved sleep (Richards et al, 2003).*
- Teach relaxation techniques. **EBN:** *A systematic review shows both cognitive and behavioral relaxation techniques have shortened time to fall asleep (Wang, Wang, & Tsai, 2005).*
- Teach complementary and alternative medicine practices as culturally congruent. *There is a growing body of research using complementary and alternative medicine that shows modalities such as tai chi, acupuncture, acupressure, yoga, and meditation have improved sleep in clinical populations (Richards et al, 2003; Carlson & Garland, 2005; Gooneratne, 2008).*
- Lower lighting in sleep area. **EB:** *Light affects hormonal secretions related to circadian rhythms of sleepiness (Bjorvatn & Pallesen, 2009).* **EBN:** *Exposure to light at night has been found to be greater in residential care settings than home settings (Chaperon, Farr, & LoChiano, 2007).*
- Mask noise in sleep area if it cannot be eliminated. **EB:** *Listening to music resulted in better sleep quality, longer sleep duration, greater sleep efficiency, shorter sleep latency, less sleep disturbance, and less daytime dysfunction (Lai & Good, 2005).* **EB:** *"White noise" (i.e., sounds covering the entire range of human hearing, e.g., ocean sounds) decreased time needed to fall asleep and nighttime awakenings in young adults (Forquer & Johnson, 2007).*

Geriatric

- Interventions discussed above may be adapted for use with geriatric clients.
- Counsel the older adult regarding normal age-related changes in sleep: **EBN:** *As people age, increased time is needed to fall asleep; frequency of waking after sleep onset increases; length of waking after sleep onset increases (which may be related to unrecognized disease/disorder); and nighttime sleep amount tends to decrease (Floyd, 2002; Cole & Richards, 2007).*
- Elicit the older adult's expectations for sleep; correct misconceptions. *The elderly person may be unduly concerned by normal age-related changes in sleep patterns, i.e., lighter sleep and occasional awakenings may be misconstrued as sleep disorders (Floyd, 2002).*
- ▲ Assess and refer as appropriate if co-existing conditions may be disrupting sleep. **EBN:** *Depression, sleep apnea, and restless leg syndrome are commonly missed co-existing conditions in the elderly (Floyd 2002; Cole & Richards, 2007; Cuellar, Strumpf, & Ratcliffe, 2007).*
- Decrease fluid intake in the evening and use diuretics early in the day unless contraindicated. *Many elderly people awaken to void during the night; increasing water intake at night or taking diuretics late in the day increases nocturia, which results in disrupted sleep (Avidan, 2005).*
- Encourage physical activities. Encourage walking unless contraindicated. Help elderly clients get outside for increased light exposure and to enjoy nature. *Exposure to natural light and social interactions influence the circadian rhythms that control sleep (Bjorvatn & Pallesen, 2009).*
- Encourage social activities. Encourage participation in group activities unless contraindicated. Help elderly clients engage with others who enjoy similar events. *Social interactions influence the circadian rhythms that control sleep (Bjorvatn & Pallesen, 2009).*

 Home Care

- The interventions discussed above may be adapted for home care use.
- Some complementary and alternative medicine interventions may be more easily tried at home than in health care facilities. **EB:** *Two studies have found the scent of lavender improved sleep (Goel, Kim, & Lao, 2005; Lewith, Godfrey, & Prescott, 2005).*
- Assess the conduciveness of the home environment for both family caregivers and care recipient's sleep. *Many factors in the home environment can promote or interfere with the sleep readiness of clients/family members (Floyd, 2002).* **EBN:** *Multicomponent sleep promotion programs improve sleep quality in family caregivers of persons with cancer (Carter, 2006).* **EB:** *New medium-firm bedding systems have been found to reduce pain and stiffness and improve sleep quality (Jacobson et al, 2008).*

Ɵvolve   See the EVOLVE website for Weblinks for client education resources.

REFERENCES

Afaghi A, O'Connor H, Chow CM: High-glycemic-index carbohydrate meals shorten sleep onset, *Am J Clin Nutr* 85(2):426–430, 2007.

Avidan AY: Sleep in the geriatric patient population, *Semin Neurol* 25(1):52, 2005.

Benca RM: Diagnosis and treatment of chronic insomnia: review, *Psychiatr Serv* 56(3):334, 2005.

Bjorvatn B, Pallesen S: A practical approach to circadian rhythm sleep disorders, *Sleep Med Rev* 13(1):47, 2009.

Campbell SS, Murphy PJ, Stauble TN: Effects of a nap on nighttime sleep and waking function in older subjects, *J Am Geriatr Soc* 53(1):48, 2005.

Carlson LE, Garland SN: Impact of mindfulness-based stress reduction (MBSR) on sleep, mood, stress and fatigue symptoms in cancer outpatients, *Int J Behav Med* 12(4):278, 2005.

Carter PA: A brief behavioral sleep intervention for family caregivers of persons with cancer, *Cancer Nurs*, 29(2):95–103, 2006.

Chaperon CM, Farr LA, LoChiano E: Sleep disturbance of residents in a continuing care retirement community, *J Gerontol Nurs* 33(10):21, 2007.

Cole C, Richards K: Sleep disruption in older adults. Harmful and by no means inevitable, it should be assessed and treated, *Am J Nurs* 107(5):40, 2007.

Cuellar NG, Strumpf NE, Ratcliffe SJ: Symptoms of restless legs syndrome in older adults: outcomes on sleep quality, sleepiness, fatigue, depression, and quality of life, *J Am Geriatr Soc* 55(9):1387, 2007.

Epstein DR, Dirksen SR: Randomized trial of a cognitive-behavioral intervention for insomnia in breast cancer survivors, *Oncol Nurs Forum* 34(5):E51, 2007.

Espie CA, MacMahon KM, Kelly HL et al: Randomized clinical effectiveness trial of nurse-administered small-group cognitive behavioral therapy for persistent insomnia in general practice, *Sleep* 30(5):574–584, 2007.

Feige B, Gann H, Brueck R et al: Effects of alcohol on polysomnographically recorded sleep in health subjects, *Alcohol Clin Exp Res* 30(9):1527–1537, 2006.

Floyd JA: Sleep and aging, *Nurs Clin North Am* 37:719, 2002.

Forquer LM, Johnson CM: Continuous white noise to reduce sleep latency and night wakings in college students, *Sleep Hypnosis* 9(2):60, 2007.

● = Independent   ▲ = Collaborative   **EBN** = Evidence-Based Nursing   **EB** = Evidence-Based

Goel N, Kim H, Lao RP: An olfactory stimulus modifies nighttime sleep in young men and women, *Chronobiol Int* 22(5):889, 2005.

Gooneratne NS: Complementary and alternative medicine for sleep disturbances in older adults, *Clin Geriatr Med* 24(1):121, 2008.

Humphries JD: Sleep disruption in hospitalized adults, *Medsurg Nurs* 17(6):391, 2008.

Jacobson BH, Wallace TJ, Smith DB et al: Grouped comparisons of sleep quality for new and personal bedding systems. *Appl Ergon* 29(2):247–254, 2008.

Lai HL, Good M: Music improves sleep quality in older adults, *J Adv Nurs* 49(3):234, 2005.

Lareau R, Benson L, Watcharotone K et al: Examining the feasibility of implementing specific nursing interventions to promote sleep in hospitalized elderly patients, *Geriatr Nurs* 29(3):197–206, 2008.

Lee KA, Ward TM: Critical components of a sleep assessment for clinical practice, *Issues Ment Health Nurs* 26:739, 2005.

Lemmer B: The sleep-wake cycle and sleep pills, *Physiol Behav* 90 (2–3):285, 2007.

Lewith GT, Godfrey AD, Prescott P: A single-blinded, randomized pilot study evaluating the aroma of Lavandula augustifolia as a treatment for mild insomnia, *J Altern Complement Med* 11(4):631–637, 2005.

Mastin DF, Bryson J, Corwyn R: Assessment of sleep hygiene using the Sleep Hygiene Index, *J Behav Med* 29(3): 223–227, 2006.

Richards K, Nagel C, Markie M et al: Use of complementary and alternative therapies to promote sleep in critical ill patients, *Crit Care Nurs Clin North Am* 15(3):329–340, 2003.

Robinson, Weitzel T, Henderson L: The Sh-h-h-h Project: nonpharmacological interventions, *Holist Nurs Pract* 19(6):263, 2005.

Roehrs T, Roth T: Caffeine: sleep and daytime sleepiness, *Sleep Med Rev* 12(2):153, 2008.

Sin CW, Ho JS, Chung JW: Systematic review on the effectiveness of caffeine abstinence on the quality of sleep, *J Clin Nurs* 18(1):13–21, 2009.

Sok SR: Sleep patterns and insomnia management in Korean-American older adult immigrants, *J Clin Nurs* 17(1):135, 2008.

Stepanski E, Wyatt J: Use of sleep hygiene in the treatment of insomnia, *Sleep Med Rev* 7(3):215, 2003.

Van Reen E, Jenni OG, Carskadon MA et al: Effects of alcohol on sleep and the sleep electroencephalogram in health young women, *Alcohol Clin Exp Res* 30(6):974–981, 2006.

Wang MY, Wang SY, Tsai PS: Cognitive behavioural therapy for primary insomnia: a systematic review, *J Adv Nurs* 50(5):553–564, 2005.

Zhang L, Samet J, Caffo B et al: Cigarette smoking and nocturnal sleep architecture, *Am J Epidem* 164(6):529, 2006.

Disturbed Sleep pattern

Judith A. Floyd, PhD, RN, FAAN, Jean D. Humphries, PhD(c), RN, and Elizabeth S. Jenuwine, PhD, MLIS

Definition

Time-limited interruptions of sleep amount and quality due to external factors

Defining Characteristics

Change in normal sleep pattern, verbal complains of not feeling well rested, dissatisfaction with sleep, decreased ability to function, reports being awakened, reports no difficulty falling asleep

Related Factors (r/t)

Ambient temperature, humidity, caregiving responsibilities, change in daylight-darkness exposure, interruptions (e.g., for therapeutics, monitoring, lab tests), lack of sleep privacy/control, lighting, noise, noxious odors, physical restraint, sleep partner, unfamiliar sleep furnishings.

 (Nursing Outcomes Classification)

Suggested NOC Outcomes

Personal Well-Being, Rest, Sleep

Example NOC Outcome with Indicators
Sleep as evidenced by the following indicators: Hours of sleep/Sleep pattern/Sleep quality/Sleep efficiency/Feels rejuvenated after sleep (Rate the outcome and indicators of **Sleep:** 1 = severely compromised, 2 = substantially compromised, 3 = moderately compromised, 4 = mildly compromised, 5 = not compromised [see Section I].)

Client Outcomes

Client Will (Specify Time Frame):

- Awaken naturally, feeling refreshed and is not fatigued during day
- Fall asleep without difficulty
- Verbalize plan to implement sleep promotion routines

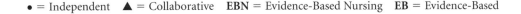

• = Independent ▲ = Collaborative **EBN** = Evidence-Based Nursing **EB** = Evidence-Based

NIC (Nursing Interventions Classification)

Suggested NIC Intervention

Sleep Enhancement

Example NIC Activities—Sleep Enhancement
Determine patient's sleep/activity pattern; Encourage patient to establish a bedtime routine to facilitate transition from wakefulness to sleep

Nursing Interventions and *Rationales*

- Obtain a sleep history including bedtime routines, noise and light levels in the sleep environment, and activities occurring in the sleep environment during hours of sleep. *Assessment of sleep–wake behavior and patterns is an important part of any health status examination (Lee & Ward, 2005; Mastin, Bryson, & Corwyn, 2006; Humphries, 2008).*
- Assess whether the client has an opportunity for adequate sleep. *During a normal night of sleep, sleepers cycle from light sleep to deep sleep to dream (i.e., REM) sleep several times. Cycles take approximately 90 to 110 minutes each. The deepest sleep is obtained during the first 2 to 3 cycles or the first 3 to 4 hours of sleep. The amount of REM sleep obtained per cycle increases over the night. Both deep sleep and REM sleep are needed for the sleeper to have adequate sleep and feel refreshed upon awakening. To obtain adequate deep sleep, the sleeper requires 3 to 4 hours of uninterrupted sleep at the beginning of the sleep period; to obtain adequate REM sleep the sleeper needs additional 90–minute blocks of sleep the second half of the night (Carskadon & Dement, 2005).*
- Assess environmental factors that interrupt sleep. *Environmental factors that most frequently interrupt sleep in all settings are related to either: (a) the physical sleep environment and/or (b) activities of others in the sleep environment (Floyd, 2002; Baynard, Dinges, & Rogers, 2005; Fang & Wang, 2007; Humphries, 2008).*
- Keep environment quiet, room lighting dim, and bedding supportive of comfortable body alignment. See Nursing Interventions and Rationales for **Readiness for enhanced Sleep**.
- Offer earplugs and eye masks if possible. **EBN:** *Although not all clients found these aids comfortable to use, and earplugs did not block all noise, some clients in critical care reported these aids improved their sleep quality (Richardson et al, 2007).*
- Establish a sleeping and waking routine with regular times for sleeping and waking including routines for preparing for sleep. See **Readiness for enhanced Sleep**.
- For hospitalized stable clients, consider instituting the following sleep protocol to a regular sleep-wake routine:
  - Night shift: Give the client the opportunity for uninterrupted sleep the first 3 to 4 hours of the sleep period. Keep environmental noise to a minimum. After major sleep period, allow 80 to 90 minutes between interruptions. (If the client must be disturbed the first 3 to 4 hours, attempt to protect 90 to 110 minute blocks of time in between awakenings.)
  - Day shift: Encourage short morning and/or after-lunch naps as needed. Promote a physical activity regimen as appropriate. Schedule newly ordered medications to avoid the need to wake the client the first few hours of the night.
  - Evening shift: Limit napping. Encourage a suitable bedtime routine. At sleep time, lower intensity of room and unit lights and keep noise and conversation on the unit to a minimum.

  Several researchers have found that the high frequency of nocturnal care interaction allows clients few uninterrupted periods for sleep that are long enough for them to complete even one 90 to 110 minute sleep cycle (Tamburri, DiBrienza, & Zozula, 2004; Lee, Low, & Twinn, 2005; Missildine, 2008). **EBN:** *Hospital clients slept worse than matched healthy community controls (Dogan, Ertekin, & Dogan, 2005).* **EBN:** *Surgical ICU clients had markedly abnormal sleep patterns with significant reductions in both deep restorative sleep and REM sleep (Friese et al, 2007).* **EBN:** *An acute-care setting had elevated light and sound levels; clients trying to sleep in the setting had markedly impaired sleep including total sleep amounts averaging less than 4 hours and frequent awakenings during the night averaging less than 30 minutes between awakenings (Missildine, 2008).*

● = Independent   ▲ = Collaborative   **EBN** = Evidence-Based Nursing   **EB** = Evidence-Based

Geriatric

- Interventions identified above are suitable for use with geriatric clients.
- See the Geriatric section of **Readiness for enhanced Sleep**.

Home Care

- Interventions identified above may be adapted for home care use.
- See the Home Care section of **Readiness for enhanced Sleep**.

Client/Family Teaching and Discharge Planning

- Teach family about sleep and the importance of uninterrupted sleep as described above.
- Teach family about signs of sleep deprivation, which may result from several environmental factors.
- See care plan for **Sleep deprivation**.

 See the EVOLVE website for Weblinks for client education resources.

REFERENCES

Baynard MD, Dinges DF, Rogers NL: Chronic sleep deprivation. In Kryger MH, Roth T, & Dement WC, editors: *Principles and practice of sleep medicine,* ed 4, Philadelphia, 2005, Elsevier.

Carskadon MA, Dement WC: Normal human sleep: an overview. In Kryger MH, Roth T, & Dement WC, editors: *Principles and practice of sleep medicine,* ed 4, Philadelphia, 2005, Elsevier.

Dogan O, Ertekin S, Dogan S: Sleep quality in hospitalized patients, *J Clin Nurs* 14(11):107, 2005.

Fang C, Wang R: Sleep quality and its associated factors among surgical intensive care unit patients, *J Evid Based Nurs* 3(1):63, 2007.

Floyd JA: Sleep and aging, *Nurs Clin North Am* 37:719, 2002.

Friese RS, Diaz-Arrastia R, McBride D et al: Quantity and quality of sleep in the surgical intensive care unit: are our patients sleeping? *J Trauma* 63(6):1210, 2007.

Humphries JD: Sleep disruption in hospitalized adults, *Medsurg Nurs* 17(6):391, 2008.

Lee CY, Low LP, Twinn S: Understanding the sleep needs of older hospitalized patients: a review of the literature, *Contemp Nurse* 20(2):212, 2005.

Lee KA, Ward TM: Critical components of a sleep assessment for clinical practice, *Issues Ment Health Nurs* 26:739, 2005.

Mastin DF, Bryson J, Corwyn R: Assessment of sleep hygiene using the Sleep Hygiene Index, *J Behav Med* 29(3):223–227, 2006.

Missildine K: Sleep and the sleep environment of older adults in acute care settings, *J Gerontol Nurs* 34(6):15, 2008.

Richardson A, Allsop M, Coghill E et al: Earplugs and eye masks: do they improve critical care patients' sleep? *Nurs Crit Care* 12(6):278–286, 2007.

Tamburri LM, DiBrienza R, Zozula R et al: Nocturnal care interactions with patients in critical care units, *Am J Crit Care* 13(2):102, 2004.

Impaired Social interaction   *Gail B. Ladwig, MSN, RN, CHTP*

NANDA-I

Definition

Insufficient or excessive quantity or ineffective quality of social exchange

Defining Characteristics

Discomfort in social situations; dysfunctional interaction with others; family report of changes in interaction (e.g., style, pattern); inability to communicate a satisfying sense of social engagement (e.g., belonging, caring, interest, or shared history); inability to receive a satisfying sense of social engagement (e.g., belonging, caring, interest, or shared history); use of unsuccessful social interaction behaviors

Related Factors (r/t)

Absence of significant others; communication barriers; deficit about ways to enhance mutuality (e.g., knowledge, skills); disturbed thought processes; environmental barriers; limited physical mobility; self-concept disturbance; sociocultural dissonance; therapeutic isolation

• = Independent   ▲ = Collaborative   **EBN** = Evidence-Based Nursing   **EB** = Evidence-Based

NOC (Nursing Outcomes Classification)

Suggested NOC Outcomes

Child Development: Middle Childhood, Adolescence, Play Participation, Role Performance, Social Interaction Skills, Social Involvement

Example NOC Outcome with Indicators
Social Involvement as evidenced by the following indicator: Interacts with close friends, neighbors, family members, and members of work groups (Rate the outcome and indicators of **Social Involvement:** I = never demonstrated, 2 = rarely demonstrated, 3 = sometimes demonstrated, 4 = often demonstrated, 5 = consistently demonstrated [see Section I].)

Client Outcomes

Client Will (Specify Time Frame):

- Identify barriers that cause impaired social interactions
- Discuss feelings that accompany impaired and successful social interactions
- Use available opportunities to practice interactions
- Use successful social interaction behaviors
- Report increased comfort in social situations
- Communicate, state feelings of belonging, demonstrate caring and interest in others
- Report effective interactions with others

NIC (Nursing Interventions Classification)

Suggested NIC Intervention

Socialization Enhancement

Example NIC Activities—Socialization Enhancement
Encourage patience in developing relationships; Help patient increase awareness of strengths and limitations in communicating with others

Nursing Interventions and *Rationales*

- Consider using a self-rating scale to assess social functioning. *Social functioning is an important dimension to assess.* **EB:** *This scale seems to be a valuable instrument for the monitoring of social functioning in psychiatric clients. It sets up the expectation of change and allows reality testing of clients' and therapists' beliefs about the presence of progress or not and to identify if therapy is working on this specific outcome domain (Zanello et al, 2006).*
- Monitor the client's use of defense mechanisms, and support healthy defenses (e.g., the client focuses on present and avoids placing blame on others for personal behavior). **EBN:** *Solution-focused techniques have been demonstrated to be beneficial. Therapy focuses on client's present and future, capitalizing on the strengths and resources of the client and significant others around them (Bowles, 2002; University of Central Lancashire: Department of Nursing, 2003).*
- Spend time with the client. **EBN:** *Being truly present was listed as one behavior that demonstrated caring (Yonge & Molzahn, 2002; Melnechenko, 2003).*
- Use active listening skills, including assessment and clarification of the client's verbal and nonverbal responses and interactions. **EBN:** *The best practice with regard to communication in palliative care could be achieved by using a sensitive assessment of how each client chooses to cope with his or her situation rather than by adopting a uniform approach to care (Dean, 2002; Lunney, 2006).*
- Identify client strengths. Have the client make a list of strengths and refer to it when experiencing negative feelings. He or she may find it helpful to put the list on a note card to carry at all times. **EBN:** *Extra stress is reduced by positive thinking (Makinen, Suominen, & Lauri, 2000).* **EB:** *Instillation of hope helps the client to see that his or her future can be better (Ruddick, 2008).*

- Have group members support each other in a group setting. **EB:** *The data in this study of clients suffering from schizophrenia suggest that each client, given enough time and support, can increase his or her own level of maturation and functioning in a group setting (Sigman & Hassan, 2006).*
- Model appropriate social interactions. Give positive verbal and nonverbal feedback for appropriate behavior (e.g., make statements such as, "I'm proud that you made it to work on time and did all the tasks assigned to you without saying that your supervisor was picking on you"; make eye contact). If not contraindicated, touch the client's arm or hand when speaking. **EBN:** *Shared feelings increased communication with stroke and aphasia clients without words (Sundin, Jansson, & Norberg, 2000).*
- Use role playing to increase social skills. **EB:** *Role playing has been demonstrated to increase social functioning with clients with schizophrenia (Bellack, Brown, & Thomas-Lohrman, 2006).*
- Use client-centered humor as appropriate. **EBN:** *This study demonstrated that client-initiated humor is important for increasing the client-caregiver communication and creating a supportive humanistic atmosphere for client care (Adamle & Turkoski, 2006).*
- Consider use of animal therapy; arrange for visitation. **EBN:** *Equine-facilitated psychotherapy, although not a new idea, is a little-known experiential intervention that offers the opportunity to achieve healing (Vidrine et al, 2002).*
- Consider the use of the Internet and email to promote socialization. **EBN:** *Use of the Internet was effective in providing social support and education for isolated rural women with chronic illness (Hill & Weinert, 2004). Email enabled engagement with a teenager with a mood disorder who had been difficult to communicate with (Roy & Gillett, 2008).*
- ▲ Refer client for behavioral interventions (life skills program) to increase social skills. **EB:** *A commercially available, facilitator-administered or self-administered behavioral training product can have significant beneficial effects on psychosocial well-being in a healthy community sample (Kirby et al, 2006).*
- Refer to care plans for **Risk for Loneliness** and **Social isolation** for additional interventions.

 ## Pediatric

- Encourage social support for clients with visual impairments. **EB:** *Research on Dutch adolescents with visual impairments indicates that social support, especially the support of peers, is important to adolescents with visual impairments (Kef, 2002).*
- Provide computers and Internet access to children with chronic disabilities that limit socialization. **EB:** *Parents who had a child with Duchenne's muscular dystrophy and were provided with a personal computer and e-mail and Internet connectivity indicated that social isolation was felt to have been reduced, and an occupation, interest, and enjoyment provided for the boys and their families (Soutter, Hamilton, & Russell, 2004).*
- Consider use of RAP therapy (therapy using rap music) in groups to advance social skills of urban adolescents. **EB:** *Findings were unequivocally in favor of the RAP therapy as a tool for advancing prosocial behavior in three adolescent groups: violent offenders, status offenders, and a control condition of high school students with no criminal history (DeCarlo & Hockman, 2003).*
- Consider residential wilderness treatment programs for adolescents with unsuccessfully treated mental health issues and antisocial behavior. *In this study 13 male adolescents in a 4–month residential wilderness program demonstrated increased self-esteem, improved social skills and problem solving skills, and less aggressive behavior (Cook, 2008).*

 ## Geriatric

- Encourage socialization through education, support groups, and programs for the elderly in the community. **EB:** *Social participation has been found to be related to better functional skills, well-being, health-related quality of life, and survival. The activities mentioned facilitate socialization (Dahan-Oliel, Gélinas, & Mazer, 2008).*
- ▲ Assess the client's potential or actual sensory problems with hearing and vision and make appropriate referrals if a problem is identified. **EB:** *Sensory problems are common experiences within the older U.S. population, and there is substantial difficulty sustaining social participation activities (Crews & Campbell, 2004).*

● = Independent   ▲ = Collaborative   **EBN** = Evidence-Based Nursing   **EB** = Evidence-Based

- Monitor for depression, a particular risk in the elderly. *Depression is one of the most common mental health problems in later life which can often stop people from enjoying spending time with their families (Sims, 2009).*
- Encourage group physical activity, such as aerobics or stretching and toning. *These activities decreased loneliness in former sedentary adults (McAuley et al, 2000).* **EB:** *Where appropriate, the development of sport and physical activity opportunities for service users should be considered by mental health professionals (Carter-Morris & Faulkner, 2003).*
- Have clients reminisce. **EBN:** *This study demonstrated that reminiscence offers a possible intervention in treatment for older women (Stinson & Kirk, 2006).*
- Refer to care plans for **Adult Failure to thrive**, **Risk for Loneliness**, and **Social isolation** for additional interventions.

Multicultural

- Assess for the effect of racism on the client's perceptions of social interactions. **EB:** *Accumulated experiences of racial discrimination by African American women constitute an independent risk factor for preterm delivery (Collins et al, 2004).*
- Approach individuals of color with respect, warmth, and professional courtesy. **EBN:** *Physicians engaged in less client-centered communication with African American clients than with Caucasian clients (Johnson et al, 2004). Minorities were significantly more likely to report being treated with disrespect or being looked down upon in the client-provider relationship (Blanchard & Lurie, 2004).*
- Validate the client's feelings regarding social interaction. **EBN:** *Research suggests that an increased risk of health pessimism among African American adults is due in part to race differences in the perception of interpersonal maltreatment (Boardman, 2004).*
- Use interpreters as needed. **EB:** *Primary care nurses act as gatekeepers to interpreting services (Gerrish et al, 2004).*
- Refer to care plan **Social isolation** for additional interventions.

Home Care

- Previously discussed interventions may be adapted for home care use.
- ▲ Refer to or support involvement with supportive groups and counseling. **EB:** *Cognitive behavioral group therapy was effective for social phobia in this group of 11 adolescent girls (Hayward et al, 2000). Group settings provide the opportunity to practice new skills (Alfano & Rowland, 2006).*

Client/Family Teaching and Discharge Planning

- ▲ Refer to appropriate social agencies for assistance (e.g., family therapy, self-help groups, crisis intervention), especially individuals who are seriously ill. **EB:** *Intensive psychotherapy may be most applicable to severely ill clients with bipolar disorder, whereas briefer treatments may be adequate for less severely ill clients (Miklowitz, 2006).*

⊖volve   See the EVOLVE website for Weblinks for client education resources.

REFERENCES

Adamle K, Turkoski B: Responding to patient-initiated humor: guidelines for practice, *Home Healthc Nurse* 24(10):638–644, 2006.

Alfano CM, Rowland JH: Recovery issues in cancer survivorship: a new challenge for supportive care, *Cancer J* 12(5):432–443, 2006.

Bellack AS, Brown CH, Thomas-Lohrman S: Psychometric characteristics of role-play assessments of social skill in schizophrenia, *Behav Ther* 37(4):339–352, 2006.

Blanchard J, Lurie N: R-E-S-P-E-C-T: patient reports of disrespect in the health care setting and its impact on care, *J Fam Pract* 53(9):721–730, 2004.

Boardman JD: Health pessimism among black and white adults: the role of interpersonal and institutional maltreatment, *Soc Sci Med* 59(12):2523–2533, 2004.

Bowles N: A solution-focused approach to engagement in acute psychiatry, *Nurs Times* 98(48):26–27, 2002.

Carter-Morris P, Faulkner G: A football project for service users: the role of football in reducing social exclusion, *J Ment Health Promot* 2(1):7, 2003.

Collins JW Jr, David RJ, Handler A et al: Very low birthweight in African American infants: the role of maternal exposure to interpersonal racial discrimination, *Am J Public Health* 94(12):2132–2138, 2004.

Cook EC: Residential wilderness programs: the role of social support in influencing self-evaluations of male adolescents, *Adolescence* 43(172):751–774, 2008.

Crews JE, Campbell VA: Vision impairment and hearing loss among community-dwelling older Americans: implications for health functioning, *Am J Pub Health* 94(5):823–829, 2004.

Dahan-Oliel N, Gélinas I, Mazer B: Social participation in the elderly: what does the literature tell us? *Crit Rev Phys Rehabil Med* 20(2):159–176, 2008.

Dean A: Talking to dying patients of their hopes and needs, *Nurs Times* 98(43):34–35, 2002.

DeCarlo A, Hockman E: RAP therapy: a group work intervention method for urban adolescents, *Soc Work Groups* 26(3):45–59, 2003.

Gerrish K, Chau R, Sobowale A et al: Bridging the language barrier: the use of interpreters in primary care nursing, *Health Soc Care Community* 12(5):407–413, 2004.

Hayward C, Varady S, Albano AM et al: Cognitive-behavioral group therapy for social phobia in female adolescents: results of a pilot study, *J Am Acad Child Adolesc Psychiatry* 39(6):721, 2000.

Hill WG, Weinert C: An evaluation of an online intervention to provide social support and health education, *Comput Inform Nurs* 22(5):282–288, 2004.

Johnson RL, Roter D, Powe NR et al: Patient race/ethnicity and quality of patient-physician communication during medical visits, *Am J Public Health* 94(12):2084–2090, 2004.

Kef S: Psychosocial adjustment and the meaning of social support for visually impaired adolescents, *J Visual Impair Blind* 96(1):22, 2002.

Kirby ED, Williams VP, Hocking MC et al: Psychosocial benefits of three formats of a standardized behavioral stress management program, *Psychosom Med* 68(6):816–823, 2006.

Lunney M: Stress overload: a new diagnosis, *Int J Nurs Terminol Classif* 17(4):165–175, 2006.

Makinen S, Suominen T, Lauri S: Self-care in adults with asthma: how they cope, *J Clin Nurs* 9(4):557, 2000.

McAuley E, Blissmer B, Marquez DX et al: Social relations, physical activity, and well-being in older adults, *Prev Med* 31(5):608, 2000.

Melnechenko KL: To make a difference: nursing presence, *Nurs Forum* 38(2):18–24, 2003.

Miklowitz DJ: An update on the role of psychotherapy in the management of bipolar disorder, *Curr Psychiatry Rep* 8(6):498–503, 2006.

Roy H, Gillett T: E-mail: a new technique for forming a therapeutic alliance with high-risk young people failing to engage with mental health services? A case study, *Clin Child Psychol Psychiatry* (1):95–103, 2008.

Ruddick F: Hope, optimism and expectation, *Ment Health Pract* 12(1):33–35, 2008.

Sigman M, Hassan S: Benefits of long-term group therapy to individuals suffering schizophrenia: a prospective 7–year study, *Bull Menninger Clin* 70(4):273–282, 2006.

Sims B: New resources fight depression, *Nurs Resident Care* 11(2):59, 2009.

Soutter J, Hamilton N, Russell P: The golden freeway: a preliminary evaluation of a pilot study advancing information technology as a social intervention for boys with Duchenne muscular dystrophy and their families, *Health Soc Care Community* 12(1):25–33, 2004.

Stinson CK, Kirk E: Structured reminiscence: an intervention to decrease depression and increase self-transcendence in older women, *J Clin Nurs* 15(2):208–218, 2006.

Sundin K, Jansson L, Norberg A: Communicating with people with stroke and aphasia: understanding through sensation without words, *J Clin Nurs* 9(4):481, 2000.

University of Central Lancashire: Department of Nursing: *Solution focused interventions* (NU3307), www.uclan.ac.uk/courses/factsheets/health/nursing/3284.pdf. Accessed January 18, 2003.

Vidrine M, Owen-Smith P, Faulkner P et al: Equine-facilitated group psychotherapy: applications for therapeutic vaulting, *Ment Health Nurs* 23(6):587, 2002.

Yonge O, Molzahn A: Exceptional nontraditional caring practices of nurses, *Scand J Caring Sci* 16(4):399, 2002.

Zanello A, Weber Rouget B, Gex-Fabry M et al: Validation of the QFS measuring the frequency and satisfaction in social behaviours in psychiatric adult population, *Encephale* 32(1 Pt 1):45–59, 2006.

Social isolation   *Mary T. Shoemaker, RN, MSN, SANE*

Definition

Aloneness experienced by the individual and perceived as imposed by others and as a negative or threatening state

Defining Characteristics

Objective

Absence of supportive significant other(s); developmentally inappropriate behaviors; dull affect; evidence of handicap (e.g., physical, mental); exists in a subculture; illness; meaningless actions; no eye contact; preoccupation with own thoughts; projects hostility; repetitive actions; sad affect; seeks to be alone; shows behavior unaccepted by dominant cultural group; uncommunicative; withdrawn

Subjective

Expresses feelings of aloneness imposed by others; expresses feelings of rejection; developmentally inappropriate interests; inadequate purpose in life; inability to meet expectations of others; expresses values unacceptable to the dominant cultural group; experiences feelings of differences from others; insecurity in public

Related Factors (r/t)

Alterations in mental status; alterations in physical appearance; altered state of wellness; factors contributing to the absence of satisfying personal relationships (e.g., delay in accomplishing developmental tasks); immature interests; inability to engage in satisfying personal relationships; inadequate personal resources; unaccepted social behavior; unaccepted social values

NOC   (Nursing Outcomes Classification)

Suggested NOC Outcomes

Loneliness Severity, Mood Equilibrium, Personal Well-Being, Play Participation, Social Interaction Skills, Social Involvement, Social Support

> ### Example NOC Outcome with Indicators
> **Social Involvement** as evidenced by the following indicator: Interacts with close friends, neighbors, family members, and members of work groups (Rate the outcome and indicators of **Social Involvement:** 1 = never demonstrated, 2 = rarely demonstrated, 3 = sometimes demonstrated, 4 = often demonstrated, 5 = consistently demonstrated [see Section I].)

Client Outcomes

Client Will (Specify Time Frame):

- Identify feelings of isolation
- Practice social and communication skills needed to interact with others
- Initiate interactions with others; set and meet goals
- Participate in activities and programs at level of ability and desire
- Describe feelings of self-worth

NIC   (Nursing Interventions Classification)

Suggested NIC Intervention

Socialization Enhancement

> ### Example NIC Activities—Socialization Enhancement
> Encourage patience in developing relationships; Help patient increase awareness of strengths and limitations in communicating with others

Nursing Interventions and *Rationales*

- Establish a therapeutic relationship by being emotionally present and authentic. *Being emotionally present and authentic fosters growth in relationships and decreases isolation (Jordan, 2000).* **EBN:** *Being truly present was listed as one behavior that demonstrated caring (Yonge & Molzahn, 2002).*
- Observe for barriers to social interaction (e.g., illness; incontinence; decreasing ability to form relationships; lack of transportation, money, support system, or knowledge). **EBN:** *Causes of social isolation may be different for each individual; assessment of the barriers is crucial to appropriate treatment (Holley, 2007).*
- Note risk factors (e.g., membership in ethnic/cultural minority, chronic physiological or psychological illness or deformities, advanced age). **EBN:** *Clients with these risk factors may be at risk for social isolation. Young adults with mental illness identify social isolation as their main concern (Mostafanejad, 2006).*
- Discuss/assess causes of perceived or actual isolation. **EBN:** *The individual's experience of illness; the circumstances of everyday living that influence quality of life; and emotions, fears, and concerns all have a bearing on the way illness is managed (McPherson, Smith-Lovin, & Brashears, 2006).*

• = Independent   ▲ = Collaborative   **EBN** = Evidence-Based Nursing   **EB** = Evidence-Based

- Establish trust one on one and then gradually introduce the client to others. Allow the client opportunities to introduce issues and to describe his or her daily life. **EBN:** *Permitting the client to describe individuality and allowing that individuality to determine interpersonal approaches and health-illness management needs and actions managed (McPherson, Smith-Lovin, & Brashears, 2006).*
- Promote social interactions. Support the expression of feelings. Consider the use of music therapy. **EB:** *Music plays role in accessing emotion (Clements-Cortes, 2004).*
- Involve clients in writing specific outcomes, such as identifying what is most important from their viewpoint and lifestyle. **EBN:** *Women diagnosed with early breast cancer state the importance of making decisions for medical treatment is a mandatory step in designing customized decision support (Budden et al, 2003).*
- Provide positive reinforcement when the client seeks out others. **EBN:** *Receiving instrumental social support, such as practical help, advice, and feedback, significantly contributes to positive well-being (Lauder, Sharkey, & Mummery, 2004).*
- Help the client identify appropriate diversional activities to encourage socialization. *Active participation by the client is essential for behavioral changes.*
- Identify available support systems and involve these individuals in the client's care. **EB:** *Clients cope more successfully with stressful life events if they have support (Bawaskar, 2006).*
- ▲ Refer clients to support groups. **EB:** *Clients who are victims of domestic violence often endure social isolation imposed by significant others and benefit from support groups (Larance & Porter, 2004).*
- Encourage liberal visitation for a client who is hospitalized or in an extended care facility. **EBN:** *Visits from those in an emotionally close network were associated with perceived support, and this was associated with a decrease in isolation (Wilkinson & McAndrew, 2008).*
- Help the client identify role models and interactions with others with similar interests. *Sometimes the client needs someone to model the appropriate behavior (Sadler, 2007).*
- See the care plan for **Risk for Loneliness**.

Pediatric

- ▲ Refer obese adolescents for diet, exercise, and psychosocial support. *Obese teens in this study reported shame and social isolation related to their obesity (Sjoberg, Nilsson & Leppert, 2005).*
- See the care plan for **Risk for Loneliness**.

Geriatric

- Assess physical and mental status to establish a firm basis for planning social activities. **EBN:** *Socialization is important throughout the life span. Older adults living alone and with spouses continue to desire social interaction at levels similar to their participation in earlier life stages (Tomaka, 2006).*
- Assess for hearing deficit. Provide aids and use adaptive techniques. **EB:** *The odds of demonstrating auditory processing abnormality for average older participants increased by 4% to 9% per year of age. Men were approximately twice as likely as women to demonstrate this abnormality (Golding et al, 2006).*
- Encourage physical closeness (e.g., use touch) if appropriate. **EBN:** *Touch helps with integration and fosters social relatedness. Tactile stimulation benefits the older adult's psychological well-being (Routasalo et al, 2009).*
- Involve client in goal setting and planning activities. Assist them to identify five activities in which they would like to participate. **EBN:** *Involvement in participation of goal setting and planning of social activities enhanced both their anticipation and their participation in the activities (Toofany, 2008).*
- Involve nonprofessionals in activities, projects, and goal setting with the client. Practice interdisciplinary management for unit-based activities: engaging in arts and crafts projects, sewing, watching videos, reading large-print books, reading magazines, playing games, playing musical instruments, and using assistive listening devices. **EBN:** *Nursing assistants are important caregivers in long-term care agencies. Understanding their perspective offers insight in creating environments in which safe, compassionate and cost-effective care co-exist (Secrest, Iorio, & Martz, 2005).* **EBN:** *In a study of the use of calming music and hand massage, physically nonaggressive behaviors decreased during each of the interventions (Remington, 2002).*

• = Independent   ▲ = Collaborative   **EBN** = Evidence-Based Nursing   **EB** = Evidence-Based

- Offer the client a choice of activities and persons with whom to sit and socialize. Introductions to strangers may need to be repeated several times. **EBN:** *A recognized intervention for loneliness is to provide opportunities and assistance for making choices, setting goals, and making decisions. Cognitively impaired clients may require several repetitions (Routasalo et al, 2009).*
- Put clients in groups according to activity preferences, abilities, age, life situations, personal and cultural characteristics, and social networks. **EB:** *In this study psychosocial group rehabilitation was associated with lower mortality and less use of health services (Pitkala et al, 2009).*
- Provide physical activity, either aerobic or stretching and toning. **EB:** *Physical activity increased social support in a group of older, formerly sedentary adults (McAuley et al, 2000).*
- Provide music with active participation, such as drum and rhythm circles. **EBN:** *There is no active participation for many residents when the music programs they experience are limited to attendance at concerts and sing-alongs. Drum circles and rhythm circles actively involve residents, even those who are cognitively impaired (Rozon, Hagens, & Martin, 2004).*
- Consider the use of simulated presence therapy (see the care plan for **Hopelessness**). **EBN:** *Simulated presence therapy appears to be the most effective therapy for treating social isolation (Woods & Ashley, 1995).*
- ▲ Refer to programs such as Foster Grandparents and Senior Companions. **EB:** *Altruistic activity has a positive effect on older persons (Dulin & Hill, 2003).*
- Consider using computers and the Internet to alleviate or reduce loneliness and social isolation. **EBN:** *Participants age 65 years and older living alone used the computer to combat loneliness (Clark, 2002). Internet use was found to decrease loneliness and depression significantly, while perceived social support and self-esteem increased significantly (Shaw & Gant, 2002; Sum et al, 2009).*

Multicultural

- Acknowledge racial/ethnic differences at the onset of care. **EBN:** *Acknowledgment of race/ethnicity issues will enhance communication, establish rapport, and promote positive treatment outcomes (D'Avanzo & Naegle, 2001).*
- Assess for the influence of cultural beliefs, norms, and values on the client's perception of social activity and relationships. **EBN:** *What the client considers normal social interaction may be based on cultural perceptions (Leininger & McFarland, 2002).*
- Approach individuals of color with respect, warmth, and professional courtesy. **EBN:** *Instances of disrespect and lack of caring have special significance for individuals of color and may impede efforts to increase social outlets (D'Avanzo & Naegle, 2001).*
- Assess personal space needs, communication styles, acceptable body language, attitude toward eye contact, perception of touch, and paraverbal messages when communicating with the client. **EBN:** *Nurses need to consider these aspects when interpreting verbal and nonverbal messages (Purnell, 2000). Native American clients may consider avoiding direct eye contact to be a sign of respect and asking questions to be rude and intrusive (Seideman et al, 1996).*
- Use a family-centered approach when working with Latino, Asian American, African American, and Native American clients. **EBN:** *Latinos may perceive the family as source of support, solver of problems, and source of pride. Asian Americans may regard the family as the primary decision maker and primary influence on individual family members (D'Avanzo & Naegle, 2001).*
- Promote a sense of ethnic attachment. **EBN:** *Older Korean clients with strong ethnic attachments had higher levels of social involvement than others (Kim, 1999).*
- Validate the client's feelings regarding social isolation. **EBN:** *Validation lets the client know that the nurse has heard and understood what was said, and it promotes the nurse-client relationship (Heineken, 1998). A study of African American men found a sense of family in the AIDS-dedicated nursing home, making it potentially a valuable source of needed social support, which decreased social isolation (Fields & Jemmot, 2003).*
- Assist refugees who are relocated to access health care; support their connections with cultural, social, and religious groups. *Sub-Saharan refugees in Australia are isolated when they relocate and do not know where or how to seek health care services (Sheikh-Mohammed et al, 2006).*

Home Care

- The interventions described previously may be adapted for home care use.
- Confirm that the home setting has a telephone. Obtain one if necessary for medical safety. If the client lives alone, set up a Lifeline safety system that requires the client to answer the telephone. *The telephone can be used to achieve continuity of care and successful client-family interaction (Skinner, 2001).*
- Consider the use of the computer and Internet to decrease isolation. **EBN:** *Pregnant women on home bed rest for preterm labor stated that their participation in a virtual online peer support group was valuable and beneficial in helping them to cope with the hardships of bed rest (Adler & Zarchin, 2002). Homebound older adults found that the Internet and e-mail were excellent sources of support and enjoyment (Nahm & Resnick, 2001).* **EB:** *These studies demonstrated computer social support for rural women with chronic illness. The women declared the computer-based social support to have positive effects (Hill, Weinert, & Cudney, 2006).*
- Assess options for living that allow the client privacy but not isolation (e.g., boarding home, congregate living, assertive community treatment programs). **EB:** *Adults with schizophrenia described their relationships with other mental health clients in primarily positive terms, yet several participants expressed dissatisfaction and desired greater integration into mainstream social networks (Angell, 2003).*
- Assist clients to interact with neighbors in the community when they move to supported housing. *Without the personal contact between the mentally ill person and the neighbors, there may be a risk that the integration will fail (Hogberg, Magnusson, & Lutzen, 2006).*

 Client/Family Teaching and Discharge Planning

- Teach role playing (practicing communication skills in specific situations). *Role playing may help clients develop social interaction skills and identify feelings associated with their isolation.*
- Encourage the client to initiate contacts with self-help groups, counselors, and therapists. **EBN:** *If adjustment is to be successful and maintained, management of a chronic illness cannot occur in isolation; it requires a complex interaction of resources (Bawaskar, 2006).*
- Provide information to the client about senior citizen services, house sharing, pets, day care centers, churches, and community resources. **EBN:** *The well-documented negative effect of social isolation suggests that clients without confidants and supportive others must be referred to alternative sources, such as cardiac rehabilitation programs, support groups, and community agencies (McCauley, 1995).* **EB:** *This study indicated that accomplishment of social roles is, for the majority of participants, more significant than daily activities (Levasseur, St-Cyr Tribble, & Desrosiers, 2009).*
- ▲ Refer socially isolated caregivers to appropriate support groups as well. *Identification and recognition of the overwhelming task of caregiving are needed so that caregivers do not suffer in silence (Bergman-Evans, 1994). (See the care plan for* **Caregiver role strain.***)*

ⓔvolve   See the EVOLVE website for Weblinks for client education resources.

REFERENCES

Adler CL, Zarchin YR: The "virtual focus group": using the Internet to reach pregnant women on home bed rest, *J Obstet Gynecol Neonatal Nurs* 31(4):418, 2002.

Angell B: Contexts of social relationship development among assertive community treatment clients, *Ment Health Serv Res* 5(1):13, 2003.

Bawaskar HS: The many stigmas of mental illness, *Lancet* 367(9520):533–534, 2006.

Bergman-Evans BF: Alzheimer's and related disorders: loneliness, depression, and social support of spousal caregivers, *J Gerontol Nurs* 20:6, 1994.

Budden LM, Pierce PF, Hayes BA et al: Australian women's prediagnostic decision-making styles, relating to treatment choices for early breast cancer treatment, *Res Theory Nurs Pract* 17(2):117–136, 2003.

Clark DJ: Older adults living through and with their computers, *Comput Inform Nurs* 20(3):117, 2002.

Clements-Cortes A: The use of music in facilitating emotional expression in the terminally ill, *Am J Hosp Palliat Care* 21(4):255–260, 2004.

D'Avanzo CE, Naegle MA: Developing culturally informed strategies for substance-related interventions. In Naegle MA, D'Avanzo CE, editors: *Addictions and substance abuse: strategies for advanced practice nursing*, St Louis, 2001, Mosby.

Dulin PL, Hill RD: Relationships between altruistic activity and positive and negative affect among low-income older adult service providers, *Aging Ment Health* 7(4):294–299, 2003.

• = Independent   ▲ = Collaborative   **EBN** = Evidence-Based Nursing   **EB** = Evidence-Based

Fields SD, Jemmott LS: The love and belonging health care needs of HIV infected African-American men upon admission to an AIDS dedicated nursing home, *J Natl Black Nurses Assoc* 14(1):38–44, 2003.

Golding M, Taylor A, Cupples L et al: Odds of demonstrating auditory processing abnormality in the average older adult: the Blue Mountains Hearing Study, *Ear Hear* 27(2):129–138, 2006.

Heineken J: Patient silence is not necessarily client satisfaction: communication in home care nursing, *Home Healthc Nurse* 16(2):115, 1998.

Hill W, Weinert C, Cudney S: Influence of a computer intervention on the psychological status of chronically ill rural women: preliminary results, *Nurs Res* 55(1):34–42, 2006.

Hogberg T, Magnusson A, Lutzen K: Living by themselves? Psychiatric nurses' views on supported housing for persons with severe and persistent mental illness, *J Psychiatr Ment Health Nurs* 13(6):735–741, 2006.

Holley U: Social isolation: a practical guide for nurses assisting clients with chronic illness, *Rehab Nurs* 32(2):51–56, 2007.

Jordan JV: The role of mutual empathy in relational/cultural therapy, *J Clin Psychol* 56(8):1005, 2000.

Kim O: Mediation effect of social support between ethnic attachment and loneliness in older Korean immigrants, *Res Nurs Health* 22(2):169, 1999.

Larance LY, Porter ML: Observations from practice: support group membership as a process of social capital formation among female survivors of domestic violence, *J Interpers Violence* 19(6):676–690, 2004.

Lauder W, Sharkey S, Mummery K: A community survey of loneliness, *J Adv Nurs* 46(1):88–94, 2004.

Leininger MM, McFarland MR: *Transcultural nursing: concepts, theories, research and practices,* ed 3, New York, 2002, McGraw-Hill.

Levasseur M, St-Cyr Tribble D, Desrosiers J: Meaning of quality of life for older adults: importance of human functioning components, *Arch Gerontol Geriatr* 49(2):e91–100, 2009.

McAuley E, Blissmer B, Marquez DX et al: Social relations, physical activity, and well-being in older adults, *Prev Med* 31(5):608, 2000.

McCauley K: Assessing social support in patients with cardiac disease, *J Cardiovasc Nurs* 10:73, 1995.

McPherson M, Smith-Lovin L, Brashears M: Social isolation in America: changes in core discussion networks over two decades, *Am Sociol Rev* 71(3):353–375, 2006.

Mostafanejad K: Reducing the isolation of young adults living with a mental illness in rural Australia, *Int J Ment Health Nurs* 15(3):181–188, 2006.

Nahm ES, Resnick B: Homebound older adults' experiences with the Internet and e-mail, *Comput Nurs* 19(6):257, 2001.

Pitkala KH, Routasalo P, Kautiainen H et al: Effects of psychosocial group rehabilitation on health, use of health care services, and mortality of older persons suffering from loneliness: a randomized, controlled trial, *J Gerontol A Biol Sci Med Sci* 64(7):792–800, 2009.

Purnell L: A description of the Purnell model for cultural competence, *J Transcult Nurs* 11(1):40, 2000.

Remington R: Calming music and hand massage with agitated elderly, *Nurs Res* 51(5):317, 2002.

Routasalo PE, Tilvis RS, Kautiainen H et al: Effects of psychosocial group rehabilitation on social functioning, loneliness and well-being of lonely, older people: randomized controlled trial, *J Adv Nurs* 65(2):297–305, 2009.

Rozon L, Hagens C, Martin LS: Music programs that create a sense of community: music therapy for even the most severe cognitively impaired resident, *Can Nurs Home* 15(1):57–59, 2004.

Sadler C: Ending the isolation, *Nurs Stand* 21(52):24–25, 2007.

Secrest J, Iorio DH, Martz W: The meaning of work for nursing assistants who stay in long-term care, *J Clin Nurs* 4(8B):90–97, 2005.

Seideman RY, Jacobson S, Primeaux M et al: Assessing American Indian families, *MCN Am J Matern Child Nurs* 21(6):274, 1996.

Shaw LH, Gant LM: In defense of the Internet: the relationship between Internet communication and depression, loneliness, self-esteem, and perceived social support, *Cyberpsychol Behav* 5(2):157, 2002.

Sheikh-Mohammed M, Macintyre CR, Wood NJ et al: Barriers to access to health care for newly resettled sub-Saharan refugees in Australia, *Med J Aust* 85(11–12):594–597, 2006.

Sjoberg RL, Nilsson KW, Leppert J: Obesity, shame, and depression in school-aged children: a population-based study, *Pediatrics* 116(3): e389–e92, 2005.

Skinner D: Intimacy and the telephone, *Caring* 20(2):28, 2001.

Sum S, Mathews RM, Pourghasem M et al: Internet use as a predictor of sense of community in older people, *Cyberpsychol Behav* 12(2):235–239, 2009.

Tomaka J: The relation of social isolation, loneliness, and social support to disease outcomes among the elderly, *J Aging Health* 18(3):359, 2006.

Toofany S: How to promote a healthier tomorrow, *Nurs Older People* 20(2):17–20, 2008.

Wilkinson & McAndrew: "I'm not an outsider, I'm his mother!" A phenomenological enquiry into carer experiences of exclusion from acute psychiatric settings, *Int J Ment Health Nurs* 17(6):392–401, 2008.

Woods P, Ashley J: Simulated presence therapy: using selected memories to manage problem behaviors in Alzheimer's disease patients, *Geriatr Nurs* 16(1):9–14, 1995.

Yonge O, Molzahn A: Exceptional nontraditional caring practices of nurses, *Scand J Caring Sci* 16(4):399, 2002.

Chronic Sorrow   *Betty J. Ackley, MSN, EdS, RN*

NANDA-I

Definition

Cyclical, recurring, and potentially progressive pattern of pervasive sadness experienced (by parent, caregiver, individual with chronic illness or disability) in response to continual loss throughout the trajectory of an illness or disability

Defining Characteristics

Expresses negative feelings (e.g., anger, being misunderstood, confusion, depression, disappointment, emptiness, fear, frustration, guilt, helplessness, hopelessness, loneliness, low self-esteem, overwhelmed,

● = Independent   ▲ = Collaborative   **EBN** = Evidence-Based Nursing   **EB** = Evidence-Based

recurring loss, self-blame); expresses feelings of sadness (e.g., periodic, recurrent); expresses feelings that interfere with ability to reach highest level of personal well-being; expresses feelings that interfere with ability to reach highest level of social well-being

Related Factors (r/t)

Death of a loved one; experiences chronic disability (e.g., physical or mental); experiences chronic illness (e.g., physical or mental); crises in management of the illness; crises related to developmental stages; missed opportunities; missed milestones; unending caregiving

 (Nursing Outcomes Classification)

Suggested NOC Outcomes

Acceptance: Health Status, Depression Level, Depression Self-Control, Grief Resolution, Hope, Mood Equilibrium

---

Example **NOC Outcome with Indicators**

Grief Resolution with plans for a positive future as evidenced by the following indicators: Describes meaning of loss or death/Reports decreased preoccupation with loss/Reports adequate nutritional intake/Reports adequate sleep/ Expresses positive expectations about the future (Rate the outcome and indicators of **Grief Resolution:** I = never demonstrated, 2 = rarely demonstrated, 3 = sometimes demonstrated, 4 = often demonstrated, 5 = consistently demonstrated [see Section I].)

Client Outcomes

Client Will (Specify Time Frame):

- Express appropriate feelings of guilt, fear, anger, or sadness
- Identify problems associated with sorrow (e.g., changes in appetite, insomnia, nightmares, loss of libido, decreased energy, alteration in activity levels)
- Seek help in dealing with grief-associated problems
- Plan for future one day at a time
- Function at normal developmental level

 (Nursing Interventions Classification)

Suggested NIC Interventions

Grief Work Facilitation, Grief Work Facilitation: Perinatal Death

---

Example **NIC Activities—Grief Work Facilitation**

Encourage client to verbalize memories of loss, both past and current; Assist client in identifying personal coping strategies

---

Nursing Interventions and *Rationales*

- Assess the client's degree of sorrow. Use the Burke/NCRS Chronic Sorrow Questionnaire for the individual or caregiver as appropriate. *This questionnaire is designed to determine the occurrence of chronic sorrow, cues that trigger sorrow, coping strategies, and factors that direct health care personnel to deal with the sorrowful client or caregiver (Isaksson, Gunnarsson, & Ahlstrom, 2007; Isaksson & Ahlstrom, 2008).*
- Identify problems of eating and sleeping; ensure that basic human needs are being met. **EBN:** *Bereaved individuals, irrespective of whether they had counseling for grief resolution or not, had a moderate risk for poor nutrition (Johnson, 2002).*
- Develop a trusting relationship with the client by using empathetic therapeutic communication techniques. **EB:** *An empathetic person who takes the time to listen, offers support and reassurance, recognizes and focuses on feelings, and appreciates the uniqueness of each individual and family is helpful to clients experiencing chronic sorrow (Isaksson, Gunnarsson, & Ahlstrom, 2007; Isaksson & Ahlstrom, 2008).*

• = Independent   ▲ = Collaborative   **EBN** = Evidence-Based Nursing   **EB** = Evidence-Based

- Help the client to understand that sorrow may be ongoing. No timetable exists for grieving, despite popular thought. After loss, life is characterized by good times and bad times when sorrow is triggered by events. **EBN:** *Loss of a child results in lifelong grief (Arnold & Gemma, 2008). Studies have demonstrated that feelings of sadness, guilt, anger, frustration, and fear occur periodically throughout the lives of people experiencing chronic loss resulting in chronic sorrow (Isaksson & Ahlstrom, 2008).*
- Help the client recognize that, although sadness will occur at intervals for the rest of his or her life, it will become bearable. **EBN:** *In time the client may develop a relationship with grief that is lifelong but livable, and as much filled with comfort as it is with sorrow (Moules et al, 2007). A study showed that the common belief about the need for resolving grief is not helpful to the bereaved, but rather, grief's presence may contribute to a new relationship with the deceased over time (Moules et al, 2004). As the grief resolves there can be times of satisfaction and even happiness (Clements et al, 2004).*
- Encourage the use of positive coping techniques:
  - Taking action: Suggested strategies include keeping busy, keeping personal interests, going away, getting out of the house, doing something to gain a feeling of control over life.
  - Cognitive coping: Techniques include concentrating on the positive aspects of life, having a "can do" attitude, taking 1 day at a time, and taking responsibility for the quality of one's own life. Encourage the client to write about the experience.
  - Interpersonal coping: Techniques include talking to a close friend, a health care professional, or someone with the same condition or circumstance. Joining a support group can also help the sorrowful person to cope.
  - Emotional coping: Encourage the client to express feelings both to other people, and to write out feelings, cry as desired, give thanks, and pray if desired.
  Clients with chronic sorrow have found these coping techniques helpful (Isaksson & Ahlstrom, 2008).
- Expect the client to meet responsibilities; give positive reinforcement for planning how to meet responsibilities, and for accomplishing responsibilities.
- ▲ Encourage the client to make time to talk to family members about the loss with the help of professional support as needed and without criticizing or belittling each other's feelings about the loss. *Once these feelings are shared, family members can better begin to accept the chronic loss and hopefully develop coping strategies.* **EBN:** *A study found that supportive family members were very helpful to clients with chronic sorrow from multiple sclerosis (Isaksson & Ahlstrom, 2008). A study analyzing the grief and coping of mothers who had lost children under the age of 7 years found that the spouse, children, grandparents, next of kin, friends, and colleagues were the main sources of support (Laakso & Paunonen-Ilmonen, 2002).*
- Help the client determine the best way and place to find social support. *Social support is shown to help bereaved individuals as they put their lives back together and find new meaning in life (Isaksson & Ahlstrom, 2008).*
- ▲ Identify available community resources, including grief counselors or support groups available for specific losses (e.g., Multiple Sclerosis Society). **EBN:** *Psychoeducational, group activity and self-assessment caused suicide rates to decrease among elderly females in a Japanese culturally sensitive intervention study (Oyama et al, 2005).*
- ▲ Identify whether the client is experiencing depression, suicidal tendencies, or other emotional disorders. Refer for counseling as appropriate. *Counseling with therapeutic goal setting has been shown to be helpful (Clements et al, 2004).*

 Pediatric/Parent

- Treat the child with respect, give him or her the opportunity to talk about their concerns, and answer questions honestly. *Children know much more than adults realize. They are very observant and generally know if a parent or loved one is dying, or cause of death, even if they have not been told (Schuurman, 2008).*
- Listen to the child's expression of grief. *The best thing to be done to help a child is to listen with our ears, eyes, hearts, and souls, and recognize that we do not have to have answers (Schuurman, 2008; Brown, 2009).*
- Help parents recognize that the grieving child does not have to be "fixed," instead they need support going through an experience of grieving just as adults. *The role of the nurse, parent, and friends is to support and assist, not to help them "get over it" (Schuurman, 2008).*

● = Independent ▲ = Collaborative **EBN** = Evidence-Based Nursing **EB** = Evidence-Based

- Consider the use of art for children in hospice care who are dying or dealing with the death of a parent, sibling, or other family member. **EBN:** *The arts are being recognized as a powerful tool for psychological, emotional, and spiritual support. Through an "ART is the heART" approach, children learn to use the arts as a healthy and effective coping strategy (Rollins & Riccio, 2002).*
- ▲ Refer grieving children and parents to a program to help facilitate grieving if desired, especially if the death was traumatic. **EBN:** *When a child dies, the parent embarks on a lifelong grief for the loss, and sharing the grief can help the parent (Arnold & Gemma, 2008).* **EB:** *A study demonstrated treatment for children and parents with grief associated with trauma helped decrease symptoms of post-traumatic stress disorder (Cohen, Mannarino, & Knudsen, 2004).*
- Help the adolescent determine sources of support and how to use them effectively. **EBN:** *In a study of adolescents dealing with the death of a loved one, the most important factors that helped adolescents cope with the grief were self-help and support from parents, relatives, and friends (Rask, Kaunonen, & Paunonen-Ilmonen, 2002).*
- ▲ Encourage parents in chronic sorrow to seek mental health services as needed, learn stress reduction, and take good care of their health. **EB:** *A study demonstrated that there was an association between chronic sorrow and situational depression (Hobdell, 2004). Parents of children with intellectual disabilities, and mental health problems, often experienced helplessness and despair (Faust & Scior, 2008).* **EBN:** *A study analyzing the grief and coping of mothers who had lost children under the age of 7 years found that the spouse, remaining children, grandparents, next of kin, friends, and colleagues were the main sources of support (Laakso & Paunonen-Ilmonen, 2002).*

Geriatric

- ▲ Use reminiscence therapy in conjunction with the expression of emotions. Refer to a reminiscence group if available. **EBN and EB:** *Two studies demonstrated that participation in a reminiscence group reduced symptoms of depression (Jones, 2003; Zauszniewski et al, 2004).*
- Identify previous losses and assess the client for depression. *In older age, losses and changes often occur in rapid succession without adequate recovery time.*
- Evaluate the social support system of the elderly client. If the support system is minimal, help the client determine how to increase available support. *The elderly who do not live with family members and have a minimal support system are more vulnerable to depression from grief. The support of family (especially children) and friends is a common way for elderly people to cope with a loss.*

Multicultural

- Assess for the influence of cultural beliefs, norms, and values on the client's expressions of sorrow. **EBN:** *Expressions of sorrow may be based on cultural perceptions (Leininger & McFarland, 2002). African Americans may be expected to act "strong" and go on with the business of life after a death; Native Americans may not talk about the death because of beliefs that such talk will detract from spirituality and bring bad luck; Latinos may wear black and act subdued during their luto (mourning) period; Southeast Asian families may wear white when mourning. Korean family caregivers' experiences in making the decision to place a family member with dementia in a long-term care facility showed a pattern of deep sorrow (Park, Butcher, & Moss, 2004). Sorrow is one of the seven emotions identified by Eastern philosophies of Buddhism, Taoism, and traditional Chinese medicine (Chan, Ho, & Chow, 2001).*

Home Care

- The interventions described previously may be adapted for home care use.
- ▲ Assess the client for depression. Refer for mental health services as indicated. *Sadness is part of the syndrome of depression. Increase in mood is unlikely unless the underlying depression is treated. Counseling services provide an opportunity for expression of feelings, increase coping skills, and provide respite for caregivers.*
- ▲ When sorrow is focused around loss of a pregnancy, encourage the client to follow through on a counseling referral. **EBN:** *Parents with a history of perinatal loss are at higher risk for depressive*

symptoms and pregnancy-specific anxiety during subsequent pregnancies, particularly before the third trimester. Mothers had a higher level of symptoms than fathers (Armstrong, 2002).

- Encourage the client to participate in activities that are diversionary and uplifting as tolerated (e.g., outdoor activities, hobby groups, church-related activities, pet care). *Diversionary activities decrease the time spent in sorrow, can give meaning to life, and provide a sense of well-being.*
- Encourage the client to participate in support groups appropriate to the area of loss or illness (e.g., Crohn's disease support group or Widow to Widow). *Support groups can increase an individual's sense of belonging. Group activity helps the client to identify alternative ways to problem solve.*
- Provide psychological support for family/caregivers. *Family/caregivers who feel supported are often able to provide greater and more consistent support to the affected person.*
- ▲ In the presence of a psychiatric disorder, refer for psychiatric home health care services for client reassurance and implementation of a therapeutic regimen.
- ▲ See the care plans for **Chronic low Self-Esteem**, **Risk for Loneliness**, and **Hopelessness.**

ⓔvolve   See the EVOLVE website for Weblinks for client education resources.

REFERENCES

Armstrong DS: Emotional distress and prenatal attachment in pregnancy after perinatal loss, *J Nurs Scholarsh* 34:339, 2002.

Arnold J, Gemma PB: The continuing process of parental grief, *Death Stud* 32:658–673, 2008.

Brown E: Helping bereaved children and young people, *Br J School Nurs* 4(2):69–73, 2009.

Chan C, Ho PS, Chow E: A body-mind-spirit model in health: an Eastern approach, *Soc Work Health Care* 34(3–4):261–282, 2001.

Clements PT, DeRanieri JT, Vigil GJ et al: Life after death: grief therapy after the sudden traumatic death of a family member, *Perspect Psychiatr Care* 40(4):149, 2004.

Cohen JA, Mannarino AP, Knudsen K: Treating childhood traumatic grief: a pilot study, *J Am Acad Child Adolesc Psychiatry* 43(10):171, 2004.

Faust H, Scior K: Mental health problems in young people with intellectual disabilities: the impact on parents, *J Appl Res Intellect Disabil* 21(5):414–424, 2008.

Hobdell E: Chronic sorrow and depression in parents of children with neural tube defects, *J Neurosci Nurs* 36(2):82, 2004.

Isaksson A, Ahlstrom G: Managing chronic sorrow: experiences of patients with multiple sclerosis, *J Neurosci Nurs* 40(3):180–192, 2008.

Isaksson A, Gunnarsson L, Ahlstrom GL: The presence and meaning of chronic sorrow in patients with multiple sclerosis, *J Nurs Healthc Chronic Illn* 10(11):1365–2702, 2007.

Johnson CS: Nutritional considerations for bereavement and coping with grief, *J Nutr Health Aging* 6(3):171, 2002.

Jones ED: Reminiscence therapy for older women with depression: effects of nursing intervention classification in assisted-living long-term care, *J Gerontol Nurs* 29(7):26–33, 2003.

Laakso H, Paunonen-Ilmonen M: Mothers' experience of social support following the death of a child, *J Clin Nurs* 11(2):176, 2002.

Leininger MM, McFarland MR: *Transcultural nursing: concepts, theories, research and practices*, ed 3, New York, 2002, McGraw-Hill.

Moules NJ, Simonson K, Fleiszer AR et al: The soul of sorrow work: grief and therapeutic interventions with families, *J Fam Nurs* 13(1):114–141, 2007.

Moules NJ, Simonson K, Prins M et al : Making room for grief: walking backwards and living forward, *Nurs Inq* 11(2):99–107, 2004.

Oyama H, Watanabe N, Ono Y et al: Community-based suicide prevention through group activity for the elderly successfully reduced the high suicide rate for females, *Psychiatry Clin Neurosci* 59(3):337–344, 2005.

Park M, Butcher HK, Maas ML: A thematic analysis of Korean family caregivers' experiences in making the decision to place a family member with dementia in a long-term care facility, *Res Nurs Health* 27(5):345–356, 2004.

Rask K, Kaunonen M, Paunonen-Ilmonen M: Adolescent coping with grief after the death of a loved one, *Int J Nurs Pract* 8(3):137, 2002.

Rollins JA, Riccio LL: ART is the heART: a palette of possibilities for hospice care, *Pediatr Nurs* 28(4):355, 2002.

Schuurman DL: The club no one wants to join: a dozen lessons I've learned from grieving children and adolescents, www.grief.org.au/child_support.html. Accessed May 20, 2008.

Zauszniewski JA, Eggenschwiler K, Preechawong S et al: Focused reflection reminiscence group for elders: implementation and evaluation, *Appl Gerontol* 23(4):429, 2004.

Spiritual distress   *Lisa Burkhart, PhD, RN*

NANDA-I

Definition

Impaired ability to experience and integrate meaning and purpose in life through connectedness with self, others, art, music, literature, nature, and/or a power greater than oneself

Defining Characteristics

Connections to Self

Anger; expresses lack of acceptance; expresses lack of courage; expresses lack of self-forgiveness; expresses lack of hope; expresses lack of love; expresses lack of meaning in life; expresses lack of purpose in life; expresses lack of serenity (e.g., peace); guilt; poor coping

• = Independent   ▲ = Collaborative   **EBN** = Evidence-Based Nursing   **EB** = Evidence-Based

Connections with Others

Expresses alienation; refuses interactions with significant others; refuses interactions with spiritual leaders; verbalizes being separated from support system

Connections with Art, Music, Literature, Nature

Disinterest in nature; disinterest in reading spiritual literature; inability to express previous state of creativity (e.g., singing/listening to music/writing)

Connections with Power Greater than Oneself

Expresses being abandoned; expresses having anger toward God; expresses hopelessness; expresses suffering; inability to be introspective; inability to experience the transcendent; inability to participate in religious activities; inability to pray; requests to see a religious leader; sudden changes in spiritual practices

Related Factors (r/t)

Self-alienation; loneliness/social isolation; anxiety; sociocultural deprivation; death and dying of self or others; pain; life change; chronic illness of self or others

NOC   (Nursing Outcomes Classification)

Suggested NOC Outcomes

Coping, Dignified Life Closure, Grief Resolution, Hope, Spiritual Health, Stress Level

Example **NOC** Outcome with Indicators
Spiritual Health as evidenced by the following indicators: Quality of faith, hope, meaning, and purpose in life/ Connectedness with inner-self and with others to share thoughts, feelings, and beliefs (Rate each indicator of **Spiritual Health:** 1 = severely compromised, 2 = substantially compromised, 3 = moderately compromised, 4 = mildly compromised, 5 = not compromised [see Section I].)

Client Outcomes

Client Will (Specify Time Frame):

- Express sense of connectedness with self, others, arts, music, literature, or power greater than one-self
- Express meaning and purpose in life
- Express sense of hope in the future
- Express ability to forgive
- Express acceptance of health status
- Discuss personal response to dying
- Discuss personal response to grieving

NIC   (Nursing Interventions Classification)

Suggested NIC Interventions

Active Listening, Forgiveness Facilitation, Grief Work Facilitation, Hope Inspiration, Humor, Music Therapy, Presence, Referral, Reminiscence Therapy, Self Awareness Enhancement, Simple Guided Imagery, Simple Massage, Simple Relaxation Therapy, Spiritual Support, Therapeutic Touch, Touch

Example **NIC** Activities—**Spiritual Support**
Encourage use of spiritual resources if desired; Be available to listen to client's expression of feelings

Nursing Interventions and *Rationales*

- Observe the client for loss of meaning, purpose, and hope in life. **EB:** *In a randomized-control trial with cancer clients, female gender, old age, years of education, performance status, and radiotherapy treatment contributes to the prediction of client's; spiritual beliefs and attitudes (Mystakidou et al,*

 = Independent   ▲ = Collaborative   **EBN** = Evidence-Based Nursing   **EB** = Evidence-Based

2008). In a qualitative study of young adult daughters with parents experiencing cancer identified exploring meaning as a theme (Puterman & Cadell, 2008). **EBN:** *In a quantitative study of 156 clients with cancer and 68 caregivers, Taylor (2006) found that one of the most prevalent spiritual needs was finding meaning. A qualitative study of family/caregivers for those in hospice identifies the search for meaning and caring presence as part of the mourning process (Clukey, 2008). In a phenomenological study, spirituality is one theme for women undergoing breast biopsy (Demir et al, 2008). In a grounded theory study, spiritual care begins by recognizing a client cue for needing spiritual care (Burkhart & Hogan, 2008).*

- Respect the client's beliefs; avoid imposing your own spiritual beliefs on the client. Be aware of your own belief systems and accept the client's spirituality. Allow for self-disclosure. Promote a sense of love, caring, and compassion. **EBN:** *In a quantitative study of 156 clients with cancer and 68 caregivers, Taylor (2006) found that one of the most prevalent spiritual needs was giving love to others. A program evaluating an end-of-life Integrated Care Pathway found that spiritual care involves individualizing interventions based on spiritual practices (Lhussier, Carr, & Wilcockson, 2007). Taylor & Mamier (2005) that most cancer clients and caregivers welcomed interventions that were less intimate, commonly used, and not overtly religious.*

- Monitor and promote supportive social contacts. **EBN:** *In a qualitative study of stroke caregivers, interacting with family and friends emerged as a theme (Pierce et al, 2008). Prince-Paul (2008) found spiritual well-being and social well-being accounted for 52.6% of the variance of quality of life for those at end-of-life.*

- Integrate family into spiritual practices as appropriate. **EBN:** *Qualitative study of 20 Caucasian women who had just completed the diagnostic process of breast cancer found their personal strength and connection to God or their spiritual beliefs were important. When overwhelmed, they sought out loved ones for support and diversion (Logan, Hackbusch-Pinto, & De Grasse, 2006). In a qualitative study of stroke caregivers, interacting with family and friends emerged as a theme (Pierce et al, 2008). Prince-Paul (2008) found spiritual well-being and social well-being accounted for 52.6% of the variance of quality of life for those at end-of-life. In a heurmineutic qualitative study, spiritual care is one type of relational or dialogic practice among families, particularly when discussing meaning related to suffering (McLeod & Wright, 2008). In a grounded theory study, spiritual care included promoting connectedness between client and family/friends (Burkhart & Hogan, 2008).*

- ▲ Refer the client to a support group or counseling. **EBN:** *Pierce et al. (2008) qualitatively studied a Web-based support and education intervention.*

- Coordinate or encourage attending spiritual retreats, courses, or programming. **EB:** *In a study with 128 male clients, expressed interest in attending an informational intervention, topics included spirituality (Manii & Ammerman, 2008).*

- Be physically present and actively listen to the client. **EB:** *In a qualitative study of young adult daughters with parents experiencing cancer identified being present as a theme (Puterman & Cadell, 2008). In a grounded theory study, spiritual care included promoting client connectedness with self (Burkhart & Hogan, 2008).*

- Support meditation, guided imagery, therapeutic touch, journaling, relaxation, and involvement in art, music, or poetry. Support outdoor activities. **EB:** *In a randomized control trial, a spiritual meditation intervention was associated with fewer migraine headaches, less anxiety and a greater pain tolerance, headache-related self-efficacy, daily spiritual experiences, and existential well-being (Wachholtz & Pargament, 2008).* **EBN:** *In a qualitative study of stroke caregivers, being one with nature emerged as a theme (Pierce et al, 2008). In a qualitative survey of chronically ill individuals, participants wanted access to a garden, a quiet space available in hospital to think through decision, spiritual help or guidance, swimming, and a choice of genres of music available (Dale & Hunt, 2008).*

- Offer or suggest visits with spiritual and/or religious advisors. **EBN:** *In a qualitative study of stroke caregivers, feeling the presence of a greater power and practicing rituals emerged as two themes (Pierce et al, 2008). In a grounded theory study, spiritual care included promoting connectedness with others, including chaplains (Burkhart & Hogan, 2008).*

- Help the client find a reason for living and be available for support. Promote hope. **EB:** *In a qualitative study of young adult daughters with parents experiencing cancer identified hope and spirituality as themes (Puterman & Cadell, 2008).* **EBN:** *In a quantitative study of 156 clients with cancer and 68 caregivers, Taylor (2006) found that one of the most prevalent spiritual needs was keeping a positive perspective.*

• = Independent   ▲ = Collaborative   **EBN** = Evidence-Based Nursing   **EB** = Evidence-Based

- Listen to the client's feelings about suffering and/or death. Be nonjudgmental and allow time for grieving. **EBN:** *Qualitative research has found that individuals at end-of-life have viewed spirituality as a central theme when coping with disease and treatment (Logan, Hackbusch-Pinto, & De Grasse, 2006). In a cross-sectional, retrospective, survey of parents of children who have died, participants identified spirituality and religion as shaping their perspective of the grief process (Arnold & Gemma, 2008).*
- Provide privacy or a "sacred space." **EBN:** *In a qualitative survey of chronically ill individuals, participants wanted access to a garden, a quiet space available in hospital to think through decision, spiritual help or guidance, swimming, and a choice of genres of music available (Dale & Hunt, 2008).*
- Allow time and a place for prayer. **EBN:** *In a descriptive study of 84 women with breast cancer, Meraviglia (2006) also found that participants used prayer more often and found that spiritual health and prayer correlated with more meaning in life and psychological well-being and less physical symptom distress. In a quantitative study of 156 clients with cancer and 68 caregivers, Taylor (2006) found that one of the most prevalent spiritual needs was understanding or relating to God. In a qualitative survey of chronically ill individuals, religious participants wanted prayer over meditation (Dale & Hunt, 2008). Cancer clients and their families frequently use prayer as a spiritual resource (Taylor & Mamier, 2005). In a grounded theory study, spiritual care included promoting religious rituals and prayer (Burkhart & Hogan, 2008).*

Geriatric

- Discuss personal definitions of spiritual wellness with the client. **EB:** *In a cross-sectional study of older adults, intrinsic religious activity was associated with older age, being female, and living situation (Yohannes et al, 2008).* **EBN:** *Narayanasamy (2006) found that nurses identified client needs in older clients by assessing religious beliefs and practice (prayer), absolution, seeking connection, comfort and reassurance, healing or searching for meaning or purpose.*
- Identify the client's past sources of spirituality. Help the client explore his or her life and identify those experiences that are noteworthy. Clients may want to read the Bible or other religious text or have it read to them. **EB:** *A cross-sectional study of individuals living in the community revealed that as people age, spirituality is more important (Trouillet & Gana, 2008.) In a cross-sectional study of older adults, religious attendance was associated with positive general health perception, and inversely associated with pack/year smoked, and severity of illness (Yohannes et al, 2008).* **EBN:** *In a qualitative study of stroke caregivers, interacting with family and friends emerged as a theme (Pierce et al, 2008).*

Multicultural

- Assess for the influence of cultural beliefs, norms, and values on the client's ability to cope with spiritual distress. **EB:** *Arab American immigrants are fatalistic in that they believe that cancer is a punishment from God and prognosis was determined by God (Shah et al, 2008). In a semistructured interview with Hawaiian women in churches, integrating religious and spiritual practices in health promotion were viewed as important in promoting breast cancer screening (Ka'opua, 2008).*
- Encourage spirituality as a source of support. **EBN:** *African Americans and Latinos may identify spirituality, religiousness, prayer, and church-based approaches as coping resources (Simoni, Frick, & Huang, 2006). Descriptive study with 178 low-income, abused African American women revealed that spiritual well-being was associated with readiness to change (Bliss et al, 2008). A qualitative study with African Americans living in rural areas revealed that spirituality/religion/prayer were helpful in coping, encouraged healthy lifestyles, and helps care providers (Jones et al, 2006).*
- Validate the client's spiritual concerns and convey respect for his or her beliefs. **EBN:** *In a meta-analysis of qualitative research on domestic violence survivors, spirituality and religiosity plays an important role and that role may differ based on culture (Yick, 2008).*

Home Care

- All of the nursing interventions described previously apply in the home setting.

ⓔvolve   See the EVOLVE website for Weblinks for client education resources.

● = Independent   ▲ = Collaborative   **EBN** = Evidence-Based Nursing   **EB** = Evidence-Based

REFERENCES

Arnold J, Gemma PB: The continuing process of parental grief, *Death Stud* 32:658–673, 2008.

Bliss JJ, Ogley-Oliver E, Jackson E et al: African American women's readiness to change abusive relationships, *J Family Violence* 23:161–171, 2008.

Burkhart L, Hogan N: An experiential theory of spiritual care in nursing practice, *Qual Health Res* 18(7):928–938, 2008.

Clukey L: Anticipatory mourning: processes of expected loss in palliative care, *Int J Palliat Nurs* 14(7):316–325, 2008.

Dale H, Hunt J: Perceived need for spiritual and religious treatment options in chronically ill individuals, *J Health Psychol* 13:712–718, 2008.

Demir F, Donmez YC, Ozsaker E et al: Patients' lived experiences of excisional breast biopsy: a phenomenological study, *J Clin Nurs* 17:744–751, 2008.

Jones RA, Utz S, Wenzel J et al: Use of complementary and alternative therapies by rural African Americans with Type 2 Diabetes, *Alt Ther* 12(5):34–38, 2006.

Ka'opua LS: Developing a culturally responsive breast cancer screening promotion with native Hawaiian women in churches, *Health Soc Work* 33(3):169–177, 2008.

Lhussier M, Carr SM, Wilcockson J: The evaluation of an end-of-life integrated care pathway, *Int J Palliat Nurs* 13(2):74–81, 2007.

Logan J, Hackbusch-Pinto R, De Grasse CE: Women undergoing breast diagnostics: the lived experience of spirituality, *Oncol Nurs Forum* 33(1):121–126, 2006.

Manii D, Ammerman D: Men and cancer: a study of the needs of male cancer patients in treatment, *J Psychosoc Oncol* 26(2):87–102, 2008.

McLeod DL, Wright LM: Living the as-yet unanswered: spiritual care practices in family systems nursing, *J Family Nurs* 14(1):118–141, 2008.

Meraviglia M: Effects of spirituality in breast cancer survivors, *Oncol Nurs Forum* 33(1):E1–E7, 2006.

Mystakidou K, Tsilika E, Parpa E et al: Demographic and clinical predictors of spirituality in advanced cancer patients: a randomized control study, *J Clin Nurs* 17(13):1779–1785, 2008.

Narayanasamy A: The impact of empirical studies of spirituality and culture on nurse education, *J Clin Nurs* 15:840–851, 2006.

Pierce LL, Steiner V, Havens H et al: Spirituality expressed by caregivers of stroke survivors, *West J Nurs Res* 30(5):606–619, 2008.

Prince-Paul M: Relationships among communicative acts, social well-being, and spiritual well-being on the quality of life at the end of life in patients with cancer enrolled in hospice, *J Palliat Med* 11(1):20–25, 2008.

Puterman J, Cadell S: Timing is everything: the experience of parental cancer for young adult daughters—a pilot study, *J Psychosoc Oncol* 26(2):103–121, 2008.

Shah SM, Ayash C, Pharaon NA et al: Arab American immigrants in New York: health care and cancer knowledge, attitudes, and beliefs, *J Immigr Min Health* 10:429–436, 2008.

Simoni JM, Frick PA, Huang BA: Longitudinal evaluation of a social support model of medication adherence among HIV-positive men and women on antiretroviral therapy, *Health Psychol* 25(1):74–81, 2006.

Taylor EJ: Prevalence and associated factors of spiritual needs among patients with cancer and family caregivers, *Oncol Nurs Forum* 33(4):729–735, 2006.

Taylor EJ, Mamier I: Spiritual care nursing: what cancer patients and family caregivers want, *J Adv Nurs* 49(3):260–267, 2005.

Trouillet R, Gana K: Age differences in temperament, character and depressive mood: a cross-sectional study, *Clin Psychol Psychother* 1:266–275, 2008.

Wachholtz AB, Pargament KI: Migraines and meditation: does spirituality matter? *J Behav Med* 31(4):351–366, 2008.

Yick AG: A metasynthesis of qualitative findings on the role of spirituality and religiosity among culturally diverse domestic violence survivors, *Qual Health Res* 18(9):1289–1306, 2008.

Yohannes AM, Koenig HG, Baldwin RC et al: Health behaviour, depression and religiosity in older patients admitted to intermediate care, *Int J Geriatr Psychiatry* 23:735–740, 2008.

Risk for Spiritual distress   *Betty J. Ackley, MSN, EdS, RN*

NANDA-I

Definition

At risk for an impaired ability to experience and integrate meaning and purpose in life through connectedness with self, others, art, music, literature, nature, and/or a power greater than oneself

Risk Factors

Developmental

Life changes

Environmental

Environmental changes; natural disasters

Physical

Chronic illness; physical illness; substance abuse

Psychosocial

Anxiety; blocks to experiencing love; change in religious rituals; change in spiritual practices; cultural conflict; depression; inability to forgive; loss; low self-esteem; poor relationships; racial conflict; separated support systems; stress

• = Independent   ▲ = Collaborative   **EBN** = Evidence-Based Nursing   **EB** = Evidence-Based

NOC, NIC, Client Outcomes, Nursing Interventions, *Rationales*, and References

Refer to care plan for **Spiritual distress.**

Readiness for enhanced Spiritual well-being   *Lisa Burkhart, PhD, RN*

NANDA-I

Definition

Ability to experience and integrate meaning and purpose in life through connectedness with self, others, art, music, literature, nature, and/or a power greater than oneself that can be strengthened

Defining Characteristics

Connections to Self

Expresses desire for enhanced acceptance; expresses desire for enhanced coping; expresses desire for enhanced courage; expresses desire for enhanced forgiveness of self; expresses desire for enhanced hope; expresses desire for enhanced joy; expresses desire for enhanced love; expresses desire for enhanced meaning in life; expresses desire for enhanced satisfying philosophy of life; expresses desire for enhanced surrender; expresses desire for enhanced serenity (e.g., peace); meditation

Connections with Others

Provides service to others; requests interactions with significant others; requests interaction with spiritual leaders; requests forgiveness of others

Connections with Art, Music, Literature, Nature

Displays creative energy (e.g., writing, poetry, singing); listens to music; reads spiritual literature; spends time outdoors

Connection with a Power Greater than Self

Expresses awe; expresses reverence; participates in religious activities; prays; reports mystical experiences

Related Factors (r/t)

Health-seeking behaviors; empathy; self-care; self-awareness; desire for harmonious interconnectedness; desire to find meaning and purpose in life

NOC   (Nursing Outcomes Classification)

Suggested NOC Outcomes

Personal Health Status, Coping, Dignified Life Closure, Grief Resolution, Hope, Personal Health Status, Psychosocial Adjustment: Life Change, Quality of Life, Social Involvement, Spiritual Health

Example NOC Outcome with Indicators
Hope as evidenced by the following indicators: Expresses expectation of a positive future orientation/Faith/Optimism/ Belief in self/Sense of meaning in life/Belief in others/Inner peace (Rate each indicator of **Hope:** 1 = never demonstrated, 2 = rarely demonstrated, 3 = sometimes demonstrated, 4 = often demonstrated, 5 = constantly demonstrated [see Section I].)

Client Outcomes

Client Will (Specify Time Frame):

- Express hope
- Express sense of meaning and purpose in life
- Express peace and serenity
- Express acceptance

• = Independent   ▲ = Collaborative   **EBN** = Evidence-Based Nursing   **EB** = Evidence-Based

- Express surrender
- Express forgiveness of self and others
- Express satisfaction with philosophy of life
- Express joy
- Express courage
- Describe being able to cope
- Describe use of spiritual practices
- Describe providing service to others
- Describe interaction with spiritual leaders, friends, and family
- Describe appreciation for art, music, literature, and nature

NIC (Nursing Interventions Classification)

Suggested NIC Interventions

Active Listening, Coping Enhancement, Counseling, Crisis Intervention, Decision-Making Support, Grief Work Facilitation, Hope Instillation, Meditation Facilitation, Mutual Goal Setting, Presence, Religious Ritual Enhancement, Imagery, Simple Relaxation Therapy, Socialization Enhancement, Spiritual Growth Facilitation, Spiritual Support, Support System Enhancement, Touch, Values Clarification

Example NIC Activities—Spiritual Support

Encourage use of spiritual resources if desired; Be available to listen to client's feelings

Nursing Interventions and *Rationales*

- Perform a spiritual assessment that includes the client's relationship with God, meaning and purpose in life, religious affiliation, and any other significant beliefs. **EBN:** *Descriptive study with 178 low-income, abused African American women revealed that spiritual well-being was associated with readiness to change (Bliss et al, 2008).*
- Be present and actively listen to the client. **EBN:** *In a grounded theory study, spiritual care included promoting client connectedness with self (Burkhart & Hogan, 2008).*
- Encourage the client to pray, setting the example by praying with and for the client. **EB:** *Spiritual practices are a coping mechanism to promote wellness and are part of leisure activity (Heintzman, 2008).* **EBN:** *Meraviglia (2006) found that prayer was associated with higher psychological well-being.*
- Encourage spiritual meditation exercises. **EB:** *Controlled study with 84 college students revealed that a spiritual mediation exercise significantly decreased anxiety and increased positive mood, spiritual health, spiritual experiences, and pain tolerance (Wachholtz & Pargament, 2005). Spiritual practices are a coping mechanism to promote wellness and are part of leisure activity (Heintzman, 2008).*
- Coordinate or encourage attending spiritual retreats or courses. **EB:** *Controlled study pre-post test design of 46 students who attended a spirituality course significantly increased their spiritual well-being (Bethel, 2004). Spiritual practices are a coping mechanism to promote wellness and are part of leisure activity (Heintzman, 2008).*
- Promote hope. **EBN:** *Descriptive study of 130 older adults in a suburban senior center correlated spiritual health with more well-being and hope (Davis, 2005).*
- Encourage clients to reflect on what is meaningful to them in life. **EBN:** *Reflection & storytelling among adolescents helps find meaning in bereavement therapy and can lead to spiritual growth (Leighton, 2008).*
- Encourage involvement in group religious practices. **EBN:** *Spiritual practices are a coping mechanism to promote wellness and are part of leisure activity (Heintzman, 2008).*
- Encourage increased quality of life through social support and family relationships. **EBN and EB:** *In a heurmineutic qualitative study, spiritual care is one type of relational or dialogic practice among families, particularly when discussing meaning related to suffering (McLeod & Wright, 2008).*
- Assist the client in identifying religious or spiritual beliefs that encourage integration of meaning and purpose in the client's life. **EBN:** *Spiritual practices are a coping mechanism to promote wellness and are part of leisure activity (Heintzman, 2008).*

● = Independent   ▲ = Collaborative   **EBN** = Evidence-Based Nursing   **EB** = Evidence-Based

- Encourage the client to engage regularly in bibliotherapy. **EBN:** *Spiritual practices are a coping mechanism to promote wellness and are part of leisure activity (Heintzman, 2008).*
- Support meditation, guided imagery, therapeutic touch, journaling, relaxation, and involvement in art, music, or poetry. Support outdoor activities. **EB:** *In a randomized control trial, a spiritual meditation intervention was associated with fewer migraine headaches, less anxiety and a greater pain tolerance, headache-related self-efficacy, daily spiritual experiences, and existential well-being (Wachholtz & Pargament, 2008).* **EBN:** *In a qualitative study of stroke caregivers, being one with nature emerged as a theme (Pierce et al, 2008). In a qualitative survey of chronically ill individuals, participants wanted access to a garden, a quiet space available in hospital to think through decision, spiritual help or guidance, swimming, and a choice of genres of music available (Dale & Hunt, 2008).*
- Encourage expressions of spirituality. **EBN:** *In a sample of 203 African American professional women, 97% rated spirituality as a coping mechanism to deal with stress (Bacchus, 2008). A phenomenology study revealed that spirituality helps women with end-stage renal disease accept, understand, and control emotions, and provide inner strength in living with renal disease (Tanyi & Werner, 2008).*
- Encourage integration of spirituality in healthy lifestyle choices. **EBN:** *Descriptive study of 256 high school students correlated spiritual health with better self care initiative and responsibility (Callaghan, 2005).*

Geriatric

- Discuss personal definitions of spiritual wellness with the client. **EB:** *In a cross-sectional study of older adults, intrinsic religious activity was associated with older age, being female, and living situation (Yohannes et al, 2008).* **EBN:** *Narayanasamy (2006) found that nurses identified client needs in older clients by assessing religious beliefs and practice (prayer), absolution, seeking connection, comfort and reassurance, healing or searching for meaning or purpose.*
- Identify the client's past sources of spirituality. Help the client explore his or her life and identify those experiences that are noteworthy. Clients may want to read the Bible or other religious text or have it read to them. **EB:** *A cross-sectional study of individuals living in the community revealed that as people age, spirituality is more important (Trouillet & Gana, 2008). In a cross-sectional study of older adults, religious attendance was associated with positive general health perception, and inversely associated with pack/year smoked, and severity of illness (Yohannes et al, 2008).* **EBN:** *In a qualitative study of stroke caregivers, interacting with family and friends emerged as a theme (Pierce et al, 2008).*

Multicultural

- Assess for the influence of cultural beliefs, norms, and values on the client's ability to cope with spiritual distress. **EB:** *Arab American immigrants are fatalistic in that they believe that cancer is a punishment from God and prognosis was determined by God (Shah et al, 2008). In a semistructured interview with Hawaiian women in churches, integrating religious and spiritual practices in health promotion were viewed as important in promoting breast cancer screening (Ka'opua, 2008).*
- Encourage spirituality as a source of support. **EBN:** *African Americans and Latinos may identify spirituality, religiousness, prayer, and church-based approaches as coping resources (Simoni, Frick, & Huang, 2006). Descriptive study with 178 low-income, abused African American women revealed that spiritual well-being was associated with readiness to change (Bliss et al, 2008). A qualitative study with African Americans living in rural areas revealed that spirituality/religion/prayer were helpful in coping, encouraged healthy lifestyles, and helps care providers (Jones et al, 2006).* **EBN:** *Spirituality is a significant cultural experience and belief that influences the health behaviors of African Americans (Lewis, 2008).*
- Validate the client's spiritual concerns and convey respect for his or her beliefs. **EBN:** *In a meta-analysis of qualitative research on domestic violence survivors, spirituality and religiosity plays an important role and that role may differ based on culture (Yick, 2008).*

Home Care

- All of the nursing interventions described previously apply in the home setting.

evolve   See the EVOLVE website for Weblinks for client education resources.

• = Independent   ▲ = Collaborative   **EBN** = Evidence-Based Nursing   **EB** = Evidence-Based

REFERENCES

Bacchus DN: Coping with work-related stress: a study of the use of coping resources among professional black women, *J Ethnic Cult Divers Soc Work* 17(1):60–81, 2008.

Bethel JC: Impact of social work spirituality courses on student attitudes, values, and spiritual wellness, *J Relig Spirituality Soc Work* 23(4):27–45, 2004.

Bliss JJ, Ogley-Oliver E, Jackson E et al: African American women's readiness to change abusive relationships, *J Family Violence* 23:161–171, 2008.

Burkhart L, Hogan N: An experiential theory of spiritual care in nursing practice, *Qual Health Res* 18(7):928–938, 2008.

Callaghan DM: The influence of spiritual growth on adolescents' initiative and responsibility for self-care, *Pediatr Nurs* 31(2):91–95, 115, 2005.

Dale H, Hunt J: Perceived need for spiritual and religious treatment options in chronically ill individuals, *J Health Psychol* 13:712–718, 2008.

Davis B: Mediators of the relationship between hope and well-being in older adults, *Clin Nurs Res* 14(3):253–272, 2005.

Heintzman P: Leisure-spiritual coping: a model for therapeutic recreation and leisure services, *Ther Rec J* 42(1):56–73, 2008.

Jones RA, Utz S, Wenzel J et al: Use of complementary and alternative therapies by rural African Americans with type 2 diabetes, *Alt Ther* 12(5):34–38, 2006.

Ka'opua LS: Developing a culturally responsive breast cancer screening promotion with native Hawaiian women in churches, *Health Soc Work* 33(3):169–177, 2008.

Leighton S: Bereavement therapy with adolescents: facilitating a process of spiritual growth, *J Child Adolesc Psychiatr Nurs* 21(1):24–34, 2008.

Lewis LM: Spiritual assessment in African-Americans: a review of measures of spirituality used in health research, *J Relig Health* 47(4):458–475, 2008.

McLeod DL, Wright LM: Living the as-yet unanswered: spiritual care practices in family systems nursing, *J Family Nurs* 14(1):118–141, 2008.

Meraviglia M: Effects of spirituality in breast cancer survivors, *Oncol Nurs Forum* 33(1):E1–E7, 2006.

Narayanasamy A: The impact of empirical studies of spirituality and culture on nurse education, *J Clin Nurs* 15:840–851, 2006.

Pierce LL, Steiner V, Havens H et al: Spirituality expressed by caregivers of stroke survivors, *West J Nurs Res* 30(5):606–619, 2008.

Shah SM, Ayash C, Pharaon NA et al: Arab American immigrants in New York: health care and cancer knowledge, attitudes, and beliefs, *J Immigr Min Health* 10:429–436, 2008.

Simoni JM, Frick PA, Huang BA: Longitudinal evaluation of a social support model of medication adherence among HIV-positive men and women on antiretroviral therapy, *Health Psychol* 25(1):74–81, 2006.

Tanyi RA, Werner JS: Women's experience of spirituality within end-stage renal disease and hemodialysis, *Clin Nurs Res* 17(1):32–49, 2008.

Trouillet R, Gana K: Age differences in temperament, character and depressive mood: a cross-sectional study, *Clin Psychol Psychother* 1:266–275, 2008.

Wachholtz AB, Pargament KI: Migraines and meditation: does spirituality matter? *J Behav Med* 31(4):351–366, 2008.

Yick AG: A metasynthesis of qualitative findings on the role of spirituality and religiosity among culturally diverse domestic violence survivors, *Qual Health Res* 18(9):1289–1306, 2008.

Yohannes AM, Koenig HG, Baldwin RC et al: Health behaviour, depression and religiosity in older patients admitted to intermediate care, *Int J Geriatr Psychiatry* 23:735–740, 2008.

Stress overload   June M. Como, RN, MSA, MS, CCRN, CCNS   ⓔvolve

NANDA-I

Definition

Excessive amounts and types of demands that require action

Defining Characteristics

Demonstrates increased feelings of anger; demonstrates increased feelings of impatience; expresses difficulty in functioning; expresses a feeling of pressure; expresses a feeling of tension; expresses increased feelings of anger; expresses increased feelings of impatience; expresses problems with decision making; reports negative impact from stress (e.g., physical symptoms, psychological distress, feeling of being sick or of going to get sick); reports excessive situational stress (e.g., rates stress level as 7 or above on a 10–point scale)

Related Factors (r/t)

Inadequate resources (e.g., financial, social, education/knowledge level); intense stressors (e.g., family violence, chronic illness, terminal illness); multiple coexisting stressors (e.g., environmental threats/demands; physical threats/demands; social threats/demands); repeated stressors (e.g., family violence, chronic illness, terminal illness)

NOC   (Nursing Outcomes Classification)

Suggested NOC Outcomes

Acceptance Health Status, Family Coping, Stress Level, Coping

• = Independent   ▲ = Collaborative   **EBN** = Evidence-Based Nursing   **EB** = Evidence-Based

Client Outcomes

Client Will (Specify Time Frame):

- Review the amounts and types of stressors in daily living
- Identify stressors that can be modified or eliminated
- Mobilize social supports to facilitate lower stress levels
- Reduce stress levels through use of health promoting behaviors and other strategies

 (Nursing Interventions Classification)

Suggested NIC Interventions

Active Listening, Anger Control Assistance, Anxiety Reduction, Aroma Therapy, Counseling, Crisis Intervention, Emotional Support, Family Integrity Promotion, Presence, Support System Enhancement

Example NIC Activities—Support System Enhancement
Assess psychological response to situation and availability of support system; Determine adequacy of social networks; Explain to concerned others how they can help; Refer to a self-help group, as appropriate; Provide services in a caring and supportive manner

Nursing Interventions and *Rationales*

- Assist client in identification of stress overload during vulnerable life events. **EB:** *Women with breast cancer who were involved in group therapy focusing on stress reduction and muscle relaxation were 56% less likely to succumb to the disease and 45% less likely to experience a recurrence (Andersen et al, 2008). Men with high stress have higher all-cause mortality, the effects being more pronounced among middle-aged men (Nielsen et al, 2008). A review of the literature from 1970 through 2006 suggests that 80% of all illnesses are stress induced (Walling, 2006).*
- Listen actively to descriptions of stressors and the stress response. **EBN:** *Developing nurse-client partnerships is the best way to obtain valid & reliable information related to stress overload (Lunney, 2006). In a qualitative study of older African American women the researcher found that descriptions of lifelong and recent incidents of stress were perceived by the respondents as having contributed to their current early-stage heart disease (Warren-Findlow, 2006).*
- In younger adult women, assess interpersonal stressors. **EB:** *Complex posttraumatic stress disorders and related extreme stress was assessed in a qualitative/quantitative study of 14 assaulted women with a mean age of 38. A high sense of coherence enabled these women to leave their abusive relationships (Scheffer & Renck, 2008).*
- Categorize stressors as modifiable or nonmodifiable. **EBN:** *Removing or minimizing some stressors, changing responses to stressors, and modifying the long-term effects of stress are all actions that can assist those with diabetes and stress (Lloyd, Smith, & Weinger, 2005).*
- Help clients modify or mitigate stressors identified as modifiable. **EBN:** *There are numerous possible strategies to modify stressors, including time management, improved organizational skills, problems solving, changing perceptions of stress, breathing, relaxation techniques, visual imagery, soothing rituals (Motzer & Hertig, 2004; Lloyd, Smith, & Weinger, 2005). Interventions that are person-directed (cognitive-behavioral approaches) versus work-directed may result in reductions in stress, burnout, and anxiety in health care workers (Marine et al, 2006).*
- Help clients distinguish between short-term, chronic, and secondary stressors. **EBN:** *Caregiver role overload exacerbates secondary stressors whereas socioeconomic support may ameliorate those stressors (Gaugler et al, 2008). Social support is a critical dimension of health and health promotion and serves as a buffer in the stress response (Pender, Murtaugh, & Parsons, 2006).* **EB:** *The frequency of stressful*

health-related events, not health-unrelated events, is associated with all-cause mortality (Phillips, Der, & Carroll, 2008).

- Provide information as needed to reduce stress responses to acute and chronic illnesses. **EBN:** *Information provided to critical care clients through the use of tactile touch interventions led to significantly lower levels of anxiety as evident by reductions in circulatory parameters (Henricson et al, 2008). Supporting the individual adaptation through facilitation of cognitive processes that help the person achieve congruence in meaning mediates the threatening effects of incongruence between situational and global meaning (Skaggs & Barron, 2006).*

- Explore possible therapeutic approaches such as cognitive behavior therapy, biofeedback, neurofeedback, acupuncture, pharmacologic agents, and complementary and alternative therapies. **EBN:** *Neurofeedback promotes optimum functioning of the central nervous system, induces relaxation, and supports healthy balance, flexibility, and resilience (Brown, 2007). Adults who had experienced hospitalizations of at least 5 days said that spirituality strengthened their coping ability (Cavendish et al, 2006). Therapeutic techniques such as acupuncture may improve levels of wellness through direct homeostatic stabilization of the autonomic nervous system (Walling, 2006).*

- Help the client to reframe his or her perceptions of some of the stressors. **EB:** *Study findings of 73 people with rheumatoid arthritis suggests that individuals high in personal mastery may be more susceptible to the effects of stress, experiences of pain, and fatigue (Younger et al, 2008). Supporting stressed families with children in addition to recommending health promoting behavior may reduce the risk for childhood obesity (Koch, Sepa, & Ludvigsson, 2008).*

- Assist the client to mobilize social supports for dealing with recent stressors. **EBN:** *Emotional support in Taiwanese caregivers is suggested as a moderator of stressors experienced by caregivers of clients with Alzheimer's disease or stroke, particularly in caregivers with lower household incomes (Huang et al, 2009). **EB:** Social support moderates the impact of recent but not chronic life stress on physical symptom reporting (Cropley & Steptoe, 2005). In a secondary analysis of data caregivers who maintained balance in their lives by taking breaks from the caregiving role experience a decrease in caregiving stressors (Knussen et al, 2008).*

Pediatric

- With children, nurses should work with parents to help them to reduce children's stressors. **EB:** *A comprehensive review of research on stress and coping in childhood showed that parents can have profound effects on reducing the stressors of childhood (Power, 2004). **EBN:** School-related stressors are one of the most significant sources of stress overload (Ryan-Wenger, Sharrer, & Campbell, 2005).*

- Help children to manage their feelings related to self-concept. **EBN:** *Events that affected self-concept were shown to be significant stressors for children (Ryan-Wenger, Sharrer, & Campbell, 2005).*

- Help children to deal with bullies and other sources of violence in schools and neighborhoods. **EBN:** *Violence in schools and neighborhoods has significant effects on children's stress. Children can be taught how to deal with bullies (Ryan-Wenger, Sharrer, & Campbell, 2005).*

- Help young children to identify and mitigate the experience of "feeling sick." **EBN:** *"Feeling sick" is described most often as a stressor. This was related to children's lack of knowledge and experience with illnesses (Taxis et al, 2004).*

- Help children to manage the complexities of chronic illnesses. **EBN:** *Teenagers who had recently been diagnosed with diabetes described high levels of stress that often related to the complexities of managing the illness (Davidson et al, 2004).*

Geriatric

- Assess for chronic stress with older adults and provide a variety of stress relief techniques. *With advancing age, stressors are more likely to be chronic and may have negative effects on memory and cognitive decline; thus, chronic stressors should be reduced through a variety of strategies (Vondras et al, 2005).*

- Encourage social support for older adults. **EB:** *Bereavement-related major depression differs from major depression seen in other stressful life events only in relation to older age at onset, individuals are more likely to be female, lower levels of treatment-seeking, higher levels of guilt, fatigue, and loss of* *interest and therefore should not be excluded from a diagnosis of major depression (Kendler, Myers, & Zisook, 2008).*

Multicultural

- Review cultural beliefs and acculturation level in relation to perceived stressors. **EBN:** *In a study of Arab migrant workers in Germany it was found that 90% were psychologically stressed. High stress scores were associated with older age, less education, number of children, country of origin, length of time in Germany, health status, and negative perceptions of immigrant status (Irfaeya, Maxwell, & Kramer, 2008).* **EB:** *Group treatment that includes cognitive differentiation and restructuring, identity reframing, depersonalization discrimination, faulty beliefs rejection, and psychosocial education is an effective approach to working with individuals dealing with race-related stressors (Loo, Ueda, & Morton, 2007).*
- Assess families for whether they experience high stress or low stress. **EBN:** *High stress in Lebanese families, often related to war and other community-based factors, was associated with family health (Farhood, 2004).* **EB:** *Stress related to racial microaggressions experienced by African Americans may have a negative cumulative effect on health outcomes (Sue et al, 2009).*
- Support social connectedness among cultural groups. **EBN:** *High social connectedness was associated with low stress in children (Taxis et al, 2004).*

Home Care

- The above interventions may be adapted for home care use.
- Develop community-based programs for stress management as needed for groups with increased risk of stress overload (e.g., firefighters, policeman, military personnel, and nurses). **EB:** *Some situations have higher risks of stress overload. Stress management interventions may prevent or modify the experience of stress overload (McNulty, 2005).*
- Support and encourage neighborhood stability. **EB:** *A "significant proportion of health differentials across neighborhoods is due to disparate stress levels across [Detroit] neighborhoods" and neighborhood stability was a buffer to reduce the negative effects of high stress (Boardman, 2004).*

Client/Family Teaching and Discharge Planning

- Diagnose the possibility of stress overload before teaching.
- Establish readiness for learning.
- Provide manageable amounts of information at the appropriate educational level.
- Evaluate the need for additional teaching and learning experiences.

ⓔvolve   See the EVOLVE website for Weblinks for client education resources.

REFERENCES

Andersen B, Yang H, Farrar WB et al: Psychologic intervention improves survival for breast cancer, *Cancer* 113(12):3450–3458, 2008.

Boardman JD: Stress and physical health: the role of neighborhoods as mediating and moderating mechanisms, *Soc Sci Med* 58(12):2473–2483, 2004.

Brown V: *KARMA or DHARMA: three acronyms that can clarify the core of neurofeedback training, at least in Neurocare.* Paper presented at Conference on Future Health, January 2007, Palm Springs, CA.

Cavendish R, Naradovy L, Como J et al: Patients' perceptions of spirituality and the nurse as a spiritual care provider, *Holistic Nurs Pract* 20:41–47, 2006.

Cropley M, Steptoe A: Social support, life events and physical symptoms: a prospective study of chronic and recent life stress in men and women, *Psychol Health Med* 10:317–325, 2005.

Davidson M, Penney ED, Muller B et al: Stressors and self-care challenges faced by adolescents living with type 1 diabetes, *Appl Nurs Res* 2:72–80, 2004.

Farhood LF: The impact of high and low stress on the health of Lebanese families, *Res Theory Nurs Pract* 18(2–3):197–212, 2004.

Gaugler JE, Linder J, Given CW et al: The proliferation of primary cancer caregiving stress to secondary stress, *Cancer Nurs* 31(2):116–123, 2008.

Henricson M, Resson A, Maatta S et al: The outcome of tactile touch on stress parameters in intensive care: a randomized controlled trial, *Complement Ther Clin Pract* 14(4):244–254, 2008.

Huang C, Sousa VD, Perng S et al: Stressors, social support, depressive symptoms and general health status of Taiwanese caregivers of persons with stroke or Alzheimer's disease, *J Clin Nurs* 18(4):502–511, 2009.

Irfaeya M, Maxwell AE, Kramer A: Assessing psychological stress among Arab migrant women in the city of Cologne/Germany using the Community Oriented Primary Care (COPC) approach, *J Immigrant Minority Health* 10(4):337–344, 2008.

• = Independent   ▲ = Collaborative   **EBN** = Evidence-Based Nursing   **EB** = Evidence-Based

Kendler K, Myers J, Zisook MD: Does bereavement-related major depression differ from major depression associated with other stressful life events? *Am J Psychiatry* 165(11):1449–1455, 2008

Knussen C, Tolson D, Brogan CA et al: Family caregivers of older relatives; ways of coping and change in distress: *Psychol Health Med* 13(3):274–290, 2008.

Koch F, Sepa A, Ludvigsson J: Psychological stress and obesity, *J Ped* 153(6):839–844, 2008.

Lloyd C, Smith J, Weinger K: Stress and diabetes: a review of the links, *Diabetes Spectr* 18(2):121–127, 2005.

Loo CM, Ueda SS, Morton RK: Group treatment for race-related stresses among minority Vietnam veterans, *Transcult Psychiatry* 44(1):115–135, 2007.

Lunney M: Stress overload: a new diagnosis, *Int J Nrs Term Class*17 (4):165–176, 2006.

Marine A, Ruotsalainen JH, Serra C et al: Preventing occupational stress in healthcare workers, *Cochrane Database Syst Rev* (4):CD002892, 2006.

McNulty PAF: Reported stressors and health care needs of active duty Navy personnel during three phases of deployment in support of the war in Iraq, *Mil Med* 170:530–535, 2005.

Motzer SA, Hertig V: Stress, stress response and health, *Nurs Clin North Am* 39:1–17, 2004.

Nielsen NR, Kristensen TS, Schnohr P et al: Perceived stress and cause-specific mortality among men and women: results from a prospective cohort study, *Am J Epidemiol* 168(5):492–496, 2008.

Pender NJ, Murtaugh CL, Parsons MA: *Health promotion in nursing practice*, ed 5, Upper Saddle River, NJ, 2006, Prentice Hall.

Phillips AC, Der G, Carroll D: Stressful life-events exposure is associated with 17–year mortality, but it is health-related events that prove predictive, *Br J Health Psychol* 13(Pt 4):647–657, 2008.

Power TG: Stress and coping in childhood: the parents' role, *Parenting: Sci Pract* 4:271–317, 2004.

Ryan-Wenger NA, Sharrer VW, Campbell KK: Changes in children's stressors over the past 30 years, *Pediatr Nurs* 31(4):282–291, 2005.

Scheffer LM, Renck B: "It is still so deep seated, the fear": psychological stress reactions as consequences of intimate partner violence, *J Psychiatr Ment Health Nurs* 15(3):219–226, 2008.

Skaggs BG, Barron CR: Searching for meaning in negative events: Concept analysis, *J Adv Nurse* 53(5):559–570, 2006.

Sue DW, Capodilupo CM, Torino GC et al: Racial microaggressions in everyday life, *Amery Psychol* 62(4):271–286, 2009.

Taxis JC, Rew L, Jackson K et al: Protective resources and perceptions of stress in a multi-ethnic sample of school-age children, *Pediatr Nurs* 30:477–487, 2004.

Vondras DD, Powless MR, Olson AK et al: Differential effects of everyday stress on the episodic memory test performances of young, mid-life, and older adults, *Aging Ment Health* 9(1):60–70, 2005.

Walling A: Therapeutic modulation of psychoneuroimmune system by medical acupuncture creates feelings of well-being, *J Am Acad Nurse Pract* 18(4):135–143, 2006.

Warren-Findlow J: Weathering: stress and heart disease in African American women living in Chicago, *Qual Health Res* 16(2):221–237, 2006.

Younger J, Finan P, Zautra A et al: Personal mastery predicts pain, stress, fatigue, and blood pressure in adults with rheumatoid arthritis, *Psychol Health* 23(5):515–535, 2008.

Risk for Suffocation   *Nadine M. Aktan, PhD, RN, FNP-BC, and Betty J. Ackley, MSN, EdS, RN*

 NANDA-I

Definition

Accentuated risk of accidental suffocation (inadequate air available for inhalation)

Risk Factors

External

Discarding refrigerators without removing doors; eating large mouthfuls of food; hanging a pacifier around infant's neck; household gas leaks; inserting small objects into airway; leaving children unattended in water; low-strung clothesline; pillow placed in infant's crib; playing with plastic bags; propped bottle placed in infant's crib; smoking in bed; use of fuel-burning heaters not vented to outside; vehicle warming in closed garage

Internal

Cognitive difficulties; disease process; emotional difficulties; injury process; lack of safety education; lack of safety precautions; reduced motor abilities; reduced olfactory sensation

 NOC   **(Nursing Outcomes Classification)**

Suggested NOC Outcomes

Knowledge: Child Physical Safety, Personal Safety, Parenting: Adolescent Physical Safety, Early/Middle Childhood Physical Safety, Infant/Toddler Physical Safety, Risk Control, Risk Detection, Safe Home Environment, Substance Addiction Consequences

---

• = Independent   ▲ = Collaborative   **EBN** = Evidence-Based Nursing   **EB** = Evidence-Based

---

Example **NOC** Outcome with Indicators
Knowledge: Child Physical Safety as evidenced by the following indicators: Strategies to prevent choking/Appropriate activities for child's developmental level/First aid techniques (Rate the outcome and indicators of **Knowledge: Child Physical Safety:** 1 = no knowledge, 2 = limited knowledge, 3 = moderate knowledge, 4 = substantial knowledge, 5 = extensive knowledge [see Section I].)

Client Outcomes

Client Will (Specify Time Frame):

- Undertake appropriate measures to prevent suffocation
- Demonstrate correct techniques for emergency rescue maneuvers (e.g., Heimlich maneuver, rescue breathing, cardiopulmonary resuscitation [CPR]) and describe situations that require them

 NIC   (Nursing Interventions Classification)

Suggested NIC Interventions

Aspiration Precautions, Environmental Management: Safety, Infant Care, Positioning, Security Enhancement, Surveillance, Surveillance: Safety, Teaching: Infant Safety

Example **NIC** Activities—Environmental Management: Safety
Identify safety hazards in the environment (i.e., physical, biological, and chemical); Remove hazards from the environment, when possible

Nursing Interventions and *Rationales*

- Identify hospitalized clients at particular risk for suffocation, including the following:
  - Clients with altered levels of consciousness
  - Infants or young children
  - Clients with developmental delays
  - Clients with mental illness, especially schizophrenia

  Institute safety measures such as proper positioning and feeding precautions. See the care plans for **Risk for Aspiration** *and* **Impaired Swallowing** *for additional interventions. Vigilance and special protective measures are necessary for clients at greater risk for suffocation.* **EB:** *Mental health clients have an increased incidence of choking and suffocation incidents (Corcoran & Walsh, 2003).*

 Pediatric

- Counsel families on the following:
  - Follow general safety practices such as not smoking in bed, not smoking during pregnancy, not smoking in the presence of an infant, properly disposing of large appliances, using properly functioning heating systems and ventilation, having functional smoke and carbon monoxide detectors, and opening garage doors when warming up a car.
  - Position infants on their back to sleep; do not position them in the prone position. **EB:** *Research has demonstrated that the prone position for sleeping infants is a risk factor for sudden infant death syndrome (SIDS) (Li et al, 2003; Malloy & Freeman, 2004). Population studies have demonstrated a striking trend in decreased incidence of SIDS since parents have been taught to not place infants in the prone position (Dwyer & Ponsonby, 2009).*
  - Avoid use of loose bedding such as blankets and sheets for sleeping. If blankets are used, they should be tucked in around the crib mattress so the infant's face is less likely to become covered by bedding. The blanket should end at the level of the infant's chest (American Academy of Pediatrics, 2000). *A study of infants who were found dead in bassinetts found that soft bedding was found in 74% of the cases (Pike & Moon, 2008).*
- Place the infant in an approved crib for sleeping, not on an adult bed, sofa, chair, or playpen. *Babies can suffocate when their faces become wedged against or buried in a mattress, pillow, infant cushion, or other soft bedding or when someone in the same bed rolls over onto them (Safe Kids, USA, 2008).*

● = Independent   ▲ = Collaborative   **EBN** = Evidence-Based Nursing   **EB** = Evidence-Based

- Teach parents not to sleep with an infant, especially if alcohol or medications/illicit drugs are used by the parents. **EB:** *Mothers who consumed three or more alcoholic drinks in the past 24 hours increased the risk of SIDS when bed sharing with an infant (Carpenter et al, 2004). The rates of accidental suffocation and strangulation in children in bed have quadrupled since 1984 (Shapiro-Mendoza et al, 2009).* **EBN:** *In a study of mothers of 3–month-old infants, 39 of almost 300 mothers reported incidences when they had rolled partially or fully over the infant in the bed (Ateah & Hamelin, 2008).*
- Assess for signs and symptoms of abuse such as Munchausen syndrome by proxy (MSBP). **EB:** *Suffocation in MSBP is one important differential diagnosis in suspected cases of SIDS (Vennemann et al, 2005).*
- Conduct risk factor identification, noting special circumstances in which preventive or protective measures are indicated. Note the presence of environmental hazards, including the following: plastic bags (e.g., dry cleaner's bags, bags used for mattress protection)/cribs with slats wider than 2 inches/ill-fitting crib mattresses that can allow the infant to become wedged between the mattress and crib/pillows in cribs/abandoned large appliances such as refrigerators, dishwashers, or freezers/clothing with cords or hoods that can become entangled/bibs, pacifiers on a string, drapery cords, pull-toy strings. *Suffocation by airway obstruction is a leading cause of death in children younger than 6 years of age. Families need to be taught child protection.*
- Counsel families to not serve these foods to the child younger than 4 years of age: hot dogs, popcorn, nuts, pretzels, chips, chunks of meat, hard pieces of fruit or vegetables, raisins, whole grapes, hard candies, marshmallows *Hot dogs are the most common item associated with fatal choking incidences in children (Kliegman, Behrman, & Jenson, 2007).* **EB:** *Children between the ages of 4 and 36 months of age are at risk for suffocation by hollow, semi-rigid hemispherical/ellipsoidal objects through suction formation and complete airway obstruction (Nakamura, Pollack-Nelson, & Chidekel, 2003).*
- Counsel families to keep these items away from infants and toddlers: balloons/coins/marbles/toys with small parts, or toys that can be compressed to fit entirely into a child's mouth, small balls, pen or market caps, small button-type batteries, and medicine syringes (Safe Kids, USA, 2008).
- Provide information to parents about obtaining the small parts tester, also known as a choke tube; if an object fits in the tube, it is too small to give to a child (Safe Kids, USA, 2007). **EB:** *Rigid items that are of a spherical or cylindrical shape can cause upper airway occlusion (Nakamura, Pollack-Nelson, & Chidekel, 2003). Accidental suffocation can result from the aspiration of a foreign body with airway occlusion (Bajanowski et al, 2005).*
- Stress water and pool safety precautions, including vigilant, uninterrupted parental supervision. *An intense drive for exploration combined with a lack of awareness of danger makes drowning a threat to small children. A child's high center of gravity and poor coordination make buckets and toilets a threat because a child looking inside can fall over and become lodged (Kliegman, Behrman, & Jenson, 2007). Pools should be surrounded completely by fencing that is difficult to climb and that does not allow direct access to the house, and gates should have self-closing latches (Schnitzer, 2006).*
- Underscore the necessity of not allowing children to play with or near electric garage doors and of keeping garage door openers out of the reach of young children. *Children close to the ground may not be large enough to trigger reversal mechanisms on the door and may become trapped.*
- For adolescents, watch for signs of depression that could result in suicide by suffocation. **EB:** *For adolescents 10 to 19 years of age, suffocation by hanging is the second most common method of suicide (CDC, 2004).*

Geriatric

- Assess the status of the swallow reflex. Offer appropriate foods and beverages accordingly. *The elderly, especially those receiving antipsychotic medications, have an increased incidence of choking.*
- Observe the client for pocketing of food in the side of the mouth; remove food as needed.
- Position the client in high Fowler's position when eating and for 1 hour afterward. *Elderly clients may be at risk for suffocation that results from dysphagia.*
- Use care in pillow placement when positioning frail elderly clients who are on bed rest. *Frail elderly clients are at risk for suffocation if the head becomes lodged against pillows and the client cannot reposition them because of weakness.*

Home Care

- Assess the home for potential safety hazards in systems that are not likely to be fixed (e.g., faulty pilot lights or gas leaks in gas stoves, carbon monoxide release from heating systems, kerosene fumes from portable heaters). Assist the family in having these areas assessed and making appropriate safety arrangements (e.g., installing detectors, making repairs). *Assessment and correction of system problems prevent accidental suffocation.*

Client/Family Teaching and Discharge Planning

- Recommend that families who are seeking day care or in-home care for children, geriatric family members, or at-risk family members with developmental or functional disabilities inspect the environment for hazards and examine the first aid preparation and vigilance of providers. *Many working families must trust others to care for family members.*
- Involve family members in learning and practicing rescue techniques, including treatment of choking and lack of breathing, as well as CPR. Initiate referral to formal training classes. *Family members need adequate preparation to deal with emergency situations and should take part in the American Heart Association Basic Lifesaving Course or the American Red Cross Infant/Child CPR Course (CDC, 2002).*

ⓔvolve See the EVOLVE website for Weblinks for client education resources.

REFERENCES

American Academy of Pediatrics, Task Force on Infant Sleep Position and Sudden Infant Death Syndrome: Changing concepts of sudden infant death syndrome: implications for infant sleeping environment and sleep position, *Pediatrics* 105(3):650, 2000.

Ateah CA, Hamelin KJ: Maternal bedsharing practices, experiences, and awareness of risks, *J Obstet Gynecol Neonatal Nurs* 37(3):274–281, 2008.

Bajanowski T, Vennemann B, Bohnert M et al: Unnatural causes of sudden unexpected deaths initially thought to be SIDS, *Int J Legal Med* 119:213–216, 2005.

Carpenter RG, Irgens LM, Blair PS et al: Sudden unexplained infant death in 20 regions in Europe: case control study, *Lancet* 363(9404):185, 2004.

Centers for Disease Control and Prevention (CDC): Methods of suicide among persons aged 10–19 years—United States, 1992–2001, *MMWR Morb Mort Wkly Rep* 53(22):471, 2004.

Centers for Disease Control and Prevention (CDC): Nonfatal choking-related episodes among children—United States, 2001, *MMWR Morb Mort Wkly Rep* 51(42):945–948, 2002.

Corcoran E, Walsh D: Obstructive asphyxia: a cause of excess mortality in psychiatric patients, *Ir J Psychol Med* 20(3):88–90, 2003.

Dwyer T, Ponsonby AL: Sudden infant death syndrome and prone sleeping position. *Ann Epidemiol* 19(4):245–249, 2009.

Kliegman RM, Behrman R, Jenson HB: *Nelson textbook of pediatrics*, ed 18, Philadelphia, 2007, Saunders.

Li DK, Petitti DB, Willinger M et al: Infant sleeping position and the risk of sudden infant death syndrome in California, 1997–2000, *Am J Epidemiol* 157(5):446, 2003.

Malloy MH, Freeman DH: Age at death, season, and day of death as indicators of the effect of the back to sleep program on sudden infant death syndrome in the United States, 1992–1999, *Arch Pediatr Adolesc Med* 158(4):359–365, 2004.

Nakamura S, Pollack-Nelson C, Chidekel A: Suction-type suffocation incidents in infants and toddlers, *Pediatrics* 111(1):12–16, 2003.

Pike J, Moon RY. Bassinet use and sudden unexpected death in infancy, *J Pediatr* 153(4):509–512, 2008.

Safe Kids, USA. Toy Safety. http://sk.convio.net/site/PageNavigator/Campaigns/ToySafety/campaignToySafetyGuide, 2007. Accessed May 29, 2009.

Safe Kids, USA. Protecting Kids from Choking, Suffocation and Strangulation, 2008, www.usa.safekids.org/tier3_cd.cfm?folder_id=301&content_item_id=26551. Accessed May 29, 2009.

Schnitzer PG: Prevention of unintentional childhood injuries, *Am Fam Physician* 74(11):1864–1869, 2006.

Shapiro-Mendoza CK, Kimball M, Tomashek KM et al: US infant mortality trends attributable to accidental suffocation and strangulation in bed from 1984 through 2004: are rates increasing? *Pediatrics* 123(2):533–539, 2009.

Vennemann B, Bajanowski T, Karger B et al: Suffocation and poisoning—the hard hitting side of Munchausen syndrome by proxy, *Int J Legal Med* 119:98–102, 2005.

Risk for Suicide   *Kathleen L. Patusky, PhD, APRN-BC*   ⓔvolve

 NANDA-I

Definition

At risk for self-inflicted, life-threatening injury

• = Independent   ▲ = Collaborative   **EBN** = Evidence-Based Nursing   **EB** = Evidence-Based

Related Factors (r/t)

Behavioral

Buying a gun; changing a will; giving away possessions; history of prior suicide attempt; impulsiveness; making a will; marked changes in attitude; marked changes in behavior; marked changes in school performance; stockpiling medicines; sudden euphoric recovery from major depression

Demographic

Age (e.g., elderly people, young adult males, adolescents); divorced; male gender; race (e.g., white, Native American); widowed

Physical

Chronic pain; physical illness; terminal illness

Psychological

Childhood abuse; family history of suicide; guilt; homosexual youth; psychiatric disorder; psychiatric illness; substance abuse

Situational

Adolescents living in nontraditional settings (e.g., juvenile detention center, prison, half-way house, group home); economic instability; institutionalization; living alone; loss of autonomy; loss of independence; presence of gun in home; relocation; retired

Social

Cluster suicides; disrupted family life; disciplinary problems; grief; helplessness; hopelessness; legal problems; loneliness; loss of important relationship; poor support systems; social isolation

Verbal

States desire to die; threats of killing oneself

NOC (Nursing Outcomes Classification)

Suggested NOC Outcomes

Depression Level, Impulse Self-Control, Loneliness Severity, Mood Equilibrium, Risk Detection, Suicide Self-Restraint

Example **NOC** Outcome with Indicators
Suicide Self-Restraint as evidenced by the following indicators: Expresses feelings/Refrains from attempting suicide/ Verbalizes suicidal ideas/Controls impulses (Rate the outcome and indicators of **Suicide Self-Restraint:** 1 = never demonstrated, 2 = rarely demonstrated, 3 = sometimes demonstrated, 4 = often demonstrated, 5 = consistently demonstrated [see Section I].)

Consider using one of the measures of suicide risk that are available for clients: Nurses' Global Assessment of Suicide Risk (NGASR) (Cutcliffe & Barker, 2004); Center for Epidemiological Studies Depression Scale (CES-D) measures depressed mood level (Chiu et al, 2009); Beck Suicide Intent Scale (SIS) identifies a strong intent to die (Astruc et al, 2004); Suicide Assessment Checklist (SAC) (Rogers, Lewis & Subich, 2002)

Client Outcomes

Client Will (Specify Time Frame):

- Not harm self
- Maintain connectedness in relationships
- Disclose and discuss suicidal ideas if present; seek help
- Express decreased anxiety and control of impulses
- Talk about feelings; express anger appropriately
- Refrain from using mood-altering substances

• = Independent   ▲ = Collaborative   **EBN** = Evidence-Based Nursing   **EB** = Evidence-Based

- Obtain no access to harmful objects
- Yield access to harmful objects
- Maintain self-control without supervision

NIC   (Nursing Interventions Classification)

Suggested NIC Interventions

Anxiety Reduction, Coping Enhancement, Crisis Intervention, Delusion Management, Mood Management, Substance Use Prevention, Suicide Prevention, Support System Enhancement, Surveillance

Example NIC Activities—Suicide Prevention
Determine presence and degree of suicidal risk; Encourage patient to seek out care providers to talk as urge to harm self occurs

Nursing Interventions and *Rationales*

- NOTE: Before implementing interventions in the face of suicidal behavior, nurses should examine their own emotional responses to incidents of suicide to ensure that interventions will not be based on countertransference reactions. **EBN:** *Medical nurses reported that they could not understand why people harm themselves, and they felt they did not have the skills to deal with suicidal clients (Valente & Saunders, 2004). Emergency Department nurses reported that they made prior judgments about the "genuineness" of clients' suicide attempts (Doyle, Keogh, & Morrissey, 2007).*
- Assess for suicidal ideation when the history reveals the following: depression, substance abuse; bipolar disorder, schizophrenia, panic disorder, posttraumatic stress disorder, dissociative disorder, eating disorder, antisocial or other personality disorders; attempted suicide, current or past; recent stressful life events (divorce and/or separation, relocation, problems with children); recent unemployment; recent bereavement; adult or childhood physical or sexual abuse; gay, lesbian, or bisexual gender orientation; family history of suicide, history of chronic trauma. *Clinicians should be alert for suicide when the aforementioned factors are present in asymptomatic persons (American Psychiatric Association, 2005).* **EBN and EB:** *Thirty-two percent of successful suicides had contact with mental health services in the preceding year, 75% had contact with primary care providers. Primary care providers could be effective in preventing suicide, particularly among older adults and women (Luoma, Martin & Pearson, 2002). First episode psychosis is a particular risk factor for suicide; early intervention has been shown to be helpful (Gonzalez-Pinto et al, 2007). (Additional relevant research: Bell & Nye, 2007; Links et al, 2007; Weaver et al, 2007; Zivin et al, 2007; Dutra et al, 2008; Hardt et al, 2008; Innamorati et al, 2008.)*
- Assess all medical clients and clients with chronic illnesses, traumatic injuries, or pain for their perception of health status and suicidal ideation. **EBN and EB:** *Clients with chronic pain, medical problems, and depression expressed suicidal ideation (Cooper et al, 2005). Medical clients who perceived their health to be poor or who were in chronic pain were significantly more likely to report current suicidal ideation (Tang & Crane, 2006). (Additional relevant research: Turner et al, 2006; Edwards et al, 2007; Simpson & Tate, 2007; Miller et al, 2008; Misono et al, 2008; Ratcliffe et al, 2008; Schneider & Shenassa, 2008; Walker et al, 2008; Woolley et al, 2008.)*
- Assess the client's ability to enter into a no-suicide contract. Contract (verbally or in writing) with the client for no self-harm if the client is appropriate for a contract; recontract at appropriate intervals. *Discussing feelings of self-harm with a trusted person provides relief for the client. A contract gets the subject out in the open and places some of the responsibility for safety with the client. Some clients are not appropriate for a contract: those under the influence of drugs or alcohol or unwilling to abstain from substance use, and those who are isolated or alone without assistance to keep the environment safe (Hauenstein, 2002). If the client will not contract, the risk of suicide should be considered higher.* **EB:** *The lack of willingness to self-disclose has been shown to discriminate the serious suicide attempter from the client with suicidal ideation or the mild attempter (Apter et al, 2001).* **EBN:** NOTE: *Although contracting is a common practice in psychiatric care settings, research has suggested that self-harm is not prevented by contracts. Thorough, ongoing assessment of suicide risk is necessary, whether or not the client has entered into a no-self-harm contract. Contracts may not be appropriate in community settings (McMyler & Pryjmachuk, 2008).*

● = Independent   ▲ = Collaborative   **EBN** = Evidence-Based Nursing   **EB** = Evidence-Based

- Be alert for warning signs of suicide: making statements such as, "I can't go on," "Nothing matters anymore," "I wish I were dead"; becoming depressed or withdrawn; behaving recklessly; getting affairs in order and giving away valued possessions; showing a marked change in behavior, attitudes, or appearance; abusing drugs or alcohol; suffering a major loss or life change. *Suicide is rarely a spontaneous decision. In the days and hours before people kill themselves, clues and warning signs usually appear (Befrienders International, 2007).*
- Take suicide notes seriously and ask if a note was left in any previous suicide attempts. Consider themes of notes in determining appropriate interventions. **EBN:** *Clients who left a suicide note were found to be at higher risk of future completed suicide in the future. A note should be viewed as indication of a failed but serious attempt (Barr, Leitner, & Thomas, 2007).* **EB:** *A theme of "apology/shame" was present in suicide notes, suggesting that alternative solutions to dilemmas may have been welcomed. Cognitive therapy techniques, particularly problem solving, would be useful (Foster, 2003).*
- Question family members regarding the preparatory actions mentioned. *Clinicians should be alert for suicide when these factors are present in asymptomatic persons (American Psychiatric Association, 2005).*
- Determine the presence and degree of suicidal risk. A number of questions will elicit the necessary information: Have you been thinking about hurting or killing yourself? How often do you have these thoughts and how long do they last? Do you have a plan? What is it? Do you have access to the means to carry out that plan? How likely is it that you could carry out the plan? Are there people or things that could prevent you from hurting yourself? What do you see in your future a year from now? Five years from now? What do you expect would happen if you died? What has kept you alive up to now? *Using the acronym SAL, the nurse can evaluate the client's suicide plan for its Specificity (how detailed and clear is the plan?), Availability (does the client have immediate access to the planned means?), and Lethality (could the plan be fatal, or does the client believe it would be fatal?). Assessment of reasons for living is another important part of evaluating suicidal clients (Malone et al, 2000).*
- Observe, record, and report any changes in mood or behavior that may signify increasing suicide risk and document results of regular surveillance checks. **EB:** *Suicidal ideation often is not continuous; it may decrease, then increase in response to negative thinking or exposure to stressors (e.g., family visits). Documentation of surveillance will alert all members of the health care team to changes in the client's potential risk for suicide so they may be prepared to respond in the event of suicidal behavior (McNiel et al, 2008; Neuner et al, 2008).*
- Develop a positive therapeutic relationship with the client; do not make promises that may not be kept. *Be aware that some clients may offer to self-disclose if the nurse will promise not to tell anyone what they have said. Clarify with the client that anything they share will be communicated only to other staff but that secrets cannot be kept.* **EBN:** *Nurses reconnect suicidal clients with humanity by guiding the client, helping them learn how to live, and helping them connect appropriately with others (Cutliffe et al, 2006; Lakeman & FitzGerald, 2008).*
- ▲ Refer for mental health counseling and possible hospitalization if evidence of suicidal intent exists, which may include evidence of preparatory actions (e.g., obtaining a weapon, making a plan, putting affairs in order, giving away prized possessions, preparing a suicide note). **EB:** *Clients vary in the preparation for suicide attempts, and professional assessment is required to determine the need for hospitalization (Conner et al, 2007; Minnix et al, 2007). Interventions below may be instituted.*
- Assign a hospitalized client to a room located near the nursing station. *Close assignment increases ease of observation and availability for a rapid response in the event of a suicide attempt.*
- Search the newly hospitalized client and the client's personal belongings for weapons or potential weapons and hoarded medications during the inpatient admission procedure, as appropriate. Remove dangerous items. *Client's intent on suicide may bring the means with them. Action is necessary to maintain a hazard-free environment and client safety.*
- Limit access to windows and exits unless locked and shatterproof, as appropriate. *Suicidal behavior may include attempts to jump out of windows or to escape the unit to find other means of suicide (e.g., gaining roof access for a jump). Hospitals should ensure that exits are secure.*
- Monitor the client during the use of potential weapons (e.g., razor, scissors). *Clients with suicidal intent may take advantage of any opportunity to harm themselves.*

● = Independent   ▲ = Collaborative   **EBN** = Evidence-Based Nursing   **EB** = Evidence-Based

- Increase surveillance of a hospitalized client at times when staffing is predictably low (e.g., staff meetings, change of shift report, periods of unit disruption). *Clients who remain intent on suicide will be watchful of periods when staff surveillance lessens to permit completion of a suicide plan.*
- ▲ If imminent suicide is suspected or an attempt has occurred, call for assistance and do not leave the client alone. *Client and staff safety will be served by assistance in the response. The client may attempt additional self-harm if left alone.*
- Place the client in the least restrictive, safe, and monitored environment that allows for the necessary level of observation. Assess suicidal risk at least daily and more frequently as warranted. *Close observation of the client is necessary for safety as long as intent remains high. Suicide risk should be assessed at frequent intervals to adjust suicide precautions and limitations on the client's freedom of movement and to ensure that restrictions continue to be appropriate.* **EB:** *Inpatient root cause analyses of suicide attempts and environmental safety checklists for units can be helpful in maintaining safety (Mills et al, 2008).*
- Consider strategies to decrease isolation and opportunity to act on harmful thoughts (e.g., use of a sitter). **EBN:** *Clients have reported feeling safe and having their hope restored in response to close observation (Bowers & Park, 2001).*
- Explain suicide precautions and relevant safety issues to the client and family (e.g., purpose, duration, behavioral expectations, and behavioral consequences). **EBN:** *Suicide precautions may be viewed as restrictive. Clients have reported the loss of privacy as distressing (Bowers & Park, 2001).*
- ▲ Refer for treatment and participate in the management of any psychiatric illness or symptoms that may be contributing to the client's suicidal ideation or behavior. *Psychiatric disorders have been associated with suicidal behavior. Symptoms of the disorder may require treatment with antidepressant, antipsychotic, or antianxiety medications.* **EB:** *A systematic review has shown a highly significant effect for cognitive behavior therapy in reducing suicidal behavior (Tarrier, Taylor, & Gooding, 2008).*
- ▲ Verify that the client has taken medications as ordered (e.g., conduct mouth checks after medication administration). *The client may attempt to hoard medications for a later suicide attempt.*
- ▲ Maintain increased surveillance of the client whenever use of an antidepressant has been initiated or the dose increased. Antidepressant medications take anywhere from 2 to 6 weeks to achieve full efficacy. *During that period the client's energy level may increase, although the depression has not yet lifted, which increases the potential for suicide.*
- Involve the client in treatment planning and self-care management of psychiatric disorders. *Self-care management promotes feelings of self-efficacy (Lorig et al, 2001), particularly for clients with depression (Ellis, 2004). Suicidal ideation may occur in response to a sense of hopelessness, a sense that the client has no control over life circumstances. The more clients participate in their own care, the less powerless and hopeless they feel.* Refer to the care plan for **Powerlessness**.
- Explore with the client all circumstances and motivations related to the suicidality. Listen to the client's own views on his or her problems. **EB:** *Primary reasons for suicide attempts were found to be feelings of loneliness and mental illness/psychological problems. Men more often cited socioeconomic problems, whereas women more often reported psychological problems and interpersonal relationship difficulties. A high number of suicide attempters were never married/single, with poor social networks and depressive symptoms. Hopelessness was associated with a wish to die, and escape motives (Skogman & Ojehagen, 2003a, 2003b). Major depression and social maladaptation were found to have significant predictive value for repeat suicide attempts (Chandrasekaran & Gnanaselane, 2008).*
- Explore with the client all perceived consequences that could act as a barrier to suicide (e.g., effect on family, religious beliefs). **EBN:** *The most common barrier to suicide is consequences to family members (Bell, 2000).*
- Avoid repeated discussion of the client's suicide history by keeping discussion oriented to the present and future. **EB:** *Clients under stress have difficulty focusing their thoughts, which leads to a sense of being overwhelmed by problems. Focusing on the present and future helps the client to address problem solving with regard to current stressors, while avoiding secondary gain from idealizing past behavior (Coleman & Casey, 2007).*
- Discuss plans for dealing with suicidal ideation in the future (e.g., how to identify precipitating factors, whom to contact, where to go for help, how to respond to desire for self-harm). **EB:** *Clients are supported in self-care management when they are helped to identify actions they can take if suicidal ideation recurs (Williams et al, 2006).*

- Assist the client in identifying a network of supportive persons and resources (e.g., clergy, family, care providers). **EB:** *Clients who are suicidal often feel alienated from others and benefit from actions that facilitate support of the client by family and friends (deCastro & Guterman, 2008).*

▲ Refer family members and friends to local mental health agencies and crisis intervention centers if the client has suicidal ideation or a suspicion of suicidal thoughts exists. *Clients at risk should receive evaluation and help (American Psychiatric Association, 2005).*

▲ Document client behavior in detail to support outpatient commitment or an overnight psychiatric observation program for an actively suicidal client. *Involuntary outpatient commitment can improve treatment, reduce the likelihood of hospital readmission, and reduce episodes of violent behavior in persons with severe psychiatric illnesses (Torrey & Zdanowicz, 2001). Overnight psychiatric observation followed by outpatient referral also can be an effective alternative to traditional hospitalization without leading to an increase in suicide gestures or attempts (Francis et al, 2000).*

- Cognitive behavioral techniques help the client to modify thinking styles that promote depression, hopelessness, and a belief that suicide is a valid means of escaping the current situation. *Suicide has been shown to be associated with constriction in cognitive style, leading to decreased problem solving and information processing (Sheehy & O'Connor, 2002).* **EBN:** *Cognitive behavioral techniques and the promotion of problem-solving skills, combined with the therapeutic relationship, have been posited as key interventions when dealing with the hopelessness inherent to suicidal ideation (Collins & Cutcliffe, 2003).*

- Group interventions can be useful to address recurrent suicide attempts. **EB:** *Group therapy was shown to decrease suicidality (Burns et al, 2005).*

- With the client's consent, facilitate family-oriented crisis intervention. *Family-oriented crisis intervention can clarify stresses and allow assessment of family dynamics.* **EBN:** *Families of suicidal clients reported potential burnout from being on guard day and night, maintaining ADLs, and trying to create a nurturing environment. Families need support in preparing to accept clients back into the home (Nosek, 2008; Sun & Long, 2008).*

- Involve the family in discharge planning (e.g., illness/medication teaching, recognition of increasing suicidal risk, client's plan for dealing with recurring suicidal thoughts, community resources). *Suicidal clients often are ambivalent about hurting themselves; they may not want to die so much as to escape an intolerable situation. Consequently they often leave clues about their state of mind.* **EBN:** *Family members must learn before clients leave the hospital how to respond to clues early, support the treatment regimen, and encourage the client to initiate the emergency plan. Nurses help in guiding families through the process (Nosek, 2008; Sun & Long, 2008).*

▲ Before discharge from the hospital, ensure that the client has a supply of ordered medications, has a plan for outpatient follow-up, understands the plan or has a caregiver able and willing to follow the plan, and has the ability to access outpatient treatment. *Clients may be discharged before they have recovered substantial functional ability and may have difficulty concentrating on the plan for follow-up. They may need the assistance of others to ensure that prescriptions are filled, that they attend appointments, or that they have transportation to the outpatient care setting.* **EB:** *Nonresponse to treatment of depression has been associated with the clinical factor of suicidal ideation, socioeconomic factors (unemployment) not usually addressed by medical intervention, and medication nonadherence (Sherbourne et al, 2004).*

▲ In the event of successful suicide, refer the family to a therapy group for survivors of suicide. *Recommended clinical interventions include addressing psychological distress, normalizing denial as an effective coping strategy, working with concerns about family disintegration, and helping families deal with stigmatization (Kaslow & Aronson, 2004).* **EBN and EB:** *Survivors of suicide may be reluctant to contact health care professionals, out of fear that they will be blamed or stigmatized. Group counseling addresses the blame, anger, guilt, shame, and search for a reason for the suicide that occurs in suicide survivors (Barlow & Morrison, 2002). Psychoeducational support group participants found relief in sharing a personal narrative of their suicide bereavement with others (Feigelman & Feigelman, 2008). Internet support groups for suicide survivors may also be helpful for bereavement (Feigelman et al, 2008).*

- See the care plans for **Risk for self-directed Violence**, **Hopelessness**, and **Risk for Self-Mutilation**. **EBN:** *Clients with suicidal ideation often are reacting to a feeling of hopelessness (Koehn & Cutliffe, 2007).*

● = Independent   ▲ = Collaborative   **EBN** = Evidence-Based Nursing   **EB** = Evidence-Based

Pediatric

- The above interventions may be appropriate for pediatric clients.
- Use brief self-report measures to improve clinical management of at-risk cases. *The Risk of Suicide Questionnaire (RSQ) is available for children and adolescents (Horowitz et al, 2001).*
- Assess for both medical and psychiatric disturbances that may contribute to suicidality. *The process leading to suicide in young people often involves untreated depression (Houston, Hawton, & Shepperd, 2001). Epilepsy has a fourfold risk increase of suicide, particularly documented in children and adolescents (Muzina, 2004).*
- Recognize that the developmental issues of childhood and adolescence may heighten suicide risks and involve different issues from those with adults. *Assessment of suicidality in children is difficult. Lethality of an action may be misperceived; motivation varies greatly among children. Reuniting with a lost loved one may be more dangerous than gaining attention or other motivations more common at an older age (Fritz, 2004). Physically aggressive behavior learned in early childhood may translate into suicide risk (Tremblay, 2004). The rates of attempted suicide are particularly higher during adolescence. Puberty, social, and cognitive changes can lead to greater unhappiness. Rage, hopelessness, despair, and guilt are common with suicide attempts, with greater variability of suicide timing, impulsivity, and mood (Spirito & Overholser, 2003).*
- Assess specific stressors for the adolescent client. *Adolescents tend to experience concerns about personal issues, school pressures, and relationships. Poor familial communications and lack of a parental confidant may be present. Key interventions include improving family communications, addressing psychosocial issues, teaching problem-solving skills, and fostering decreased impulsivity (Webb, 2002).*
- Assess for exposure to suicide of a significant other. **EB:** *Among risk factors of previous psychiatric history, poor psychosocial function, dysphoric mood and psychomotor restlessness, suicide of a significant other was shown to create risk for adolescents diagnosed with adjustment disorder (Pelkonen et al, 2005).*
- Evaluate for the presence of self-mutilation and related risk factors. Refer to care plan for **Risk for Self-Mutilation** for additional information. **EBN:** *Self-mutilation is common and suicide is possible for boys who have been sexually abused (Valente, 2005).*
- Be aware that complete overlap does not exist between suicidal behavior and self-mutilation. The motivation may be different (ending life rather than coping with difficult feelings), and the method is usually different. **EB:** *In one study, about half of the participants reported both attempted suicide and self-mutilation; in the other half there was no overlap in types of acts (Bolognini et al, 2003).*
- Assess for the presence of an eating disorder. *Suicidal behavior was shown to be more common among adolescents with dependence issues (drug abuse and eating disorders) (Bolognini et al, 2003). The thought processes of adolescents with an eating disorder were found to center on themes of feeling undeserving of receiving help, feeling helpless and hopeless in dealing with the eating disorder itself, difficulty with recognizing and expressing feelings, and ambivalence regarding treatment along with mistrust of health care providers (Manley & Leichner, 2003).*
- Involve the adolescent in multimodal treatment programs. **EB:** *Thorough assessment and multiple modes of treatment, including family sessions, were found to improve psychosocial functioning and self-image in a program for adolescent inpatients (Hintikka et al, 2006).*
- Before discharge from the hospital, ensure that the client's parent has a supply of ordered medications, has a plan for outpatient follow-up, has a caregiver who understands the plan or is able and willing to follow the plan, and has the ability to access outpatient treatment. *Lack of adequate follow-up has been associated with repeated suicide attempts among adolescents (Hulten et al, 2001).* **EB:** *A compliance enhancement intervention (including contracting interviews with parent and adolescent, and telephone contacts) improved attendance at follow-up appointments only when barriers to service were controlled (e.g., delays in getting appointments, placement on a waiting list, inability to switch therapists, problems with insurance coverage) (Spirito et al, 2002).*
- Parental education groups can influence suicide risk factors. **EB:** *A program of parent education groups focused on improved communication skills and relationships with adolescents. Students in the intervention group reported increased maternal care, decreased conflict with parents, decreased substance abuse, and decreased delinquency (Toumbourou & Gregg, 2002).*
- Support the implementation of school-based suicide prevention programs. *School nurses can be key to early intervention.* **EBN:** *An intervention study by school nurses on providing coping skills training*

• = Independent ▲ = Collaborative **EBN** = Evidence-Based Nursing **EB** = Evidence-Based

and emotional support yielded a 55% decrease in suicidal ideation (Houck, Darnell, & Lussman, 2002). **EB:** *A test of the effectiveness of the Signs of Suicide (SOS) prevention program found that suicide attempts decreased, knowledge-based awareness increased, and adaptive attitudes toward depression and suicide were observed (Aseltine & DeMartino, 2004).*

- Encourage family meals. **EB:** *Frequency of family meals was inversely associated with tobacco, alcohol, and marijuana use; low grade point average; depressive symptoms; and suicide involvement (Eisenberg et al, 2004).*

Geriatric

- Evaluate the older client's mental and physical health status and financial stressors. *The possibility of reversible/medical causes of depression, including medical or neurological disorders, as well as psychomimetic reactions to medications, should inform nursing observations (Hall, Hall, & Chapman, 2003).*
- Explore with client any concerns or pressures (physical and financial) regarding ability to secure support of medical care, especially perceived pressures about being a burden on family. **EB:** *The suicide notes of older adults were more likely than those of younger adults to contain the theme "burden to others" (Foster, 2003).*
- When assessing suicide risk factors, incorporate a higher degree of risk for older men and for some older adults who have lost a loved one in the previous year. **EB:** *Although mortality for oldest old adults (80+) has increased, the suicide mortality has not decreased. In one study, oldest old men had the highest increase in suicide risk after death of a partner (more so than oldest old women) and took a longer time to recover from the death of a spouse (Erlangsen et al, 2004). Suicide rate may be rising among men over age 65, and marriage may no longer be the protective factor it was once considered to be (Lamprecht et al, 2005).*
- Explore triggers of and barriers to suicidal behavior, with particular attention to real and perceived losses (e.g., professional role, health). **EB:** *For adults 75 years of age or older, predictors of suicide included family conflict, serious physical illness, and both major and minor depressions. For adults 65 to 74 years of age, but not for the older group, economic problems were predictive of suicide (Waern, Rubenowitz, & Wilhelmson, 2003).* **EBN:** *A study of older Caucasian men revealed that losing connections initiated a process of loss and depression and triggered a decision point that could include suicidal ideation. Triggers included death of a spouse, emotional pain, health problems, and feelings of uselessness or hopelessness. A strong barrier was consequences to family members. Religion and social isolation were not relevant (Bell, 2000).*
- An older adult who shows self-destructive behaviors should be evaluated for dementia. **EB:** *In a study of nursing home residents, self-destructive behaviors were common; these behaviors were more likely related to dementia than to depression and were only weakly associated with suicidal intent (Draper et al, 2002).*
- Anticipate overall responsiveness to treatment, but monitor for early relapse. **EB:** *Older adults had high remission rates after antidepressant treatment, whether they had suicidal ideation or not. However, older adults with suicidal ideation had a higher relapse rate and a greater need for adjunctive psychotropic medications (Szanto et al, 2001).*
- ▲ Advocate for the older client with other professionals in securing treatment for suicidal states. Primary care physicians have been noted to underrecognize and undertreat older adult clients with depression. **EB:** *Older adults above age 75 with major or minor depression were less likely than those ages 65 to 74 to receive depression treatment (Waern et al, 2003).*
- Encourage physical activity in older adults. **EB:** *Evidence-based research supports the argument that Qigong improves cardiovascular-respiratory function and lipid profile, decreases blood sugar, and relieves anxiety and depression for elders (Hung & Chen, 2009).* **EB:** *A study testing response to exercise, sertraline, or exercise plus sertraline found that the exercise-only group experienced the lowest depression levels, with the benefit of exercise continuing after the intervention period (Babyak et al, 2000).*
- Assist the older adult to identify protective factors that serve as resources to mitigate against suicidal ideation. *Internal and external factors that can serve as resources for the older adult include the ability to learn from experience and accept help, a sense of humor and interest in social concerns, a*

sense of purpose or meaning in life, a history of successful coping, caring and available family and a supportive community network, and membership in a religious community (Holkup, Tang, & Titler, 2003).

- Collaborative care management of older adults in primary care settings is a growing area for nursing intervention. **EB:** *A wide-scale study of individualized care provided by "depression care managers" (social workers, nurses, psychologists) in collaboration with physicians yielded a faster decline of suicidal ideation in the intervention group, along with a greater degree and speed of depression symptom reduction (Bruce et al, 2004).*
- Telephone contacts can serve as an effective intervention for suicidal older adults. **EBN:** *Nurse telehealth care, involving an average of 10 calls over 16 weeks to answer questions, offer support, and discuss overall health, reduced depressive symptoms more than did usual physician care (Hunkeler et al, 2000).* **EB:** *A protocol of twice-weekly support calls resulted in significantly fewer suicide deaths among women but not among men. The researchers concluded that outreach, continuity of care, and increased emotional support provided protection against suicide, at least for women (De Leo, Della Buono, & Dwyer, 2002).*

 ### Multicultural

- Assess for the influence of cultural beliefs, norms, and values on the individual's perceptions of suicide. **EBN:** *What the individual believes about suicide may be based on cultural perceptions (Leininger & McFarland, 2002). Among Hispanics, the largest proportion of suicides occurred among young persons; suicide rates were higher among males; and the most common method of suicide was by firearms (CDC, 2004).*
- Identify and acknowledge the stresses unique to culturally diverse individuals. *Financial difficulties and maintaining cultural values are two of the most common family stressors cited by women of color (Majumdar & Ladak, 1998). Suicide rates among African American male teenagers increased 105% from 1980 to 1986 (Surgeon General, 1999), with "suicide by cop" speculated to have increased these rates (Daugherty, 1999). A high rate of suicidal ideation has been reported as a result of the social discrimination experienced by gay and bisexual Latino men in the United States (Diaz et al, 2001). There may be a relationship between the possible relationship between rapid social change and the increasing rates of suicide among Alaska Natives (Richards, 2004).*
- Identify and acknowledge unique cultural responses to stressors in determining sensitive interventions to prevent suicide. **EBN:** *In a study of African American, Hispanic/Latina, and Caucasian adolescent girls, the Hispanic/Latina girls had a significantly higher percentage of suicide attempts. Relationships were found between recent suicide attempts and family history of suicide attempts, friend's history of suicide attempt, history of physical or sexual abuse, and environmental stress. For all three groups, rate of recent suicide attempts was also associated with stress level, social connectedness, and religious influence (Rew et al, 2001). A recent study found African-American men committed suicide at rates much lower than those for Caucasians, but they do so at much younger ages (Garlow, Purselle, & Heninger, 2005).*
- Encourage physical activity as intervention to decrease suicidal behavior. **EB:** *Increased physical activity was associated with lower suicidal feelings and suicidal behaviors in Hispanic and non-Hispanic boys (Brosnahan et al, 2004).*
- Encourage family members to demonstrate and offer caring and support to each other. **EB:** *In this study of urban African American youth individual and family protective variables emerged as powerful sources of resilience. (Li, Nussbaum, & Richards, 2007). Family closeness is strong resiliency factor of suicidal behavior in African American and Hispanic youths (O'Donnell et al, 2004).*
- Foster the client's use of available family and religious supports. **EB:** *Christian religious roots and family closeness, although eroding among many young African Americans, traditionally have worked against suicidal behavior among African Americans (Neeleman, Wessely, & Lewis, 1998).*
- Validate the individual's feelings regarding concerns about the current crisis and family functioning. *Validation lets the client know that the nurse has heard and understood what was said, and it promotes the nurse-client relationship (Giger & Davidhizar, 2008).*

Home Care

- Communicate the degree of risk to family and caregivers; assess the family and caregiving situation for ability to protect the client and to understand the client's suicidal behavior. Provide the family and caregivers with guidelines on how to manage self-harm behaviors in the home environment. *Client safety between home visits is a nursing priority. Family and caregivers may become frightened by the client's suicidal ideation, may be angry at the client's perceived lack of self-control, or may feel as if they are walking on eggshells awaiting another suicide attempt.*
- If the client's suicidal ideation intensifies, or if a suicide plan with access to means becomes evident, institute an emergency plan for mental health intervention. *Over a quarter (29%) of clients who had previously self-harmed died within 3 months of discharge from psychiatric care and 36% had missed their last service appointment. Measures that may prevent suicide pacts in the mentally ill include the effective treatment of depression and closer supervision in both inpatient and community settings (Hunt et al, 2009).*
- Counsel parents and homeowners to restrict unauthorized access to potentially lethal prescription drugs and firearms within the home. *Identifying teens at high risk of firearm suicide and limiting access to firearms are public health interventions likely to be successful in preventing firearm suicides (Shah et al, 2000).*
- Identify the client's concerns and implement interventions to address the consequences of disability in a client with medical illness. **EB:** *In a study of cancer clients being cared for at home, primary factors influencing vulnerability to suicide were identified as real or feared loss of autonomy and independence, concerns about being a burden on others, hopelessness about the health condition, and fear of suffering (Filiberti et al, 2001). Hopelessness and demoralization in conjunction with dependence have been noted as precursors to suicidal ideation in palliative care clients (Kissane, Clarke, & Street, 2001).* Refer to the care plans for **Hopelessness** and **Powerlessness**.
- ▲ Refer for homemaker or psychiatric home health care services for respite, client reassurance, and implementation of a therapeutic regimen. *Respite decreases the high degree of caregiver stress that goes with the responsibility of caring for a person at risk for suicide.* **EB:** *In a study of community-integrated, home-based treatment for depression, depressive symptoms were significantly reduced in elderly participants, and improved health status was noted in chronically medically ill older adults with minor depression and dysthymia (Ciechanowski et al, 2004).*
- ▲ If the client is on psychotropic medications, assess the client's and family's knowledge of medication administration and side effects. Teach as necessary. *Knowledge of the medical regimen promotes compliance and promotes safe use of medications.*
- ▲ Evaluate the effectiveness and side effects of medications and adherence to the medication regimen. Review with the client and family all medications kept in the home; encourage discarding of old prescriptions. Monitor the amount of medications ordered/provided by the physician; limiting the amount of medications to which the client has access may be necessary. *Accurate clinical feedback improves the physician's ability to prescribe an effective medical regimen specific to the client's needs. At home, clients may have greater access to medications, including old prescriptions that may be used to overdose.*

 Client/Family Teaching and Discharge Planning

- Establish a supportive relationship with family members. **EBN:** *Family members experience a great deal of stress around suicidal ideation and benefit from nurses' support (Sun & Long, 2008).*
- Explain all relevant symptoms, procedures, treatments, and expected outcomes for suicidal ideation that is illness based (e.g., depression, bipolar disorder). **EBN:** *The Health Belief Model identifies perceived barriers and perceived susceptibility to disease, as powerful predictors of clients' motivation in taking action to prevent disease and participate in self-care management (Pender, Murdaugh, & Parsons, 2005).*
- Teach the family how to recognize that the client is at increased risk for suicide (changes in behavior and verbal and nonverbal communication, withdrawal, depression, or sudden lifting of depression). **EB and EBN:** *A client may be at peace because a suicide plan has been made and the client has the energy to carry it out. Therefore when depression lifts, increased vigilance is necessary (Rouget & Aubrey, 2007; Sun & Long, 2008).*

- Provide written instructions for treatments and procedures for which the client will be responsible. **EBN:** *A written record provides a concrete reference so that the client and family can clarify any verbal information that was given (Sun & Long, 2008).*
- Instruct the client in coping strategies (assertiveness training, impulse control training, deep breathing, progressive muscle relaxation). **EBN:** *Suicidal ideation may be triggered by stress and painful emotions. Once clients are able to identify these triggers, they need to learn how to respond to them more effectively through assertiveness, impulse control, or relaxation techniques, as appropriate (Lakeman & Fitzgerald, 2008).*
- Role play (e.g., say, "Tell me how you will respond if a friend asks why you were in the hospital"). **EB:** *Role playing is a technique to decondition the anxiety that arises from interpersonal encounters by allowing the client to practice how he or she might respond in a given situation. Suicide survivors reported they have difficulty talking with others about the suicide (McMenamy, Jordan, & Mitchell, 2008).*
- Teach cognitive behavioral activities, such as active problem solving, reframing (reappraising the situation from a different perspective), or thought stopping (in response to a negative thought, picturing a large stop sign and replacing the image with a prearranged positive alternative). Teach the client to confront his or her own negative thought patterns (or cognitive distortions), such as catastrophizing (expecting the very worst), dichotomous thinking (perceiving events in only one of two opposite categories), or magnification (placing distorted emphasis on a single event). *Cognitive behavioral activities address clients' assumptions, beliefs, and attitudes about their situations and foster modification of these elements to be as realistic and optimistic as possible. Through cognitive behavioral interventions, clients become more aware of their cognitive choices in adopting and maintaining their belief systems and thereby exercise greater control over their own reactions (Hagerty & Patusky, 2008).*
- Provide the client and family with phone numbers of appropriate community agencies for therapy and counseling. *Continuous follow-up care should be implemented; therefore the method to access this care must be given to the client (Rouget & Aubrey, 2007; Sun & Long, 2008).*

⊝volve See the EVOLVE website for Weblinks for client education resources.

REFERENCES

American Psychiatric Association-Medical Specialty Society: *Practice guideline for the assessment and treatment of patients with suicidal behaviors.* www.psychiatryonline.com/pracGuide/loadGuidelinepdf.aspx?file=SuicidalBehavior. Accessed December 29, 2009.

Apter A, Horesh N, Gothelf D et al: Relationship between self-disclosure and serious suicidal behavior, *Compr Psychiatry* 42(1):70, 2001.

Aseltine RH Jr, DeMartino R: An outcome evaluation of the SS suicide prevention program, *Am J Public Health* 94:446, 2004.

Astruc B, Torres S, Jollant F et al: A history of major depressive disorder influences intent to die in violent suicide attempters, *J Clin Psychiatr* 65:690, 2004.

Babyak M, Blumenthal JA, Herman S et al: Exercise treatment for major depression: maintenance of therapeutic benefit at 10 months, *Psychosom Med* 62:633, 2000.

Barlow CA, Morrison H: Survivors of suicide. Emerging counseling strategies, *J Psychosoc Nurs Ment Health Serv* 40(1):28, 2002.

Barr W, Leitner M, Thomas J: Self-harm or attempted suicide? Do suicide notes help us decide the level of intent in those who survive? *Accid Emerg Nurs* 15:122, 2007.

Befrienders International: *The warning signs of suicide.* http://befrienders.org/support/index.asp?PageURL_warningSigns.php. Accessed April 24, 2007.

Bell JB, Nye EC: Specific symptoms predict suicidal ideation in Vietnam combat veterans with chronic post-traumatic stress disorder, *Military Med* 172:1144, 2007.

Bell MA: *Losing connections: a process of decision-making in late-life suicidality* [doctoral dissertation], Tucson, 2000, University of Arizona.

Bolognini M, Plancherel B, Laget J et al: Adolescents' self-mutilation: relationship with dependent behaviour, *Swiss J Psychol* 62(4):241, 2003.

Bowers L, Park A: Special observation in the care of psychiatric inpatients: a literature review, *Issues Ment Health Nurs* 22:769, 2001.

Brosnahan J, Steffen LM, Lytle L et al: The relation between physical activity and mental health among Hispanic and non-Hispanic white adolescents, *Arch Pediatr Adolesc Med* 158(8):818–823, 2004.

Bruce ML, Ten Have TR, Reynolds CF III et al: Reducing suicidal ideation and depressive symptoms in depressed older primary care patients: a randomized controlled trial, *JAMA* 291:1081, 2004.

Burns J, Dudley M, Hazell P et al: Clinical management of deliberate self-harm in young people: the need for evidence-based approaches to reduce repetition, *Aus NZ J Psychiatry* 39:121, 2005.

Centers for Disease Control and Prevention (CDC): Suicide among Hispanics—United States, 1997–2001, *MMWR Morb Mort Wkly Rep* 53(22):478–481, 2004.

Chandrasekaran R & Gnanaselane J: Predictors of repeat suicidal attempts after first-ever attempt: a two-year follow-up study, *Hong Kong J Psychiatry* 18:131, 2008.

Chiu S, Webber MP, Zeig-Owens R et al: Validation of the Center for Epidemiologic Studies Depression Scale in screening for major depressive disorder among retired firefighters exposed to the World Trade Center disaster, *J Affect Disord*, 2009 [Epub ahead of print].

Ciechanowski P, Wagner E, Schmaling K et al: Community-integrated home-based depression treatment in older adults: a randomized controlled trial, *JAMA* 291(13):1569, 2004.

● = Independent ▲ = Collaborative **EBN** = Evidence-Based Nursing **EB** = Evidence-Based

Coleman D, Casey JT: Therapeutic mechanisms of suicidal ideation: The influence of changes in automatic thoughts and immature defenses, *Crisis: J Crisis Interven & Suicide* 28:198, 2007.

Collins S, Cutcliffe JR: Addressing hopelessness in people with suicidal ideation: building upon the therapeutic relationship utilizing a cognitive behavioural approach, *J Psychiatr Ment Health Nurs* 10:175, 2003.

Conner KR, Duberstein PR, Beckman A et al: Planning of suicide attempts among depressed inpatients ages 50 and over, *J Affect Disord* 97:123, 2007.

Cooper J, Kapur N, Webb R et al: Suicide after deliberate self-harm: a 4–year cohort study, *Am J Psychiatry* 162:297, 2005.

Cutcliffe JR, Barker P: The Nurses' Global Assessment of Suicide Risk (NGASR): developing a tool for clinical practice, *J Psychiatr Ment Health Nurs* 11(4):393, 2004.

Cutliffe JR, Stevenson C, Jackson S et al: A modified grounded theory study of how psychiatric nurses work with suicidal people, *Int J Nurs Stud* 43:791, 2006.

Daugherty M: Suicide by cop, *J Calif Alliance Ment Ill* 10(2):79, 1999.

DeCastro S, Guterman JT: Solution focused therapy for families coping with suicide, *J Marital Fam Ther* 34:93, 2008.

De Leo D, Della Buono M, Dwyer J: Suicide among the elderly: the long-term impact of a telephone support and assessment intervention in northern Italy, *Br J Psychiatr* 181:226, 2002.

Diaz RM, Ayala G, Bein E et al: The impact of homophobia, poverty, and racism on the mental health of gay and bisexual Latino men: findings from 3 U.S. cities, *Am J Public Health* 91:927, 2001.

Doyle L, Keogh B, Morrissey J: Caring for patients with suicidal behaviour: an exploratory study, *Br J Nurs* 16:1218, 2007.

Draper B, Brodaty H, Low LF et al: Self-destructive behaviors in nursing home residents, *J Am Geriatr Soc* 50:354, 2002.

Dutra L, Callahan, K, Forman E et al: Core schemas and suicidality in a chronically traumatized population, *J Nerv Ment Dis* 196:71, 2008.

Edwards RR, Magyar-Russell G, Thomb G et al: Acute pain at discharge from hospitalization is a prospective predictor of long-term suicidal ideation after burn injury, *Arch Phys Med Rehab* 88(S2):S36, 2007.

Eisenberg ME, Olson RE, Neumark-Sztainer D et al: Correlations between family meals and psychosocial well-being among adolescents, *Arch Pediatr Adolesc Med* 158(8):792–796, 2004.

Ellis TE: Collaboration and a self-help orientation in therapy with suicidal clients, *J Contemp Psychother* 34(1):41, 2004.

Erlangsen A, Jeune B, Bille-Brahe U et al: Loss of partner and suicide risks among oldest old: a population-based register study, *Age Ageing* 33(4):378–383, 2004.

Feigelman B, Feigelman W: Surviving after suicide loss: the healing potential of suicide survivor support groups, *Illn Crisis Loss* 16:185, 2008.

Feigelman W, Gorman BS, Beal KC et al: Internet support groups for suicide survivors: a new mode for gaining bereavement assistance, *Omega* 57:217, 2008.

Filiberti A, Ripamonti C, Totis A et al: Characteristics of terminal cancer patients who committed suicide during a home palliative care program, *J Pain Symptom Manage* 22:544, 2001.

Foster T: Suicide note themes and suicide prevention, *Int J Psychiatry Med* 33(4):323, 2003.

Francis E, Marchand W, Hart M et al: Utilization and outcome in an overnight psychiatric observation program at a Veterans Affairs medical center, *Psychiatr Serv* 51:92, 2000.

Fritz GK: Suicide in young children (editorial), *Brown Univ Child Adolesc Behav Lett* 20(7):8, 2004.

Garlow SJ, Purselle D, Heninger M: Ethnic differences in patterns of suicide across the life cycle, *Am J Psychiatry* 162(2):319–323, 2005.

Giger, J, Davidhizar, R: *Transcultural nursing: assessment and intervention*, St Louis, 2008, Mosby.

Gonzalez-Pinto A, Aldama A, Gonzalez C et al: Predictors of suicide in first-episode affective and nonaffective psychotic inpatients: five-year follow-up of patients from a catchment area in Vitoria, Spain, *J Clin Psychiatry* 68:242, 2007.

Hagerty B, Patusky K: Mood disorders: depression and mania. In Fortinash KM, Holoday-Worret PA, editors: *Psychiatric mental health nursing*, ed 4, St Louis, 2008, Mosby.

Hall RCW, Hall RCW, Chapman MJ: Identifying geriatric patients at risk for suicide and depression, *Clin Geriatr* 11(10):36, 2003.

Hardt J, Sidor A, Nickel R et al: Childhood adversities and suicide attempts: a retrospective study, *J Fam Violence* 23:713, 2008.

Hauenstein EJ: Case finding and care in suicide: children, adolescents, and adults. In Boyd MA, editor: *Psychiatric nursing: contemporary practice*, ed 2, Philadelphia, 2002, Lippincott Williams & Wilkins.

Hintikka U, Marttunen M, Pelkonen M et al: Improvement in cognitive and psychosocial functioning and self-image among adolescent inpatient suicide attempters, *BMC Psychiatry* 6:58, 2006.

Holkup PA, Tang JH, Titler MG: Evidence-based protocol elderly suicide—secondary prevention, *J Gerontol Nurs* 29(6):6, 2003.

Horowitz LM, Wang PS, Koocher GP et al: Detecting suicide risk in a pediatric emergency department: development of a brief screening tool, *Pediatrics* 107:1133, 2001.

Houck GM, Darnell S, Lussman S: A support group intervention for at-risk female high school students, *J School Nurs* 18(4):212, 2002.

Houston K, Hawton K, Shepperd R: Suicide in young people aged 15–24: a psychological autopsy study, *J Affect Disord* 63(1–3):159, 2001.

Hulten A, Jiang GX, Wasserman D et al: Repetition of attempted suicide among teenagers in Europe: frequency, timing and risk factors, *Eur Child Adolesc Psychiatry* 10:161, 2001.

Hung HM, Chen KM: [Scientific and holistic therapy perspectives on Qigong practice for elders with cardiovascular disease risk factors] [article in Chinese], *Hu Li Za Zhi* 56(1):73–78, 2009.

Hunkeler EM, Meresman JF, Hargreaves WA et al: Efficacy of nurse telehealth care and peer support in augmenting treatment of depression in primary care, *Arch Fam Med* 9:700, 2000.

Hunt IM, While D, Windfuhr K et al: Suicide pacts in the mentally ill: a national clinical survey *Psychiatry Res* 15;167(1–2):131–138, 2009.

Innamorati M, Pompili M, Masotti V et al: Completed versus attempted suicide in psychiatric patients: a psychological autopsy study, *J Psychiatr Pract* 14:216, 2008.

Kaslow NJ, Aronson SG: Recommendations for family interventions following a suicide, *Prof Psychol Res Pract* 35(3):240, 2004.

Kissane DW, Clarke DM, Street AF: Demoralization syndrome-relevant psychiatric diagnosis for palliative care, *J Palliat Care* 17(1):12, 2001.

Koehn CV, Cutliffe JR: Hope and interpersonal psychiatric/mental health nursing: a systematic review of the literature—part one, *J Psychiatr Ment Health Nurs* 14:134, 2007.

Lakeman R, FitzGerald M: How people live with or get over being suicidal: a review of qualitative studies, *J Adv Nurs* 64:114, 2008.

Lamprecht HC, Pakrasi S, Gash A et al: Deliberate self-harm in older people revisited, *Int J Geriatr Psychiatry* 20:1090, 2005.

Leininger MM, McFarland MR: *Transcultural nursing: concepts, theories, research and practices*, ed 3, New York, 2002, McGraw-Hill.

Li ST, Nussbaum KM, Richards MH: Risk and protective factors for urban African-American youth, *Am J Community Psychol.* 39(1–2):21–35, 2007.

Links PS, Eynan R, Heisel MJ et al: Affective instability and suicidal ideation and behavior in patients with borderline personality disorder, *J Pers Disord* 21:72, 2007.

Lorig KR, Ritter P, Stewart AL et al: Chronic disease self-management program: 2–year health status and health care utilization outcomes, *Med Care* 39:1217, 2001.

Luoma JB, Martin CE, Pearson JL: Contact with mental health and primary care providers before suicide: a review of the evidence, *Am J Psychiatry* 159:909, 2002.

Majumdar B, Ladak S: Management of family and workplace stress experienced by women of color from various cultural backgrounds, *Can J Public Health* 89(1):48, 1998.

Malone KM, Oquendo MA, Haas GL et al: Protective factors against suicidal acts in major depression: reasons for living, *Am J Psychiatry* 157:1084, 2000.

Manley RS, Leichner P: Anguish and despair in adolescents with eating disorders: helping to manage suicidal ideation and impulses, *Crisis* 24(1):32, 2003.

McMenamy JM, Jordan JR, Mitchell AM: What do suicide survivors tell us they need? Results of a pilot study, *Suicide & Life-Threat Behav* 38:375, 2008.

McMyler C, Pryjmachuk S: Do "no-suicide" contracts work? *J Psychiatr Ment Health Nurs* 15:512, 2008.

McNiel DE, Fordwood SR, Weaver CM et al: Effects of training on suicide risk assessment, *Psychiatric Serv* 59:1462, 2008.

Miller M, Mogun H, Azrael D et al: Cancer and the risk of suicide in older Americans, *J Clin Oncol* 26:4720, 2008.

Mills PD, DeRosier JM, Ballot BA et al: National patient safety goals. Inpatient suicide and suicide attempts in Veterans Affairs hospitals, *Joint Comm J Qual Patient Saf* 34:482, 2008.

Minnix JA, Romero C, Joiner TE et al: Change in "resolved plans" and "suicidal ideation" factors of suicidality after participation in an intensive outpatient treatment program, *J Affect Disord* 103:63, 2007.

Misono S, Weiss NS, Fann JR et al: Incidence of suicide in persons with cancer, *J Clin Oncol* 26:4731, 2008.

Muzina DJ: What physicians can do to prevent suicide, *Cleveland Clinic J Med* 71(3):242, 2004.

Neeleman J, Wessely S, Lewis G: Suicide acceptability in African and white Americans: the role of religion, *J Nerv Ment Dis* 186:12, 1998.

Neuner T, Schmid R, Wolfersdorf et al: Predicting inpatient suicide attempts by using clinical routine data? *Genl Hosp Psychiatry* 30:324, 2008.

Nosek CL: Managing a depressed and suicidal loved one at home: impact on the family, *J Psychosoc Nurs Ment Health Serv* 46:36, 2008.

O'Donnell L, O'Donnell C, Wardlaw DM et al: Risk and resiliency factors influencing suicidality among urban African American and Latino youth, *Am J Community Psychol* 33(1–2):37–49, 2004.

Pelkonen M, Marttunen M, Henriksson M et al: Suicidality in adjustment disorder: clinical characteristics of adolescent outpatients, *Eur Child Adolesc Psychiatry* 14:174, 2005.

Pender NJ, Murdaugh CL, Parsons MA: *Health promotion in nursing practice*, ed 5, Upper Saddle River, NJ, 2005, Prentice-Hall.

Ratcliffe GE, Enns MW, Belik S et al: Chronic pain conditions and suicidal ideation and suicide attempts: an epidemiological perspective, *Clin J Pain* 24:204, 2008.

Rew L, Thomas N, Horner SD et al: Correlates of recent suicide attempts in a triethnic group of adolescents, *J Nurs Scholarsh* 33:361, 2001.

Richards B: From respect to rights to entitlement, blocked aspirations and suicidal behavior, *Int J Circumpolar Health* (Suppl 1):19–24, 2004.

Rogers JR, Lewis MM, Subich LM: Validity of the Suicide Assessment Checklist in an emergency crisis center, *J Counsel Develop* 80:493, 2002.

Rouget BW, Aubrey JM: Efficacy of psychoeducational approaches on bipolar disorders: a review of the literature, *J Affect Disord* 98:11, 2007.

Schneider KL, Shenassa E: Correlates of suicide ideation in a population-based sample of cancer patients, *J Psychosoc Oncol* 26:49, 2008.

Shah S, Hoffman RE, Wake L et al: Adolescent suicide and household access to firearms in Colorado: results of a case-control study, *J Adolesc Health* 26(3):157, 2000.

Sheehy N, O'Connor RC: Cognitive style and suicidal behaviour: implications for therapeutic intervention, research lacunae and priorities, *Br J Guidance Counsel* 30(4):353, 2002.

Sherbourne C, Schoenbaum M, Wells KB et al: Characteristics, treatment patterns, and outcomes of persistent depression despite treatment in primary care, *Gen Hosp Psychiatry* 26:106, 2004.

Simpson G & Tate R: Suicidality in people surviving a traumatic brain injury: prevalence, risk factors and implications for clinical management, *Brain Injury* 21:1335, 2007.

Skogman K, Ojehagen A: Motives for suicide attempts—the views of the patient, *Arch Suicide Res* 7:193, 2003a.

Skogman K, Ojehagen A: Problems of importance for suicide attempts—the patients' views, *Arch Suicide Res* 7:207, 2003b.

Spirito A, Boergers J, Donaldson D et al: An intervention trial to improve adherence to community treatment by adolescents after a suicide attempt, *J Am Acad Child Adolesc Psychiatry* 41(4):435, 2002.

Spirito A, Overholser J: The suicidal child: assessment and management of adolescents after a suicide attempt, *Child Adolesc Psychiatric Clin North Am* 12:649, 2003.

Sun F, Long A: A theory to guide families and carers of people who are at risk of suicide, *J Clin Nurs* 17:1939, 2008.

Surgeon General: *The Surgeon General's call to action to prevent suicide, 1999*, www.surgeongeneral.gov/library/calltoaction/default.htm. Accessed April 24, 2007.

Szanto K, Mulsant BH, Houck PR et al: Treatment outcome in suicidal vs. non-suicidal elderly patients, *Am J Geriatr Psychiatry* 9(3):261, 2001.

Tang NK, Crane C: Suicidality in chronic pain: a review of the prevalence, risk factors, and psychological links, *Psychol Med* 36:575, 2006.

Tarrier N, Taylor K, Gooding P: Cognitive-behavioral interventions to reduce suicidal behavior, *Behav Modif* 32:77, 2008.

Torrey EF, Zdanowicz M: Outpatient commitment: what, why, and for whom, *Psychiatr Serv* 52(3):337, 2001.

Toumbourou JW, Gregg ME: Impact of an empowerment-based parent education program on the reduction of youth suicide risk factors, *J Adolesc Health* 31:277, 2002.

Tremblay RE: Physical aggression during early childhood: trajectories and predictors, *Pediatrics* 114(1):43, 2004.

Turner AP, Williams RM, Bowen JD et al: Suicidal ideation in multiple sclerosis, *Arch Phys Med Rehab* 87:1073, 2006.

Valente S, Saunders JM: Barriers to suicide risk management in clinical practice: a national survey of oncology nurses, *Issues Ment Health Nurs* 25:629, 2004.

Valente SM: Sexual abuse of boys, *JCAPN* 18:10, 2005.

Waern M, Rubenowitz E, Wilhelmson K: Predictors of suicide in the old elderly, *Gerontology* 49:328, 2003.

Walker J, Waters RA, Murray G et al: Better off dead: suicidal thoughts in cancer patients, *J Clin Oncol* 26:4725, 2008.

Weaver TL, Allen JA, Hopper E et al: Mediators of suicidal ideation within a sheltered sample of raped and battered women, *Health Care Women Int* 28:478, 2007.

Webb L: Deliberate self-harm in adolescence: a systematic review of psychological and psychosocial factors, *J Adv Nurs* 38(3):235, 2002.

Williams JM, Duggan DS, Crane C et al: Mindfulness-based cognitive therapy for prevention of recurrence of suicidal behavior, *J Clin Psychol* 62:201, 2006.

Woolley SB, Fredman L, Goethe JW et al: Headache complaints and the risk of suicidal thoughts or behaviors, *J Nerv Ment Dis* 196:822, 2008.

Zivin K, Kim M, McCarthy JF et al: Suicide mortality among individuals receiving treatment for depression in the Veterans Affairs Health System: associations with patient and treatment setting characteristics, *Am J Public Health* 97:2193, 2007.

Delayed Surgical recovery
DeLancey Nicoll, SN, and Leslie H. Nicoll, PhD, MBA, RN, BC ⊖volve

NANDA-I

Definition

Extension of the number of postoperative days required to initiate and perform activities that maintain life, health, and well-being

Defining Characteristics

Difficulty in moving about; evidence of interrupted healing of surgical area (e.g., red, indurated draining, immobilized); fatigue; loss of appetite with nausea; loss of appetite without nausea perception that more time is needed to recover; postpones resumption of work/employment activities; requires help to complete self-care; report of discomfort; report of pain

Related Factors (r/t)

Extensive surgical procedure; obesity; pain; postoperative surgical site infection; preoperative expectations; prolonged surgical procedure

NOC (Nursing Outcomes Classification)

Suggested NOC Outcomes

Endurance, Infection Severity, Mobility, Pain Control, Self-Care: Activities of Daily Living (ADLs), Wound Healing: Primary Intention

Example NOC Outcome with Indicators
Wound Healing: Primary Intention as evidenced by the following indicators: Skin approximation/Scar formation (Rate the outcome and indicators of **Wound Healing as: Primary Intention: 1** = none, **2** = limited, **3** = moderate, **4** = substantial, **5** = extensive [see Section I].)

Client Outcomes

Client Will (Specify Time Frame):

- Have surgical area that shows evidence of healing: no redness, induration, draining, or immobility
- State that appetite is regained
- State that no nausea is present
- Demonstrate ability to move about
- Demonstrate ability to complete self-care activities
- State that no fatigue is present
- State that pain is controlled or relieved after nursing interventions
- Resume employment activities/activities of daily living (ADLs)

NIC (Nursing Interventions Classification)

Suggested NIC Interventions

Incision Site Care, Nutrition Management, Pain Management, Self-Care Assistance

Example NIC Activities—Incision Site Care
Teach the patient and/or the family how to care for the incision, including signs and symptoms of infection; Inspect the incision site for redness, swelling, or signs of dehiscence or evisceration

Nursing Interventions and *Rationales*

- Perform a thorough assessment of the client, including risk factors. Allow time to be with the client. **EBN:** *Assessment of clients preoperatively by nursing and medical staff is an important part of the surgical experience to ensure that appropriate interventions are used and recovery from surgery is as*

• = Independent   ▲ = Collaborative   **EBN** = Evidence-Based Nursing   **EB** = Evidence-Based

quick as possible (Layzell, 2008). There may not be a relationship between vital-signs collection and the occurrence or detection of complications (Zeitz & McCutcheon, 2006).

- Assess for the presence of medical conditions and treat appropriately before surgery. If the client is diabetic, maintain normal blood glucose levels before surgery. **EB:** *High blood glucose levels slow healing and increase risk of infection. The American Diabetes Association recommends that blood glucose should be less than 180 mg/dL for people in the hospital or having surgery. For some, the goal is less than 110 mg/dL (Anonymous, 2005). Comorbidities require additional management and comprehensive documentation. The complex care that comorbities require is a role for all nurses to integrate in the client's care plan (Williams, Dunning, & Manias, 2007). Risks involved with surgery increase when a client suffers from diabetes. Those risks can be avoided by meticulous assessment of the client's condition, careful planning of timing of the operation and anesthesia technique, and good control of blood glucose levels before, during, and after surgery (Ritmala-Castérn, 2007).*

- Carefully assess client's use of dietary supplements such as feverfew, ginkgo biloba, garlic, ginseng, ginger, valerian, kava, St. John's wort, ephedra (Ma huang or metabolite), and echinacea. It is recommended that all clients be advised to stop all dietary supplements at least 1 week before major surgical or diagnostic procedures. *Certain dietary supplements can react or interact with frequently used surgical medications—including anesthesia—and may cause serious unforeseen consequences or complications. Arrhythmias, poor wound healing, bleeding, photosensitivity reaction, and prolonged sedation are among the serious reactions during and after surgical and diagnostic procedures that have been attributed to these products (Ciocon, Ciocon, & Galindo, 2004).* **EB:** *Herbal remedies are common in clients presenting for anesthesia. Because of the potential interactions between anesthetic drugs or techniques and such medication it is important for anesthetists to be aware of their use (Baillard et al, 2007).*

- Assess and treat for depression and anxiety in a client complaining of continuing fatigue after surgery. **EB:** *Fatigue is common after major surgery and delays recovery. The results of this study indicate that psychological processes may well be relevant in the etiology of postoperative fatigue (Rubin, Cleare, & Hotopf, 2004).*

- Play music of the client's choice preoperatively, intraoperatively, and postoperatively. **EBN:** *Listening to self-selected music during the preoperative period can effectively reduce anxiety levels and should be a useful tool for preoperative nursing (Arslan, Özer, & Özyurt, 2008).* **EBN:** *Outpatient orthopedic clients indicate that participants overwhelmingly felt that music listening was a positive addition to traditional pain and anxiety management (Lukas, 2004).*

- Consider using healing touch in the perianesthesia setting and other mind-body-spirit interventions such as stress control and imagery. **EBN:** *Research showed that stress management, imagery, and touch therapy all produced reductions in reported worry, as compared with standard therapy (Seskevich, Crater, & Lane, 2004). Hypnosis is a behavioral technique that can reduce pain as part of a comprehensive pain-management plan. As an analgesic, it provides rest, relaxation, and comfort, without negative side effects (Valente, 2006).*

- Use warmed cotton blankets to reduce heat loss during surgery. **EB:** *Warming helps a client maintain normothermia and appears to decrease client anxiety (Wagner, Byrne, & Kolcaba, 2006). Normothermia is associated with low postoperative infection rates (Leaper, 2006).*

- Use careful aseptic technique when caring for wounds. **EBN:** *Client safety when performing aseptic technique is of the highest importance. There is a relationship between standards of aseptic technique and rise in hospital infection (Preston, 2005).*

- Suggest the use of a semipermeable dressing and suction drainage for selected orthopedic clients. **EB:** *This form of postoperative wound management appears to retain the nursing and hygiene advantages of suction drainage while preventing client discomfort and possibilities of wound infection associated with deep internal drainage (Panousis, Grigoris, & Strover, 2004).*

- Clients should be allowed to shower after surgery to maintain cleanliness if not contraindicated because of the presence of pacemaker wires. **EB:** *In a prospective randomized study early water contact was allowed in order to test postoperative wound healing, regardless of whether the wounds were kept dry or had water contact with or without shower foam from the second postoperative day; no infection was registered (Neues & Haas, 2000).*

- Promote early ambulation and deep breathing. Consider use of a transcutaneous electrical nerve stimulation (TENS) unit for pain relief. **EBN:** *Both high and low frequency TENS significantly decreased postoperative pain intensity using the numeric rating scale, pain rating index, and number of*

• = Independent   ▲ = Collaborative   **EBN** = Evidence-Based Nursing   **EB** = Evidence-Based

words chosen compared with placebo TENS (Desantana, Sluka, & Lauretti, 2009). Early ambulation after hip fracture surgery accelerates functional recovery and is associated with more discharges directly home and less to high-level care (Oldmeadow et al, 2006).

- The client should be provided with a complete, balanced therapeutic diet after the immediately postoperative period (24-48 hours). **EB:** *Improvement in nutritional status can improve outcomes of wound healing (Thomas, 2006).* **EBN:** *Good nutrition is important for effective wound healing (Anderson, 2005).*

- Provide 20-minute foot and hand massage (5 minutes to each extremity), 1 to 4 hours after a dose of pain medication. **EBN:** *The clients who had foot and hand massage experienced moderate pain after they received pain medications. This pain was reduced by the intervention, thus supporting the effectiveness of foot and hand massage in postoperative pain management (Wang & Keck, 2004).*

- ▲ Carefully consider the use of alternative therapy with a physician's order, such as application of aloe vera or aqueous cream to promote wound healing. **EBN:** *Aloe vera gel did not significantly reduce radiation-induced skin side effects in breast cancer clients. Aqueous cream was useful in reducing dry desquamation and pain related to radiation therapy (Heggie et al, 2002).*

- Consider the use of noetic therapies: stress management, imagery, and touch therapy. **EBN:** *Studies of therapeutic touch, healing touch, and reiki are quite promising; however, at this point, they can only suggest that these healing modalities have efficacy in reducing anxiety; improving muscle relaxation; aiding in stress reduction, relaxation, and sense of well-being; promoting wound healing; and reducing pain (Engebretson & Wardell, 2007).* **EB:** *Touch therapies may have a modest effect in pain relief (So, Jiang, & Qin, 2008).*

- Encourage the client to use prayer as a form of spiritual coping if this is comfortable for the client. **EB:** *Hierarchical multiple regression analyses showed that preoperative positive religious coping styles and optimism contributed to reduced physical fatigue, controlling for postoperatively confirmed prayer coping and such covariates as severe injury (Ai et al, 2006).*

- See the care plans for **Anxiety, Acute Pain, Fatigue, Risk for deficient Fluid volume, Risk for perioperative positioning Injury, Impaired physical Mobility,** and **Nausea.**

Pediatric

- Support information the parents have gotten from the Internet regarding their child's condition. **EB:** *The Internet is a useful educational tool in teaching parents about their child's condition. Parental use of the Internet is already widespread and may need to be specifically addressed during consultation and preoperative teaching (Sim, Kitteringham, & Spitz, 2007).*

- Teach imagery and encourage distraction for children for postsurgical pain relief. **EBN:** *Distraction decreases pain in children undergoing painful procedures (Stubenrauch, 2007).* **EBN:** *Imagery using distraction was helpful in decreasing the use of analgesics for pain in a group of 7– to 12–year-olds who had had tonsillectomy and/or adenoidectomy (Huth, 2002).*

- Children who are at normal risk for aspiration/regurgitation should be allowed fluids prior to anesthesia. **EB:** *This study demonstrated that there is no evidence that children who are not permitted oral fluids for more than 6 hours preoperatively benefit in terms of intraoperative gastric volume and pH over children permitted unlimited fluids up to 2 hours preoperatively. Children permitted fluids have a more comfortable preoperative experience in terms of thirst and hunger (Brady et al, 2005).*

Geriatric

- Perform a thorough preoperative assessment, including a cardiac and social support assessment. **EB:** *Better preoperative risk assessment and preparation of the client have helped to improve outcomes in geriatric clients (Dharmarajan, Unnikrishnan, & Dharmarajan, 2003).* **EBN:** *Older clients, those with preoperative comorbidities, and those without a caregiver at home experience delays in functional recovery and discharge. These findings support the addition of functional recovery and social support risk items to the preoperative cardiac surgery risk assessment (Anderson et al, 2006).*

- Assess for pain. **EBN:** *Often pain is undermanaged in older people. There is a need for individualized assessment (Brown, 2004).*

- Carefully evaluate the client's temperature. Know what is normal and abnormal for each client. Check baseline temperature and monitor trends. **EB:** *Older subjects have mean oral body temperatures lower than 98.6° F. Relatively few even achieve this temperature (Gomolin et al, 2005).*
- Teach guided imagery for pain relief. **EBN:** *Elderly clients with hip replacements demonstrated positive outcomes for pain relief, decreased anxiety, and decreased length of stay with guided imagery (Antall & Kresevec, 2004).*
- Offer spiritual support. **EB:** *Religious activities, attitudes, and spiritual experiences are prevalent in older hospitalized clients and are associated with greater social support, better psychological health, and to some extent, better physical health. Awareness of these relationships may improve health care (Koenig, George, & Titus, 2004).*

Home Care

- The above interventions may be adapted for the home setting.
- Provide supportive telephone calls from nurse to client as a means of decreasing anxiety and providing the psychosocial support necessary for recovery from surgery. **EBN:** *The clients who had had surgery for breast cancer show that the telephone intervention 1 week after surgery was helpful and the timing was appropriate. The intervention group showed significantly better body image; they worried less about the future and had less postoperative side effects than the control group did (Salonen et al, 2009).*

Client/Family Teaching and Discharge Planning

- Provide preoperative teaching by a nurse to decrease postoperative problems of anxiety, pain, nausea, and lack of independence. **EBN:** *Explanations of hospital routines, facilities and procedures, along with information about forthcoming treatment and specific aftercare can reduce the feelings of anxiety (Theofanidis, 2006). One helpful intervention is to simplify information provision, including the use of reinforcement techniques and being specific about details (Gilmartin & Wright, 2007).*
- Provide preoperative information in verbal and written form. **EB:** *Clients increasingly expect written information; however, amount, quality, and timeliness vary considerably. Combining commercially produced information with standard hospital information may be to the client's benefit (Sheard & Garrud, 2006).*
- Teach systematic muscle relaxation for pain relief. **EBN:** *Unrelieved pain after surgery can lead to complications, prolonged hospital stay, and delayed recovery. Substantial reductions in the sensation and distress of pain were found when postoperative clients used systematic relaxation (Roykulcharoen & Good, 2004).*
- Provide individualized teaching plans for the client with an ostomy. Consider basic needs: (1) maintenance of a pouching seal for a consistent, predictable wear time; (2) maintenance of peristomal skin integrity; and (3) social and professional support of the client. **EB:** *Guiding the client to the ostomy management system suited to his or her lifestyle can play a vital role toward achieving individual quality-of-life goals. Teaching plans should be individualized and customized to reflect and accommodate the phase of rehabilitation and client-defined quality-of-life goals at the time the nurse interacts with the client (Turnbull, Colwell, & Erwin-Toth, 2004).*

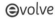 See the EVOLVE website for Weblinks for client education resources.

REFERENCES

Ai AL, Peterson C, Tice TN et al: Faith Differential effects of faith-based coping on physical and mental fatigue in middle-aged and older cardiac patients, *Int J Psychiatry Med* 36(3):351–365, 2006.

Anderson B: Nutrition and wound healing: the necessity of assessment, *Br J Nurs* 14(19):S30, S32, S34, 2005.

Anderson JA, Petersen NJ, Kistner C et al: Determining predictors of delayed recovery and the need for transitional cardiac rehabilitation after cardiac surgery, *J Am Acad Nurse Pract* 18(8):386–392, 2006.

Anonymous: Diabetes in the hospital: taking charge, *Diabetes Spectrum* 18(1):49–50, 2005.

Antall GF, Kresevic D: The use of guided imagery to manage pain in an elderly orthopaedic population, *Orthop Nurs* 23(5):335–340, 2004.

Arslan S, Özer N, Özyurt F: Effect of music on preoperative anxiety in men undergoing urogenital surgery, *Aus J Adv Nurs* 26(2):46–54, 2008.

Baillard C, Bianchi A, Gehan G et al: Anaesthetic preoperative assessment of chronic medications and herbal medicine use: a multicenter survey, *Ann Fr Anesth Reanim* 26(5):468–469, 2007.

• = Independent   ▲ = Collaborative   **EBN** = Evidence-Based Nursing   **EB** = Evidence-Based

Brady M, Kinn S, O'Rourke K et al: Preoperative fasting for preventing perioperative complications in children, *Cochrane Database Syst Rev* (2):CD005285, 2005.

Brown D: A literature review exploring how healthcare professionals contribute to the assessment and control of postoperative pain in older people, *J Clin Nurs* 13(6b):74–90, 2004.

Ciocon JO, Ciocon DG, Galindo DJ: Dietary supplements in primary care. Botanicals can affect surgical outcomes and follow-up, *Geriatrics* 59(9):20–24, 2004.

Desantana JM, Sluka KA, Lauretti GR: High and low frequency TENS reduce postoperative pain intensity after laparoscopic tubal ligation: a randomized controlled trial, *Clin J Pain* 25(1):12–19, 2009.

Dharmarajan TS, Unnikrishnan D, Dharmarajan L: Preparing the older adult for surgery, *Hosp Physician* 39(11):45–54, 2003.

Engebretson J, Wardell DW: Energy-based modalities, *Nurs Clin North Am* 42(2):243–259, 2007.

Gilmartin J, Wright K: The nurse's role in day surgery: a literature review, *Int Nurs Rev* 54(2): 183–190, 2007.

Gomolin IH, Aung MM, Wolf-Klein G et al: Older is colder: temperature range and variation in older people, *J Am Geriatr Soc* 53(12):2170–2172, 2005.

Heggie S, Bryant GP, Tripcony L et al: A phase III study on the efficacy of topical aloe vera gel on irradiated breast tissue, *Cancer Nurs* 25(6):442–451, 2002.

Huth MM: *Imagery to reduce children's postoperative pain* [doctoral dissertation], Cleveland, OH, 2002, Case Western Reserve University.

Koenig HG, George LK, Titus P: Religion, spirituality, and health in medically ill hospitalized older patients, *J Am Geriatr Soc* 52(4):554–562, 2004.

Layzell M: Current interventions and approaches to postoperative pain management, *Brit J Nurs* 17(7):414–419, 2008.

Leaper D: Effects of local and systemic warming on postoperative infections, *Surg Infect (Larchmt)* (Suppl 2):S101–S103, 2006.

Lukas LK: Orthopedic outpatients' perception of perioperative music listening as therapy, *J Theory Construct Testing* 8(1):7–12, 2004.

Neues C, Haas E: [Modification of postoperative wound healing by showering] [article in German], *Chirurg* 71(2):234–236, 2000.

Oldmeadow LB, Edwards ER, Kimmel LA et al: No rest for the wounded: early ambulation after hip surgery accelerates recovery, *ANZ J Surg* 76(7):607–611, 2006.

Panousis K, Grigoris P, Strover AE: Suction dressings in total knee arthroplasty—an alternative to deep suction drainage, *Acta Orthop Belg* 70(4):349–354, 2004.

Preston R: Aseptic technique: evidence-based approach for patient safety, *Br J Nurs* 14(10):540–544, 2005.

Ritmala-Castérn M: [Diabetic patient in surgery] [article in Finnish], *Sairaanhoitaja* 80(4):28–30, 2007.

Roykulcharoen V, Good M: Systematic relaxation to relieve postoperative pain, *J Adv Nurs* 48(2):140–148, 2004.

Rubin GJ, Cleare A, Hotopf M: Psychological factors in postoperative fatigue, *Psychosom Med* 66(6):959–964, 2004.

Salonen P, Tarkka MT, Kellokumpu-Lehtinen PL et al: Telephone intervention and quality of life in patients with breast cancer, *Cancer Nurs* 32(3):177–190, 2009.

Seskevich JE, Crater SW, Lane JD: Beneficial effects of noetic therapies on mood before percutaneous intervention for unstable coronary syndromes, *Nurs Res* 53(2):116–121, 2004.

Sheard C, Garrud P: Evaluation of generic patient information: effects on health outcomes, knowledge and satisfaction, *Patient Educ Couns* 61(1):43–47, 2006.

Sim NZ, Kitteringham L, Spitz L: Information on the World Wide Web—how useful is it for parents? *J Pediatr Surg* 42(2):305–312, 2007.

So PS, Jiang Y, Qin Y: Touch therapies for pain relief in adults, *Cochrane Database Syst Rev.* 8;(4):CD006535, 2008.

Stubenrauch J: Striving for distraction, *AJN* 107(3):94–95, 2007.

Theofanidis D: Stress and the hospitalized patient: can we deal with it? *ICUS Nurs Web J* 27, 2006.

Thomas DR: Prevention and treatment of pressure ulcers, *J Am Med Dir Assoc* 42(5):46–59, 2006.

Turnbull GB, Colwell J, Erwin-Toth P: Quality of life: pre, post, and beyond ostomy surgery: clinician strategies for helping people with a stoma lead healthy, productive lives, *Ostomy Wound Manage* 50(7): S2, 2004.

Valente SM: Hypnosis for pain management, *J Psychosoc Nurs* 44(2):22–30, 2006.

Wagner D, Byrne M, Kolcaba K: Effects of comfort warming on preoperative patients, *AORN J* 84(3):427–448, 2006.

Wang H, Keck JF: Foot and hand massage as an intervention for postoperative pain, *Pain Manage Nurs* 5(2):59–65, 2004.

Williams A, Dunning T, Manias E: Continuity of care and general well-being of patients with comorbidities requiring joint replacement, *J Adv Nurs* 57(3):244–256, 2007.

Zeitz K, McCutcheon H: Observations and vital signs: ritual or vital for the monitoring of postoperative patients? *Appl Nurs Res* 19(4):204–211, 2006.

Impaired Swallowing   *Betty J. Ackley, MSN, EdS, RN*   ⊝volve

NANDA-I

Definition

Abnormal functioning of the swallowing mechanism associated with deficits in oral, pharyngeal, or esophageal structure or function

Defining Characteristics

Esophageal phase impairment: Abnormality in esophageal phase by swallow study; acidic smelling breath; bruxism; complaints of "something stuck"; epigastric pain; food refusal; heartburn or epigastric pain; hematemesis; hyperextension of head (e.g., arching during or after meals); nighttime awakening; nighttime coughing; observed evidence of difficulty in swallowing (e.g., stasis of food in oral cavity, coughing/choking); odynophagia; regurgitation of gastric contents (wet burps); repetitive swallowing; unexplained irritability surrounding mealtime; volume limiting; vomiting; vomitus on pillow

Oral phase impairment: Abnormality in oral phase of swallow study; choking, coughing, or gagging before a swallow; drooling; food falls from mouth; food pushed out of mouth; inability to clear

• = Independent   ▲ = Collaborative   **EBN** = Evidence-Based Nursing   **EB** = Evidence-Based

oral cavity; incomplete lip closure; lack of chewing; lack of tongue action to form bolus; long meals with little consumption; nasal reflux; piecemeal deglutition; pooling in lateral sulci; premature entry of bolus; sialorrhea; slow bolus formation; weak suck resulting in inefficient nippling

Pharyngeal phase impairment: abnormality in pharyngeal phase by swallowing study; altered head position; choking, coughing, or gagging; delayed swallow; food refusal; gurgly voice quality; inadequate laryngeal elevation; multiple swallows; nasal reflux; recurrent pulmonary infections; unexplained fevers

Related Factors (r/t)

Congenital Defects

Behavioral feeding problems; conditions with significant hypotonia; congenital heart disease; failure to thrive; history of tube feeding; mechanical obstruction (e.g., edema, tracheostomy tube, tumor); neuromuscular impairment (e.g., decreased or absent gag reflex, decreased strength or excursion of muscles involved in mastication, perceptual impairment, facial paralysis); protein energy malnutrition; respiratory disorders self-injurious behavior; upper airway anomalies

Neurological Problems

Achalasia; acquired anatomic defects; cerebral palsy; cranial nerve involvement; developmental delay; esophageal defects; gastroesophageal reflux disease; laryngeal abnormalities; laryngeal defects; nasal defects; nasopharyngeal cavity defects; oropharynx abnormalities; prematurity; tracheal defects; traumas; traumatic head injury; upper airway anomalies

NOC (Nursing Outcomes Classification)

Suggested NOC Outcomes

Swallowing Status, Swallowing Status: Esophageal Phase, Oral Phase, Pharyngeal Phase

Example NOC Outcome with Indicators
Swallowing Status as evidenced by the following indicators: Delivery of bolus to hypopharynx is timed with swallow reflex/Ability to clear oral cavity/Number of swallows appropriate for bolus size and texture/Voice quality/Choking, coughing, gagging/Normal swallow effort (Rate the outcome and indicators of **Swallowing Status:** 1 = severely compromised, 2 = substantially compromised, 3 = moderately compromised, 4 = mildly compromised, 5 = not compromised [see Section I].)

Client Outcomes

Client Will (Specify Time Frame):

- Demonstrate effective swallowing without choking or coughing
- Remain free from aspiration (e.g., lungs clear, temperature within normal range)

NIC (Nursing Interventions Classification)

Suggested NIC Interventions

Aspiration Precautions, Swallowing Therapy

Example NIC Activities—Swallowing Therapy
Assist client to sit in erect position (as close to 90 degrees as possible) for feeding/exercise; Instruct client not to talk during eating, if appropriate

Nursing Interventions and *Rationales*

- Determine the client's readiness to eat. The client needs to be alert, able to follow instructions, able to hold the head erect, able to swallow, and able to move the tongue in the mouth. *If one of these elements is missing, it may be advisable to withhold oral feeding and use enteral feeding for nourishment (Wieseke, Bantz, & Siktberg, 2008).*

• = Independent ▲ = Collaborative **EBN** = Evidence-Based Nursing **EB** = Evidence-Based

- Observe for signs associated with swallowing problems (e.g., coughing, choking, spitting of food, drooling, difficulty handling oral secretions, double swallowing or major delay in swallowing, watering eyes, nasal discharge, wet or gurgly voice, decreased ability to move the tongue and lips, decreased mastication of food, decreased ability to move food to the back of the pharynx, slow or scanning speech) (Wieseke, Bantz, & Siktberg, 2008). **EB:** *A study demonstrated that voice analysis could accurately predict the clients with dysphagia by presence of perturbation, shimmer percentage, noise-to-harmonic ratio, and voice turbulence as tested by videofluoroscopic swallowing studies (Ryu, Park, & Choi, 2004).*

▲ If the client has impaired swallowing, do not feed until an appropriate diagnostic workup is completed. Refer to a speech pathologist for bedside evaluation, and videofluoroscopy to determine swallowing problems and solutions as soon as possible. Ensure that the client is seen by a speech pathologist within 48 hours after admission if the client has had a CVA. Ensure proper nutrition by consulting with a physician regarding enteral feedings, preferably using a percutaneous endoscopic gastrostomy (PEG) tube in most cases. **EBN:** *Early referral of CVA clients to a speech pathologist, along with early initiation of nutritional support, can result in decreased length of hospital stay, shortened recovery time, and reduced overall health costs (Runions et al, 2004).* **EB:** *Enteral feedings via PEG tube are generally preferable to nasogastric tube feedings, but further studies are needed (Bath, Bath-Hextrall, & Smithard, 2005). A referral for a formal swallowing evaluation is indicated in preventing aspiration pneumonia (Hammond & Goldstein, 2006).*

▲ To manage impaired swallowing, use a dysphagia team composed of a rehabilitation nurse, speech pathologist, dietitian, physician, and radiologist who work together. *The dysphagia team can help the client learn to swallow safely and maintain a good nutritional status Feeding a client who cannot adequately swallow results in aspiration and possibly death (Wieseke, Bantz, & Siktberg, 2008).*

- Assess ability to swallow by positioning the thumb and index finger on the client's laryngeal protuberance. Ask the client to swallow; feel the larynx elevate. Note the length of time needed for the larynx to elevate, a prolonged time is associated with impaired swallowing. Ask the client to cough, and test for a gag reflex on both sides of the posterior pharyngeal wall (lingual surface) with a tongue blade. Do not rely on the presence of a gag reflex to determine when to feed. *Clients can aspirate even if they have an intact gag reflex (Wieseke, Bantz, & Siktberg, 2008).* **EB:** *CVA clients with prolonged pharyngeal transit times (prolonged swallowing) have an increased chance of developing aspiration pneumonia (Marik & Kaplan, 2003).*

- Consider the use of the Massey Bedside Swallowing Screen to screen for swallowing dysfunction. **EBN:** *The Massey Bedside Swallowing Screen demonstrated high sensitivity and specificity in predicting dysphagia, compared with assessment by experts in the field (Massey & Jedlicka, 2002).*

- Recognize that impaired swallowing may be caused by the medications the client is taking. Side effects of medications include xerostomia (antidepressants, anticholinergics, antihistamines, bronchodilators, antineoplastic, anti-Parkinson), CNS depression (anticonvulsants, benzodiazepines, antispasmodics, antidepressants, antipsychotics), myopathy (corticosteroids, lipid-lowering agents, colchicines), and esophageal sphincter tone decrease (antihistamines, diuretics, opiates, antipsychotics, antihypertensives, anticholinergics). *Medications can cause impaired swallowing in multiple ways. For more information about medications, refer to these references (Wieseke, Bantz, & Siktberg, 2008; Gallagher & Naidoo, 2009).*

- If client is not eating a sufficient amount of food, recognize that the immune system may be impaired with resultant increased risk of infection. **EB:** *A study comparing elderly clients with dysphagia who were tube fed versus others who were orally fed, the orally fed clients had much lower CD4 cell counts, as well as a low CD4/CD8 ratio (Leibovitz et al, 2004).*

- If the client has an intact swallowing reflex, attempt to feed. Observe the following feeding guidelines:
  - Position the client upright at a 90–degree angle with the chin tucked forward at a 45–degree angle if this has been determined to be helpful (Metheny, 2007). *The chin tuck is protective for most people with dysphagia, because the epiglottis forms a protective shelf over the vocal folds as the client swallows (West & Redstone, 2004).*
  - Ensure that the client is awake, alert, and able to follow sequenced directions before attempting to feed. *As the client becomes less alert, the swallowing response decreases, which increases the risk of aspiration.*
  - Begin by feeding the client one third of a teaspoon of applesauce. Provide sufficient time to masticate and swallow.

● = Independent ▲ = Collaborative **EBN** = Evidence-Based Nursing **EB** = Evidence-Based

- Place the food on the unaffected side of the tongue.
- During feeding, give the client specific directions (e.g., "Open your mouth, chew the food completely, and when you are ready, tuck your chin to your chest and swallow").
- Avoid rushing or forcing feeding.
- Ensure client is kept in an upright posture for an hour after eating. *An upright posture after eating has been associated with a decreased incidence of pneumonia in the elderly (Coleman, 2004; Metheny, 2007).*

▲ Watch for uncoordinated chewing or swallowing; coughing immediately after eating or delayed coughing, which may indicate silent aspiration; pocketing of food; wet-sounding voice; sneezing when eating; delay of more than 1 second in swallowing; or a change in respiratory patterns. If any of these signs is present, put on gloves, remove all food from the oral cavity, stop feedings, and consult with a speech and language pathologist and a dysphagia team. *These are signs of impaired swallowing and possible aspiration (Wieseke, Bantz, & Siktberg, 2008).*

● If the client tolerates single-textured foods such as pudding, hot cereal, or strained baby food, advance to a soft diet with guidance from the dysphagia team. Avoid foods such as hamburgers, corn, and pastas that are difficult to chew. Also avoid sticky foods such as peanut butter and white bread. *The dysphagia team should determine the appropriate diet for the client based on progression in swallowing and need to ensure that the client is nourished and hydrated.*

▲ Avoid providing liquids until the client is able to swallow effectively. Add a thickening agent to liquids as ordered based on a swallowing study to obtain a soft consistency that is similar to nectar, honey, or pudding, depending on the degree of swallowing problems. *Liquids can be easily aspirated; thickened liquids form a cohesive bolus that the client can swallow with increased efficiency (Wieseke, Bantz, & Siktberg, 2008). The majority of clients with swallowing difficulties received liquids thickened to nectar-syrup consistency (60%), 33% received honey consistency, and only 6% received pudding consistency thickened fluids (Castellanos et al, 2004). NOTE: Several studies have shown that clients receiving thickened fluids do not meet daily fluid requirements, and may become dehydrated (Campbell-Taylor, 2008).*

▲ Work with the client on swallowing exercises prescribed by the dysphagia team (e.g., touching the palate with the tongue, stimulating the tonsillar arch and soft palate with a cold metal examination mirror [thermal stimulation], labial/lingual range-of-motion exercises). *Swallowing exercises, including both motor and sensory stimulation, can improve the client's ability to swallow (Hagg & Larsson, 2004). Exercises need to be done at intervals, which necessitates nursing involvement).* **EB:** *Clients who received a high-intensity swallowing intervention versus usual care or a low-intensity swallowing intervention were more likely to return to a normal diet and recover swallowing ability by 6 months (Carnaby, Hankey, & Pizzi, 2006).*

▲ For many adult clients, avoid the use of straws if recommended by the speech pathologist. *Use of straws can increase the risk of aspiration, because straws can result in spilling of a bolus of fluid rapidly in the posterior pharynx.* **EB:** *A reduction in airway protection with use of a straw was shown for drinking in the older men as compared with the younger men (Daniels et al, 2004).*

● If needed, provide meals in a quiet environment away from excessive stimuli, such as a community dining room for some clients who are easily distracted. *A noisy environment can be an aversive stimulus and can decrease effective chewing and swallowing.*

● Ensure that there is adequate time for the client to eat. *Clients with swallowing impairments often take longer than others to eat, if they are being fed. Often, food is offered rapidly to speed up the task, which can increase the chance of aspiration (Metheny, 2007).*

● Recognize that the client can aspirate oral feedings, even if there are no symptoms of coughing or distress. *This phenomenon is called silent aspiration and is common (Easterling & Robbins, 2008). Studies have shown that most individuals aspirate their own saliva during sleep. What determines if the client develops pneumonia is the ability of the immune system to control bacteria and the amount of contamination of the oropharynx (Campbell-Taylor, 2008).*

● Have suction equipment available during feeding. If choking occurs and suctioning is necessary, discontinue oral feeding until the client is safely assessed with a videofluoroscopic swallow study.

● Check the oral cavity for proper emptying after the client swallows and after the client finishes the meal. Provide oral care at the end of the meal. It may be necessary to manually remove food from the client's mouth. If this is the case, use gloves and keep the client's teeth apart with a padded tongue blade. *Food may become pocketed on the affected side and cause stomatitis, tooth decay, and possible later aspiration.*

- Praise the client for successfully following directions and swallowing appropriately. *Praise reinforces behavior and sets up a positive atmosphere in which learning takes place.*
- Keep the client in an upright position for 45 minutes to an hour after a meal. **EB:** *A study demonstrated that the number of elderly clients developing a fever was significantly reduced when clients were kept sitting upright after eating (Matsui et al, 2002).*
- ▲ Watch for signs of aspiration and pneumonia. Auscultate lung sounds after feeding. Note new onset of crackles or wheezing, and note elevated temperature. Notify the physician as needed. *The presence of an increased respiratory rate, new crackles or wheezing, an elevated temperature or white blood cell count, a change in sputum, and also new onset of delirium could indicate aspiration of food or onset of pneumonia (Metheny, 2007).* **EB:** *Bronchial auscultation of lung sounds was shown to be specific in identifying clients at risk for aspirating (Shaw et al, 2004).*
- Watch for signs of malnutrition and dehydration. Keep a record of food intake. *Malnutrition is common in dysphagic clients (Wieseke, Bantz, & Siktberg, 2008). Clients with dysphagia are at serious risk for malnutrition and dehydration, which can lead to aspiration pneumonia resulting from depressed immune function and weakness, lethargy, and decreased cough.*
- ▲ Weigh the client weekly to help evaluate nutritional status. Evaluate nutritional status daily. If the client is not adequately nourished, work with the dysphagia team to determine whether the client needs therapeutic feeding only or needs enteral feedings until the client can swallow adequately. **EB:** *Dysphagic stroke clients who received thickened fluid dysphagia diets failed to meet their needs for fluids, whereas a group receiving enteral feeding and IV fluid did meet fluid requirements (Finestone et al, 2001).*
- ▲ If client has a tracheostomy, ask for referral to speech pathologist for swallowing studies before attempting to feed. After evaluation, the decision should be made to have cuff either inflated or deflated when client eats. **EB:** *Studies have shown that use of speaking valves for the client with a tracheostomy may reduce risk of aspiration when the client eats (Baumgartner, Bewyer, & Bruner, 2008). A study found that tracheostomy was not associated with increased aspiration (Sharma et al, 2007).*

Pediatric

- ▲ Refer to a physician and a dietician a child who has difficulty swallowing and symptoms such as difficulty manipulating food, delayed swallow response, and pocketing of a bolus of food. **EB:** *Adequate nutrition is extremely important for children to ensure sufficient growth and development of all body systems (Morgan, Ward, & Murdoch, 2004).*
- ▲ Provide oral motor stimulation that increases oral-sensory awareness by waking the mouth using exercises that focus on temperature, taste, and texture. *Many of these infants require supplemental tube feedings and special nipples or bottles to boost oral intake.*
- For infants with poor sucking and swallowing, support the cheeks and jaw to increase sucking skills; pace or rhythmically move the bottle, which encourages better suck-swallow-breathe synchrony.
- Watch for indicators of aspiration: coughing, a change in web vocal quality while feeding, perspiration and color changes during feeding, sneezing, and increased heart rate and breathing.
- Watch for warning signs of reflux: sour-smelling breath after eating, sneezing, lack of interest in feeding, crying and fussing extraordinarily when feeding, pained expressions when feeding, and excessive chewing and swallowing after eating. *Many premature and medically fragile children experience growth deficits and respiratory problems from an underlying dysphagia. Some infants may need to work harder to breathe than others and as a result develop a decreased tolerance for food intake. They also demonstrate inconsistent arousal and poor/uncoordinated suck-swallow-breath synchrony. Many of these infants require supplemental tube feedings and the use of special nipples or bottles to boost oral intake.*

Geriatric

- Recognize that being elderly does not necessarily result in dysphagia, but having medical problems including such things as cerebrovascular and other neurological disease along with chronic medical

---

● = Independent   ▲ = Collaborative   **EBN** = Evidence-Based Nursing   **EB** = Evidence-Based

problems can result in dysphagia. *There are changes in physiological function associated with aging that can affect swallowing, but the effects are more pronounced when superimposed on disease (Easterling & Robbins, 2008).*

- Recognize that the loss of teeth can cause problems with chewing and swallowing. *Missing teeth and poorly fitting dentures predispose the client for aspiration, because of inadequate chewing and swallowing (Metheny, 2007).*

▲ Evaluate medications the client is presently taking, especially if elderly. Consult with the pharmacist for assistance in monitoring for incorrect doses and drug interactions that could result in dysphagia. *Most elderly clients take numerous medications, which when taken individually can slow motor function, cause anxiety and depression, and reduce salivary flow. When taken together, these medications can interact, resulting in impaired swallowing function. Drugs that reduce muscle tone for swallowing and can cause reflux include calcium channel blockers and nitrates. Drugs that can reduce salivary flow include antidepressants, antiparkinsonism drugs, antihistamines, antispasmodics, antipsychotic agents or major tranquilizers, antiemetics, antihypertensives, and drugs for treating diarrhea and anxiety (Wieseke, Bantz, & Siktberg, 2008; Gallagher & Naidoo, 2009).*

- Recognize that the elderly client with dementia needs a longer time to eat. *The dementia client has decreased ability to smell, decreased cognition, distractibility, and decreased efficiency in chewing and is likely to have problems with swallowing (Easterling & Robbins, 2008).*

- For the client with dementia, hydration and nutrition can be optimized using the following techniques:
  - Good oral hygiene
  - Encouraging six small meals and hydration breakers per day
  - Offering foods that are sweet, spicy, or sour to increase sensory input
  - Allowing clients to touch food, and self-feed, with their hands if necessary
  - Eliminating from the tray or table nonfoods such as salt and pepper, or anything that can be distracting
  - Keeping desserts out of sight until the end of the meal
  - Offering finger foods to the client who has trouble holding still to eat
  - Not making clients wait when they come for the meal

  Dementia clients are often impulsive, and easily distracted. These techniques can help increase nutrition (Easterling & Robbins, 2008)

- Recognize that the client with advanced dementia, who is unable to swallow, may or may not benefit from enteral tube feedings. *Some dementia clients enter into a catabolic state with negative protein balance, and it may be irreversible. In addition there is often an increased risk for aspiration pneumonia in the tube fed client (Easterling & Robbins, 2008).*

Home Care

▲ Refer to speech therapy. Speech therapists can work with clients to enhance swallowing ability.

Client/Family Teaching and Discharge Planning

▲ Teach the client and family exercises prescribed by the dysphagia team.
▲ Teach the client a systematic method of swallowing effectively as prescribed by the dysphagia team.
- Educate the client, family, and all caregivers about rationales for food consistency and choices. *It is common for family members to disregard necessary dietary restrictions and give the client inappropriate foods that predispose to aspiration*
- Teach the family how to monitor the client to prevent and detect aspiration during eating.

Ⓔvolve   See the EVOLVE website for Weblinks for client education resources.

REFERENCES

Bath PM, Bath-Hextrall FJ, Smithard EG: Interventions for dysphagia in acute stroke, *Cochrane Database Syst Rev* (2): CD000323, DJ9, 2005.

Baumgartner CA, Bewyer E, Bruner D: Management of communication and swallowing in intensive care: the role of the speech pathologist, *AACN Adv Crit Care* 19(4):433–443, 2008.

Campbell-Taylor I: Oropharyngeal dysphagia in long-term care: misperceptions of treatment efficacy, *J Am Med Dir Assoc*, 9(7):523–531, 523–531, 2008.

Carnaby G, Hankey G, Pizzi J: Behavioral intervention for dysphagia in acute stroke: a randomized controlled trial, *Lancet Neurol* 5:31–7, 2006.

Castellanos VH et al: Use of thickened liquids in skilled nursing facilities, *J ADA Assoc* 104(8):1222, 2004.

Coleman PR: Pneumonia in the long-term care setting: etiology, management, and prevention, *J Gerontol Nurs* 30(4):14, 2004.

Daniels S, Corey D, Hadskey et al: Mechanism of sequential swallowing during straw drinking in healthy young and older adults, *J Speech Lang Hearing Res* 47:33–45, 2004.

Easterling CS, Robbins E: Dementia and dysphagia, *Geriatr Nurs* 29(4):275–285, 2008.

Finestone H, Foley N, Woodbury MG et al: Quantifying fluid intake in dysphagic stroke patients: a preliminary comparison of oral and nonoral strategies, *Arch Phys Med Rehabil* 82:1744–1746, 2001.

Gallagher L, Naidoo P: Prescription drugs and their effects on swallowing, *Dysphagia* 24(2):159–166, 2009.

Hagg, Larsson B: Effects of motor and sensory stimulation in stroke patients with long-lasting dysphagia, *Dysphagia* 19(4):219, 2004.

Hammond CA, Goldstein LB: Cough and aspiration of food and fluids due to oral-pharyngeal dysphagia: ACCP evidence-based clinical practice guidelines, *Chest*, 129:154–68, 2006.

Leibovitz A et al: CD4 lymphocyte count and CD4/CD8 ratio in elderly long-term care clients with oropharyngeal dysphagia: comparison between oral and tube enteral feedings, *Dysphagia* 19(2):83, 2004.

Marik PE, Kaplan D: Aspiration pneumonia and dysphagia in the elderly, *Chest* 124(1):328, 2003.

Massey R, Jedlicka D: The Massey Bedside Swallowing Screen, *J Neurosci Nurs* 34(5):252, 2002.

Matsui T et al: Sitting position to prevent aspiration in bed-bound patients, *Gerontology* 48:194, 2002.

Metheny NA: Try this: best practices in nursing care to older adults. Preventing aspiration in older adults with dysphagia, *Medsurg Nurs* 16(4):271–272, 2007.

Morgan A, Ward E, Murdoch B: Clinical characteristics of acute dysphagia in pediatric patients following traumatic brain injury, *J Head Trauma Rehabil* 19(3):226–240, 2004.

Runions S, Rodrigue N, White C: Practice on an acute stroke until after implementation of a decision-making algorithm for dietary management of dysphagia, *J Neurosci Nurse* 36(4): 200, 2004.

Ryu JS, Park SR, Choi KH: Prediction of laryngeal aspiration using voice analysis, *Am J Phy Med Rehabil* 83(10):753, 2004.

Sharma OP, Oswanski MF, Singer D et al: Swallowing disorders in trauma patients: impact of tracheostomy, *Am Surg* 73(11):1117–1121, 2007.

Shaw JL et al: Bronchial auscultation: an effective adjunct to speech and language therapy bedside assessment when detecting dysphagia and aspiration? *Dysphagia* 19(4):211, 2004.

West JF, Redstone F: Feeding the adult with neurogenic disorders, *Top Geriatr Rehabil* 20(2):131–134, 2004.

Wieseke A, Bantz D, Siktberg L: Assessment and early diagnosis of dysphagia, *Geriatric Nursing* 29(6):376–383, 2008.

Ineffective family Therapeutic regimen management
Dawn Fairlie, ANP, FNP, GNP, DNS(c)

NANDA-I

Definition

Pattern of regulating and integrating into family processes a program for treatment of illness and its sequelae that is unsatisfactory for meeting specific health goals

Defining Characteristics

Acceleration of illness symptoms of a family member; inappropriate family activities for meeting health goals; failure to take actions to reduce risk factors; lack of attention to illness; verbalizes desire to manage the illness; verbalizes difficulty with therapeutic regimen

Related Factors (r/t)

Complexity of health care system; complexity of therapeutic regimen; decisional conflicts; economic difficulties; excessive demands; family conflict

NOC   (Nursing Outcomes Classification)

Suggested NOC Outcomes

Family Health-Status, Knowledge: Treatment Regimen, Family Participation in Professional Care

• = Independent   ▲ = Collaborative   **EBN** = Evidence-Based Nursing   **EB** = Evidence-Based

Example NOC Outcome with Indicators
Knowledge: Treatment Regimen as evidenced by the following indicator: Description of prescribed medication, activity, exercise, and specific disease process (Rate the outcome and indicators of **Knowledge: Treatment Regimen:** 1 = no knowledge, 2 = limited knowledge, 3 = moderate knowledge, 4 = substantial knowledge, 5 = extensive knowledge [see Section I].)

Family Outcomes

Family Will (Specify Time Frame):

- Make adjustments in usual activities (e.g., diet, activity, stress management) to incorporate therapeutic regimens of its members
- Reduce illness symptoms of family members
- Desire to manage therapeutic regimens of its members
- Describe a decrease in the difficulties of managing therapeutic regimens
- Describe actions to reduce risk factors

 (Nursing Interventions Classification)

Suggested NIC Interventions

Family Involvement Promotion, Family Mobilization, Teaching: Disease Process

Example NIC Activities—Family Involvement Promotion
Identify and respect coping mechanisms used by family members; Provide crucial information to family members about the patient in accordance with client's preference

Nursing Interventions and *Rationales*

- Base family interventions on knowledge of the family, family context, and family function. **EBN:** *Family research has established that families differ widely from one another, even within cultures (Wright & Leahey, 2005). Family context includes all aspects of the larger societal systems. In a literature review, family functioning was shown to have positive effects on self-management (Grey, Knafl, & McCorkle, 2006).*
- Use a family approach when helping an individual with a health problem that requires therapeutic management. **EBN:** *In studies of self-management, family support was found to be a predictor of positive self-management (Leong, Molassiotis, & Marsh, 2004; Whittemore, Melkus, & Grey, 2005).*
- Review with family members the congruence and incongruence of family behaviors and health-related goals. **EBN:** *To attain the motivation needed for changes in health habits, family members should understand the relation of daily habits to health-related goals (Wright & Leahey, 2005).*
- Acknowledge the challenge of integrating therapeutic regimens with family behaviors. **EBN:** *Therapeutic regimens require modifications of daily activities that have already been established based on family values and beliefs. Acknowledging the difficulty of changing family habits supports families through the process (Wright & Leahey, 2005).*
- Review the symptoms of specific illness(es) and work with the family toward development of greater self-efficacy in relation to these symptoms. **EBN:** *Knowledge of symptoms improves the ability of family members to adjust behaviors to prevent and manage symptoms (Lubkin & Larsen, 2006).*
- Support family decisions to adjust therapeutic regimens as indicated. **EBN:** *Sometimes families do not have access to health providers and should make independent decisions because of side effects or adverse effects of therapeutic regimens. Family members need to make informed decisions in their best interests (Wright & Leahey, 2005).*
- Advocate for the family in negotiating therapeutic regimens with health providers. **EB:** *Illness regimens generally are neither arbitrary nor absolute; therefore, modifications can be discussed as needed to fit with the family lifestyle (Wright & Leahey, 2005).*
- Help the family mobilize social supports. **EBN:** *Increased social support helps families to meet health-related goals (Pender, Murdaugh, & Parsons, 2006).*

• = Independent   ▲ = Collaborative   **EBN** = Evidence-Based Nursing   **EB** = Evidence-Based

- Help family members modify perceptions as indicated. **EBN:** *Individual perceptions of the seriousness of, susceptibility to, and threat of illness may be distorted or inaccurate and may be modified with new information (Pender, Murdaugh, & Parsons, 2006).*
- Use one or more theories of family dynamics to describe, explain, or predict family behaviors (e.g., theories of Bowen, Satir, and Minuchin). **EBN:** *Family systems may not be understood by the nurse without adequate knowledge of family theory (Wright & Leahey, 2005).*
- ▲ Collaborate with expert nurses or other consultants regarding strategies for working with families. **EBN:** *Family systems are complex and challenging (Wright & Leahey, 2005); expert nurses can assist with problem solving and planning.*
- Promote and support public health programs to support families. **EB:** *Because the burden of family care is significant, a national effort is underway to support family caregivers, the National Family Caregiver Support Program. One study showed that 10 states have begun development of such programs (Feinberg & Newman, 2004).*
- Coaching methods can be used to help families improve their health. **EB:** *Coaching processes were shown to improve family outcomes related to improved nutrition and physical activity (Heimendinger et al, 2007).*

Pediatric

- Support kangaroo care for infants at risk at birth. Keep infants in an upright position in skin-to-skin contact until they no longer tolerate it. **EB:** *Kangaroo Mother Care has a positive impact on family and home environment. The results of this study also suggest, first, that both parents should be involved as direct caregivers in the Kangaroo Mother Care procedure and secondly, that this intervention should be directed more specifically at infants who are more at risk at birth (Tessier et al, 2009).*

Geriatric

- Recommend that clients use the "Ask Me 3" program when communicating with their pharmacist (What is my main problem?, What do I need to do?, Why is it important for me to do this?). **EB:** *The Ask Me 3 program is a practical tool that creates awareness and reinforces principles of clear health communication with pharmacists and community dwelling well-elder seniors who participated in this study (Miller et al, 2008).*

Multicultural

- Acknowledge racial and ethnic differences at the onset of care. **EBN:** *Acknowledgment of race and ethnicity issues enhances communication, establishes rapport, and promotes treatment outcomes (Leininger & McFarland, 2006; Giger & Davidhizar, 2008).*
- Ensure that all strategies for working with the family are congruent with the culture of the family. **EBN:** *Many nursing studies among people of a variety of cultures show that cultural variations exist in the management of therapeutic regimens, and these differences should be taken into account when working with families (Leininger & McFarland, 2006; Hanley, 2008).*
- Approach families of color with respect, warmth, and professional courtesy. **EBN:** *Instances of disrespect and lack of caring have special significance for families of color (Degazon, 2006).*
- Support religious beliefs and the comfort role of religion. **EBN:** *Studies have shown a strong relation between religion and subjective health and that subjective health is predictive of health outcomes (Harvey, 2006).*
- Use a family-centered approach when working with Latino, Asian, African American, and Native American clients. **EBN:** *Latinos may perceive the family as a source of support, solver of problems, and source of pride. Asian Americans may regard the family as the primary decision maker and influence on individual family members. Native American families may have extended structures and exert powerful influences over functioning (Leininger & McFarland, 2006; Hanley, 2008). Findings in this study suggest that incorporating family norms is critical when developing interventions to increase formal health service utilization among African Americans (Barksdale & Molock, 2009).*

• = Independent   ▲ = Collaborative   **EBN** = Evidence-Based Nursing   **EB** = Evidence-Based

- Facilitate modeling and role playing for the family regarding healthy ways to communicate and interact. **EBN:** *It is helpful for families and the client to practice communication skills in a safe environment before trying them in a real-life situation (Wright & Leahey, 2005; Degazon, 2006).*
- Use the nursing intervention of cultural brokerage to help families deal with the health care system. **EBN:** *Cultural brokerage helps individuals and families integrate their cultural values, beliefs, and traditions with health care decision making (Degazon, 2006).*

Client/Family Teaching and Discharge Planning

- Teach about all aspects of therapeutic regimens. Provide as much knowledge as family members will accept, adjust instruction to account for what the family already knows, and provide information in a culturally congruent manner.
- Teach ways to adjust family behaviors to include therapeutic regimens, such as safety in taking medications and teaching family members to act as self-advocates with health providers who prescribe therapeutic regimens.

⊖volve See the EVOLVE website for Weblinks for client education resources.

REFERENCES

Barksdale CL, Molock SD: Perceived norms and mental health help seeking among African American college students, *J Behav Health Serv Res* 36(3):285–299, 2009.

Degazon C: Cultural influences in nursing in community health. In Stanhope M, Lancaster J, editors: *Foundations of nursing in the community: community-oriented practice,* ed 2, St Louis, 2006, Mosby.

Feinberg LF, Newman SL: A study of 10 states since passage of the national family caregiver support program: policies, perceptions, and program development, *Gerontologist* 44:760–769, 2004.

Giger JN, Davidhizar R: *Transcultural nursing: assessment and intervention,* ed 5, St Louis, 2008, Mosby.

Grey M, Knafl K, McCorkle R: A framework for the study of self- and family management of chronic conditions, *Nurs Outlook* 54:278–286, 2006.

Hanley K: Navajos. In Giger JN, Davidhizar R: *Transcultural nursing: assessment and intervention,* ed 5, St Louis, 2008, Mosby.

Harvey IS: Self management of a chronic illness: an exploratory study on the role of spirituality among older African American women, *J Women Aging* 18(3):75–88, 2006.

Heimendinger J, Uyeki T, Andhara A et al: Coaching process outcomes of a family visit nutrition and physical activity intervention, *Health Educ Behav* 34:71–89, 2007.

Leininger MM, McFarland MR: *Culture care diversity and universality: a worldwide nursing theory,* ed 2, Boston, 2006, Jones & Bartlett.

Leong J, Molassiotis A, Marsh H: Adherence to health recommendations after a cardiac rehabilitation programme in post-myocardial infarction patients: the role of heath beliefs, locus of control and psychological status, *Clin Eff Nurs* 8(1):26–38, 2004.

Lubkin IM, Larsen PD: *Chronic illness: impact and interventions,* ed 6, Boston, 2006, Jones and Bartlett.

Miller MJ, Abrams MA, McClintock B et al: Promoting health communication between the community-dwelling well-elderly and pharmacists: the Ask Me 3 program, *J Am Pharm Assoc* 48(6):784–792, 2008.

Pender NJ, Murdaugh CL, Parsons MA: *Health promotion in nursing practice,* ed 5, Upper Saddle River, NJ, 2006, Prentice Hall.

Tessier R, Charpak N, Giron M et al: Kangaroo Mother Care, home environment and father involvement in the first year of life: a randomized controlled study, *Acta Paediatr.* Epub ahead of print, Jun 4, 2009.

Whittemore R, Melkus GD, Grey M: Metabolic control, self management and psychosocial adjustment in women with type 2 diabetes, *J Clin Nurs* 14:195–204, 2005.

Wright LM, Leahey M: *Nurses and families: a guide to family assessment and intervention,* ed 4, Philadelphia, 2005, F.A. Davis.

Ineffective Thermoregulation *Betty J. Ackley, MSN, EdS, RN*

NANDA-I

Definition

Temperature fluctuation between hypothermia and hyperthermia

Defining Characteristics

Cool skin; cyanotic nail beds; fluctuations in body temperature above and below the normal range; flushed skin; hypertension; increased respiratory rate; mild shivering; moderate pallor; piloerection; reduction in body temperature below normal range; seizures; slow capillary refill; tachycardia; warm to touch

Related Factors (r/t)

Aging; fluctuating environmental temperature; illness; immaturity; trauma

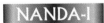 • = Independent ▲ = Collaborative **EBN** = Evidence-Based Nursing **EB** = Evidence-Based

(Nursing Outcomes Classification)

Suggested NOC Outcomes

Thermoregulation, Thermoregulation: Newborn

Example NOC Outcome with Indicators
Thermoregulation as evidenced by the following indicators: Body temperature/Skin temperature/Skin color changes/ Hydration/Reported thermal comfort (Rate the outcome and indicators of **Thermoregulation:** 1 = severely compromised, 2 = substantially compromised, 3 = moderately compromised, 4 = mildly compromised, 5 = not compromised [see Section I].)

Client Outcomes

Client Will (Specify Time Frame):

- Maintain temperature within normal range
- Explain measures needed to maintain normal temperature
- Explain symptoms of hypothermia or hyperthermia

 (Nursing Interventions Classification)

Suggested NIC Interventions

Temperature Regulation, Temperature Regulation: Inoperative

Example NIC Activities—Temperature Regulation
Institute use of a continuous core temperature–monitoring device, as appropriate; Promote adequate fluid and nutritional intake

Nursing Interventions and *Rationales*

- Measure and record the client's temperature using an oral or rectal thermometer every 1 to 4 hours depending on severity of the situation or whenever a change in condition occurs (e.g., chills, change in mental status). **EBN and EB:** *Oral temperature measurement provides a more accurate temperature than tympanic measurement, axillary measurement, or use of a chemical dot thermometer (Frommelt, Ott, & Hays, 2008; Hill, 2004; Fallis, Hamelin, & Wang, 2006; Devrim et al, 2007). Research has demonstrated the accuracy of temperature measurement from most accurate to least accurate: intravascular, esophageal, bladder thermistor, rectal, oral, tympanic membrane. Axillary, temporal artery, and chemical dot thermometers are less accurate and should be avoided in caring for the critically ill adult client (O'Grady et al, 2008).*
- Use the same site and method (device) for temperature measurement for a given client so that temperature trends are assessed accurately; record site of temperature measurement. **EBN and EB:** *There are significant differences in temperature depending on the site (oral, rectal, axillary, or temporal artery) (Devrim et al, 2007; Frommelt, Ott, & Hays, 2008; O'Grady et al, 2008).*
- Evaluate the significance of a decreased or increased temperature. *Normal adult temperature is usually identified as 98.6° F (37° C), but in actuality the normal temperature fluctuates throughout the day. In the early morning it may be as low as 96.4° F (35.8° C) and in the late afternoon or evening as high as 99.1° F (37.3° C) (Bickley & Szilagyj, 2007). Disease, injury, or pharmacological agents may impair regulation of body temperature (Fauci et al, 2008).*
- ▲ Notify the physician of temperature according to institutional standards or written orders, or when temperature reaches 100.5° F (38.3° C) and above (O'Grady et al, 2008). Also notify the physician of the presence of a change in mental status. *A change in mental status may indicate the onset of septic shock (Sepsis, 2007).*

Hypothermia

- Take vital signs frequently, noting changes associated with hypothermia: first, increased blood pressure, pulse, and respirations; then, decreased values as hypothermia progresses. *Mild hypothermia activates the sympathetic nervous system, which can increase the levels of vital signs; as hypothermia progresses, the heart becomes suppressed, with decreased cardiac output and lowering of vital sign readings (Fauci et al, 2008).*

- Monitor the client for signs of hypothermia (e.g., shivering, cool skin, piloerection, pallor, slow capillary refill, cyanotic nailbeds, decreased mentation, dysrhythmias) (Elliott, 2004).
- Maintain a consistent room temperature (72° F [22.2° C]). *A consistent temperature limits environmental effects on thermoregulation.*
- Keep the surgical suite at a consistent room temperature to prevent hypothermia of surgical clients. **EBN:** *The ambient temperature in a surgical suite is the main factor preventing hypothermia with deleterious effects in surgical clients; in a study the majority of surgical nurses were not aware of this reality (Burns, Wojnowski, & Cooper, 2008).*
- Promote adequate nutrition and hydration. *These measures help maintain a normal body temperature.*
- See the care plan for **Hypothermia** as appropriate.

Hyperthermia

- Note changes in vital signs associated with hyperthermia: rapid, bounding pulse; increased respiratory rate; and decreased blood pressure, accompanied by orthostatic hypotension (Fauci et al, 2008). *Consistent monitoring promotes prevention and early intervention in clients with altered cardiopulmonary status associated with hyperthermia.*
- Monitor the client for signs of hyperthermia (e.g., headache, nausea and vomiting, weakness, absence of sweating, delirium, and coma). *Monitoring for the defining characteristics of hyperthermia allows for early intervention.*
- Adjust clothing to facilitate passive warming or cooling as appropriate.
- See the care plan for **Hyperthermia** as appropriate.

Pediatric

- For routine measurement of temperature, use an electronic thermometer in the axilla in infants under the age of 4 weeks; for a child up to 5 years of age, use an electronic thermometer in the axilla, or an infrared tympanic thermometer. **EBN:** *Oral and rectal routes should not be used routinely to measure the temperature of infants to children of 5 years of age (Xue, 2008; National Collaborating Centre for Women's and Children's Health, 2007).*
- Recognize that pediatric clients have a decreased ability to adapt to temperature extremes. Take the following actions to maintain body temperature in the infant/child:
  - Keep the head covered.
  - Use blankets to keep the client warm.
  - Keep the client covered during procedures, transport, and diagnostic testing.
  - Keep the room temperature at 72° F (22.2° C).
  The combination of a relatively smaller body surface area, smaller body fluid volume, less well-developed temperature control mechanisms, and smaller amount of protective body fat limits the infant's and child's ability to maintain normal temperatures (Hockenberry, 2005).
- Recognize that the infant and small child are both vulnerable to develop heat stroke in hot weather; ensure they receive sufficient fluids and are protected from hot environments. *Infants and young children are at risk for heat stroke for many reasons including a decreased thermoregulatory ability in the young body and the inability to obtain their own fluids.*

Geriatric

- Do not allow an elderly client to become chilled. Keep the client covered when giving a bath and offer socks to wear in bed. Be aware of factors such as room temperature (heating/air conditioning), clothing (layered/loose), and fluid intake. *Older adults have a decreased ability to adapt to temperature extremes and need protection from extreme environmental temperatures. The response to cold environment is also compromised with the cutaneous vasoconstrictor response, the shivering process being less effective, and decreased ability to feel cold (McLafferty, Farley, & Hendry, 2009). Research indicates that this can be traced in part to medications used to treat chronic age-associated diseases.*

● = Independent ▲ = Collaborative **EBN** = Evidence-Based Nursing **EB** = Evidence-Based

- Recognize that the elderly client may have an infection without a rise in body temperature. *Febrile response to infection was found to be reduced with increasing age, and baseline temperatures were generally lower in older clients (Barakzai & Fraser, 2008; Heckenberg, 2008).*
- Ensure that elderly clients receive sufficient fluids during hot days and stay out of the sun. *The elderly may have trouble walking independently to obtain fluids, have decreased thirst sensation, and have chronic illnesses that predispose them to heat stroke.*
- Assess the medication profile for the potential risk of drug-related altered body temperature. *Anesthetics, barbiturates, salicylates, nonsteroidal antiinflammatory drugs, diuretics, antihistamines, anticholinergics, beta-blockers, and thyroid hormones have been linked to altered body temperature (Elliott, 2004).*

Home Care

Prevention of Hypothermia in Cold Weather

- Instruct the client to avoid prolonged exposure outdoors. When outdoors, the client should wear gloves, a coat, and a cap on the head.
- Keep the room temperature at 68° to 72° F (20° to 22.2° C). Bring a thermometer to the home to check the temperature in the home as needed.
- ▲ Ensure an adequate source of heat. Refer to social services if the client/family has a low income and the heat could be turned off.
- Help the elderly client locate a warm environment to which the client can go for safety in cold weather if the home environment is no longer warm.

Prevention of Hyperthermia in Hot Weather

- Encourage the client to wear lightweight cotton clothing. Help the elderly client remove the usual sweater.
- Ensure that the client drinks adequate amounts of fluids (2000 mL/day). Monitor elderly clients for deficient fluid volume carefully, noting new onset of weakness, dizziness, and postural hypotension. *Older adults have a higher osmotic point for thirst sensation and a diminished sensitivity to thirst, relative to younger adults (Wotton, Crannitch, & Munt, 2008).*
- During warm weather, help the client obtain a fan or an air conditioner to increase evaporation, as needed.
- Take the temperature of the elderly client in hot weather. *Elderly clients may not be able to tell that they are hot because of decreased sensation.*
- Help the elderly client locate a cool environment to which the client can go for safety in hot weather.

Client/Family Teaching and Discharge Planning

- Teach the client and family the signs of hypothermia and hyperthermia and appropriate actions to take if either condition develops.
- Teach the client and family an age-appropriate method for taking the temperature.
- Teach the client to avoid alcohol and medications that depress cerebral function. *When the client is sedated or under the influence of alcohol, mentation is depressed, which results in decreased activities to maintain an adequate body temperature.*

Ⓔvolve   See the EVOLVE website for Weblinks for client education resources.

REFERENCES

Barakzai MD, Fraser D: Assessment of infection in older adults: signs and symptoms in four body systems, *J Gerontol Nurs* 34(1):7–13, 2008.

Bickley LS, Szilagyj PJ: *Bate's guide to physical examination and history taking*, ed 9, Philadelphia, 2007, JB Lippincott.

Burns SM, Wojnowski M, Cooper K: Promoting thermal balance: a team approach, *AANA J* 76(5):366, 2008.

Devrim I, Kara A, Ceyhan M et al: Measurement accuracy of fever by tympanic and axillary thermometry, *Pediatr Emerg Care* 23(1): 16–19, 2007.

Elliott F: You'd better watch out, *Occup Health Saf* 73(11):76, 2004.

Fallis WM, Hamelin K, Wang X: A multimethod approach to evaluate chemical dot thermometers for oral temperature measurement, *J Nurs Meas* 14(3):151–161, 2006.

Fauci A, Braunwald E, Kasper D et al: *Harrison's principles of internal medicine*, ed 17, New York, 2008, McGraw-Hill.

Frommelt T, Ott C, Hays V: Accuracy of different devices to measure temperature, *Medsurg Nurs* 17(3):171–177, 2008.

Heckenberg G: *Febrile response: management. Evidence Summaries—* Joanna Briggs Institute, July 28, 2008.

Hill PD: *A comparison of tympanic and oral temperature readings in adults* [dissertation], Gonzaga University, Washington (UMI No. 1420518), 2004.

Hockenberry MJ: *Wong's essentials of pediatric nursing*, ed 7, St Louis, 2005, Mosby.

McLafferty E, Farley A, Hendry C: Prevention of hypothermia, *Nurs Older People* 21(4):34–38, 2009.

National Collaborating Centre for Women's and Children's Health (UK): Feverish illness in children: assessment and initial management in children younger than 5 years, *National Institute for Health and Clinical Excellence (NICE) Clinical Guideline 47,* London, May 2007, NICE.

O'Grady NP, Barie PS, Bartlett JG et al: Guidelines for evaluation of new fever in critically ill adult patients: 2008 update from the American College of Critical Care Medicine and the Infectious Diseases Society of America, *Crit Care Med* 36(4):1330–1349, 2008.

Sepsis: Fremont-Rideout Health Group launches groundbreaking programs for the treatment of shock, *Blood Weekly,* Dec 20, 466, 2007.

Wotton K Crannitch K, Munt R: Prevalence, risk factors and strategies to prevent dehydration in older adults, *Contemp Nurse* 31(1):44–56, 2008.

Xue Y: *Febrile response management*, Joanna Briggs Institute. May 5, 2008.

Impaired Tissue integrity   *Sharon Baranoski, MSN, RN, CWCN, APN, FAAN*   ⊖volve

NANDA-I

Definition

Damage to mucous membrane, corneal, integumentary, or subcutaneous tissues

Defining Characteristics

Damaged tissue (e.g., cornea, mucous membrane, integumentary or subcutaneous tissue); destroyed tissue

Related Factors (r/t)

Altered circulation; chemical irritants; fluid deficit; fluid excess; impaired physical mobility; knowledge deficit; mechanical factors (e.g., pressure, shear, friction); nutritional factors (e.g., deficit or excess); radiation; temperature extremes

NOC   (Nursing Outcomes Classification)

Suggested NOC Outcomes

Tissue Integrity: Skin & Mucous Membranes, Wound Healing: Primary Intention, Secondary Intention

Example NOC Outcome with Indicators
Intact **Tissue Integrity: Skin & Mucous Membranes** as evidenced by the following indicators: Skin intactness/Skin lesions absent/Tissue perfusion/Skin temperature (Rate the outcome and indicators of **Tissue Integrity: Skin & Mucous Membranes:** 1 = severely compromised, 2 = substantially compromised, 3 = moderately compromised, 4 = mildly compromised, 5 = not compromised [see Section I].)

Client Outcomes

Client Will (Specify Time Frame):

- Report any altered sensation or pain at site of tissue impairment
- Demonstrate understanding of plan to heal tissue and prevent reinjury
- Describe measures to protect and heal the tissue, including wound care
- Experience a wound that decreases in size and has increased granulation tissue

NIC   (Nursing Interventions Classification)

Suggested NIC Interventions

Incision Site Care, Pain Management, Pressure Ulcer Care, Risk Identification, Skin Care: Topical Treatments, Skin Surveillance, Wound Care, Wound Irrigation

• = Independent   ▲ = Collaborative   **EBN** = Evidence-Based Nursing   **EB** = Evidence-Based

> **Example NIC Activities—Pressure Ulcer Care**
>
> Monitor color of wound bed, temperature, edema, errythema, moisture, and appearance of surrounding skin; Note characteristics of any drainage

Nursing Interventions and *Rationales*

- Assess the site of impaired tissue integrity and determine the cause (e.g., acute or chronic wound, burn, dermatological lesion, pressure ulcer, leg ulcer, skin failure). **EB:** *The etiology or cause of the wound must be determined before appropriate interventions can be implemented. This provides the basis for additional testing and evaluation to start the assessment process (Langemo & Brown, 2006; Baranoski & Ayello, 2008).*
- Determine the size and depth of the wound (e.g., full-thickness wound, deep tissue injury, stage III or IV pressure ulcer). **EB:** *Serial wound assessments are more reliable when performed by the same caregiver, with the client in the same position, and using the same techniques (Ankrom et al, 2005; Black, 2005; Romero, Treston, & O'Sullivan, 2006).*
- Classify pressure ulcers in the following manner (NPUAP, 2009).
  - **Category/Stage III:** Full-thickness tissue loss. Subcutaneous fat may be visible but bone, tendon, or muscle are not exposed. Some slough may be present. May include undermining and tunneling. The depth of a Category/Stage III pressure ulcer varies by anatomical location. The bridge of the nose, ear, occiput and malleolus do not have (adipose) subcutaneous tissue and can be shallow. In contrast, areas of significant adiposity can develop extremely deep pressure ulcers. Bone/tendon is not visible or directly palpable (NPUAP, 2009).
  - **Category/Stage IV:** Full-thickness tissue loss with exposed bone, tendon, or muscle. Slough or eschar may be present. Often include undermining and tunneling. The depth of a Category/Stage IV pressure ulcer varies by anatomical location. The bridge of the nose, ear, occiput, and malleolus do not have (adipose) subcutaneous tissue and can be shallow. Category IV ulcers can extend into muscle and/or supporting structures (e.g. fascia, tendon, or joint capsule) making osteomyelitis or osteitis likely to occur. Exposed bone/muscle is visible or directly palpable (NPUAP, 2009).
  - **Suspected Deep Tissue Injury:** Purple or maroon localized area of discolored intact skin or blood-filled blister due to damage of underlying soft tissue from pressure and/or shear. The area may be preceded by tissue that is painful, firm, mushy, boggy, warmer, or cooler as compared to adjacent tissue. Deep tissue injury may be difficult to detect in individuals with dark skin tones. Evolution may include a thin blister over a dark wound bed. The wound may further evolve and become covered by thin eschar. Evolution may be rapid exposing additional layers of tissue even after treatment (NPUAP, 2009).
  - **Unstageable/Unclassified:** Full thickness tissue loss in which actual depth of the ulcer is completely obscured by slough (yellow, tan, gray, green, or brown) and/or eschar (tan, brown, or black) in the wound bed. Until enough slough and/or eschar is removed to expose the base of the wound, the true depth cannot be determined; however, it will be either a Category/Stage III or Category/Stage IV (NPUAP, 2009).
- Monitor the site of impaired tissue integrity at least once daily for color changes, redness, swelling, warmth, pain, or other signs of infection. Determine whether the client is experiencing changes in sensation or pain. Pay special attention to all high-risk areas such as bony prominences, skin folds, sacrum, and heels. *Systematic inspection can identify impending problems early.* **EBN:** *Pain secondary to dressing changes can be managed by interventions aimed at reducing trauma and other sources of wound pain (Ayello & Braden, 2002; Rastinehad, 2006; WUWHS, 2007).*
- Monitor the status of the skin around the wound. Monitor the client's skin care practices, noting type of soap or other cleansing agents used, temperature of water, and frequency of skin cleansing. *Individualize the plan according to the client's skin condition, needs, and preferences. Avoid harsh cleansing agents, hot water, extreme friction or force, or too-frequent cleansing (Bergstrom et al, 1994; Rodeheaver, 2007).*
- Monitor the client's continence status and minimize exposure of the skin impairment site and other areas to moisture from urine or stool, perspiration, or wound drainage. *If the client is incontinent, implement an incontinence management plan to prevent exposure to chemicals in urine and*

● = Independent　▲ = Collaborative　**EBN** = Evidence-Based Nursing　**EB** = Evidence-Based

stool that can strip or erode the skin. Refer to a continence care specialist, urologist, or gastroenterologist for incontinence assessment (WOCN, 2003; Ratcliff, 2005). **EB:** *Implementing an incontinence prevention plan with the use of a skin or cleanser protectant can significantly decrease skin breakdown and pressure ulcer formation (Fantl, 1996).*

- Monitor for correct placement of tubes, catheters, and other devices. Assess the skin and tissue affected by the tape that secures these devices. *Mechanical damage to skin and tissues as a result of pressure, friction, or shear is often associated with external devices (Faller & Beitz, 2007).*

- In an orthopedic client, check every 2 hours for correct placement of foot boards, restraints, traction, casts, or other devices, and assess skin and tissue integrity. Be alert for symptoms of compartment syndrome (refer to the care plan for **Risk for Peripheral neurovascular dysfunction**). *Mechanical damage to skin and tissues (pressure, friction, or shear) is often associated with external devices.*

- For a client with limited mobility, use a risk-assessment tool to assess immobility-related risk factors systematically. **EBN and EB:** *A validated risk assessment tool such as the Norton or Braden scale should be used to identify clients at risk for immobility-related skin breakdown (Ayello & Braden, 2002; Braden & Maklebust, 2005). Targeting variables (e.g., age and Braden Scale risk category) can focus assessment on particular risk factors (e.g., pressure) and help guide the plan of prevention and care (WOCN, 2003, 2009; Ratcliff, 2005; Magnan & Maklebust, 2009).*

- Implement a written treatment plan for the topical treatment of the skin impairment site. *A written treatment plan ensures consistency in care and documentation (Baranoski & Ayello, 2008).*

- ▲ Identify a plan for debridement if necrotic tissue (eschar or slough) is present and if consistent with overall client management goals. **EB:** *Debride devitalized tissue within the wound bed or edge of pressure ulcers when appropriate to individual's condition and consistent with overall goals of care (NPUAP, 2009).* **EB:** *Do not debride stable, hard, dry eschar in ischemic limbs (NPUAP, 2009).*

- Select a topical treatment that maintains a moist, wound-healing environment and also allows absorption of exudate and filling of dead space. *No single wound care product provides the optimal environment for healing all wounds.* **EBN:** *Choose dressings that provide a moist environment, keep periwound skin dry, and control exudate and eliminate dead space (WOCN, 2003, 2009; Ayello, 2006; Brett, 2006; Baranoski & Ayello, 2008; NPUAP, 2009).*

- Do not position the client on the site of impaired tissue integrity. *If it is consistent with overall client management goals, turn and position the client at least every 2 hours, and transfer the client carefully to avoid adverse effects of external mechanical forces (pressure, friction, and shear) (WOCN, 2003, 2009; NPUAP, 2009).*

- Evaluate for the use of specialty mattresses, beds, or devices as appropriate (Fleck, 2007; Brienza et al, 2008).

- If the goal of care is to keep the client comfortable (e.g., for a terminally ill client), turning and repositioning may not be appropriate. *Maintain the head of the bed at the lowest degree of elevation possible to reduce shear and friction and use lift devices, pillows, foam wedges, and pressure-reducing devices in the bed (WOCN, 2003, 2009; Krasner, Rodeheaver, & Sibbald, 2007; Baranoski & Ayello, 2008; NPUAP, 2009).*

- Avoid massaging around the site of impaired tissue integrity and over bony prominences. **EB:** *Panel for the Prediction and Prevention of Pressure Ulcers in Adults, 1992).*

- ▲ Assess the client's nutritional status; refer for a nutritional consultation and/or institute use of dietary supplements. **EB:** *The benefit of nutritional evaluation and intensive nutritional support in clients at risk for and with pressure ulcers is not supported by rigorous clinical trials. Despite this lack of evidence, the National Pressure Ulcer Advisory Panel endorses the application of reasonable nutritional assessment and treatment for clients at risk for and with pressure ulcers (NPUAP, 2009).*

- ▲ A comprehensive plan of care includes a thorough wound assessment, treatment interventions, support surfaces, nutritional products, adjunctive therapies, and evaluation of the outcome of care. *Documentation of these essential elements is paramount to establishing a framework for quality care (Baranoski, 2006).*

Home Care

- Some of the interventions previously described may be adapted for home care use.

● = Independent   ▲ = Collaborative   **EBN** = Evidence-Based Nursing   **EB** = Evidence-Based

▲ Assess the client's current phase of wound healing (inflammation, proliferation, maturation) and stage of injury; initiate appropriate wound management. **EB:** *Accurate understanding of tissue status combined with knowledge of underlying diagnoses and product validity provide a basis for determining appropriate treatment objectives (Baranoski & Ayello, 2008).*

• Instruct and assist the client and caregivers in understanding how to change dressings and in the importance of maintaining a clean environment. Provide written instructions and observe them completing the dressing change.

▲ Initiate a consultation in a case assignment with a wound specialist or wound, ostomy, and continence nurse to establish a comprehensive plan as soon as possible. Plan case conferencing to promote optimal wound care. *Case conferencing ensures that cases are regularly reviewed to discuss and implement the most effective wound care management to meet client needs.*

▲ Consultation with other health care disciplines provides a thorough, comprehensive assessment. *Consider referring to a dietitian, physical therapist, occupational therapist, and social worker as needed.*

Client/Family Teaching and Discharge Planning

• Teach skin and wound assessment and ways to monitor for signs and symptoms of infection, complications, and healing. *Early assessment and intervention help prevent serious problems from developing.*

• Teach the client why a topical treatment has been selected. Explain wound bed changes that the caregiver can expect to see. Instruct on when the dressing needs to be changed. **EBN:** *The type of wound dressing needed may change over time as the wound heals and/or deteriorates (Brett, 2006; Baranoski & Ayello, 2008).*

▲ If it is consistent with overall client management goals, teach how to turn and reposition the client at least every 2 hours. **EB:** *If the goal of care is to keep the client comfortable (e.g., for a terminally ill client), turning and repositioning may not be appropriate (Krasner, Rodeheaver, & Sibbald, 2007).*

• Teach the use of pillows, foam wedges, and pressure-reducing devices to prevent pressure injury. *The use of effective pressure-reducing seat cushions for elderly wheelchair users significantly prevented sitting-acquired pressure ulcers (Brienza et al, 2008).*

ⓔvolve   See the EVOLVE website for Weblinks resources for client education resources.

REFERENCES

Ankrom MA, Bennett RG, Sprigle S et al: Pressure related deep tissue injury under intact skin and the current pressure ulcer staging system, *Adv Skin Wound Care* 18(1):35–42, 2005.

Ayello EA, Braden B: How and why to do pressure ulcer risk assessment, *Adv Skin Wound Care* 15(3):125, 2002.

Ayello EA: New evidence for an enduring wound-healing concept: moisture control, *J Wound Ostomy Continence Nurs* 33(6S):S1–S2, 2006.

Baranoski S: Pressure ulcers: a renewed awareness, *Nursing* 36(8):36–41, 2006.

Baranoski S, Ayello EA, editors: *Wound care essentials: practice principles,* ed 2, Ambler, PA, 2008, Lippincott Williams & Wilkins.

Bergstrom N, Allman R, Alvarez OM et al: *Treatment of pressure ulcers: clinical practice guideline no. 15,* Rockville, MD, 1994, U.S. Department of Health and Human Services.

Black JM, National Pressure Ulcer Advisory Panel: Moving toward a consensus on deep tissue injury and pressure ulcer staging, *Adv Skin Wound Care* 18(8):415–421, 2005.

Braden B, Maklebust J: Wound wise: preventing pressure ulcers with the Braden scale, *AJN* 105 (6):70–72, 2005.

Brett DW: A review of moisture-control dressings in wound care, *J Wound Ostomy Continence Nurse* 33(6S):S3–S7, 2006.

Brienza DM, Geyer MJ, Springle S et al: Pressure redistribution: seating, positioning, and support surfaces. In Baranoski S, Ayello EA, editors: *Wound care essentials: practice principles,* ed 2, Ambler, PA, 2008, Lippincott, Williams & Wilkins.

Faller N, Beitz J: When a wound isn't a wound: tubes, drains, fistulas and draining wounds. In Krasner D, Rodeheaver G, Sibbald RG, editors: *Chronic wound care: a clinical source book for healthcare professionals,* ed 4, Malvern, PA, 2007, HMP Communications.

Fantl JA et al: *Urinary incontinence in adults: acute and chronic management,* Clinical Practice Guideline No 2, 1996 Update, Agency for Health Care Policy and Research, Pub No 96, Rockville, MD, 1996, Public Health Service, U.S. Department of Health and Human Services.

Fleck D: Support surfaces: criteria and selection. In Krasner D, Rodeheaver G, Sibbald RG, editors: *Chronic wound care: a clinical source book for healthcare professionals,* ed 4, Malvern, PA, 2007, HMP Communications.

Krasner D, Rodeheaver G, Sibbald RG, editors: *Chronic wound care: a clinical source book for healthcare professionals,* ed 4, Malvern, PA, 2007, HMP Communications.

Langemo DK, Brown G: Skin fails too: acute, chronic and end-stage skin failure, *Adv Skin Wound Care* 19(4)206–211, 2006.

Magnan MA, Maklebust J: The nursing process and pressure ulcer prevention: making the connection, *Adv Skin Wound Care* 22(2):83–91, 2009.

National Pressure Ulcer Advisory Panel (NPUAP): *The new international guideline consensus on implementation,* 11th Annual Biennial Conference, Washington, DC, Feb 2009.

● = Independent   ▲ = Collaborative   **EBN** = Evidence-Based Nursing   **EB** = Evidence-Based

Panel for the Prediction and Prevention of Pressure Ulcers in Adults: *Pressure ulcers in adults: prediction and prevention, clinical practice guideline no 3,* Rockville, MD, 1992, U.S. Department of Health and Human Services.

Rastinehad D: Pressure ulcer pain, *J Wound Ostomy Continence Nurs* 33(3):252–257, 2006.

Ratcliff CR: WOCN's evidence-based pressure ulcer guideline, *Adv Skin Wound Care* 18(4):204–208, 2005.

Rodeheaver GT: Wound cleansing, wound irrigation wound disinfection. In Krasner D, Rodeheaver G, Sibbald RG, editors: *Chronic wound care: a clinical source book for healthcare professionals,* ed 4, Malvern, PA, 2007, HMP Communications.

Romero DV, Treston J, O'Sullivan AL: Raising awareness of pressure ulcer prevention and treatment, *Adv Skin Wound Care* 19(7):398–404, 2006.

World Union of Wound Healing Societies (WUWHS) Initiative: Principles of best practice, minimizing pain at dressing-related procedures: "Implementation of pain relieving strategies," *WoundPedia*, 2007.

Wound, Ostomy, and Continence Nurses Society (WOCN): *Guideline for prevention and management of pressure ulcers, WOCN Clinical Practice Guideline Series 2,* Glenview, IL, 2003, Wound, Ostomy, and Continence Nurses Society.

Wound, Ostomy, and Continence Nurses Society: *Pressure ulcer assessment: best practice for clinicians,* Mt Laurel, NJ, 2009, The Society.

Impaired Transfer ability   *Brenda Emick-Herring, RN, MSN, CRRN*

Definition

Limitation of independent movement between two nearby surfaces

Defining Characteristics

Inability to transfer: between uneven levels; from bed to chair; from chair to bed; on or off a toilet; on or off a commode; in or out of tub; in or out of shower; from chair to car; from car to chair; from chair to floor; from floor to chair; from standing to floor; from floor to standing; from bed to standing; from standing to bed; from chair to standing; from standing to chair

Related Factors (r/t)

Cognitive impairment; insufficient muscle strength; musculoskeletal impairment (e.g., contractures); neuromuscular impairment; obesity; pain

NOTE: Specify level of independence using a standardized functional scale

NOC   (Nursing Outcomes Classification)

Suggested NOC Outcomes

Balance, Body Positioning: Self-Initiated, Transfer Performance

Example NOC Outcome with Indicators
Transfer Performance as evidenced by the following indicators: Transfers from bed to chair and back/Transfers from wheelchair to toilet and back/Transfers from wheelchair to vehicle and back (Rate the outcome and indicators of **Transfer Performance:** 1 = severely compromised, 2 = substantially compromised, 3 = moderately compromised, 4 = mildly compromised, 5 = not compromised [see Section I].)

Client Outcomes

Client Will (Specify Time Frame):
- Transfer from bed to chair and back successfully
- Transfer from chair to chair successfully
- Transfer from wheelchair to toilet and back successfully
- Transfer from wheelchair to car and back successfully

NIC   (Nursing Interventions Classification)

Suggested NIC Interventions

Exercise Promotion: Strength Training, Exercise Therapy: Muscle Control

 = Independent   ▲ = Collaborative   **EBN** = Evidence-Based Nursing   **EB** = Evidence-Based

Example NIC Activities—Exercise Promotion: Strength Training
Obtain medical clearance for initiating a strength-training program, as appropriate; Assist to set realistic short- and long-term goals and to take ownership of the exercise plan

Nursing Interventions and *Rationales*

▲ Request consult for a physical and/or occupational therapist (PT and OT) to develop exercise and strengthening program early in the client's recovery. *Leg/trunk strength are key for standing transfers; arm/trunk strength are key for slide-board transfers. A minimum of three resistive exercise sessions/ week involving three sets per exercise over 30 to 40 minutes, unless fairly uncomfortable, was recommended by The Gerontological Nursing Interventions Research Center (Mobily & Mobily, 2004).* **EB:** *Latham and colleagues (2003) via a Cochrane review, reported progressive resistance strength training of disabled elders effectively increased muscle strength and yielded some increased gait speed in older hospitalized clients.*

▲ Obtain a consult for a PT, OT, or orthotist to evaluate and fit clients with proper orthoses, braces, collars, and walking aids before helping them stand. *Equipment helps clients move and function safely, comfortably, and independently (Hoeman et al, 2008). Walking devices improve stability and balance (Lyons, 2004).*

• Help client don/doff collars, braces, prostheses, antiembolism stockings, and abdominal binders while in bed. *Such devices stabilize and align body parts during motion. Antiembolism stockings prevent DVT, and stockings and abdominal binders help prevent orthostatic hypotension; the binder must be put on and taken off in bed to ensure hemodynamic stability.* **EBN:** *A literature review reported knee-high stockings were as effective as above-the-knee stockings in preventing DVT in immobile medical/surgical inpatients and compliance was better (Ingram, 2003).*

• Assess clients' dependence, weight, strength, balance, tolerance to position change, cooperation, fatigue level, and cognition plus available equipment and staff ratio/experience to decide whether to do a manual or device-assisted transfer (U.S. Department of Veterans Affairs, 2005; Nelson, Harwood, et al, 2008).

▲ Collaborate with PT and use algorithms to identify technological aids to handle and transfer dependent and obese clients; do not use under-axilla method (U.S. Department of Labor, 2005). *Powered stand-assist devices, mechanical lifts, stretchers to chairs, and friction-reducing devices prevent musculoskeletal injuries of staff and safe client handling (Baptiste et al, 2008).* **EBN:** *A multifaceted ergonomic program for client handling tasks effectively reduced staff musculoskeletal injury, saved facility costs, and increased two nursing job satisfaction subscales (Nelson et al, 2006). Results of an exploratory study indicated a safe client handling program (ergonomic assessments, handling assessment criteria, handling devices, etc.) improved client depression, urinary continence, engagement in activities, and morning alertness, and lessened risk of falls (Nelson, Collins, et al, 2008).*

• Implement and document type of transfer (such as slide board, pivot), weight-bearing status (non-weight-bearing, partial), equipment (walker, sling lift), and level of assistance (standby, moderate) on care plan and white board in room. *Team consistency is critical for clients' motor (re)learning, progress, and for staff safety. (U.S. Department of Veterans Affairs, 2005; APTA, ARN, VHA Task Force, 2005).* **EBN:** *Kjellberg, Lagerstrom & Hagberg (2004) found a positive relation between nurses' skill in performing client transfers, and quality of care (clients' feeling of safety and comfort during lifts and transfers).*

• Apply a gait belt with handles before transferring clients with partial weight-bearing abilities; keep the belt and client close to provider during the transfer. *If used incorrectly, such as at arm's length, it prevents support of client and places staff at risk for back and arm injuries (U.S. Department of Veterans Affairs, 2005).*

• Help clients don shoes with nonskid soles and socks/hose. *Proper shoes help prevent slips/pain/pressure and improve balance.* **EB:** *Results of a descriptive study of elders showed those wearing athletic/ canvas shoes had lower risk of falling (Koepsell et al, 2004).*

• Nursing staff should wear positive-grip shoe covers or nonslip shoes when transferring clients off shower chairs on tile floors. **ENB:** *Results from a small quality improvement study indicated nurses did not slip or fall when wearing such shoe products (Staal, White, & Brasser, 2004).*

• = Independent   ▲ = Collaborative   **EBN** = Evidence-Based Nursing   **EB** = Evidence-Based

- Remove or swivel wheelchair armrests, leg rests, and footplates to the side, especially with squat or slide board transfers. *This gives clients and nurses feet space to maneuver in and provides fewer obstacles to trip over.*
- Adjust transfer surfaces so they are similar in height. For example, lower a hospital bed to about an inch higher than commode height. **EB:** *Similar heights between seat surfaces require less upper extremity muscular effort during transfers (Hoeman et al, 2008).*
- Place wheelchair and commode at a slight angle toward the surface onto which client will transfer. *The two surfaces are close together yet allow room for the caregiver to adjust the client's movements during the transfer (Hoeman et al, 2008).*
- Teach client to consistently lock brakes on wheelchair/commode/shower chair before transferring. *Wheels will roll if not locked, thus creating risk for falls. Pneumatic wheelchair tires must be adequately inflated for brakes to lock effectively.*
- Give clear simple instructions, allow client time to process information, and let him or her do as much of the transfer as possible. *Over-assistance by staff and family may decrease client learning and self-esteem.* **EB:** *In a descriptive study, McAuley et al (2005) found a close relationship between physical activity/self-efficacy and self-esteem.*
- ▲ Remind clients to comply with weight-bearing restrictions ordered by their physician. *Weight bearing may retard healing in fractured bones.*
- Place client in set position before standing him or her; for example, sitting on edge of surface with bilateral weight bearing on buttocks and hips, with knees flexed, balls of feet aligned under knees, and head in midline. *This position prepares individuals for bearing weight and permits shifting of weight from pelvis to feet as the center of gravity changes while rising.*
- Support and stabilize client's weak knee(s) by placing one or both of your knees next to or encircling client's knee(s), rather than blocking them. *This allows client to flex his or her knee(s) and lean forward to stand and transfer.*
  - Squat transfer: client leans well forward, slightly raises flexed hips off the surface, pivots, and sits down on new surface. *This is beneficial for clients with slight weight-bearing ability.*
  - Standing pivot transfer: client leans forward with hips flexed and pushes up with hands from seat surface (or arms of chair), then stands erect, pivots, and sits down on new surface. *This is beneficial for clients who have fair weight-bearing ability.*
  - Slide board transfer: client should have on pants or have a pillowcase over the board. Remove arm and leg rest from wheelchair on one side then slightly angle chair toward new surface. Help client lean sideways, thus shifting his or her weight so transfer board can be placed well under the upper thigh of the leg next to new surface. Make sure board is safely angled across both surfaces. Help client to sit upright and place one hand on board and the other hand on surface. Remind and help client perform a series of pushups with arms while leaning slightly forward and lifting (not sliding) hips in small increments across board with each pushup. *This benefits clients with little to no weight-bearing ability (Hoeman et al, 2008).*
- Position walking aids logistically so a standing client can grasp and use them once he or she is upright. *These aids help provide support, balance, and stability to help client stand and step safely (Lyons, 2004).*
- Reinforce to clients who use walkers, to place one hand on walker and push with opposite hand against chair arm or surface from which they are arising to stand up. *Placing both hands on the walker may cause it to tip and the client to lose balance and fall.*
- Use ceiling-mounted or bedside mechanical bariatric lifts to transfer dependent bariatric (extremely obese) clients. *Equipment prevents client/staff injury and is essential for clients who require a moderate/maximum assist transfer (Dionne, 2005).*
- ▲ Assist therapists to transfer bariatric clients who can support their own weight with minimal assistance. Position locked beds against a corner wall. Before sitting client, inflate air mattress overlay if applicable and place a friction-reducing sheet underneath client, then 'flat spin' client with the transfer sheet so he/she is laying supine perpendicular to the bed. Deflate all air devices and pad bed edge where posterior thighs will dig in if skin is fragile. Place both knees level with thighs (put feet on a footstool if needed) while client is still supine and assist client to arise to sitting. If client starts sliding, lay client back supine. *The wall helps prevent bed movement. Level knees are essential to prevent feet (and weight) from drifting and sliding downward as client sits up; laying a client supine stops the slide (Dionne, 2005).*

• = Independent   ▲ = Collaborative   **EBN** = Evidence-Based Nursing   **EB** = Evidence-Based

- Use bariatric devices, such as 60–inch-long gait belt or two regular belts buckled together, slide board, wheelchair, and commode during transfers (Dionne, 2005; Saffari, 2007).
- Place a mechanical lift sling in the wheelchair preventatively. Place two transfer sheets or a slide board under bariatric client. Reinforce head forward and level hips/knees and help hold wheelchair in place as therapists directs/helps client with a scoot transfer. *Client may be too fatigued to do a manual transfer back to bed after sitting so sling/lift can be used; if one sheet slips out, one is still available for staff; leaning forward unweights the client's gluteal structures; level hips prevent downward weight shift/fall (Dionne, 2005).*
- Perform initial and subsequent fall risk assessment. *Fall assessments quickly identify persons at risk so prevention and protection measures can be implemented (Morse, 2006).*
- ▲ Collaborate with PT, OT, and pharmacy for individualized preventative/postfall plans, for example, scheduled toileting, balance and strength training, removal of hazards, chair alarms, call system/phone in reach, and review of medications (Browne et al, 2004; Resnick & Junlapeeya, 2004). **EB:** *Results from a study showed low-intensity exercise and incontinence care in residents in nursing homes reduced falls (Messecar, 2003). Results of a clinical trial demonstrated supervised group exercise and home exercises reduced risk of falls and improved balance (Barnett et al, 2003). Lyons (2004) concluded that taking numerous meds every day and that sedatives, hypnotics, antidepressants, antipsychotics, neuroleptics, diuretics, benzodiazepines, antiarrhythmics, cardioglycosides, and antidiabetic agents placed elders at risk for falls.*

Home Care

- ▲ Obtain referral for OT and PT to teach home exercises and balance as well as fall prevention and recovery. They also evaluate for potential modifications such as an entry ramp, elevated toilet seat/toilevator (raised base under toilet), tub seat or shower chair, need for shower stall with built in seat or wheel-in shower stall without a curb/threshold, hand-held flexible shower head, lever type facets, pull out drawers with loop handles versus cupboards, standing lift, etc. *Safety and accessibility helps prevent falls; bathroom tasks and transfers are often dangerous due to clothing adjustment and wet floors/bodies (McCullagh, 2006; Valenza, 2007).* **EB:** *A Cochrane review of numerous clinical trials indicated muscle strengthening and balance training supervised by health professionals at home reduced falls or fallers in the elderly (Gillespie, Gillespie, & Robertson, 2003). Petersson et al (2008) reported study subjects self-ratings for everyday life, especially in terms of safety and less difficulty in the bathroom and transfers in/out of the home, increased after home modifications.*
- Assess for adequate lighting and hazards such as throw/area rugs, clutter, cords, and unfitted bedspreads. Suggest safe floor surfaces, such as use of adhesive nonslip strips in tubs/thresholds/areas where floor height changes; removal of wax from slippery floors; and installing low-pile carpet/nonglazed or nonglossy tiles/wood/linoleum coverings. Stress relocating commonly used items to shelves/drawers in reach, applying remote controls to appliances, and optimizing furniture placement for function, maneuverability, and stability. *Barrier removal promotes safety and accessibility; steady furniture can be used to steady or pull oneself up with if a fall occurs (McCullagh, 2006).* EB: *Results from a controlled study reported removal of home barriers improved elderly subjects' occupational performance (Stark, 2004).*
- ▲ Involve social worker or case manager to educate clients about potential assistive technology, financial cost and benefits, regulations of payers, and local resources. *Information helps clients understand options and cost of services and aids.*
- ▲ Implement approaches for home care staff and family to safely handle and transfer clients. *Risk of injury is high because people often work alone, without mechanical aids or adjustable beds and in crowded spaces while giving care (Long, 2008).*
- For further information, refer to care plans for **Impaired physical Mobility** and **Impaired Walking**.

Client/Family Teaching and Discharge Planning

- Assess for readiness to learn and use teaching modalities conducive to personal learning styles including written instructions for home use. *Learning varies but may be enhanced with visual, auditory, tactile, and cognitive stimulus (Ignatavicius & Workman, 2006).* **EB:** *A Cochrane review* *recommended both written/verbal methods of communicating discharge information/ cares to clients and their caregivers (Johnson, Sanford, & Tyndall, 2003).*

- Supervise practice sessions in which client and family apply items such as gait belts, braces, and orthoses. and check skin once aids are removed. *Repetition reinforces motor learning for safety and sound skin integrity.*
- Teach and monitor client/family for consistent use of safety precautions for transfers (e.g. nonskid shoes, correctly placed equipment/chairs, locked brakes, leg rests swiveled away, and so forth) and for correct performance of transfer or use of lifts/slings. *Promotes safety.*
- Teach client/family how to check brakes on chairs to ensure they engage and how to check tires for adequate air pressure; advise routine inspection and annual tune-up of devices. *Long-term use may loosen brakes or cause them to slip; brakes work only if they make sound contact with tire or wheel. Pneumatic tires must be adequately inflated.*
- Offer information on safe use of shower and commode chairs to prevent discomfort, pressure, and falls during transfer, transport, care, and hygiene.
- For further information, refer to the care plans for **Impaired physical Mobility**, **Impaired Walking**, and **Impaired wheelchair Mobility**.

⊝volve See the EVOLVE website for Weblinks for client education resources.

REFERENCES

American Physical Therapy Association, Association of Rehabilitation Nurses and Veterans Health Administration Task Force: Strategies to improve patient and healthcare provider safety in patient handling and movement tasks, *Rehabil Nurs* 30(3):80–83, 2005.

Baptiste A, McCleerey M, Matz M et al: Proper sling selection and application while using patient lifts, *Rehabil Nurs* 33(1):22–32, 2008.

Barnett A, Smith B, Lord SR et al: Community-based group exercise improves balance and reduces falls in at risk older people: a randomized controlled trial, *Age Ageing* 32(4):407–414, 2003.

Bonham P, Flemister B: Guidelines for management of wounds in patients with lower extremity arterial disease, *Clinical practice guidelines* (Series No.1), Glenview, IL: Wound Ostomy Continence Nurses Society, 2002.

Browne JA, Covington BG, Davila Y et al: Using information technology to assist in redesign of a fall prevention program, *J Nurs Care Qual* 19(3):218, 2004.

Dionne M: Watch your back. *Rehabil Manag* 18(6):30, 32–33, 50, 2005.

Gillespie LD, Gillespie WJ, Robertson MC: Interventions for preventing falls in elderly people. *Cochrane Database Syst Rev* (4):CD000340, 2003.

Hoeman SP, Liszner L, Alverzo J: Functional mobility with activities of daily living. In Hoeman SP, editor: *Rehabilitation nursing: process, application, and outcomes*, ed 4, St Louis, 2008, Mosby.

Ingram JE: A review of thigh-length vs knee-length antiembolism stockings. *Br J Nurs* 12(14):845–851, 2003.

Ignatavicius DD, Workman ML, editors: *Medical-surgical nursing: critical thinking for collaborative care*, ed 5, Philadelphia, 2006, Saunders.

Johnson A, Sanford J, Tyndall J: Written and verbal information versus verbal information only for patients being discharged from acute hospital settings to home, *Cochrane Database Syst Rev* (4):CD003716, 2003.

Kjellberg K, Lagerstrom M, Hagberg M: Patient safety and comfort during transfers in relation to nurses' work technique, *J Adv Nurs* 47(3):251, 2004.

Koepsell TD, Wolf ME, Buchner DM et al: Footwear style and risk of falls in older adults. *J Am Geriatr Soc* 52(9):1495–1501, 2004.

Latham N, Anderson C, Bennett D et al: Progressive resistance strength training for physical disability in older people, *Cochrane Database Syst Rev* (2):CD002759, 2003.

Long F: Safe lift strategy, *Rehabil Manag* 21(6):28–30, 2008.

Lyons SS: *Fall prevention for older adults*. University of Iowa Gerontological Nursing Interventions Research Center (UIGN). Iowa City, IA, Feb, 2004, Research Dissemination Core.

McAuley E, Elavsky S, Motl RW: Physical activity, self-efficacy, and self esteem: Longitudinal relationships in older adults, *J Gerontol B Psychol Sci Soc Sci* 60(5):268–275, 2005.

McCullagh MC: Home modification. *Am J Nurs* 106(10):54–63, 2006.

Messecar D: An exercise and incontinence intervention did not reduce the incidence or cost of acute conditions in nursing home residents, *Evid Based Nurs* 6(4):116–117, 2003.

Mobily K, Mobily P: *Progressive resistance training*. University of Iowa Gerontological Nursing Interventions Research Center (UIGN), Iowa City, IA: Research Dissemination Core. Feb 2004.

Morse JM: The safety of safety research: the case of patient fall research, *Can J Nurs Res* 38(2):74, 2006.

Nelson A, Matz M, Chen F et al: Development and evaluation of a multifaceted ergonomics program to prevent injuries associated with patient handling tasks, *Int J Nurs Stud* 43(6):717– 733, 2006.

Nelson A, Collins J, Siddharthan K et al: Link between safe patient handling and patient outcomes in long-term care, *Rehabil Nurs* 33(1):33–43, 2008.

Nelson A, Harwood KJ, Tracey CA et al: Myths and facts about safe patient handling in rehabilitation, *Rehabil Nurs* 33(1):10–17, 2008.

Petersson I, Lilja M, Hammel J et al: Impact of home modification services on ability in everyday life for people ageing with disabilities, *J Rehabil Med* 40:253–260, 2008.

Resnick B, Junlapeeya P: Falls in a community of older adults: findings and implications for practice, *Appl Nurs Res* 17(2):81, 2004.

Saffari M: Special care for special needs: bariatric rehabilitation presents challenges for both patients and their caretakers, *Rehabil Manag* 20(1):22–29, 2007.

Staal C, White B, Brasser B: Reducing employee slips, trips, and falls during employee-assisted patient activities, *Rehabil Nurs* 29(6):211, 2004.

Stark S: Removing environmental barriers in the homes of older adults with disabilities improves occupational performance. *OTJR: Occupation, Participation and Health* 24(1):32–39, 2004.

U.S. Department of Labor, Occupational Safety and Health Administration: *Guidelines for nursing homes: Ergonomics for the prevention of*

• = Independent ▲ = Collaborative **EBN** = Evidence-Based Nursing **EB** = Evidence-Based

musculoskeletal disorders, 2005. www.osha.gov/ergonomics/
guidelines/nursinghome/final_nh_guidelines.pdf. Accessed
March 25, 2009.

U.S. Department of Veterans Affairs: *Safe patient handling and movement: Patient care ergonomics resource guide:* Ergo guide, Part 1, Chap
6, The Veterans Integrated Service Network 8 (visn8) Patient Safety

Center of Inquiry, Tampa, FL, 2005. www.visn8.med.va.gov/
patientsafetycenter/resguide/ErgoGuidePtone.pdf. Accessed
April 3, 2009.

Valenza T: Home sweet home modification, *Rehabil Manag* 20(5):12–19,
2007.

Risk for Trauma   *Amy Brown, APRN, MSN*

NANDA-I

Definition

Accentuated risk of accidental tissue injury (e.g., wound, burn, fracture)

Risk Factors

External

Accessibility of guns; bathing in very hot water (e.g., unsupervised bathing of young children); bathtub without antislip equipment; children playing with dangerous objects; children playing without gates at top of stairs; children riding in the front seat in car; contact with corrosives; contact with intense cold; contact with rapidly moving machinery; defective appliances; delayed lighting of gas appliances; driving a mechanically unsafe vehicle; driving at excessive speeds; driving while intoxicated; driving without necessary visual aids; entering unlighted rooms; experimenting with chemicals; exposure to dangerous machinery; faulty electrical plugs; flammable children's clothing; flammable children's toys; frayed wires; grease waste collected on stoves; high beds; high-crime neighborhood; inappropriate call-for-aid mechanisms for bed-resting client; inadequate stair rails; inadequately stored combustibles (e.g., matches, oily rags); inadequately stored corrosives (e.g., lye); knives stored uncovered; lack of protection from heat source; large icicles hanging from the roof; misuse of necessary headgear; misuse of seat restraints; non-use of seat restraints; obstructed passageways; overexposure to radiation; overloaded electrical outlets; overloaded fuse boxes; physical proximity to vehicle pathways (e.g., driveways, lanes, railroad tracks); playing with explosives; pot handles facing toward front of stove; potential ignition of gas leaks; slippery floors (e.g., wet or highly waxed); smoking in bed; smoking near oxygen; struggling with restraints; unanchored electric wires; unanchored rugs; unsafe road; unsafe walkways; unsafe window protection in homes with children; use of cracked dishware; use of unsteady chairs; use of unsteady ladders; wearing flowing clothes around open flame

Internal

Balancing difficulties; cognitive difficulties; emotional difficulties; history of previous trauma; insufficient finances; lack of safety education; lack of safety precautions; poor vision; reduced hand-eye coordination; reduced muscle coordination; reduced sensation; weakness

Related Factors (r/t)

See Risk Factors.

NOC   (Nursing Outcomes Classification)

Suggested NOC Outcomes

Risk Control, Fall Prevention Behavior

Example **NOC** Outcome with Indicators
Accomplishes **Risk Control** as evidenced by the following indicators: Monitors environmental risk factors/Develops effective risk control strategies/Modifies lifestyle to reduce risk (Rate the outcome and indicators of **Risk Control:** 1 = never demonstrated, 2 = rarely demonstrated, 3 = sometimes demonstrated, 4 = often demonstrated, 5 = consistently demonstrated [see Section I].)

● = Independent   ▲ = Collaborative   **EBN** = Evidence-Based Nursing   **EB** = Evidence-Based

Client Outcomes

Client Will (Specify Time Frame):

- Remain free from trauma
- Explain actions that can be taken to prevent trauma

NIC   (Nursing Interventions Classification)

Suggested NIC Interventions

Environmental Management: Safety, Skin Surveillance

Example NIC Activities—Environmental Management
Provide family/significant other with information about making home environment safe for patient; Remove harmful objects from the environment

Nursing Interventions and *Rationales*

- Screen clients with a fall risk factor assessment tool to identify those at risk for falls. *A major strategy of all fall prevention programs is the identification of clients at risk of falling. This is most commonly performed with the aid of a fall-risk assessment tool (Kim et al, 2007).* **EBN:** *A recent study has shown that the development and implementation of a fall-risk assessment tool that involves a collaborative and multidisciplinary approach increased the identification of high-risk clients and slightly lowered fall rates (Williams et al, 2007).*
- Provide vision aids for visually impaired clients. *A client that suffers from one or more sensory alteration impairs their ability to function and relate effectively within the environment safely is impaired; therefore the visually impaired client must use vision aids (Potter & Perry, 2007).*
- Help the client with ambulation. Allow the client to use assistive devices in ADLs as needed. *Assistive devices can augment the client's ability to perform ADLs. The client with sensory alterations requires a complete orientation to the immediate environment (Potter & Perry, 2007). One study suggested it is equally important to consider the impact of environmental factors. When designing a unit, features should include a decrease in long, confusing corridors, providing safe and consistent floor surfaces, furnishings, good lighting that reduces glare and clear signage (Neno, 2008).*
- Educate and provide clients and family with hip protector devices. **EB:** *One recent study has shown that the use of hip protectors in care homes with clients identified as high risk for falls had a slight decrease rate of hip fractures, which is a great cause of morbidity and mortality in the geriatric population (Oliver et al, 2006). A Garfinkel et al (2008) study supports the use of hip protectors specifically in clients with dementia. They found that when appropriately introduced and used, hip protectors have a high efficacy in preventing hip fractures.*
- Have a family member evaluate water temperature for the client. *Clients with tactile sensory alterations are at risk for injury if their living environments are not safe (Potter & Perry, 2007).*
- Assess the client for causes of impaired cognition. **EB:** *Cognitive impairment and depression have been identified as significant factors that impact the likelihood of falling. This study also showed that a multifactorial, multidisciplinary falls prevention program could be effective in reducing the incidence of risk of falling (Conn, 2007). Older adults with certain chronic conditions and activity limitations had higher rates of trauma from falls compared with older adults that did not (Schiller, Bramarow, & Dey, 2007).*
- Provide assistive devices in bathrooms (e.g., hand rails, nonslip decals on the floor of the shower and bathtub). **EB:** *Handheld shower heads; secure, easily seen grab bars; nonslip colored adhesive tape on the bottom of the tub; elevated toilet set with armrests; and nonslip strips on the floor in front of the toilet have been proven to reduce the risk of falls (McCullagh, 2006).*
- Ensure that call light systems are functioning and that the client is able to use them in conjunction with the nurse making hourly rounds. **EBN:** *The preliminary results of a study conducted by the Alliance for Health Care Research concludes that hourly checks ensure availability of the call light while saving nursing time and energy by reducing call light use (Trinsey, 2006).*
- Use a nightlight after dark to assist in orientation and improve visual acuity. *Adequate lighting reduces physical hazards by illuminating areas in which a person moves. Night-lights in dark halls and bathrooms help older adults maintain safety by reducing the risk of falls (Potter & Perry, 2007).*

● = Independent   ▲ = Collaborative   **EBN** = Evidence-Based Nursing   **EB** = Evidence-Based

- Teach the client to observe safety precautions in high-crime neighborhoods (e.g., lock doors, do not leave home at night without a companion, keep entryways well lighted). *Utilizing bright lighting in the garage, walkways, and doorways will help to discourage intruders and violence in the home area (Potter & Perry, 2007). Clients who sustain violent trauma are frequently poor or in marginalized population with limited access to health care, and lack education on safety precautions and other opportunities (Sommers, 2006).* **EB:** *In trauma prevention, scientists identified community health education initiatives to reduce trauma in high-violence areas (Sommers, 2006).*
- ▲ Instruct the client not to drive under the influence of alcohol or drugs. Assess for a substance abuse problem and refer to appropriate resources for drug and alcohol education. **EB:** *Alcohol consumption is an important factor in unintentional injuries such as motor vehicle crashes, and in violent crime behavior. Alcohol impairs both judgment and reaction times (Ray et al, 2008).*
- ▲ Review drug profile for potential side effects that may inhibit performance of ADLs. **EB:** *A study by Liperoti et al (2007) has shown a direct correlation between the effects of antipsychotic medications and the likelihood of a decreased ability for clients to carry out certain ADLs. This study also showed a need for caution in the use of this type of medication with the high risk for falls geriatric population.*
- See care plans for **Risk for Aspiration**, **Impaired Home maintenance**, **Risk for Injury**, **Risk for Poisoning**, and **Risk for Suffocation**.

Pediatric

- Assess the client's socioeconomic status. **EB:** *Pediatric clients living in poverty are at higher risk for injury (Shenassa, Stubbendick, & Brown, 2004).*
- Assess family interests in safety topics to identify priority areas for counseling. **EB:** *Soliciting parents' interest before counseling may help identify priority areas for counseling as well as dispel myths and unfounded fears regarding childhood injury risk (McDonald et al, 2006).*
- Never leave young children unsupervised around water or cooking areas. *Young children are at risk for drowning even in small amounts of water. Heat and fire from cooking are a hazard to young children (Potter & Perry, 2007).*
- Keep flammable and potentially flammable articles out of the reach of young children.
- Lock up harmful objects such as guns. *Increased access to guns and limited parental supervision significantly increase the risk of youths' exposure to gun violence (Slovak, Brewer, & Carlson, 2008).*

Geriatric

- Assess the geriatric client's cognitive level of functioning both at admission and periodically. **EB:** *Delirium after Day 7 of inpatient care; sleeping disturbances; and male sex were associated with inpatient falls. Intervention programs should include prevention and treatment of delirium and sleep disturbances as well as increased supervision of male clients (Stenvall et al, 2006).*
- Assess for routine eye examinations and use of appropriate prescription glasses. *Poor vision reduces postural stability and significantly increases the risk of fall and fractures in older people (Lord, 2006).*
- Perform a home safety assessment and recommend the following preventive measures: keep electrical cords out of the flow of traffic; remove small rugs or make sure they are slip resistant; increase lighting in hallways and other dark areas; place a light in the bathroom; keep towels, curtains, and other items that might catch fire away from the stove; store harmful products away from food products; provide at least one grab bar in tubs and showers; check prescribed medications for appropriate labels; and store medications in original containers or in a dispenser of some type (e.g., egg carton, 7–day plastic dispenser). If the client cannot administer medications according to directions, secure someone to administer medications. **EB:** *Home hazard assessment and modification are personal safety measures to prevent falls (Gillespie et al, 2009). Identifying risks and implementing changes decrease risk of injury (National Center for Disease Control and Prevention, 2006).*
- Mark stove knobs with bright colors (yellow or red) and outline the borders of steps. *Easily visible markings are helpful for clients with decreased depth perception (Potter & Perry, 2007).*
- Discourage driving at night. *A decline in depth perception and night blindness are common in the elderly, making night driving a difficult and unsafe task.*

• = Independent   ▲ = Collaborative   **EBN** = Evidence-Based Nursing   **EB** = Evidence-Based

- Encourage the client to participate in resistance and impact exercise programs as tolerated. **EB:** *Muscle strengthening and balance retraining are beneficial in preventing falls (Gillespie et al, 2009). Structured, group-based exercise programs offered by community organizations can successfully increase balancing ability among community-dwelling older adults concerned about falls (Robitaille et al, 2005).*
- Implement fall and injury prevention strategies in residential care facilities. **EB:** *An interdisciplinary and multifactorial prevention program targeting residents, staff, and the environment may reduce falls and femoral fractures (Jensen et al, 2002).*
- Attend a fall prevention screening clinic. **EB:** *Clients who attended a fall prevention screening clinic demonstrated improved confidence during ADLs and reduced falls (Perell et al, 2006).*

Client/Family Teaching and Discharge Planning

- Educate the family regarding age-appropriate child safety precautions, environmental safety precautions, and intervention in an emergency. **EB:** *The developmental stage of the child creates a significant threat to safety due to the factors of mobility status, sensory impairments and safety awareness (Potter & Perry, 2007). Home safety education, especially with the provision of safety equipment, is effective in increasing some thermal injury prevention practices (Kendrick et al, 2009).*
- Teach the family to assess the childcare provider's knowledge regarding child safety, environmental safety precautions, and assistance of a child in an emergency. **EB:** *Accidents involving infants and toddlers are most likely preventable, but caregivers need to be educated on safety precautions for each level of development (Potter & Perry, 2007).*
- Educate the client and family regarding helmet use during recreation and sports activities. *Fatalities from bicycles accidents are related to head injuries; therefore children need to understand the importance of wearing a properly fitted helmet (Potter & Perry, 2007).*
- Encourage the use of proper car seats and safety belts. *Every state requires that children ride buckled up; using a car safety seat or belt correctly can prevent injuries to children (American Academy of Pediatrics, 2007).*
- Teach parents to restrict nighttime driving after 10 PM for young drivers. **EB:** *The risk of motor vehicle accidents is higher among 16- to 19-year-old drivers than any other age group (Potter & Perry, 2007).*
- Teach how to plan safe prom and graduation parties. *Adolescents under the influence appear more vulnerable and are more likely to engage in dangerous activities. Alcohol decreases the adolescents' ability to evaluate the consequences of their actions (Hustmyre & Dixit, 2009).*
- Teach parents the importance of monitoring youths after school. *Avoid placing yourself in dangerous environments and be aware of your surroundings at all time. Location is a key factor in avoiding street violence and crimes (Hustmyre & Dixit, 2009).*
- Teach firearm safety. Encourage the family to keep firearms and ammunition in locked storage. **EB:** *One study suggests proactive and preventive measures of a routine firearm assessment to be done in the home, as well as safety counseling occurring with all contacts with any health care providers will increase awareness of the dangers of firearms (Slovak et al, 2008).*
- ▲ Educate that the use of psychotropic medications may increase the risk of falls and that withdrawal of psychotropic medications should be considered. **EB:** *One study should a risk of falls within the elderly population who were on multiple drugs including antianxiety and antidepressants medications (Stark et al, 2008).*
- For further information, refer to care plans for **Risk for Aspiration**, **Impaired Home maintenance**, **Risk for Injury**, **Risk for Poisoning**, and **Risk for Suffocation**.

ⓔvolve   See the EVOLVE website for Weblinks for client education resources.

REFERENCES

American Academy of Pediatrics: *Car safety seats: a guide for families*, 2007. www.aap.org/family/carseatguide.htm. Accessed April 3, 2009.

Conn L: Mind your step! A falls prevention program designed to reduce falls in those over 75 years, *Qual Ageing Policy* 8(1):10–22, 2007.

Garfinkel D, Radmislsky Z, Jamal S et al: High efficacy for hip protectors in the prevention of hip fractures among elderly people with dementia, *J Am Med Dir Assoc* 9(5):313–318, 2008.

Gillespie LD, Robertson MC, Gillespie WJ et al: Interventions for preventing falls in older people living in the community, *Cochrane Database Syst Rev* (2):CD007146, 2009.

Hustmyre C, Dixit J: Marked for mayhem, *Psychol Today* 10(4):80–85, 2009.

Jensen J, Lundin-Olsson L, Nyberg L et al: Fall and injury prevention in older people living in residential care facilities, *Ann Intern Med* 136(10):733, 2002.

Kendrick D, Smith S, Sutton AJ et al: The effect of education and home safety equipment on childhood thermal injury prevention: meta-analysis and meta-regression, *Inj Prev* 15(3):197–204, 2009.

Kim E, Mordiffi S, Bee W et al: Evaluation of three fall-risk assessment tools in the acute care setting, *J Adv Nurs* 60(4):427–435, 2007.

Liperoti R, Onder G, Lapane K et al: Conventional or atypical antipsychotics and the risk of femur fracture among elderly patients: result of a case-control study, *J Clin Psychiatry* 68(6): 929–934, 2007.

Lord SR: Visual risk factors for falls in older people, *Age Ageing* 35(2):1142–1145, 2006.

McCullagh, M: Home modification: how to help patients make their homes safer and more accessible as their abilities change, *Am J Nurs* 106(10):54–56, 2006.

McDonald EM, Solomon BS, Shields WC et al: Do urban parents' interests in safety topics match their children's injury risks? *Health Promot Pract* 7(4):388–395, 2006.

National Center for Disease Control and Prevention: Injury Center: *Preventing falls among older adults*, 2006. www.cdc.gov/ncipc/preventadultfalls.htm. Accessed April 25, 2007.

Neno, R: The of falls research, *Nurs Older People* 20(6):8–9, 2008.

Oliver D, Connell J, Victor C et al: Strategies to prevent falls and fractures in hospitals and care homes and effect of cognitive impairment: systematic review and meta-analyses, *BMJ* 334(7584):82–90, 2006.

Perell KL, Manzano ML, Weaver R et al: Outcomes of a consult fall prevention screening clinic, *Am J Phys Med Rehabil* 85(11):882–888, 2006.

Potter P, Perry A: *Fundamentals of nursing*, St Louis, 2007, Mosby.

Ray J, Rahim M, Bell C et al: Alcohol sales and risk of serious assault, *PLoS Med* 5(5):55–62, 2008.

Robitaille Y, Laforest S, Fournier M et al: Moving forward in fall prevention: an intervention to improve balance among older adults in real-world settings, *Am J Public Health* 95(11):2049–2056, 2005.

Schiller J, Bramarow E, Dey A: Fall injury episodes among noninstitutionalized older adults, United States 2001–2003, *Adv Data* 392:1–16, 2007.

Shenassa E, Stubbendick A, Brown M: Social disparities in housing and related pediatric injury: a multilevel study, *Am J Pub Health* 94(4):633–640, 2004.

Slovak K, Brewer T, Carlson, K: Client firearm assessment and safety counseling: the role of social workers, *Nat Assoc Soc Workers* 53(4):358–366, 2008.

Sommers M: Injury as a global phenomenon of concern in nursing science, *J Nurs Scholarsh* 38(4):314–320, 2006.

Stark A, Gray DB, Hollingsworth H et al: A subjective measure of environmental facilitators and barriers to participation for people with mobility limitations, *Disabil Rehabil* 30(6):434–457, 2008.

Stenvall M, Olofsson B, Lundstrom M et al: Inpatient falls and injuries in older patients treated for femoral neck fracture, *Arch Gerontol Geriatr* 43(3):389–399, 2006.

Trinsey M: Hourly rounds keep call lights quiet, *Nursing* 36(2):33, 2006.

Williams T, King G, Hill A et al: Evaluation of a falls prevention program in an acute tertiary care hospital, *J Clin Nurs* 16: 316–324, 2007.

Risk for vascular Trauma   *Emilia Campos de Carvalho, RN, PhD*

NANDA-I

Definition

At risk for damage to a vein and its surrounding tissues related to the presence of a catheter and/or infused solutions

Risk Factors

Catheter type; catheter width; impaired ability to visualize the insertion site; inadequate catheter fixation; infusion rate; insertion site; length of insertion time; nature of solution (e.g. concentration, chemical irritant, temperature, pH)

NOC   (Nursing Outcomes Classification)

Suggested NOC Outcomes

Risk Control, Tissue Integrity: Skin and Mucous Membranes

Example NOC Outcome with Indicators
Accomplishes **Risk Control** as evidenced by the following indicators: Acknowledges risk/Develops effective risk-control strategies/Follows selected risk control strategies (Rate the outcome and indicators of **Risk Control**: 1 = never demonstrated; 2 = rarely demonstrated; 3 = sometimes demonstrated; 4 = often demonstrated; 5 = consistently demonstrated [see Section I].)

• = Independent   ▲ = Collaborative   **EBN** = Evidence-Based Nursing   **EB** = Evidence-Based

Client Outcomes

Client Will (Specify Time Frame):

- Remain free from vascular trauma
- Remain free from signs and symptoms that indicate vascular trauma
- Remain free from impaired tissue and/or skin
- Maintain skin integrity, tissue perfusion, usual tissue temperature, color and pigment
- Report any altered sensation or pain
- State site is comfortable

NIC   (Nursing Interventions Classification)

Suggested NIC Interventions

Intravenous (IV) Therapy, Medication Administration: Intravenous (IV)

Example NIC Activities—Intravenous (IV) Therapy
Monitor intravenous flow rate and intravenous site during infusion; Perform IV site care according to agency protocol

Nursing Interventions and *Rationales*

Client Preparation

▲ Verify objective and estimate duration of treatment. Check physician's order. *Verify if client will remain hospitalized during the whole treatment or will go home with the device (Phillips, 2005).*
- Assess client's clinical situation when venous infusion is indicated. *Consider possible clinical conditions that cause changes in temperature, color and sensitivity of the possible venous access site. Verify situations that alter venous return (e.g., mastectomy, stroke) (Phillips, 2005).*
- Assess if client is prepared for an IV procedure. Explain the procedure if necessary to decrease stress. *Stress may cause vasoconstriction that can interfere in the visualization of the vein and flow of the infused solution (Wells, 2008).*
- Provide privacy and make the client comfortable during the intravenous insertion. *Privacy and comfort help to decrease stress (Phillips, 2005; Gabriel, 2008).*
- Teach the client what symptoms of possible vascular trauma they should be alert to and to immediately inform staff if they notice any of these symptoms. *Prompt attention to adverse changes decreases chance of adverse effects from complications (Dougherty, 2008).*

Insertion

- Wash hands before touching the client. Use gloves and always reduce the number of staff present in the environment during the procedure if possible. **EB:** *These measures reduce the risk of infection (Couzigou et al, 2005; Ingram & Lavery, 2007).*
- Assess the condition of the client's veins, possible age-related influence, and previous intravenous site use. *The tunica (intima, media, and adventitia) that form the vessel wall can be damaged when a catheter is placed. Multiple puncture attempts or transfixation can lead to vascular trauma such as phlebitis (Trim, 2005).*
- In cases of hard-to-access veins, consider strategies such as the use of ultrasound (US) to assist in vein localization and safe venipuncture. *The use of ultrasound guidance by nursing staff for safe placement of lines in hard-to-access veins, both in adult and pediatric clients, has been successfully reported in the literature (Nichols & Doellman, 2007).* **EB:** *In a recent study, after a brief tutorial, the ENs had a high success rate (87%) with few complications (4%) when using US for IV access in many clients with difficult access sites. The need for central venous access and physician involvement in peripheral line placement was low (Brannam et al, 2004).*
- Avoid areas of joint flexion or bony prominences. *Movement in these sites can cause mechanical trauma in veins (Macklin, 2003; RCN, 2005; Gabriel, 2008).*
- Choose an appropriate Vascular Access Device (VAD) based on the types and characteristics of the devices and insertion site. Consider the following:
  - **Peripheral Cannulae:** short devices that are placed into a peripheral vein; can be straight, winged, or ported and winged
  - **Midline Catheters or Peripherally Inserted Catheters (PICs)** with ranges from 7.5 to 20 cm

• = Independent   ▲ = Collaborative   **EBN** = Evidence-Based Nursing   **EB** = Evidence-Based

- **Central Venous Access Devices (CVADs):** terminated in the central venous circulation; are available in a range of gauge sizes; they can be non-tunneled catheters, skin-tunneled catheters, implantable injection ports, or peripherally inserted central catheters/PICC (Gabriel, 2008; Scales, 2008)
  - **Polyurethane Venous Devices** cause less friction and consequently less risk of mechanical phlebitis compared to the polytetrafluoroethylene devices (Macklin, 2003; Ingram & Lavery, 2007; Lavery & Smith, 2007)

  CVADs made from silicone rubber minimize irritation of the lining of the vein, reducing the potential for phlebitis and thrombosis (Gabriel, 2008); choosing the wrong device can delay or interrupt the application of therapy (Mickler, 2008); verify if device size is compatible with the localization of selected vein (Phillips, 2005)

▲ Choose a device with consideration of the nature, volume, and flow of prescribed solution. **EBN:** *Choosing the right gauge size reduces the risk of vascular trauma (Dougherty & Lister, 2004; Trim, 2005). Verify if the osmolarity of the solution to be infused is compatible with the available access site and device (Phillips, 2005).*

- If possible, choose the venous access site considering the client's preference.
- Select the gauge of the venous device according to the purpose of the procedure and the size of the vein. *Emergency situations require short, large-bore cannulae. Hydration fluids and antibiotics can be delivered through much smaller cannulae (Trim, 2005; Scales, 2008). Select the smallest gauge necessary to achieve the prescribed flow rate, in order to minimize the potential for catheter–vein wall contact (Macklin, 2003).*
- Verify if client is allergic to fixation or device material.
- Disinfect the venipuncture site. *Assess that skin is dry before puncturing.*
- Provide a comfortable, safe, hypoallergenic, easily removable stabilization dressing, allowing for visualization of the access site (Gabriel et al, 2005). *Catheter stabilization shall be used to preserve the integrity of the access device and to prevent catheter migration and loss of access (INS, 2006). Some peripheral cannulae have stabilization wings (that increase the external surface area) and/or ports (that are used to administer bolus medication) incorporated into their design (Gabriel, 2008). Catheter stabilization shall be performed using aseptic technique (INS, 2006).*
- Apply a sterile, transparent dressing on the access device (Scales, 2008). *The dressing can remain for 72 hours if it is intact, clean, and dry (RCN, 2005). The use of a transparent occlusive dressing can facilitate regular monitoring by visually inspecting the vascular access device (Lavery & Ingram, 2006).*
- Document insertion date, site, type of vascular access device (VADs), number of punctures performed, other occurrences, and measures/arrangements taken.
- Always decontaminate the device before infusing medication or manipulating IV equipment (Scales, 2008).

▲ Verify the sequence of drugs to be administrated. *Vesicants should always be administrated first in a sequence of drugs (Dougherty, 2008).*

Monitoring Infusion

- Monitor permeability and flow rate at regular intervals.
- Monitor catheter-skin junction and surrounding tissues at regular intervals, observing possible appearance of burning, pain, erythema, altered local temperature, infiltration, extravasation, edema, secretion, tenderness or induration. Remove promptly. *The infusion should be discontinued at the first sign of infiltration or extravasation (INS, 2006).*

▲ Replace device according to institution protocol. **EB:** *The use of hospital-wide written guidelines for short peripheral venous catheter (SPVC) insertion on the frequency of local catheter-related complications was considered negatively associated (OR 0.31, 95%CI = 0.09 – 0.97) (Couzigou et al, 2005).* Note: *There are variations regarding catheter permanence time in the literature. Recommended catheter permanence time varies from 72 (Scales, 2008) to 96 hours or less if there are any clinical signs (Ingram & Lavery, 2007).* **EB:** *In randomized controlled trials, carriers of peripheral intravenous cannulae replaced periodically every 72 hours (control group) in comparison to carriers of catheter replaced when presenting clinical signs (intervention group) did not present statistical differences regarding the occurrence of phlebitis or infiltration (Webster et al, 2008) or duration of peripheral cannulation;*

• = Independent   ▲ = Collaborative   **EBN** = Evidence-Based Nursing   **EB** = Evidence-Based

nevertheless significantly more re-sites occurred in the control group (p=0.222) and higher cost of cannula in the intervention group (Webster et al, 2007).

▲ Flush vascular access according to organizational policies and procedures, and as recommended by the manufacturer. *Vascular access devices shall be flushed at established intervals to promote and maintain patency and prevent the mixing of incompatible medications and solutions (INS, 2006). 0.9% sodium chloride or heparinized sodium chloride have been applied in peripheral IV cannulae, although there are controversies regarding the best choice (Tripathi, Kaushik, & Singh, 2008).*

• Remove catheter upon suspected contamination or when no longer required. *A PICC shall be removed immediately upon suspected contamination, unresolved complication, or therapy discontinuation (INS, 2006). A peripheral-short catheter in the adult client shall be removed every 72 hours and immediately upon suspected contamination, complication, or therapy discontinuation (INS, 2006). Replace any SPVC inserted under emergency conditions within 24 hours (Couzigou et al, 2005).*

Pediatric

• The above interventions may be adapted for the pediatric client.

• Inform the client and family about the IV procedure, obtain permissions, maintain client's comfort and perform appropriate assessment prior to venipuncture. *Assess the client for any allergies or sensitivities to tape, antiseptics, or latex. Choose a healthy vein and appropriate site for insertion of selected device (Mickler, 2008).*

• The use of an appropriate device to obtain blood samples reduces discomfort in the pediatric client. However, this procedure needs to be effective and safe. *Lumen diameters of PICCs are extremely small; with volumes of less than 1 mL, the need for conscientious nursing care is clear. Therefore, PICCs are at increased risk of malfunctioning or occluding if used for viscous solutions, such as blood, TPN, or frequent blood specimen withdrawals, without adhering to strict flushing protocols (Thibodeau, Riley, & Rouse, 2007).* **EBN:** *A study with 204 children was carried out using catheter 3 French PICC. Blood sampling was successful more than 98% of the time from all clients in the blood sampling group; the higher occlusion rate in the blood sampling group did not reach statistical significance; there was no significant difference between the groups in terms of infection or mechanical complication rate (Knue et al, 2005).* **EB:** *The duration of patency of the cannula had a significant positive correlation with the age of the child. The patency of cannulations was significantly longer with a 22-gauge cannula (48.6 to 20.8 hours) versus a 24-size cannula (42.1 to 20.3 hours) at (P < .05 by the Student test) (Tripathi, Kaushik, & Singh, 2008).*

• Avoid areas of joint flexion or bony prominences. *A recent study with children demonstrated that cannulae inserted away from joints survived significantly longer (Tripathi, Kaushik, & Singh, 2008).*

▲ Consider if sedation or the use of local anesthetic is suitable for insertion of a catheter taking into consideration the age of the pediatric client. *Use diversion while carrying out the procedure to reduce anxiety (Willock et al, 2004; Earhart, Jorgensen, & Kaminski, 2007; Mickler, 2008).*

Geriatric

• Above interventions may be adapted for the geriatric client.

• Use strict aseptic technique for venipuncture of older clients. **EB:** *Older clients are at a higher risk of nosocomial and other health care complications due to defective host defenses that compromise their ability to ward off infectious agents. The odds of local SPVC-related complications in those aged 73 to 99 years were six times higher than that in those aged 10 to 20 years (Couzigou et al, 2005).*

Home Care

• Some devices can be kept after discharge. Inform client and family members about care of the selected device.

• Help in the choice of actions that support self-care. *The nurse can provide valuable information that can be used to guide decision making to maximize the self-care abilities of clients receiving home infusion therapy (O'Halloran, El-Masri, & Fox-Wasylyshyn, 2008).*

• Select, with the client, the insertion site most compatible with the development of activities of daily living.

• = Independent ▲ = Collaborative **EBN** = Evidence-Based Nursing **EB** = Evidence-Based

- Avoid the use of the dominant hands as an IV placement site. **EBN:** *A prospective nonexperimental cohort design, conducted on a convenience sample of 92 clients receiving home IV therapy delivered, observed that clients who had the VAD placed in their dominant hands reported greater dependence in ability to perform their self-care ADLs than those who had it in their nondominant hands (O'Halloran, El-Masri, & Fox-Wasylyshyn, 2008).*
- Minimize the use of continuous IV therapy whenever possible. **EBN:** *Clients who received intermittent IV therapy via a saline lock were more independent with regard to ability to perform self-care ADLs than those who received continuous IV therapy. The need for assistive mobility devices was also an independent predictor of ability to perform self-care ADLs (O'Halloran, El-Masri, & Fox-Wasylyshyn, 2008).*

ⓔvolve   See the EVOLVE website for Weblinks for client education resources.

REFERENCES

Brannam L, Blaivas M, Lyon M et al: Emergency nurses' utilization of ultrasound guidance for placement of peripheral intravenous lines in difficult-access patients, *Acad Emerg Med* 11(12):1331–1336, 2004.

Couzigou C, Lamory J, Salmon-Ceron D et al: Short peripheral venous catheters: effect of evidence-based guidelines on insertion, maintenance and outcomes in a university hospital, *J Hosp Infect* 59(1):197–204, 2005.

Dougherty L: IV therapy: recognizing the differences between infiltration and extravasations, *Br J Nurs* 17(14):896–901, 2008.

Dougherty L, Lister S, editors: *The Royal Marsden Hospital manual of clinical nursing procedure*, ed 6, Oxford, 2004, Blackwell.

Earhart A, Jorgensen C, Kaminski D: Assessing pediatric patients for vascular access and sedation, *J Infus Nurs* 30(4):226–231, 2007.

Gabriel J: Infusion therapy part one: minimising the risks, *Nurs Stand* 22(31):51–56, 2008.

Gabriel J, Bravery K, Dougherty L et al: Vascular access: indications and implications for patient care, *Nurs Stand* 19(26):45–52, 2005.

Infusion Nurses Society (INS): Infusion nursing standards of practice, *J Infus Nurs* 29(1S):S1 – S92, 2006.

Ingram P, Lavery I: Peripheral intravenous cannulation safe insertion and removal technique, *Nurs Stand* 22(1):44–48, 2007.

Knue M, Doellman D, Rabin K et al: The efficacy and safety of blood sampling through peripherally inserted central catheter devices in children, *J Infus Nurs* 28(1):30–35, 2005.

Lavery I, Ingram P: Prevention of infection in peripheral intravenous devices, *Nurs Stand* 20(49):49–56, 2006.

Lavery I, Smith E: Peripheral vascular access devices: risk prevention and management. *Br J Nurs* 16(22):1378–1383, 2007.

Macklin D: Phlebitis: a painful complication of peripheral IV catheterization that may be prevented, *Amer J Nurs* 103(2):155–160, 2003.

Mickler PA: Neonatal and pediatric perspectives in PICC placement, *J Infus Nurs* 31(5):282–285, 2008.

Nichols I, Doellman D: Pediatric peripherally inserted central catheter placement- application of ultrasound technology, *J Infus Nurs* 30(6):351–356, 2007.

O'Halloran L, El-Masri MM, Fox-Wasylyshyn SM: Home intravenous therapy and the ability to perform self-care activities of daily living, *J Infus Nurs* 31(6):367–373, 2008.

Phillips L: *Manual of IV therapeutics*, ed 4, Philadelphia, 2005, Davis.

Royal College of Nursing (RCN): *Standards for infusion therapy*, London, 2005, RCN.

Scales K: Intravenous therapy: a guide to good practice, *Br J Nurs*- IV Supplement, 17(19):S4–S10, 2008.

Thibodeau S, Riley J, Rouse KB: Effectiveness of a new flushing and maintenance policy using peripherally inserted central catheters for adults, *J Infus Nurs* 30(5):287–292, 2007.

Trim JC: Peripheral intravenous catheters: considerations in theory and practice, *Br J Nurs* 14(12):654–658, 2005.

Tripathi S, Kaushik V, Singh V: Peripheral IVs: factors affecting complications and patency—a randomized controlled trial, *J Infus Nurs* 31(3):182–188, 2008.

Webster J, Clarke S, Paterson D et al: Routine care of peripheral intravenous catheters versus clinically indicated replacement: randomised controlled trial, *BMJ* 337:157–160, 2008.

Webster J, Lloyd S, Hopkins T et al: Developing a research base for intravenous peripheral cannula re-sites (DRIP trial). A randomized controlled trial of hospital in-patients, *Int J Nurs Stud* 44:664–671, 2007.

Wells S: Venous access in oncology and haematology patients: part one *Nurs Stand* 22(52):39–46, 2008.

Willock J, Richardson J, Brazier A et al: Peripheral venipuncture in infants and children, *Nurs Stand* 18(27):42–50, 2004.

Impaired Urinary elimination   *Mikel Gray, PhD, CUNP, CCCN, FAANP, FAAN*   ⓔvolve

NANDA-I

Definition

Disturbance in urine elimination

NOTE: This broad diagnosis may be used to describe many dysfunctional voiding conditions. Refer to **Functional urinary Incontinence, Reflex urinary Incontinence, Stress urinary Incontinence, Urge urinary Incontinence,** and **Urinary retention** for information on these more specific diagnoses.

Defining Characteristics

The term *lower urinary tract symptoms* (LUTS) is now used to describe the variety of complaints associated with disorders of bladder filling/storage or altered patterns of urine elimination (Abrams

• = Independent   ▲ = Collaborative   **EBN** = Evidence-Based Nursing   **EB** = Evidence-Based

et al, 2002). Bothersome bladder filling/storage symptoms include diurnal frequency (voiding more than every 2 hours), infrequent urination (voiding less then every 6 hours), and nocturia (arising from sleep more than twice to urinate). Our understanding of the physiologic desire is incomplete, but the term *urgency* has been defined as "a sudden and strong desire to urinate that is not easily deferred" (Abrams et al, 2002). Lower urinary tract pain may present as dysuria (pain associated with micturition), burning, pressure, or cramping discomfort during bladder filling and storage. Voiding symptoms may include reduced force of the urinary stream, intermittency, hesitancy, and the need to strain to evacuate the bladder. Other voiding symptoms are postvoid dribbling, feelings of incomplete bladder emptying, or the total inability to urinate (acute urinary retention).

Urinary incontinence is the uncontrolled loss of urine of sufficient magnitude to constitute a problem for the client, family, or caregivers (Abrams et al, 2002). Stress urinary incontinence is the loss of urine with physical exertion. Urge urinary incontinence is the loss of urine associated with overactive detrusor contractions and a precipitous desire to urinate. It is part of a larger symptom syndrome called *overactive bladder*. The overactive bladder is characterized by bothersome urgency and typically associated with frequent daytime voiding and nocturia. Approximately 37% of clients with overactive bladder dysfunction experience urge urinary incontinence (Stewart et al, 2003).

Reflex urinary incontinence is urine loss associated with neurogenic detrusor overactivity, diminished or absent sensations of bladder filling, and dyssynergia between the detrusor and striated urethral sphincter muscles. Functional urinary incontinence is urine loss associated with deficits of mobility, dexterity, cognition, or environmental barriers to timely toileting. Urine loss from an extraurethral source can be defined as total incontinence, and urinary retention is the condition where the client is unable to completely evacuate urine from the bladder despite micturition. Chronic urinary retention is defined as the inability to completely evacuate urine from the bladder after voiding, and acute urinary retention is the inability to urinate (Gray, 2000).

Related Factors (r/t)

Bothersome LUTS (urological disorders, neurological lesions, gynecological conditions, dysfunction of bowel elimination); incontinence (refer to specific diagnosis); urinary retention (refer to specific diagnosis); acute urinary retention (refer to **Urinary retention**)

 (Nursing Outcomes Classification)

Suggested NOC Outcomes

Urinary Continence, Urinary Elimination

Example NOC Outcome with Indicators
Urinary Continence as evidenced by the following indicators: Has no urine loss leakage with increased abdominal pressure (e.g., sneezing, laughing, lifting)/Voids in appropriate receptacle/Gets to toilet between urge and passage of urine/Keeps underclothing dry during day/Keeps underclothing or bedding dry during night (Rate the outcome and indicators of **Urinary Continence**: 1 = never demonstrated, 2 = rarely demonstrated, 3 = sometimes demonstrated, 4 = often demonstrated, 5 = consistently demonstrated [see Section I].)

Client Outcomes

Client Will (Specify Time Frame):

- Demonstrate diurnal frequency no more than every 2 hours
- Demonstrate nocturia two times or less per night
- Be able to postpone voiding until toileting facility is accessed and clothing is removed
- Be able to perceive and recognize cues for toileting, move to toilet or use urinal or portable toileting apparatus, and remove clothing as necessary for toileting
- Demonstrate postvoiding residual volumes less than 150 mL to 200 mL or 25% of total bladder capacity
- State absence of pain or excessive urgency during bladder storage or during urination

| NIC | (Nursing Interventions Classification) |

Suggested NIC Intervention

Urinary Elimination Management

Example NIC Activities—Urinary Elimination Management
Monitor urinary elimination, including frequency, consistency, odor, volume, and color, as appropriate; Teach patient signs and symptoms of urinary tract infection

Nursing Interventions and *Rationales*

- Routinely screen all adult women and aging men for urinary incontinence or LUTS including bothersome urgency. *Urinary incontinence and overactive bladder dysfunction are prevalent problems, particularly among women and aging males in the sixth decade of life or older (Hunskaar et al, 2005). Routine screening is justified because urinary incontinence is prevalent, negatively affects physical health and psychosocial function, and is amenable to treatment (Gray, 2003).*
- ▲ Assess bladder function using the following techniques:
  - Take a focused history including duration of bothersome LUTS, characteristics of symptoms, patterns of diurnal and nocturnal urination, frequency and volume of urine loss, alleviating and aggravating factors, and exploration of possible causative factors.
  - In close consultation with a physician or advanced practice nurse, administer a validated questionnaire querying lower urinary symptoms, associated bowel elimination symptoms, and symptoms of pelvic organ prolapse in women.
  - Perform a focused physical assessment of perineal skin integrity, evaluation of the vaginal vault, evaluation of urethral hypermobility, and neurological evaluation including bulbocavernosus reflex and perineal sensations.
  - Review results of urinalysis for the presence of urinary infection, polyuria, hematuria, proteinuria, and other abnormalities, or obtain urine for analysis.

  A focused history and physical examination are essential elements of the initial evaluation of impaired urine elimination (Staskin et al, 2005). **EBN:** *There is limited evidence to support the diagnostic value of the physical examination in the diagnosis of urinary incontinence and differential diagnosis of stress versus urge incontinence in elderly women (van Gerwen & Lagro-Janssen, 2006). There are 23 validated tools for the evaluation of lower urinary tract symptoms, bowel elimination symptoms, and symptoms associated with pelvic organ prolapse in women. These instruments can assist the clinician to differentiate the primary type of incontinence, distinguish urgency from pelvic pain, and identify associated bowel elimination disorders and pelvic organ prolapse (Avery et al, 2007).*

- Complete a more detailed assessment on selected clients including a bladder log and functional/cognitive assessment. (Refer to **Functional urinary Incontinence, Reflex urinary Incontinence, Stress urinary Incontinence, Overflow urinary Incontinence,** and **Urge urinary Incontinence**.)
- Assess the client for urinary retention. (Refer to **Urinary retention.**)
- Teach the client general guidelines for bladder health:
  - Clients should avoid dehydration and its irritative effects on the bladder; fluid consumption for the ambulatory, normally active adult should be approximately 30 mL/kg of body weight (0.5 oz per pound per day).
  - Clients with storage LUTS, overactive bladder dysfunction, or urinary incontinence should consider reducing or eliminating caffeine intake (Gray, 2001; Milne, 2008).
  - Clients with lower urinary tract pain or interstitial cystitis should be encouraged to eliminate potential bladder irritants: caffeine, alcohol, aspartame, carbonated beverages, alcohol, citrus juices, chocolate, vinegar, and highly spiced foods such as those flavored with curries or peppers (Interstitial Cystitis Association, 2009). These foods should be reintroduced singly to the diet to determine their effect (if any) on bothersome LUTS. *Although the pathophysiology is not well understood, more than 90% of clients with interstitial cystitis report that one of more of these types of foods exacerbate associated symptoms (Shorter et al, 2007).*

● = Independent   ▲ = Collaborative   **EBN** = Evidence-Based Nursing   **EB** = Evidence-Based

- All clients should be counseled about measures to alleviate or prevent constipation including adequate consumption of dietary fluids, dietary fiber, exercise, and regular bowel elimination patterns.
- All clients should be strongly advised to stop smoking; it is associated with an increased risk of bladder cancer (Bjerregaard et al, 2006), urinary incontinence (Danforth et al, 2006), and bothersome lower urinary tract symptoms in men (Haidinger et al, 2000). *Dehydration increases irritating voiding symptoms and may enhance the risk of urinary infection. Constipation predisposes the individual to urinary retention, and it increases the risk of urinary infection. Smoking may increase the severity and risk of stress incontinence, and it is clearly linked with an increased risk for bladder cancer (Lodovici & Bigagli, 2009).* **EBN:** *Client education, alteration of fluid volume intake, reduction of caffeine consumption, and bladder training and pelvic floor muscle training administered by generic and advanced practice nurses reduce the frequency of urinary incontinence, pad use, and perceived severity of bothersome LUTS (Sampselle et al, 2000; Borrie et al, 2002; Dougherty et al, 2002).*
- ▲ Consult the physician for culture and sensitivity testing and antibiotic treatment in the individual with evidence of a symptomatic urinary tract infection. *UTI is a transient, reversible conditions that is sometimes associated with urgency or urge urinary incontinence (French et al, 2009). Although the precise nature of this relationship remains unclear, it is known that eradication of UTI will alleviate or reverse LUTS, including suprapubic pressure and discomfort, urgency, daytime voiding frequency, and dysuria (French et al, 2009).*
- ▲ Refer the individual with chronic lower urinary tract pain to a urologist or specialist in the management of pelvic pain. *Bladder pain and storage symptoms, in the absence of an acute urinary infection, may indicate the presence of interstitial cystitis, a chronic condition requiring ongoing treatment (Gray, Hufstuttler, & Albo, 2002).*
- Teach the client to recognize symptoms of UTI (dysuria that crescendos as the bladder nears complete evacuation; urgency to urinate followed by micturition of only a few drops; suprapubic aching discomfort; malaise; voiding frequency; sudden exacerbation of urinary incontinence with or without fever, chills, and flank pain). *There are a variety of typical and unexpected symptoms in women with a history of recurring UTI (French et al, 2009).*
- Teach colleagues that a cloudy or malodorous urine, in the absence of other lower urinary tract symptoms, does not indicate the presence of a urinary tract infection and that asymptomatic bacteriuria, in the elderly, does not justify the need for a course of antibiotics. *Nurses are more likely than physicians to interpret presence of cloudy urine as indicating the presence of a UTI in the frail elder. Asymptomatic bacteriuria may be associated with cloudy or malodorous urine, but these signs alone do not justify antimicrobial therapy when balanced against the potential adverse effects of treatment including adverse side effects of the various antibiotics and encouragement of colonization of the urine with antibiotic-resistant bacterial strains (Midthun et al, 2005).*
- Teach the client to recognize hematuria and to seek help promptly if hematuria occurs. *Hematuria in the presence of irritative voiding symptoms typically indicates urinary infection; however, gross or microscopic, in the absence of an existing UTI it raises the risk for urinary system tumor and requires further investigation (Kincaid-Smith & Fairley, 2005).*
- Assist the individual with urinary leakage to select a product that adequately contains urine, avoids soiling clothing, is not apparent when worn under clothing, and protects the underlying skin.
- Teach perineal care including judicious use of soaps and use of vaginal douches only under special circumstances.

Geriatric

- Provide an environment that encourages toileting for the elderly client cared for in the home or in acute care, long-term care, or critical care units. *Insufficient toileting opportunities, medications, acute or chronic illnesses, and environmental factors may contribute to functional incontinence or exacerbate other forms of urinary leakage in the elderly client (Thompson, 2006).*
- Perform urinalysis in all elderly persons who experience a sudden change in urine elimination patterns, lower abdominal discomfort, acute confusion, or a fever of unclear origin. *Elderly persons often experience atypical symptoms with a UTI or pyelonephritis (Inouye, 2006).*

- Encourage elderly women to drink at least 10 oz of cranberry juice daily, regularly consume one to two servings of fresh blueberries, or supplement the diet with cranberry concentrate capsules (usually taken in 500 mg doses with each meal). **EBN:** *Systematic literature review reveals that consumption of 400 mg of cranberry tablets, 8 to 10 oz of cranberry juice, or an equivocal portion of foods containing whole cranberries or blueberries exerts a bacteriostatic effect on* Escherichia coli, *the most common pathogen associated with urinary infection among community-dwelling adult women. Mixed evidence tends to support a reduction in UTI risk among community-dwelling women, although no beneficial effect has been found in clients with neurogenic bladder dysfunction who are managed by intermittent or indwelling catheters (Gray, 2002; Masson et al, 2009).*
- Encourage clients with spinal cord injury and neurogenic bladder dysfunction to consume cranberry extract tablets or cranberry juice on a daily basis. *Limited evidence suggests that regular consumption of cranberry extract tablets and a robust glomerular filtration rate (≥ 75 mL/min) experience fewer UTIs than clients who do not routinely consume cranberry extract tablets (Hess et al, 2008).*

Client/Family Teaching and Discharge Planning

- Teach the client/family that urinary incontinence is not a normal part of aging and that incontinence can be corrected or managed with proper evaluation and care.
- Teach all persons the signs and symptoms of UTI and its management.
- Teach all persons to recognize hematuria and to promptly seek care if this symptom occurs.

⊖volve   See the EVOLVE website for Weblinks for client education resources.

REFERENCES

Abrams P, Cardozo L, Fall M et al: The standardization of terminology of lower urinary tract function: report from the Standardization Subcommittee of the International Continence Society, *Am J Obstet Gynecol* 187(1):116–126, 2002.

Avery KN, Bosch JL, Gotoh M et al: Questionnaires to assess urinary and anal incontinence: review and recommendations, *J Urol* 177(1):39–49, 2007.

Bjerregaard BK, Raaschou-Nielsen O, Sorensen M et al: Tobacco smoke and bladder cancer—in the European Prospective Investigation into Cancer and Nutrition, *Int J Cancer* 119(10):2412–2416, 2006.

Borrie MJ, Bawden M, Speechley M et al: Interventions led by nurse continence advisers in the management of urinary incontinence: a randomized controlled trial, *Can Med Assoc J* 166(10):1267–1273, 2002.

Danforth KN, Townsend MK, Lifford K et al: Risk factors for urinary incontinence among middle-aged women, *Am J Obst Gynecol* 194(2):339–345, 2006.

Dougherty MC, Dwyer JW, Pendergast JF et al: A randomized trial of behavioral management for continence with older rural women, *Res Nurs Health* 25:3–13, 2002.

French L, Phelps K, Pothula NR et al: Urinary problems in women, *Prim Care* 36(1):53–71, 2009.

Gray M: Urinary retention. Management in the acute care setting. Part 1, *Am J Nurs* 100(7):40–47, 2000.

Gray M: Caffeine and urinary incontinence, *J Wound Ostomy Continence Nurs* 28:66–69, 2001.

Gray M: Are cranberry juice or cranberry products effective in the prevention or management of urinary tract infection? *J Wound Ostomy Continence Nurs* 29:122–126, 2002.

Gray M: The importance of screening, assessing and managing urinary incontinence in primary care, *J Am Acad Nurse Practitioners* 15(3):102, 2003.

Gray M, Hufstuttler S, Albo M: Interstitial cystitis: a guide to recognition, evaluation and management for the nurse practitioner, *J Wound Ostomy Continence Nurs* 29:93–102, 2002.

Haidinger G, Temml G, Schatzl G, Brüssner C et al: Risk factors for lower urinary tract symptoms in elderly men. For the Prostate Study Group of the Austrian Society of Urology. *Eur Urol* 37(4):413–420, 2000.

Hess MJ, Hess PE, Sullivan MR et al: Evaluation of cranberry tablets for the prevention of urinary tract infections in spinal cord injured patients with neurogenic bladder, *Spinal Cord* 46(9):622–626, 2008.

Hunskaar S et al: Epidemiology of urinary (UI) and fecal incontinence (FI) and pelvic organ prolapse (POP). In Abrams P, Cardozo L, Khoury S et al, editors: *3rd International consultation on incontinence,* ed 3, Plymouth, UK, 2005, Plymbridge, Health Publications.

Inouye SK: Current concepts: delirium in older persons, *N Engl J Med* 354(11):1157–1165, 1217–1220, 2006.

Interstitial Cystitis Association: *IC/PBS guidelines.* www.ichelp.org/LivingwithIC/Diet/tabid/247/Default.aspx. Accessed July 4, 2009.

Kincaid-Smith P, Fairley K: The investigation of hematuria, *Semin Nephrol* 25(3):127–135, 2005.

Lodovici M, Bigagli E: Biomarkers of induced active and passive smoking damage, *Int J Environ Res Public Health* 6(3):874–888, 2009.

Masson P, Matheson S, Webster AC et al: Meta-analyses in prevention and treatment of urinary tract infections, *Infect Dis Clin North Am* 23(2):355–385, 2009.

Midthun S, Paur R, Bruce AW et al: Urinary tract infections in the elderly: a survey of physicians and nurses, *Geriatr Nurs* 26(4):245–251, 2005.

Milne JL: Behavioral therapies for overactive bladder: making sense of the evidence, *J Wound Ostomy Continence Nurs* 35(1):93–101, 2008.

Sampselle CM, Wyman JF, Thomas KK et al: Continence for women: evaluation of AWHONN's third research utilization project. Association of Women's Health Obstetric and Neonatal Nurses, *J Obstet Gynecol Neonatal Nurs* 29(1):9–17, 2000.

Shorter B, Lesser M, Moldwin RM et al: Effect of comestibles on symptoms of interstitial cystitis, *J Urol* 178(1):145–152, 2007.

Staskin D, Hilton P, Emmanuel A et al: Initial assessment of incontinence. In Abrams P, Cardozo, L, Khoury S et al, editors: *Incontinence: 3rd international consultation on incontinence,* ed 3, Plymouth, UK, 2005, Plymbridge, Health Publications.

● = Independent   ▲ = Collaborative   **EBN** = Evidence-Based Nursing   **EB** = Evidence-Based

Stewart WF, Van Rooyen JB, Cundiff GW et al: Prevalence and burden of overactive bladder in the United States, *World J Urol* 20(6):327–336, 2003.

Thompson DL: Pathology and management of functional factors contributing to incontinence. In Doughty DB, editor: *Urinary and fecal incontinence*, St Louis, 2006, Mosby.

van Gerwen M, Lagro-Janssen AL: [Diagnostic value of patient history and physical examination in elderly patients with urinary incontinence; a literature review] [article in Dutch], *Ned Tijdschr Geneeskd* 150(32):1771–1775, 2006.

Readiness for enhanced Urinary elimination   *Mikel Gray, PhD, CUNP, CCCN, FAANP, FAAN*

Definition

A pattern of urinary functions that is sufficient for meeting eliminatory needs and can be strengthened

Defining Characteristics

Amount of output is within normal limits; expresses willingness to enhance urinary elimination; fluid intake is adequate for daily needs; positions self for emptying of bladder; specific gravity is within normal limits; urine is odorless; urine is straw colored

 (Nursing Outcomes Classification)

Suggested NOC Outcomes

Urinary Continence, Urinary Elimination

Example **NOC Outcome with Indicators**
Urinary Continence as evidenced by the following indicators: Voids >150 mL each time/Empties bladder completely/Absence of postvoid residual/Postvoid residual <100 to 200 mL (Rate the outcome and indicators of **Urinary Continence:** 1 = never demonstrated, 2 = rarely demonstrated, 3 = sometimes demonstrated, 4 = often demonstrated, 5 = consistently demonstrated [see Section I].)

Client Outcomes

Client Will (Specify Time Frame):

- Eliminate or reduce incontinent episodes
- Recognize sensory stimulus indicating readiness for urine elimination
- Respond to prompts for toileting

NIC **(Nursing Interventions Classification)**

Suggested NIC Intervention

Urinary Elimination Management

Example **NIC Activities—Urinary Elimination Management**
Monitor urinary elimination, including frequency, consistency, odor, volume, and color, as appropriate; Teach patient signs and symptoms of urinary tract infection

Nursing Interventions and *Rationales*

- Assess the client for readiness for improving urine elimination patterns, focusing on need for physical assistance to access toilet, cognitive awareness of sensations indicating readiness for urine elimination, and current continence status (bladder management strategy, frequency of incontinent episodes). *Urinary continence has been identified as a quality indicator within the Nursing Home Quality Initiative (NHQI). Individualized assessment, and establishment of a bladder management program that maximizes continence is an essential component of individual care and the NHQI (Palmer, 2008).*

• = Independent   ▲ = Collaborative   **EBN** = Evidence-Based Nursing   **EB** = Evidence-Based

- Use data from the Minimum Data Set (MDS) and the Resident Assessment Protocol (RAP) to assist in identification of urinary incontinence in nursing home clients, and to assist in designing an individualized care plan to maximize continence. *Completing the CHAMMP (Continence History, Assessment, Medications, Mobility Plan) tool assists nurses to identify nursing home residents who are likely to respond to toileting programs, and it is essential data for the MDS and RAP (Bucci, 2007). Individualized assessment of clients and identification of clients who experience occasional urinary incontinence can reduce the frequency of incontinence episodes among nursing home residents (Morgan et al, 2008).*
- Ask the client to complete a bladder diary of diurnal and nocturnal urine elimination patterns and patterns of urinary leakage. **EB:** *A study demonstrated that women over estimated daytime urinary frequency from recall. Use of a bladder diary results in increased accuracy of reporting of bladder symptoms (Stav, Dwyer, & Rosamilia, 2009).*
- Begin a scheduled toileting program (usually every 2 to 3 hours) for the client who has mild to moderately impaired cognition and who requires some physical assistance to access the toilet. **EBN:** *Elders with no to moderate cognitive impairment, who are able to cooperate with toileting, and who have adequate mobility to toilet with minimal or moderate assistance are ideal candidates for scheduled toileting (Jirovec & Templin, 2001).*
- Remove environmental barriers to toilet access.
- Provide a urinal or bedside toilet as indicated.
- Assist client to remove clothing, transfer to the toilet, cleanse the perineal skin, and redress as indicated.
- Ensure that toileting opportunities are offered both during daytime hours and during hours of sleep. *Certain clients who are homebound or reside in a long-term care facility have the potential for continence but experience urine loss because they lack adequate physical assistance needed to access the toilet, remove clothing, and redress after toileting is finished. The level of assistance varies significantly and depends on the client's mobility and dexterity, as well as the availability of bedside toileting aids (Palmer, 2008).*
- For the client experiencing urinary incontinence who has mild cognitive deficits, begin a prompted voiding program or patterned urge–response toileting program. Begin a prompted toileting program based on the results of bladder log over a period of 2 to 3 days, using a check-and-change system as indicated.
  - Approach the client and briefly explain that it is time to toilet.
  - Assist the client to the toilet, provide assistance removing clothing and urine-containment devices (pads, adult urine-containment briefs), and check for urinary leakage since the last scheduled toileting.
  - Praise the client when toileting occurs with prompting.
  - If the client does not toilet or has evidence of an incontinence episode, refrain from praise, gently inform the client of the urine loss, remove and replace the soiled containment device, and assist the client to redress and rejoin activities or return to bed.

  EBN: *There is weak evidence that prompted voiding increases successful, self-initiated voiding episodes and diminishes incontinent episodes (Eustice, Roe, & Paterson, 2000).*
- Institute regular use of incontinence-containment devices combined with a structured perineal skin care program for the client with severe cognitive impairment, significant functional impairment, or no reduction in urinary incontinence frequency or severity with a scheduled or prompted toileting program. *Urine-containment products include a variety of absorptive pads, incontinent briefs, under-pads for bedding, absorptive inserts that fit into specially designed undergarments, and condom catheters. Careful selection of an absorptive device and education concerning its use maximizes its effectiveness in controlling urine loss in a particular individual (Fader, Cottenden, & Getliffe, 2008).*
- Encourage elderly women to drink at least 10 oz of cranberry juice daily, regularly consume one to two servings of fresh blueberries, or supplement the diet with cranberry concentrate capsules (usually taken in 500 mg doses with each meal). **EBN:** *Systematic literature review reveals that consumption of 400 mg of cranberry tablets, 8 to 10 oz of cranberry juice, or an equivocal portion of foods containing whole cranberries or blueberries exerts a bacteriostatic effect on* Escherichia coli, *the most common pathogen associated with urinary infection among community-dwelling adult women. Mixed evidence tends to support a reduction in UTI risk among community-dwelling women, although no*

beneficial effect has been found in clients with neurogenic bladder dysfunction who are managed by intermittent or indwelling catheters (Gray, 2002; Masson et al, 2009).

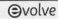 See the EVOLVE website for Weblinks for client education resources.

REFERENCES

Bucci AT: Be a continence champion: use the CHAMMP tool to individualize the plan of care, *Geriatr Nurs* 28(2):120–124, 2007.

Eustice S, Roe B, Paterson J: Prompted voiding for the management of urinary incontinence in adults, *Cochrane Database Syst Rev* (2): CD002113, 2000.

Fader M, Cottenden AM, Getliffe K: Absorbent products for moderate-heavy urinary and/or faecal incontinence in women and men, *Cochrane Database Syst Rev* (4):CD007408, 2008.

Gray M: Are cranberry juice or cranberry products effective in the prevention or management of urinary tract infection? *J Wound Ostomy Continence Nurs* 29:122–126, 2002.

Jirovec MM, Templin T: Predicting success using individualized scheduled toileting for memory-impaired elders at home, *Res Nurs Health* 24(1):1–8, 2001.

Masson P, Matheson S, Webster AC et al: Meta-analyses in prevention and treatment of urinary tract infections, *Infect Dis Clin North Am* 23(2):355–385, 2009.

Morgan C, Endozoa N, Paradiso C et al: Enhanced toileting program decreases incontinence in long term care, *Joint Com J Qual Patient Safety* 34(4):206–208, 2008.

Palmer MH: Urinary incontinence quality improvement in nursing homes: where have we been? Where are we going? *Urol Nurs* 28(6):439–444, 453, 2008.

Pfister SM: Bladder diaries and voiding patterns in older adults, *J Gerontol Nurs* 25(3):36–41, 1999.

Stav K, Dwyer PL, Rosamilia A: Women overestimate daytime urinary frequency: the importance of the bladder diary, *J Urol* 181(5):2176–2180, 2009.

Urinary retention *Mikel Gray, PhD, CUNP, CCCN, FAANP, FAAN* evolve

NANDA-I

Definition

Incomplete emptying of the bladder

Defining Characteristics

Measured urinary residual greater than 150 to 250 mL or 25% of total bladder capacity; voiding and postmicturition LUTS (slow stream, intermittency of stream, hesitancy of urination, postvoid dribbling, feelings of incomplete bladder emptying); often accompanied by storage LUTS (urgency, day and nighttime voiding frequency); occasionally accompanied by overflow incontinence (dribbling urine loss caused when intravesical pressure overwhelms the sphincter mechanism)

Related Factors (r/t)

Bladder outlet obstruction (benign prostatic hyperplasia [BPH], prostate cancer, prostatitis, acute prostatic congestion and inflammation after implantation of irradiated seeds, urethral stricture, bladder neck dyssynergia, bladder neck contracture, detrusor striated sphincter dyssynergia, high-tone pelvic floor muscle dysfunction, obstructing cystocele, urethral tumor, urethral polyp, posterior urethral valves, postoperative complication)

Deficient detrusor contraction strength (sacral level spinal lesions, cauda equina syndrome, peripheral polyneuropathies, herpes zoster or simplex affecting sacral nerve roots, injury or extensive surgery causing denervation of pelvic plexus, medication side effect, complication of illicit drug use, impaction of stool)

Defining characteristics and related factors adapted from the work of NANDA-I.

NOC (Nursing Outcomes Classification)

Suggested NOC Outcome

Urinary Elimination

Example NOC Outcome with Indicators

Urinary Elimination as evidenced by the following indicators: Empties bladder completely/Absence of urinary leakage between catheterizations or containment of micturition by condom catheter and drainage bag/Absence of UTI (negative leukocytes and bacterial growth negative or <100,000 CFU/mL (Rate the outcome and indicators of **Urinary Elimination Continence:** 1 = severely compromised, 2 = Substantially compromised, 3 = moderately compromised, 4 = mildly compromised, 5 = not compromised [see Section I].)

Client Outcomes

Client Will (Specify Time Frame):

- Demonstrate consistent ability to urinate when desire to void is perceived or via timed schedule; measured urinary residual volume is <200 to 250 mL or 25% of total bladder capacity (voided volume plus urinary residual volume)
- Experience correction or relief from voiding and postvoid LUTS
- Experience correction or alleviation of storage LUTS
- Be free of upper urinary tract distress (renal function remains sufficient; febrile urinary infections are absent)

 NIC   **(Nursing Interventions Classification)**

Suggested NIC Interventions

Urinary Catheterization, Urinary Retention Care

Example NIC Activities—Urinary Retention Care

Perform a comprehensive urinary assessment focusing on incontinence (e.g., urinary output, urinary voiding pattern, cognitive function, and preexistent urinary problems); Use the power of suggestion by running water, or flushing toilet; Provide enough time for bladder emptying; Use double voiding technique

Nursing Interventions and *Rationales*

- Obtain a focused urinary history emphasizing the character and duration of lower urinary tract symptoms. Query the client about episodes of acute urinary retention (complete inability to void) or chronic retention (documented elevated postvoid residual volumes). *Although the presence of obstructive or irritative lower urinary tract symptoms is not diagnostic of urinary retention (Roehrborn et al, 2002), a focused nursing history can provide clues to the likely cause of retention and its management (Gray, 2000a).*
- Question the client concerning specific risk factors for urinary retention including:
  - Disorders affecting the sacral spinal cord such as spinal cord injuries of vertebral levels T12–L2, disk problems, cauda equina syndrome, tabes dorsalis
  - Acute neurological injury causing sudden loss of mobility such as spinal shock or ischemic stroke
  - Metabolic disorders such as diabetes mellitus, chronic alcoholism, and related conditions associated with polyuria and peripheral polyneuropathies
  - Herpetic infection involving the sacral skin and underlying spinal dermatomes
  - Heavy-metal poisoning (lead, mercury) causing peripheral polyneuropathies
  - Advanced stage human immunodeficiency virus (HIV)
  - Medications including antispasmodics/parasympatholytics, alpha-adrenergic agonists, antidepressants, sedatives, narcotics, psychotropic medications, illicit drugs
  - Recent surgery requiring general or spinal anesthesia
  - Vaginal delivery within the past 48 hours
  - Bowel elimination patterns, history of fecal impaction, encopresis
  - Recent surgical procedures
  - Recent prostatic biopsy or brachytherapy therapy

  Urinary retention is related to multiple factors affecting either detrusor contraction strength or urethral resistance to urinary outflow (Gray, 2000a; Acheson & Mudd, 2004; Darabi et al, 2004; Gehrich et al,

• = Independent   ▲ = Collaborative   **EBN** = Evidence-Based Nursing   **EB** = Evidence-Based

2005; Thomas et al, 2005; Ohashi et al, 2006; Feliciano et al, 2008; Ismail & Emery, 2008). **EBN:** *Multiple factors in the surgical client are associated with an increased risk of postoperative urinary retention including preoperative voiding difficulty, advanced age, total amount of fluid replacement during a 24–hour postoperative period, type of anesthesia, pain management medications, and route and length of medication administration (Baldini et al, 2009).*

▲ Perform a focused physical assessment or review results of a recent physical including perineal skin integrity; inspection, percussion, and palpation of the lower abdomen for obvious bladder distention; a neurological examination including perineal skin sensation and the bulbocavernosus reflex; and vaginal vault examination in women and digital rectal examination in men. *The physical assessment provides clues to the likely cause of urinary retention and its management (Selius & Subedi, 2008).*

▲ Determine the urinary residual volume by catheterizing the client immediately after urination or by obtaining a bladder ultrasound after micturition. *Although catheterization provides the most accurate method to determine urinary residual volume, it is invasive, produces discomfort, and carries a risk of infection (Gray, 2000b).* **EBN:** *Postvoid bladder ultrasound performed by registered nurses provided reasonable estimates of postvoid residual bladder volumes in clients treated in acute care and geriatric rehabilitation units (Borrie et al, 2001; O'Farrell et al, 2001). The results of the ultrasonic measurement changed nursing practice by 51% of instances, reducing unneeded catheterizations by 32% (O'Farrell et al, 2001).*

• Complete a bladder log including patterns of urine elimination, urine loss (if present), nocturia, and volume and type of fluids consumed for a period of 3 to 7 days. *The bladder log provides an objective verification of urine elimination patterns and allows comparison of fluids consumed versus urinary output during a 24–hour period (Nygaard & Holcomb, 2000).*

▲ Consult with the physician concerning eliminating or altering medications suspected of producing or exacerbating urinary retention. *Observational studies suggest that medications may play a role in approximately 10% of all cases of urinary retention. The most commonly implicated drug classes include antipsychotics, antidepressants, anticholinergic respiratory agents, opioid analgesics alpha-adrenoceptor agonists, benzodiazepines, nonsteroidal antiinflammatory drugs, antimuscarinics, and calcium channel blockers (Verhamme et al, 2008).*

• Teach the client with mild to moderate obstructive symptoms to double void by urinating, resting in the bathroom for 3 to 5 minutes, and then trying again to urinate. *Double voiding promotes more efficient bladder evacuation by allowing the detrusor to contract initially and then rest and contract again (Gray, 2000b).*

• Teach the client with urinary retention and infrequent voiding to urinate by the clock. *Timed or scheduled voiding may reduce urinary retention by preventing bladder overdistention (Gray, 2000b).*

• Advise the male client with urinary retention related to BPH to avoid risk factors associated with acute urinary retention as follows:
  ▪ Avoid over-the-counter cold remedies containing a decongestant (alpha-adrenergic agonist) or antihistamine such as diphenhydramine, which has anticholinergic effects.
  ▪ Avoid taking over-the-counter dietary medications (frequently contain alpha-adrenergic agonists).
  ▪ Discuss voiding problems with a health care provider before beginning new prescription medications.
  ▪ After prolonged exposure to cool weather, warm the body before attempting to urinate.
  ▪ Avoid overfilling the bladder by regular urination patterns and refrain from excessive intake of alcohol.

These modifiable factors predispose the client to acute urinary retention by overdistending the bladder and compromising detrusor contraction strength or by increasing outlet resistance (Gray, 2000b).

• Teach the client who is unable to void specific strategies to manage this potential medical emergency as follows:
  ▪ Attempt urination in complete privacy.
  ▪ Place the feet solidly on the floor.
  ▪ If unable to void using these strategies, take a warm sitz bath or shower and void (if possible) while still in the tub or shower.

- Drink a warm cup of caffeinated coffee or tea to stimulate the bladder, which may promote voiding.
- If unable to void within 6 hours or if bladder distention is producing significant pain, seek urgent or emergency care.

Attempting urination in complete privacy and placing the feet solidly on the floor help relax the pelvic muscles and may encourage voiding. Warm water also stimulates the bladder and may produce voiding; the cooling experienced by leaving the tub or shower may again inhibit the bladder (Gray, 2000b).

▲ Remove the indwelling urethral catheter at midnight in the hospitalized client to reduce the risk of acute urinary retention. **EBN:** *Removal of indwelling catheters in clients undergoing urologic surgery at midnight offers several advantages to "morning removal," including a larger initial voided volume and earlier hospital discharge with no increased risk for readmission compared with those undergoing morning removal (Griffiths, Fernandez, & Murie, 2004).*

▲ Consult the physician about bladder stimulation in the client with urinary retention caused by deficient detrusor contraction strength. **EBN:** *High-frequency transvaginal electrical stimulation of the bladder neck has been shown to be beneficial in a small case series involving women with chronic urinary retention owing to deficient detrusor contraction strength (Bernier & Davila, 2000).*

▲ Perform sterile or clean intermittent catheterization as directed for clients with urinary retention. **EBN:** *Clients managed with intermittent catheterization using clean technique had no more symptomatic UTI than those managed by intermittent catheterization using sterile technique (Moore, Burt, & Voaklander, 2006).*

▲ Teach the client with significant urinary retention to perform clean, self-intermittent catheterization as directed. **EBN:** *Intermittent catheterization allows regular, complete bladder evacuation without serious complications (Robinson, 2006). Intermittent catheterization can be mastered by clients with mild cognitive dysfunction associated with neurological conditions such as multiple sclerosis, enabling them to maintain adequate bladder emptying without resorting to an indwelling catheter (Vahter et al, 2009).*

- Advise clients who undergo intermittent catheterization that bacteria are likely to colonize the urine but that this condition does not indicate a clinically significant urinary tract infection. *Bacteriuria frequently occurs in the client undergoing intermittent catheterization; only symptoms producing infections warrant treatment (Wyndaele, 2002).*
- Insert an indwelling catheter for the individual with urinary retention who is not a suitable candidate for intermittent catheterization. *An indwelling catheter provides continuous drainage of urine; however, the risks of serious urinary complications with prolonged use are significant (Weld et al, 2000).*
- Advise clients with indwelling catheters that bacteria in the urine is an almost universal finding after the catheter has remained in place for a period of 30 days or longer and that only symptomatic infections warrant treatment. *The long-term indwelling catheter is inevitably associated with bacterial colonization. Most bacteriuria does not produce significant infection, and attempts to eradicate bacteriuria often produce subsequent morbidity because resistant bacteria are encouraged to reproduce while more easily managed strains are eradicated (Gray, 2004). Intermittent catheterization was preferred in a rehabilitation setting because it improves client quality of life and diminishes the time required to recover spontaneous voiding with a postvoid residual volume <150 mL (Tang et al, 2006).*
- Use the following strategies to reduce the risk for catheter-associated UTIs whenever feasible:
  - Insert the indwelling catheter only when indicated.
  - Remove the indwelling catheter as soon as possible; acute care facilities should institute a policy for regular review of the necessity of an indwelling catheter, beginning 3–4 days after insertion.
  - Insert a silver alloy catheter for short-term indwelling catheterization (<14 days).
  - Maintain a closed drainage system whenever feasible.
  - Regularly cleanse the urethral meatus with a gentle cleanser to remove apparent soiling.
  - Change the long-term catheter every 4 weeks whenever possible; more frequent catheter changes should be reserved for clients who experience catheter encrustation and blockage.
  - Place clients managed in an acute or long-term care facility with a catheter-associated UTI in a separate room from others managed by an indwelling catheter to reduce the risk of spreading the offending pathogen.

• = Independent   ▲ = Collaborative   **EBN** = Evidence-Based Nursing   **EB** = Evidence-Based

■ Educate staff about the risks of catheter-associated UTIs and specific strategies to reduce this risk.

EBN: *These strategies are supported by sufficient evidence to recommend routine use (Parker et al, 2009; Willson et al, 2009). Strategies that lack sufficient evidence to support routine use include (1) strict aseptic technique when replacing a long-term indwelling catheter; (2) application of antimicrobial ointments during routine meatal care; (3) application of antimicrobial ointments or creams to the urethral meatus; (4) adding hydrogen peroxide or silver sulfadiazine or slow-releasing silver ions to the catheter drainage bag; (5) frequent drainage bag changes; or (6) one-way catheter valves (Willson et al, 2009).*

 ### Geriatric

- Aggressively assess elderly clients, particularly those with dribbling urinary incontinence, UTI, and related conditions for urinary retention. *Elderly women (and men) may experience urinary retention with few or no apparent symptoms; a urinary residual volume and related assessments are necessary to determine the presence of retention in this population (Ostaszkiewicz, O'Connell, & Ski, 2008).*
- Assess elderly clients for impaction when urinary retention is documented or suspected. *Fecal impaction and urinary retention frequently coexist in elderly clients and, unless reversed, may lead to acute delirium, UTI, or renal insufficiency (Waale, Bruijns, & Dautzenberg, 2001; Waardenburg, 2008).*
- Assess elderly male clients for retention related to prostatic enlargement (BPH or prostate cancer). *Prostate enlargement in elderly men increases the risk of acute and chronic urinary retention (Loh & Chin, 2002).*

 ### Home Care

- The interventions listed previously may be adapted for home care use.
- Encourage the client to report any inability to void. *Pathophysiological factors of urinary retention require follow-up.*
- Maintain an up-to-date medication list; evaluate side effect profiles for risk of urinary retention. *New medications or changes in dose may cause urinary retention.*
- ▲ Refer the client for physician evaluation if urinary retention occurs. *Identification of cause is important. Left untreated, urinary retention may lead to UTI or kidney failure.*

 ### Client/Family Teaching and Discharge Planning

- Teach techniques for intermittent catheterization including use of clean rather than sterile technique, washing using soap and water or a microwave technique, and reuse of the catheter.
- Teach the client with an indwelling catheter to assess the tube for patency, maintain the drainage system below the level of the symphysis pubis, and routinely cleanse the bedside bag.
- Teach the client with an indwelling catheter or undergoing intermittent catheterization the symptoms of a significant urinary infection including hematuria, acute-onset incontinence, dysuria, flank pain, or fever.

⊖volve   See the EVOLVE website for Weblinks for client education resources.

REFERENCES

Acheson J, Mudd D: Acute urinary retention attributable to sacral herpes zoster, *Emerg Med J* 21(6):752–753, 2004.

Baldini G, Bagry H, Aprikian A et al: Postoperative urinary retention: anesthetic and perioperative considerations, *Anesthesiology* 110(5):1139–1157, 2009.

Bernier F, Davila GW: The treatment of nonobstructive urinary retention with high-frequency transvaginal electrical stimulation, *Urol Nurs* 20(4):261–264, 2000.

Borrie MJ, Campbell K, Arcese ZA et al: Urinary retention in patients in a geriatric rehabilitation unit: prevalence, risk factors, and validity of bladder scan evaluation, *Rehab Nurs* 26(5):187–191, 2001.

Darabi K, Segal AM, Torres G: Herpes zoster infection: a rare cause of urinary retention, *Can J Urol* 11(4):2314, 2004.

Feliciano T, Montero J, McCarthy M et al: A retrospective, descriptive, exploratory study evaluating incidence of postoperative urinary retention after spinal anesthesia and its effect on PACU discharge, *J Perianesth Nurs* 23(6):394–400, 2008.

Gehrich AP, Aseff JN, Iglesia CB et al: Chronic urinary retention and pelvic floor hypertonicity after surgery for endometriosis: a case series, *Am J Obst Gynecol* 193(6):2133–2137, 2005.

Gray M: Urinary retention. Management in the acute care setting. Part 1, *Am J Nurs* 100(7):40–47, 2000a.

 ● = Independent   ▲ = Collaborative   **EBN** = Evidence-Based Nursing   **EB** = Evidence-Based

Gray M: Urinary retention: Management in the acute care setting. II, *Am J Nurs* 100(8):36–43, 2000b.

Gray M: What nursing interventions reduce the risk of symptomatic urinary tract infection in the patient with an indwelling catheter? *J Wound Ostomy Continence Nurs* 31(1):3–13, 2004.

Griffiths RD, Fernandez RS, Murie P: Removal of short-term indwelling urethral catheters: the evidence, *J Wound, Ostomy Continence Nurs* 31(5):299–308, 2004.

Horsley JA, Crane J, Reynolds MA: *Clean intermittent catheterization: conduct and utilization of research in nursing project,* New York, 1982, Grune & Stratton.

Ismail SIMF, Emery SJ: The prevalence of silent postpartum retention of urine in a heterogeneous cohort, *J Obstet Gynaecol* 28(5):504–507, 2008.

Loh SY, Chin CM: A demographic profile of patients undergoing transurethral resection of the prostate for benign prostate hyperplasia and presenting in acute urinary retention, *Br J Urol Int* 89(6):531–533, 2002.

Moore KN, Burt J, Voaklander DC: Intermittent catheterization in the rehabilitation setting: a comparison of clean and sterile technique, *Clin Rehabil* 20(6):461–468, 2006.

Narayan P, Tewari A: A second phase III multicenter placebo study of 2 dosages of modified release tamsulosin in patients with symptoms of benign prostatic hyperplasia. United States 93–01 study group, *J Urol* 160:1701–1706, 1998.

Nygaard I, Holcomb R: Reproducibility of the seven day voiding diary in women with stress urinary incontinence, *Int Urogynecol J Pelvic Floor Dysfunct* 11:15–17, 2000.

O'Farrell B, Vandervoort MK, Bisnaire D et al: Evaluation of portable bladder ultrasound: accuracy and effect on nursing practice in an acute neuroscience unit, *J Neurosci Nurs* 33(6):301–309, 2001.

Ohashi T, Yorozu A, Toya K et al: Predictive factors of acute urinary retention requiring catheterization following 125I prostate brachytherapy, *Jpn J Clin Oncol* 36(5):285–289, 2006.

Ostaszkiewicz J, O'Connell B, Ski CP: A guideline for the nursing assessment and management of urinary retention in elderly hospitalised patients, *Aust Nz Continence J* 14(3):76–83, 2008.

Parker D, Callan L, Harwood J et al: Nursing interventions to reduce the risk of catheter-associated urinary tract infection. Part 1: catheter selection, *J Wound Ostomy Continence Nurs* 36(1):23–34, 2009.

Robinson J: Intermittent self-catheterization: principles and practice, *Br J Community Nurs* 11(4):144, 146, 148 passim, 2006.

Roehrborn CG, McConnell JD, Saltzman B et al: Storage (irritative) and voiding (obstructive) symptoms as predictors of benign prostatic hyperplasia progression and related outcomes, *Eur Urol* 42(1):1–6, 2002.

Selius BA, Subedi R: Urinary retention in adults: diagnosis and initial management, *Am Fam Physician* 77(5):643–650, 2008.

Tang MW, Kwok TC, Hui E et al: Intermittent versus indwelling urinary catheterization in older female patients, *Maturitas* 53(3):274–281, 2006.

Thomas AW, Cannon A, Bartlett E et al: The natural history of lower urinary tract dysfunction in men: minimum 10–year urodynamic follow-up of untreated bladder outlet obstruction, *BJU Int* 96(9):1301–1306, 2005.

Vahter L, Zopp I, Kreegipuu M, et al: Clean intermittent self-catheterization in persons with multiple sclerosis: the influence of cognitive dysfunction, *Mult Scler* 15(3):379–384, 2009.

Verhamme KM, Sturkenboom MC, Stricker BH et al: Drug-induced urinary retention: incidence, management, and prevention. *Drug Saf* 31(5):373–388, 2008.

Waale WH, Bruijns E, Dautzenberg PJ: Delirium due to urinary retention: confusing for both the patient and the doctor, *Tijdschr Gerontol Geriatr* 32(3):100–103, 2001.

Waardenburg IE: Delirium caused by urinary retention in elderly people: a case report and literature review on the "Cystocerebral syndrome," *J Am Geriatr Soc* 56(12):2371–2372, 2008.

Weld KJ, Wall BM, Mangold TA et al: Influences on renal function in chronic spinal cord injured patients, *J Urol* 164(5):1490–1493, 2000.

Willson M, Wilde M, Webb ML et al: Nursing interventions to reduce the risk of catheter-associated urinary tract infection: part 2: staff education, monitoring, and care techniques, *J Wound Ostomy Continence Nur* 36(2):137–54, 2009.

Wyndaele JJ: Complications of intermittent catheterization: their prevention and treatment, *Spinal Cord* 40(10):536, 2002.

Impaired spontaneous Ventilation   *Elizabeth A. Henneman, RN, PhD, CCNS, FAAN*

NANDA-I

Definition

Decreased energy reserves result in an individual's inability to maintain breathing adequate to support life

Defining Characteristics

Apprehension; decreased cooperation; decreased P_{O_2}; decreased Sa_{O_2}; decreased tidal volume; dyspnea; increased heart rate; increased metabolic rate; increased P_{CO_2}; increased restlessness; increased use of accessory muscles

Related Factors (r/t)

Metabolic factors; respiratory muscle fatigue

NOC   (Nursing Outcomes Classification)

Suggested NOC Outcomes

Neurological Status: Central Motor Control, Respiratory Status: Gas Exchange, Ventilation

 V

● = Independent   ▲ = Collaborative   **EBN** = Evidence-Based Nursing   **EB** = Evidence-Based

Example NOC Outcome with Indicators

Achieves appropriate **Respiratory Status: Ventilation** as evidenced by the following indicators: Respiratory rate/Respiratory rhythm/Depth of inspiration/Symmetrical chest expansion/Ease of breathing/Moves sputum out of airway/Accessory muscle use not present/Adventitious breath sounds not present/Chest retraction not present/Tidal volume/Vital capacity (Rate the outcome and indicators of **Respiratory Status: Ventilation:** 1 = severe deviation from normal range, 2 = substantial deviation from normal range, 3 = moderate deviation from normal range, 4 = mild deviation from normal range, 5 = no deviation from normal range [see Section I].)

Client Outcomes

Client Will (Specify Time Frame):

- Maintain arterial blood gases within safe parameters
- Remain free of dyspnea or restlessness
- Effectively maintain airway
- Effectively mobilize secretions

NIC   (Nursing Interventions Classification)

Suggested NIC Interventions

Artificial Airway Management, Mechanical Ventilation: Invasive, Respiratory Monitoring, Resuscitation: Neonate, Ventilation Assistance, Mechanical Ventilation Management: Noninvasive

Example NIC Activities—Mechanical Ventilation Management: Invasive

Monitor for conditions indicating a need for ventilation support (e.g., respiratory muscle fatigue, neurological dysfunction second to trauma, anesthesia, drug overdose, refractory respiratory acidosis); Consult with other health care personnel in selection of a ventilator mode

Nursing Interventions and *Rationales*

- ▲ Collaborate with the client, family, and physician regarding possible intubation and ventilation. Ask whether the client has advanced directives and, if so, integrate them into the plan of care with clinical data regarding overall health and reversibility of the medical condition. **EB:** *Client preferences must be acknowledged when planning care. Advanced directives protect client autonomy and help to ensure that the client's wishes are respected (Baggs et al, 2007; Burns, 2007).*
- • Assess and respond to changes in the client's respiratory status. Monitor the client for dyspnea, increase in respiratory rate, use of accessory muscles, retraction of intercostal muscles, flaring of nostrils, decrease in O_2 saturation, and subjective complaints (Schultz, 2005). **EBN:** *It is essential to monitor for these signs of impending respiratory failure or inability to tolerate ventilator setting/weaning process (Burns, 2005).*
- • Have the client use a numerical scale (0–10) to rate dyspnea before and after interventions (if appropriate). **EBN:** *The numerical rating scale is a valid measure of dyspnea and has been found to be easiest for clients to use. This allows measurement of the intensity, progression, and resolution of dyspnea (Gift & Narsavage, 1998; Powers & Bennett, 1999).*
- • Assess for history of chronic respiratory disorders when administering oxygen. *With chronic obstructive pulmonary disease (COPD) the respiratory drive is primarily in response to hypoxia, not hypercarbia; oxygenating too aggressively can result in respiratory depression. When managing acute respiratory failure in clients with COPD, use caution in administering oxygen because hyperoxygenation can lead to respiratory depression.*
- ▲ Collaborate with the physician and respiratory therapists in determining the appropriateness of noninvasive positive pressure ventilation (NPPV) for the decompensated client with COPD.
- ▲ Assist with implementation, client support, and monitoring if NPPV is used. **EB:** *In a client with exacerbation of COPD, NPPV can be as effective as intubation with use of a ventilator. It can also be used if the client has other complications, such as hypotension or severely impaired mental status (Perkins & Shortall, 2000; Pierson, 2002). The use of continuous positive airway pressure (CPAP) and bi-*

• = Independent   ▲ = Collaborative   **EBN** = Evidence-Based Nursing   **EB** = Evidence-Based

level positive airway pressure (bi-PAP) has been shown to improve oxygenation and decrease the rate of endotracheal intubation in clients with acute pulmonary edema (Park et al, 2004).

- If the client has apnea, pH <7.25, Paco$_2$ >50 mm Hg, Pao$_2$ <50 mm Hg, respiratory muscle fatigue, or somnolence, prepare the client for possible intubation and mechanical ventilation. **EBN:** *These indicators may predict the need for invasive mechanical ventilation (Burns, 2005; Burns 2007).*

Ventilator Support

- ▲ Explain the intubation and mechanical ventilation process to the client and family as appropriate, and during intubation administer sedation for client comfort according to the physician's orders. **EBN:** *Explanation of the procedure decreases anxiety and reinforces information; premedication allows for a more controlled intubation with decreased incidence of insertion problems (Burns, 2005; St. John & Seckel, 2007).*

- Secure the endotracheal tube in place using either tape or a commercially available device, auscultate bilateral breath sounds, use a CO$_2$ detector, and obtain a chest radiograph to confirm endotracheal tube placement. **EBN:** *Secure taping is needed to prevent inadvertent extubation. Nursing studies have shown conflicting results regarding the preferable way to secure the endotracheal tube (Clarke et al, 1998).* **EB:** *Auscultation alone is an unreliable method for checking endotracheal tube placement (Takeda et al, 2003). A CO$_2$ detector can be used to confirm tube placement in the trachea (Takeda et al, 2003); however, correct position of the endotracheal tube in the trachea (3 to 5 cm above the carina) must be confirmed by chest radiograph (Burns, 2005; Henneman, Ellstrom, & St. John, 1998; St. John & Seckel, 2007). Calormetric CO$_2$ detectors have also been used successfully to detect inadvertent airway intubation during gastric tube placement (Burns et al, 2004).*

- Ensure that ventilator settings are appropriate to meet the client's minute ventilation requirements. *Ventilator settings should be adjusted to prevent hyperventilation or hypoventilation. A variety of new modes of ventilation are currently available that are responsive to client effort (pressure support). Little data is available to support the best use of these ventilator modes or their effect on client outcome (Burns, 2008).*

- ▲ Suction as needed and hyperoxygenate according to unit policy. Refer to the care plan **Ineffective Airway clearance** for further information on suctioning.

- Check that monitor alarms are set appropriately at the start of each shift. *This action helps ensure client safety (Burns, 2005).*

- Respond to ventilator alarms promptly. If unable to immediately locate the source/cause of an alarm, use a manual self-inflating resuscitation bag to ventilate the client while waiting for assistance. *Common causes of a high-pressure alarm include secretions, condensation in the tubing, biting of the endotracheal tube, decreased compliance of the lungs, and compression of the tubing. Common causes of a low-pressure alarm are ventilator disconnection, leaks in the circuit, and changing compliance. Using a manual self-inflating resuscitation bag with supplemental oxygen, the nurse can provide immediate ventilation and oxygenation as needed (Burns, 2005).*

- Prevent unplanned extubation by maintaining stability of endotracheal tube and using soft wrist restraints on the client if needed and ordered. *Use only when other methods are ineffective, such as orienting client and allowing family at bedside.*

- Drain collected fluid from condensation out of ventilator tubing as needed. *This action reduces the risk of infection by decreasing inhalation of contaminated water droplets (Burns, 2005).*

- Note ventilator settings of flow of inspired oxygen, peak inspiratory pressure, tidal volume, and alarm activation at intervals and when removing the client from the ventilator for any reason. *Checking the settings ensures that safety measures are taken and that the client is not left on 100% oxygen after suctioning (Burns, 2007).*

- ▲ Administer analgesics and sedatives as needed to facilitate client comfort and rest. Pain and sedation scales provide a consistent way of monitoring sedation levels and ensuring that therapeutic outcomes are being met (Consensus Conference on Sedation Assessment, 2004) **EBN:** *An earlier study demonstrated that a nurse-implemented sedation protocol decreased the number of days of intubation, the need for a tracheotomy, and the length of hospital stay (Brook et al, 1999), although new evidence suggests that protocols may be unnecessary when nurses are autonomous and skilled in managing ventilator processes such as weaning (Rose et al, 2007).* **EB:** *Avoid oversedation; use of continuous IV sedative infusions is associated with longer duration of mechanical ventilation compared with bolus sedation (Kollef et al, 1998; Brook et al, 1999; Kress et al, 2000). It has been suggested that clients*

• = Independent   ▲ = Collaborative   **EBN** = Evidence-Based Nursing   **EB** = Evidence-Based

receiving continuous sedative infusions should undergo once daily interruptions of the medication to assess the client's level of anxiety and need for medication (Kress et al, 2000). These daily interruptions (often termed "sedation vacations") require close monitoring by the nurse and should not be conducted unless the nurse is able to be physically present at the bedside. Oral intubation and inadequate sedation have been noted to be indicators for unplanned extubation (Chevron et al, 1998).

- Tools as the Riker Sedation-Agitation Scale, the Motor Activity Assessment Scale, the Ramsey Scale, or the Richmond Agitation-Sedation Scale may be useful in monitoring levels of sedation. **EB:** *Each of these instruments has established reliability and validity and can be used to monitor the effect of sedative therapy (Ely et al, 2003; Jacobi et al, 2003). However, recent research suggests that the use of sedation and pain scales may not decrease duration of mechanical ventilation (Williams et al, 2008).*

- Alternatives to medications for decreasing anxiety should be attempted, such as music therapy with selections of the client's choice played on headphones at intervals. **EBN:** *Music therapy has been reported to decrease anxiety and reduce heart and respiratory rate in critically ill and intubated clients (Chlan, 1998; White, 2000).*

- Analyze and respond to arterial blood gas results, end-tidal CO_2 levels, and pulse oximetry values. *Ventilatory support must be closely monitored to ensure adequate oxygenation and acid-base balance.* **EBN:** *End-tidal CO_2 monitoring is best used as an adjunct to direct client observation and is used to monitor a client's ventilatory status and pulmonary blood flow (Good, 2005; St. John & Seckel, 2007).*

- Use an effective means of verbal and nonverbal communication with the client. Barriers to communication include endotracheal tubes, sedation, and general weakness associated with a critical illness. Basic technologies should be readily available to the client, including eyeglasses and hearing aids (Henneman, 2009). Inadequate communication with the client and family may increase the risk for medical errors and adverse events (Kleinpell et al, 2008). A variety of communication devices are available, including electronic voice output communication aids, alphabet boards, picture boards, computers, and writing slate. Ask the client for input into their care as appropriate. **EBN:** *Inability to communicate can lead to client frustration, insecurity, and sometimes panic (Happ, 2001). Clients have reported a high level of frustration in communicating their needs while being mechanically ventilated (Patak et al, 2004) and believe the use of a communication board would have decreased this frustration (Patak et al, 2006).* **EB:** *Use of a voice-output communication device was shown to be effective in a group of intubated surgery clients (Costello, 2000).* **EBN:** *Practitioner behaviors reported to facilitate communication include being kind, informative, and physically present at the bedside (Patak et al, 2004).*

- Move the endotracheal tube from side to side every 24 hours, and tape it or secure it with a commercially available device. Assess and document client's skin condition, and ensure correct tube placement at lip line. *These steps help prevent skin breakdown at the lip line resulting from endotracheal tube pressure (St. John & Seckel, 2007).*

- Implement steps to prevent ventilator associated pneumonia (VAP), including continuous removal of subglottic secretions, elevation of the head of bed to 30 to 45 degrees unless medically contraindicated, change of the ventilator circuit no more than every 48 hours, and handwashing before and after contact with each client (Tablan et al, 2004; Berry et al, 2007). See details in the sections that follow.

- Use endotracheal tubes that allow for the continuous aspiration of subglottic secretions (CASS) (if available). **EB:** *The accumulation of contaminated oropharyngeal secretions above the endotracheal tube may contribute to the risk of aspiration. Two studies have suggested a decrease in the rate of VAP in clients requiring mechanical ventilation for >3 days when CASS was used (Mahul et al, 1992; Valles et al, 1995). This practice is recommended by the Centers for Disease Control and Prevention (Tablan et al, 2004).*

- Position the client in a semirecumbent position with the head of the bed at a 30– to 45–degree angle to decrease the aspiration of gastric secretions. **EB:** *Studies have shown that mechanically ventilated clients have a decreased incidence of pneumonia if the client is placed in a 30– to 45–degree semirecumbent position as opposed to a supine position (Torres et al, 1992; Drakulovic et al, 1999; Collard, Saint, & Matthay, 2003).*

- Perform handwashing using both soap and water (if hands are visibly soiled) or alcohol-based solution before and after all client contact (Tablan et al, 2004). **EB:** *Handwashing with an alcohol-based solution decreases bacterial counts (Girou et al, 2002; Lucet et al, 2002; Trick et al, 2003).*

● = Independent ▲ = Collaborative **EBN** = Evidence-Based Nursing **EB** = Evidence-Based

- Provide routine oral care using tooth brushing and oral rinsing with an antimicrobial agent if needed. **EB:** *Most episodes of VAP are thought to result from aspiration of oropharyngeal secretions containing potentially pathogenic organisms (Berry et al, 2007). The optimal method of providing oral hygiene has not been established. Experts have recommended tooth brushing (versus use of sponge toothettes) to remove plaque (Munro & Grap, 2004). The use of an oral rinse of chlorhexidine has been shown to be effective in preventing nosocomial pneumonia in clients after cardiac surgery (Houston et al, 2002).*
- Reposition the client as needed. Use rotational bed therapy in clients for whom side-to-side turning is contraindicated or difficult. **EBN:** *Changing position frequently decreases the incidence of atelectasis, pooling of secretions, and resultant pneumonia (Burns, 2005).* **EB and EBN:** *Continuous, lateral rotational therapy has been shown to improve oxygenation and decrease the incidence of VAP (Wang et al, 2003).*
- ▲ If the client is intubated and is stable, consider getting the client up to sit at the edge of the bed, transfer to a chair, or walk as appropriate, if an effective interdisciplinary team is developed to keep the client safe. *For every week of bedrest, muscle strength can decrease 20%, early ambulation helped clients develop a positive outlook (Perme & Chandrashekar, 2009).*
- Assess bilateral anterior and posterior breath sounds every 2 to 4 hours and PRN; respond to any relevant changes.
- Assess responsiveness to ventilator support; monitor for subjective complaints and sensation of dyspnea (Burns, 2005).
- ▲ Collaborate with the interdisciplinary team in treating clients with acute respiratory failure (Grap et al, 2003). **EB:** *A collaborative approach to caring for mechanically ventilated clients has been demonstrated to reduce length of time on the ventilator and length of stay in the ICU (Henneman et al, 2001, 2002). The mechanical ventilator is usually a temporary support until the underlying pathology can be effectively resolved.*

Geriatric

- Recognize that older adults have a high rate of morbidity when mechanically ventilated. *Implement such interventions as positioning and nutrition maintenance early to prevent decline (Phelan, Cooper, & Sangkachand, 2002).*

Home Care

- ▲ Some of the interventions listed previously may be adapted for home care use. Begin discharge planning as soon as possible with the case manager or social worker to assess the need for home support systems, assistive devices, and community or home health services.
- ▲ With help from a medical social worker, assist the client and family to determine the fiscal affect of care in the home versus an extended care facility.
- Assess the home setting during the discharge process to ensure the home can safely accommodate ventilator support (e.g., adequate space and electricity).
- Have the family contact the electric company and place the client residence on a high-risk list in case of a power outage. *Some home-based care requires special conditions for safe home administration.*
- Assess the caregivers for commitment to supporting a ventilator-dependent client in the home.
- Be sure that the client and family or caregivers are familiar with operation of all ventilation devices, know how to suction secretions if needed, are competent in doing tracheostomy care, and know schedules for cleaning equipment. Have the designated caregiver or caregivers demonstrate care before discharge. *Some home-based care involves specialized technology and requires specific skills for safe and appropriate care.*
- Assess client and caregiver knowledge of the disease, client needs, and medications to be administered via ventilation-assistive devices. Avoid analgesics. Assess knowledge of how to use equipment. Teach as necessary. *A client receiving ventilation support may not be able to articulate needs. Respiratory medications can have side effects that change the client's respiration or level of consciousness.*
- Establish an emergency plan and criteria for use. Identify emergency procedures to be used until medical assistance arrives. Teach and role play emergency care. *A prepared emergency plan reassures the client and family and ensures client safety.*

● = Independent   ▲ = Collaborative   **EBN** = Evidence-Based Nursing   **EB** = Evidence-Based

Client/Family Teaching and Discharge Planning

- Explain to the client the potential sensations that will be experienced, including relief of dyspnea, the feeling of lung inflations, the noise of the ventilator, and the reality of alarms. **EBN:** *Knowledge of potential sensations and experiences before they are encountered can decrease anxiety. Administration of sedatives or narcotics may be needed to provide adequate oxygenation and ventilation in some clients (Burns, 2005).*

- Explain to the client and family about being unable to speak, and work out an alternative system of communication. See previously mentioned interventions.

- Demonstrate to the family how to perform simple procedures, such as suctioning secretions in the mouth with a tonsil-tip catheter, providing range-of-motion exercises, and reconnecting the ventilator immediately if it becomes disconnected. *Families are a critical part of the client's care, may be present at the bedside for prolonged periods of time, and need information about the plan of care (Henneman & Cardin, 2002; Burns, 2005; Davidson, 2009).*

- Offer both the client and family explanations of how the ventilator works and answer any questions. *Having questions answered is often cited as an important need of clients and families when a client is on a ventilator (Burns, 2005).*

ⓔvolve   See the EVOLVE website for Weblinks for client education resources.

REFERENCES

Baggs JG, Norton SA, Schmitt M et al: Intensive care unit cultures and end-of-life decision making, *J Crit Care* 22:159–168, 2007.

Berry AM, Davidson PM, Masters J et al: Systematic literature review of oral hygiene practices for intensive care patients receiving mechanical ventilation, *AJCC* 16(6):552–563, 2007.

Boland D, Sims S: Family care giving at home as a solitary journey, *Image* 28:1, 1996.

Brook AD, Ahrens TS, Schaiff R et al: Effect of a nursing-implemented sedation protocol on the duration of mechanical ventilation, *Crit Care Med* 27(12):2609, 1999.

Burns SM: Ventilatory management—volume and pressure modes. In Lynn-McHale DJ, Carlson KK, editors: *AACN Procedure Manual for Critical Care,* ed 4, Philadelphia, 2005, Saunders.

Burns SM: Weaning from mechanical ventilation. In Burns SM, editor: *AACN protocols for practice: care of mechanically ventilated patients,* ed 2, Sudbury, MA, 2007, Jones & Bartlett.

Burns SM: Pressure modes of mechanical ventilation: the good the bad, and the ugly, *AACN Adv Crit Care* 19(4):399–411, 2008.

Burns SM, Carpenter R, Smith C et al: Identifying inadvertent airway intubation during gastric tube insertion using a disposable colormetric CO_2 detector and variables that affect placement, *Crit Care Med* 32(12):A92, 2004.

Chevron V, Menard JF, Richard JC et al: Unplanned extubation risk factors of development and predictive criteria for reintubation, *Crit Care Med* 26(6):1049, 1998.

Chlan L: Effectiveness of a music therapy intervention on relaxation and anxiety for patients receiving ventilatory assistance, *Heart Lung* 27(3):169, 1998.

Clarke T, Evans S, Way P et al: A comparison of two methods of securing an endotracheal tube, *Aust Crit Care* 11(2):45, 1998.

Collard HR, Saint S, Matthay MA: Prevention of ventilator-associated pneumonia: an evidence-based systemic review, *Ann Intern Med* 138(6):494, 2003.

Consensus conference on sedation assessment. Abbott Laboratories, American Association of Critical Care Nurses, St. Thomas Health System, *Crit Care Nurse* 24:33, 2004.

Costello JM: AAC intervention in the intensive care unit: the Children's Hospital Boston model, *Augment Altern Commun* 16(3):137–153, 2000.

Davidson JE: Family-centered care: Meeting the needs of patient's families and helping families adapt to critical illness. *Critical Care Nurse* 29(3):28–34, 2009.

Drakulovic MB, Torres A, Bauer TT et al: Supine body position as a risk factor for nosocomial pneumonia in mechanically ventilated patients: a randomized trial, *Lancet* 354(9193):1851, 1999.

Ely EW, Truman B, Shintani A et al: Monitoring sedation status over time in ICU patients: reliability and validity of the Richmond Agitation-Sedation Scale (RASS), *JAMA* 289(22):2983–2991, 2003.

Gift A, Narsavage G: Validity of the numeric rating scale as a measure of dyspnea, *Am J Crit Care* 7(3):200, 1998.

Girou E, Loyeau S, Legrand P et al: Efficacy of hand rubbing with alcohol based solution versus standard handwashing with antiseptic soap: randomized, clinical trial, *BMJ* 325:362, 2002.

Good VS: Continuous end-tidal carbon-dioxide monitoring. In Lynn-McHale DJ, Carlson KK, editors: *AACN procedure manual for critical care,* ed 4, Philadelphia, 2005, WB Saunders.

Grap MJ, Strickland D, Tormey L et al: Collaborative practice: development, implementation and evaluation of a weaning protocol for patients receiving mechanical ventilation, *Am J Crit Care* 12:454–460, 2003.

Happ MB: Communicating with mechanically ventilated patients: state of the science, *AACN Clin Issues* 12(2):247, 2001.

Henneman EA: Patient safety and technology, *AACN Adv Crit Care* 20(2):128–132, 2009.

Henneman EA, Cardin C: Family centered critical care: a practical approach to making it happen, *Crit Care Nurse* 22(6):12–19, 2002.

Henneman EA, Dracup K, Ganz T et al: Effect of a collaborative weaning plan on patient outcome in the critical care setting, *Crit Care Med* 29:297, 2001.

Henneman EA, Dracup K, Ganz T et al: Using a collaborative weaning plan to decrease duration of mechanical ventilation and length of stay in the intensive care unit for patients receiving long-term ventilation, *Am J Crit Care* 11:132, 2002.

Henneman EA, Ellstrom KE, St. John RE: *Airway management.* In *AACN practice protocol.* Aliso Viejo, CA, 1998, American Association of Critical Care Nursing.

Houston S, Hougland P, Anderson JJ et al: Effectiveness of 0.12% chlorhexidine gluconate oral rinse in reducing prevalence of nosocomial pneumonia in patients undergoing heart surgery, *Am J Crit Care* 11(6):567–570, 2002.

Jacobi J, Fraser GL, Coursin DB et al: Clinical practice guidelines for the sustained use of sedatives and analgesics in the critically ill adult, *Crit Care Med* 30 (1):119–141, 2003.

Kleinpell RM, Patak L, Wilson-Stronks A et al: Communication in the ICU, *Advance for Nurses,* Last updated December 10, 2008. http://nursing.advanceweb.com/Article/Communication-in-the-ICU-2.aspx. Accessed September 30, 2009.

Kollef MH, Levy NT, Ahrens TS et al: The use of continuous IV sedation is associated with prolongation of mechanical ventilation, *Chest* 114(2):541, 1998.

Kress JP, Pohlman AS, O'Connor MF et al: Daily interruption of sedative infusions in critically ill patients undergoing mechanical ventilation, *N Eng J Med* 342:1471, 2000.

Lucet JC, Rigaud MP, Menter F et al: Hand contamination before and after different hygiene techniques: a randomized clinical trial, *J Hosp Infect* 50:276–280, 2002.

Mahul P, Auboyer C, Jospe R et al: Prevention of nosocomial pneumonia in intubated patients: respective role of mechanical sub-glottic secretions drainage and stress ulcer prophylaxis, *Intensive Care Med* 18:20, 1992.

Munro CL, Grap MJ: Oral health and care in the intensive care unit: state of the science, *Am J Crit Care* 13(1):25–33, 2004.

Park M, Sangean MC, Volpe MS et al: Randomized, prospective trial of oxygen, continuous positive airway pressure and bilevel positive airway pressure by face mask in acute cardiogenic pulmonary edema, *Crit Care Med* 32:2407, 2004.

Patak L, Gawlinski A, Fung NI et al: Patient's reports of healthcare practitioner interventions that are related to communication during mechanical ventilation, *Heart Lung* 33:308, 2004.

Patak L, Gawlinski A, Fung NI et al: Communication boards in critical care: patient's views. *Appl Nurs Res* 19:182–190, 2006.

Perkins LA, Shortall SP: Ventilation without intubation, *RN* 63(1):34, 2000.

Perme C, Chandrashekar R: Early mobility and walking program for patients in intensive care units: creating a standard of care, *Am J Crit Care* 18(3):212–220, 2009.

Phelan BA, Cooper DA, Sangkachand P: Prolonged mechanical ventilation and tracheostomy in the elderly, *AACN Clin Issues* 13:1, 2002.

Pierson DJ: Indications for mechanical ventilation in adults with acute respiratory failure, *Respir Care* 47:3, 2002.

Powers J, Bennett SJ: Measurement of dyspnea in patients treated with mechanical ventilation, *Am J Crit Care* 8(4):254–261, 1999.

Rose L, Nelson S, Johnson L et al: Decisions made by critical care nurses during mechanical ventilation and weaning in an Australian intensive care unit, *Am J Crit Care* 16(5):434–446, 2007.

Schultz SL: Oxygen saturation monitoring by pulse oximetry. In Lynn-McHale DJ, Carlson KK, editors: *AACN procedure manual for critical care,* ed 4, Philadelphia, 2005, WB Saunders.

St. John RE, Seckel MA: Airway management. In Burns SM, editor: *AACN protocols for practice: care of mechanically ventilated patients,* ed 2, Sudbury, MA, 2007, Jones & Bartlett.

Tablan O, Anderson L, Besser R et al: Guidelines for preventing health-care–associated pneumonia, 2003. Recommendations of CDC and the Healthcare Infection Control Practices Advisory Committee, *MMWR Recomm Rep* 53(RR-3):1–36, 2004.

Takeda T, Tanigawa K, Tanaka H et al: The assessment of three methods to verify tracheal tube placement in the emergency setting, *Resuscitation* 56(2):153–157, 2003.

Torres A, Serra-Batlles J, Ros E et al: Pulmonary aspiration of gastric contents in patients receiving mechanical ventilation: the effect of body position, *Ann Intern Med* 116:540, 1992.

Trick W, Vernon M, Hayes R et al: Impact of ring wearing on hand contamination and comparison of hand hygiene agents in a hospital, *Clin Infect Dis* 36:1383–1390, 2003.

Valles J, Artigas A, Rello J et al: Continuous aspiration of subglottic secretions in preventing ventilator-associated pneumonia, *Ann Intern Med* 122:179, 1995.

Wang JY, Chuang PY, Lin CJ et al: Continuous lateral rotational therapy in the medical intensive care unit, *J Formos Med Association* 102:788, 2003.

White JM: State of the science of music interventions: critical care and perioperative practice, *Crit Care Nurs Clin North Am* 12(2):219–225, 2000.

Williams TA, Martin S, Leslie G et al: Duration of mechanical ventilation in an adult intensive care unit after introduction of sedation and pain scales, *Am J Crit Care* 17(4):349–356, 2008.

Dysfunctional Ventilatory weaning response   *Elizabeth A. Henneman, RN, PhD, CCNS, FAAN*

NANDA-I

Definition

Inability to adjust to lowered levels of mechanical ventilator support that interrupts and prolongs the weaning process

Defining Characteristics

Mild

Breathing discomfort; expressed feelings of increased need for oxygen; fatigue; increased concentration on breathing; queries about possible machine malfunction; restlessness; slight increase of respiratory rate from baseline; warmth

Moderate

Apprehension; baseline increase in respiratory rate (<5 breaths/min); color changes; decreased air entry on auscultation; diaphoresis; hypervigilance to activities; inability to cooperate; inability to respond to coaching; pale; slight cyanosis; slight increase from baseline blood pressure (<20 mm Hg);

• = Independent   ▲ = Collaborative   **EBN** = Evidence-Based Nursing   **EB** = Evidence-Based

slight increase from baseline heart rate (<20 beats/min); light respiratory accessory muscle use; wide-eyed look

Severe

Adventitious breath sounds; agitation; asynchronized breathing with the ventilator; audible airway secretions; cyanosis; decreased level of consciousness; deterioration in arterial blood gases from current baseline; full respiratory accessory muscle use; gasping breaths; increase from baseline blood pressure (greater than or equal to 20 mm Hg); increase from baseline heart rate (greater than or equal to 20 breaths per minute) paradoxical abdominal breathing; profuse diaphoresis; respiratory rate increases significantly from baseline; shallow breaths

Related Factors (r/t)

Physiological

Inadequate nutrition; ineffective airway clearance; sleep pattern disturbance; uncontrolled pain

Psychological

Anxiety; decreased motivation; decreased self-esteem; fear; hopelessness; insufficient trust in the nurse; knowledge deficit of the weaning process; client-perceived inefficacy about ability to wean; powerlessness

Situational

Adverse environment (e.g., noisy, active environment; negative events in the room; low nurse : client ratio, unfamiliar nursing staff; history of ventilator dependence >4 days; inadequate social support; inappropriate pacing of diminished ventilator support; uncontrolled episodic energy demands

 (Nursing Outcomes Classification)

Suggested NOC Outcomes

Respiratory Status: Gas Exchange, Ventilation

Example NOC Outcome with Indicators
Achieves appropriate **Respiratory Status: Ventilation** as evidenced by the following indicators: Respiratory rate/ Respiratory rhythm/Depth of inspiration/Symmetrical chest expansion/Ease of breathing/Moves sputum out of airway/Accessory muscle use not present/Adventitious breath sounds not present/Chest retraction not present/Tidal volume/Vital capacity (Rate the outcome and indicators of **Respiratory Status: Ventilation:** 1 = severe deviation from normal range, 2 = substantial deviation from normal range, 3 = moderate deviation from normal range, 4 = mild deviation from normal range, 5 = no deviation from normal range [see Section I].)

Client Outcomes

Client Will (Specify Time Frame):

• Wean from ventilator with adequate arterial blood gases
• Remain free of unresolved dyspnea or restlessness
• Effectively clear secretions

 (Nursing Interventions Classification)

Suggested NIC Interventions

Mechanical Ventilation Management: Invasive, Mechanical Ventilatory Weaning

Example NIC Activities—Mechanical Ventilatory Weaning
Monitor for optimal fluid and electrolyte status; Monitor to assure patient is free of significant infection prior to weaning

Nursing Interventions and *Rationales*

• Assess client's readiness for weaning as evidenced by the following:

• = Independent   ▲ = Collaborative   **EBN** = Evidence-Based Nursing   **EB** = Evidence-Based

- Physiological readiness (Cook et al, 2000). *There has been little research devoted to the study of psychological readiness to wean.* **EBN:** *An in-depth qualitative nursing research study suggests that three key criteria give an indication of a client's psychological readiness: (1) being orientated, (2) mental ease, and (3) a positive attitude (Logan & Jenny, 1997).*
- Resolution of initial medical problem that led to ventilator dependence
- Hemodynamic stability
- Normal hemoglobin levels
- Absence of fever
- Normal state of consciousness
- Metabolic, fluid, and electrolyte balance
- Adequate nutritional status with serum albumin levels >2.5 g/dL
- Adequate sleep
- Adequate pain management and sedation

EB: *Adequate respiratory parameters include the following: adequate gas exchange (Pao_2/Fio_2 ratio >200), respiratory rate ≤35 breaths/min, a negative inspiratory pressure <20 cm, positive expiratory pressure >30 cm H_2O, spontaneous tidal volume >5 mL/kg, vital capacity >10 to 15 mL/kg.* **EBN:** *These respiratory predictors of weaning success have limited value in the management of clients receiving long-term mechanical ventilation (Burns, 2007).*

- For best results ensure that the client is in an optimal physiological and psychological state before introducing the stress of weaning (Earven et al, 2004; MacIntyre, 2004; Burns, 2007). *For more information on weaning assessment, please refer to the Burns Weaning Assessment Program (Burns, 2007).*
- Involve family as appropriate to help the client provide a maximal effort during weaning readiness measurements (Burns, 2005).
- Provide adequate nutrition to ventilated clients, using enteral feeding when possible. **EB:** *Protein malnutrition results in decreased muscle strength, which will impair the weaning process. Enteral nutrition is preferred to total parenteral nutrition because it provides an equal number of calories at lower cost and with fewer complications, while preserving gut integrity (McClave et al, 2009). The use of a nutrition management program has been shown to decrease the number of days on a ventilator (Barr et al, 2004). Parenteral nutrition should be initiated in any client in whom enteral nutrition cannot be utilized because of gut dysfunction (Simpson & Doig, 2005; McClave et al, 2009).*
- Use evidence-based weaning and extubation protocols as appropriate. **EBN and EB:** *Protocol-directed weaning has been demonstrated to be safe and effective but not superior to other weaning methods that used structured rounds and other processes that allow for timely and ongoing clinical decision making by expert nurses and physicians (Rose et al, 2007; Arias-Rivera et al, 2008; Navalesi et al, 2008; Robertson et al, 2008).*
- Identify reasons for previous unsuccessful weaning attempts, and include that information in development of the weaning plan. **EBN:** *Analyzing client responses after each weaning attempt prevents repeated unsuccessful weaning trials (Henneman et al, 2001; Henneman, 2001; Henneman et al, 2002; Burns, 2004).*
- ▲ Collaborate with an interdisciplinary team (physician, nurse, respiratory therapist, physical therapist, and dietician) to develop a weaning plan with a time line and goals; revise this plan throughout the weaning period. Use a communication device, such as a weaning board or flow sheet. **EBN:** *Effective interdisciplinary collaboration can positively affect client outcomes (Grap et al, 2003). Collaborative weaning plans using dry-erase boards and flow sheets have been demonstrated to decrease the number of days on a ventilator and length of stay in the intensive care unit (Henneman et al, 2001; Henneman et al, 2002). Decisions related to weaning trials should be made in conjunction with members of the interdisciplinary team (Burns, 2005).*
- Assist client to identify personal strategies that result in relaxation and comfort (e.g., music, visualization, relaxation techniques, reading, television, family visits). Support implementation of these strategies. **EBN:** *A study found that use of music was beneficial as a relaxation technique for clients if they were willing to accept it, and were able to choose the selection of music (Chan et al, 2009).*
- Provide a safe and comfortable environment. Stay with the client during weaning if possible. If unable to stay, make the call light button readily available and assure the client that needs will be

---

• = Independent   ▲ = Collaborative   **EBN** = Evidence-Based Nursing   **EB** = Evidence-Based

met responsively. **EBN:** *A client who feels safe and trusts the health care providers can focus on the immediate work of weaning; support from the nurse helps decrease anxiety (Burns, 2005).*

▲ Coordinate pain and sedation medications to minimize sedative effects. **EB:** *Appropriate levels of sedation may be key to successful weaning. The use of sedation is associated with longer duration of mechanical ventilation, weaning time, and length of stay in the ICU (Arroliga et al, 2005). Nonetheless, this does not mean to imply that sedation, when used judiciously, is not in the best interest of the client. The use of continuous IV sedation is associated with longer duration of mechanical ventilation compared with bolus sedation (Brook et al, 1999; Kress et al, 2000).* **EBN:** *Nursing implemented sedation protocols have been used effectively to improve the probability of successful extubation (Arias-Rivera et al, 2008). Of note is that a recent study in Australia reported that sedation and analgesia scales did not reduce the duration of mechanical ventilation (Williams et al, 2008). This may be due, in part, to the nurses' autonomy in making decisions about the appropriate level of sedation for any given client.*

• Schedule weaning periods for the time of day when the client is most rested. Cluster care activities to promote successful weaning. Avoid other procedures during weaning: keep the environment quiet and promote restful activities between weaning periods. *It is important that the client receive adequate rest between weaning periods. Control of external noises and stimuli can promote restful periods (Cropp et al, 1994).*

• Promote a normal sleep-wake cycle, allowing uninterrupted periods of nighttime sleep. *Limit visitors during weaning to close and supportive persons; ask visitors to leave if they are negatively affecting the weaning process.*

• During weaning, monitor the client's physiological and psychological responses; acknowledge and respond to fears and subjective complaints. Validate the client's efforts during the weaning process. **EBN:** *Weaning is a stressful experience that requires active participation by the client. The client's work needs to be understood and supported by clinicians to facilitate recovery from mechanical ventilation and weaning (Blackwood, 2000; Burns, 2005).*

• Monitor subjective and objective data (breath sounds, respiratory pattern, respiratory effort, heart rate, blood pressure, oxygen saturation per oximetry, amount and type of secretions, anxiety, and energy level) throughout weaning to determine client tolerance and responses (Burns, 2005).

• Involve the client and family in the weaning plan. Inform them of the weaning plan and possible client responses to the weaning process (e.g., potential feelings of dyspnea). *Knowledge of anticipated sensory experiences reduces anxiety and distress (Burns, 2005).*

• Coach the client through episodes of increased anxiety. Remain with the client or place a supportive and calm significant other in this role. Give positive reinforcement, and with permission use touch to communicate support and concern. *It is not unusual for a client with lung disease to experience self-limiting episodes of increased shortness of breath. Supporting and coaching a client through such episodes allows weaning to continue.*

• Terminate weaning when the client demonstrates predetermined criteria or when the following signs of weaning intolerance occur:
  ▪ Tachypnea, dyspnea, or chest and abdominal asynchrony
  ▪ Agitation or mental status changes
  ▪ Decreased oxygen saturation: Sao_2 <90%
  ▪ Increased $PaCO_2$ or $ETCO_2$
  ▪ Change in pulse rate or blood pressure or onset of new dysrhythmias
  Discontinue weaning trial when client intolerance leads to fatigue and possible cardiovascular failure (Burns, 2005).

▲ If the dysfunctional weaning response is severe, consider slowing weaning to brief periods (e.g., 5 minutes). Continue to collaborate with the team to determine whether an untreated physiological cause for the dysfunctional weaning pattern remains. Consult with physician regarding use of noninvasive ventilation immediately after discontinuing ventilation. Consider an alternative care setting (subacute, rehabilitation facility, home) for clients with prolonged ventilator dependence as a strategy that can positively affect outcomes. *Use of noninvasive ventilation has been effective for the client who is difficult to wean from a ventilator (Epstein, 2009).* **EB:** *One study indicated that half of the clients admitted to a rehabilitation facility were weaned from the ventilator (Modawal et al, 2002).*

Geriatric

- Recognize that older clients may require longer periods to wean. **EBN:** *A study demonstrated that older clients required a longer period to wean, especially if they were older than 80 years (Epstein, El-Modadem, & Peerless, 2002).*

Home Care

- Weaning from a ventilator at home should be based on client stability and comfort of the client and caregivers under an intermittent care plan. *Generally the client will be safer weaning in a hospital environment.*

⊝volve   See the EVOLVE website for Weblinks for client education resources.

REFERENCES

Arias-Rivera S, del Mar Sanchez-Sanchez M, Santos-Diaz R et al: Effect of a nursing-implemented sedation protocol on weaning outcome, *Crit Care Med* 36(7):2054–2060, 2008.

Arroliga A, Frutos-Vivar F, Hall J et al: Use of sedatives and neuromuscular blockers in a cohort of patients receiving mechanical ventilation, *Chest* 128(2):496–506, 2005.

Baggs JG, Schmitt MH, Mushlin AI et al: Nurse-physician collaboration and satisfaction with the decision-making process in three critical care units, *Am J Crit Care* 6:393–399, 1997.

Baggs JG, Schmitt MH, Mushlin AI et al: The association between nurse-physician collaboration and patient outcomes in three intensive care units, *Crit Care Med* 27(9):1991–1998, 1999.

Barr J, Hecht M, Flavin KE et al: Outcomes in critically ill patients before and after the implementation of an evidence-based nutritional management protocol, *Chest* 125(4):1446–1457, 2004.

Blackwood B: The art and science of predicting patient readiness for weaning from mechanical ventilation, *Int J Nurs Stud* 37:145, 2000.

Brook AD, Ahrens TS, Schaiff R et al: Effect of a nursing-implemented sedation protocol on the duration of mechanical ventilation, *Crit Care Med* 27:2609, 1999.

Burns SM: The science of weaning: when and how? *Crit Care Nurs Clin North Am* 16:379, 2004.

Burns SM: Weaning process. In Lynn-McHale DJ, Carlson KK, editors: *AACN procedure manual for critical care,* ed 4, Philadelphia, 2005, WB Saunders.

Burns SM: Weaning from mechanical ventilation. In Burns SM, editor: *AACN protocols for practice: care of mechanically ventilated patients,* ed 2, Sudbury, MA, 2007, Jones & Bartlett.

Chan MF, Chung YFL, Chung SWA et al: Investigating the physiological responses of patients listening to music in the intensive care unit, *J Clin Nurs* 18(9):1250–1257, 2009.

Cook D, Meade M, Guyatt G et al: *Criteria for weaning from mechanical ventilation. Evidence Report/Technology Assessment Number 23.* Agency for Healthcare Research and Quality. 2000. www.ncbi.nlm.nih.gov/bookshelf/br.fcgi?book=hserta&part=A31811. Accessed May 31, 2009.

Cropp AJ, Woods LA, Raney D et al: Name that tone: the proliferation of noise in the intensive care unit, *Chest* 105:1217, 1994.

Earven S, Fisher C, Lewis R et al: The experience of four outcomes managers: an institutional approach to weaning patients from long-term mechanical ventilation, *Crit Care Nurs Clin North Am* 16:395, 2004.

Epstein CD, El-Modadem N, Peerless JR: Weaning older patients from long-term mechanical ventilation: a pilot study, *Am J Crit Care* 11:4, 2002.

Epstein SK: Weaning from ventilatory support, *Curr Opin Crit Care* 15(1):36–43, 2009.

Grap MJ, Strickland D, Tormey L et al: Collaborative practice: development, implementation, and evaluation of a weaning protocol for patients receiving mechanical ventilation, *Am J Crit Care* 12(5):454–460, 2003.

Henneman EA: Liberating patients from mechanical ventilation, a team approach, *Crit Care Nurs* 21(3):25, 2001.

Henneman EA, Dracup K, Ganz T et al: Effect of a collaborative weaning plan on patient outcome in the critical care setting, *Crit Care Med* 29:297, 2001.

Henneman EA, Dracup K, Ganz T et al: Using a collaborative weaning plan to decrease duration of mechanical ventilation and length of stay in the intensive care unit for patients receiving long-term ventilation, *Am J Crit Care* 11:132, 2002.

Kress JP, Pohlman AS, O'Connor MF et al: Daily interruption of sedative infusions in critically ill patients undergoing mechanical ventilation, *N Engl J Med* 342:1471, 2000.

Logan J, Jenny J: Qualitative analysis of patients' weaning work during mechanical ventilation and weaning, *Heart Lung* 26:140, 1997.

MacIntyre NR: Evidence-based guidelines for weaning and discontinuing ventilatory support, *Respir Care* 47(1):69, 2004.

McClave S, Martindale R, Vanek V et al: Guidelines for the provision and assessment of nutrition support therapy in the adult critically ill patient. Aspen Clinical Guidelines, *J Parenteral Enteral Nutr* 33(3):277–316, 2009.

Modawal A, Candadai NP, Mandell KM et al: Weaning success among ventilator-dependent patients in a rehabilitation facility, *Arch Phys Med Rehabil* 83(2):154, 2002.

Navalesi P, Frigerio P, Moretti MP et al: Rate of reintubation in mechanically ventilated neurosurgical and neurologic patients: evaluation of a systematic approach to weaning and extubation, *Crit Care Med* 36(11):2986–2992, 2008.

Robertson TE, Mann HJ, Hyzy R et al: Multicenter implementation of a consensus-developed, evidence-based, spontaneous breathing trial protocol, *Crit Care Med* 36(10):2753–2762, 2008.

Rose L, Nelson S, Johnson L et al: Decisions made by critical care nurses during mechanical ventilation and weaning in an Australian intensive care unit, *AJCC* 16(5):434–446, 2007.

Simpson F, Doig GS: Parenteral vs enteral nutrition in the critically ill patient: a meta-analysis if trials using the intention to treat principle, *Intens Care Med* 31(1):12–23, 2005.

Williams TA, Martin S, Leslie G et al: Duration of mechanical ventilation in an adult intensive care unit after introduction of sedation and pain scales, *Am J Crit Care* 17(4): 349–356, 2008.

Risk for other-directed Violence   *Kathleen L. Patusky, PhD, APRN-BC*

NANDA-I

Definition

At risk for behaviors in which an individual demonstrates that he or she can be physically, emotionally, and/or sexually harmful to others

Risk Factors

Availability of weapon(s); body language (e.g., rigid posture, clenching of fists and jaw, hyperactivity, pacing, breathlessness, threatening stances) cognitive impairment (e.g., learning disabilities, attention deficit disorder, decreased intellectual functioning); cruelty to animals; fire setting; history of childhood abuse; history of indirect violence (e.g., tearing off clothes, ripping objects off walls, writing on walls, urinating on floor, defecating on floor, stamping feet, temper tantrum, running in corridors, yelling, throwing objects, breaking a window, slamming doors, making sexual advances); history of substance abuse; history of threats of violence (e.g., verbal threats against property, verbal threats against person, social threats, cursing, threatening notes/letters, threatening gestures, sexual threats); history of witnessing family violence; history of violence against others (e.g., hitting someone, kicking someone, spitting at someone, scratching someone, throwing objects at someone, biting someone, attempted rape, rape, sexual molestation, urinating/defecating on someone); history of violent antisocial behavior (e.g., stealing, insistent borrowing, insistent demanding of privileges, insistent interrupting of meetings, refusal to eat, refusal to take medication, ignoring instructions); impulsivity; motor vehicle offenses (e.g., frequent traffic violations, use of a motor vehicle to release anger); neurological impairment (e.g., positive EEG, CAT, or MRI; positive neurological findings; head trauma; pathological intoxication; seizure disorders); perinatal/prenatal complications; psychotic symptomatology (e.g., auditory, visual, command hallucinations; paranoid delusions; loose, rambling, or illogical thought processes); motor vehicle offenses (e.g., frequent traffic violations, use of a motor vehicle to release anger); suicidal behavior

NOC   (Nursing Outcomes Classification)

Suggested NOC Outcomes

Abuse Cessation, Abusive Behavior Self-Restraint, Aggression Self-Control, Distorted Thought Self-Control, Impulse Self-Control, Risk Detection

Example NOC Outcome with Indicators
Aggression Self-Control as evidenced by the following indicators: Refrains from harming others/Expresses/Vents needs and negative feelings in a nondestructive manner/Identifies when angry (Rate the outcome and indicators of **Aggression Self-Control:** 1 = never demonstrated, 2 = rarely demonstrated, 3 = sometimes demonstrated, 4 = often demonstrated, 5 = consistently demonstrated [see Section I].)

Client Outcomes

Client Will (Specify Time Frame):

- Stop all forms of abuse (physical, emotional, sexual; neglect; financial exploitation)
- Have cessation of abuse reported by victim
- Display no aggressive activity
- Refrain from verbal outbursts
- Refrain from violating others' personal space
- Refrain from antisocial behaviors
- Maintain relaxed body language and decreased motor activity
- Identify factors contributing to abusive/aggressive behavior
- Demonstrate impulse control or state feelings of control
- Identify impulsive behaviors
- Identify feelings/behaviors that lead to impulsive actions

• = Independent   ▲ = Collaborative   **EBN** = Evidence-Based Nursing   **EB** = Evidence-Based

- Identify consequences of impulsive actions to self or others
- Avoid high-risk environments and situations
- Identify and talk about feelings; express anger appropriately
- Express decreased anxiety and control of hallucinations as applicable
- Displace anger to meaningful activities
- Communicate needs appropriately
- Identify responsibility to maintain control
- Express empathy for victim
- Obtain no access or yield access to harmful objects
- Use alternative coping mechanisms for stress
- Obtain and follow through with counseling
- Demonstrate knowledge of correct role behaviors

Victim (and Children If Applicable) Will (Specify Time Frame):

- Have safe plan for leaving situation or avoiding abuse
- Resolve depression or traumatic response

Parent Will (Specify Time Frame):

- Monitor social/play contacts
- Provide supervision and nurturing environment
- Intervene to prevent high-risk social behaviors

NIC   (Nursing Interventions Classification)

Suggested NIC Interventions

Abuse Protection Support, Anger Control Assistance, Behavior Management, Calming Technique, Coping Enhancement, Crisis Intervention, Delusion Management, Dementia Management, Distraction, Environmental Management: Violence Prevention, Mood Management, Physical Restraint, Seclusion, Substance Use Prevention

---

Example NIC Intervention—Environmental Management: Violence Prevention

Remove other individuals from the vicinity of a violent or potentially violent patient; Provide ongoing surveillance of all patient access areas to maintain patient safety and therapeutically intervene as needed

---

Nursing Interventions and *Rationales*
Client Violence

▲ Monitor the environment, evaluate situations that could become violent, and intervene early to deescalate the situation. Know and follow institution's policies and procedures concerning violence. Consider that family members or other staff may initiate violence in all settings. Enlist support from other staff rather than attempting to handle the situation alone. **EBN:** *APNA guidelines (2008) warn that workplace violence can occur in all settings, from a variety of sources. Nurses need to be aware and informed of department policies and procedures. Policies should be developed, and training programs should be provided in proper use and application of restraints. All nursing units should develop a proactive plan for dealing with violent situations.*

- Assess causes of aggression: social versus biological. **EBN:** *Knowing the client, having experience with similar clients, paying attention, and planning interventions are expert practices used by nurses to predict and respond to aggressive behavior effectively (Pryor, 2006).*

- Assess the client for risk factors of violence, including those in the following categories: personal history (e.g., past violent behavior); psychiatric disorders (particularly psychoses, paranoid or bipolar disorders, substance abuse, PTSD, antisocial personality or borderline personality disorder); neurological disorders (e.g., head injury, temporal lobe epilepsy, CVA, dementia or senility), medical disorders (e.g., hypoxia, hypo- or hyperglycemia), psychological precursors (e.g., low tolerance for stress, impulsivity), coping difficulties (e.g., inability to plan solutions or see long-term consequences of behavior), and childhood or adolescent disorders (e.g., conduct disorders, hyperactivity, autism, learning disability). **EBN and EB:** *All of these risk factors have been implicated in aggressive,*

● = Independent   ▲ = Collaborative   **EBN** = Evidence-Based Nursing   **EB** = Evidence-Based

agitated, or violent behavior (APNA, 2008; Fountoulakis, Leucht, & Kaprinis, 2008; Temcheff et al, 2008).

- The Broset Violence Checklist (BVC) has been developed for short-term prediction of violence in psychiatric inpatients. *Some false-positive cases were met with preventive measures, which may have avoided violence (Abderhalden et al, 2004). The Alert Assessment Form may be used to identify potentially aggressive clients with moderate (71%) sensitivity and high (94%) specificity (Kling et al, 2006). The Attempted and Actual Assaults Scale (Attacks), completed after a violent incident, measures the nature and severity of an assault (Bowers, Nijman, & Palmstierna, 2007). The Domestic Violence Survivor Assessment (DVSA) measures survivor progress toward a lifestyle free from violence over time (Dienemann et al, 2007). The Caregiver Psychological Elder Abuse Behavior Scale may be used to identify elder abuse behavior (Wang, 2005).*

- Assess the client with a history of previous assaults. Listen to and acknowledge feelings of anger, observe for increased motor activity, and prepare to intervene if the client becomes aggressive. **EB:** *In this study of mentally disordered offenders the most significant risk factor for physical violence was a past history of physically aggressive behavior (Amore et al, 2008).*

- Assess the client for physiological signs and external signs of anger. *Internal signs of anger include increased pulse rate, respiration rate, and blood pressure; chills; prickly sensations; numbness; choking sensation; nausea; and vertigo. External signs include increased muscle tone, changes in body posture (clenched fists, set jaw), eye changes (eyebrows lower and drawn together, eyelids tense, eyes assuming a "hard" appearance), lips pressed together, flushing or pallor, goose bumps, twitching, and sweating.* **EBN:** *Anger is an early warning sign of possible violence (Puskar et al, 2008).*

- Assess for the presence of hallucinations. **EB:** *Command hallucinations may direct the client to behave violently (Shawyer et al, 2008).*

- Apply STAMPEDAR as an acronym for assessing the immediate potential for violence. **EB:** *A study of nurses experienced in workplace violence identified the following as factors and behaviors indicating the likelihood of a violent episode: Staring, Tone of voice, Anxiety, Mumbling, Pacing, Emotions, Disease process, Assertive/non-assertive behavior and Resources (Chapman et al, 2009).*

- Determine the presence and degree of homicidal or suicidal risk. A number of questions will elicit the necessary information. "Have you been thinking about harming someone? If yes, who? How often do you have these thoughts, and how long do they last? Do you have a plan? What is it? Do you have access to the means to carry out that plan? What has kept you from hurting the person until now?" Refer to the care plan for **Risk for Suicide.** *Psychotherapists are required to report harm or threats of harm to another person, referred to as the duty to warn. State laws and mental health codes should be checked to determine local mandates for threat reporting by specific health care professionals.*

- Take action to minimize personal risk: Use nonthreatening body language. Respect personal space and boundaries. Maintain at least an arm's length distance from the client; do not touch the client without permission (unless physical restraint is the goal). Do not allow the client to block access to an exit. If speaking with the client alone, keep the door to the room open. Be aware of where other staff is at all times. Notify other staff of where you are at all times. Take verbal threats seriously and notify other staff. Wear clothing and accessories that are not restricting and that will not be dangerous (e.g., sandals or shoes with heels can lead to twisted ankles; necklaces or dangling earrings could be grabbed). **EBN:** *Programs for violence prevention have been implemented that reduce workplace violence. For OSHA guidelines, visit www.osha.gov/SLTC/workplaceviolence/index.html (Lipscomb et al, 2006).*

- Remove potential weapons from the environment. Be prepared to remove obstructions to staff response from the environment. Search the client and his or her belongings for weapons or potential weapons on admission to the hospital as appropriate. *Clients prone to violence may use available weapons opportunistically. If client restraint becomes necessary, environmental hazards (e.g., chairs, wastebaskets) should be moved out of the way to prevent injuries.*

- Inform the client of unit expectations for appropriate behavior and the consequences of not meeting these expectations. Emphasize that the client must comply with the rules of the unit. Give positive reinforcement for compliance. Increase surveillance of the hospitalized client at smoking, meal, and medication times. **EBN:** *Clients benefit from clear guidance and positive reinforcement regarding behavioral expectations and consequences, providing much-needed structure and emphasizing client responsibility for his or her own behavior (APNA, 2007a). The unit serves as a microcosm of*

• = Independent   ▲ = Collaborative   **EBN** = Evidence-Based Nursing   **EB** = Evidence-Based

the client's outside world, so adherence to social norms while on the unit models adherence upon discharge and provides the client with staff support to learn appropriate coping skills and alternative behaviors.

• Assign a single room to the client with a potential for violence toward others. *The client will be able to take time away from unit stimulation to calm self as needed. Another client will not be placed at risk as a roommate.* **EBN:** *Research suggests lack of single-bed rooms may reduce rest and privacy and increase the risk of overstimulation (Stolker, Nijman, & Zwanikken, 2006).*

• Maintain a calm attitude in response to the client. Provide a low level of stimulation in the client's environment; place the client in a safe, quiet place, and speak slowly and quietly. *Anxiety is contagious.* **EBN:** *Maintenance of a calm environment contributes to the prevention of aggression (APNA, 2007a).*

• Redirect possible violent behaviors into physical activities (e.g., walking, jogging) if the client is physically able. *Using a punching bag or hitting a pillow is not indicated, because they are not calming activities and they continue patterning violent behavior. However, activities that distract while draining excess energy help to build a repertoire of alternative behaviors for stress reduction.*

• Provide sufficient staff if a show of force is necessary to demonstrate control to the client. *When staff responds to an escalating or violent situation, it can reassure clients that they will not be allowed to lose control. On the other hand, leave immediately if the client becomes violent and you are not trained to handle it.*

• Protect other clients in the environment from harm. Remove other individuals from the vicinity of a violent or potentially violent client. Follow safety protocols of the department. *The risk of a violent client to others in the area (other clients, visitors) should be anticipated, even as efforts proceed to de-escalate the situation with the client.*

• Maintain a secluded area for the client to be placed when violent. Ensure that staff are continuously present and available to client during seclusion. **EBN:** *Clients perceived seclusion to be punishment; however, the main negative effect reported by clients was that seclusion intensified preexisting feelings of exclusion, rejection, abandonment, and isolation. Staff presence is necessary to prevent the harmful effects of social isolation and to honor clients' motivation to connect with staff (Holmes, Kennedy, & Perron, 2004).*

▲ Recognize legal requirements that the least restrictive alternative of treatment should be used with aggressive clients. The hierarchy of intervention is: promote a milieu that provides structure and calmness, with negotiation and collaboration taking precedence over control; maintain vigilance of the unit and respond to behavioral changes early; talk with client to calm and promote understanding of emotional state; use chemical restraints as ordered; increase to manual restraint if needed; increase to mechanical restraint and seclusion as a last resort. **EBN:** *APNA guidelines (2007a, 2007b) support early assessment and intervention to prevent aggression, with nursing actions to reduce stimulation, divert client from aggressive thought patterns, set appropriate limits on behavior, and provide medications as needed.*

▲ Use mechanical restraints if ordered and as necessary. *Physical restraint can be therapeutic to keep the client and others safe.* **EBN:** *Restraint skill training, audits of adverse events, and examination of the safe use of restraints and medications are important to safe restraint practices (Ryan & Bowers, 2006).*

▲ Follow the institution's protocol for releasing restraints. Observe the client closely, remain calm, and provide positive feedback as the client's behavior becomes controlled. *The period during which restraints are removed can be dangerous for staff if they do not recognize that the client may choose to reinitiate violence. Protocols will specify safe procedures for removing restraints.*

▲ After a violent event on a unit, debriefing and support of both staff and clients should be made available. *Allowing discussion of a violent episode, either individually or in a group, among other clients present reveals clients' responses to the event and provides the opportunity for staff to offer reassurance and support. Clients may have concerns that staff will attempt to restrain them without reason or may feel uncertain whether staff can keep them safe.* **EBN:** *A study of the impact of serious events on psychiatric units found that staff reported a variety of negative emotional responses; levels of containment increased; the provision of care could be affected; and client reactions were largely ignored (Bowers et al, 2006; APNA, 2008).*

• Form a therapeutic alliance with the client, remaining calm, identifying the source of anger as external to both nurse and client, and using the therapeutic relationship to prevent the need for seclu-

• = Independent   ▲ = Collaborative   **EBN** = Evidence-Based Nursing   **EB** = Evidence-Based

sion or restraint. *The development of a therapeutic relationship before aggressive behavior occurs provides an alternative for working through anger and frustration. Assisting the client to identify a source of anger or frustration that is external to both the nurse and client prevents the need for defensiveness by both and directs energy at solving an external problem.* **EBN:** *One study concluded that, although most client aggressiveness was verbal rather than physical, the resulting fear could lead to increased use of seclusion or restraint (Foster, Bowers, & Nijman, 2007).*

- Allow, encourage, and assist the client to verbalize feelings appropriately either one-on-one or in a group setting. Actively listen to the client; explore the source of the client's anger, and negotiate resolution when possible. Teach healthy ways to express feelings/anger, appropriate gender roles, and how to communicate needs appropriately. **EBN:** *When clients' feelings are not addressed, when an individual feels threatened, or when gratification is delayed or denied, violence may be used as a manifestation of the internal feeling state (APNA, 2008).*
- Identify with client the stimuli that initiate violence and the means of dealing with the stimuli. Have the client keep an anger diary and discuss alternative responses together. Teach cognitive-behavioral techniques. *Assisting the client to identify situations and people that upset him or her provides information needed for problem solving. The client may then identify alternative responses (e.g., leaving the stimulus; using relaxation techniques, such as deep breathing; initiating thought stopping; initiating a distracting activity; responding assertively rather than aggressively).* **EB:** *Use of a coping questionnaire to assess client preferences for dealing with agitation was part of a successful program to decrease restraint and seclusion at a psychiatric hospital (Hellerstein, Staub, & Lequesne, 2007).*
- ▲ Initiate and promote staff attendance at aggression management training programs. **EBN and EB:** *Multiple studies have supported the positive influence of aggression management training programs on the ability and confidence of nurses in responding to aggressive or violent behavior (Meehan et al, 2006; Hills, 2008; Oostrom & Mierlo, 2008).*

Intimate Partner Violence (IPV)/Domestic Violence

NOTE: Before implementation of interventions in the face of domestic violence, nurses should examine their own emotional responses to abuse, their knowledge base about abuse, and systemic elements within the emergency department (ED) to ensure that interventions will be compassionate and appropriate. **EBN and EB:** *Barriers to domestic violence screening in the ED, and attitudes about violence against women, are influenced by lack of education and instruction about how to ask about abuse, the nurse's personal or family history of abuse, and lack of a sense of self-efficacy, as well as gender and culture-based factors (Hollingsworth & Ford-Gilboe, 2006; Yonaka et al, 2007; Smith et al, 2008; Flood & Pease, 2009).*

- Screen for possible abuse in women or children with a pattern of multiple injuries, particularly if any suspicion exists that the physical findings are inconsistent with the explanation of how the injuries were incurred. **EBN:** *IPV/domestic violence is recognized as a nationwide public health issue. In one study, nurses cited insufficient evidence as a reason for not reporting IPV. Nurses with a personal history of IPV were more likely to report (Smith et al, 2008).*
- ▲ Report suspected child abuse to Child Protective Services. Refer women suspected of being in a spousal abuse situation to an area crisis center and provide phone number of area crisis hotline. *Rapid screening tools are helpful to identify intimate partner violence. All nurses are required by law to report suspected child abuse.* **EB:** *Child and spouse maltreatment often occur together; all family members should be evaluated and provided with assistance as needed (Taylor et al, 2009).*
- Assess for physical and mental concerns of women, including risk of HIV. **EB:** *Major health needs of women with a history of IPV were found to include chronic pain, chronic diseases, and mental illness, as well as concerns regarding risk of HIV. Barriers to health care created by the IPV may prevent these concerns from being addressed (Wilson et al, 2007; Cole, Logan, & Shannon, 2008; Macy, Ferron, & Crosby, 2009).*
- Assist the client in negotiating the health care system and overcoming barriers. **EBN:** *Victims of IPV were found to experience barriers, including inappropriate responses from providers, when attempting to access health care services (Robinson & Spilsbury, 2008).*
- With women who repeatedly experience injuries from domestic violence, maintain a nonjudgmental approach and continue to offer resources/referrals. If the woman voices a willingness to leave her situation, assist with developing an emergency plan that will consider all contingencies possible (e.g., safe location, financial resources, care of children, when to leave safely) (Amar & Cox, 2006). *A woman in a domestic violence situation may change her mind several times before actually leaving.*

● = Independent   ▲ = Collaborative   **EBN** = Evidence-Based Nursing   **EB** = Evidence-Based

Proactive organization of an emergency plan helps to increase the possibility that women will be able to leave safely. The most dangerous time of a domestic violence situation is when the spouse tries to leave.

- Maintain a nonjudgmental response when clients return to husbands or refuse to leave them. *Women have many reasons for remaining in an abusive relationship, including economic concerns (especially with children), socialization about the women's role, political or legal obstacles, powerlessness, and a realistic fear of retaliation or death). Refer to the care plan for* **Powerlessness.** **EBN:** *Experienced nurses working with abused women came to redefine success as client personal growth over time, rather than leaving the relationship (Webster et al, 2006).*

- Focus on providing support, insuring safety, and promoting self-efficacy while encouraging disclosure about IPV events. **EBN:** *A review of evidence concluded that nursing care should focus on providing physical, psychological, and emotional support; ensuring safety of the client and family; and promoting the self-efficacy of the woman (Olive, 2007).* **EB:** *Women were more willing to disclose abuse when health care providers were probing (asking more than one question), asking open-ended questions, giving opportunities to talk, and being responsive to women's clues about psychosocial issues (Rhodes et al, 2007).*

- Screen pregnant women for the potential for domestic violence during pregnancy, especially with teenage pregnancies. **EBN:** *In a study of high-risk teen mothers, IPV was reported by 61% of the participants, with 37.5% reporting IPV during pregnancy (Mylant & Mann, 2008). Psychological health was found to be predicted by a history of abuse among women in a high-risk prenatal care clinic (Svavarsdottir & Orlygsdottir, 2008). Pregnant women will remain in an abusive relationship if they perceive it to be in the best interest of the child, part of a process of "double-binding" with child and abusive spouse (Libbus et al, 2006; Lutz et al, 2006). Systematic screening of pregnant women is recommended, and choking is a danger that should be added to routine screening (Bullock et al, 2006; Jeanjot, Barlow, & Rozenberg, 2008). Women afraid of IPV before and during pregnancy had poorer physical and psychological outcomes (Brown, McDonald, & Krastev, 2008).*

- Screen women and children for effects of domestic violence during the postpartum period. **EB:** *Less educated women, women who reported substance abuse by spouse, and women who reported unwanted pregnancies were at risk of IPV both during and after pregnancy. Violence during pregnancy predicted postpartum violence. U.S. women employed during pregnancy were most likely to leave an abusive partner at 1 year postpartum (Charles & Perreira, 2007). In cases of high IPV, less than optimal infant health and difficult temperament were found (Burke, Lee, & O'Campo, 2008).*

- Women with physical or mental disabilities require extended assessment, including a comprehensive functional assessment, with attention to cultural issues, the nature of the disability, and needed resources. Women with disabilities may experience abuse from multiple sources, and particular attention should be paid to the additional emotional stressors present. *Difficulties leaving home, physical needs that shelter may not be able to accommodate, and the undesirability of nursing home placement are just a few stressors. Personal assistance providers may be abusive or take advantage financially.* **EBN:** *Women with disabilities may follow a unique model of IPV progression, requiring adaptation of the usual interventions, and may be slower in returning to usual routines (Copel, 2006; Focht-New et al, 2008). Women with schizophrenia are especially vulnerable and have complex needs (Rice, 2006; Bengtsson-Tops & Tops, 2007).*

- ▲ Referral for spiritual counseling may be considered, but be aware that clergy vary in their helpfulness. **EBN:** *Survivors of sexual violence described being able to cope with their situation through Spiritual Connection, Spiritual Journey, and Spiritual Transformation (Knapik, Martsolf, & Draucker, 2008). A study of women in abusive relationships who sought spiritual guidance from male clergy revealed themes of spiritual suffering, devaluation, loss, and powerlessness consistent with old societal biases. The authors noted that conclusions could not be drawn regarding the helpfulness of female clergy (Copel, 2008).*

- Identify risk factors such as ongoing mental illness by a parent, and monitor family closely. **EBN:** *Concern for the children of parents with a mental illness has been identified in light of the potential for family dysfunction and violence among the mentally ill (Copeland, 2007; Mason, Subedi, & Davis, 2007).*

- ▲ In cases where spouse or child abuse accompanies substance abuse, refer the abusive client to a substance abuse treatment program. Refer the spouse receiving abuse to Al-Anon and the children to Alateen. **EB:** *Use of drugs or alcohol may decrease impulse control and aggravate abusive behavior, depending on specific drug used and culture (Caetano, Ramisetty-Mikler, & Harris, 2008; Stalans & Ritchie, 2008).*

▲ In cases where an adult reveals a history of unresolved/untreated sexual abuse as a child, referral to a local Adults Molested as Children (AMAC) group may be helpful. **EB:** *Childhood sexual abuse has been associated with adult depression, attempted suicide, self-harm, and higher risk for later interpersonal violence (Murrell, Christoff, & Henning, 2007). Interventions tailored to the AMAC experience may be helpful.* Refer to the care plans for **Risk for Suicide**, **Self-Mutilation**, and **Risk for Self-Mutilation**.

▲ Intervention may include referral to a number of programs available, including parenting classes or a parental counseling support group. **EBN:** *Theraplay (Bennett, Shiner, & Ryan, 2006) and IN-SIGHT (Zust, 2006) address domestic violence issues.*

▲ Referral of women for psychiatric/psychological treatment should be considered as an appropriate intervention. **EBN:** *Treatment needs to address the relationship between shame and depression that perpetuates an abusive relationship. Overcoming shame, building a stable sense of identity, and becoming less dependent on others' approval should be addressed, along with physical health and PTSD symptoms (Smith & Randall, 2007; Woods et al, 2008).* **EB:** *In a study of 3429 women enrolled in an HMO, 46% reported a lifetime history and 14.7% reported a history within the previous 5 years of physical, sexual, and/or nonphysical abuse, with posttraumatic disorder a potential outcome (Dutton, 2009). Self-blame was associated with all factors involved in IPV, with outcomes of PTSD, depression, suicidality, and substance abuse (Campbell, Dworkin, & Cabral, 2009).*

▲ Referral of children for psychiatric/psychological treatment should be considered as an appropriate intervention. **EBN:** *Older children in particular were found to be at highest risk for behavior disorders, depression, and anxiety (McFarlane et al, 2007).* **EB:** *Children living with domestic violence were found to express fear and anxiety, self-esteem issues, ambivalent relationships with the abuser, and a sense of a lost childhood (Buckley, Holt, & Whelan, 2007).*

▲ Batterer intervention programs are often available and may be court mandated. **EBN:** *Batterers believe behaviors toward them are not justified, and their behaviors toward others are justified and minimized. Treatment should include emotional skills training that address these areas (Smith, 2007).*

Social Violence

● Assess for acute stress disorder (ASD) and posttraumatic stress disorder (PTSD) among victims of violence. **EB:** *In the acute phase following an assault, women reported high rates of ASD symptoms. Four months after an attack, dissatisfaction with previous life, prior mental health problems, recent life events, and earlier abuse were risk factors for PTSD (Renck, 2006).*

▲ Assess the support network of women who become victims of violent crime and refer for appropriate levels of assistance. **EB:** *In a national study of female crime victims, three help-seeking strategies were identified: (1) minimal or no help seeking, (2) family and friend help seeking, and (3) substantial help seeking (from family, friends, psychiatrists, social service providers, and police) (Kaukinen, 2004). Of particular concern would be women who do not have family or friends to provide support or who have difficulty accessing other types of assistance.*

● Be aware that hate crime is increasing, particularly toward gay and transgendered individuals, and it requires support and advocacy for victims. **EBN:** *Gay men who experienced antigay abuse reported that the events affected their self-image. In addition to verbal and physical abuse, spiritual abuse emerged as the men internalized schemas of Outcast and Sinner (Lucies & Yick, 2007).*

▲ Victims of violence seen in the ED should receive an assessment for needed services and assignment to case management. *Establishment of linkages with social service agencies can provide important services for referral.* **EB:** *An ED study provided linkages with internal services, such as primary care, gang-related tattoo removal, psychiatric services, substance abuse treatment, and dental care; and with a social service agency providing such services as programs in personal development and education, comprehensive employment preparation, computer skills, and others. Outside agencies were also used for legal assistance, spiritual counseling, GED classes, and financial assistance. With case management initiated in the ED as the key element, the number of resources used by young victims of interpersonal violence as compared with controls was significantly increased (Zun, Downey, & Rosen, 2003).*

● = Independent   ▲ = Collaborative   **EBN** = Evidence-Based Nursing   **EB** = Evidence-Based

Rape-Trauma Syndrome

- Approach client with sensitivity. **EBN:** *Using Peplau's theory of nursing roles, researchers found that the roles of counselor and technical expert were most helpful, with interpersonal sensitivity important to clients (Courey et al, 2008).*
- ▲ Monitor for paradoxical drug reactions, and report any to the physician. *Violent behavior can be stimulated by a medication intended to calm the client.*
- Assess for brain insults, such as recent falls or injuries, strokes, or transient ischemic attacks. *Clients with brain injuries may respond to stimulus control, problem solving, social skills training, relaxation training, and anger management to reduce aggressive behaviors. Brain injuries, lowered impulse control, and reduced coping can cause violent reactions to self or others. Brain injury symptoms may be mistaken for mental illness.*
- Decrease environmental stimuli if violence is directed at others. *Removal of the client to a quiet area can reduce violent impulses. Use a calm voice to "talk down" the client.*
- Assess holistic needs of the client. **EBN:** *Risk factors for negative mental health outcomes following sexual violence were found to be low income, low education level, lack of social support, and poor health promotion (Vandemark & Mueller, 2008).*
- Discuss with client her wishes regarding use of an emergency contraceptive. **EBN:** *If emergency contraception were offered to every female victim of sexual assault, researchers concluded that unintended pregnancies would decline. However, the findings are limited, as only 15% of women who are raped seek health care promptly (Womack, 2008).*
- ▲ If abuse or neglect of an elderly client is suspected, report the suspicion to an adult protective services agency with jurisdiction over the geographical area where the client lives.

Pediatric

- Be alert for both shaken baby syndrome and exposure of children to violence. *Nurse practitioners can play an important role in identifying shaken baby syndrome and educating others about prevention (Walls, 2006). Approaches for addressing children exposed to family violence include the Ploeger Model of enhanced maternal and child health (Edgecombe & Ploeger, 2006) and the Health Promotion Model for Violence Prevention (Skybo & Polivka, 2007).*
- Assess for dating violence among adolescent girls. Additional assessments may be required for sexually transmitted diseases and pregnancy. **EB:** *Adolescent girls who have been intentionally hurt by a date in the previous year were found to be more likely to experience sexual health risks and pregnancy (Silverman, Raj, & Clements, 2004). A high rate of dating violence by both male and female university students has been found worldwide (Straus, 2004).*
- Pregnant teens should be assessed for abuse, particularly if they are with an older partner. **EBN:** *In a study of predominantly African American pregnant teens, 13% reported domestic violence during pregnancy. Teens with adult partners (4 or more years older) were twice as likely to report abuse as teens with similar age partners (Harner, 2004).*
- ▲ When physical abuse by parents is present, parent-child interaction therapy (PCIT) may be helpful. **EB:** *PCIT is an empirically supported treatment that has been shown to reduce abuse (Chambless & Ollendick, 2000; Chaffin et al, 2004).*
- ▲ In the case of child abuse or neglect, refer for early childhood home visitation. **EB:** *Home visits during a child's first 2 years of life have been found to be effective in preventing child abuse and neglect (Hahn et al, 2003).*

Geriatric

- Be alert to the potential for elder abuse in clients, including the possibility of psychological abuse. *Abuse may occur along a continuum, from neglect to physical or sexual abuse. Family and strangers may commit financial exploitation. Look for signs of bruising, malnutrition, and fearful responses to or around caregivers.* **EBN:** *Female caregivers, those with more education, and those with greater burdens showed more severe psychologically abusive behavior (Wang, Lin, & Lee, 2006).*
- Assess for changes in physiological functions (e.g., constipation, dehydration) or impairment of the ability to meet basic needs (e.g., inadequate toileting, decreased mobility). Observe for signs of fear,

anxiety, anger, and agitation, and intervene immediately. *In older adults subtle physiological changes, interruptions of or changes in routine, or fears about medical disorders or potential loss of independence can be transformed into anger, irritability, or agitation.* **EB:** *Agitation in nursing home clients was predicted independently by cognitive impairment, vision and hearing impairment, and gender. Individuals with significant hearing impairment were more likely to become agitated than less impaired individuals (Vance et al, 2003).*

- Observe for dementia and delirium. *Clients with dementia or delirium may strike out if they are frustrated or if they have the sense that their personal space is being violated. However, this may not occur within a cognitive capacity that permits discussion of the behavior.*
- Assess sensory impairments, physical illness, etc and the influence they may have on the client's behavior. **EB:** *In this study associations between various conditions and the development of aggressive behavior in elderly people with dementia were found, including the contributions of degrees of cognitive impairment, personality, sensory change, physical illness, language impairment, brain pathology, affective and psychotic disorders (Hall & O'Connor, 2004).*
- Be alert for the potential of sexual abuse of elders. *Nurses are in the position not only to provide acute care intervention, but also to collect forensic evidence and report suspected cases to the authorities (Burgess et al, 2006).* **EB:** *Sensitive assessment and intervention is called for, to overcome the marginalization of elders who may experience inadequate response to issues of violence and power (Burgess & Clements, 2006; Jones & Powell, 2006).* Refer to care plan for **Rape-Trauma syndrome.**

Multicultural

- Exercise cultural competence when dealing with domestic violence. *Within the demands and difficulties of an increasingly diverse health care environment, increased need exists for awareness, education, cultural sensitivity, and action in responding to multicultural issues of family violence (Anderson & Aviles, 2006; Hindin, 2006; Sumter, 2006).* **EBN:** *Battered Latina women voiced equal fear of the abuser and of disclosing the abuse to health care professionals, based on the consequences, but wanted to be asked about abuse and receive help (Kelly, 2006).*

Home Care

- Be alert to the potential for violent behavior in the home setting. Respond to verbal aggression with interventions to de-escalate negative emotional states. *Violence is a process that can be recognized early. De-escalation involves reducing client stressors, responding to the client with respect, acknowledging the client's feeling state, and assisting the client to regain control. If de-escalation does not work, the nurse should leave the home (Distasio, 2000).* **EB:** *Verbal aggression was shown to be a predictor of negative psychological outcomes (Bussing & Hoge, 2004).*
- Assess family members or caregivers for their ability to protect the client and themselves. *The safety of the client between home visits is a nursing priority. Caregivers often need assistance with recognizing or admitting fear of or danger from a loved one.*
- Include an initial and ongoing assessment and evaluation of potential abuse and neglect. Photograph evidence of abuse or neglect when possible. *Victims of abuse perceive themselves to be powerless to change the situation. Indeed, the abuser fosters this perception and may threaten violence or death if the victim attempts to leave. Chronic abuse and neglect by a spouse or other family among the elderly is often hidden until home care is actively involved.* Refer to the care plan for **Powerlessness.**
- ▲ If neglect or abuse is suspected, identify an emergency plan that addresses the problem immediately, ensures client safety, and includes a report to the appropriate authorities. Discuss when to use hotlines and 911. Role play access to emergency resources with the client and caregivers. *Client safety is a nursing priority. An emergency plan should address either immediate removal to a safe environment or identification of appropriate steps to take in the event of abuse and the securing of resources for the anticipated action (e.g., available phone, packed bag, alternative living arrangements). Reporting is a legal requirement of health care workers.*
- Encourage appropriate safety behaviors in abused women; call the client at intervals during a 6–month period to determine whether safety behaviors are being carried out. **EBN:** *A study of telephone contacts to women who sought help through the district attorney's office demonstrated that safety behaviors increased dramatically. Safety behaviors included hiding money; hiding an extra set*

● = Independent   ▲ = Collaborative   **EBN** = Evidence-Based Nursing   **EB** = Evidence-Based

of house and car keys; establishing a code for abuse occurrence with family or friends; asking neighbors to call police if violence occurs; removing weapons; keeping available family social security numbers, rent and utility receipts, family birth certificates, identification or driver licenses, bank account numbers, insurance policies and numbers, marriage license, valuable jewelry, important phone numbers, and a hidden bag with extra clothing (McFarlane et al, 2002).

- Assess the home environment for harmful objects. Have the family remove or lock objects as able. *The safety of the client and caregivers is a nursing priority.*
- ▲ Refer for homemaker or psychiatric home health care services for respite, client reassurance, and implementation of a therapeutic regimen. *Responsibility for a person who may become violent provides high caregiver stress. Respite decreases caregiver stress. The presence of caring individuals is reassuring to both the client and caregivers, especially during periods of client anxiety. Individuals exhibiting violent behaviors can respond to the interventions described previously, modified for the home setting.*
- ▲ If the client is taking psychotropic medications, assess client and family knowledge of medication and its administration and side effects. Teach as necessary. *Knowledge of the medical regimen supports compliance.*
- ▲ Evaluate effectiveness and side effects of medications. *Accurate clinical feedback improves the physician's ability to prescribe an effective medical regimen specific to a client needs.*
- If client displays mildly intensifying aggressive behavior, attempt to diffuse anger or violence (e.g., ask for a glass of water to distract client). Later in the visit explain that aggressive behavior is not acceptable and present consequences of continued aggressive behavior (i.e., right of agency to discontinue services). *Mild aggression can be diffused safely. Confronting the client before severe aggression is evident places responsibility on the client and family for respectful partnership in care.*
- Document all acts or verbalizations of aggression. *Safety of the staff is a primary responsibility of home health agencies. Law enforcement intervention may be necessary.*
- ▲ If client verbalizes or displays threatening behavior, notify your supervisor and plan to make joint visits with another staff person or a security escort. *Having a second person at the visit is a show of power and control used to subdue aggressive behavior.*
- If the client's behavior is not overtly threatening but makes the nurse uncomfortable, a meeting may be held outside the home in sight of others (e.g., front porch). *The nurse should trust a "gut" reaction that prompts concern regarding the client's potential for aggressive or violent behavior. Such intuitive reactions are often the result of subliminal cues that are not readily voiced.*
- Never enter a home or remain in a home if aggression threatens your well-being.
- ▲ Never challenge a show of force, such as a gun threat. Leave and notify your supervisor and the appropriate authorities. Document the incident. *Safety of the staff is a primary responsibility of home health agencies. Law enforcement intervention may be necessary.*
- ▲ If client behaviors intensify, refer for immediate mental health intervention. *The degree of disturbance and ability to manage care safely at home determines the level of services needed to protect the client.*

Client/Family Teaching and Discharge Planning

- Instruct victims of IPV in the dynamics and prognosis of domestic violence behavior. **EB:** *A study of 220 male defendants found that failure to comply with domestic violence treatment and additional reports of new criminal activity predicted recidivism for domestic violence offenders, and emphasized the need for court supervision of defendant behavior to promote victim safety (Kindness et al, 2009).*
- Instruct victims of IPV in the outcomes for children who witness or are victims of domestic violence. **EB:** *Children exposed to violence often have difficulties with violence as adults. Boys were more likely to commit domestic violence as adults when they witnessed IPV as children; boys who were abused were more likely as adults to abuse children (Murrell, Christoff, & Henning, 2007).*
- Teach relaxation and exercise as ways to release anger and deal with stress. **EB:** *IPV and parenting stress were found to be risk factors for child maltreatment (Taylor et al, 2009).*
- Teach cognitive-behavioral activities, such as active problem solving, reframing (reappraising the situation from a different perspective), or thought stopping (in response to a negative thought, picture a large stop sign and replace the image with a prearranged positive alternative). Teach the client to confront his or her own negative thought patterns (or cognitive distortions), such as catastrophizing (expecting the very worst), dichotomous thinking (perceiving events in only one of two

opposite categories), magnification (placing distorted emphasis on a single event), or unrealistic expectations (e.g., "I should get what I want when I want it."). *Cognitive-behavioral activities address clients' assumptions, beliefs, and attitudes about their situations, fostering modification of these elements to be as realistic as possible. Through cognitive-behavioral interventions, clients become more aware of their cognitive choices in adopting and maintaining their belief systems, thereby exercising greater control over their own reactions (Hagerty & Patusky, 2007).*

▲ Refer to individual or group therapy.

• Teach the adolescent client violence prevention, and encourage him or her to become involved in community service activities. *School programs that couple community service with classroom health instruction can have a measurable effect on violent behaviors of young adolescents at high risk for being both the perpetrators and victims of peer violence. Community service programs may be a valuable part of multicomponent violence-prevention programs (O'Donnell et al, 1999).*

• Teach the use of appropriate community resources in emergency situations (e.g., hotline, community mental health agency, ED, 911 in most places in the United States, the toll-free National Domestic Violence Hotline [1–800–799–SAFE]). *Internet resources are increasing and should be made available to clients. It is necessary to get immediate help when violence occurs.*

• Encourage the use of self-help groups in nonemergency situations.

• Inform the client and family about medication actions, side effects, target symptoms, and toxic reactions.

ⓔvolve See the EVOLVE website for Weblinks for client education resources.

REFERENCES

Abderhalden C, Needham I, Miserez B et al: Predicting inpatient violence in acute psychiatric wards using the Broset violence checklist: a multicenter prospective cohort study, *J Psychiatr Ment Health* 11(4);422, 2004.

Amar AF, Cox CW: Intimate partner violence: implications for critical care nursing, *Crit Care Nurs Clin North Am* 18:287, 2006.

Amore M, Menchetti M, Tonti C et al: Predictors of violent behavior among acute psychiatric patients: clinical study, *Psychiatry Clin Neurosci* 62(3):247–55, 2008.

Anderson TR, Aviles AM: Diverse faces of domestic violence, *ABNF J* 17:129, 2006.

American Psychiatric Nurses Association (APNA): Position statement on seclusion and restraint, 2007a. www.apna.org/i4a/pages/index.cfm?pageid=3729. Accessed on July 6, 2009.

APNA: Seclusion and restraints standards of practice, 2007b. www.apna.org/files/public/APNA_SR_Standards-Final.pdf. Accessed on July 6, 2009.

APNA: Position statement on workplace violence, 2008. www.apna.org/i4a/pages/index.cfm?pageid=3786. Accessed on July 6, 2009.

Bengtsson-Tops A, Tops D: Self-reported consequences and needs for support associated with abuse in female users of psychiatric care, *Int J Ment Health Nurs* 16:35, 2007.

Bennett LR, Shiner SK, Ryan S: Using Theraplay in shelter settings with mothers & children who have experienced violence in the home, *J Psychosoc Nurs Ment Health Serv* 44:38, 2006.

Bowers L, Nijman H, Palmstierna T: The Attempted and Actual Assault Scale (Attack), *Intl J Methods Psychiatr Res* 16:171, 2007.

Bowers L, Simpson A, Eyres S et al: Serious untoward incidents and their aftermath in acute inpatient psychiatry: the Tompkins Acute Ward study, *Int J Ment Health Nurs* 15:226, 2006.

Brown SJ, McDonald EA, Krastev AH: Fear of an intimate partner and women's health in early pregnancy: findings from the Maternal Health Study, *BIRTH* 35:293, 2008.

Buckley H, Holt S, Whelan S: Listen to me! Children's experiences of domestic violence, *Child Abuse Rev* 16:296, 2007.

Bullock L, Bloom T, Davis J et al: Abuse disclosure in privately and Medicaid-funded pregnant women, *J Midwifery Womens Health* 51:361, 2006.

Burgess AW, Clements PT: Information processing of sexual abuse in elders, *J Forensic Nurs* 2:113, 2006.

Burgess AW, Watt ME, Brown KM et al: Management of elder sexual abuse cases in critical care settings, *Crit Care Nurs Clin North Am* 18:313, 2006.

Burke J, Lee L, O'Campo P: An exploration of maternal intimate partner violence experiences and infant general health and temperament, *Matern Child Health J* 12:172, 2008.

Bussing A, Hoge T: Aggression and violence against home care workers, *J Occup Health Psychol* 9(3):206, 2004.

Caetano R, Ramisetty-Mikler S, Harris TR: Drinking, alcohol problems and intimate partner violence among White and Hispanic couples in the U.S.: longitudinal associations, *J Fam Violence* 23:37, 2008.

Campbell R, Dworkin E, Cabral G: An ecological model of the impact of sexual assault on women's mental health, *Trauma, Violence, & Abuse* 10:225, 2009.

Chaffin M, Silovsky JF, Funderburk B et al: Parent-child interaction therapy with physically abusive parents: efficacy for reducing future abuse reports, *J Consult Clin Psychol* 72(3):500, 2004.

Chambless DL, Ollendick TH: Empirically supported psychological interventions: controversies and evidence, *Annu Rev Psychol* 52:685, 2000.

Chapman R, Perry L, Styles I et al: Predicting patient aggression against nurses in all hospital areas, *Br J Nurs* 18:476, 2009.

Charles P, Perreira KM: Intimate partner violence during pregnancy and 1–year postpartum, *J Fam Violence* 22:609, 2007.

Cole J, Logan TK, Shannon L: Self-perceived risk of HIV among women with protective orders against male partners, *Health & Soc Work* 33:287, 2008.

Copel LC: Partner abuse in physically disabled women: a proposed model for understanding intimate partner violence, *Perspect Psychiatr Care* 42:114, 2006.

Copel LC: The lived experience of women in abusive relationships who sought spiritual guidance, *Issues Ment Health Nurs* 29:115, 2008.

Copeland DA: Conceptualizing family members of violent mentally ill individuals as a vulnerable population, *Issues Ment Health Nurs* 28:943, 2007.

• = Independent   ▲ = Collaborative   **EBN** = Evidence-Based Nursing   **EB** = Evidence-Based

Courey TJ, Martsolf DS, Draucker CB et al: Hildegard Peplau's theory and the health care encounters of survivors of sexual violence, *J Am Psychiatr Nurses Assoc* 14:136, 2008.

Dienemann J, Glass N, Hanson G et al: The Domestic Violence Survivor Assessment (DVSA): A tool for individual counseling with women experiencing intimate partner violence, *Issues Ment Health Nurs* 28:913, 2007.

Distasio CA: Violence against home care providers. Stop it before it starts, *Caring* 19(10):14, 2000.

Dutton M: Pathways linking intimate partner violence and posttraumatic stress disorder, *Trauma, Violence & Abuse* 10:211, 2009.

Edgecombe G, Ploeger H: Working with families experiencing violence: the Ploeger Model of enhanced maternal and child health nursing practice, *Contemp Nurse* 21:287, 2006.

Flood M, Pease B: Factors influencing attitudes to violence against women, *Trauma, Violence, & Abuse* 10:125, 2009.

Focht-New G, Barol B, Clements PT et al: Persons with developmental disability exposed to interpersonal violence and crime: Approaches for intervention, *Perspect Psychiatr Care* 44:89, 2008.

Foster C, Bowers L, Nijman H: Aggressive behaviour on acute psychiatric wards: prevalence, severity and management, *J Adv Nurs* 58:140, 2007.

Fountoulakis KN, Leucht S, Kaprinis GS: Personality disorders and violence, *Curr Opin Psychiatry* 21:84, 2008.

Hagerty B, Patusky K: Mood disorders: depression and mania. In Fortinash KM, Holoday-Worret PA, editors: *Psychiatric mental health nursing*, ed 4, St Louis, 2008, Mosby.

Hahn RA, Bilukha OO, Crosby A et al: First reports evaluating the effectiveness of strategies for preventing violence: early childhood home visitation, *MMWR Recomm Rep* 52(RR-14):1, 2003.

Hall KA, O'Connor DW: Correlates of aggressive behavior in dementia. *Int Psychogeriatr* 16(2):41–58, 2004.

Harner HM: Domestic violence and trauma care in teenage pregnancy: does paternal age make a difference? *J Obstet Gynecol Neonatal Nurs* 33(3):312, 2004.

Hellerstein DJ, Staub AB, Lequesne E: Decreasing the use of restraint and seclusion among psychiatric inpatients, *J Psychiatr Practice* 13:308, 2007.

Hills D: Relationships between aggression management training, perceived self-efficacy and rural general hospital nurses' experiences of patient aggression, *Contemp Nurs* 31(1):20, 2008.

Hindin PK: Intimate partner violence screening practices of certified nurse-midwives, *J Midwifery Womens Health* 51:216, 2006.

Hollingsworth E, Ford-Gilboe M: Registered nurses' self-efficacy for assessing and responding to woman abuse in emergency department settings, *Can J Nurs Res* 38:54, 2006.

Holmes D, Kennedy SL, Perron A: The mentally ill and social exclusion: a critical examination of the use of seclusion from the patient's perspective, *Issues Ment Health Nurs* 25:559, 2004.

Jeanjot I, Barlow P, Rozenberg S: Domestic violence during pregnancy: survey of patients and healthcare providers, *J Womens Health* 17:557, 2008.

Jones H, Powell JL: Old age, vulnerability and sexual violence: implications for knowledge and practice, *Int Nurs Rev* 53:211, 2006.

Kaukinen C: The help-seeking strategies of female violent crime victims, *J Interpers Violence* 19(9):967, 2004.

Kelly U: "What will happen if I tell you?" Battered Latina women's experiences of health care, *Can J Nurs Res* 38:78, 2006.

Kindness A, Kim H, Alder et al: Court compliance as a predictor of postadjudication recidivism for domestic violence offenders, *J Interpers Violence* 24:1222, 2009.

Kling R, Corbiere M, Milord R et al: Use of a violence risk assessment tool in an acute care hospital: effectiveness in identifying violent patients, *AAOHN J* 54:481, 2006.

Knapik GP, Martsolf DS, Draucker CB: Being delivered: spirituality in survivors of sexual violence, *Issues Ment Health Nurs* 29:335, 2008.

Libbus MK, Bullock LF, Neltson T et al: Abuse during pregnancy: current theory and new contextual understandings, *Issues Ment Health Nurs* 27:927, 2006.

Lipscomb J, McPhaul K, Rosen J et al: Violence prevention in the mental health setting: the New York state experience, *Can J Nurs Res* 38:96, 2006.

Lucies C, Yick AG: Images of gay men's experiences with antigay abuse: object relations theory reconceptualized, *J Theory Construct Test* 11:55, 2007.

Lutz KE, Curry MA, Robrecht LC et al: Double binding, abusive intimate partner relationships, and pregnancy, *Can J Nurs Res* 38(4):118–134, 2006.

Macy RJ, Ferron J, Crosby C: Partner violence and survivors' chronic health problems: Informing social work practice, *Soc Work* 54:29, 2009.

Mason C, Subedi S, Davis RB: Clients with mental illness and their children: Implications for clinical practice, *Issues Ment Health Nurs* 28:1105, 2007.

McFarlane J, Malecha A, Gist J et al: An intervention to increase safety behaviors of abused women: results of a randomized clinical trial, *Nurs Res* 51:347, 2002.

McFarlane J, Malecha A, Watson K et al: Intimate partner physical and sexual assault & child behavior problems, *Amer J MCN* 32:74, 2007.

Meehan T, Fjeldsoe K, Stedman T et al: Reducing aggressive behaviour and staff injuries: a multi-strategy approach, *Aus Health Rev* 30(2):203–210, 2006.

Murrell AR, Christoff KA, Henning KR: Characteristics of domestic violence offenders: Associations with childhood exposure to violence, *J Fam Violence* 22:523, 2007.

Mylant M, Mann C: Current sexual trauma among high-risk teen mothers, *J Child Adol Psychiatr Nurs* 21:164, 2008.

O'Donnell L, Stueve A, San Doval A et al: Violence prevention and young adolescents' participation in community youth service, *J Adolesc Health* 24(1):28, 1999.

Olive P: Care for emergency department patients who have experienced domestic violence: A review of the evidence base, *J Clin Nurs* 16:1736, 2007.

Oostrom JK, Mierlo, H: An evaluation of an aggression management training program to cope with workplace violence in the healthcare sector, *Res Nurs Health* 4:320, 2008.

Pryor J: What do nurses do in response to their predictions of aggression? *J Neurosci Nurs* 38:177, 2006.

Puskar K, Ren D, Bernardo LM et al: Anger correlated with psychosocial variables in rural youth, *Issues Compr Pediatr Nurs* 31(2):71, 2008.

Renck B: Psychological stress reactions of women in Sweden who have been assaulted: acute response and four-month follow-up, *Nurs Outlook* 54:312, 2006.

Rhodes KV, Frankel RM, Levinthal N et al: "You're not a victim of domestic violence, are you?" Provider-patient communication about domestic violence, *Ann Intern Med* 147:620, 2007.

Rice E: Schizophrenia and violence: the perspective of women, *Issues Ment Health Nurs* 27:961, 2006.

Robinson L, Spilsbury K: Systematic review of the perceptions and experiences of accessing health services by adult victims of domestic violence, *Health Soc Care Community* 16:16, 2008.

Ryan CJ, Bowers L: An analysis of nurses' post-incident manual restraint reports, *J Psychiatr Ment Health Nurs* 13:527, 2006.

Shawyer F, Mackinnon A, Farhall J et al: Acting on harmful command hallucinations in psychotic disorders: an integrative approach, *J Nerv Ment Dis* 196:390, 2008.

● = Independent   ▲ = Collaborative   **EBN** = Evidence-Based Nursing   **EB** = Evidence-Based

Silverman JG, Raj A, Clements K: Dating violence and associated sexual risk and pregnancy among adolescent girls in the United States, *Pediatrics* 114(2):220, 2004.

Skybo T, Polivka B: Health promotion model for violence prevention and exposure, *J Clin Nurs* 16:38, 2007.

Smith JS, Rainey SL, Smith KR et al: Barriers to the mandatory reporting of domestic violence encountered by nursing professionals, *J Trauma Nurs* 15:9, 2008.

Smith ME: Self-deception among men who are mandated to attend a batterer intervention program, *Perspect Psychiatr Care* 43:193, 2007.

Smith ME, Randall EJ: Batterer intervention program: The victim's hope in ending the abuse and maintaining the relationship, *Issues Ment Health Nurs* 28:1045, 2007.

Stalans LJ, Ritchie J: Relationship of substance use/abuse with psychological and physical intimate partner violence: variations across living situations, *J Fam Violence* 23:9, 2008.

Stolker JJ, Nijman HL, Zwanikken PH: Are patients' views on seclusion associated with lack of privacy in the ward? *Arch Psychiatr Nurs* 20:282, 2006.

Straus MA: Prevalence of violence against dating partners by male and female university students worldwide, *Violence Against Women* 10(7):790, 2004.

Sumter M: Domestic violence and diversity: a call for multicultural services, *J Health Hum Serv Adm* 29:173, 2006.

Svavarsdottir EK, Orlygsdottir B: Effect of abuse by a close family member on health, *J Nurs Schol* 40:311, 2008.

Taylor CA, Guterman NB, Lee SJ et al: Intimate partner violence, maternal stress, nativity, and risk for maternal maltreatment of young children, *Am J Public Health* 99:175, 2009.

Temcheff CE, Serbin LA, Martin-Storey A et al: Continuity and pathways from aggression in childhood to family violence in adulthood: a 30–year longitudinal study, *J Fam Violence* 23:231, 2008.

Vance DE, Burgio LD, Roth DL et al: Predictors of agitation in nursing home residents, *J Gerontol* 58B(2):P129, 2003.

Vandemark LM, Mueller M: Mental health after sexual violence: the role of behavioral and demographic risk factors, *Nurs Res* 57:175, 2008.

Walls C: Shaken baby syndrome education: a role for nurse practitioners working with families of small children, *J Pediatr Health Care* 20:304, 2006.

Wang JJ: Psychological abuse behavior exhibited by caregivers in the care of the elderly and correlated factors in long-term care facilities in Taiwan, *Nurs Res* 13:271, 2005.

Wang JJ, Lin JN, Lee FP: Psychologically abusive behavior by those caring for the elderly in a domestic context, *Geriatr Nurs* 27:284, 2006.

Webster F, Bouck MS, Wright BL et al: Nursing the social wound: public health nurses' experience of screening for woman abuse, *Can J Nurs Res* 38:136, 2006.

Wilson KS, Silberberg MR, Brown AJ et al: Health needs and barriers to healthcare of women who have experienced intimate partner violence, *J Women's Health* 16:1485, 2007.

Womack KA: Emergency contraception to avoid unintended pregnancy following sexual assault, *Womens Health Care* 7:10, 2008.

Woods SJ, Hall RJ, Campbell JC et al: Physical health and posttraumatic stress disorder symptoms in women experiencing intimate partner violence, *J Midwifery Womens Health* 53:538, 2008.

Yonaka L, Yoder MK, Darrow JB et al: Barriers to screening for domestic violence in the emergency department, *J Contin Educ Nurs* 38:37, 2007.

Zun LS, Downey LV, Rosen J: Violence prevention in the ED: linkage of the ED to a social service agency, *Am J Emerg Med* 21(6):454, 2003.

Zust BL: Meaning of INSIGHT participation among women who have experienced intimate partner violence, *Issues Ment Health Nurs* 27:775, 2006.

Risk for self-directed Violence   Kathleen L. Patusky, PhD, APRN-BC

NANDA-I

Definition

At risk for behaviors in which an individual demonstrates that he/she can be physically, emotionally and/or sexually harmful to self

Risk Factors

Age 15–19; age over 45; behavioral clues (e.g., writing forlorn love notes, directing angry messages at a significant other who has rejected the person, giving away personal items, taking out a large life insurance policy); conflictual interpersonal relationships; emotional problems (e.g., hopelessness, despair, increased anxiety, panic, anger, hostility); employment problems (e.g., unemployed, recent job loss/failure); engagement in autoerotic sexual acts; family background (e.g., chaotic or conflictual, history of suicide); history of multiple suicide attempts; lack of personal resources (e.g., poor achievement, poor insight, affect unavailable and poorly controlled); lack of social resources (e.g., poor rapport, socially isolated, unresponsive family); physical health problems (e.g., hypochondriasis, chronic or terminal illness); marital status (single, widowed, divorced); mental health problems (e.g., severe depression, psychosis, severe personality disorder, alcoholism, or drug abuse); occupation (executive, administrator/owner of business, professional, semiskilled worker); sexual orientation (bisexual [active], homosexual [inactive]); suicidal ideation; suicidal plan; verbal clues (e.g., talking about death, "better off without me," asking questions about lethal dosages of drugs)

NOC, NIC, Client Outcomes, Nursing Interventions, Client/Family Teaching and Discharge Planning, *Rationales,* **and References**

Refer to care plans for **Risk for Suicide**, **Self-Mutilation**, and **Risk for Self-Mutilation**.

Impaired Walking   *Brenda Emick-Herring, RN, MSN, CRRN*

NANDA-I

Definition

Limitation of independent movement within the environment on foot (or artificial limb)

Defining Characteristics

Impaired ability to: climb stairs, walk on uneven surface, walk required distances, walk on even surfaces, walk on an incline or decline, navigate curbs

Related Factors (r/t)

Cognitive impairment; deconditioning; depressed mood; environmental constraints (e.g., stairs, inclines, uneven surfaces, unsafe obstacles, distances, lack of assistive devices or person, restraints); fear of falling; impaired balance; impaired vision; insufficient muscle strength; lack of knowledge; limited endurance; musculoskeletal impairment (e.g., contractures); neuromuscular impairment; obesity; pain

NOC   (Nursing Outcomes Classification)

Suggested NOC Outcomes

Ambulation, Mobility

Example NOC Outcome with Indicators
Ambulation as evidenced by the following indicators: Walks with effective gait/Walks at moderate pace/Walks up and down steps/Walks moderate distance (Rate the outcome and indicators of **Ambulation:** 1 = severely compromised, 2 = substantially compromised, 3 = moderately compromised, 4 = mildly compromised, 5 = not compromised [see Section I].)

Client Outcomes/Goals

Client Will (Specify Time Frame):
- Demonstrate optimal independence and safety in walking
- Demonstrate the ability to direct others on how to assist with walking
- Demonstrate the ability to properly and safely use and care for assistive walking devices

NIC   (Nursing Interventions Classification)

Suggested NIC Intervention

Exercise Therapy: Ambulation

Example NIC Activities—Exercise Therapy: Ambulation
Assist patient to use footwear that facilitates walking and prevents injury; Encourage to sit in bed, on side of bed ("dangle"), or in chair, as tolerated

Nursing Interventions and *Rationales*

- Progressively mobilize clients (gradual elevation of head of bed, sitting in reclined chair, standing, etc.). *Helps clients adapt to and tolerate upright position changes/postures.*
- Assist clients to apply orthosis, immobilizers, splints, and braces before walking. *Maintain joint stability, immobilization, support and/or alignment during motion.*

• = Independent   ▲ = Collaborative   **EBN** = Evidence-Based Nursing   **EB** = Evidence-Based

- Apply thromboembolic deterrent stockings (TEDs) and/or elastic leg wraps and abdominal binders; raise head of bed (HOB) slowly in small increments to sitting, have clients move feet/legs up and down then stand slowly; avoid prolonged standing, eat frequent small, low carbohydrate meals, and maintain partial head elevation when resting in bed for orthostatic hypotension. *Enhances circulatory redistribution so blood doesn't pool in legs/feet; low carbohydrate meals help prevent postprandial hypotension, and HOB elevation stimulates baroreceptors and decreases nocturnal diuresis (Johnson & Psustian, 2005; Sclater & Alagiakrishnan, 2006; Weimer & Zadeh, 2009).*

▲ Compare morning lying/sitting/standing blood pressures. If systolic pressure falls 20 mm Hg or diastolic pressure falls 10 mm Hg from lying to standing within 3 minutes, and/or if light-headedness, dizziness, syncope, or unexplained falls occur, consult a physician (Irvin & White, 2004; Weimer & Zadeh, 2009). *Detection of orthostatic hypotension is key to fall prevention.* **EB:** *Persons with orthostatic hypotension are often symptomatic and have postprandial (after-meal) hypotension/heart rate variability (Ejaz et al, 2004).*

▲ Give prescribed hydration and medications to treat orthostatic hypotension. *Cerebral hypoperfusion is a common cause of orthostatic intolerance and hypotension (Weimer & Zadeh, 2009). Water has a pressor effect in those with autonomic orthostatic hypotension (Shannon et al, 2002).* **EB:** *A small group of seated persons with severe orthostatic postprandial hypotension had elevated blood pressures after rapid ingestion of 500 mL of water (Shannon et al, 2002).*

- Screen for deep vein thrombosis (DVTs), vigilantly apply compression stockings (TEDs), and give medications as prescribed to persons at risk for/with (DVT). *Screening for risk, using mechanical devices to prevent stasis, and medications prevent/treat blood clots (Crowther, 2008).* Refer to care plan for **Ineffective peripheral tissue Perfusion.**

▲ Apply compression stockings and assist persons with DVT to walk as ordered. *Such stockings stimulate fibrinolysis with acute DVT and should be used long term to help prevent postthrombotic syndrome (Crowther, 2008).* **EB:** *Results from a meta-analysis and a descriptive study (Trujillo-Santos et al, 2004, 2005), and a clinical trial (Romera et al, 2005), concluded that ambulating persons with DVT did not produce higher rates of pulmonary emboli. Via a clinical trial, Prandoni and colleagues (2004) showed that wearing compression stockings for 2 years following DVT decreased the risk of postthrombotic syndrome by half.*

▲ Reinforce correct use of prescribed mobility devices and remind clients of weight-bearing restrictions. *Devices give stability and help compensate for poor balance (Lyons, 2004). Canes provide stability in persons with hemiparesis; standard walkers assist those with generalized weakness and wheeled walkers assist with low endurance; crutches may be used with restricted/non–weight-bearing status (Kreger, 2006; Hoeman, Liszner, & Alverzo, 2008). Full weight bearing may retard bone healing in fractured limbs.* **EB:** *Older adults living in a residential facility who were physically active and used walking aids had fewer falls (Graafmans et al, 2003). Use of two-wheeled walkers allowed persons with leg amputations and prosthetics to walk faster and halt less often than when four-footed walkers were used (Tsai et al, 2003).*

- Teach clients with leg amputations to correctly don stump socks, liner, immediate postoperative prostheses (IPOP) or traditional prosthesis before standing/walking. *IPOPs often reduce pain, healing time, knee flexion contractures and promote early ambulation (Olson, 2008). A thin nylon sheath prevents the limb from turning in the socket of the prosthesis. A stump sock establishes proper fit between limb and socket. The liner helps prevent pressure ulcers.* **EB:** *Researchers found clients with transtibial amputations had improved wound healing as evidenced by an average of 58 days for those with prefabricated polyethylene rigid removable dressings until custom fitting for the prosthesis, compared to 84 days with soft dressings (Ladenheim, Oberti-Smith, & Tablada, 2007).*

- Emphasize the importance of wearing properly fitting, low-heeled shoes with nonskid soles, and socks/hose, and of seeking medical care for foot pain or problems with abnormal toenails, corns, calluses, or diabetes. *Proper footwear may help balance and prevent falls, pressure ulcers, impaired circulation, and pain (Bonham & Flemister, 2002).*

▲ Use a snug gait belt with handles and assistive devices while walking clients, as recommended by the physical therapist (PT). *Belts help staff steady clients (U.S. Department of Veterans Affairs, 2005).*

- Walk clients frequently with an appropriate number of people; have one team member state short, simple motor instructions. *Standing/weight bearing benefits gut motility, spasticity, and respiratory/bowel/bladder function, and promotes muscle stretching (Meyer, 2008).* **EB:** *Stroke survivors engaging in a verbal task while walking had poorer balance and gait velocity (Bowen et al, 2001).*

● = Independent ▲ = Collaborative **EBN** = Evidence-Based Nursing **EB** = Evidence-Based

- Cue and manually guide clients with neglect as they walk in corridors, etc. *Prevents clients bumping into objects/people.* **EB:** *Research subjects with left neglect, when driving a powered wheelchair veered left, whereas when walking, subjects veered right (Turton et al, 2009).*
- Document the number of helpers, level of assistance (maximum, standby, etc.), type of assistance, and devices needed on the care plan and room white board. *Communication and consistency promote client learning/safety and helps prevent staff injury (U.S. Department of Veterans Affairs, 2005).*
▲ Take pulse rate/rhythm and pulse oximetry before walking clients, and reassess within 5 minutes of walking, then ongoing as needed. If either are abnormal, have the client sit 5 minutes, then re-measure. If still abnormal, walk clients more slowly and with more help, or for a shorter time or notify physician. If uncontrolled diabetes/angina/arrhythmias/tachycardia (≥100 bpm) or resting SBP ≥200 mm Hg or DBP ≥110 mg Hg occur, do not initiate walking exercise. *Pulse rate and arterial blood oxygenation indicate cardiac/exercise tolerance; pulse oximetry identifies hypoxia early on so oxygen order can be obtained (Grimes, 2007; Schmitz, 2007).*
▲ Monitor the client's tolerance for walking. Initiate a 5–minute rest period if persistent dyspnea, pain or severe claudication, pale/diaphoretic skin, dizziness, syncope, or mental confusion occurs. If signs persist, stop walking therapy and notify the physician (Grimes, 2007). Refer to the care plan for **Activity intolerance**.
▲ Perform initial/ongoing screening for risk of falling and perform postfall assessments including meds and lab assays to prevent further falls. *Fall-assessment tools help identify persons at risk so prevention and protection measures can be implemented (Morse, 2006).* **EB:** *A study showed a nurse-led fall program that used the Morse Scale to identify high-risk clients significantly reduced multiple falls (Schwendimann et al, 2006).* **EBN:** *A study demonstrated that a 30-item post fall–assessment tool identified causes of falls and guided future nursing interventions (Gray-Miceli et al, 2006).*
- Individualize interventions to prevent falls such as scheduled toileting, balance/strength training, sleep hygiene, education on risk of medication/alcohol use, and removal of hazards (Browne et al, 2004; Resnick & Junlapeeya, 2004). **EBN:** *Assessment and root cause analysis indicated that inpatients who fell had gait problems, were confused, and were self-toileting; individualizing preventions decreased fall rates (Gowdy & Godfrey, 2003). Messecar (2003) reported results from a randomized blinded study that low-intensity exercise and incontinence care in residents in nursing homes reduced falls.* **EB:** *Following metaanalysis of clinical trials, Chang et al (2004), reported multifactorial fall-risk assessment/management was the most effective intervention for fall prevention.*

Geriatric

▲ Assess for swaying, poor balance, weakness, and fear of falling while elders stand/walk. If present, refer to physical therapy (PT). *Fear of falling and repeat fallers are common. Balance rehabilitation provides individualized treatment for persons with various diseases/deficits (Studer, 2008).*
▲ Review medications for polypharmacy and those that place elders at risk for falls, consult with pharmacy as needed. *Lyons (2004) reported the following medications increase risk for falls: sedatives/hypnotics, antidepressants, antipsychotics, neuroleptics, benzodiazepines, diuretics, antiarrhythmics, cardioglycosides, and antidiabetic agents.*
- Teach compensatory strategies for orthostatic hypotension. *Older adults develop arterial stiffness and reduced autonomic nervous system functioning. Their baroreceptors respond slowly so they are less able to maintain blood pressure when standing (Sclater & Alagiakrishnan, 2006).*
- Encourage walking while recognizing that older adults often walk slowly. *Slow gait may be related to fear of falling; decreased strength in hip extensors, hip abductors, or plantar flexor muscles, reduced balance or visual acuity, knee-flexion contractures and foot pain (Jones, 2001).*
- Assess risk, then implement fall precautions, such as using a visual identifier on clients starting exercise/education programs, clearing obstacles, and reviewing medication. *Previous falls, physiological changes, and adverse effects from multiple medications put elders at risk for falls (Radwanski, 2008).* **EB:** *A systematic review of studies concluded that strength training had many benefits, including reducing falls and symptoms of some prevalent chronic diseases in the elderly (Seguin & Nelson, 2003).*

Home Care

- Establish a support system for emergency and contingency care (e.g., Lifeline). *Impaired walking may pose a life threat during a crisis (e.g., fall, fire, orthostatic episode).*
- Assess for and modify any barriers to walking in the home environment. *Promotes safety.* **EB:** *Results from a study reported removal of home barriers improved elderly subjects occupational performance (Stark, 2004).*
- Stress the importance of adequate lighting and handrails, tacking down carpet edges, removing cords/clutter/throw/area rugs or using nonskid backings on rugs; adding adhesive nonslip strips to shower stalls/tubs/thresholds/steps/floors where coverings change height; applying nonskid wax to floors or installing nonglossy and nonglazed tiles, wood, linoleum, or low-pile carpeted surfaces. *Prophylaxis and removal of hazards may prevent falls (McCullagh, 2006).*
- ▲ Obtain orders for PT home visits for individualized strength, balance retraining, and an exercise plan. **EB:** *A Cochrane review indicated muscle strengthening and balance training supervised by health professional at home, was an intervention that helped reduce falls/fallers (Gillespie, Gillespie, & Robertson, 2003).*
- ▲ Make referrals for home health services for support and assistance with activities of daily living (ADLs). *This is a key component of discharge planning.* **EBN and EB:** *Results of systematic reviews indicated that access to health/social services was problematic (Naylor et al, 2005); low usage may relate to lack of awareness of availability (Brodaty et al, 2005) and could affect caregiver distress (Given & Sherwood, 2006).*
- ▲ Listen to and support client/caregivers; refer to support groups that meet or are online. Refer to care plan for **Caregiver role strain**.

Client/Family Teaching and Discharge Planning

- Teach clients to routinely check devices, e.g. remove dirt from and replace rubber tips of walkers and canes; check pushbutton locks on walkers with telescoping legs; and inspect prostheses for cracks, rough spots inside the socket, odd noises, and movement at joints or the foot. *Keeps devices in safe working order.*
- Teach diabetics that they are at risk for foot ulcers and train them in preventative interventions. **EB:** *Systematic literature review of diabetics indicated clients should be assessed/educated on risk factors for foot ulcers, foot care interventions, prescription footwear, podiatric care, and evaluation for surgical intervention (Singh, Armstrong, & Lipsky, 2005).*
- ▲ Instruct men/women at risk for osteoporosis or hip fractures to bear weight, walk, take calcium and vitamin D supplements, drink milk, stop smoking, and consult a physician for antiresorptive therapy. **EB:** *Older men surviving hip fractures rarely received antiresorptive therapy, or calcium or vitamin D supplements (Kiebzak et al, 2002). A review of clinical trials showed a 20% reduction for risk of falls in persons taking Vitamin D (Bischoff-Ferrari et al, 2004) and fewer falls occurred in subjects with intake of more than 500 mg calcium daily when taking alfacalcidol (Dukas et al, 2004).*
- For more information, please refer to the care plans for **Impaired Transfer ability** and **Impaired wheelchair Mobility**.

ⓔvolve   See the EVOLVE website for Weblinks for client education resources.

REFERENCES

Bischoff-Ferrari HA, Dawson-Hughes B, Willet WC et al: Effect of Vitamin D on falls: a meta-analysis. *J Am Med Assoc* 291(16):1999–2006, 2004.

Bonham P, Flemister, B: Guidelines for Management of Wounds in Patients with Lower Extremity Arterial Disease, *Clinical practice guidelines* (Series No 1), Glenview, IL, Wound Ostomy Continence Nurses Society, 2002.

Bowen A, Wenman R, Mickelborough J et al: Dual-task effects of talking while walking on velocity and balance following stroke, *Age Ageing* 30(4):319, 2001.

Brodaty H, Thomson C, Thompson C et al: Why caregivers of people with dementia and memory loss don't use services, *Int J Geriatr Psychiatry* 20(6):537–546, 2005.

Browne JA, Covington BG, Davila Y et al: Using information technology to assist in redesign of a fall prevention program, *J Nurs Care Qual* 19(3):218, 2004.

Chang JT, Morton SC, Rubenstein LZ et al: Interventions for the prevention of falls in older adults: Systematic review and meta-analysis of randomized clinical trials, *Br Med J* 328(7441):680, 2004.

● = Independent   ▲ = Collaborative   **EBN** = Evidence-Based Nursing   **EB** = Evidence-Based

Crowther M: Deep vein thrombosis: treatment. In Ackley BJ, Ladwig GB, Swan BA, editors: *Evidence-based nursing care guidelines: Medical-surgical interventions,* St Louis, 2008, Mosby.

Dukas L, Bischoff HA, Lindpaintner LS et al: Alfacalcidol reduces number of fallers in a community-dwelling elderly population with a minimum calcium intake of 500 mg daily, *J Am Geriatr Soc* 52(2):230–236, 2004.

Ejaz AA, Haley WE, Wasiluk A et al: Characteristics of 100 consecutive patients presenting with orthostatic hypotension, *Mayo Clin Proc* 79(7):890, 2004.

Gillespie LD, Gillespie WJ, Robertson MC: Interventions for preventing falls in elderly people, *Cochrane Database Syst Rev* (4):CD000340, 2003.

Given B, Sherwood PR: Family care for the older person with cancer, *Semin Oncol Nurs* 22(1):43–50, 2006.

Gowdy M, Godfrey S: Using tools to assess and prevent inpatient falls, *Jt Comm J Qual Saf* 29(7):363, 2003.

Graafmans WC, Lips P, Wijlhuizen GJ et al: Daily physical activity and the use of a walking aid in relation to falls in elderly people in a residential care setting, *Z Gerontol Geriatr* 36(1):23, 2003.

Gray-Miceli DL, Strumpf NE, Johnson J et al: Psychometric properties of the Post-Fall Index, *Clin Nurs Res* 15(3):157–176, 2006.

Grimes K: Heart disease. In O'Sullivan SB, Schmitz JT, editors: *Physical rehabilitation,* ed 5, Philadelphia, 2007, F.A. Davis Company.

Hoeman SP, Liszner K, Alverzo J: Functional mobility with activities of daily living. In Hoeman SP, editor: *Rehabilitation nursing: prevention, intervention, & outcomes,* ed 4, St Louis, 2008, Mosby.

International Food Information Council Foundation (IFIC): *IFIC review: physical activity, nutrition and bone health,* Washington, DC, April 2002. http://ific.org/publications/reviews/bonehealthir.cfm. Accessed March 18, 2009.

Irvin DJ, White M: The importance of accurately assessing orthostatic hypotension, *Geriatr Nurs* 25(2):99, 2004.

Johnson JJ, Psustian C: Guidelines for management of wounds in patients with lower extremity venous disease. In Wound, Ostomy, and Continence Nurses Society (WOCN): *Clinical practice guidelines* (Series No 4). Glenview, IL, 2005, Wound Ostomy and Continence Nurses Society.

Jones DA: Successful aging: maintaining mobility in a geriatric patient population, *Rehabil Manag* 14(9):46, 2001.

Kiebzak GM, Beinart GA, Perser K et al: Undertreatment of osteoporosis in men with hip fracture, *Arch Intern Med* 162(19):2217, 2002.

Kreger A: Choosing mobility, *Rehabil Manag* 19(3):34, 2006.

Ladenheim E, Oberti-Smith K, Tablada G: Results of managing transtibial amputations with a prefabricated polyethylene rigid removable dressing, *J Prosthet Orthot* 19(1):2–4, 2007.

Lyons SS: *Fall prevention for older adults,* University of Iowa Gerontological Nursing Interventions Research Center, Research Dissemination Core, Iowa City, IA, 2004, University of Iowa.

McCullagh MC: Home Modification, *Am J Nurs* 106(10):54–63, 2006.

Messecar D: An exercise and incontinence intervention did not reduce the incidence or cost of acute conditions in nursing home residents, *Evid Based Nurs* 6(4):116–117, 2003.

Meyer A: Stand for health, *Rehabil Manag* 21(7):16–20, 2008.

Morse JM: The safety of safety research: the case of patient fall research, *Can J Nurs Res* 38(2):74, 2006.

Naylor MD, Stephens C, Bowles KH et al: Cognitively impaired older adults: from hospital to home, *Am J Nurs* 105(2):52–61, 2005.

Olson RS: Muscle and skeletal function. In Hoeman SP, editor: *Rehabilitation nursing: prevention, intervention, & outcomes,* ed 4, St Louis, 2008, Mosby.

Prandoni P, Lensing AW, Prins MH et al: Below-knee elastic compression stockings to prevent the post-thrombotic syndrome: a randomized, controlled trial, *Ann Intern Med* 141(4):249–256, 2004.

Radwanski ML: Gerontological rehabilitation nursing. In Hoeman SP, editor: *Rehabilitation nursing: Prevention, intervention, & outcomes,* ed 4, St Louis, 2008, Mosby.

Resnick B, Junlapeeya P: Falls in a community of older adults: findings and implications for practice, *Appl Nurs Res* 17(2):81, 2004.

Romera A, Vila R, Perez-Piqueras A et al: Early mobilization in patients with acute deep vein thrombosis: Does it increase the incidence of symptomatic pulmonary embolism? *Phlebology* 20(3):141, Abstract, 2005.

Schmitz TJ: Vital signs. In O'Sullivan SB, Schmitz TJ, editors: *Physical Rehabilitation,* ed 5, Philadelphia, 2007, F.A. Davis Company.

Schwendimann R, Milisen K, Buhler H et al: Fall prevention in a Swiss acute care hospital setting: Reducing multiple falls, *J Gerontol Nurs* 32(3):13–22, 2006.

Sclater A, Alagiakrishnan K: Orthostatic hypotension: a primary care primer for assessment and treatment, *Geriatrics* 59(8):22, 2006.

Seguin R, Nelson M: The benefits of strength training for older adults, *Am J Prev Med* 25(3 Suppl 2):141–149, 2003.

Shannon JR, Diedrich A, Biaggioni I et al: Water drinking as a treatment for orthostatic syndromes, *Am J Med* 112(5):355, 2002.

Singh N, Armstrong DG, Lipsky BA: Preventing foot ulcers in patients with diabetes, *J Am Med Assoc* 293(2):217–228, 2005.

Stark S: Removing environmental barriers in the homes of older adults with disabilities improves occupational performance, *OTJR: Occupation, Participation and Health* 24(1):32–39, 2004.

Studer M: Keep it moving: advances in gait training techniques help clients reduce balance issues, *Rehabil Manag* 21(5):10–15, 2008.

Trujillo-Santos AJ, Martos-Perez F, Perea-Milla E et al: Bed rest or early mobilization as treatment of deep vein thrombosis: a systematic review and meta-analysis, *Med Clin (Barc)* 122(17):641–647, 2004.

Trujillo-Santos AJ, Perea-Milla E, Mimenez-Puente A et al: Bed rest or ambulation in the initial treatment of patients with acute deep vein thrombosis or pulmonary embolism: Findings from the RIETE registry, *Chest* 127(5):1631–1636, 2005.

Tsai HA, Kirby RL, MacLeod DA et al: Aided gait of people with lower-limb amputations: comparisons of 4–footed and 2–wheeled walkers, *Arch Phys Med Rehabil* 84(4):584, 2003.

Turton AJ, Dewar SJ, Lievesley A et al: Walking and wheelchair navigation in patients with left visual neglect, *Neuropsychol Rehabil* 19(2):274–290, 2009.

U. S. Department of Veterans Affairs: *Safe patient handling and movement: Patient care ergonomics resource guide: Ergo guide,* Part 1, Chap 6, The Veterans Integrated Service Network 8 Patient Safety Center of Inquiry, Tampa FL, 2005. www.visn8.med.va.gov/patientsafetycenter/resguide/ErgoGuidePtone.pdf. Accessed April 3, 2009.

Weimer LH, Zadeh P: Neurological aspects of syncope and orthostatic intolerance. *Med Clin North Am* 93(2):427–449, 2009.

Wandering   *Donna Algase, PhD*

NANDA-I

Definition

Meandering; aimless or repetitive locomotion that exposes the individual to harm; frequently incongruent with boundaries, limits, or obstacles

Defining Characteristics

Frequent or continuous movement from place to place, often revisiting the same destinations; persistent locomotion in search of "missing" or unattainable people or places; haphazard locomotion; locomotion in unauthorized or private spaces; locomotion resulting in unintended leaving of a premise; long periods of locomotion without an apparent destination; fretful locomotion or pacing; inability to locate significant landmarks in a familiar setting; locomotion that cannot be easily dissuaded or redirected; following behind or shadowing a caregiver's locomotion; trespassing; hyperactivity; scanning, seeking, or searching behaviors; periods of locomotion interspersed with periods of nonlocomotion (e.g., sitting, standing, sleeping); getting lost

Related Factors (r/t)

Cognitive impairment, specifically memory and recall deficits, disorientation, poor visuoconstructive (or visuospatial) ability, and language (primarily expressive) defects; cortical atrophy; premorbid behavior (e.g., outgoing, sociable personality); separation from familiar people and places; sedation; emotional state, especially fear, anxiety, boredom, or depression (agitation); overstimulating/understimulating social or physical environment; physiological state or need (e.g., hunger/thirst, pain, urination, constipation); time of day

NOC   (Nursing Outcomes Classification)

Suggested NOC Outcomes

Caregiver Home Care Readiness, Fall Prevention Behavior, Falls Occurrence

Example NOC Outcome with Indicators
Caregiver Home Care Readiness as evidenced by the following indicators: Knowledge of recommended treatment regimen/Knowledge of prescribed activity/Knowledge of emergency care/Confidence in ability to manage care at home (Rate the outcome and indicators of **Caregiver Home Care Readiness:** 1 = not adequate, 2 = slightly adequate, 3 = moderately adequate, 4 = substantially adequate, 5 = totally adequate [see Section I].)

Client Outcomes

Client Will (Specify Time Frame):

- Decrease incidence of falls (preferably free of falls)
- Decrease incidence of elopements
- Maintain appropriate body weight

Caregiver Will (Specify Time Frame):

- Be able to explain interventions he or she can use to provide a safe environment for a care receiver who displays wandering behavior

NIC   (Nursing Interventions Classification)

Suggested NIC Intervention

Dementia Management

• = Independent   ▲ = Collaborative   **EBN** = Evidence-Based Nursing   **EB** = Evidence-Based

Example NIC Activities—Dementia Management
Place identification bracelet on the patient; Provide space for safe pacing and wandering

Nursing Interventions and *Rationales*

- Assess and document the amount (frequency and duration), percentage of hours with wandering, pattern (random, lapping, or pacing), and 24–hour distribution of wandering behavior over 3 days. **EBN:** *Assessment over time provides a baseline against which behavior change can be evaluated (Algase et al, 1997, 2009). Such assessment can also reveal the time of day when wandering is greatest and when surveillance or other precautionary measures are most necessary. Extremes in rate, duration, and percentage of hours with wandering distinguish three types of wanderers: classic, moderate, and subclinical, who also vary by degree of cognitive impairment (worse for classics), mobility (best for classics, and general and specific health parameters (worse for classics) (Algase et al, in press).*
- Document particular aspects of wandering that are troubling. **EBN:** *Such instruments as the Algase Wandering Scale (Long-Term Care or Community Version) (Algase et al, 2004; Algase, Moore et al, 2007) can indicate whether the behavior is persistent, spatially disordered, or prone to elopement. The Everyday Spatial Questionnaire (Chiu et al, 2005) or the Wayfinding Effectiveness Scale (Algase, Son et al, 2007) can be used to assess the nature of navigational deficits. Information from such instruments can direct caregivers toward more appropriate intervention strategies.*
- Obtain a history of personality characteristics and behavioral responses to stress. **EBN and EB:** *Information about long-standing behavioral tendencies may reveal circumstances under which wandering will occur and can aid in interpreting both positive and negative meanings of wandering behavior of the client (Kolanowski, Strand, & Whall, 1997; Thomas, 1997; Song & Algase, 2008).*
- Evaluate for neurocognitive strengths and limitations, particularly language, attention, visuospatial skills, and perseveration. **EBN:** *Wanderers may have expressive language deficits that hamper their ability to communicate needs (Algase, 1992).* **EBN and EB:** *Knowledge of attentional and visuospatial deficits, which may account for certain patterns of wandering or way-finding deficits, can lead to identification of appropriate environmental modifications that could enhance functional ambulation, such as elimination of distractions and enhancement of cues marking desired destinations (Henderson, Mack & Williams, 1989; Fischer, Marterer & Danielczyk, 1990; Passini et al, 2000; Kavcic & Duffy, 2003; Mapstone, Steffenella & Duffy, 2003; Monacelli, Cushman, & Kavcic, 2003, Algase et al, 2004; Chiu et al, 2004).* **EB:** *The presence of perseveration may indicate that the wanderer is unable to voluntarily stop his or her behavior (Passini et al, 1995; Ryan et al, 1995), thus calling for nursing judgment as to when wandering should be interrupted to enhance the wanderer's safety, comfort, or wellbeing.*
- Assess for physical distress or needs, such as hunger, thirst, pain, discomfort, or elimination. **EBN:** *Although physical needs have not been documented in relation to wandering, the Need-Driven Dementia-Compromised Model hypothesizes this relationship (Algase et al, 1996).*
- Assess for emotional or psychological distress, such as anxiety, fear, or feeling lost. **EB:** *Anxiety and depression frequently accompany wandering (Teri et al, 1999).*
- Observe wandering episodes for antecedents and consequences. **EBN and EB:** *People, events, or circumstances surrounding the onset or conclusion of wandering may provide clues about triggers or rewards that are stimulating or reinforcing wandering behavior (Hirst & Metcalf, 1989; Heard & Watson, 1999).*
- Observe the location where and environmental conditions in which wandering is occurring and modify those that appear to induce wandering. **EBN:** *In a recent observational study wanderers were less likely to wander from where the likelihood of social interaction was greater (i.e., activities room, dayroom, staff area); where the environment was more soothing (i.e., their own room); or where rooms had a designated purpose (e.g., dayrooms, the wanderer's own room, activities and staff areas) (Algase, Beattie, & Antonakos, in review). In the same study, wandering was less likely when lighting was low and variation in sound levels was small.*
- Apply observed consequences of wandering, such as personal attention, food, and so forth, at times when the person is not wandering, and withhold them while the person is wandering. **EB:** *Differential reinforcement of other behavior (nonwandering) can reduce wandering episodes by 50% to 80% (Heard & Watson, 1999).*

- = Independent   ▲ = Collaborative   **EBN** = Evidence-Based Nursing   **EB** = Evidence-Based

- Assess regularly for the presence of or potential for negative outcomes of wandering, such as declining social skills, falls, elopement, and getting lost. **EB:** *Wanderers are at greater risk for falls than other cognitively impaired persons (Kippenbrock & Soja, 1993; Rowe & Bennet, 2003; Rowe, Feinglass & Wiss, 2004). Wanderers have also shown greater loss in social skills over time than nonwandering counterparts (Cornbleth, 1977).*

- Weigh the client at defined intervals to detect onset of weight loss, and watch for symptoms associated with inadequate food intake, including constipation, dehydration, muscle wasting, and starvation. *Wandering behavior can affect the client's ability to eat, when the client is unable to sit at a table for the time needed to eat a meal (Beattie & Algase, 2002).*

- For the client who displays wandering behavior during mealtimes, use behavioral interventions to shape behavior, including verbal statements, nonverbal social behavior, and systematic extinguishing of undesirable client behavior. **EBN:** *Results of a study using behavior interventions demonstrated that they were effective in increasing the time the client sat at the table, and the amount of food the client ate (Beattie, Algase & Song, 2004).*

- Provide for safe ambulation with comfortable and well-fitting clothes, shoes with nonskid soles and foot support, and any necessary walking aids (e.g., a cane, walker, or Merry Walker). *Wanderers are at increased risk for falls (Katz et al, 2004).*

- Provide safe and secure surroundings that deter accidental elopements, using perimeter control devices, camouflage, or electronic tracking systems. **EBN:** *Eloping can have hazardous outcomes, including death (Rowe & Glover, 2001).* **EB:** *Perimeter control devices can effectively reduce or prevent exiting behavior (Negley, Molla, & Obenchain, 1990).* **EBN and EB:** *However, under some circumstances, these devices are viewed as unnecessarily restrictive, and more passive means, such as camouflage, have been substituted. Camouflage techniques, such as masking the doorknob or creating striped floor patterns in front of exits, have been used with success (Hussian & Brown, 1987; Namazi, Rosner, & Calkins, 1989), particularly in subjects with Alzheimer's disease (Hewewasam, 1996), but the effectiveness may be mitigated by other architectural features of the setting (Chafetz, 1990; Hamilton, 1993). A Cochrane review found that no randomized controlled trials have been done to validate the effectiveness of subjective barriers to prevent wandering in cognitively impaired clients (Price, Hermans, & Grimley Evans, 2000). Newer electronic monitoring and tracking systems are highly effective and reduce caregiver burden (Altus et al, 2000; Nelson et al, 2004; Siders et al, 2004).*

- During periods of inactivity, position the wanderer so that desirable destinations (e.g., bathroom) are within the client's line of vision and undesirable destinations (e.g., exits or stairwells) are out of sight. **EBN and EB:** *Functional, nonwandering ambulation is possible even into late-stage dementia and may be facilitated by keeping appropriate visual cues accessible (Passini et al, 2000; Algase, 1999).*

- If wandering takes a random or haphazard route, reduce environmental distractions and increase relevant environmental cues. Note and eliminate stimuli that distract the wanderer while in route. Provide afternoon rest periods if assessment reveals that random-pattern wandering worsens as the day progresses. **EBN:** *Random-pattern wandering may be affected by environmental stimuli (Algase, 1999). The proportion of wandering that is random increases as the day progresses (Algase et al, 1997; Algase, 1999) and may indicate fatigue.*

- Enhance institutional settings with areas that provide interesting views and opportunities to sit. **EB:** *Enhanced environments can improve mood, and they encourage wanderers to linger or sit more than purely institutional surroundings do (Cohen-Mansfield & Werner, 1998).*

- Engage wanderers in social interaction and structured activity, especially when wanderers appear distressed or otherwise uncomfortable, or their wandering presents a challenge to others in the setting. **EBN and EB:** *Wandering and social interaction are inversely related. Wanderers often have an outgoing or sociable personality and also have deficits in expressive language skills. Thus although they may prefer social interaction, their ability to initiate it may be compromised (Algase, 1992; Thomas, 1997).*

- If wandering has a pacing quality, attempt to identify and address any underlying problems or concerns. Offer stress-reducing approaches, such as music, massage, or rocking. Attempts to distract or redirect the pacing wanderer may worsen wandering. **EBN:** *Pacing, as a wandering pattern, is not associated with level of cognitive impairment and may reflect anxiety, agitation, pain, or another internal process (Gerdner, 2000; Algase, Beattie, & Therrien, 2001).*

• = Independent ▲ = Collaborative **EBN** = Evidence-Based Nursing **EB** = Evidence-Based

- If wandering is a recently acquired behavior or if it increases in intensity over previous levels, evaluate for constipation, pneumonia, or acute physical problems. **EBN and EB:** *Persons who first exhibit wandering within 3 months after admission to a nursing home are more likely than others to have developed physical problems that stimulate wandering (Keily, Morris, & Algase, 2000).*

- If wandering has a lapping or circuitous pattern, signs or labels may be effective. Substitute another repetitive activity, such as folding or rocking, if lapping becomes problematic or excessive. **EBN:** *Not all wanderers display lapping-pattern wandering, and when it does occur, it tends to occur early in the day or to follow rest periods. Thus it may be a more functional pattern than random wandering and may indicate a slightly better level of cognitive function for the individual, even if transient. Thus wanderers who lap may be better able to use information in the environment (Algase, Beattie, & Therrien, 2001).* **EB:** *However, this pattern of wandering may also be a form of perseveration, and therefore the person may be unable to disengage voluntarily (Passini et al, 1995; Ryan et al, 1995).*

- Provide a regularly scheduled and supervised exercise or walking program, particularly if wandering occurs excessively during the night or at times that are inconvenient in the setting. **EBN and EB:** *Although exercise or walking programs do not reduce daytime wandering, they have been shown to reduce or eliminate nighttime wandering (Robb, 1987; Carillon Nursing and Rehabilitation Center, 2000) and to decrease general agitation levels (Holmberg, 1997).*

- Use slow-stroke, hand, or foot massage before the times of day or events that induce wandering. **EBN and EB:** *Various massage techniques have been shown to reduce wandering and diffuse agitation in persons with dementia (Malaquin-Pavan, 1997; Kilstoff & Chenoweth, 1998; Rowe & Alfred, 1999; Sutherland, Reakes, & Bridges, 1999).*

 Multicultural

- Recognize that wandering occurs with little variation in expression among individuals with dementia regardless of culture or ethnicity. **EB:** *Wandering has been reported in multiple populations and varies little by cultural group (Song et al, 2003; Chiu et al, 2004; Greiner et al, 2007; Young et al, 2008).*

- Assess for the influence of cultural beliefs, norms, and values on the family's understanding of wandering behavior. **EBN:** *Latina caregivers of people with dementia delay institutionalization significantly longer than female Caucasian caregivers. In addition, Latino cultural values and positive views of the caregiving role are important factors that may significantly influence their decision to institutionalize loved ones with dementia (Mausbach et al, 2004). Another study found that black and Latino community-dwelling clients with moderate to severe dementia have a higher prevalence of wandering and other dementia-related behaviors (Sink et al, 2004).*

- ▲ Refer the family to social services or other supportive services to assist with the impact of caregiving for the wandering client.

- Encourage the family to use support groups or other service programs.

 Home Care

- Help the caregiver set up a plan to deal with wandering behavior using the interventions mentioned earlier.

- Assess the home environment for modifications that will protect the client and prevent elopement. *Security devices are available to notify the caregiver of the client's movements (e.g., alarms at doors, bed alarms).*

- Assist the family to set up a plan of exercise for the client, including safe walking. *Walking is a valuable source of exercise, even for clients with dementia (Oddy, 2004).*

- Enroll wanderers in the Safe Return Program of the Alzheimer's Association, and help the caregiver develop a plan of action to use if the client elopes. **EBN:** *The Safe Return Program has assisted in locating numerous persons who have eloped from their homes or other residential care settings. Mortality rates are high if there is failure to locate elopers within the first 24 hours (Rowe & Glover, 2001).*

- Help the caregiver develop a plan of action to use if the client elopes.

- ▲ Refer for homemaker or psychiatric home health care services for respite, client reassurance, and implementation of a therapeutic regimen. Refer to the care plan for **Caregiver role strain**. *Responsibility for a person at high risk for wandering provides high caregiver stress. Respite care decreases*

• = Independent   ▲ = Collaborative   **EBN** = Evidence-Based Nursing   **EB** = Evidence-Based

caregiver stress. The presence of caring individuals is reassuring to both the client and caregivers, especially during periods of client anxiety. Wandering behavior can make use of the interventions described previously, modified for the home setting.

Client/Family Teaching and Discharge Planning

- Inform the client and family of the meaning of and reasons for wandering behavior. *An understanding of wandering behavior will enable the client and family to provide the client with a safe environment.*
- Teach the caregiver/family methods to deal with wandering behavior using the interventions mentioned in Nursing Interventions and Rationales.

ⓔvolve   See the EVOLVE website for Weblinks for client education resources.

REFERENCES

Algase D, Antonakos C, Beattie E et al: Empirical derivation and validation of a wandering typology, *J Am Geriatr Soc* in press.

Algase DL: Cognitive discriminants of wandering among nursing home residents, *Nurs Res* 41(2):78, 1992.

Algase DL: Wandering: a dementia-compromised behavior, *J Gerontol Nurs* 25(9):10, 1999.

Algase DL, Antonakos C, Beattie ERA et al: New parameters for daytime wandering, *Res Gerontol Nurs* 2(1):58–68, 2009.

Algase DL, Beattie E, Antonakos C: Wandering and the physical environment, in review.

Algase DL, Beattie ER, Bogue EL et al: The Algase Wandering Scale: initial psychometrics of a new caregiver reporting tool, *Am J Alzheimers Dis Other Demen* 16(3):141–152, 2001.

Algase DL, Beattie ERA, Therrien B: Impact of cognitive impairment on wandering behavior, *West J Nurs Res* 23:283, 2001.

Algase DL, Beck C, Kolanowski A et al: Need-driven dementia-compromised behavior: an alternative view of disruptive behavior, *Am J Alzheimers Dis Other Demen* 11(6):10–19, 1996.

Algase DL, Kupferschmid B, Beel-Bates CA et al: Estimates of stability of daily wandering behavior among cognitively impaired long-term care residents, *Nurs Res* 46(3):172–178, 1997.

Algase DL, Moore HD, Gavin-Dreschnack D et al: Wandering definitions and terms. In Nelson AL, Algase DL, editors: *Evidence-based protocols for managing wandering behaviors*, New York, 2007, Springer.

Algase DL, Son GR, Beattie E et al: The interrelatedness of wandering and wayfinding in a community sample of persons with dementia, *Dement Geriatr Cogn Disord* 17(3):231–239, 2004b.

Algase DL Son GR, Beel-Bates C et al: Initial psychometric evaluation of the wayfinding effectiveness scale, *West J Nurs Res,* 29(8):1015–1032, 2007.

Altus DE, Mathews RM, Xaverius PK et al: Evaluating an electronic monitoring system for people who wander, *Am J Alzheimers Dis* 15(2):121–125, 2000.

Beattie ERA, Algase DL: Improving table-sitting behavior of wanderers via theoretic substruction, *J Gerontol Nurs* 28(10):6, 2002.

Beattie ERA, Algase DL, Song J: Keeping wandering nursing home residents at the table: improving food intake using a behavior communication intervention, *Aging Ment Health* 8(2):109, 2004.

Carillon Nursing and Rehabilitation Center: Nature walk: from aimless wandering to purposeful walking, *Nurs Homes Long Term Care Manage* 49(11):50, 2000.

Chafetz PK: Two dimensional grid is ineffective against demented patients' exiting through glass doors, *Psychol Aging* 5:146, 1990.

Chiu Y, Algase D, Whall A et al: Getting lost: directed attention and executive function in early Alzheimer's disease patients, *Dement Geriatr Cogn Disord* 17(3):174–180, 2004.

Chiu YC, Algase D, Liang J et al: Conceptualization and measurement of getting lost behavior in persons with early dementia, *Int J Geriatr Psychiatry* 20(8):760–768, 2005.

Cohen-Mansfield J, Werner P: The effects of an enhanced environment on nursing home residents who pace, *Gerontologist* 38(2):199, 1998.

Cornbleth T: Effects of a protected hospital ward area on wandering and non-wandering geriatric patients, *J Gerontol* 32:573, 1977.

Fischer P, Marterer A, Danielczyk W: Right-left disorientation in dementia of the Alzheimer's type, *Neurology* 40:1619, 1990.

Gerdner LA: Effects of individualized versus classical "relaxation" music on the frequency of agitation in elderly persons with Alzheimer's disease and related disorders, *Int Psychogeriatr* 12(1):49, 2000.

Greiner C, Makimoto K, Suzuki M et al: Feasibility study of the integrated circuit tag monitoring system for dementia residents in Japan, *Am J Alzheimers Dis Other Demen* 22(2):129–136, 2007.

Hamilton C: *The use of tape patterns as an alternative method for controlling wanderers' exiting behavior in a dementia care unit* [unpublished master's thesis], Blacksburg, VA, 1993, Virginia Polytechnic Institute and State University.

Heard K, Watson TS: Reducing wandering by persons with dementia using differential reinforcement, *J Appl Behav Anal* 32(9):381, 1999.

Henderson V, Mack W, Williams BW: Spatial disorientation in Alzheimer's disease, *Arch Neurol* 46:391, 1989.

Hewewasam L: Floor patterns limit wandering of people with Alzheimer's, *Nurs Times* 92:41, 1996.

Hirst ST, Metcalf BJ: Whys and whats of wandering, *Geriatr Nurs* 10(5):237, 1989.

Holmberg SK: Evaluation of a clinical intervention for wanderers on a geriatric nursing unit, *Arch Psychiatr Nurs* 11:21, 1997.

Hussian RA, Brown DC: Use of two dimensional grid patterns to limit hazardous ambulation in demented patients, *J Gerontol* 42:558, 1987.

Katz IR, Rupnow M, Kozma C et al: Risperidone and falls in ambulatory nursing home residents with dementia and psychosis or agitation: secondary analysis of a double-blind, placebo-controlled trial, *Am J Geriatr Psychiatry* 12(5):499–508, 2004.

Kavcic V, Duffy CJ: Attentional dynamics and visual perception: mechanisms of spatial disorientation in Alzheimer's disease, *Brain* 126 (pt 5):1173–1181, 2003.

Keily DK, Morris JN, Algase DL: Resident characteristics associated with wandering in nursing homes, *Int J Geriatr Psychiatry* 15:1013, 2000.

Kilstoff K, Chenoweth L: New approaches to health and well-being for dementia day-care clients, family carers and day care staff, *Int J Nurs Pract* 4(2):72, 1998.

Kippenbrock T, Soja M: Preventing falls in the elderly: interviewing patients who have fallen, *Geriatr Nurs* 14:205, 1993.

Kolanowski AM, Strand G, Whall A: A pilot study of the relation in premorbid characteristics to behavior in dementia, *J Gerontol Nurs* 23:21, 1997.

Malaquin-Pavan E: Therapeutic benefit of touch-massage in the overall management of demented elderly, *Rech Soins Infirm* 49:11, 1997.

Mapstone M, Steffenella TM, Duffy CJ: A visuospatial variant of mild cognitive impairment: getting lost between aging and AD, *Neurology* 60(5):802–808, 2003.

Mausbach BT, Coon DW, Depp C et al: Ethnicity and time to institutionalization of dementia patients: a comparison of Latina and Caucasian female family caregivers, *J Am Geriatr Soc* 52(7):1077–1084, 2004.

Monacelli AM, Cushman LA, Kavcic V: Spatial disorientation in Alzheimer's disease: the remembrance of things passed, *Neurology* 61(11):1491–1497, 2003.

Namazi KH, Rosner TT, Calkins MP: Visual barriers to prevent ambulatory Alzheimer's patients from exiting through an emergency door, *Gerontologist* 29:699, 1989.

Negley E, Molla PM, Obenchain J: No exit: the effects of an electronic security system on confused patients, *J Gerontol Nurs* 16:21, 1990.

Nelson A, Powell-Cope G, Gavin-Dreschnack D et al: Technology to promote safe mobility in the elderly, *Nurs Clin North Am* 39(3):649–671, 2004.

Oddy R: Walk this way: assisted exercise for all people with dementia, *J Dement Care* 12(1):21, 2004.

Passini R, Pigot H, Rainville C et al: Wayfinding in a nursing home for advanced dementia of the Alzheimer's type, *Environ Behav* 32(5):684–710, 2000.

Passini R, Rainville C, Marchand N et al: Wayfinding in dementia of the Alzheimer's type: planning abilities, *J Clin Exp Neuropsychol* 17(6):820–832, 1995.

Price JC, Hermans DG, Grimley Evans J: Subjective barriers to prevent wandering of cognitively impaired people, *Cochrane Database Syst Rev* (4):CD001932, 2000.

Robb SS: Exercise treatment for wandering. In Altman HJ, editor: *Alzheimer's disease: problems, prospects, and perspectives,* New York, 1987, Plenum.

Rowe M, Alfred D: The effectiveness of slow stroke massage in diffusing agitated behaviors in individuals with Alzheimer's disease, *J Gerontol Nurs* 25(6):22, 1999.

Rowe MA, Bennett V: A look at deaths occurring in persons with dementia lost in the community, *Am J Alzheimers Dis Other Demen* 18(6):343–348, 2003.

Rowe MA, Feinglass NG, Wiss ME: Persons with dementia who become lost in the community: a case study, current research, and recommendations, *Mayo Clin Proc* 79(11):1417–1422, 2004.

Rowe MA, Glover JC: Antecedents, descriptions and consequences of wandering in cognitively-impaired adults and the Safe Return (SR) program, *Am J Alzheimers Dis* 16(6):344, 2001.

Ryan JP, McGowan J, McCaffrey N et al: Graphomotor perseveration and wandering in Alzheimer's disease, *J Geriatr Psychiatry Neurol* 8(4):209–212, 1995.

Siders C, Nelson A, Brown LM et al: Evidence for implementing nonpharmacological interventions for wandering, *Rehabil Nurs* 29(6):195–206, 2004.

Sink KM, Covinsky KE, Newcomer R et al: Ethnic differences in the prevalence and pattern of dementia-related behaviors, *J Am Geriatr Soc* 52(8):1277–1283, 2004.

Song JA, Algase DL: Premorbid characteristics and wandering behavior in persons with dementia, *J Psychos Nurs* 22(6):318–327, 2008.

Song J, Algase DL, Beattie ERA et al: Comparison of U.S., Canadian and Australian participants' performance on the Algase Wandering Scale-version 2 (AWS-V2), *Res Theory Nurs Pract* 17:241–256, 2003.

Sutherland JA, Reakes J, Bridges C: Foot acupressure and massage for patients with Alzheimer's disease and related dementias, *J Nurs Sch* 31(4):34, 1999.

Teri L, Ferretti LE, Gibbons LE et al: Anxiety of Alzheimer's disease: prevalence and comorbidity, *J Gerontol A Biol Sci Med Sci* 54(7):M348–M342, 1999.

Thomas DW: Understanding the wandering patient: a continuity of personality perspective, *J Gerontol Nurs* 23(1):16, 1997.

Yang CH, Hwang JP, Tsai S J, et al: Wandering and associated factors in psychiatric inpatients with dementia of Alzheimer's type in Taiwan: Clinical implications for management, *Journal of Nervous Mental Disorder* 187(11):695–697, 1999

Young ML, Son GR, Song JA, et al: Factors affecting burden of family caregivers of community-dwelling ambulatory elders with dementia in Korea, *Archives of Psychiatric Nursing* 22(4):226–234, 2008.

Nursing Diagnoses Arranged by Maslow's Hierarchy of Needs

Because human beings adapt in many ways to establish and maintain the self, health problems are much more than simple physical matters. Maslow's Hierarchy of Needs (see diagram below) is a system of classifying human needs. Maslow's hierarchy is based on the idea that lower-level physiological needs must be met before higher-level, abstract needs can be met.

For nurses, Maslow's hierarchy has special significance in decision making and planning for care. By considering need categories as you identify client problems, you will be able to provide more holistic care. For example, a client who demands frequent attention for a seemingly trivial matter may require help with self-esteem needs. Need levels vary from client to client. If a client is short of breath, the client is probably not interested in or capable of discussing spirituality. In addition, a client's need level may change throughout planning and intervention, so you will need to be vigilant in your assessment.

Read the descriptions of each category in the diagram and see how you would relate them to nursing diagnoses. Compare your evaluation with how the authors categorized the nursing diagnoses according to this hierarchy. Be sure to assess clients for potential problems at all levels of the pyramid, regardless of their initial complaint.

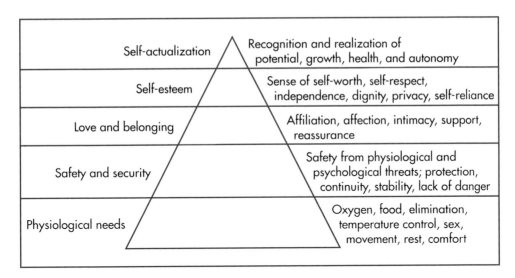

Reprinted with permission from *Nursing diagnosis reference manual,* copyright 1991, Springhouse Corp. All rights reserved.

Physiological Needs

Activity intolerance
Activity intolerance, risk for
Airway clearance, ineffective
Allergy response, latex
Aspiration, risk for
Bleeding, risk for
Body temperature, imbalanced, risk for
Bowel incontinence
Breastfeeding, effective
Breastfeeding, ineffective
Breastfeeding, interrupted
Breathing pattern, ineffective
Cardiac output, decreased
Comfort, impaired
Comfort, readiness for enhanced
Constipation
Constipation, perceived
Constipation, risk for
Dentition, impaired
Diarrhea
Electrolyte imbalance, risk for
Fatigue
Feeding pattern, infant, ineffective
Fluid balance, readiness for enhanced
Fluid volume, deficient
Fluid volume, excess
Fluid volume, deficient, risk for
Fluid volume, imbalanced, risk for
Gas exchange, impaired
Glucose level, blood, unstable, risk for
Hyperthermia
Hypothermia
Immunization status, readiness for
    enhanced

Incontinence, urinary, functional
Incontinence, urinary, overflow
Incontinence, urinary, reflex
Incontinence, urinary, stress
Incontinence, urinary, urge
Incontinence, urinary, urge, risk for
Infant behavior, disorganized
Infant behavior, disorganized, risk for
Infant behavior, organized, readiness
    for enhanced
Insomnia
Intracranial adaptive capacity,
    decreased
Jaundice, neonatal
Liver function, impaired, risk for
Mobility, bed, impaired
Mobility, physical, impaired
Mobility, wheelchair, impaired
Motility, gastrointestinal, dysfunctional
Motility, gastrointestinal, dysfunctional,
    risk for
Nausea
Nutrition: less than body requirements,
    imbalanced
Nutrition: more than body require-
    ments, imbalanced
Nutrition: more than body require-
    ments, imbalanced, risk for
Oral mucous membrane, impaired
Pain, acute
Pain, chronic
Perfusion, renal, ineffective, risk for
Perfusion, tissue, cardiac, decreased,
    risk for

Perfusion, tissue, cerebral, ineffective,
    risk for
Perfusion, tissue, gastrointestinal, inef-
    fective, risk for
Perfusion, tissue, peripheral, ineffective
Protection, ineffective
Self-Care deficit, bathing
Self-Care deficit, dressing
Self-Care deficit, feeding
Self-Care deficit, toileting
Sensory perception, disturbed (specify):
    visual, auditory, kinesthetic, gusta-
    tory, tactile, olfactory
Sexual dysfunction
Sexuality pattern, ineffective
Shock, risk for
Skin integrity, impaired
Skin integrity, impaired, risk for
Sleep deprivation
Sleep, readiness for enhanced
Surgical recovery, delayed
Swallowing, impaired
Thermoregulation, ineffective
Tissue integrity, impaired
Transfer ability, impaired
Trauma, vascular, risk for
Urinary elimination, impaired
Urinary elimination, readiness for
    enhanced
Urinary retention
Ventilation, spontaneous, impaired
Ventilatory weaning response,
    dysfunctional
Walking, impaired

Safety and Security Needs

Allergy response, latex, risk for
Anxiety
Anxiety, death
Autonomic dysreflexia
Autonomic dysreflexia, risk for
Communication, readiness for
    enhanced
Communication, verbal, impaired
Confusion, acute
Confusion, acute, risk for
Confusion, chronic
Contamination
Contamination, risk for
Death syndrome, infant, sudden,
    risk for
Disuse syndrome, risk for

Environmental interpretation syn-
    drome, impaired
Falls, risk for
Family processes, dysfunctional
Fear
Grieving
Grieving, complicated
Grieving, complicated, risk for
Growth, disproportionate, risk for
Health maintenance, ineffective
Home maintenance, impaired
Infection, risk for
Injury, risk for
Injury, positioning, perioperative,
    risk for
Knowledge, deficient

Knowledge, readiness for enhanced
Memory, impaired
Neglect, self
Neglect, unilateral
Peripheral neurovascular dysfunction,
    risk for
Poisoning, risk for
Religiosity, impaired
Religiosity, impaired, risk for
Resilience, compromised, risk for
Sorrow, chronic
Suffocation, risk for
Therapeutic regimen management,
    family, ineffective
Trauma, risk for
Wandering

Love and Belonging Needs

Anxiety
Attachment, impaired, risk for
Caregiver role strain
Caregiver role strain, risk for
Conflict, parental role
Coping, family, compromised
Coping, family, disabled
Coping, family, readiness for enhanced

Coping, readiness for enhanced
Failure to thrive, adult
Family processes, interrupted
Family processes, readiness for
   enhanced
Grieving
Loneliness, risk for
Maternal/Fetal dyad, disturbed, risk for

Parenting, impaired
Parenting, impaired, risk for
Parenting, readiness for enhanced
Relationship, readiness for enhanced
Relocation stress syndrome
Relocation stress syndrome, risk for
Social interaction, impaired
Social isolation

Self-Esteem Needs

Behavior, health, risk-prone
Body image, disturbed
Conflict, decisional
Coping, community, ineffective
Coping, community, readiness for
   enhanced
Coping, defensive
Coping, ineffective
Decision-Making, readiness for
   enhanced
Denial, ineffective

Dignity, human, compromised, risk for
Diversional activity, deficient
Hope, readiness for enhanced
Hopelessness
Identity, personal, disturbed
Noncompliance
Post-Trauma syndrome
Post-Trauma syndrome, risk for
Power, readiness for enhanced
Powerlessness
Powerlessness, risk for

Rape-Trauma syndrome
Role performance, ineffective
Self-Esteem, low, chronic
Self-Esteem, low, situational
Self-Esteem, low, situational, risk for
Self-Mutilation
Self-Mutilation, risk for
Suicide, risk for
Violence, other-directed, risk for
Violence, self-directed, risk for

Self-Actualization Needs

Activity planning, ineffective
Childbearing process, readiness for
   enhanced
Development, delayed, risk for
Energy field, disturbed

Growth and development, delayed
Lifestyle, sedentary
Nutrition, readiness for enhanced
Religiosity, readiness for enhanced
Self-Care, readiness for enhanced

Self-Concept, readiness for enhanced
Spiritual distress
Spiritual distress, risk for
Spiritual well-being, readiness for
   enhanced

Nursing Diagnoses Arranged by Gordon's Functional Health Patterns

Diagnoses currently accepted by NANDA-International (North American Nursing Diagnosis Association, new/revised diagnoses are indicated by *).

Health-Perception—Health-Management Pattern

Risk-prone health Behavior
Contamination
Risk for Contamination
Disturbed Energy field
Risk for Falls
Ineffective Health maintenance
Ineffective self Health management

Readiness for enhanced Immunization
   status
Risk for Infection
Risk for Injury
Risk for perioperative positioning
   Injury
Self Neglect

Noncompliance
Risk for Poisoning
Ineffective Protection
Readiness for enhanced Self Health
   management
Risk for Suffocation
Risk for Trauma

Nutritional-Metabolic Pattern

Latex Allergy response
Risk for Aspiration
Risk for imbalanced Body temperature
Effective Breastfeeding
Ineffective Breastfeeding
Interrupted Breastfeeding
Impaired Dentition
Risk for Electrolyte imbalance
Adult Failure to thrive
Ineffective infant Feeding pattern
Readiness for enhanced Fluid balance
Deficient Fluid volume
Risk for deficient Fluid volume

Excess Fluid volume
Risk for imbalanced Fluid volume
Risk for unstable blood Glucose level
Hypothermia
Neonatal Jaundice
Risk for impaired Liver function
Dysfunctional gastrointestinal
   Motility
Risk for dysfunctional gastrointestinal
   Motility
Nausea
Imbalanced Nutrition: less than body
   requirements

Imbalanced Nutrition: more than body
   requirements
Risk for imbalanced Nutrition: more
   than body requirements
Readiness for enhanced Nutrition
Impaired Oral mucous membrane
Risk for ineffective gastrointestinal
   tissue Perfusion
Impaired Skin integrity
Risk for impaired Skin integrity
Impaired Swallowing
Ineffective Thermoregulation
Impaired Tissue integrity (specify type)

Elimination Pattern

Bowel Incontinence
Constipation
Perceived Constipation
Risk for Constipation
Diarrhea
Functional urinary Incontinence

Overflow urinary Incontinence
Reflex urinary Incontinence
Stress urinary Incontinence
Urge urinary Incontinence
Risk for urge urinary Incontinence

Risk for ineffective renal Perfusion
Readiness for enhanced Urinary
   elimination
Impaired Urinary elimination
Urinary retention

Activity-Exercise Pattern

Activity intolerance
Risk for Activity intolerance
Ineffective Airway clearance
Autonomic dysreflexia
Risk for Autonomic dysreflexia
Risk for Bleeding
Ineffective Breathing pattern
Decreased Cardiac output
Risk for sudden infant Death syndrome
Risk for delayed Development
Risk for Disuse syndrome

Deficient Diversional activity
Fatigue
Impaired Gas exchange
Delayed Growth and development
Risk for disproportionate Growth
Impaired Home maintenance
Disorganized Infant behavior
Risk for disorganized Infant behavior
Readiness for enhanced organized
   Infant behavior
Sedentary Lifestyle

Impaired bed Mobility
Impaired physical Mobility
Impaired wheelchair Mobility
Risk for decreased cardiac tissue
   Perfusion
Ineffective peripheral tissue Perfusion
Risk for Peripheral neurovascular
   dysfunction
Readiness for enhanced Self-Care
Bathing Self-Care deficit
Dressing Self-Care deficit

Feeding Self-Care deficit
Toileting Self-Care deficit
Risk for Shock
Delayed Surgical recovery
Impaired Transfer ability

Risk for vascular Trauma
Impaired spontaneous Ventilation
Dysfunctional Ventilatory weaning
    response

Impaired Walking
Wandering

Sleep-Rest Pattern

Insomnia
Sleep deprivation

Disturbed Sleep pattern

Readiness for enhanced Sleep

Cognitive-Perceptual Pattern

Ineffective Activity planning
Impaired Comfort
Readiness for enhanced Comfort
Decisional Conflict
Acute Confusion
Risk for acute Confusion
Chronic Confusion

Readiness for enhanced Decision-
    Making
Impaired Environmental interpretation
    syndrome
Decreased Intracranial adaptive capacity
Deficient Knowledge
Readiness for enhanced Knowledge

Impaired Memory
Unilateral Neglect
Acute Pain
Chronic Pain
Risk for ineffective cerebral tissue
    Perfusion
Disturbed Sensory perception

Self-Perception—Self-Concept Pattern

Anxiety
Death Anxiety
Disturbed Body image
Risk for compromised human Dignity
Fear
Readiness for enhanced Hope

Hopelessness
Disturbed personal Identity
Risk for Loneliness
Readiness for enhanced Power
Powerlessness
Risk for Powerlessness

Readiness for enhanced Self-Concept
Chronic low Self-Esteem
Situational low Self-Esteem
Risk for situational low Self-Esteem
Risk for self-directed Violence

Role-Relationship Pattern

Risk for impaired Attachment
Caregiver role strain
Risk for Caregiver role strain
Readiness for enhanced
    Communication
Impaired verbal Communication
Dysfunctional Family processes
Interrupted Family processes

Readiness for enhanced Family processes
Grieving
Complicated Grieving
Risk for complicated Grieving
Risk for disturbed Maternal/Fetal dyad
Impaired Parenting
Risk for impaired Parenting
Readiness for enhanced Parenting

Readiness for enhanced Relationship
Relocation stress syndrome
Risk for Relocation stress syndrome
Ineffective Role performance
Impaired Social interaction
Social isolation
Chronic Sorrow
Risk for other-directed Violence

Sexuality-Reproductive Pattern

Readiness for enhanced Childbearing
    process

Risk for distrubed Maternal/Fetal dyad
Rape-Trauma syndrome

Sexual dysfunction
Ineffective Sexuality pattern

Coping—Stress-Tolerance Pattern

Risk-prone health Behavior
Ineffective community Coping
Readiness for enhanced community
    Coping
Defensive Coping
Compromised family Coping
Disabled family Coping

Readiness for enhanced family Coping
Ineffective Coping
Readiness for enhanced Coping
Ineffective Denial
Moral Distress
Post-Trauma syndrome
Risk for Post-Trauma syndrome

Risk for compromised Resilience
Impaired individual Resilience
Readiness for enhanced Resilience
Self-Mutilation
Risk for Self-Mutilation
Stress overload*
Risk for Suicide

Value-Belief Pattern

Impaired Religiosity
Risk for impaired Religiosity
Readiness for enhanced Religiosity

Spiritual distress
Risk for Spiritual distress

Readiness for enhanced Spiritual well-being

APPENDIX C

Wellness-Oriented Diagnostic Categories

This is a list of NANDA-I diagnoses in a wellness format. When available, readiness diagnoses are listed first in each category. Risk diagnoses are listed next. The goal is to support wellness, prevent illness, and intervene when illness is present.

Diagnoses are arranged first by priority according to the ABCs (airway, breathing, circulation). They are then arranged according to possible priority physiological needs and then psychosocial needs. Diagnoses dealing with family, infant, and child are grouped together. It is the responsibility of the nurse to individualize and reorder based on the patient's assessment data.

Adult: (asterisked diagnoses have pediatric interventions in care plans**)

Physiological

Airway/Breathing

- Risk for Aspiration
- Risk for Suffocation
- Impaired Swallowing
- Ineffective Airway clearance
- Ineffective Breathing pattern
- Impaired Gas exchange
- Impaired spontaneous Ventilation
- Dysfunctional Ventilatory weaning response

Circulation

- Risk for Bleeding
- Risk for decreased cardiac tissue Perfusion
- Risk for ineffective cerebral tissue Perfusion
- Risk for ineffective gastrointestinal tissue Perfusion
- Risk for Peripheral neurovascular dysfunction
- Risk for ineffective renal Perfusion
- Risk for Shock
- Decreased Cardiac output
- Ineffective peripheral tissue Perfusion

Cognition/Sensory Perception

- Risk for acute Confusion
- Risk for Autonomic dysreflexia
- Ineffective Activity planning
- Autonomic dysreflexia
- Decreased Intracranial adaptive capacity
- Disturbed Sensory perception
- Acute Confusion
- Chronic Confusion
- Impaired Environmental interpretation syndrome
- Impaired Memory

Injury: Falls/Infection/Poisoning/Trauma

- Readiness for enhanced Immunization status**
- Risk for Contamination
- Risk for Falls
- Risk for Injury**
- Risk for Infection**
- Risk for latex Allergy response
- Risk for perioperative positioning Injury
- Risk for Poisoning**
- Risk for Trauma
- Risk for Vascular trauma**
- Acute Pain** (psychosocial)
- Chronic Pain** (psychosocial)
- Contamination
- Delayed Surgical recovery
- Ineffective Protection
- Latex Allergy response
- Rape-Trauma syndrome

Homeostasis

- Risk for impaired Liver function
- Risk for unstable Blood glucose level
- Risk for imbalanced Body temperature**
- Risk for Electrolyte imbalance
- Adult Failure to thrive
- Disturbed Energy field**
- Hyperthermia
- Hypothermia**
- Ineffective Thermoregulation

Fluid/Nutrition/Gastrointestinal/Oral/Dental Management

- Readiness for enhanced Fluid balance
- Readiness for enhanced Nutrition

- Risk for dysfunctional gastrointestinal Motility
- Risk for imbalanced Nutrition: more than body requirements
- Risk for imbalanced Fluid volume
- Risk for deficient Fluid volume
- Dysfunctional gastrointestinal Motility
- Nausea
- Imbalanced Nutrition: more than body requirements
- Imbalanced Nutrition: less than body requirements
- Deficient Fluid volume**
- Excess Fluid volume
- Impaired Oral mucous membrane
- Impaired Dentition

Elimination
Urinary Elimination

- Readiness for enhanced Urinary elimination
- Impaired Urinary elimination
- Urinary retention

Incontinence, Bowel

- Bowel incontinence

Incontinence, Bladder

- Risk for urge urinary Incontinence
- Functional urinary Incontinence
- Overflow urinary Incontinence
- Reflex urinary Incontinence
- Stress urinary Incontinence
- Urge urinary Incontinence

Bowel Elimination
Constipation

- Risk for Constipation

- Perceived Constipation
- Constipation

Diarrhea

- Diarrhea**

Activity/Movement/Self-Care

- Readiness for enhanced Self-Care
- Risk for Activity intolerance
- Risk for Disuse syndrome
- Sedentary Lifestyle**
- Deficient Diversional activity**
- Activity intolerance

- Fatigue
- Impaired physical Mobility
- Bathing Self-Care deficit
- Dressing Self-Care deficit
- Feeding Self-Care deficit
- Toileting Self-Care deficit
- Self Neglect
- Impaired Walking
- Impaired Transfer ability
- Impaired bed Mobility
- Impaired wheelchair Mobility
- Unilateral Neglect
- Wandering

Skin/Tissue

- Risk for impaired Skin integrity
- Impaired Skin integrity
- Impaired Tissue integrity

Sleep

- Readiness for enhanced Sleep
- Disturbed Sleep Pattern
- Insomnia
- Sleep deprivation

Psychosocial

Comfort

- Readiness for enhanced Comfort
- Impaired Comfort
- Acute Pain** (Physiological)
- Chronic Pain** (Physiological)

Communication/Healthy Behaviors/Therapeutic Regimen/Knowledge
Individual

- Readiness for enhanced Communication**
- Readiness for enhanced Self Health management
- Readiness for enhanced Knowledge**
- Risk-prone health Behavior
- Impaired verbal Communication**
- Ineffective self Health management
- Deficient Knowledge**
- Ineffective Health maintenance

Family

- Ineffective family Therapeutic regimen management

Spirituality/Religious Beliefs

- Readiness for enhanced Spiritual well-being
- Readiness for enhanced Religiosity**
- Readiness for enhanced Hope
- Risk for Spiritual distress
- Risk for impaired Religiosity
- Impaired Religiosity
- Spiritual distress
- Hopelessness

Harm: Self and Others

- Risk for Suicide
- Risk for Self-Mutilation
- Risk for other-directed Violence
- Risk for self-directed Violence
- Self-Mutilation

Anxiety/Stress

- Readiness for enhanced Decision making
- Risk for Relocation stress syndrome
- Risk for compromised human Dignity
- Anxiety
- Death Anxiety
- Ineffective Denial
- Decisional Conflict
- Dysfunctional Family processes **
- Fear**
- Noncompliance
- Relocation stress syndrome**
- Stress overload

Coping
Individual

- Readiness for enhanced Coping**
- Readiness for enhanced Power
- Readiness for enhanced Resilience
- Risk for Caregiver role strain
- Risk for Powerlessness
- Risk for Loneliness**
- Risk for Post-Trauma syndrome**
- Ineffective Activity planning
- Defensive Coping

- Ineffective Coping
- Caregiver role strain
- Impaired individual Resilience
- Impaired Social interaction
- Post-Trauma syndrome
- Powerlessness
- Ineffective Role performance**
- Social isolation

Community

- Readiness for enhanced community Coping
- Ineffective community Coping

Sexuality/Body Image

- Disturbed Body image
- Sexual dysfunction
- Ineffective Sexuality pattern**

Grief/Sorrow

- Risk for complicated Grieving**
- Grieving**
- Complicated Grieving**
- Chronic Sorrow

Self-concept/Self-esteem/Personal Identity

- Readiness for enhanced Self-Concept**
- Risk for situational low Self-Esteem
- Disturbed personal Identity
- Situational low Self-Esteem
- Chronic low Self-Esteem

Family/Infant/Child

Sudden Infant Death

- Risk for sudden infant Death syndrome

Development/Growth

- Risk for delayed Development
- Risk for disproportionate Growth
- Delayed Growth and development

Neonate

- Neonatal Jaundice

Infant Care

- Readiness for enhanced organized Infant behavior
- Readiness for enhanced Immunization status
- Risk for disorganized Infant behavior

- Risk for impaired Attachment
- Disorganized Infant behavior
- Ineffective infant Feeding pattern

Parenting

- Readiness for enhanced Parenting
- Risk for impaired Parenting
- Impaired Parenting
- Parental role Conflict

Breastfeeding

- Effective Breastfeeding
- Interrupted Breastfeeding
- Ineffective Breastfeeding

Coping/Family

- Readiness for enhanced family Coping
- Readiness for enhanced Relationship

- Risk for disturbed Maternal/Fetal dyad
- Compromised family Coping
- Disabled family Coping
- Ineffective family Therapeutic regimen management

Family Processes

- Readiness for enhanced Childbearing process
- Readiness for enhanced Family processes
- Interrupted Family processes
- Dysfunctional Family processes

INDEX

Boldface entries indicate care plan titles; page numbers in *italics* indicate care plan locations.

A

Abdominal distention, 14
Abdominal hysterectomy, 14
Abdominal pain, 14
Abdominal surgery, 14. *See also* Aortic aneurysm
    repair
  aneurysm, 21
Abdominal trauma, 14
Ablation, radiofrequency catheter (usage), 14
Abnormal dehiscence, 41
Abortion, induced, 14
Abortion, spontaneous, 14
Abruptio placentae, 14–15
Abscess Formation, 15
Absent bowel sounds, 27
Absent gag reflex, 51
Abuse. *See* Children; Elder abuse; Parents; Physical abuse;
    Significant other; Spouse
Accessory muscle, usage, 15
Accident prone, 15
Achalasia, 15
Acid-base imbalances, 15
Acidosis. *See* Metabolic acidosis; Respiratory acidosis
Acne, 15
Acquired immunodeficiency syndrome (AIDS), 15, 18
  dementia, 18
Acromegaly, 15
Activity intolerance, 24, 33, *119–125*
  risk for, *124–125*
Activity planning, ineffective, *125–128*
Acute abdominal pain, 16
Acute alcohol intoxication, 16
Acute back, 16
Acute coronary syndrome (ACS), 15
Acute lymphocytic leukemia (ALL), 16, 19
Acute myocardial infarction (AMI), 20
Acute renal failure, 97
Acute respiratory distress syndrome (ARDS), 16, 23
Acute respiratory infection, 97. *See also* Children
Acute tubular necrosis (ATN), 24, 77
Acyanotic disease/anomaly, 37
Adams-Stokes syndrome, 16
Addiction, 16
Addison's disease, 16
Adenoidectomy, 16
Adhesions, lysis, 16
Adjustment
  disorder, 16
  impairment, 16

Adolescents
  maturational issues, 71
  pregnant, 16
  sexuality, 102
  substance abuse, 106
  terminal illness, 109
Adoption. *See* Children
Adrenocortical insufficiency, 17
Adults. *See* Older adult
  inflammatory bowel disease, 61
  seizure disorders, 101
  terminal illness, 109
Advance directives, 17
Affective disorders, 17
Age-related macular degeneration (AMD), 17, 20, 23
Aggressive behavior, 17
Aging, 17–18
Agitation, 18
Agoraphobia, 18
Agranulocytosis, 18
Airway clearance, ineffective, *128–133*
Airway obstructions/secretions, 18
  Alcohol withdrawal, 18–19, 115
Alcoholic ketoacidosis, 64
Alcoholism, 19
Alkalosis, 19. *See also* Metabolic alkalosis
ALL. *See* Acute lymphocytic leukemia
Allergies, 19
Allergy response, latex, *134–139*
  risk for, *140–142*
Alopecia, 19
ALS. *See* Amyotrophic lateral sclerosis
Altered mental status. *See* Mental status
Alzheimer's disease, 19
AMD. *See* Age-related macular degeneration
Amenorrhea, 20
AMI. *See* Acute myocardial infarction
Amnesia, 20
Amniocentesis, 20
Amnionitis, 20
Amniotic membrane rupture, 20
Amputation, 20
Amyotrophic lateral sclerosis (ALS), 19, 20
Anal fistula, 20
Anaphylactic shock, 20
Anasarca, 20
Anemia, 20. *See also* Aplastic anemia; Pernicious anemia;
    Pregnancy
  sickle cell. *See* Sickle cell anemia

2009-2011 NANDA-I Nursing Diagnoses